| | ANTIBODIES | | | | | | | | |
|---|---|---|---|---|---|---|---|---|---|
| | Serology | | Comp. Binding | Immunogloblin Class | | Optimum Temperature | Clinical Significance | | |
| Stimulation | Saline | AHG | | IgM | IgG | | HTR | | |
| RBC | occ | yes | no | occ | yes | warm | yes | yes | Very rarely IgA anti-D may be produced; however, this is invariable with IgG. |
| RBC | occ | yes | no | occ | yes | warm | yes | yes | |
| RBC/NRBC | occ | yes | no | occ | yes | warm | yes | yes | Anti-E may often occur without obvious immune stimulation. |
| RBC | occ | yes | no | occ | yes | warm | yes | yes | |
| RBC | occ | yes | no | occ | yes | warm | yes | yes | Warm autoantibodies often appear to have anti-e-like specificity. |
| RBC | occ | yes | no | occ | yes | warm | yes | ? | |
| RBC | occ | yes | no | occ | yes | warm | yes | yes | |
| RBC/NRBC | occ | yes | no | occ | yes | warm | yes | yes | Anti-C$^w$ may often occur without obvious immune stimulation. |
| RBC | occ | yes | no | occ | yes | warm | yes | yes | |
| RBC | occ | yes | no | occ | yes | warm | yes | yes | Antibodies to V and VS present problems only in the black population, where the antigen frequencies are in the order of 20 to 25. |
| RBC | occ | yes | no | occ | yes | warm | yes | yes | |
| RBC | occ | yes | some | occ | yes | warm | yes | yes | Some antibodies to Kell system have been reported to react poorly in low ionic media. |
| RBC | no | yes | no | no | yes | warm | yes | yes | |
| RBC | no | yes | no | no | yes | warm | yes | yes | Kell system antigens are destroyed by AET and by ZZAP. |
| RBC | no | yes | no | no | yes | warm | yes | yes | |
| RBC | no | yes | no | no | yes | warm | yes | yes | Anti-K1 has been reported to occur following bacterial infection. |
| RBC | no | yes | no | no | yes | warm | yes | yes | |
| RBC | no | yes | no | occ | yes | warm | yes | yes | The lack of Kx expression on RBCs and WBCs has been associated with the McLeod phenotype and CGD. |
| RBC | rare | yes | some | rare | yes | warm | yes | yes | Fy(a) and (b) antigens are destroyed by enzymes. Fy(a–b–) cells are resistant to invasion by P. vivax merozoites, a malaria-causing parasite. |
| RBC | rare | yes | some | rare | yes | warm | yes | yes | |
| RBC | no | yes | ? | no | yes | warm | ? | yes | FY3, 4, and 5 are not destroyed by enzymes. |
| RBC | no | yes | some | no | yes | warm | | | |
| RBC | no | yes | ? | no | yes | warm | | | FY5 may be formed by interaction of Rh and Duffy gene products. |
| RBC | no | yes | ? | ? | yes | warm | ? | ? | FY6 antibody reacts with most human red cells except Fy(a–b–) and is responsible for susceptibility of cells to penetration by P. vivax. |

(Continued on inside back cover)

# MODERN BLOOD BANKING AND TRANSFUSION PRACTICES

## FOURTH EDITION

### Denise M. Harmening, PhD, MT(ASCP), CLS(NCA)

Chair and Professor
Department of Medical and Research
Technology
University of Maryland, Baltimore
School of Medicine
Baltimore, Maryland

 **F.A. DAVIS COMPANY • Philadelphia**

F. A. Davis Company
1915 Arch Street
Philadelphia, PA 19103

Printed in the United States of America

Last digit indicates print number: 10 9 8 7 6 5 4 3

*Publisher:* Jean-François Vilain
*Developmental Editor:* Crystal Spraggins
*Production Editor:* Jessica Howie Martin
*Cover Designer:* Louis J. Forgione

As new scientific information becomes available through basic and clinical research, recommended treatments and drug therapies undergo changes. The author and publisher have done everything possible to make this book accurate, up to date, and in accord with accepted standards at the time of publication. The author, editors, and publisher are not responsible for errors or omissions or for consequences from application of the book, and make no warranty, expressed or implied, in regard to the contents of the book. Any practice described in this book should be applied by the reader in accordance with professional standards of care used in regard to the unique circumstances that may apply in each situation. The reader is advised always to check product information (package inserts) for changes and new information regarding dose and contraindications before administering any drug. Caution is especially urged when using new or infrequently ordered drugs.

### Library of Congress Cataloging-in-Publication Data

Modern blood banking and transfusion practices / [edited by] Denise M.
    Harmening. — 4th ed.
        p.   cm.
    Includes bibliographical references and index.
    ISBN 0-8036-0419-X (hard cover)
    1. Blood banks.   2. Blood—Transfusion.   I. Harmening, Denise.
    [DNLM: 1. Blood Banks.   2. Blood Transfusion.   3. Blood Grouping
and Crossmatching.   WH 460 M688 1999]
RM172.M62 1999
615'.39—dc21
DNLM/DLC
for Library of Congress                                    98–54477
                                                              CIP

To all students—full-time, part-time, past, present, and future—who have touched and will continue to touch the lives of so many educators . . . It is to you this book is dedicated in the hope of inspiring an unquenchable thirst for knowledge and love of humankind.

# FOREWORD

Blood transfusion science is one of the newest branches of medical laboratory science. Blood groups were discovered only approximately 95 years ago, and most of them have been recognized only in the last 45 years. Although transfusion therapy was used soon after the ABO blood groups were discovered, it was not until after World War II that blood transfusion science really started to become an important branch of medical science in its own right. Thus, compared with many subdisciplines of medicine, blood transfusion science is an infant, growing fast, changing continually, and presenting a great potential for research and future development.

To be able to grow, our young infant needs to be nurtured with a steady flow of new knowledge generated from research. This knowledge then has to be applied at the bench. To understand and best take advantage of the continual flow of new information being generated by blood transfusion scientists, and to apply it to everyday work in the blood bank, technologists and pathologists need to have a good understanding of basic immunology, genetics, biochemistry (particularly membrane chemistry), and the physiology and function of blood cells. To apply new concepts, they need technical expertise and enough flexibility to reject old dogma when necessary and accept new ideas when they are supported by sufficient scientific data.

High standards are always expected and strived for by technologists who are working in blood banks or transfusion services. I strongly believe that technologists should understand the principles behind the tests they are performing, rather than perform tasks as a machine does. Because of this, I do not think that "cookbook" technical manuals have much value in *teaching* technologists; they do have a place as reference books in the laboratory. During the years (too many to put in print) that I have been involved in teaching medical technologists, it has been very difficult to select one book to cover all that technologists in training need to know above blood transfusion science, without confusing them. Classic texts used regularly in teaching SBB students and pathology residents often contain too much information for the average medical technologist, especially those in training. They contain certain sections that can, and perhaps should, be read, but sometimes these sections confuse learners rather than help and stimulate them. Some of them are written to be encyclopedic reference tomes, and others contain a great deal of clinical material or esoterica that are unnecessary for medical technologists who are not yet greatly experienced in blood transfusion practice.

Dr. Denise Harmening has produced a single volume that covers everything a student of medical technology needs to know about blood transfusion science. She has been involved in teaching medical technologists for most of her career, and after seeing how she has arranged this book, I would guess that her teaching philosophies are close to my own. She has gathered together a group of experienced scientists and teachers who, along with her, cover all the important areas of blood transfusion science.

The chapters on the basic principles of cell preservation, genetics, and immunology provide a firm base for the learner to understand the practical and technical importance of the other chapters. The chapters on the blood groups and transfusion practice provide enough information for medical technologists without overwhelming them with esoterica and clinical details.

Although this book was primarily designed for medical technologists, I believe that it is admirably suited to pathology residents, hematology fellows, and others who want to review any aspect of modern blood transfusion science.

**George Garratty, PhD, FIMLS, MRC Path**
Scientific Director
American Red Cross Blood Services
Los Angeles, California

# PREFACE

This book is designed to provide the medical technologist, blood bank specialist, or resident with a concise and thorough guide to transfusion practices and immunohematology. A perfect "crossmatch" of theory and practice, this text provides the reader with a working knowledge of modern routine blood banking.

Twenty color plates provide a means for standardizing the reading of agglutination reactions. They also aid in the comprehension of difficult concepts not routinely illustrated in other texts. Thirty-nine contributors from across the country have shared their knowledge and expertise in 27 comprehensive chapters.

Several features of this textbook offer great appeal to students and educators. There are comprehensive outlines and educational objectives at the beginning of each chapter, extensive glossary that provides easy access for defining immunohematologic terms, and study guide questions. A blood group antibody characteristic chart is also provided on the inside cover of the book to aid in retention of the vast amount of information and to serve as an easy access and guide to the characteristics of the blood group systems. Summary charts at the end of each chapter identify for students the most important information to know for clinical rotations.

The introduction to the historical aspects of blood transfusion and preservation is a prelude to an overview of red cell and platelet metabolism as well as current and future approaches to blood storage. Basic concepts of genetics, blood group immunology, and routine serologic testing introduce a thorough and current overview of blood group systems.

The next section of the book focuses on routine blood bank practices, including donor selection and component preparation, detection and identification of antibodies, compatibility testing, transfusion therapy, and apheresis. A chapter on transfusion safety and federal regulations clarifies the required quality assurance and inspection procedures. New to the fourth edition is Chapter 15, "Quality in Blood Banking." Chapter 13, "Orientation to the Routine Blood Bank Laboratory," introduces the common organizational divisions of a routine blood bank laboratory, allowing the student to prepare for clinical rotations. Certain clinical situations that are particularly relevant to blood banking are discussed in detail, including transfusion reactions, hemolytic disease of the newborn, autoimmune and drug-induced hemolytic anemia, transfusion-transmitted viruses, human leucocyte antigens (HLA), and paternity testing. Chapter 25, "Informational Systems in the Blood Bank," helps prepare the blood banker for the responsibility of operating and maintaining a blood bank informaton system.

Unique to *Modern Blood Banking and Transfusion Practices* are Chapter 26, "Medicolegal and Ethical Aspects of Providing Transfusion Services," and the Cybertest, a computerized test bank of questions that can be used for examinations. Questions can be selected by chapter number and level of difficulty.

This book is a culmination of the tremendous efforts of a number of dedicated professionals who participated in this project by donating their time and expertise because they care about the blood bank profession. The book's intention is foster improved patient care by providing the reader with a basic understanding of the function of blood, the involvement of blood group antigens and antibodies, the principles of transfusion therapy, and the adverse effects of blood transfusion. It has been designed to generate an "unquenchable thirst for knowledge" in all medical technologists, blood bankers, and practitioners whose education, knowledge, and skills provide the public with excellent health care.

**Denise M. Harmening, PhD, MT(ASCP), CLS(NCA)**

# CONTRIBUTORS

**William Bernard, MT(ASCP)SBB**
St. John's Hospital Transfusion Services
Department of Laboratory Medicine
Springfield, Illinois

**Lucia M. Berte, MA, MT(ASCP) SBB, DLM, CQA(ASQ)**
Quality Systems Consultant
Elmhurst, Illinois

**Loni Calhoun, MT(ASCP)SBB**
Senior Technical Specialist, Education and
    Immunohematology
Division of Transfusion Medicine
UCLA Medical Center
Los Angeles, California

**Linda Comeaux, MT(ASCP)**
Arapahoe Community College
Department Chair/Program Director
Medical Laboratory Technology
Littleton, Colorado

**Lloyd O. Cook, MD**
Medical Director, Blood Bank and Transfusion Medicine
Assistant Professor, Department of Pathology
Medical College of Georgia
Augusta, Georgia

**Deirdre DeSantis, MS, MT(ASCP)SBB, CLS(NCA)**
Education and Development Coordinator
Transfusion Medicine Division
Johns Hopkins Hospital
Baltimore, Maryland

**Aamir Ehsan, MD**
Hematopathology Fellow
Department of Pathology
The University of Texas
Health Science Center at San Antonio
San Antonio, Texas

**Deborah Firestone, MA, MT(ASCP)SBB**
Chair, Clinical Laboratory Science
Stony Brook Health Sciences Center
School of Health Technology & Management
Division of Diagnostic & Therapeutic Sciences
State University of New York at Stony Brook
Stony Brook, New York

**Frankie Gillen Gibbs, MS, MT(ASCP)SBB**
Quality Assurance for Transfusion Services
Intermountain Health Care (or IHC) Laboratories
    Services
Murray, Utah

**Ralph E. B. Green, BAppSci, FAIMS, MACE**
Associate Professor
Faculty Director of Teaching Quality
Department of Medical Laboratory Science
RMIT University
Melbourne, Australia

**Pamela Ellis Hall, MA, MT(ASCP)SBB**
MLT Program Education Coordinator
Alamance Community College
Graham, North Carolina

**Denise M. Harmening, PhD, MT(ASCP),
    CLS(NCA)**
Chair and Professor
Department of Medical and Research
    Technology
University of Maryland School of Medicine
Baltimore, Maryland

**Chantal Ricaud Harrison, MD**
Medical Director
Medical Center Blood Bank
Associate Professor, Department of Pathology
University of Texas-Health Center
San Antonio, Texas

**Virginia C. Hughes, MS, MT(ASCP)**
Anne Arundel Medical Center
Laboratory Services
Annapolis, Maryland

**Melanie S. Kennedy, MD**
Director, Transfusion Service Laboratory
The Ohio State University Medical Center
Associate Professor, Department of Pathology
The Ohio State University
Columbus, Ohio

**Patricia Joyce Larison, MA, MT(ASCP)SBB**
Blood Bank Supervisor
Associate Professor, Department of Medical Technology
Medical College of Georgia
Augusta, Georgia

**Larry Lasky, MD**
Director, Division of Transfusion Medicine
Associate Professor of Pathology & Internal Medicine
The Ohio State University
Columbus, Ohio

**Perthena Latchaw, MS, MT(ASCP)**
MLT Program Director
Seminole State College
Seminole, Oklahoma

**Veronica Nichols Lewis, MS, MT(ASCP)SBB**
Research Assistant Professor
Medical Laboratory Sciences
School of Biomedical & Health Information Sciences
College of Health and Human Development Sciences
University of Illinois at Chicago
Chicago, Illinois

**Beth Lingenfelter, MS, MT(ASCP)SBB**
Director of Quality Assurance and Regulatory Affairs
Myriad Genetic Laboratories
Salt Lake City, Utah

**Bonnie Lupo, MS, SBB(ASCP)**
Director, Technology
Department of Science & Technology
New York Blood Center
New York, New York

**Sharon Martin, EdD, MT(ASCP)**
Coordinator of Instructional Technology Design
Central Virginia Community College
Lynchburg, Virginia

**JoAnn M. Moulds, PhD**
University of Texas Health Science Center
Division of Rheumatology
Houston, Texas

**Mary P. Nix, MS, MT(ASCP)SBB**
Technical Supervisor, Blood Bank
Department of Pathology and Laboratory Medicine
Hospital of the University of Pennsylvania
Philadelphia, Pennsylvania

**Donna L. Phelan, BA, CHS(ABHI), MT(HEW)**
Technical Supervisor, HLA Laboratory
Barnes-Jewish Hospital
St. Louis, Missouri

**Herbert F. Polesky, MD**
Medical Director
Memorial Blood Center of Minnesota
Minneapolis, Minnesota

**Lee Ann Prihoda, MEd, MT(ASCP), SBB**
Manager, Education and SBB School
Gulf Coast Regional Blood Center
Houston, Texas

**Francis R. Rodwig, Jr., MD, MPH**
Medical Director, Blood Bank
Ochsner Medical Institutions
New Orleans, Louisiana

**Kathleen Sazama, MD, JD, MS, MT(ASCP)**
Professor and Division Director, Laboratory Medicine
Allegheny University of the Health Sciences
Philadelphia, Pennsylvania

**Peggy Perkins Simpson, MS, MT(ASCP)**
MLT Program Director
Alamance Community College
Graham, North Carolina

**Steven D. Sosler, MS, SBB(ASCP)**
Assistant Professor and Associate Director
Transfusion Medicine Research and Education
University of Illinois at Chicago
Chicago, Illinois

**Judith Ann Sullivan, MGA, BS, MT(ASCP)SBB**
Independent Blood Bank Consultant
Silver Spring, Maryland

**Mitra Taghizadeh, MS, MT(ASCP)**
Clinical Assistant Professor
Department of Medical and Research Technology
University of Maryland School of Medicine
Baltimore, Maryland

**Ann Tiehen, MT(ASCP)SBB**
Manager, Blood Center
Rush-Presbyterian-St. Luke's Medical Center
Chicago, Illinois

**Mary Ann Tourault, MA, MT(ASCP)SBB**
Regulatory and Quality Assurance Consulting
Silver Spring, Maryland

**Abdul Waheed, MS, MT(ASCP)SBB**
Supervisor
Reference and Prenatal Laboratory
Transfusion Service
The Ohio State University Medical Center
Columbus, Ohio

**Phyllis S. Walker, MS, MT(ASCP)SBB**
Reference Laboratory Supervisor
Irwin Memorial Blood Centers
San Francisco, California

**Merilyn Wiler, MA Ed, MT(ASCP)SBB**
Director, Quality Engineering
Belle Bonfils Memorial Blood Center
Denver, Colorado

**Patricia A. Wright, BA, MT(ASCP)SBB**
Production Manager
American Red Cross
National Testing Laboratories
Dedham, Massachusetts

# REVIEWERS

**Pamela Ellis Hall, MA, MT(ASCP)SBB**
MLT Program Education Coordinator
Alamance Community College
Medical Laboratory Technology Program
Graham, North Carolina

**Virginia C. Hughes, MS, MT(ASCP)**
Anne Arundel Medical Center
Laboratory Services
Annapolis, Maryland

**Yvonne M. Kros, MT(ASCP)BB**
Blood Bank Teaching Coordinator
University of Nebraska Medical Center
Transfusion and Transplantation
Omaha, Nebraska

**Elizabeth F. Williams, MT(ACSP)SBB, CLS(NCA)**
Associate Professor of Clinical Medical Technology
Louisiana State University
Department of Medical Technology
School of Allied Health
New Orleans, Louisiana

# CONTENTS

# PLATES 1 THROUGH 20

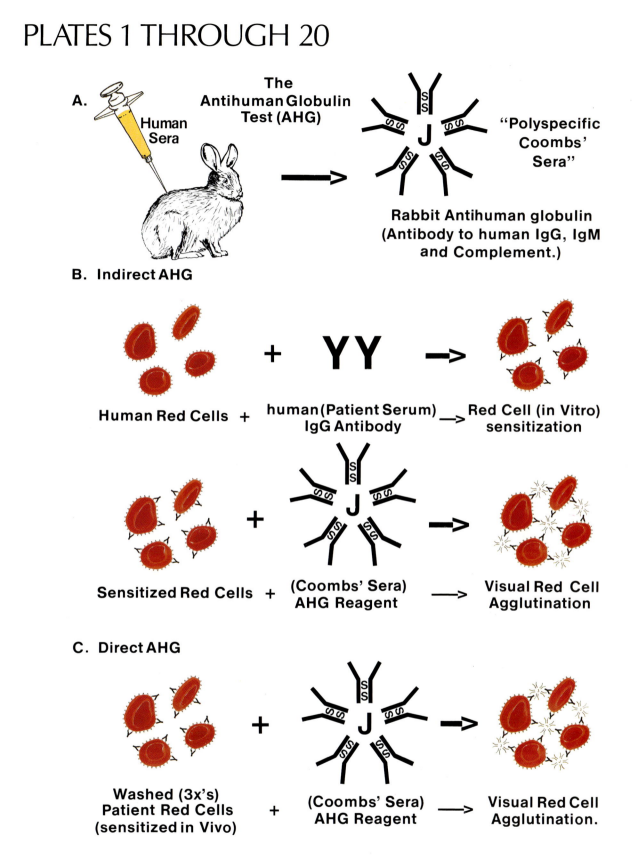

**A.** The Antihuman Globulin Test (AHG)

Human Sera

"Polyspecific Coombs' Sera"

Rabbit Antihuman globulin (Antibody to human IgG, IgM and Complement.)

**B. Indirect AHG**

Human Red Cells + human (Patient Serum) IgG Antibody ⟶ Red Cell (in Vitro) sensitization

Sensitized Red Cells + (Coombs' Sera) AHG Reagent ⟶ Visual Red Cell Agglutination

**C. Direct AHG**

Washed (3x's) Patient Red Cells (sensitized in Vivo) + (Coombs' Sera) AHG Reagent ⟶ Visual Red Cell Agglutination.

**Plate 1.** The antihuman globulin (AHG) test (primary immunization). Note: The AHG reagents currently sold are the products of subsequent immunizations and contain primarily IgG rabbit antibody.

Color Plate 2

# RED CELL ANTIGEN-
## SEROLOGIC
### MACROSCOPIC

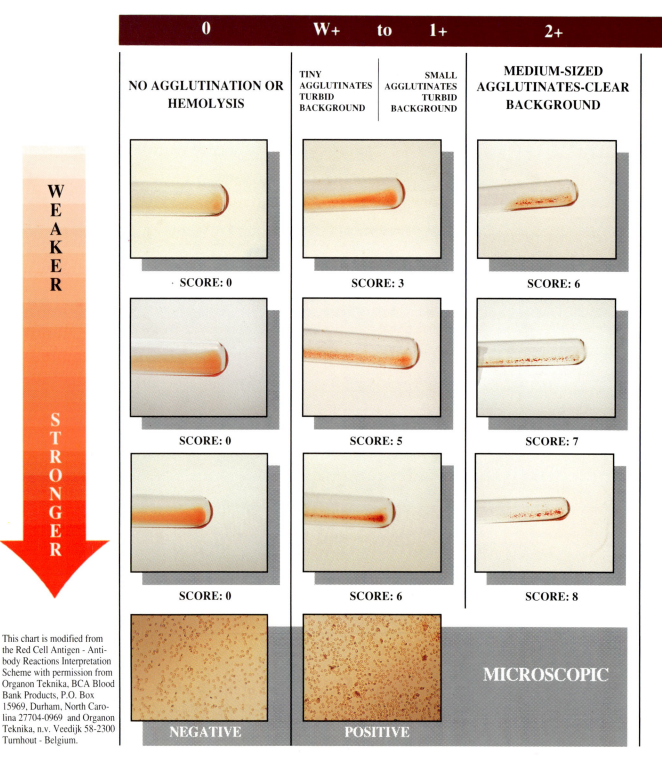

Plate 2. Red cell antigen-antibody reactions: serologic grading and macroscopic evaluation.

# ANTIBODY REACTIONS
## GRADING
## EVALUATION

| 3+ | 4+ |
|---|---|
| **SEVERAL LARGE AGGLUTINATES-CLEAR BACKGROUND** | **ONE SOLID AGGLUTINATE** |

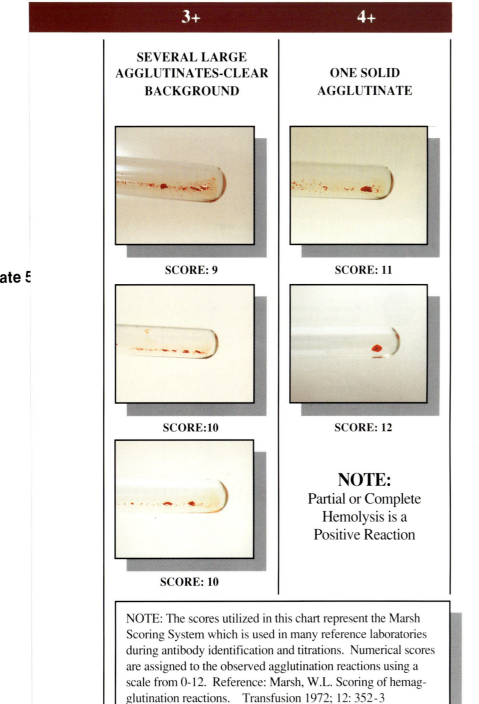

SCORE: 9

SCORE: 11

SCORE:10

SCORE: 12

SCORE: 10

**NOTE:**
Partial or Complete Hemolysis is a Positive Reaction

NOTE: The scores utilized in this chart represent the Marsh Scoring System which is used in many reference laboratories during antibody identification and titrations. Numerical scores are assigned to the observed agglutination reactions using a scale from 0-12. Reference: Marsh, W.L. Scoring of hemagglutination reactions. Transfusion 1972; 12: 352-3

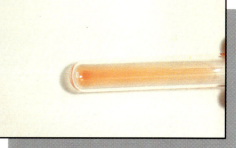

**NEGATIVE: NO AGGREGATES**

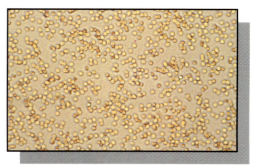

**NEGATIVE: NO AGGREGATES (Microscopic)**

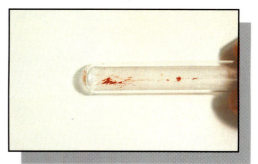

**PSEUDOAGGLUTINATION OR STRONG ROULEAUX (2+)**

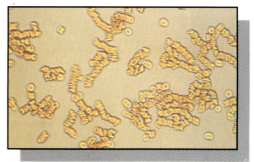

**ROULEAUX:Microscopic (original magnification x10; enlarged 240%) NOTE: The "stack of coins" appearance of the agglutinates**

Plate 5

Plate

# D-Galactose: Immunodominant Sugar responsible for "B" specificity

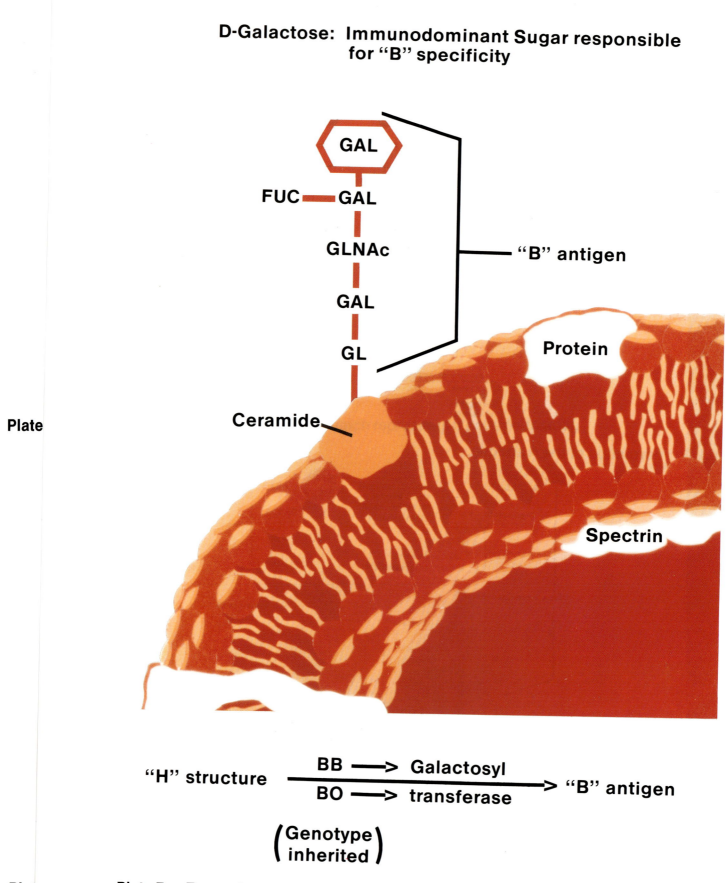

"B" antigen

"H" structure

$$\text{"H" structure} \xrightarrow[\text{BO} \longrightarrow]{\text{BB} \longrightarrow} \begin{array}{l}\text{Galactosyl}\\ \text{transferase}\end{array} \longrightarrow \text{"B" antigen}$$

$\left(\begin{array}{c}\text{Genotype}\\ \text{inherited}\end{array}\right)$

Plate 7. Formation of the B antigen.

**Genotype: Se se**
**AB**
**HH**

water soluble secretions
produced by tissue cells

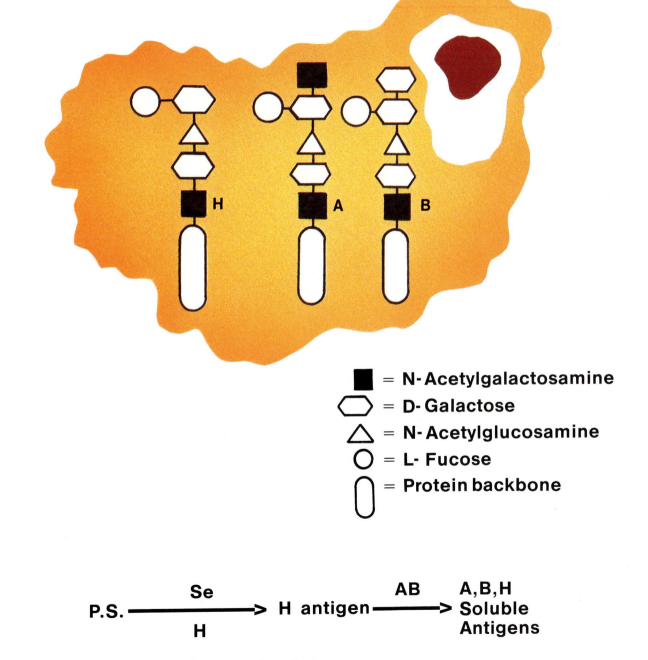

■ = **N-Acetylgalactosamine**
⬡ = **D-Galactose**
△ = **N-Acetylglucosamine**
○ = **L-Fucose**
▯ = **Protein backbone**

P.S. $\xrightarrow[\text{H}]{\text{Se}}$ H antigen $\xrightarrow{\text{AB}}$ A,B,H Soluble Antigens

**Plate 8.  Secretor ABH glycoprotein substances.**

**A**

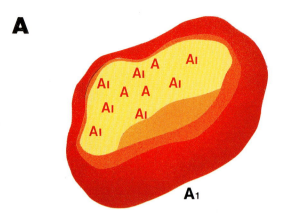
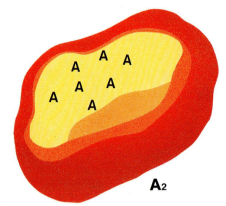

$A_1$

$A_2$

Reactions of Patient's Red Cells with

| Blood Group | Antigens present | Anti A (from B sera) | Anti-A₁ lectin |
|---|---|---|---|
| $A_1$ | $A_1$  A | + | + |
| $A_2$ | A | + | neg |

**B**

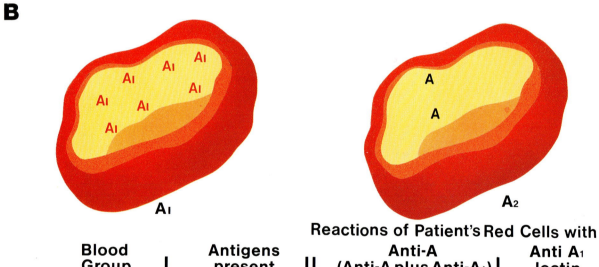

$A_1$

$A_2$

Reactions of Patient's Red Cells with

| Blood Group | Antigens present | Anti-A (Anti-A plus Anti-A₁) | Anti A₁ lectin |
|---|---|---|---|
| $A_1$ | $A_1$ | + | + |
| $A_2$ | A | + | neg |

**Plate 9.**   (A) $A_1$ versus $A_2$ phenotypes. (B) $A_1$ versus $A_2$ phenotypes (alternative conceptual presentation).

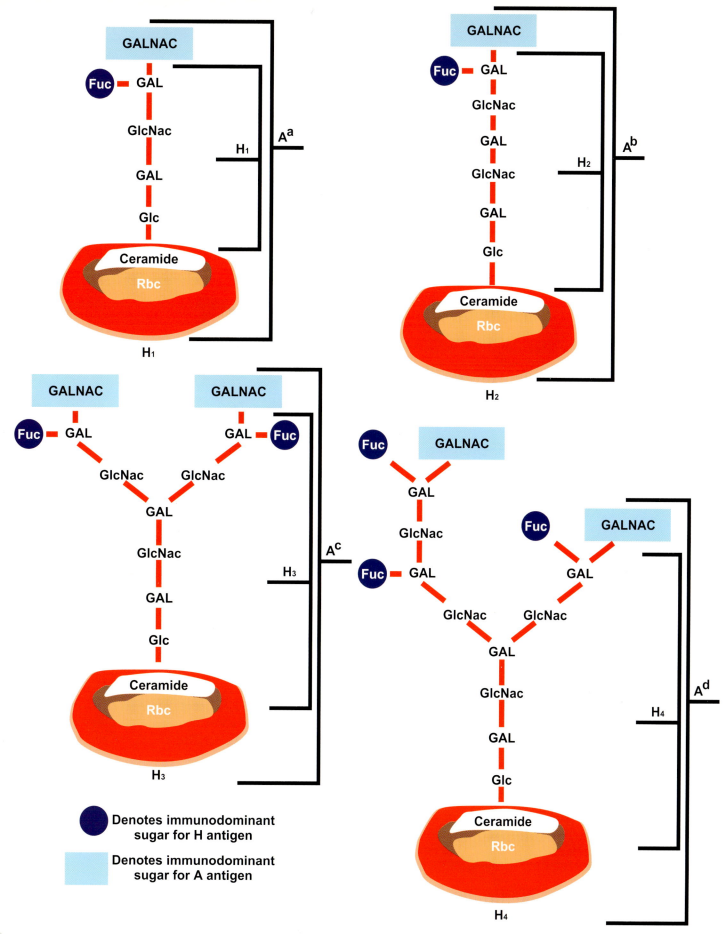

**Plate 10. H-active antigenic structures**

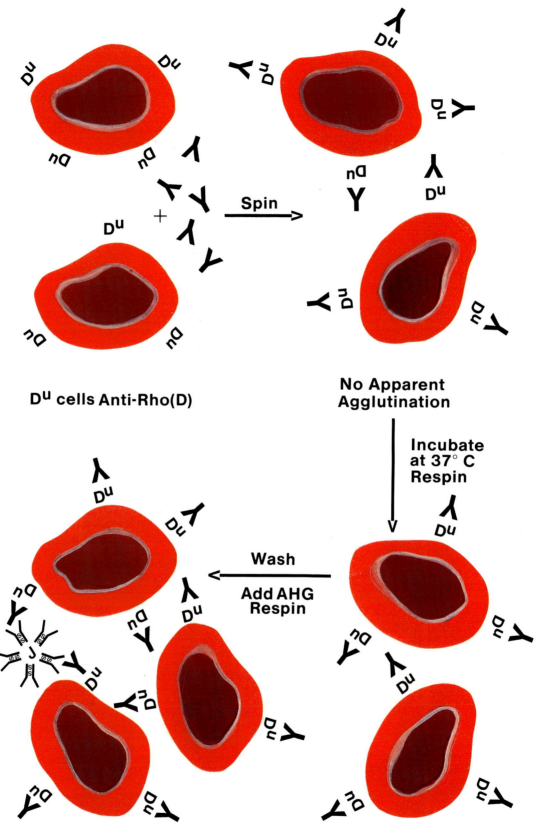

D$^u$ cells Anti-Rho(D)

Spin

No Apparent
Agglutination

Incubate
at 37° C
Respin

Wash

Add AHG
Respin

Visual Agglutination (D$^u$ Positive)

**Plate 11.** D$^u$ testing.

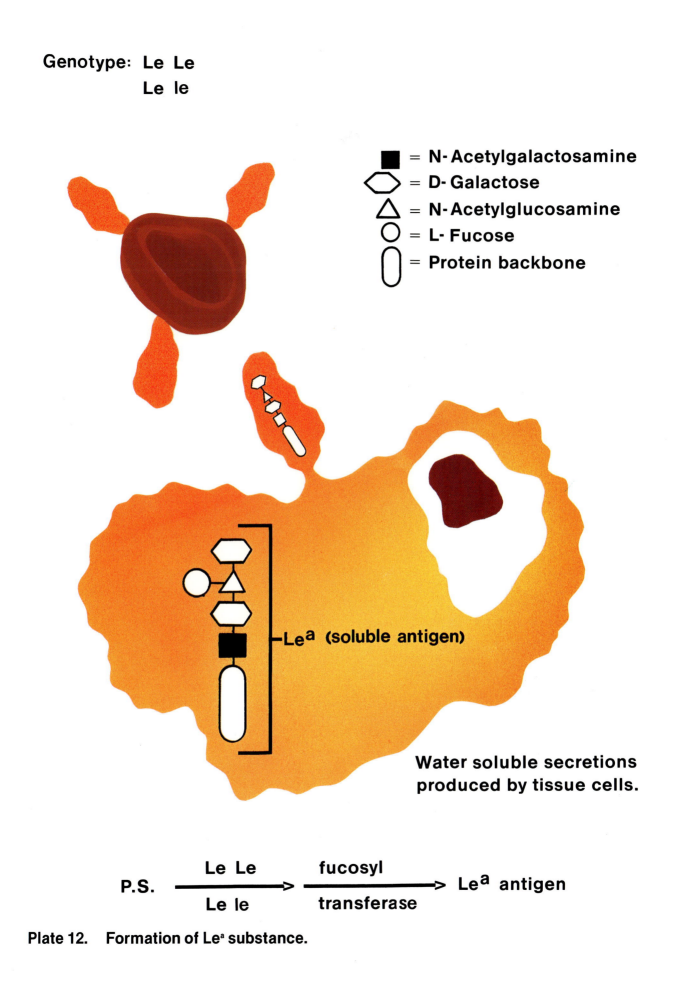

Genotype: Le Le
Le le

■ = N- Acetylgalactosamine
⬡ = D- Galactose
△ = N- Acetylglucosamine
○ = L- Fucose
⬭ = Protein backbone

Le$^a$ (soluble antigen)

Water soluble secretions
produced by tissue cells.

P.S. $\xrightarrow{\dfrac{\text{Le Le}}{\text{Le le}}}$ $\xrightarrow{\dfrac{\text{fucosyl}}{\text{transferase}}}$ Le$^a$ antigen

Plate 12.   Formation of Le$^a$ substance.

**Genotype: Le**
**Se**

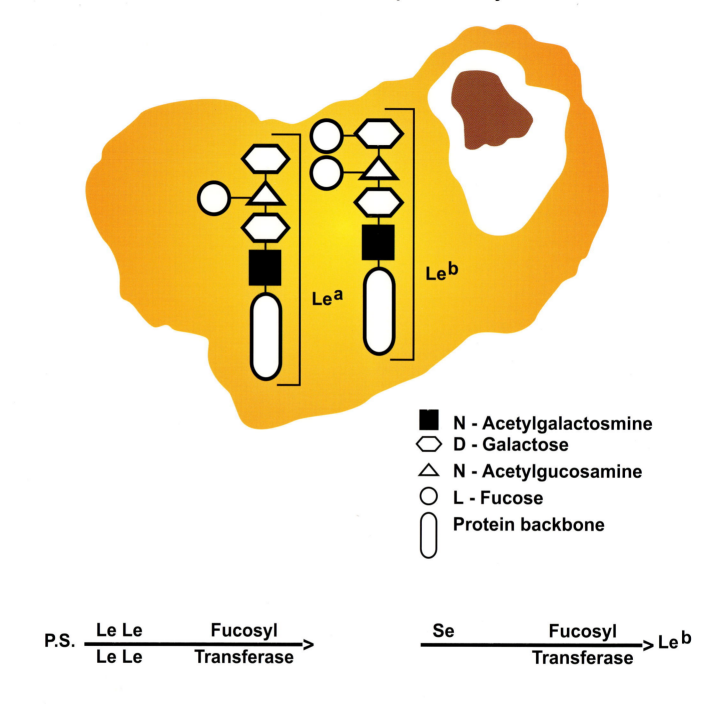

■ N - Acetylgalactosmine
⬡ D - Galactose
△ N - Acetylgucosamine
○ L - Fucose
▢ Protein backbone

P.S. $\dfrac{\text{Le Le}}{\text{Le Le}}$ $\xrightarrow{\begin{array}{c}\text{Fucosyl}\\ \text{Transferase}\end{array}}$ $\xrightarrow[\text{Transferase}]{\begin{array}{c}\text{Se} \qquad \text{Fucosyl}\end{array}}$ Le$^{b}$

Le gene elicits L-fucosyl transferase which adds L-fucose to form Le$^a$. Se gene
elicits L-fucosyl transferase which adds L-fucose to the last sugar D-galactose
forming Le$^b$.

Plate 13. Formation of Le$^b$ substance.

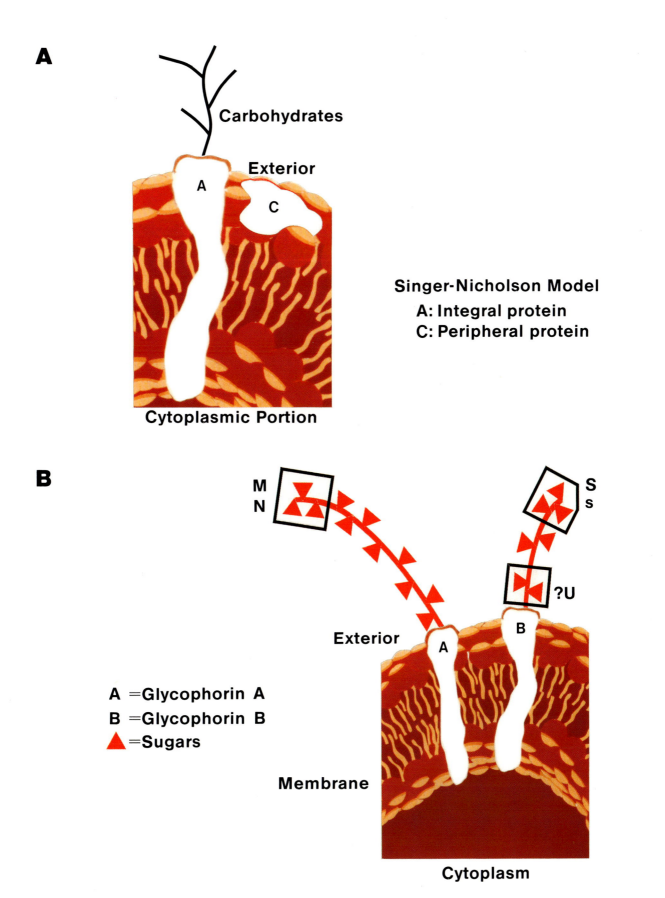

**A**

Carbohydrates

Exterior

A

C

Singer-Nicholson Model
A: Integral protein
C: Peripheral protein

Cytoplasmic Portion

**B**

M
N

S
s

?U

Exterior

A

B

A = Glycophorin A
B = Glycophorin B
▲ = Sugars

Membrane

Cytoplasm

Plate 14.   Theoretical structure of the MNSs antigens.  (A) Singer-Nicholson model of the red blood cell membrane. (B) MNSsU red cell antigens.

**Mother:  Rh negative and Immunized**
**Baby:  Rh positive**

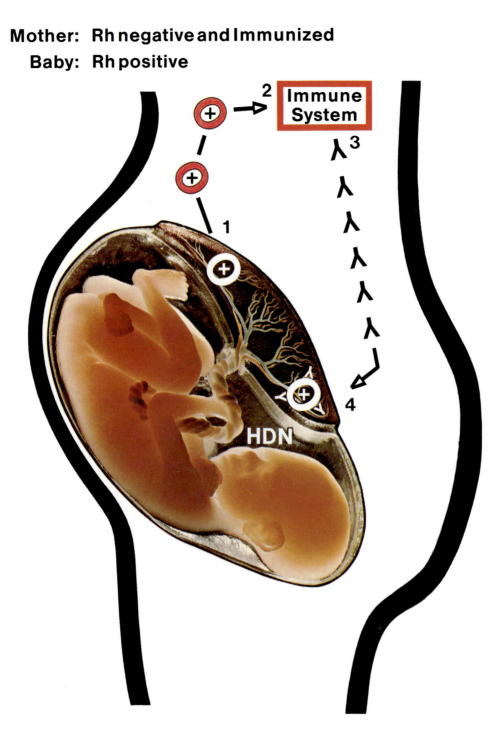

1. Fetal red cells enter maternal circulation at birth.
2. Red cells are recognized by the mother's immune system.
3. Mother is sensitized and produces antibody.
4. Antibody crosses the placenta and causes HDN.

**Plate 15.    Hemolytic disease of the newborn.**

# RhIG: Prevention of Antigenic Sensitization

**Untreated:**

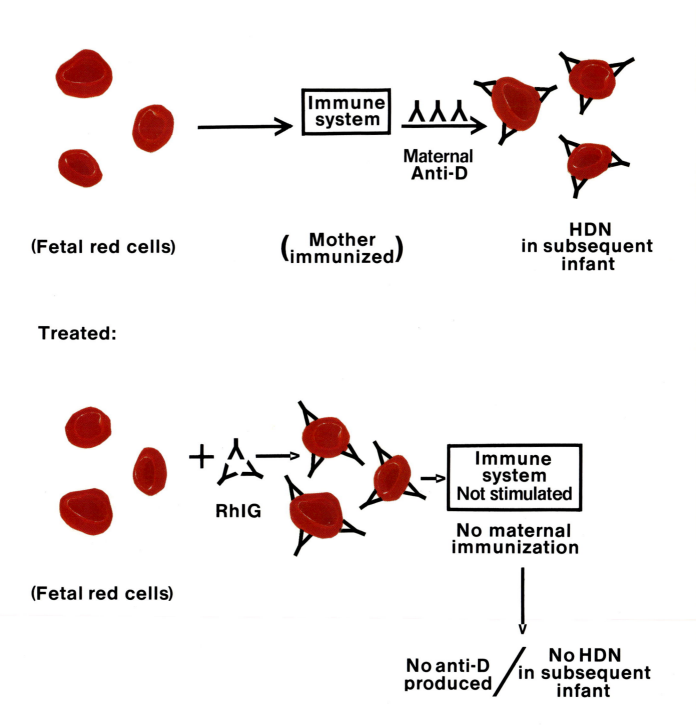

**(Fetal red cells)**

Immune system

Maternal Anti-D

$\left(\begin{array}{c}\text{Mother}\\\text{immunized}\end{array}\right)$

HDN in subsequent infant

**Treated:**

**(Fetal red cells)**

RhIG

Immune system Not stimulated

No maternal immunization

No anti-D produced / No HDN in subsequent infant

Plate 16.    Rh immune globulin (RhIG).

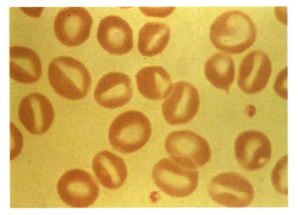

**17**

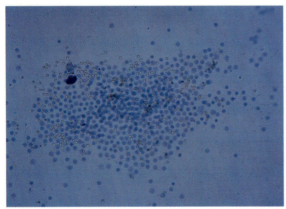

**18(A)**

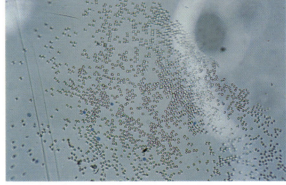

**18(B)**

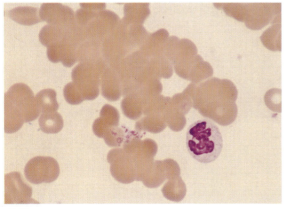

**19**

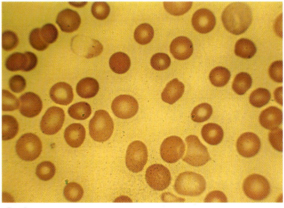

**20**

Plate 17.    Stomatocytosis (original magnification × 100; enlarged 230%).

Plate 18.    (A) Positive cytotoxic reaction. (B) Negative cytotoxic reaction.

Plate 19.    Cold agglutinin disease (peripheral blood). (From Pittiglio, DH and Sacher, RS: *Clinical Hematology and Fundamentals of Hemostasis.* FA Davis, Philadelphia, 1987, with permission.)

Plate 20.    Autoimmune hemolytic anemia (peripheral blood). (From Pittiglio, DH and Sacher, RS: *Clinical Hematology and Fundamentals of Hemostasis,* FA Davis Company, Philadelphia, 1987, with permission.)

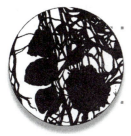

# CHAPTER 1

# BLOOD PRESERVATION: HISTORICAL PERSPECTIVES, REVIEW OF METABOLISM, AND CURRENT TRENDS

Denise M. Harmening, PhD, MT(ASCP), CLS(NCA),
Larry Lasky, MD,
and Perthena Latchaw, MS, MT(ASCP)

## OBJECTIVES

*On completion of this chapter, the learner
should be able to:*

1 List the areas of red blood cell (RBC) metabolism that are crucial to normal RBC survival and functions.

2 Describe the chemical composition of the RBC membrane in terms of percentage of lipids, proteins, and carbohydrates.

3 List the two most important RBC membrane proteins and describe their function and the characteristics of deformability and permeability.

4 List the various metabolic pathways involved in RBC metabolism, stating the specific function of each one.

5 List the globin chains found in HbA, $HbA_2$, HbF, and glycosylated hemoglobin and their respective concentrations (in percent) found in vivo.

6 Describe hemoglobin function in terms of the oxygen dissociation curve.

7 Define $P_{50}$ and state normal in vivo levels.

8 List the approved preservative solutions and the blood storage time for each.

9 List four areas of blood preservation research.

10 Describe the following terms: additive solutions, RBC freezing, and rejuvenation.

11 List the currently licensed additive solutions and the storage time.

**12** List the advantages and disadvantages of RBC freezing.

**13** State the currently licensed storage period for frozen cells.

**14** List the types of hemoglobin-based oxygen carriers.

**15** Define stroma-free hemoglobin solution (SFHS).

**16** Define perfluorochemicals and their use as a blood substitute.

**17** List the advantages and disadvantages of perfluorochemicals.

**18** Describe the metabolism and function of platelets.

**19** List the currently licensed storage times and temperatures for platelet concentrates.

**20** List at least one type of platelet substitute.

## HISTORICAL ASPECTS

People have always been fascinated by blood: ancient Egyptians bathed in it, aristocrats drank it, authors and playwrights used it as themes, and modern humanity transfuses it. The road to an efficient, safe, and uncomplicated transfusion technique has been rather difficult, but great progress has been made.

In 1492 blood was taken from three young men and given to the stricken Pope Innocent VII in the hope of curing him; unfortunately, all four died. Although the outcome of this event was unsatisfactory, it is the first time a blood transfusion was duly recorded in history. The path to the successful transfusions so familiar today is marred by many reported failures, but our physical, spiritual, and emotional fascination with blood is primordial. Why did success elude experimenters for so long?

Clotting was the principal obstacle to overcome. Attempts to find a nontoxic anticoagulant began in 1869, when Braxton Hicks recommended sodium phosphate. This was perhaps the first example of blood preservation research. Karl Landsteiner in 1901 discovered the ABO blood groups and explained the serious reactions that occur in humans as a result of incompatible transfusions. His work early in the twentieth century won a Nobel Prize.

Next came appropriate devices designed for performing the transfusions. Edward E. Lindemann was the first to succeed. He carried out vein-to-vein transfusion of blood by using multiple syringes and a special cannula for puncturing the vein through the skin. However, this time-consuming, complicated procedure required many skilled assistants. It was not until Unger designed his syringe-valve apparatus that transfusions from donor to patient by an unassisted physician became practical.

An unprecedented accomplishment in blood transfusion was achieved in 1914, when Hustin reported the use of sodium citrate as an anticoagulant solution for transfusions. Later, in 1915, Lewisohn determined the minimum amount of citrate needed for anticoagulation and demonstrated its nontoxicity in small amounts. Transfusions became more practical and safer for the patient.

The development of preservative solutions to enhance the metabolism of the red cell followed. Glucose was tried as early as 1916 when Rous and Turner introduced a citrate-dextrose solution for the preservation of blood. However, the function of glucose in red cell metabolism was not understood until the 1930s. Therefore, the common practice of using glucose in the preservative solution was delayed.

World War II stimulated blood preservation research because the demand for blood and plasma increased. The pioneer work of Charles Drew during World War II on developing techniques in blood transfusion and blood preservation led to the establishment of a widespread system of blood banks. In February of 1941, Dr. Drew was appointed director of the first American Red Cross Blood Bank at Presbyterian Hospital. The pilot program Dr. Drew established became the model for the national volunteer blood donor program of the American Red Cross.[1] In 1943, Loutit and Mollison of England introduced the formula for the preservative acid-citrate-dextrose (ACD). Efforts in several countries resulted in the landmark publication of the July 1947 issue of the *Journal of Clinical Investigation*, which devoted nearly a dozen papers to blood preservation. Hospitals responded immediately, and in 1947 blood banks were established in many major cities of the United States; subsequently, transfusion became commonplace. The daily occurrence of transfusions led to the discovery of numerous blood group systems. Antibody identification surged to the forefront as sophisticated techniques were developed. The interested student can review historic events during World War II in Kendrick's *Blood Program in World War II, Historical Note.*[2] In 1957, Gibson introduced an im-proved preservative solution, citrate-phosphate-dextrose (CPD), which was less acidic and eventually replaced ACD as the standard preservative used for blood storage.

Frequent transfusions and the massive use of blood soon resulted in new problems, such as circulatory overload. Component therapy has solved these problems. Before, a single unit of whole blood could serve only one patient. With component therapy, however, one unit may be used for multiple transfusions. Today, physicians can select the specific component for their patient's particular needs without risking the inherent hazards of whole blood transfusions. Physicians can transfuse only the required fraction in the concentrated form, without overloading the circulation. Appropriate blood component therapy now provides more effective treatment and more complete use of blood products. Extensive use of blood during this period, coupled with component separation, led to increased comprehension of erythrocyte metabolism and a new awareness of the problems associated with red cell storage. Today approximately 23 million units of blood components are transfused into 4 million recipients every year in the United States.[3] These units are donated by less than 5 percent of healthy Americans who are eligible to donate each year, primarily through blood drives conducted at their place of work. Individuals can also donate at community blood centers (which collect approximately 88 percent of the nation's blood) or hospital-based donor centers (which collect approximately 12 percent of the nation's blood supply). Volunteer donors (who are *not* paid) provide nearly all of the blood used for transfusion in the United States. Each unit of whole blood collected contains approximately 450 ml of blood (one pint) and 63 ml of anticoagulant-preservative solution, which is present in the commercially available blood collection bags.

The total blood volume of most adults is 10 to 12 pints, and donors can replenish the fluid lost from the donation of 1 pint in 24 hours. The donor red cells are replaced within 1 to 2 months after donation. A volunteer donor can donate whole blood every 8 weeks. Most of the whole blood collected is separated into components. A total of 4 components may be prepared from 1 unit of blood; these include packed red cells, platelets, plasma, and other clotting factors, such as cryoprecipitated antihemophilic factor (AHF) (refer to Chapter 10). A unit of blood may be stored for 21 to 42 days, depending on the preservative solution used. Although most people assume that donated blood is free—and, indeed, most blood-collecting organizations are nonprofit—a fee is still charged for each unit to cover the costs associated with collecting, storing, testing, and transfusing blood! The national average for the cost of processing a unit of red cells is approximately $75.

The donation process consists of three steps or processes: (1) educational reading materials, (2) the donor health history questionnaire, and (3) the abbreviated physical examination (Table 1–1). The donation process, especially steps (1) and (2), has been refined over time to allow carefully for the rejection of donors who may be at risk for transmission of transfusion-associated disease. For a more detailed description of donor screening and processing, the reader should refer to Chapter 10.

The nation's blood supply is safer than it has ever

**Table 1–2.** Donor Screening Tests for Infectious Diseases

| Test | Date Test Required |
|---|---|
| Human immunodeficiency virus 24 antigen (HIV) | 1996 |
| Human immunodeficiency virus antibodies (anti-HIV-2) | 1992 |
| Hepatitis C virus antibodies (anti-HCV) | 1990 |
| Human T-cell lymphotropic virus antibody (HTLV-1) | 1989 |
| Hepatitis B core antibody (anti-HBc) | 1986 |
| Human immunodeficiency virus antibodies (anti-HIV-1) | 1985 |
| Hepatitis B surface antigen (HBsAg) | 1972 |
| Syphilis (Rapid Plasma Reagin [RPR] test) | 1945 |

been because of the donation process and extensive laboratory screening (testing) of blood. Currently, eight screening tests for infectious disease are performed on each unit of donated blood (Table 1–2). A study by Screiber and colleagues has estimated that the aggregate risk of the transmission of virus—specifically, human immunodeficiency virus (HIV), human T-lymphotropic virus (HTLV), hepatitis B and hepatitis C viruses—by the transfusion of screened blood is 1 in 34,000.[4] Refer to Chapter 19 for a detailed discussion of transfusion-transmitted viruses.

## RED CELL BIOLOGY AND PRESERVATION

Three areas of red blood cell (RBC) biology are crucial for normal erythrocyte survival and function:

1. Normal chemical composition and structure of the RBC membrane
2. Hemoglobin structure and function
3. RBC metabolism

Defects in any or all of these areas will result in RBC survival of less than the normal 120 days in circulation.

### Red Cell Membrane

The red cell membrane represents a semipermeable lipid bilayer supported by a protein meshlike cytoskeleton structure (Fig. 1–1).[5] Phospholipids, the main lipid components of the membrane, are arranged

**Table 1–1.** The Donation Process

*Step 1: Educational Reading Materials*
Educational material (such as the AABB pamphlet, "An Important Message to All Blood Donors") that contains information on the risks of infectious diseases transmitted by blood transfusion, including the symptoms and sign of AIDs, is given to each prospective donor to read.

*Step 2: The Donor Health History Questionnaire*
A uniform donor history questionnaire designed to ask questions that protect the health of both the donor and the recipient is given to every donor. The health history questionnaire is used to identify donors who have been exposed to other diseases (e.g., malaria, babesiosis, or Chagas' disease).

*Step 3: The Abbreviated Physical Examination*
The abbreviated physical examination for donors includes blood pressure, pulse, and temperature readings.

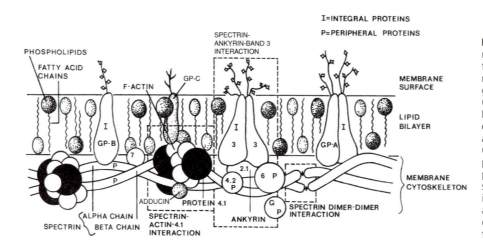

**Figure 1–1.** Schematic illustration of red blood cell membrane depicting the composition and arrangement of red cell membrane proteins. GP-A = glycophorin A; GP-B = glycophorin B; GP-C = glycophorin C; G = globin. Numbers refer to pattern of migration of SDS (sodium dodecyl sulfate) poly-acrylamide gel pattern stained with Coomassie brilliant blue. Relations of protein to each other and to lipids are purely hypothetical; however, the positions of the proteins relative to the inside or outside of the lipid bilayer are accurate. (Note: Proteins are not drawn to scale and many minor proteins are omitted.)

**Table 1–3.** Red Cell Membrane Integral and Peripheral Proteins

| Integral Proteins | Peripheral Proteins |
| --- | --- |
| Glycophorin A | Spectrin |
| Glycophorin B | Actin (band 5) |
| Glycophorin C | Ankyrin (band 2.1) |
| Anion-exchange-channel protein (band 3) | Band 4.1 and 4.2 |
| | Band 6 |
| | Adducin |

in a bilayer structure comprising the framework in which globular proteins traverse and move. Proteins that extend from the outer surface and span the entire membrane to the inner cytoplasmic side of the RBC are termed "integral" membrane proteins. Beneath the lipid bilayer, a second class of membrane proteins, called "peripheral" proteins, is located and limited to the cytoplasmic surface of the membrane forming the red cell cytoskeleton (Table 1–3).[5] Both proteins and lipids are organized asymmetrically within the red cell membrane. Lipids are not equally distributed in the two layers of the membrane. The external layer is rich in glycolipids and choline phospholipids.[6] The internal cytoplasmic layer of the membrane is rich in amino phospholipids.[6] The biochemical composition of the red cell membrane is approximately 52 percent protein, 40 percent lipid, and 8 percent carbohydrate.[7]

As mentioned previously, the normal chemical composition and the structural arrangement and molecular interactions of the erythrocyte membrane are crucial to the normal length of red cell survival in circulation of 120 days. In addition, they maintain a critical role in two important RBC characteristics: deformability and permeability.

### Deformability

To remain viable, normal RBCs must also remain flexible, deformable, and permeable. The loss of adenosine

triphosphate (ATP) (energy) levels leads to a decrease in the phosphorylation of spectrin and, in turn, a loss of membrane deformability.[6] An accumulation or increase in deposition of membrane calcium also results, causing an increase in membrane rigidity and loss of pliability. These cells are at a marked disadvantage when they pass through the small (3 to 5 μm in diameter) sinusoidal orifices of the spleen, an organ that functions in extravascular sequestration and removal of aged, damaged, or less deformable RBCs or fragments of their membrane. The loss of RBC membrane is exemplified by the formation of "spherocytes" (cells with a reduced surface-to-volume ratio) (Fig. 1–2) and "bite cells," in which the removal of a portion of membrane has left a permanent indentation in the remaining cell membrane (Fig. 1–3). The survival of these forms is also shortened.

### Permeability

The permeability properties of the RBC membrane and the active RBC cation transport prevent colloid hemolysis and control the volume of the red cell. Any abnormality that increases permeability or alters cationic transport may lead to decrease in RBC survival.

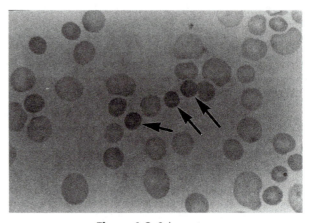

**Figure 1–2.** Spherocytes.

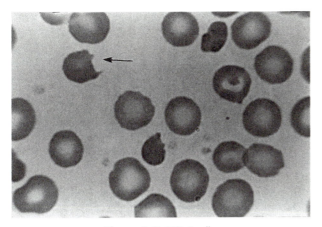

**Figure 1–3.** "Bite" cells.

The RBC membrane is freely permeable to water and anions. Chloride ($Cl^-$) and bicarbonate ($HCO_3^-$) can traverse the membrane in less than a second. It is speculated that this massive exchange of ions occurs through a large number of exchange channels located in the RBC membrane. The RBC membrane is relatively impermeable to cations such as sodium ($Na^+$) and potassium ($K^+$). Red blood cell volume and water homeostasis are maintained by controlling the intracellular concentrations of sodium and potassium. The erythrocyte intracellular-to-extracellular ratios for sodium and potassium are 1:12 and 25:1, respectively. The 300 cationic pumps, which actively transport sodium out of the cell and potassium into the cell, require energy in the form of ATP. Calcium ($Ca^{2+}$) is also actively pumped from the interior of the RBC through energy-dependent calcium-ATPase pumps. Calmodulin, a cytoplasmic calcium-binding protein, is speculated to control these pumps and to prevent excessive intracellular calcium buildup, which changes the shape and makes the RBC more rigid.

When RBCs are ATP-depleted, calcium and sodium are allowed to accumulate intracellularly, and potassium and water are lost, resulting in a dehydrated, rigid cell subsequently sequestered by the spleen, resulting in a decrease in RBC survival.

## Metabolic Pathways

The red cell's metabolic pathways that produce ATP are mainly anaerobic, because the function of the red cell is to deliver oxygen, not to consume it. Because the mature erythrocyte has no nucleus and there is no mitochondrial apparatus for oxidative metabolism, energy must be generated almost exclusively through the breakdown of glucose.

Red cell metabolism may be divided among the anaerobic glycolytic pathway and three ancillary pathways that serve to maintain the function of hemoglobin (Fig. 1–4). All of these processes are essential if the erythrocyte is to transport oxygen and to maintain critical physical characteristics for its survival.

Glycolysis generates about 90 percent of the ATP needed by the RBC. Approximately 10 percent is provided by the pentose phosphate pathway. The activity of this pathway increases following increased oxidation of glutathione or decrease in activity of the glycolytic pathway.

When the pentose phosphate pathway is functionally deficient, the amount of reduced glutathione becomes insufficient to neutralize intracellular oxidants. The result is denaturation and precipitation of globin as aggregates (Heinz bodies) within the cell. The formation of Heinz bodies makes the RBC less deformable than a normal red cell and may cause the red cell to be caught in the spleen or capillaries, damaging the membrane. If membrane damage is sufficient, cell destruction occurs.

The methemoglobin reductase pathway is another important pathway of red cell metabolism. This pathway is necessary to maintain the heme iron of hemoglobin in the ferrous ($Fe^{2+}$) functional state. In the absence of the enzyme methemoglobin reductase and the action of nicotinamide adenine dinucleotide (NAD), there is an accumulation of methemoglobin, which results from a conversion of ferrous iron to the ferric form ($Fe^{3+}$). Methemoglobin represents a nonfunctional form of hemoglobin and a loss of oxygen transport capabilities, inasmuch as metheme cannot bind with oxygen. To illustrate the efficiency of this system, normal healthy individuals have no more than 1 percent methemoglobin circulating in their red cells. A defect in the methemoglobin reductase pathway is, therefore, significant to red cell posttransfusion survival and function.

Another pathway that is crucial to red cell function is the Luebering-Rapaport shunt. This pathway permits the accumulation of another important red cell organic phosphate, 2,3-diphosphoglycerate (2,3-DPG). The large amount of 2,3-DPG found within red cells has a significant effect on the affinity of hemoglobin for oxygen.

## Hemoglobin Structure and Function

Hemoglobin makes up approximately 95 percent of the dry weight of a red cell or approximately 33 percent of its weight by volume.[8] Because of its multichain structure, hemoglobin, which has a molecular weight of 68,000, is capable of considerable allosteric change as it loads and unloads oxygen. Normal hemoglobin consists of globin (a tetramer of two pairs of polypeptide chains) and four heme groups, each of which contains a protoporphyrin ring plus iron ($Fe^{2+}$).

### Hemoglobin Synthesis

Normal hemoglobin production is dependent on three processes:

1. Adequate iron delivery and supply
2. Adequate synthesis of protoporphyrins (the precursor of heme)
3. Adequate globin synthesis

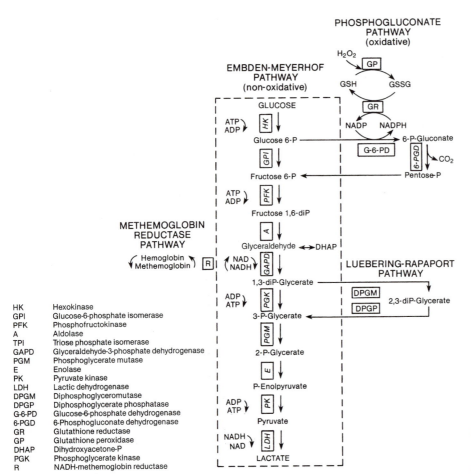

**Figure 1–4.** Red cell metabolism. (From Hillman, RF, and Finch, CA: Red Cell Manual, ed 7, FA Davis, Philadelphia, 1996, p 15, with permission.)

All adult normal hemoglobins are formed as tetramers consisting of two alpha chains plus two (nonalpha) globin chains. Normal adult RBCs contain the following types of hemoglobin:

92 to 95 percent of the hemoglobin is HbA, which consists of two alpha, two beta ($\alpha_2\beta_2$) chains.

2 to 3 percent of the hemoglobin is HbA$_2$, which consists of two alpha, two delta ($\alpha_2\delta_2$) chains.

1 to 2 percent of the hemoglobin is fetal hemoglobin (HbF), which consists of two alpha, two gamma ($\alpha_2\gamma_2$) chains.

Each synthesized globin chain links with heme (ferroprotoporphyrin 9) to form hemoglobin, which normally consists of two alpha chains, two beta chains, and four heme groups.

The rate of globin synthesis is directly related to the rate of porphyrin synthesis, and vice versa: protoporphyrin synthesis is reduced when globin synthesis is impaired.

### Hemoglobin Function

Hemoglobin's primary function is gas transport: oxygen delivery to the tissues and carbon dioxide excretion. One of the most important controls of hemoglobin affinity for oxygen is the RBC organic phosphate 2,3-DPG. The unloading of oxygen by hemoglobin is accompanied by widening of a space between beta chains and the binding of 2,3-DPG on a mole-for-mole basis, with the formation of anionic salt bridges between the chains. The resulting conformation of the deoxyhemoglobin molecule is known as the tense (T) form, which has a lower affinity for oxygen. When hemoglobin loads oxygen and becomes oxyhemoglobin, the established salt bridges are broken and beta chains are pulled together, expelling 2,3-DPG. This is the relaxed (R) form of the hemoglobin molecule, which has a higher affinity for oxygen.

These allosteric changes that occur as the hemoglobin loads and unloads oxygen are referred to as the *respiratory movement*. The dissociation and binding of oxygen by hemoglobin are not directly proportional to the partial pressure of oxygen ($Po_2$) in its environment but, instead, exhibit a sigmoid-curve relationship, known as the hemoglobin-oxygen dissociation curve (Figure 1–5). The shape of this curve is very important physiologically because it permits a considerable amount of oxygen to be delivered to the tissues with a small drop in oxygen tension. For example, in the environment of the lungs, where the oxygen ($Po_2$) tension, measured in millimeters of mercury (mm Hg), is nearly 100 mm

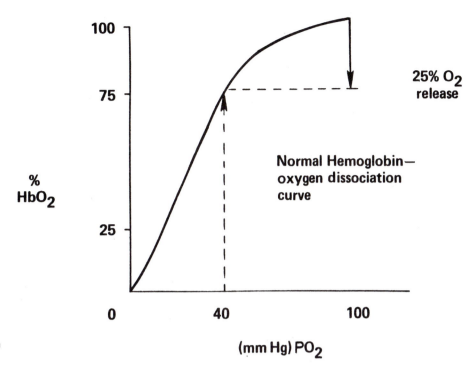

**Figure 1–5.** Hemoglobin-oxygen dissociation curve.

Hg, the hemoglobin molecule is almost 100 percent saturated with oxygen. As the red cells travel to the tissues, where the $PO_2$ drops to an average 40 mm Hg (mean venous oxygen tension), the hemoglobin saturation drops to approximately 75 percent saturation, releasing approximately 25 percent of the oxygen to the tissues.

This is the normal situation of oxygen delivery at basal metabolic rate. The normal position of the oxygen dissociation curve depends on three different ligands normally found within the red cell: $H^+$ ions, $CO_2$, and organic phosphates. Of these three ligands, 2,3-DPG plays the most important physiologic role. The dependence of normal hemoglobin function on

2,3-DPG levels in the red cell has been well documented.[9–12] In situations such as hypoxia, a compensatory "shift to the right" of the hemoglobin-oxygen dissociation curve occurs to alleviate a tissue oxygen deficit (Fig. 1–6). This rightward shift of the curve, mediated by increased levels of 2,3-DPG, results in a decrease in hemoglobin's affinity for the oxygen molecule and an increase in oxygen delivery to the tissues. Note in Figure 1–6 that the oxygen saturation of hemoglobin in the environment of the tissues (40 mm Hg $PO_2$) is now 50 percent; the other 50 percent of the oxygen is being released to the tissues. The RBCs thus have become more efficient in terms of oxygen delivery.

Therefore, a patient who is suffering from an anemia

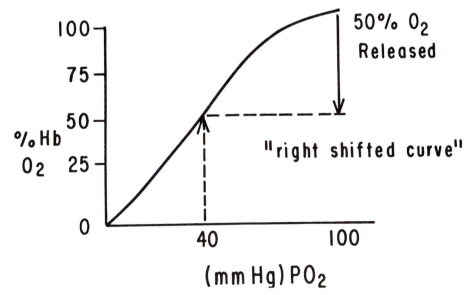

**Figure 1–6.** "Shift to the right" of the hemoglobin-oxygen dissociation curve.

caused by loss of RBCs may be able to compensate by shifting the oxygen dissociation curve to the right, making the RBCs, although few in number, more efficient. Some patients may be able to tolerate anemia better than others because of this compensatory mechanism. A shift to the right may also occur in response to acidosis or a rise in body temperature. The shift to the right of the hemoglobin-oxygen dissociation curve is only one way in which patients may compensate for various types of hypoxia. Other ways include an increase in total cardiac output and an increase in the production of red cells (erythropoiesis).

A "shift to the left" of the hemoglobin-oxygen dissociation curve results, conversely, in an increase in hemoglobin-oxygen affinity and a decrease in oxygen delivery to the tissues (Fig. 1–7). With such a dissociation curve, RBCs are much less efficient because only 12 percent of the oxygen can be released to the tissues. Among the conditions that can shift the oxygen dissociation curve to the left are alkalosis; increased quantities of abnormal hemoglobins, such as methemoglobin and carboxyhemoglobin; increased quantities of hemoglobin F; or multiple transfusions of 2,3-DPG–depleted stored blood (attesting to the importance of 2,3-DPG in oxygen release).

Hemoglobin-oxygen affinity can also be expressed by $P_{50}$ values, which designate the $PO_2$ at which hemoglobin is 50 percent saturated with oxygen under standard in vitro conditions of temperature and pH. The $P_{50}$ of normal blood is 26 to 30 mm Hg. An increase in $P_{50}$ represents a decrease in hemoglobin-oxygen affinity, or a shift to the right of the oxygen dissociation curve. A decrease in $P_{50}$ represents an increase in hemoglobin-oxygen affinity, or a shift to the left of the oxygen dissociation curve. In addition to the reasons listed previously for shifts in the curve, inherited abnormalities of the hemoglobin molecule can result in either situation; these abnormalities are described by the $P_{50}$ measurements. Abnormalities in hemoglobin structure or function can therefore have profound effects on the ability of the RBCs to provide oxygen to the tissues.

### Red Cell Preservation

The goal of blood preservation is to provide viable and functional blood components for patients requiring blood transfusion. Red cell viability is a measure of in vivo red cell survival following transfusion. Because blood must be stored from the time of donation until the time of transfusion, the viability of red cells must be maintained during the storage time as well. Seventy-five percent of cells that have been transfused should remain viable for 24 hours for the transfusion to be considered successful.[13] Also, as storage time increases, red cell viability decreases. To maintain optimum viability, blood is stored in the liquid state between 1°C and 6°C for a predetermined shelf life.

The loss of red cell viability has been correlated with the "lesion of storage," which is associated with various biochemical changes. These changes include a decrease in pH, a buildup of lactic acid, a decrease in glucose consumption, a decrease in ATP levels, and a loss of red cell function.[12] This loss of function is expressed as a shift to the left of the hemoglobin-oxygen dissociation curve or an increase in hemoglobin-oxygen affinity.

Because low 2,3-DPG levels profoundly influence the oxygen dissociation curve of hemoglobin,[14] 2,3-DPG-depleted red cells may have an impaired capacity to deliver oxygen to the tissues. The rate of restoration of 2,3-DPG is influenced by the acid-base status of the recipient, phosphorus metabolism, and the degree of anemia.

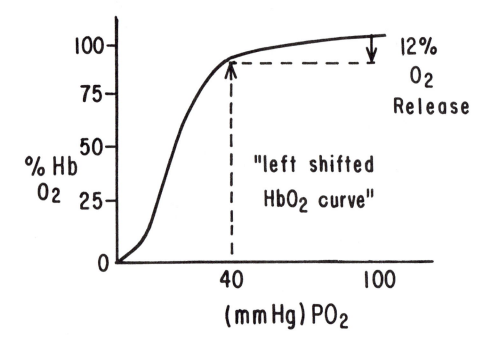

**Figure 1–7.** "Shift to the left" of the hemoglobin-oxygen dissociation curve.

As blood is stored, however, 2,3-DPG levels decrease, there is a shift to the left of the hemoglobin-oxygen dissociation curve, and less oxygen is delivered to the tissues. Therefore, an effective blood preservative must be capable of maintaining both viability reflected in ATP levels and hemoglobin function reflected by 2,3-DPG levels.

## Approved Preservative Solutions

Acid-citrate-dextrose, CPD, and CP2D are approved preservative solutions for blood storage at 1 to 6°C for 21 days[15] (Table 1–4). Because of the lower pH in ACD preservative, most of the 2,3-DPG is lost early in the first week of storage. Therefore, a substitute preservative, CPD, came into widespread use in the United States because it was superior for preserving this organic phosphate. This effect is the result of a higher pH (Table 1–5). Even in CPD, red cells become low in 2,3-DPG by the second week. Subsequent studies led to the addition of various chemicals along with the currently approved anticoagulant CPD in pursuit of a means to stimulate glycolysis.[11]

One of the chemicals, adenine, was approved for addition to CPD by the Food and Drug Administration (FDA) in August 1978. The incorporation of adenine (CPDA-1) into blood storage seems to increase ADP levels, thereby driving glycolysis toward the synthesis of ATP. CPDA-1 contains 0.25 mM of adenine plus 25 percent more glucose than CPD (see Table 1–5). Adenine-

supplemented blood can be stored at 1 to 6°C for 35 days. CP2D contains 100 percent more glucose than CPD, or 60 percent more glucose than CPDA-1. However, blood stored in all CPD preservatives also becomes depleted of 2,3-DPG by the second week of storage.

The reported pathophysiologic effects of the transfusion of red blood cells with low 2,3-DPG levels and increased affinity for oxygen include either an increase in cardiac output, a decrease in mixed venous $PO_2$ tension, or a combination of these. The physiologic importance of these effects is *not* easily demonstrated. This is a complex mechanism with numerous variables involved that are beyond the scope of this text.

Stored red cells do regain the ability to synthesize 2,3-DPG after transfusion, but levels necessary for optimal hemoglobin oxygen delivery are not reached immediately. Approximately 24 hours are required to restore normal levels of 2,3-DPG after transfusion.[12] The 2,3-DPG concentrations after transfusion have been reported to reach normal levels as early as 6 hours post-transfusion.[13] Most of these studies have been performed on normal, healthy individuals. However, evidence suggests that, in the transfused subject whose capacity is limited by an underlying physiologic disturbance, even a brief period of altered oxygen hemoglobin affinity is of great significance.[14]

It is quite clear now that 2,3-DPG levels in transfused blood are important in certain clinical conditions. Several animal studies demonstrate significantly increased mortality associated with transfusing blood that is low in 2,3-DPG levels in subjects with persistent anemia, hypotension, hypoxia, and cardiac and hemorrhagic shock. Human studies demonstrate that myocardial function improves following transfusion of blood with high 2,3-DPG levels during cardiovascular surgery.[16]

Several investigators suggest that the patient in shock who is given 2,3-DPG–depleted erythrocytes in transfusion may have already strained the compensatory mechanisms to their limits.[16–18] Perhaps for this type of patient the poor oxygen delivery capacity of 2,3-DPG–depleted cells makes a significant difference in recovery and survival.

**Table 1–4.** Approved Preservatives

| Name | Abbreviation | Storage Time (days) |
|---|---|---|
| Acid-citrate-dextrose | ACD | 21 |
| Citrate-phosphate-dextrose | CPD | 21 |
| Citrate-phosphate-adenine | CPDA-1 | 35 |
| Citrate-phosphate-double dextrose | CP2D | 21 |

**Table 1–5.** Comparison of the Composition of Acid-Citrate-Dextrose (ACD) and Citrate-Phosphate-Dextrose (CPD) Preservatives

| | ACD | CPD | CPDA-1 | CP2D |
|---|---|---|---|---|
| Trisodium citrate (g) | 22.0 | 26.30 | 26.35 | 26.35 |
| Citric acid (g) | 8.0 | 3.27 | 3.27 | 3.27 |
| Dextrose (g) | 24.5 | 25.50 | 31.90 | 51.10 |
| Monobasic sodium phosphate (g) | — | 2.22 | 2.22 | 2.22 |
| Adenine (g) | — | — | 0.27 | — |
| Water (mL) | 1000 | 1000 | 1000 | 1000 |
| Volume/100 mL blood (mL) | 15 | 14 | 14 | 14 |
| Approximate volume of preservative solution/bag (mL) | 67.5 | 63.0 | 63.0 | 63.0 |
| Initial pH of solution* | 5.0 | 5.6 | 5.6 | 5.6 |
| pH of blood on initial day drawn into storage bag* | 7.0 | 7.2 | 7.4 | 7.3 |
| Storage time (days) 1–6°C | 21 | 21 | 35 | 21 |

**Note:** Approximately 63 mL of anticoagulant preservative is mixed with approximately 450 mL of blood in each unit.
*Indicates measurement at room temperature.

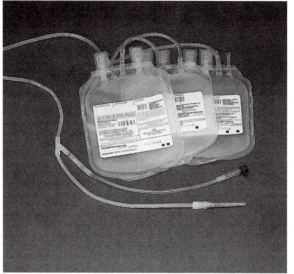

**Figure 1–8.** The Teruflex CPD/Optisol Triple blood bags with blood sampling arm. (Courtesy of Terumo Medical Corporation, Somerset, NJ.)

It is apparent that many factors may limit the viability of transfused red cells. One of these factors is the plastic material used for the storage container. The plastic must be sufficiently permeable to $CO_2$ in order to maintain higher pH levels during storage. Glass storage containers are a matter of history in the United States. Currently all blood is stored in polyvinyl chloride (PVC) plastic bags (Fig. 1–8). Another problem associated with PVC bags is the plasticizer, di(ethylhexyl)-phthalate (DEHP), which is used in the manufacture of the bags. It has been found to leach into the blood from the plastic into the lipids of the plasma and cell membranes during storage. The accumulation of excessive amounts of acid from glucose use, even at low storage temperatures, is also a major problem in liquid preservation of red cells. Research, therefore, has been focused on the development of an improved plastic blood bag as well as better preservative solutions. In addition to blood preservation problems, adverse effects and risks associated with blood transfusion have created concern and caution among clinicians when determining the need for blood and blood components (see Chapter 18).

## CURRENT TRENDS IN BLOOD PRESERVATION RESEARCH

Research and development in blood preservation have advanced in four directions: (1) additive solutions, (2) rejuvenation solutions, (3) red cell freezing, and (4) blood substitutes.

### Additive Solutions

Traditional anticoagulants and preservatives were developed and put into use when whole blood was the major blood product. With the advent of component therapy, red cell concentrate usage increased in the 1970s and several problems arose. Because approximately 40 percent of adenine and glucose present in standard anticoagulants was removed in the preparation of red cell concentrates, a decrease in viability was seen, particularly in the last 2 weeks of storage.[12] Red cell concentrates relatively void of plasma were also more viscous and difficult to infuse in emergency situations.

In an effect to overcome these problems, blood centers began monitoring the hematocrits of their red cell units. In general, red cell concentrates were prepared with hematocrits of less than 80 percent to allow adequate plasma to remain for red cell nourishment and improved flow properties. This, in turn, resulted in lower plasma yields, affecting fresh frozen plasma and cryoprecipitate production as well as production of plasma derivatives.

While blood centers in the United States improved the quality of red cell concentrates by adjusting the hematocrit, a new additive system concept was developed by Lovric[19] in Australia and Hogman[20] in Sweden. This new blood collection system employed a primary bag containing standard anticoagulant and an accessory, or satellite, bag containing an additional nutrient solution. After the plasma was removed from a unit of whole blood, the additive solution was added to the red cells, thus providing nutrients for improved viability.

Additive systems were routinely used in Sweden (Hogman) and in Australia (Lovric) before their introduction in the United States.[21] In general, the additive solutions employed in the systems were composed of standard ingredients used intravenously: saline, dextrose, and adenine. The systems described by Hogman and Lovric differ only slightly in their approach. Hogman's system uses the standard CPD anticoagulant in the primary bag with an additive solution containing saline, adenine, and glucose (SAG).[20] This system was modified further with the addition of mannitol (SAGM), which protected against spontaneous storage hemolysis.[20] Lovric doubled the dextrose concentration in the primary anticoagulant (CP2D) and used it in connection with an additive solution composed of saline, adenine, glucose, trisodium citrate, citric acid, and sodium phosphate.[19]

Three additive solutions are licensed in the United States: (1) Adsol (AS-1) (Fenwal Laboratories), (2) Nutricel (AS-3) (Medsep Corporation, formerly Cutter Biological), and (3) Optisol (AS-5) (Terumo Corporation). Adsol solution contains buffered adenine, glucose, and mannitol to retard hemolysis. It is coupled with CPD as the primary bag anticoagulant. Nutricel employs CP2D for the primary bag anticoagulant-preservative and 100 mL of buffered adenine glucose solution for RBC viability. Optisol contains adenine, glucose, and mannitol and uses CPD in the primary bag. All of these additive solutions are approved for 42 days of storage. Table 1–6 lists the currently approved

**Table 1–6.** Additive Solutions

| Name | Abbreviation | Storage Time (days) |
|---|---|---|
| Adsol (Fenwal Laboratories) | AS-1 | 42 |
| Nutricel (Medsep Corporation) | AS-3 | 42 |
| Optisol (Terumo Corporation) | AS-5 | 42 |

**Table 1–7.** Formulations of Additive Solutions

| | AS-1 | AS-3 | AS-5 |
|---|---|---|---|
| Adenine (mM) | 2.00 | 2.22 | 2.22 |
| Glucose (mM) | 111.00 | 55.51 | 45.41 |
| Mannitol (nM) | 41.20 | — | 28.82 |
| NaCl (mM) | 154.00 | 70.15 | 150.04 |
| $Na_2HPO_4$ (mM) | — | 23.00 | — |
| Primary bag anticoagulant | CPD | CP2D | CPD |

additive solutions and Table 1–7 describes formulations for each one.[15]

In clinical trials, conflicting data regarding red cell survivals on AS-1–stored red cells resulted in the FDA convening a workshop on AS-1 and other additive solutions in 1985. The consensus of the FDA Advisory Panel resulted in (1) changing the approval of AS-1 from 49 days to 42 days, which is the storage limit for all additive solutions in the United States; and (2) raising the minimum average acceptable survival requirements for additive solutions from 70 percent to 75 percent. In clinical studies, red cells stored for 42 days in AS-5, AS-3, or AS-1 demonstrated a mean posttransfusion survival greater than 75 percent.

Table 1–8 shows the biochemical characteristics of red cells stored in the three additive solutions after 42 days of storage.[15,22] Poststorage survival rates of greater than 80 percent were demonstrated (safely above the minimum 75 percent level required) with less than 1 percent hemolysis. Additive system red cells are indicated for use in the same patient population receiving standard red cell transfusions.[23]

None of the additive solutions maintains 2,3-DPG throughout the storage time, and one should be aware of the metabolic load the patient must handle in the

**Table 1–8.** Additive Red Cells: Biochemical Characteristics

| | AS-1 | AS-3 | AS-5 |
|---|---|---|---|
| Storage period | 42.00 | 42.00 | 42.00 |
| pH (measured at 37°C) | 6.6 | 6.5 | 6.5 |
| 24-hour survival* (%) | 83.00 | 85.1 | 80.0 |
| ATP (% initial) | 68.00 | 67.0 | 68.5 |
| 2,3-DPG (% initial) | 6.0 | 6.0 | 5.0 |
| Hemolysis (%) | 0.5 | 0.7 | 0.6 |

*Survival studies reported are from selected investigators and do not include an average of all reported survivals.

blood stored in these additive solutions (see Table 1–8). Therefore, blood stored in additive solutions is *not* routinely given to newborn infants and should be evaluated in light of the patient's underlying condition.

In summary, all currently FDA-approved additive solutions provide 42-day storage of red cells with greater than 80 percent posttransfusion survival.[23] This facilitates better inventory control of blood as well as wider use of autologous red cells in elective surgical procedures.[23] In addition, the use of additive solutions allows extraction of increased volumes of fresh plasma for optimal production of platelets, factor VIII yields, and fresh frozen plasma components.[23] Additive solutions allow the storage of whole blood at room temperature for up to 8 hours, which allows increased time for the preparation of blood components and thereby improves overall work flow.[23]

## Rejuvenation Solutions

Solutions containing phosphate, inosine, glucose, pyruvate, and adenine (PIGPA), incubated with outdated erythrocytes, can regenerate both ATP and 2,3-DPG levels in red cells stored in CPD, CPDA-1, or AS-1.[24] Valeri[25] and coworkers have been the forerunners in these rejuvenation studies on outdated blood. Subsequent investigations have led to the removal of glucose from the original mixture, and the resulting solution is designated PIPA.[26] Currently, Rejuvesol (Cytosol Laboratories) is the only FDA-approved rejuvenation solution sold in the United States and contains the same chemicals as the original PIPA solution.[15] Generally, red cells stored in the liquid state for fewer than 3 days after their outdate[26] can be rejuvenated by incubation for 1 to 4 hours at 37°C with this solution. The red cells are washed before transfusion to remove the rejuvenation mixture and deleterious amounts of extracellular potassium. Because the blood bag has been open for the washing procedure, usually by mechanical devices, federal regulations require the unit to be used within 24 hours to minimize the risk of bacterial contamination.[15] Rejuvesol is used in some blood centers primarily to regenerate ATP and 2,3-DPG levels before red cell freezing, most often in autologous units that could not be frozen within the first 6 days of storage. The rejuvenation process is expensive and time consuming; therefore, it is not used often but is invaluable for preserving selected autologous and rare units of blood for later use.

## Red Cell Freezing

Red cell freezing is primarily used for autologous units and the storage of rare blood types. Autologous transfusion allows individuals to donate blood for their own (autologous) use in meeting their needs for blood transfusion (see Chap. 16).

The procedure for freezing a unit of packed red cells is simple. Basically, it involves the addition of a cryoprotective agent to red cells that are less than 6 days old. Glycerol is used most commonly and is added to the red cells slowly with vigorous shaking, thereby enabling the glycerol to permeate the red cells. The cells are then rapidly frozen and stored in a freezer. The usual storage temperature is below $-65°C$, although storage (and freezing) temperature depends on the concentration of glycerol used.[14] Two concentrations of glycerol have been used to freeze red cells: a high-concentration glycerol (40 percent weight in volume [w/v]) and a low-concentration glycerol (20 percent w/v) in the final concentration of the cryopreservative.[22] Most blood banks that freeze red cells use the high-concentration glycerol technique. Table 1–9 lists the advantages of the high glycerol technique in comparison with low glycerol. The reader is referred to Chapter 10 for a detailed description of the red cell freezing procedure.

Transfusion of frozen cells must be preceded by a deglycerolization process; otherwise the thawed cells would be accompanied by hypertonic glycerol when infused. Removal of glycerol is achieved by systematically replacing the cryoprotectant with decreasing concentrations of saline. The usual protocol involves washing with 12 percent saline, followed by 1.6 percent saline, with a final wash of 0.2 percent dextrose in normal saline.[22] A commercially available cell-washing system, such as one of those manufactured by several companies, can be used in the deglycerolizing process.

Excessive hemolysis is monitored by noting the hemoglobin concentration of the wash supernatant. Osmolality of the unit should also be monitored to ensure adequate deglycerolization. Because the unit of blood is entered to incorporate the glycerol (before freezing) or the saline solutions (for deglycerolization), the outdating period of thawed red cells stored at 1 to 6°C is 24 hours. However, sterile connecting devices or suitably configured multiple plastic storage bags allow freezing and deglycerolization in a closed system with possible extension of the storage period at

1 to 6°C using an additive solution. Generally, red cells are glycerolized and frozen within 6 days of whole blood collection in CPD or CPDA-1 anticoagulants. Red blood cells stored in additive solutions such as AS-1 and AS-3 have been frozen up to 42 days after liquid storage. In addition, after biochemical rejuvenation RBCs can be frozen for prolonged storage.

Currently, the FDA licenses frozen red cells for a period of 10 years from the date of freezing; that is, frozen red cells may be stored up to 10 years before thawing and transfusion.[15] Once thawed, these cells demonstrate function and viability near those of fresh blood. Experience has shown that 10-year storage periods do not adversely affect viability and function.[14] Table 1–10 lists the advantages and disadvantages of red cell freezing.

## Blood Substitutes

Another area of blood research deals with the development of blood substitutes such as hemoglobin-based oxygen carriers and the perfluorochemicals (PFCs).[27,28] A common feature among all of these products is their ability to carry oxygen in the absence of intact red cells. Advantages and disadvantages of blood substitutes are presented in Tables 1–11 and 1–12.

Despite more than 30 years of research for acceptable blood substitutes, an alternative to a unit of red cells is still not approved for human use. Originally developed to be used in trauma situations such as accidents, combat, and surgery, red cell substitutes have fallen short of meeting requirements for this application. Owing to major complicating side effects, blood substitutes are still not in routine use today, although several companies have Investigational New Drug (IND) applications on file at the FDA and are in various phases of clinical trials (Table 1–13).

**Table 1–9.** Advantages of High-Concentration Glycerol Technique Used by Most Blood Banks over Low-Concentration Glycerol Technique

| Advantage | High Glycerol | Low Glycerol |
|---|---|---|
| 1. Initial freezing temperature | $-80°C$ | $-196°C$ |
| 2. Need to control freezing rate | No | Yes |
| 3. Type of freezer | Mechanical | Liquid nitrogen |
| 4. Maximum storage temperature | $-65°C$ | $-120°C$ |
| 5. Shipping requirements | Dry ice | Liquid nitrogen |
| 6. Effect of changes in storage temperature | Can be thawed and refrozen | Critical |

**Table 1–10.** Advantages and Disadvantages of Red Cell Freezing

| Advantages | Disadvantages |
|---|---|
| Long-term storage (10 years) | A time-consuming process |
| Maintenance of red cell viability and function | Higher cost of equipment and materials |
| Low residual leukocytes and platelets | Storage requirements ($-65°C$) |
| Removal of significant amounts of plasma proteins | Higher cost of product |

**Table 1–11.** Advantages and Disadvantages of Stroma-free Hemoglobin Solutions

| Advantages | Disadvantages |
| --- | --- |
| Long shelf life | Short intravascular half-life |
| Very stable | Possible toxicity |
| No antigenicity (unless bovine) | Increased $O_2$ affinity |
| No requirement for blood-typing procedures | Increased oncotic effect |

**Table 1–12.** Advantages and Disadvantages of Perfluorochemicals

| Advantages | Disadvantages |
| --- | --- |
| Biologic inertness | Adverse clinical effects |
| Lack of immunogenicity | High $O_2$ affinity |
| Easily synthesized | Retention in tissues |
| | Requirement for $O_2$ administration when infused |
| | Deep-freeze storage temperatures |

## Hemoglobin-based Oxygen Carriers

Hemoglobin-based oxygen carriers include stroma-free hemoglobin solution (SFHS), chemically modified hemoglobin solutions, recombinant hemoglobin, and encapsulated hemoglobins. Stroma-free hemoglobin solution has been considered for use as a medium to carry oxygen for many years.[29] These solutions can be prepared by hemolyzing outdated red blood cells and removing all of the contaminating stroma, which may be toxic to the kidney. These solutions have several shortcomings.[30] One is their short intravascular persistence, inasmuch as hemoglobin solutions are very quickly eliminated in the urine. The intravascular half-life of native stroma-free hemoglobin is approximately 2 to 4 hours.[30] Another factor that poses problems is the high oxygen affinity of native stroma-free hemoglobin. The hemoglobin-oxygen dissociation curve shows a shift to the left, and $P_{50}$ values range from 12 to 17 mm Hg.[29] In unmodified hemoglobin, the hemoglobin tetramers dissociate into dimers and monomers and lose their relationship with 2,3-DPG.[31] High oncotic effect is the third problem associated with unmodified hemoglobin. As a result, significant toxicity characterized by renal dysfunction, systemic vasoconstriction, and gastrointestinal stress has been demonstrated in previous clinical trials.[30]

Chemical modification of the hemoglobin can be used to address some of these problems. Cross-linking and/or polymerizing the hemoglobin chains can increase dwell time by enlarging the molecule and inhibiting its breakup into smaller subunits, which are easily filtered by the kidney.[32,33] This decreases the osmotic load. Depending on how the chemical modifications are made, oxygen affinity can also be altered, as can the change in affinity related to 2,3-DPG concentration.[34] These chemical modifications can be made using conventional chemical reactions or by making the hemoglobin with an altered amino acid sequence from raw materials. The latter has been accomplished and is being tested clinically by one company.[35] The hemoglobin is made using modified human genes expressed in bacterial cells. Chemically modified human and bovine hemoglobin also are at various stages of development and testing (see Table 1–13).

**Table 1–13.** Commercially Prepared Blood Substitutes Currently in Clinical Trials

| Blood Substitutes | Product Name | Indications for Use | Manufacturer |
| --- | --- | --- | --- |
| Pyridoxylated human Hb conjugated to polyoxyethylene | PHP | Septic shock | Apex Biosciences |
| Human Hb internally cross-linked with bis(3,5 dibromosalicyl) fumarate (DBBF) | HemAssist | Hemorrhagic shock Surgery | Baxter Healthcare |
| Glutaraldehyde-polymerized bovine Hb | Hemopure | Hemodilution Sickle cell disease | Biopure |
| Bovine Hb conjugated to polyethylene glycol | PEG-Hemoglobin | Radiosensitization of solid tumors | Enzon |
| o-Raffinose cross-linked and polymerized human Hb | Hemolink | Surgery Hemodilution | Hemosol |
| Glutaraldehyde-polymerized human Hb | PolyHeme | Trauma Surgery | Northfield Laboratories |
| Recombinant di-alpha human Hb | Optro | Hemodilution Erythropoiesis | Somatogen |
| Emulsified perflubron | Oxygent | Hemodilution Cardiopulmonary bypass | Alliance Pharmaceutical |
| Emulsified perfluorodichlorooctane | Oxyfluor | Cardiopulmonary bypass | HemaGen/PFC |

Hb = hemoglobin
PHP = pyridoxylated hemoglobin polyoxyethyline
PEG = polyethylene glycol
PFC = perfluorocarbon emulsions

Another way to increase dwell time and to minimize osmotic effect is to encapsulate the hemoglobin in an artificial membrane.[36] This approach results in a close red cell analog. Inside the microparticles, an environment could be created that would allow the normal relationship between the hemoglobin tetramer and 2,3-DPG.[36] Other investigators have succeeded in enclosing hemoglobin in liposomal vesicles at concentrations equal to those in erythrocytes.[37,38] The liposome capsule consists of a bilipid layer of phospholipid and cholesterol similar to a cellular membrane but without the incorporated protein or carbohydrate that would give most cellular membranes their immunogenicity. Although this approach is still in its infancy, some hemoglobin-containing microparticles have demonstrated an oxygen affinity similar to that of normal whole blood and a hemoglobin concentration similar to that of red cells.[36] These preparations have been transfused to animals with very low apparent toxicity. However, their circulating half-life is very short.

### Perfluorochemicals

Perfluorochemicals (PFCs) have experienced a tremendous amount of research and testing, as well as publicity. Perfluorochemicals are hydrocarbon structures in which all the hydrogen atoms have been replaced with fluorine. They are chemically inert, are excellent gas solvents, and carry $O_2$ and $CO_2$ by dissolving them. Most PFCs can dissolve as much as 40 to 70 percent of oxygen per unit by volume, whereas whole blood can dissolve only about 20 percent.[39] The concentration of dissolved oxygen in the PFC solution is directly proportional to the concentration of oxygen in the environment. Because PFCs are immiscible with blood, these chemicals are injected as emulsions with albumin, fats, or other chemicals; otherwise, they may cause pulmonary embolism, asphyxia, and death.[39]

The ability of PFC to transport sufficient amounts of oxygen was first demonstrated when mice survived submersion in an oxygenated PFC. Shortly thereafter, Geyer exchanged the blood of rats with PFCs to a hematocrit of 1 percent without any sign of complication.[39] Reperfusion of the rats was also accomplished successfully. Numerous PFCs have been studied, each with different characteristics as far as emulsification capacity, ability to dissolve oxygen, circulation half-life, and tissue half-life.[39] Emulsifying agents also vary. To be considered as a possible red cell substitute, a PFC should be nontoxic, chemically inert, stable to oxygen and carbon dioxide, rapidly excreted, and readily available.[39] The particle size of the emulsion should be small, 0.1 to 0.2 $\mu$m.[39] Larger particle size emulsions are more rapidly removed from the circulation, increase the viscosity of the solution, and lessen the amount of oxygen dissolved. In addition, PFC emulsions of large size are unstable and may separate, thus causing embolization when transfused. Research needs to focus on the production of a PFC that is very stable, does not have a prolonged tissue retention time, does

not require oxygen administration for effectiveness, and has practical storage requirements. The advantages and disadvantages of perfluorochemicals are summarized in Table 1–12.

## PLATELET PRESERVATION

### Introduction

Platelets are intimately involved in *primary hemostasis,* which is the interaction of platelets and the vascular endothelium in halting bleeding following vascular injury. Platelets are cellular fragments derived from the cytoplasm of megakaryocytes present in the bone marrow. Platelets are released and circulate approximately 9 to 12 days as small, disc-shaped cells with an average diameter of 2 to 4 $\mu$m. The normal platelet count ranges from 150,000 to 300,000 $\mu$L, depending on the method employed. Approximately 30 percent of the platelets in the circulation are sequestered in the microvasculature or in the spleen as functional reserves after their release from the bone marrow.

Platelets have specific roles in the hemostatic process that are critically dependent on an adequate number of circulating thrombocytes as well as on normal platelet function. The role of platelets in hemostasis includes (1) maintenance of vascular integrity, (2) initial arrest of bleeding by platelet plug formation, and (3) stabilization of the hemostatic plug by contributing to the process of fibrin formation. Platelets, like other cells, require energy in the form of ATP for cellular movement, active transport of molecules across the membrane, biosynthetic purposes, and maintenance of a hemostatic steady state.

### Preservation of Platelets

Preservative solutions, usually designed for maintenance of red cell function and viability, also have a direct influence on platelet function and viability.

Platelet concentrates (PCs) are effectively used to treat bleeding associated with thrombocytopenia as well as other disorders in which platelets are qualitatively or quantitatively defective. In the 1950s, platelet transfusions were given as freshly drawn whole blood or platelet-rich plasma. Circulatory overload quickly developed as a major complication of this method of administering platelets. Today platelets are prepared as concentrates and still remain the only effective means of correcting thrombocytopenia, even though therapeutic responsiveness varies according to patient population and undefined consequences of platelet storage conditions.

Currently, two methods for PC preparation are available: centrifugation and apheresis (see Chaps. 10 and 17). During centrifugation, a PC can be prepared from a unit of whole blood drawn into a double or triple collection bag by separating platelet-rich plasma from the blood unit and centrifuging again to concentrate platelets. It should be noted that the unit of blood must be kept at room temperature until the platelets have been prepared, which must be done within 8 hours after collection (6 hours for certain companies' bags). Approximately 50 mL of plasma is retained on the PC, which must contain a minimum of $5.5 \times 10^{10}$ platelets, a volume between 45 and 65 mL, and a pH of at least 6.0.[40] In addition, regulations require that at least four PCs be tested monthly for pH, volume, and platelet count at the time of expiration.[15] The expiration date of the PC is determined by the collection system and type of plastics used. Platelet concentrate stored in 3-day bags must have the expiration date and time recorded on the concentrate.

Recording of the expiration date and time is not required when PCs are stored in 5-day bags. If the seal of any PC bag is broken, the platelets should be used within 4 hours if stored at 20 to 24°C.[40] Monitoring and recording of the temperature within the platelet storage area is required.

In plateletpheresis, platelets may also be obtained by drawing blood from a donor into an apheresis instrument, which separates the blood into components using centrifugation, retains the platelets, and returns the remainder of the blood to the donor. This apheresed PC contains about four to six times as many platelets as a unit of platelets obtained from whole blood, with a minimum of $3.0 \times 10^{11}$ specified by the American Association of Blood Banks (AABB) Standards of Apheresis platelets.[41]

To accommodate a common dosage of either 4 to 6 or 6 to 8 units for a bleeding patient, platelet concentrates may be pooled using a transfer bag to combine multiple units into one transfusable product. Once platelet concentrates are pooled, the expiration date changes to 4 hours.[1] Platelet concentrates are most often stored at 20 to 24°C, with continuous agitation for 5 days if prepared in a closed system.[40] Currently elliptical, flat-bed, and circular agitators are commercially available. If polyolefin storage bags are used without plasticizer, then elliptical rotators are not recommended. Fenwal Laboratories currently offers two 5-day platelet bags: PL 732, a polyolefin plastic, and PL 1240, a multipurpose plastic. Terumo Corporation markets Teruflex XT612 plastic container for 5-day platelet storage. Table 1–14 lists factors that should be considered when using 5-day platelet storage containers.[42]

By necessity, storage conditions do cause alterations in the metabolism and function of platelets. Initial pH, temperature of storage, total platelet count, volume of plasma, duration of storage, agitation during storage, and lactic acid accumulation are some of the controversial factors known to influence platelet metabolism and function.[43]

A number of other interrelated variables can also affect platelet viability and function during storage: the anticoagulant used for blood collection; the method used to prepare platelet concentrates; and the composition, surface area, and thickness of the walls of the storage container.

Several studies evaluating platelet storage at various temperatures reported that 20 to 24°C was the optimal storage temperature for platelets, rather than 4°C.[44,45] Platelets stored at 4°C are associated with an irreversible disc-to-sphere transformation. When stored for several hours at 4°C, platelets do not return to their disc shape upon rewarming and are irreversibly spherical.[44] This loss of shape in platelets stored at 4°C is probably a result of microtubule disassembly, which may also be a major contributor to decreased survival of platelets stored at 4°C.[46] The major objection to platelets stored at 4°C is their shortened life span after reinfusion, which can be marked by a decrease after only 18 hours of storage.[44]

In light of these developments, PCs are now prepared and stored at 22°C. However, even storage at 22°C for platelets has several disadvantages. One major difficulty is the regulation of pH, and another is bacterial contamination.[47–49] Virtually all units of PC demonstrate a decrease in pH from their initial value of 7.0. This decrease is primarily a result of the production of lactic acid by platelet glycolysis and, to a lesser extent, of accumulation of carbon dioxide from oxidative phosphorylation. As pH falls from 6.8 to 6.0, the platelets progressively change shape from discs to spheres. In this pH range, the changes of shape are reversible if the platelets are resuspended in plasma with physiologic pH. However, if the pH falls below 6.0, a further irreversible change occurs that renders the platelets nonviable after infusion in vivo.[13]

The loss of platelet viability has been correlated with the "lesion of storage," which is associated with various biochemical changes. Because of this correlation, every effort is being made to understand the metabolic, morphological, and functional changes that occur during platelet preservation. The ultimate goal is to increase the storage time of PCs while maintaining viability and function. Viability indicates the capacity of platelets to circulate after infusion without premature removal or destruction. Platelet viability is determined by measuring pretransfusion and multiple posttransfusion platelet counts,[50] or by determining the disappearance

**Table 1–14.** Factors to Be Considered When Using 5-Day Plastic Storage Bags

Temperature control of 20–24°C is critical during platelet preparation, equilibration, and storage.

n Careful handling of plastic bags during expression of platelet-poor plasma helps prevent the platelet button from being distributed and prevents removal of excess platelets with the platelet-poor plasma.

n Residual plasma volumes recommended for the preparation of platelet concentrates are dependent on the type of plastic bag: PL 732 container = 45–55 mL, PL 1240 container = 55–65 mL, Teruflex XT612 = 55–65 mL.

rate of transfused radiolabeled platelets. Function is defined as the ability of viable platelets to respond to vascular damage in promoting hemostasis. The template bleeding time test represents the most important assay of the functional integrity of transfused platelets. However, no one in vitro test can predict the effectiveness of a particular PC before transfusion.

Maintenance of pH appears to prevent the deleterious changes associated with platelet storage. Apparently, oxygen supply to the platelets within the plastic bag is also intimately related to pH maintenance. If the supply is sufficient, glucose will be metabolized oxidatively, resulting in carbon dioxide production, which diffuses out of the walls of the plastic storage bag. If the supply of oxygen is insufficient, glucose will be metabolized anaerobically, resulting in the production of lactic acid, which must remain within the container and thus lowers the pH. The oxygen tension within the container is governed by several factors: the concentration of platelets, which consume oxygen; the permeability of the wall of the plastic PC bag; the surface area of the container available for gas exchange; and the type of agitation used, inasmuch as this facilitates gas exchange.

Containers for platelet storage were originally constructed from PVC containing a plasticizer. Platelets stored in these "first-generation containers" had a pH below 6.0 after 3 days of storage.[43] Currently, "second-generation containers" are available that allow 5 days of storage of platelets without a significant fall in pH (e.g., Baxter's PL 732 and Terumo's XT612).[43] The second-generation containers maintain a higher pH by facilitating gas transport, thereby allowing carbon dioxide escape and increased oxygen transport.[43] The higher oxygen tension is thought to reduce the glycolytic rate by accelerating oxidative metabolism. Although these bags have the ability to store platelets for 7 days, the FDA allows storage for 5 days only, because a high frequency of septicemia related to transfusion of bacterially contaminated platelets stored at room temperature has been reported. Pooled PCs can be stored for only 4 hours before they must be transfused. A higher incidence and greater bacterial contamination has been reported in pooled PCs than in PCs not pooled.[51]

## SUMMARY

Current federal regulation licenses the storage of PCs for 5 days at 22°C and for 72 hours at 4°C.[15] Each PC must be resuspended in a sufficient volume of plasma to maintain a pH of 6.0 or greater and to maintain a minimum platelet count of $5.5 \times 10^{10}$ platelets per bag (50 to 55 mL plasma).[40] Furthermore, when PCs are stored at 22°C, continuous gentle agitation must be used to facilitate gas exchange. During transportation of a PC in insulated styrofoam boxes kept at 20 to 24°C, discontinuation of agitation should not exceed 24 hours during shipping.[40] Platform, elliptical, and circular rotators are currently in use. Platelet concentrates may be stored for 5 days at 20 to 24°C with circular or flat-bed agitators. It should be noted that elliptical rotators are not recommended in polyolefin (PL 732) bags. If the PC bag is broken or opened, the unit must be used within 24 hours when stored at 1 to 6°C and within 6 hours when stored at 20 to 24°C.

Current research is investigating the development of a synthetic storage medium to replace plasma in an attempt to provide the highest-quality platelet product that is also cost-effective.[52-54] Table 1-15 lists the main advantages of using a platelet additive solution instead of plasma for the storage of PCs.[55] Future directions for platelet research include the use of lyophilized platelets and platelet substitutes for the control of thrombocytopenic bleeding in animal models.[56-62] Two platelet substitutes—specifically, Thrombospheres (Hemosphere, Irvine, CA) and infusible platelet membranes (IPMs)—have been reported to shorten the bleeding time in thrombocytopenic rabbits.[58-61] Infusible platelet membranes have been used in clinical trials in patients at several centers.[62]

**Table 1–15.** Advantages of Using Platelet Additive Solutions

- Reduces plasma-associated transfusion side effects
- Improves platelet storage conditions
- Saves plasma for other purposes (e.g., transfusion or fractionation)
- Increases the efficiency of procedures for the decontamination of viruses and bacteria

---

**SUMMARY CHART: IMPORTANT POINTS TO REMEMBER (MT/MLT)**

n Each unit of whole blood collected contains approximately 450 mL of blood and 63 mL of anticoagulant-preservative solution.

n A donor can give blood every 8 weeks.

n Each unit of donated blood is tested by eight screening tests for infectious diseases.

n Glycolysis generates approximately 90% of the ATP needed by RBCs, and 10% is provided by the pentose phosphate pathway.

n RBCs contain 92–95% HbA, 2–3% $HbA_2$, and 1–2% HbF, and 75% posttransfusion survival of red cells is necessary for a successful transfusion.

n ACD, CPD, and CP2D are approved preservative solutions for storage of blood at 1–6°C for 21 days, and CPDA-1 is approved for 35 days.

n Additive solutions (Adsol, Nutricel, Optisol) are approved for blood storage for 42 days.

n Rejuvesol is the only FDA-approved rejuvenation solution used in some blood centers to regenerate ATP and 2,3-DPG levels before red cell freezing.

n Red cells are glycerolized and frozen within 6 days of whole blood collection in CPD or CPDA-1 and can be stored for 10 years from the date of freezing.

n Current blood substitutes include hemoglobin-based oxygen carriers and perfluorochemicals.

n Hemoglobin-based oxygen carriers include stroma-free hemoglobin solutions (SFHS), chemically modified hemoglobin solutions, recombinant hemoglobin (rHb), and encapsulated hemoglobin.

n Platelet concentrates (PCs) can be prepared by centrifugation or apheresis.

n A PC must contain a minimum of $5.5 \times 10^{10}$ platelets in a volume between 45 and 65 mL and a pH of 6.0 or greater.

n An apheresis PC contains 4–6 times as many platelets as a PC obtained from whole blood and must contain a minimum of $3.0 \times 10^{11}$ platelets.

n PC can be stored for 5 days at 20–24°C with continuous agitation and for 72 hours at 4°C.

n If the PC bag is broken or opened, the PC must be used within 6 hours when stored at 20–24°C and within 24 hours when stored at 1–6°C.

n If PC (4–6 or 6–8 units) are pooled into one transfusible product, the storage time changes to 4 hours.

---

## REVIEW QUESTIONS

1. The loss of ATP leads to:
   A. An increase in phosphorylation of spectrin and a loss of membrane deformability
   B. An increase in phosphorylation of spectrin and an increase of membrane deformability
   C. A decrease in phosphorylation of spectrin and a loss of membrane deformability
   D. A decrease in phosphorylation of spectrin and an increase of membrane deformability

2. The majority of normal adult hemoglobin consists of:
   A. Two alpha chains and two beta chains
   B. Two alpha chains and two delta chains
   C. Two alpha chains and two gamma chains
   D. Four alpha chains

3. When blood is stored, there is a "shift to the left." This means:
   A. Hemoglobin oxygen affinity increases owing to an increase in 2,3-DPG
   B. Hemoglobin oxygen affinity increases owing to a decrease in 2,3-DPG
   C. Hemoglobin oxygen affinity decreases owing to a decrease in 2,3-DPG
   D. Hemoglobin oxygen affinity decreases owing to an increase in 2,3-DPG

4. Which of the following is (are) the role(s) of platelets?

   A. Maintain vascular integrity
   B. Initial arrest of bleeding
   C. Stabilizing the hemostatic plug
   D. All of the above

5. Which of the following preservatives has a storage time of 21 days at 1 to 6°C?
   A. ACD
   B. CP2D
   C. CPD
   D. All of the above

6. What is the currently licensed storage time and temperature for platelet concentrates?
   A. 5 days at 1 to 6°C
   B. 5 days at 24 to 27°C
   C. 5 days at 20 to 24°C
   D. 7 days at 22 to 24°C

7. What is the minimum number of platelets required in a PC prepared from whole blood by centrifugation?
   A. $5.5 \times 10^{11}$
   B. $3.0 \times 10^{10}$
   C. $3.0 \times 10^{11}$
   D. $5.5 \times 10^{10}$

8. All but which one of these factors will influence platelet metabolism and function in a closed system?
   A. Total platelet count
   B. Duration of storage
   C. Temperature of storage
   D. Fibrinogen concentration

9. One of the major disadvantages of stroma-free hemoglobin solutions is:
   A. High oxygen affinity
   B. No antigenicity
   C. Long shelf life
   D. Long stability

10. Blood is stored at what temperature?
    A. 1 to 6°C
    B. 20 to 24°C
    C. 37°C
    D. 24 to 27°C

11. Additive solutions are approved for blood storage for how many days?
    A. 21 days
    B. 42 days
    C. 35 days
    D. 7 days

12. Blood can be stored in CPDA-1 at 1 to 6°C for how many days?
    A. 21
    B. 42
    C. 35
    D. 7

## ANSWERS TO REVIEW QUESTIONS

1. C (p 4)

2. A (p 6)

3. B (p 8)

4. D (p 14)

5. D (p 9, Table 1–4)

6. C (p 15)

7. D (p 15)

8. D (p 15)

9. A (p 13, Table 1–11)

10. A (p 9)

11. B (p 10)

12. C (p 11)

## REFERENCES

1. Parks, D: Charles Richard Drew, MD 1904–1950. J Natl Med Assoc 71:893–895, 1979.
2. Kendrick, DB: Blood Program in World War II, Historical Note. Washington Office of Surgeon General, Department of Army, Washington, DC, 1964, pp 1–23.
3. http://www.aabb.org, 1997.
4. Screiber, GB, et al: The risk of transfusion-transmitted viral infections. N Engl J Med 334:1685–1690, 1996.
5. Harmening, DM: Clinical Hematology and Fundamentals of Hemostasis, ed 3. FA Davis, Philadelphia, 1997, p 55.
6. Mohandas, N, and Chasis, JA: Red blood cell deformability, membrane material properties and shape: Regulation of transmission, skeletal and cytosolic proteins and lipids. Semin Hem 30:171–192, 1993.
7. Mohandas, N, and Evans, E: Mechanical properties of the genetic defects. Ann Rev Biophys Biomol Struct 23:787–818, 1994.
8. Bunn, HF: Hemoglobin structure, function and assembly. In Embury, SH, Hebbel, RP, Mohandas, N, and Steinberg, MH (eds): Sickle Cell Disease: Basic Principles and Clinical Practice. Raven Press, New York, 1994.
9. Benesch, R, and Benesch, RE: The effect of organic phosphates from the human erythrocyte on the allosteric properties of hemoglobin. Biochem Biophys Res Commun 26:162, 1967.
10. Chanutin, A, and Curnish, RF: Effect of organic and inorganic phosphates on the oxygen equilibrium of human erythrocytes. Arch Biochem Biophys 121:96, 1967.
11. Beutler, E: Red cell metabolism and storage. In Anderson, KC, and Ness, PM (eds): Scientific Basis of Transfusion Medicine. WB Saunders, Philadelphia, 1994, pp 188–202.
12. Beutler, E: Preservation of liquid red cells. In Rossi, EC, et al (eds): Principles of Transfusion Medicine, ed 2. Williams & Wilkins, Baltimore, 1996, pp 51–60.
13. Petz, LD, and Swisher, SN: Clinical Practice of Transfusion Medicine, ed 3. Churchill Livingstone, New York, 1996.
14. Valeri, CR: Frozen red blood cells. In Rossi, EC, Simon, TL, Moss, GS, and Gould, SA (eds): Principles of Transfusion Medicine, ed 2. Williams & Wilkins, Baltimore, 1996, pp 61–66.
15. The Code of Federal Regulations, 21 CFR Section of Blood Products 600–680. US Government Printing Office, Washington, DC: 1997.
16. Sowade, O, et al: Evaluation of oxygen availability with oxygen status algorithm in patients undergoing open heart surgery treated with epoetin beta. J Lab Clin Med 129(1):97–105, 1997.
17. Gramm, J, et al: Effect of transfusion on oxygen transport in critically ill patients. Shock 5(3):190–193, 1996.
18. Yu, M: Invasive and noninvasive oxygen consumption and hemodynamic monitoring in elderly surgical patients. New Horiz 4(11):443–452, 1996.
19. Lovric, VA: Modified packed red cells and the development of the circle pack. Vox Sang 51:337, 1986.
20. Hogman, CF: Additive system approach in blood transfusion birth of the SAG and Sagman systems. Vox Sang 51:337, 1986.
21. Hogman, CF: Recent advances in the preparation and storage of red cells. Vox Sang 67:243–246, 1994.
22. Technical Manual, ed 12. American Association of Blood Banks, Bethesda, 1996.
23. Yasutake, M, and Takahashi, TA: Current advances of blood preservation—development and clinical application of additive solutions for preservation of red blood cells and platelets. Nippon Rinsho 55(9):2429–2433, 1997.
24. Samuel, LH, Anderson, G, and Mintz, PD: Rejuvenation of irradiated AS-1 red cells. Transfusion 37:25–28, 1997.
25. Valeri, CR: Use of rejuvenation solutions in blood preservation. CRC Crit Rev Clin Lab Sci 17:299–374, 1982.
26. Samuel, LH, Anderson, G, and Mintz, PD. Rejuvenation of irradiated AS-1 red cells. Transfusion 37:25–28, 1997.
27. Dietz, NM, Joyner, MJ, and Warner, MA: Blood substitutes: Fluid, drugs, or miracle solutions? Anesth Analg 82:390–405, 1996.
28. Winslow, RM: Blood substitutes. Science & Medicine 4:54–63, 1997.
29. Gould, SA, Lakshman, RS, and Moss, GS: Hemoglobin solutions as an acellular oxygen carrier. In Rossi, EC, et al (eds): Principles of Transfusion Medicine, ed 2. Williams & Wilkins, Baltimore, 1996, pp 51–60.
30. Everse, J, and Hsia, N: The toxicities of native and modified hemoglobins. Free Radic Biol Med 22:1075–1099, 1997.
31. Kasper, SM, et al: Effects of a hemoglobin-based oxygen carrier (HBOC-201) on hemodynamics and oxygen transport in patients undergoing preoperative hemodilution for elective abdominal aortic surgery. Anesth Analg 83:921–927, 1996.
32. DeAngeles, DA, et al: Resuscitation from hemorrhagic shock with diaspirin cross-linked hemoglobin, blood, or hetastarch. Trauma 42(3):406–414, 1997.
33. Hughes, GS, et al: Physiology and pharmacokinetics of a novel

hemoglobin-based oxygen carrier in humans. Crit Care Med 24(5):756–764, 1996.

34. Krieter, H, et al: Isovolemic hemodilution with a bovine hemoglobin-based oxygen carrier: Effects on hemodynamics and oxygen transport in comparison with a nonoxygen-carrying volume substitute. J Cardiothorac Vasc Anesth 11(1):3–9, 1997.

35. Looker, D, et al: Expression of recombinant human hemoglobin in *Escherichia coli*. Methods Enzymol 231:364–374, 1994.

36. Cedrati, N, et al: Structure and stability of human hemoglobin microparticles prepared with a double emulsion technique. Artif Cells Blood Substit Immobil Biotechnol 25(9):457–462, 1997.

37. Takaori, M, and Fukui, A: Treatment of massive hemorrhage with liposome encapsulated human hemoglobin (NRC) and hydroxyethyl starch (HES) in beagles. Art, Cells, Blood Subs, and Immob Biotech 24(6):643–653, 1996.

38. Szebeni, J, et al: Complement activation in vitro by the red cell substitute, liposome-encapsulated hemoglobin: Mechanism of activation and inhibition by soluble complement receptor type 1. Transfusion 37:150–159, 1997.

39. Spence, RK: Perfluorocarbons. In Rossi, EC, et al (eds): Principles of Transfusion Medicine, ed 2. Williams & Wilkins, Baltimore, 1996, pp 189–196.

40. Standards, ed. 18. American Association of Blood Banks, Bethesda, 1997.

41. Kelly, DL, et al: High yield platelet concentrates attainable by continuous quality improvement reduce platelet transfusion cost and donor expense. Transfusion 37:482–486, 1997.

42. Baxter Healthcare Corporation: Preparing effective platelet concentrates in triple Blood-Pack units. July 1993.

43. Eriksson, L, Eriksson, G, and Hogman, CF: Storage of buffy coat preparations at 22°C in plastic containers with different gas permeability. Vox Sang 73(2):74–80, 1997.

44. Holme, S, et al: Studies on platelets exposed to or stored at temperatures below 20°C or above 24°C. Transfusion 37:5–11, 1997.

45. Bode, AP, and Knupp CL: Effect of cold storage on platelet glycoprotein Ib and vesiculation. Transfusion 34:690–696, 1994.

46. Winokur, R, and Hartwig, JH: Mechanism of shape change in chilled human platelets. Blood 85:1796–1804, 1994.

47. Chiu, EKW, et al: A prospective study of symptomatic bacteremia following platelet transfusion and of its management. Transfusion 34:950–954, 1994.

48. Bertolini, F, and Murphy, S: A multicenter inspection of the swirling phenomenon in platelet concentrates prepared in routine practice. Transfusion 36:128–132, 1996.

49. Leiby, DA, et al: A retrospective analysis of microbial contaminants in outdated random-donor platelets from multiple sites. Transfusion 37:259–263, 1997.

50. Eriksson, L, et al: Evaluation of platelet function using the in vitro bleeding time and corrected count increment of transfused platelets. Comparison between platelet concentrates derived from pooled buffy coats and apheresis. Vox Sang 70(2):69–75, 1996.

51. Wagner, SJ, et al: Comparison of bacteria growth in single and pooled platelet concentrates after deliberate inoculation and storage. Transfusion 35:298–302, 1995.

52. Gulliksson, H: Storage of platelets in additive solutions: The effect of citrate and acetate in vitro studies. Transfusion 33:301–303, 1993.

53. Turner, VS, et al: Inclusion of potassium in an additive solution enhances platelet storage. Trans Med 6(2):33, 1996.

54. Gulliksson, H, et al: Buffy-coat-derived platelet concentrates prepared from half-strength citrate CPD and CPD whole blood units. Comparison between three additive solutions: In vitro studies. Vox Sang 68:152–159, 1995.

55. Hogman, CF, et al: Buffy-coat-derived platelet concentrates: Swedish experience. Transfus Sci 18, 1997.

56. Bode, AP, et al: Hemostatic properties of lyophilized platelets in a thrombocytopenic rabbit model and a simulated bleeding time device. Transfusion 34(10S):74S (abstr), 1994.

57. Bode, AP, Lust, RM, and Read, MS: Lyophilized platelets correct the bleeding time test in a canine model of cardiopulmonary bypass recirculation. Thromb Haemost 63(abstr), 1997.

58. Blajchman, MA, and Lee, DH: The thrombocytopenic rabbit bleeding time model to evaluate the in vivo hemostatic efficacy of platelets and platelet substitutes. Transf Med Rev 11:95–105, 1997.

59. Lee, DH, et al: The effect of thrombospheres on the bleeding time and blood loss in thrombocytopenic rabbits (abstract). Clin Invest Med 19:S31, 1996.

60. Yen, RKC, Ho, TWC, and Blajchman, MA: A new hemostatic agent: Thrombospheres shorten the bleeding time (BT) in thrombocytopenic rabbits (abstract). Thromb Haemost 73:986, 1995.

61. Vickers, JD, Lee, DH, and Blajchman, MA: Binding of thrombospheres to chymotrypsin-treated rabbit platelets decreases phosphatidylinositol 4,5-bisphosphate (PIP$_2$) (abstract). Thromb Haemost (suppl):481, 1997.

62. Aster, RH: Infusible platelet membrane (IMPs) for the control of bleeding in thrombocytopenic bleeding in thrombocytopenic patients. In The compendium: A Selection of Short Topic Presentations. American Association of Blood Banks, Bethesda, MD, 1997.

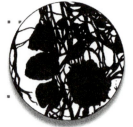

# CHAPTER 2

# CLASSIC GENETICS

JoAnn M. Moulds, PhD
With Summary Overview by
Linda F. Comeaux, MT(ASCP)

**OBJECTIVES**

*On completion of this chapter, the learner should be able to:*

1 Describe the processes of mitosis and meiosis.

2 Discuss Mendel's laws of independent segregation and of dominance.

3 Correlate Mendel's law of dominance with specific examples of the inheritance of blood group antigens.

4 Correlate the Hardy-Weinberg principle with a specific example of the inheritance of blood group antigens.

5 Interpret the inheritance pattern of a trait or gene by examination of the pedigree analysis.

6 Distinguish between X-linked and autosomal inheritances.

7 Describe the processes of replication, transcription, and translation.

8 For each of the above processes, give a specific example of how a mutation could occur.

9 Discuss the importance of restriction fragment length polymorphism analysis.

10 List the uses of polymerase chain reaction.

Today's study of blood group genetics requires not only an appreciation of classic mendelian genetics but also an understanding of the structure of deoxyribonucleic acid (DNA) and how it can be manipulated. The student of genetics must know how to interpret not only a familial inheritance pattern but also a Southern blot.

In this chapter, 130 years of genetics are reviewed. Obviously, this must be nothing more than a brief overview. Interested readers are referred to the original references as well as selected books for more in-depth reading. However, these are only suggestions, and many other good books covering genetics alone are available for the reader who desires a deeper understanding of this complex topic.

## CLASSIC GENETICS

### Mitosis and Meiosis

Genetics is the study of inheritance—the transmission of characteristics from parents to offspring. The transmission of traits was first observed by the ancients and often led to bizarre theories on the mechanism of the hereditary process. Not until 1865, when Gregor Mendel did experimental matings with garden peas, did the science of genetics come into being. His studies led to the basic understanding of how genetic traits are passed to each generation.

Within each living human cell is a central organelle called a *nucleus* that contains most of the genetic material. Under a light microscope this appears as dark-staining bands known as *heterochromatin* and lighter bands called *euchromatin*. The chromatin coils up tightly to make structures called *chromosomes*. Humans have 46 chromosomes, whereas other species possess between 10 and 50 chromosomes. The chromosomes usually occur together in pairs (one from each parent), resulting in the diploid, or 2N, species. Humans have 22 pairs of autosomes and one set of sex chromosomes (*XX* in females, *XY* in males).

As a cell divides, it must reproduce its chromosomes so that all the daughter cells are identical to the parent cell. This process is known as *mitosis*. The chromosomes are duplicated and one of each pair passes to the daughter. This process is illustrated in Figure 2–1.

Obviously, this process cannot explain the production of new individuals. If a diploid ovum and sperm combined, then the resulting cell would have 4N chromosomes; this is unacceptable. Therefore, the gamete must carry only one copy of each chromosome (haploid) so that when a diploid ovum and sperm fuse, a diploid cell results. This type of cell division is unique to reproduction or the germinal tissues and is called *meiosis* (Figure 2–2).

### Mendel's Laws

In his classic paper of 1865, Mendel demonstrated that the physical traits of an organism corresponded to

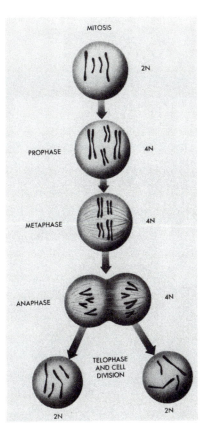

**Figure 2–1.** Cell division of mitosis leads to two daughter cells having the same number of chromosomes as the parent. (From Watson, JD, Tooze, J, and Kurtz, DT: Recombinant DNA: A Short Course. Copyright 1983 by James D. Watson, John Tooze, and David T. Kurtz. Reprinted by permission of WH Freeman and Company, New York, p 7.)

some invisible "elementen" in the cell. We now know these "elementens" as genes. Furthermore, Mendel proposed that the genes occurred in pairs and that one of each gene was passed from parent to offspring.

In one set of experiments Mendel cultivated sweet peas until they bred offspring with flowers of all one color (e.g., red or white only). He then cross-bred these two plants and obtained a first filial generation that had all red flowers. When plants from this generation were bred with each other, they produced red and white flowers in a ratio of 3:1. This is illustrated in Figure 2–3, in which the parents are homozygous for the red trait (*RR*) or the white trait (*rr*). The first filial generation are heterozygous (Rr). They carry the dominant (expressed) gene R for red color as well as the recessive (nonexpressed) gene *r*. The second filial generation then results in one homozygous red plant (*RR*), two heterozygous red plants (*Rr*), and one homozygous recessive white plant (*rr*). This illustrates Mendel's law of independent segregation as well as his law of dominance.

A slight variation of this law can occur when one trait is not dominant over the other. When the traits are codominant, both are expressed equally. Thus, in the previous example, if the genes were codominant, the

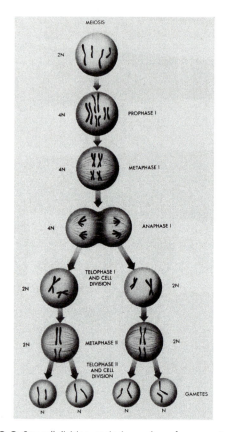

Figure 2–2. Sex-cell division, meiosis, produces four gametes having half the number of chromosomes present in the parent cell. (From Watson, JD, Tooze, J, and Kurtz, DT: Recominant DNA: A Short Course. Copyright 1983 by James D. Watson, John Tooze, and David T. Kurtz. Reprinted by permission of WH Freeman and Company, New York, p 7.)

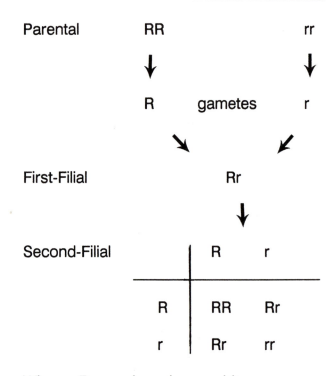

Where R = red and r = white

Figure 2–3. A schematic illustration of Mendel's law of separation.

heterozygotes (*Rr*) would be pink, whereas *RR* plants would remain red and *rr* white. An example of codominantly inherited blood group genes is seen in Figure 2–4, wherein both the M and N antigens can be detected in the heterozygous family members.

Another of Mendel's laws is the law of independent assortment. Simply stated, this means that factors for different characteristics are inherited independently from each other (if they reside on different chromosomes). Mendel ascertained this by performing dihybrid crosses—that is, crosses between strains breeding true for two characteristics. For example, if seeds that were round or wrinkled and green or yellow were bred, the parental genotypes would be *RRYY* and *rryy*. If the generations were bred as previously described, we would have gametes pairing as shown in Figure 2–5. The results of the dihybrid cross would yield the following phenotypes: round/yellow, round/green, wrinkled/yellow, and wrinkled/green in a ratio of 9:3:3:1. Of course, there are exceptions to these rules. Sometimes the genes for different traits can be carried on the same chromosome, such as the genes for *MN* and *Ss*. Because they are so close to each other physically, they are inherited as a unit, or "travel" together. In addition, the expected gene ratios may not occur if recombination has

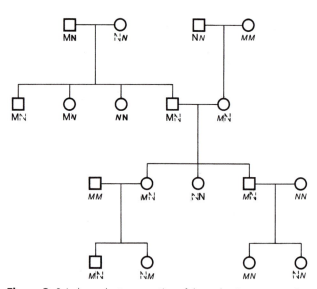

Figure 2–4. Independent segregation of the codominant genes of *M* and *N*.

happened during meiosis. This is caused by breaking the DNA strand, followed by exchange of chromosomal material, which yields new hybrid genotypes.

Mendel's laws apply to all sexually reproducing diploid organisms. In combination, they demonstrate just how immense the genetic variations can become in just a few generations. Multiply this by thousands of genes in the human genome, and it is not surprising that each individual is unique.

Parental              RRYY                    rryy
                        ↓                       ↓
                    RY      gametes      ry
                        ↘              ↙
First-Filial        RY    Ry    rY    ry
                            ↓

Second-Filial           | RY    Ry    rY    ry

                RY      | RRYY  RRYy  RrYY  RrYy
                Ry      | RRYy  RRyy  RrYy  Rryy
                rY      | RrYY  RrYy  rrYY  rrYy
                ry      | RrYy  Rryy  rrYy  rryy

Where R = round      r = wrinkled

      Y = yellow      y = green

**Figure 2–5.** A schematic illustration of Mendel's law of independent assortment.

## POPULATION GENETICS

### Hardy-Weinberg Principle

Once the principles of mendelian inheritance gained acceptance, certain questions regarding recessive alleles persisted. The question of why a recessive trait would not be lost from the population was finally answered by a mathematician, G. H. Hardy, and a German physician, W. Weinberg, who produced the Hardy-Weinberg equation. Several basic premises, however, underlie this mathematical formula:

1. The population must be large and mating must occur at random.
2. Mutations must not occur.
3. There must be no migration, differential fertility, or mortality of the genotype.

Obviously, these conditions are seldom met by human populations. Today there is a constant mixing of populations leading to "gene flow." Nevertheless, the Hardy-Weinberg formula is the best estimate we can make for population genetics.

Genetic variability is widely divergent in large populations. To determine the frequency of each allele, we count the number of persons of each phenotype. Given the two alleles $D$ and $d$, the frequency of $D$ would be the sum of $D$ alleles in each phenotype divided by the total number of alleles. This would be p in the Hardy-Weinberg equation. Similarly, counting the number of an allele gives us the figure for q. P plus q must equal 1.0. Accordingly, the ratio of homozygotes and het-

erozygotes is represented by the formula $p^2 + 2pq + q^2 = 1$.

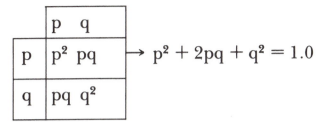

$$p^2 + 2pq + q^2 = 1.0$$

This can also be visualized in the mating sequence, which we used in Figure 2–3.

Let us look at an example using blood group gene frequencies. If we tested 1000 donors for the Rh factor and found that Rh positives ($DD$ and $Dd$) represented 84 percent of the population and Rh negatives ($dd$) 16 percent, we could then calculate the gene frequencies as follows:

p = gene frequency of $D$
q = gene frequency of $d$

$$\left.\begin{array}{l} p^2 = DD \\ 2pq = Dd \end{array}\right\} 0.84$$

$$q^2 = dd = \frac{0.16}{1.00}$$

$$q = \sqrt{0.16} = 0.4$$
$$p + q = 1$$
$$p = 1 - q$$
$$p = 1 - 0.4$$
$$p = 0.6$$

This is only a simple example of the Hardy-Weinberg equation. Blood group systems with more codominant alleles require an expansion of the binomial equation. For example, a three-allele system would be calculated using the formula $p + q + r = 1$ or $p^2 + 2pq + 2pr + q^2 + 2qr + r^2 = 1$. The interested reader is referred to other genetic textbooks for these more complex equations.

### Inheritance Patterns

To interpret pedigree analyses, we must first be familiar with some standard conventions. Males are denoted by squares and females by circles. A line joining a male and a female indicates mating, and the offspring are indicated by a vertical line. A consanguineous mating has a double line between the male and female. An abortion or stillbirth is shown as a small blackened circle; other deceased family members have a cross through them. When a particular individual is found who draws attention to the pedigree, he or she is called the propositus, or index case; this is indicated on the pedigree by an arrow. Figure 2–6 illustrates pedigrees and their inheritance patterns.

Example A is a pedigree demonstrating autosomal-recessive inheritance. Autosomal means that the trait is not carried on the sex chromosomes. A recessive trait is carried by but not expressed in the parents. When two heterozygous individuals mate, they can produce a child who inherits a recessive gene from each parent;

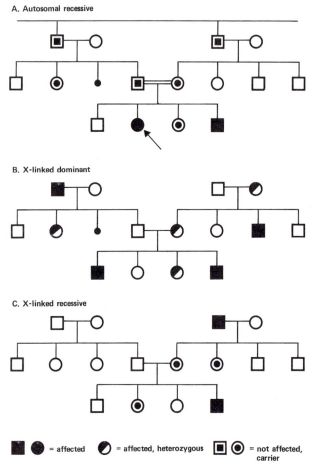

A. Autosomal recessive

B. X-linked dominant

C. X-linked recessive

■ ● = affected   ◐ = affected, heterozygous   ▣ ◉ = not affected, carrier

**Figure 2–6.** Common inheritance patterns.

thus he or she is homozygous recessive for that trait. An example of this can be found in the Rh blood group. The gene *d* can be carried by two Rh-positive parents (*Dd*), who both pass *d* to the child. The resulting genotype is *dd*, and the child's red cells type as Rh (*D*) negative.

In example B we see a dominant X-linked trait. If the father carries the trait on his X chromosome, he has no sons with the trait (because he passed his Y chromosome to his sons); however, all his daughters will express the trait. If a female carries the X-linked gene, she can be heterozygous or homozygous for the trait. In this case, transmission is identical to an autosomal dominant inheritance pattern. The Xgᵃ blood group system is an example of this type of inheritance.

Finally, in example C we see a case of X-linked recessive inheritance. Characteristically, the trait is expressed in the father but is never passed from father to son. Instead, the father passes the trait to all his daughters, who then become carriers. These females then pass the trait on to half of their sons. The trait is expressed in the hemizygous state (X'Y) and less frequently in a homozygous female (X'X').

## BIOCHEMICAL GENETICS

### Deoxyribonucleic Acid

Human chromosomes are composed of linear strands of deoxyribonucleic acid (DNA) wound around proteins called *histones,* as shown in Figure 2–7. This complex of DNA and proteins is called *chromatin.* It is this wrapping and condensing of DNA that allows so much genetic material to be stored in a small piece of the chromosome.

Deoxyribonucleic acid is composed of four nitrogenous bases, a molecule of deoxyribose, and one phosphate group. The four nitrogen-containing bases (Fig. 2–8) are the purines adenine (A) and guanine (G) and the pyrimidines thymine (T) and cytosine (C). Each base can bind to a deoxyribose sugar to form a nucleoside; the addition of the phosphate group makes the compound a nucleotide. Hydrogen bonds can form between the A and T or the C and G bases of the nucleotide, as shown in Figure 2–9. This binding together of two polymeric strands forms the DNA double helix, as first postulated by Watson and Crick.[1]

Phosphoric acid can attach to the deoxyribose sugar at either the third or the fifth carbon atom. The linkage of the purine or pyrimidine base to the sugar is at carbon one. Thus, the two strands of the double helix are antiparallel; that is, one runs 5′ to 3′, whereas the other strand runs 3′ to 5′. Usually the helix has a right-hand twist, but other studies have elucidated a left-hand configuration known as Z-DNA.[2] In the case of DNA, only one strand of the double helix is transcribed—namely, the 3′ to 5′ (left-to-right) strand.

Because there are 20 amino acids, it is readily apparent that a single nucleotide cannot code for a single amino acid. Thus, DNA uses a triplet of nucleotides known as a *codon* to specify a single amino acid. Some amino acids have more than one codon, whereas other codons are signals for stopping transcription (discussed farther on). The genetic code is shown in Table 2–1.

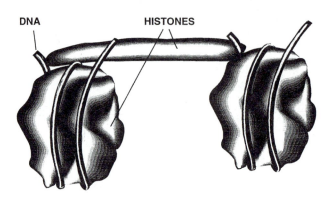

**Figure 2–7.** The nucleosome consists of a stretch of DNA wound around a group of proteins called *histones.*

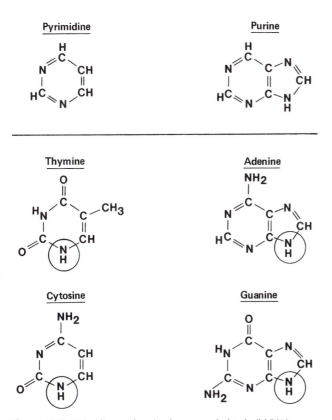

**Figure 2–8.** Pyrimidine and purine bases needed to build DNA.

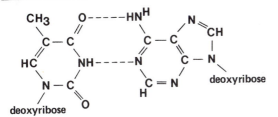

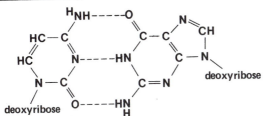

Dotted lines represent interatomic hydrogen bonds, which hold the base pairs together.

**Figure 2–9.** Base pairing in DNA.

## Replication

Following mitoses, each cell must have the correct amount of DNA; therefore, synthesis of DNA must be integrated into the cell cycle. Most DNA replication is

**Table 2–1.** The Genetic Code

| First Position | Second Position | | | | Third Position |
|---|---|---|---|---|---|
| | U | C | A | G | |
| U | PHE | SER | TYR | CYS | U |
| | PHE | SER | TYR | CYS | C |
| | LEU | SER | Stop | Stop | A |
| | LEU | SER | Stop | TRP | G |
| C | LEU | PRO | HIS | ARG | U |
| | LEU | PRO | HIS | ARG | C |
| | LEU | PRO | GLN | ARG | A |
| | LEU | PRO | GLN | ARG | G |
| A | ILE | THR | ASN | SER | U |
| | ILE | THR | ASN | SER | C |
| | ILE | THR | LYS | ARG | A |
| | MET | THR | LYS | ARG | G |
| C | VAL | ALA | ASP | GLY | U |
| | VAL | ALA | ASP | GLY | S |
| | VAL | ALA | GLU | GLY | A |
| | VAL | ALA | GLU | GLY | G |

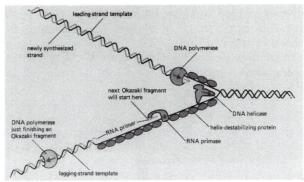

**Figure 2–10.** Some of the major proteins important for DNA replication. (From Alberts, B, et al: Molecular Biology of the Cell. Garland Publishing, New York, 1983, p 230, with permission.)

bidirectional as well as semiconservative.[3] Simply stated, this means that replication occurs on both DNA strands, and the new DNA copies contain one each of the parent DNA strands.

Many enzymes and other factors participate in the replication process; the most important are shown in Figure 2–10. When DNA replicates, the two strands must unwind or separate from each other. This is accomplished by an enzyme known as *helicase*, which is driven by the energy produced from hydrolysis of ATP. The DNA polymerase acts on the 5′ to 3′ parent strand to produce an anticomplementary duplicate strand. Replication of the 3′ to 5′ parent strand, also known as the lagging strand, is more complicated. A ribonucleic acid (RNA) primer is first produced by the enzyme primase, which must anneal to the parent strand to start the duplication process. This occurs at multiple sites along the DNA strand, producing what are called *Okasaki fragments*. These fragments are then joined together by a DNA ligase, resulting in the second identical copy of the DNA double helix. Finally the cell can proceed to divide.

## Repair

With such a complex system for the replication of DNA, it is obvious that some errors may occur. Because the integrity of the DNA is vital to the cell, a system has evolved to correct the occasional replication error. The DNA polymerases themselves have an editing function and correct wrongly incorporated bases. A second system exists to correct the rare error missed by the polymerase editing. This correction system is called *mismatch repair*. In this system, the incorrect base is removed and DNA polymerase I again has a chance to fill in the blank with the correct base.

Many other alterations can occur in DNA when it is exposed to noxious chemicals, x-rays, ultraviolet (UV) light, and so forth. Chemicals known as alkylating agents can react with guanine, resulting in depurination. This observation has become a basis for cancer treatment. Ionizing radiation and chemicals such as peroxides can cause single-stranded breaks in the DNA. Ultraviolet light can alter thymine bases, resulting in *thymine dimers*. Some antibodies, such as mitomycin C, can form covalent linkages between bases in opposite strands, thus preventing strand separation during DNA replication. Each of these defects can be corrected by one of several repair systems.

The four major repair systems include photoreactivation (PR), excision repair, recombinational repair, and SOS repair. Photoreactivation enzymatically cleaves thymine dimers when the PR enzyme is activated by visible light. Thymine dimers can also be removed by the multiple enzyme process of excision repair where the bad section of DNA is cut out. Recombinational repair uses a DNA segment from the "good" strand to fill in the strand where the error has been excised. Polymerase I and DNA ligase then fill in the other dimer strand. Finally, SOS repair can be induced following cell (and DNA) damage.

## Mutations

Even with all the proofreading and repair systems present, changes can occur in the DNA and hence in the messages contained in the genes. Mutation refers to any structural alteration of DNA in an organism (mutant) that is caused by a physical or chemical agent (mutagen). Some changes may occur in nature without spontaneous mutagenesis.

Mutations may involve only a single base or as much as an entire gene. Simple base changes are known as *point mutations* and include substitutions, insertions, and deletions. Although a base substitution changes the triplet code, it may not result in an amino acid change. For example, changing ACA to ACC still codes for thre-

|  | S antigen | s̄ antigen |
|---|---|---|
| amino acid | methionine | threonine |
| mRNA code | AUG | ACG |
| DNA code | TAC | TGC |

**Transversion**

|  | `N` antigen | He antigen |
|---|---|---|
| amino acid | leucine | tryptophan |
| mRNA code | UUG | UGG |
| DNA code | AAC | ACC |

**Figure 2–11.** Types of DNA mutations.

onine. A result of the redundancy in the genetic code, this is known as a *silent mutation*. It may also refer to an amino acid substitution, which has no detectable effect on the phenotype. A change of a purine base to another purine is known as a *transition* (Fig. 2–11). When the mutation causes a purine-to-pyrimidine change, or vice versa, it is known as a *transversion*.[4]

Other base substitutions may cause a change in the triplet code, which results in a change of the amino acid sequence. This may result in a protein that is incapable of performing its normal function. Many abnormal types of hemoglobin occur because of these "missense" mutations.[5] Sometimes there is no amino acid that corresponds to the changed triplet code. These "nonsense" mutations may be referred to as amber, ochre, or opal mutations, depending on which particular base is mutated, causing the termination of polypeptide production.

Insertions and deletions always result in a change of the triplet code and usually of the resulting amino acid sequence. These types of mutations result in a change in the reading frame and are thus called *frameshift mutations*. Recent cloning of the A, B, and O genes has shown that the DNA sequence of the O gene is identical to the A allele, except for a single base deletion at position 258.[6] This deletion shifts the reading frame and results in an entirely different but nonfunctional transferase protein.

Gross genetic changes occurring at a very low frequency can also be classified as mutations. These phenomena include duplications, recombinations, and large gene deletions. Duplications are fairly common in animal cells and may result from evolutionary pressures. Several examples are now known to exist in the world of blood groups. The glycophorin A and B genes, as well as the Rh genes *D* and *CcEe*, are thought to arise from gene duplication. The *C4* genes (the fourth component of complement) duplicated and evolved into *C4A* and *C4B*, which carry the Rodgers and Chido blood group antigens, respectively.

Recombination or crossing over takes place during meiosis in sexually reproducing organisms. The process of recombination involves breaking two double-stranded homologous DNA molecules, exchanging both strands at the break, and resolving the two duplexes (Fig. 2–12). A number of such hybrids can be found in blood group genes, especially those of the MNSs blood group system. Single and double crossover events give rise to the genes for Stones (St$^a$), Dantu, and Mi V. Recombination is probably best observed in the splicing and joining of V and J genes to produce various types of immunoglobins.

Deletion of large segments of DNA spanning several thousand base pairs is the final type of mutation to be discussed. Although some DNA mutations can revert to the original phenotype either spontaneously or induced by a mutagen, reversions are never observed in cases of gene deletions. Thus, the possibility of restoring function to a deleted gene is virtually zero. One such example is the Rodgers-negative phenotype. A deletion spanning approximately 30 kD removes the genes for both C4A (Rodgers) and 21-hydroxylase.[7] This deletion (in the homozygous state) results in the Rodgers-negative phenotype because of the complete loss of C4A protein.

## Ribonucleic Acid

Similar to DNA, ribonucleic acid (RNA) is composed of nucleotides, but it usually exists as a single strand.

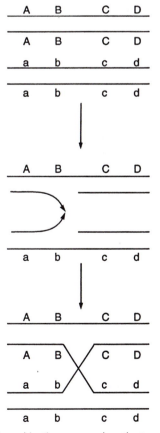

**Figure 2–12.** Recombination occurs when the two strands of DNA break and cross over as shown.

Other differences include the substitution of ribose for deoxyribose and the nitrogenous base uracil for thymine. Ribose differs from deoxyribose by the presence of a hydroxyl group at the 1' carbon. Uracil differs from thymine by its lack of a methyl group. Some viruses exist that use only RNA to store their genetic information. In humans, however, RNA is used to translate the genetic code from DNA into protein.

There are three major classes of RNA molecules: messenger RNA (mRNA), ribosomal RNA (rRNA), and transfer RNA (tRNA). All are synthesized from DNA sequences, but each has a very different function in protein synthesis. There are also significant differences in the RNA of prokaryotes versus eukaryotes. Because we are interested in human genetics, our focus will be on the eukaryotic system.

### Transcription

Messenger RNA accounts for only about 5 percent of the total RNA content of a cell; however, it has a primary role in protein production. This role is the transcription from DNA to RNA that can be translated into amino acid sequences. To begin transcription, an enzyme known as RNA polymerase II must bind to a specific region of the gene called the *promoter.* Promoters can be under the control of either positive or negative effectors, which influence the rate of transcription. Transcription starts at the 3' end of the coding DNA strand and proceeds to the 5' end.

Shortly after initiation of transcription, the 5' end of the mRNA is capped with a methyl residue. Capping may be needed to protect the mRNA from degradation by nucleases. Most mRNAs terminate at the 3' end with a series of adenines called the polyadenylate (polyA) tail. Polyadenylation is thought to increase the stability of the mRNA.

Additional processing of the mRNA occurs in eukaryotes before it is translated (Fig. 2–13). Eukaryotic mRNA characteristically contains intervening sequences (introns), which are not translated. They must be removed from the mRNA by a process known as RNA splicing. The excision of the introns leaves a mature mRNA, which contains only coding regions (exons) of the gene. Once completed, the mRNA is transported to the cytoplasm where it is translated.

### Translation

Protein synthesis occurs on intracellular particles known as *ribosomes* composed of rRNA. Translation of mRNA in eukaryotes, unlike that in prokaryotes, is monocistronic; that is, only one ribosome reads the mRNA transcript at any point in time. The process of protein production involves three major steps: initiation, elongation, and termination.

As shown in Figure 2–14, the first event of the initiation sequence is the attachment of a free molecule of methionine to a specialized transfer RNA called tRNA$^{Met}$. This requires the additional presence of the

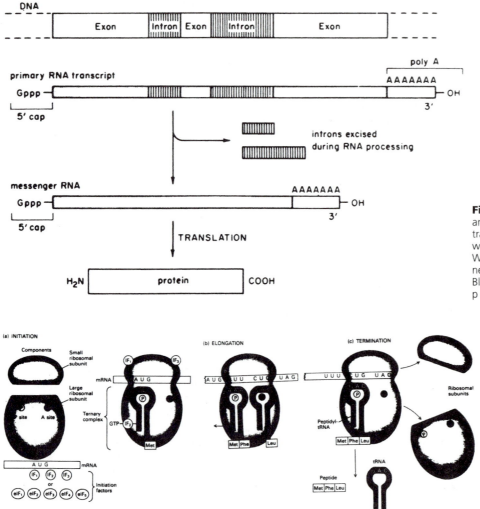

**Figure 2–13.** Transition of DNA and RNA and processing of the transcript to yield mRNA. (From Edwards-Moulds, J, and Tregellas, WM: Introductory Molecular Genetics. American Association of Blood Banks, Arlington, VA, 1986, p 59, with permission.)

**Figure 2–14.** Translation of mRNA to protein. (From Lodish, Danrell, and Baltimore: Molecular Cell Biology. Copyright 1986 by WH Freeman, New York, pp 122–123, with permission.)

high-energy molecule guanine triphosphate (GTP) and an initiation factor (IF2). In the presence of two other initiation factors, IF1 and IF3, the tRNA^Met binds to the small subunit (40S) of rRNA to form an initiation complex. A large ribosomal subunit (60S) then joins the complex hydrolyzing GPT and releases the IFs in the process.

On the large rRNA subunit are two sites: the A site and the P site. The tRNA^Met with its attached amino acid first occupies the P site. The empty and adjoining A site must next be filled with tRNA carrying the appropriately coded amino acid. There are many different tRNA molecules, but all display a similar structure (Fig. 2–15). This single strand of RNA contains two important regions. One of these is a sequence of three bases that can hydrogen-bind to the codon of the mRNA (i.e., the anticodon). The other major site is the area to which the amino acids are bound. Through a specific recognition region, a specific aminoacyl synthetase attaches the proper amino acid to the tRNA. Once charged, the tRNA can now transport its amino acid to the growing polypeptide chain. The incoming tRNA binds to the A site in the presence of an elongation fac-

tor (EF2). This complex hydrolyzes GTP to supply the energy so that the tRNA in the A site can move to the P site. At the same time, the tRNA originally in the P site is removed from its amino acid and ejected. The ribosome continues to move down the codons on the mRNA one at a time.

When the ribosome arrives at the stop codon UAG, the translation is complete. With the aid of a termination factor, the ribosomal units separate, and the polypeptide chain is ready for posttranslational processing such as glycosylation or sulfation. The mRNA may be rapidly degraded by enzymes at this point, or another 40S rRNA subunit may attach at the start site to begin the process again.

## MODERN MOLECULAR TECHNIQUES

The past 25 years have witnessed an explosion in our knowledge not only of genetic material but also of how to manipulate it. Recombinant DNA techniques have made their way into the clinical laboratory and the courtrooms alike. The project to sequence the entire

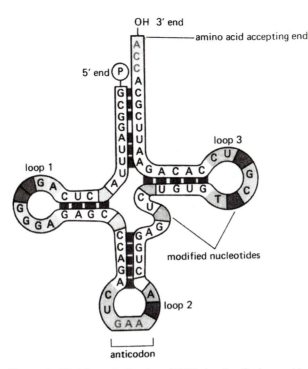

OH 3′ end
— amino acid accepting end

5′ end (P)

loop 1

loop 3

modified nucleotides

loop 2

anticodon

**Figure 2–15.** Schematic drawing of tRNA showing the base pairing and loop structures. (From Alberts, B, et al: Molecular Biology of the Cell. Garland Publishing, New York, 1983, p 109, with permission.)

Blunt Cut

5′ G T T ↓ A A C          Hpa I recognizes

3′ C A A ↑ T T G          6 base pairs

Staggered Cut

5′ G ↓ A A T T C          Eco RI recognizes

3′ C T T A A ↑ G          6 base pairs

**Figure 2–16.** Cutting the DNA by restriction techniques.

human genome is well under way. Thus, it is appropriate that such discussions be presented here.

## DNA Typing

### Restriction Fragment Length Polymorphism Analysis

One of the most used methods in molecular genetics is the Southern blotting technique first described by E. M. Southern.[8] It has been a powerful tool in analyzing the eukaryotic genome, as a preliminary analysis before gene cloning, and for the typing of blood group genes, including human leukocyte antigen (HLA). It is important, therefore, to have a basic understanding of the terminology as well as the technique.

The first step involved with Southern blotting is to obtain DNA for analysis. When RNA is substituted for DNA, the procedure is called Northern blotting. Sources of DNA can be tissues in which the gene under study is expressed, bone marrow, peripheral leukocytes, or cell cultures, to name a few. Genomic DNA is usually prepared by a salting-out technique or a procedure that uses proteinase K digestion followed by a phenol-chloroform extraction and ethanol precipitation.

Once the DNA is in hand, it must be digested (cut into smaller pieces) by restriction enzymes. Restriction endonucleases are enzymes found naturally occurring in various strains of bacteria. Each enzyme is named after its host organism (e.g., *Escherichia coli* produces an enzyme called Eco RI). Each enzyme cuts

DNA of a specific length of base pairs and at a specific site. As shown in Figure 2–16, the cut may be either blunt or staggered. A blunt cut cuts the two pieces evenly into halves, whereas a staggered cut leaves overhanging edges. The latter is useful in cloning techniques.

The fragments that result from the digestion must now be separated by running them on agarose gel electrophoresis. Because the agarose gel is too bulky to be handled easily, the separated pieces are transferred to a solid support matrix, usually nitrocellulose, before detection. Once the replica of DNA is made, it can be probed.

A *probe* is a piece of DNA having a sequence for the gene one is studying. Probes can come from several sources, including complementary DNA (cDNA), genomic DNA, or oligonucleotides. Oligonucleotide probes are artificially manufactured pieces of DNA whose sequences are based on known amino acid sequences. The probe can be labeled with a radioisotope such as [32]P or a nonradioactive substance that emits light when reacted and hybridized to the nitrocellulose blot. Matching sequences can then be visualized in a procedure known as *autoradiography*. This method involves exposing a piece of x-ray film to the blot hybridized to the labeled probe.

When the blots are fully developed, one sees a series of bands based on molecular weight. If DNA from several individuals is analyzed, one may see different banding patterns (Fig. 2–17). These restriction fragment length polymorphisms (RFLPs) result from a change in the base pair sequence of DNA, which is recognized by the restriction enzyme and results in a change in the size of the DNA fragments.

One very useful application of RFLP analysis is typing for HLA genes in transplant patients. Another is the detection of an O gene in the heterozygous state (i.e., AO or BO). Because an O gene expressed no product, it was impossible to detect its presence in the heterozygous state using serologic techniques. The base pair deletion identified in persons having an O gene

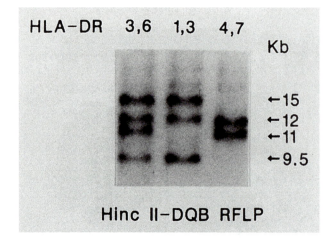

**Figure 2–17.** Southern blot analysis of genomic DNA to determine HLA–DR genotype.

## A or B Gene

5' G↓GTGACCC

3' CCACTGG↑G

### BstE II restriction site

## O Gene

deletion
#258

5' GGT-ACC↓C

3' C↑CA-TGG G

### Kpn I restriction site

**Figure 2–18.** Identification of a blood group O gene by changes in restriction enzyme sites.

(Fig. 2–18) results in the loss of a *BstE II* site and creation of a new *Kpn I* site.[6] Thus, by subjecting DNA from these individuals to Southern blot analysis, the presence of the O gene can be ascertained. This may be particularly useful in cases of disputed paternity.

## Polymerase Chain Reaction and Allele-Specific Probes

Since the first report of DNA amplification using polymerase chain reaction (PCR), the number of different applications has grown steadily. Only the applications most pertinent to the field of immunogenetic and transfusion medicine are discussed here.

The PCR is an in vitro method for the enzymatic synthesis of specific DNA sequences, using two oligonucleotide primers that hybridize to opposite DNA strands and that flank the region of interest.[9] Thus, as with most molecular techniques, one needs a source of DNA to amplify. One advantage to this technique is that only a small amount of DNA is necessary, as the reactions are typically done in small total volumes (50 to 100 µL).

The DNA is mixed with a reaction buffer, nucleotides, the appropriate oligonucleotide primers, and *Taq* enzyme. *Taq* is a thermal stable DNA polymerase obtained from the bacteria that live in hot springs (i.e., *Thermus aquaticus*). In the procedure, the target DNA is first denatured and the primers are allowed to base-pair or anneal to the DNA. The *Taq* polymerase then fills in the remainder of the new DNA strand, resulting in two molecules of DNA where originally there had been one. Because these primer extension products can serve as templates in the next cycle, the number of target DNA copies doubles at each cycle. For example, after 20 PCR cycles there is a millionfold amplification of DNA. This entire process has been automated and has become a very useful technique in many settings.

Following the amplification process, the DNA samples can be blotted onto nitrocellulose. Because the thermocycler has 96 wells, a "dot blot" of all 96 samples can be made at one time. The blot is then hybridized to an allele-specific probe and interpreted following exposure to x-ray film (Fig. 2–19).

Polymerase chain reaction has already had an impact on the field of medicine. This new technique is now being used in place of RFLP analyses for the prenatal detection of sickle cell disease, β-thalassemia, and so forth. The ability to detect DNA polymorphisms in minute biologic evidence samples using PCR has revolutionized forensic testing. Probably the most significant applications in the practice of transfusion medicine will be the use of PCR to detect small amounts of viral DNA in donor blood samples and the ability to type more accurately for the HLA antigens that are so important in transplantations.[10] Most of the hypervariable regions of the class II HLA genes have been sequenced, thus allowing allele-specific oligonucleotides to be produced. Because these oligonucleotides can be used to type individuals undergoing transplantation more accurately, it is highly likely that PCR and allele-specific oligonucleotide typing will replace conventional serologic typing for all clinical purposes.[11]

## Cloning and Sequencing

The field of blood group genetics is once again undergoing change. Recognition of blood group antigens

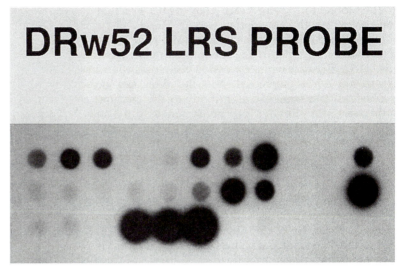

**Figure 2–19.** Dot-blot of PCR products hybridized to an allele-specific HLA probe.

was first performed serologically. Years later, biochemical analyses gave us new insights into antigenic structure and function. Today, we are attacking these questions at the gene level. Already the genes for ABO, Rh, MNSs, Gerbich, Chido, and Rodgers, to name a few, have been cloned. Thus, to understand the latest immunogenetics literature, one needs some knowledge of the basic terminology and techniques involved.

Just as with the crossmatch, many variations of gene cloning have evolved. It is impossible to discuss all of them here, so the following is a general approach to cloning a blood group gene (Fig. 2–20). First one must obtain a source of RNA for the cloning process. In the case of blood group genes, this source is reticulocytes or the fetal liver. The mRNA is selectively separated from the total RNA by passing it over an oligo-dT column. The thymines bind only to molecules of mRNA because only this type of RNA has the complementary polyA tail.

Next the single-stranded mRNA must be converted to double-stranded DNA. This procedure involves synthesis of the first strand of cDNA using the enzyme reverse transcriptase. Using this as a template, the second DNA strand can be generated using DNA polymerase I.

The double-stranded cDNA is then inserted into a cloning vector. A vector is a extrachromosomal genetic element that can carry a recombinant DNA molecule into a host bacterial cell. Vectors can be bacteriophages such as λgt11, plasmids such as pBR322, or cosmids. The cDNA is incubated with the vectors in the presence of T4 ligase, which joins the two DNA molecules together.

The vector is then transfected or transferred into the bacterial host, where it is replicated with each replication of the bacterium. Because each individual vector may contain a different mRNA, only a few vectors may contain the message of the gene being studied. This variety of vectors carrying many different mRNAs, propagated in a host bacteria, is called a cDNA library.

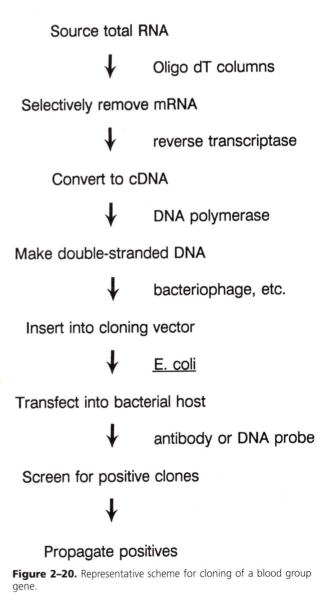

**Figure 2–20.** Representative scheme for cloning of a blood group gene.

The blood group gene is carried by the bacteria that have taken up the appropriate vector. These can be identified by screening a bacterial culture plate using a method very similar to that for Southern blotting. If the cDNA library is in an expression vector, the blood group antigen is expressed, and the filter can be probed using a conjugated antibody to the antigen. Otherwise, the library can be screened with an oligonucleotide probe based on part of a known amino acid sequence.[12] Positive clones are then picked out and propagated until a pure culture is obtained.

The cloned DNA is now ready to be purified and sequenced. Two basic methods are available for sequencing, the Maxam-Gilbert technique[13] and the Sanger dideoxy technique.[14] In the chemical degradation technique of Maxam and Gilbert,[13] a DNA fragment is first radiolabeled usually with $^{32}$P. The DNA is then partially degraded in a set of base-specific chemical reactions, resulting in removal of the derivative base and subsequent cleavage of the DNA. The series of labeled fragments is run side by side on an acrylamide gel electrophoresis followed by autoradiography. The pattern of bands on the x-ray film is read sequentially to determine the DNA sequence (Fig. 2–21).

In the enzymatic method of Sanger,[14] an oligonucleotide primer is hybridized to a single-strand DNA template. The strand is filled in, using $^{32}$P-labeled dATP, DNA polymerase, dideoxynucleotides, and normal deoxynucleotides. The result is a series of labeled bands, which can then be separated by electrophoresis as described previously. From the gene sequence it is a simple matter to deduce the amino acid sequence of its protein. In fact, presently it is often easier to sequence the gene than to determine the amino acid structure.

## SUMMARY OVERVIEW

*Linda F. Comeaux, MT(ASCP)*

This chapter gives the reader a basic introduction to classic, modern, and blood bank genetics. By understanding the basic principles, we can better appreciate the complexity of today's knowledge regarding blood groups. In addition, knowledge of the molecular techniques used today helps us to assimilate them more rapidly into the ever growing field of transfusion medicine.

A strong understanding of the theory and principles of classic genetics, such as that presented here, is advisable and valid. In addition, a knowledge of how these concepts relate to blood banking is also necessary.

All blood group systems (i.e., ABO, Rh, Kell, etc.) follow a process in which the blood group antigens are inherited. For a more detailed explanation, see the corresponding chapters for the specific blood group system. However, to aid the reader's comprehension, a few basic concepts are reviewed here.

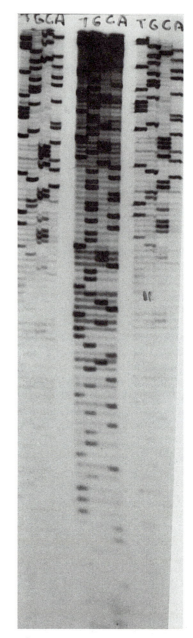

**Figure 2–21.** DNA sequencing gel.

## Terminology

Remember that each parent contributes half of the genetic information to the child in hereditary units called *genes*. These genes are precisely organized, like a string of beads, on a strand of DNA (deoxyribonucleic acid) known as a *chromosome*. Each gene occupies a specific location on the chromosome called a *locus* (plural = *loci*), and at each locus there may be several different expressions or forms of the gene, which are known as *alleles*.

In a simplified example using the ABO blood group system, the gene that codes for the A, B, or O blood type is located on the terminal portion of the long arm of chromosome 9,[15] and the allele or options for inheritance at this locus are A, B, or O. (See Chap. 5 for a more exact explanation of ABO inheritance.)

Remember, too, that the outward expression or the observation of detectable traits produced is the *phenotype*, and the notation of the actual genes inherited is known as the *genotype*.

Therefore, if an offspring inherits identical alleles from both parents (e.g., A from the mother and A from the father) the genotype is *homozygous (AA)* and the phenotype is type A blood. If, however, the offspring inherits different alleles from the parents (e.g., A from the mother and B from the father), then the genotype is considered *heterozygous (AB)*, and the phenotype is type AB blood.

Another concept that must be acknowledged here is that of the silent gene, or *amorph*. An amorph is a gene that does not produce any detectable traits, and one must necessarily be homozygous for the amorph to demonstrate any lack of blood group antigens. An example of this is found in the Rh blood group system with the D (pronounced "big D") antigen and its amorph d (pronounced "little d"). In this case, whenever an individual inherits the gene for D, D antigens appear on the surface of the red blood cells, and this individual is designated Rh-positive. However, if this person is homozygous for the amorph d, no detectable antigens are found, and he or she is Rh-negative.

Figure 2–22 shows that both parents have passed on the D gene and the offspring has a homozygous DD genotype, which results in the presence of the D antigen on the red blood cells. Therefore, this individual is designated Rh-positive.

Figure 2–23 also results in an Rh-positive individual; however, in this case the offspring has inherited one D gene from the mother and the amorphic gene d from the father. Although this person is considered heterozygous Dd, the phenotype still shows detectable D antigens on the red blood cells.

Figure 2–24 demonstrates the only possible inheritance that results in an Rh-negative individual. If the

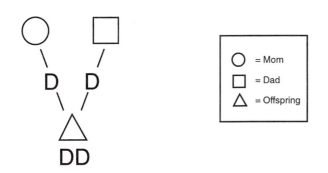

genotype = DD
phenotype = D or Rh+

**Figure 2–22.** Fundamental illustration of a homozygous *DD* genotype.

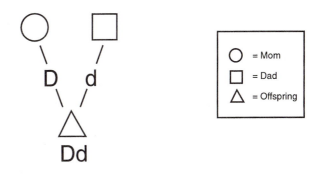

genotype = Dd
phenotype = D or Rh+

**Figure 2–23.** Fundamental illustration of a homozygous *Dd* genotype.

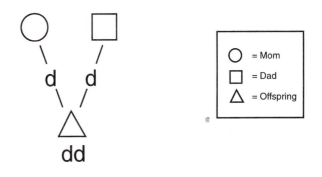

genotype = dd
phenotype = Rh negative

**Figure 2–24.** Fundamental illustration of a homozygous recessive *dd* genotype (amorph).

amorph d is inherited from both parents, there is no detectable D antigen on the red blood cell surface and the offspring is known to be Rh-negative.

Other blood groups such as the Ii, Kell, Lutheran, Duffy, and Kidd systems also encompass the principle of an amorphic allele.

## Blood Group Nomenclature

The nomenclature for blood group systems is not standardized and varies from typical mendelian genetics. Mendel's laws indicate that if a gene is *dominant*, it is denoted with a capitalized letter, and a recessive gene is symbolized by a lowercase letter.

This is not always the situation in blood group nomenclature. In some blood group systems the antigens that have detectable traits can be represented by both upper- and lowercase letters. This is seen with the concept of codominance, which means that each allele is equally expressed, even in the heterozygous condition. The Cc and Ee antigens of the Rh system are just such an example.

For instance, if a person inherits the gene for C ("big C") from the mother and the gene c ("little c") from the father, the genotype is Cc and the detectable traits on the red blood cells are both the C antigen and the c antigen. This theory of codominance applies to most blood group systems.

Additional nomenclature such as that found in the MNSs systems uses a single letter for the blood group and a plus or minus sign to indicate the presence or absence of the detectable antigen, respectively.

Finally, some blood group systems—such as Kidd, Lutheran, Lewis, or Duffy—may use two letters to denote the system; for example, in the Duffy system, a superscript a or b indicates the allele ($Fy^a$ and $Fy^b$), and the plus or minus symbol represents the allele's presence or absence ($Fy^a - Fy^b +$).

---

## SUMMARY CHART: IMPORTANT POINTS TO REMEMBER (MT/MLT)

- Genetics is defined as the study of inheritance or the transmission of characteristics from parents to offspring.
- Humans have 22 pairs of autosomes and one set of sex chromosomes (XX and XY).
- Mendel's law of independent assortment states that factors for different characteristics are inherited independent of each other if they reside on different chromosomes.
- Human chromosomes are composed of the genetic material chromatin, a complex of DNA wrapped around proteins called histones.
- Replication of DNA is accomplished via the enzyme DNA polymerase, which produces an anti-complementary duplicate strand of nucleic acid.
- Mutation refers to any structural alteration of DNA in an organism (mutant) that is caused by a physical or chemical agent (mutagen).
- Transcription is an enzymatic process whereby genetic information in a DNA strand is copied onto an mRNA complementary strand.

- Southern blotting analyzes DNA, whereas Northern blotting analyzes RNA.
- Restriction endonucleases are enzymes found in various strains of bacteria and used in molecular techniques to cut DNA at specific sites.
- A DNA probe is a piece of DNA having a sequence for the specific gene of study that can be labeled with a radioactive substance and visualized by autoradiography.
- The polymerase chain reaction (PCR) is an in vitro method for enzymatic synthesis of specific DNA sequences using two oligonucleotide primers that hybridize to opposite DNA strands and flank the region of interest.
- A cloning vector is an extrachromosomal genetic element that can carry a recombinant DNA molecule into a host bacterial cell (bacteriophages, plasmids, cosmids).
- Sources of DNA in molecular techniques may include bone marrow, peripheral leukocytes, or cell cultures; sources of RNA include reticulocytes or fetal liver.

---

## REVIEW QUESTIONS

1. Which of the following best describes mitosis?
   A. Genetic material is duplicated, equally divided among four daughter cells.
   B. Genetic material is duplicated, equally divided between two daughter cells.
   C. Genetic material is triplicated, equally divided between two daughter cells.
   D. Genetic material is halved, equally divided between two daughter cells.

2. When a recessive trait is expressed, it means that:
   A. One gene carrying the trait was present
   B. Two genes carrying the trait were present
   C. No gene carrying the trait was present
   D. The trait is present but difficult to observe

3. In a pedigree, the index case is another name for:
   A. Stillbirth
   B. Consanguineous mating
   C. Propositus
   D. Dizygotic twins
   E. Monozygotic twins

4. What four nitrogenous bases make up DNA?
   A. Adenine, leucine, guanine, thymine
   B. Alanine, cytosine, guanine, purine
   C. Adenine, cytosine, guanine, leucine
   D. Alanine, cytosine, guanine, thymine
   E. Adenine, cytosine, guanine, thymine

5. Proteins are formed on structures called:
   A. Golgi bodies
   B. Mitochondria
   C. Nuclei
   D. Ribosomes
   E. Azure bodies

6. Which phenotype could not result from the mating of a Jk(a+b+) female and a Jk(a+b+) male?

A. Jk (a+b−)
B. Jk(a+b+)
C. Jk(a−b+)
D. Jk(a−b−)

7. Exon refers to:
   A. The part of a gene that is excised when mRNA is produced
   B. The coding region of a gene
   C. The repetitive sequences at the end of the mRNA
   D. The enzymes used to cut DNA into fragments
   E. The control region of a gene

8. PCR technology can be used to:
   A. Amplify small amounts of DNA
   B. Clone fragments of RNA
   C. Digest genomic DNA into small fragments
   D. Repair broken pieces of DNA

9. Transcription can be defined as:
   A. Introduction of DNA into cultured cells
   B. Reading of mRNA by the ribosome
   C. Synthesis of RNA using DNA as a template
   D. Removal of intravening sequences to form a mature RNA molecule E.
   Production of many copies of genomic DNA

10. When a man possesses a trait that he passes to all his daughters and none of his sons, the trait is said to be:
    A. X-linked dominant
    B. X-linked recessive
    C. Autosomal dominant
    D. Autosomal recessive
    E. Balanced hemizygous

## ANSWERS TO REVIEW QUESTIONS

1. B (p 21)

2. B (pp 27–28)

3. C (p 23)

4. E (p 24)

5. D (p 27)

6. D (p 22)

7. B (p 27)

8. A (p 30)

9. C (p 27)

10. A (p 24)

## REFERENCES

1. Watson, JD, and Crick, FHC: Molecular structure of nucleic acids: A structure for deoxyribose nucleic acid. Nature 171:737, 1953.
2. Garret, RH, and Grisham, CM: Structure of nucleic acids. In Roskoski, JR: Biochemistry, ed 1. WB Saunders, Philadelphia, 1995, pp 222–224.
3. Knippers, R, and Ruff, J: The initiation of eukaryotic DNA replication. In DNA Replication and the Cell Cycle. Springer-Verlag, New York, 1992, pp 2–10.
4. Vogel, F, and Motulsky, AG: Gene mutation: Analysis at the molecular level. In Human Genetics Problems and Approaches, ed 3. Springer, New York, 1997, pp 413–414.
5. Caskey, CT, et al: Triplet repeat mutations in human disease. Science 256(5058):784–789, 1992.
6. Yamamoto, F, et al: Molecular genetic basis of the histo-blood group ABO system. Nature 345:229, 1990.
7. de Van Kim, C, et al: Molecular cloning and primary structure of the human blood group RhD polypeptide. Proc Natl Acad Sci USA 89:10929, 1992.
8. Southern, EM: Detection of specific sequences among DNA fragments separated by gel electrophoresis. J Mol Biol 98:503, 1975.
9. Vosberg, HP: The polymerase chain reaction: An improved method for analysis of nucleic acids. Hum Genet 83(1):1–15, 1989.
10. Bidwell, JL: Applications of the polymerase chain reaction to HLA class II typing. Vox Sang 63(2):81–89, 1992.
11. Pollack, MS: Class II HLA antigens: HLA-D, –DR, –DQ, and –DP. In Moulds, JM, Fawcett, KJ, and Garner, RJ (eds): Scientific and Technical Aspects of the Major Histocompatibility Complex. American Association of Blood Banks, Arlington, VA, 1989, p 47.
12. Monaco, AP: Isolation of genes from cloned DNA. Curr Opin Genet Dev 4(3):360–365, 1994.
13. Maxam, AM, and Gilbert, W: A new method for sequencing DNA. Proc Natl Acad Sci USA 74:560, 1977.
14. Szabo, PE, Mann, JR, and Forrest, G: Sequencing of PCR products. In Pfeifer, GP: Technologies for Detection of DNA Damage and Mutations. Plenum, New York, 1996, pp 351–366.
15. Cartron, JP, and Rouger, P: Blood cell biochemistry, Vol 6, Molecular Basis of Human Blood Group Antigens. Plenum, London, 1995.

## BIBLIOGRAPHY

Alberts, B, et al: Molecular Biology of the Cell. Garland Publishing, New York, 1983.
American Association of Blood Banks: Blood Group Genetics: Tech Manual, ed 12. Bethesda, MD, 1996.
American Association of Blood Banks: Molecular Biology in Transfusion Medicine: Tech Manual. Bethesda, MD, 1996.
Freifelder, D: Molecular Biology: A Comprehensive Introduction to Prokaryotes and Eukaryotes. Jones & Bartlett, Boston, 1983.
Giblett, ER: Genetic Markers in Human Blood. Blackwell Scientific, Oxford, 1969.
Maxson, LR, and Daugherty, CH: Genetics: A Human Perspective. Wm C Brown, Dubuque, IA, 1985.
Quinley, ED: Immunohematology: Principles and Practice. JB Lippincott, Philadelphia, 1993.
Race, RR, and Sanger, R: Blood Groups in Man, ed 5. Blackwell Scientific, Oxford, 1975.
Rothwell, NV: Understanding Genetics: A Molecular Approach. Wiley-Lissler, New York, 1993.
Stansfield, WD: Shchaum's Outline Series: Theory and Problems of Genetics. McGraw-Hill, New York, 1991.
Vogel, F, and Motulsky, AG: Human Genetics: Problems and Approaches. Springer, New York, 1997.

# CHAPTER 3

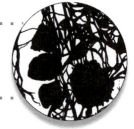

# FUNDAMENTALS OF IMMUNOLOGY FOR BLOOD BANKERS

Veronica Nichols Lewis, MS, MT(ASCP)SBB
and Sharon Martin, EdD, MT(ASCP)

## OBJECTIVES

*On completion of this chapter, the learner should be able to:*

1 Briefly describe the first, second, and third lines of defense in the immune system.

2 Name and describe the characteristics and functions of cells involved in the immune response.

3 List cytokines according to their role in the immune response.

4 Describe how the immune system is regulated by gene expression.

5 Explain how the major histocompatibility complex and human leukocyte antigen control the immune response.

6 Describe the characteristics of immunoglobulins in relation to structure, significance for blood banking, variations, and Fc receptors on effector cells.

7 Explain the activation sequence for the two major complement pathways, how complement is bound by red cell antibodies, and the preservation and destruction of complement in test systems and preserved blood products.

8 Characterize the immune response according to antigen-antibody reactions, host factors, suppression, and primary and secondary responses.

9 Discuss traditional and nontraditional laboratory techniques for detecting antigen-antibody reactions.

10 Discuss factors affecting agglutination reactions.

11 Explain the significance of certain immune-mediated diseases for blood bank testing.

## INTRODUCTION

### The Role of the Immune System

The *immune system* plays two important roles in the human body. First, it provides the defense mechanism, which protects the body against external foreign substances, and second, it plays an important role in the identification and destruction of abnormal cells. These abnormal cells include those that are malignant; those that are infected intracellularly by agents such as viruses, microorganisms, or parasites; and those that are aged or imperfect. Imperfect cells may be those that are coated with antibody or those that have abnormal shapes, as may be seen with senescent or atypical red cells. As a defense mechanism, the immune system functions first by recognizing foreign or abnormal substances and then responding by enlisting the participation of a diversity of reactions to eliminate the offending agent. Because of the numerous agents that continuously challenge the immune system, it has evolved into an extremely complex process consisting of an enormous variety of interrelated processes and mechanisms.

Historically, the blood banker's role was predominantly concerned with tests aimed at detecting blood group antigens and antibodies. As this role has expanded, especially in bone marrow and stem cell transplantation, a basic knowledge of the overall immune response is necessary in the evaluation, performance, and problem resolution of increasingly complex blood bank tests, procedures, and protocols. Because of the complexity of the immune system, this chapter should be considered an overview of fundamental concepts and current information. Readers interested in advanced topics beyond the scope of this discussion are advised to refer to the references listed at the end of this chapter.

## OVERVIEW OF THE IMMUNE SYSTEM

### Basic Concepts

All organisms are challenged by constant invasions from their environment. Many times these invasions are from other organisms trying to profit biologically at the expense of the invaded organism, or *host*. Evolution has developed defenses for living beings to provide protection, or *immunity*, from such attacks. The term "immunity" refers to the vast number of biologic mechanisms used by the body as protection against any substances that are foreign to the body. If it were not for these mechanisms, all living organisms would lack the capability to resist and to reject foreign substances and to overcome infection or disease.

One of the basic concepts in the study of immunology involves understanding how the body distinguishes between what is "self" and what is "nonself." *Self* may be defined as any substance the body identifies as "same as me" or "like me." The self of an organism is the assortment of characteristics of cell and fluid-phase molecules governed by the organism's genetic constitution. All other molecular configurations are considered foreign. *Nonself* includes any substance the body recognizes as "not me" or "not like me" or "foreign." By recognizing self from nonself, the immune system can defend itself from nonself agents. The reaction of the body to the introduction of these nonself agents, called the *immune response*, involves a highly complex network of tissues, organs, cells, and biologic mediators. This defense system's sole purpose is to recognize and reject all substances foreign to itself, or nonself, while minimizing the damage they cause. The immune response protects an organism from such foreign substances as invading pathogenic microorganisms, parasites, viruses, malignant or mutant cells, foods, chemicals, drugs, pollen, and animal hair or dander. Inasmuch as foreign substances come in a vast variety of forms, different immune response mechanisms are required to eliminate or destroy each type of agent.

The immune system has two basic components: the *cellular* component, which consists of the many types of cells, such as leukocytes and tissue cells, involved in immunity; and the *humoral* component, which is composed of soluble substances involved in immunity and which are normally present in body fluids, such as plasma.

A key element of the immune system is the *antibody*, a large protein molecule called an immunoglobulin (Ig), which is found in the globulin portion of normal plasma or serum, and which binds with molecules the body recognizes as foreign. An *antigen* is the substance that the body recognizes as foreign. Antigens can be located on the cell surface of foreign or abnormal cellular agents such as microorganisms, transfused red cells, or cancer cells. An individual antibody binds with only a very specific portion of the target antigen. Under the appropriate conditions, an antigen stimulates the production of antibodies with the corresponding identical receptors to the particular portion of the antigen, termed the *antigenic determinant* or *epitope*. The uniquely shaped molecular structure of the antigen binds like a lock and key to its specific antibody. This binding forms an antibody-antigen complex that inactivates the antigen and triggers a variety of other elaborate defensive mechanisms. The laboratory study of antibodies is called *serology*.

## Innate Immunity and Acquired Immunity

Immunity may be classified by the two major ways in which infections are prevented. The evolutionarily primitive *innate* immune process operates nonspecifically against foreign substances that threaten the body. The more advanced *acquired* immune response is a late evolutionary development, found only in vertebrates, which uses the antigen-antibody mechanism. The antigen-antibody mechanism has the singular ability to remember the infectious antigen and to improve the immune defense process upon successive exposures. This results in prevention of disease at later encounters with the same pathogen.

**Innate Immunity.** *Innate*, or *natural*, *immunity* is the primary line of defense and the simplest way to avoid foreign substances from entering the body. Two key features define the innate immune system. First, the same mechanism is used against every invasive or harmful stimulus trying to gain access to the body and is therefore considered nonspecific. This immunity exists from birth (is innate) and is always present and available to protect the individual from foreign invaders. Second, this process does not change on repeated exposure to the same antigen challenge. These defense mechanisms developed very early in evolution and consist of basic physical and biochemical barriers that prevent the entry of pathogens into the body (Table 3–1). The first line of immune defense is the skin. Intact skin and mucous membranes are impermeable to most infectious agents and are examples of the *external* component of the innate immune system located on the outside of the body. Biochemical defenses on the body's surface, such as the effects of lactic acid and fatty acids in sweat and sebaceous secretions, inhibit or destroy bacterial growth. Many body secretions contain bactericidal components such as lysozyme, one of many serum protein enzymes present in tears, nasal secretions, and saliva with the capability to destroy bacterial cell walls. The very low pH of the stomach and vagina destroys most microbes. Other effective external barriers to foreign environmental agents include mechanical defenses, such as the cough reflex (Table 3–2).

**Table 3–1.** Comparison of the Major Mechanisms of the Immune System

| Innate or Natural Immunity | Acquired or Adaptive Immunity |
| --- | --- |
| • Primary lines of defense | • Supplements protection provided by innate immunity |
| • Early evolutionary development | • Later evolutionary development—seen only in vertebrates |
| • Nonspecific<br>  • Natural—present at birth<br>  • Immediately available<br>  • May be physical, biochemical, mechanical, or a combination of defense mechanisms | • Specific<br>  • Specialized<br>  • Acquired by contact with a specific foreign substance<br>  • Initial contact with foreign substance triggers synthesis of specialized antibody proteins resulting in reactivity to that particular foreign substance |
| • Mechanism does not alter on repeated exposure to any specific antigen | • Memory<br>  • Response improves with each successive encounter with the same pathogen<br>  • Remembers the infectious agent and can prevent it from causing disease later<br>  • Immunity to withstand and resist subsequent exposure to the same foreign substance is acquired |
| FIRST LINE OF DEFENSE          SECOND LINE OF DEFENSE | THIRD LINE OF DEFENSE |

**Table 3–2.** Cellular and Humoral Components of the Immune System

| Innate or Natural Immunity | | Acquired or Adaptive Immunity |
| --- | --- | --- |
| First Line of Defense | Second Line of Defense | Third Line of Defense |
| *External Components* <br> • Physical <br>   • Intact skin <br>   • Mucous membranes <br>   • Cilia <br>   • Cough reflex <br> • Biochemical <br>   • Secretions <br>     • Sweat <br>     • Tears <br>     • Saliva <br>     • Mucus <br>   • Very low pH of vagina and stomach | *Internal Components* <br> • Cellular <br>   • Phagocytic cells <br>     • Macrophages <br>     • Monocytes <br>     • PMNs: Large granular lymphocytes <br>   • NK cells <br> • Humoral (fluid)/biochemical <br>   • Complement-alternate pathway <br>   • Cytokines <br>     • Interferons (INFs) <br>     • Interleukins (ILs) <br> • Acute inflammatory reaction | • Cellular <br>   • Lymphocytes <br>     • T cells <br>       • $T_H$ <br>       • $T_C$ <br>       • T memory cells <br>     • B cells <br>       • B memory cells <br>       • Plasma cells <br>   • APCs <br>     • Macrophages <br>     • Monocytes <br>     • Dendritic cells <br>     • B cells <br> • Humoral <br>   • Antibodies <br>   • Complement-classic pathway <br>   • Cytokines |

APCS = antigen-presenting cells.

The innate system's second line of defense is found *internal* to the body and is triggered once the foreign agent is able to penetrate the external barriers and enter the body itself. The cellular component of this second line of defense is composed of various leukocytes whose purpose is to destroy the invader. Phagocytes, the most important cells of this system, recognize various macromolecules suspended in body fluid or on particulate matter as foreign or nonself. Phagocytes may be found in fixed tissue (e.g., liver, kidney, and lung) and are part of the mononuclear phagocytic sytem (MPS) as well as circulating blood monocytes and polymorphonuclear neutrophils (PMNs). These bind to the invading foreign matter, internalize them, and then destroy them. The innate immune response is still in operation because a primitive nonspecific recognition system is used by the phagocytes to bind to a variety of macromolecular or cellular products.[1] *Opsonins* are factors that promote phagocytosis and help make foreign particles easier targets for the phagocyte. Opsonins include antibodies and various serum components of complement. (A detailed discussion of opsonins and complement may be found in this chapter under Advanced Concepts.) After ingestion by the phagocyte, the foreign substance is entrapped, stimulating lysosomes to release their powerful enzymes to digest the particle. Once these phagocytes are activated, they release soluble substances called *cytokines.* A variety of cytokines are secreted by a number of different types of cells that have assorted effects on other cells (Table 3–3). One of the functions of these polypeptide products of activated cells is to regulate the intensity and duration of an immune response.[2] (An in-depth discussion of cytokines may be found in this chapter under Advanced Concepts.) Abnormal host cells, such as those infected with a virus or tumor cells, have abnormal molecular structures on their cell membranes. These structures are recognized by natural killer (NK) cells, which use nonspecific recognition systems. (Acquired immune response cytotoxic T lymphocytes have the capacity to recognize these surface changes by using specific recognition mechanisms.) Natural killer cells are a group of large granular lymphocytes (LGLs) that probably play a role in the early stages of viral infection or tumorogenesis, before the cytotoxic T lymphocytes of the acquired immune response increase in numbers.[3] They destroy the abnormal target host cell by releasing biologically potent cytokines, such as interferon and interleukin-2. *Interferon (INF)* is an antiviral cytokine. It inhibits intracellular viral replication and is a major factor in the recovery from viral infections. The antiviral activity of INF limits the spread of the infection but is not part of the mechanism that prevents infection on subsequent exposure. *Interleukins (ILs)* are mediators made by leukocytes that "signal" to other leukocytes. *Interleukin-2* is a powerful growth factor and activator for many cells that produce cytotoxic anticancer agents.[4]

The *complement system* proteins are the major component of the humoral innate immune response.[5] The function of the complement system is the lysis of cells through interaction with antibodies, mediation of phagocytosis through opsonization, and control of inflammation. The complement system consists of a group of serum proteins that circulate in an inactive proenzyme or inactive state. These proteins can be activated by two main pathways using specific and nonspecific immune mechanisms that convert the inactive proenzymes into active enzymes. The classic pathway activates complement proenzymes by antigen-antibody

**Table 3–3.** Cytokines

| Cytokine | Source | Stimulatory Function |
|---|---|---|
| *Interleukins* | | |
| IL-1 | Mφ, fibroblasts | Proliferation-activated B cells and T cells |
| | | Induction $PGE_2$ and cytokines by Mφ |
| | | Induction neutrophil and T-cell adhesion molecules on endothelial cells |
| | | Induction IL-6, INF-β 1, and GM-CSF |
| | | Induction fever, acute phase proteins, bone resorption by osteoclasts |
| IL-2 | T | Growth-activated T cells and B cells; activation NK cells |
| IL-3 | T, MC | Growth and differentiation hematopoietic precursors |
| | | Mast cell growth |
| IL-4 | CD4, T, MC, BM stroma | Proliferation-activated B cells, T cells, mast cells, and hematopoietic precursor |
| | | Induction MHC class II and FcεR on B cells, p75 IL-2R on T cells |
| | | Isotype switch to IgG1 and IgE |
| | | Mφ APC and cytotoxic function, Mφ fusion (migration inhibition) |
| IL-5 | CD4, T, MC | Proliferation-activated B cells; production IgM and IgA |
| | | Proliferation eosinophils; expression p 55 IL-2R |
| IL-6 | CD4, T, Mφ, MC, fibroblasts | Growth and differentiation B-cell and T-cell effectors, and hemopoietic precursors |
| | | Induction acute phase proteins |
| IL-7 | BM stromal cells | Proliferation pre-B cell, CD4 cells, CD8 cells, and activated mature T cells |
| IL-8 | Monocytes | Chemotaxis and activation neutrophilis |
| | | Chemotaxis T cells |
| | | Inhibits IFNγ secretion |
| IL-9 | T | Growth and proliferation T cells |
| IL-10 | CD4, T, B, Mφ | Inhibits mononuclear cell inflammation |
| IL-11 | BM stromal cells | Induction acute phase proteins |
| IL-12 | T | Activates NK cells |
| IL-13 | T | Inhibits mononuclear phagocyte inflammation |
| *Colony Stimulating Factors* | | |
| GM-CSF | T, Mφ, fibroblasts, MC, edothelium | Growth of granulocyte and Mφ colonies |
| | | Activated Mφ, neutrophils, eosinophils |
| G-CSF | Fibroblasts, endothelium | Growth of mature granulocytes |
| M-CSF | Fibroblasts, endothelium, epithelium | Growth of macrophage colonies |
| Steel factor | BM stromal cells | Stem cell division (c-kit ligand) |
| *Tumor Necrosis Factors* | | |
| TNF-α | Mφ,T | Tumor cytotoxicity; cachexia |
| TNF-β | T | Induction acute phase proteins |
| | | Antiviral and antiparasitic activity |
| | | Activation phagocytic cells |
| | | Induction IFN-γ, TNF-α, IL-1, GM-CSF, and IL-6 |
| *Interferons* | | |
| INF-α | Leukocytes | Antiviral; expression MHCI |
| INF-β | Fibroblasts | |
| IFN-γ | T | Antiviral; Mφ activation |
| | | Expression MHC class I and II on Mφ and other cells |
| | | Differentiation of cytotoxic T cells |
| | | Synthesis IgG2a by activated B cells |
| | | Antagonism several IL-4 actions |
| *Other* | | |
| TGF-β | T, B | Inhibition IL-2R upregulation and IL-2 dependent T-cell and B-cell proliferation |
| | | Inhibition (by TGF-β1) of IL-3 and CSF induced hematopoiesis |
| | | Isotype switch to IgA |
| | | Wound repair (fibroblast chemotaxin) and angiogenesis |
| | | Neoplastic transformation of certain normal cells |
| LIF | T | Proliferation of embryonic stem cells without affecting differentiation |
| | | Chemoattraction and activation of eosinophils |

Roitt, I: Essential Immunology, ed 8. Blackwell Scientific Publications, London, 1994, with permission.
APC = antigen-presenting cells; BM = bone marrow; CSIF = cytokine synthesis inhibitory factor, FcεR = immunoglobulin Fc receptor for IgE; G-CSF = granulocyte colony stimulating factor; GM-CSF = granulocyte monocyte/macrophage colony stimulating factor; IFN = interferon; IL = interleukin; LIF = leukocyte inhibitory factor; MC = mast cell; M-CSF = monocyte colony stimulating factor; MHC = major histocompatibility complex; Mφ = macrophage; NK = natural killer cells; $PGE_2$ = prostaglandin $E_2$; T = T lymphocyte; TGF = transforming growth factor; TNF = tumor necrosis factor.

*alternate pathway*

binding through specific immune mechanisms. The alternative pathway activates complement by innate, nonspecific reactions with polysaccharides or lipopolysaccharides found on the surfaces of many microorganisms and tumor cells. (An in-depth discussion of the complement system may be found in this chapter under Advanced Concepts.)

Another major component of the body's innate immune system is the *inflammatory response*. The inflammatory response is initiated by tissue damage, which may be caused by a variety of factors such as wounds, tissue necrosis, bone fractures, burns, or infection by pathogenic microorganisms. The major function of the inflammatory response is to heal the injured tissue and assist in the establishment of its normal state. The primary events that occur in inflammation are increased blood flow, increased capillary permeability, and the influx of phagocytic cells. This nonspecific immune response is activated and completed by yet another complex series of interactions between biochemical and cellular components of the innate immune system.

**Acquired Immunity.** *Acquired*, or *adaptive*, *immunity* can be considered the third line of the defensive resistance to foreign substances[5] (see Table 3–1). This mechanism of immunity evolved relatively late and is present only in vertebrates. This type of immunity is acquired by contact with a specific invader. Although the individual is born with the ability to produce an acquired immune response, the response is not immediately available. The response is attained and available at a later time after initial contact with the foreign substance. Although innate immunity is nonspecific and uses the same defense mechanism regardless of the character of the foreign agent, acquired immunity is considered specialized in that the defense mechanism activated is specific to the character and molecular structure identified as nonself for that particular invader. Once stimulated, the acquired immune system results in the synthesis of an antibody. One of the essential features of the acquired immune system is *specificity*, the ability of this antibody to recognize and to bind only to the uniquely shaped molecular structure of the antigen that initialized its production. For example, if an individual who lacks the Kell antigen is exposed to a nonself Kell red cell antigen through transfusion or pregnancy, the immune system may be stimulated to manufacture an anti-Kell antibody. Anti-Kell does not bind with any other antigen found in nature except its *antithetical*, or corresponding, Kell antigen. As previously mentioned, the acquired immune mechanism has *memory*, the ability to remember the infectious antigen and to improve the immune defense process upon successive exposures.

*Immunization* involves the process of conferring immunity by rendering the body resistant to a specific foreign antigen by the availability of antibody with specificity against the same agent. The *acquired immune response* is triggered by the initial exposure of an antigen that stimulates the host's lymphocytes. Lymphocytes are responsible for nonself antigen recognition

and thereby initiate the acquired immune response. All lymphocytes are able to recognize antigens by means of membrane receptors specific for the foreign substance. Each lymphocyte is genetically programmed to recognize only one particular antigen. As previously discussed, this type of nonself recognition is highly specific and distinguishes subtle differences between antigens. Slight molecular differences stimulate the production of different antibodies with different specificities. The difference of a single amino acid between self and nonself molecules can trigger an adaptive immune response.[6] Lymphocytes as a whole can specifically recognize millions of antigens. Therefore, on initial exposure to a nonself antigen, lymphocytes recognizing any particular antigen represent only a very small proportion of the body's total lymphocyte population. A *clone* describes a family of cells arising from a single progenitor resulting in very large numbers of cells genetically identical to the original parent cell. When an antigen binds to the few lymphocytes that can recognize it, a process called *clonal selection* occurs. Each lymphocyte cell is activated to generate clones of its own antigen-binding cells specific for the original foreign agent recognized by the lymphocyte as nonself.

The progression of an effective immune response involves two major groups of cells: lymphocytes and antigen-presenting cells (APCs)[6,7] (see Table 3–2).

The many different types of lymphocytes in the adaptive immune system fall into two major categories: *B lymphocytes*, or *B cells*, and *T lymphocytes*, or *T cells*. As a result of antigenic activation, both B and T cells differentiate into *effector cells*, whose function results in death or elimination of foreign agents, and *memory cells*, which have the capability to recall previous contact with a foreign antigen. Once stimulated, the lymphocytes are said to have "memory." The pattern, or adaptation, of response by the lymphocyte to that particular specific antigen is permanently altered. After an infection has been overcome, some of the newly produced lymphocytes remain. These memory cells preserve the immunologic memory of the particular antigen and are available for restimulation if the antigen is encountered again. If the same antigen is subsequently encountered, the adaptive immune system "remembers" the antigen and improves its defense with a larger and more rapid response, thus eliminating the agent before it can cause any damage and preventing ensuing pathology.[8] It is the memory cells that give the body lasting immunity to a particular pathogen.

The role of B cells is to synthesize and to secrete antibodies. Antibodies interact with antigens generally found outside cells, such as when bacteria are encountered in the plasma component of the bloodstream. The B-cell receptor is an antibody molecule. When a B cell comes across an antigen for which its membrane-bound antibody is specific, the cell is activated and begins to divide rapidly. Its descendants differentiate into *plasma cells* and *memory B cells*. Memory B cells have a long lifespan and continue to express antibody on their membrane with the same specificity as the original parent cell. Plasma cells produce large quantities of antibody in a form that can be secreted into body fluids, or the humoral system. These circulating antibodies found in serum and tissue fluids recognize specific antigens structurally identical to the primary B-cell antigen receptors. Immunoglobulin (Ig) antibodies can neutralize toxic substances, or antigens, by simple binding. This renders the antigen site nonactive, facilitates phagocytosis by acting as an opsonin to coat antigens, kills microbes directly by causing cell lysis, and combines with antigens on cellular surfaces to cause destruction of antigen either extravascularly or intravascularly, in combination with complement.

T cells participate in *cell-mediated immunity (CMI)* by recognition and response to protein antigens that originate inside the cell and are presented at the surface of the host cell as small polypeptide fragments. Antibodies manufactured by B cells do not generally have access to antigens found inside cells such as blood cells internally invaded by viral agents. Cell-mediated immunity by T cells involves response against nonself protein antigens, such as fungal or viral infections, intracellular pathogens, foreign-tissue grafts, or tumors, in which antibody plays a minor role in the defense mechanism. Unlike B-cell receptors, which can recognize foreign antigen alone, T-cell receptors can recognize foreign antigen only in association with cell membrane proteins known as *major histocompatibility complex (MHC)* molecules. The adaptive immune response is therefore genetically influenced by the MHC genes, which determine the human leukocyte antigen (HLA) found on cells. MHC class I genes express HLA-A, HLA-B, or HLA-C antigens. MHC class II genes express HLA-D, HLA-DR, HLA-DQ, or HLA-DC antigens. Both class I and class II are important in the cellular recognition processes that occur during an immune reaction to a foreign substance. Major histocompatibility complex molecules are also involved in antigen presentation, which will be discussed later.

T cells have two major functions. First, they produce a series of cytokines, such as interleukins and interferons, which influence many different cells. Second, T cells have the ability to kill cells that contain foreign antigen.[9] On activation, T cells respond by secreting an array of cytokines and/or exhibiting considerably altered behavior toward other cells. The two main subgroups of T lymphocytes are *T helper ($T_H$) cells* and *T cytotoxic ($T_C$) cells*. $T_C$ cells have the distinguishing ability to kill cells, or *cytotoxicity*. $T_H$ cells recognize antigen, together with the MHC class II molecules. $T_H$ cells determine which antigens and epitopes become targets and are recognized for immune response. $T_H$ cells also select which effector mechanisms are to be directed against the selected target epitope. They aid proliferation and enhance the function of the appropriate effector cell type. Not all available effector systems are activated equally in any one immune response. When certain groups of $T_H$ cells are activated, they secrete lymphokines. Changes in the pattern of secreted lymphokines result in qualitative changes in the type of immune response that develops. For example, some lymphokines activate, or "help," the B lymphocytes divide, differentiate, and make antibody. Other $T_H$-activated cells interact with mononuclear phagocytes and help them kill intracellular pathogens. Still other $T_H$ cells stimulate $T_C$ cells to proliferate and to differentiate. The $T_C$ cells interact with MHC class I molecules. Under the influence of $T_H$-derived lymphokines, when a $T_C$ cell recognizes antigen together with MHC molecules, the $T_C$ cell proliferates to become an cytotoxic effector cell with the ability to issue a lethal strike, leading to the death of the target cell. In comparison with the $T_H$ cells, $T_C$ cells generally do not secrete many lymphokines. $T_C$ cells are responsible for the destruction of host cells that have become infected by viruses or other intracellular agents. $T_C$ cells also eliminate tumor cells and cells of foreign tissue grafts.[10]

The activation of $T_H$ cells leading to the production of lymphokines must be carefully regulated to avoid inappropriate immune responses to self-components. To ensure proper levels of stimulation, $T_H$ activation occurs only when the antigen is displayed together with MHC on the surface of specialized cells called antigen-presenting cells (APCs). Antigen-presenting cells are a heterogeneous population of leukocytes, which include monocytes and polymorphonuclear granulocytes. Additionally, other cells that are not leukocytes can acquire the ability to become APCs when stimulated by cytokines. Examples of such cells include Langerhans' cells in the skin and follicular dendritic cells in the lymph nodes. Antigen-presenting cells are primarily found in the skin, lymph nodes, spleen, and thymus. These specialized cells phagocytize and process the antigen, then re-express a part of the antigen together with the MHC molecule, presenting the processed antigen on their membrane to the lymphocyte. The $T_H$ cell then recognizes the antigen associated with the MHC molecule on the membrane of the APC.[10]

**Primary and Secondary Response and Memory Cells.** Because of the complexity of interactions required to mount an immune response to a foreign antigen, and because this response is influenced by antigen characteristics as well as by a variety of host factors, a period extending from a few days to a few months may pass before realization of a full response to an antigenic stimulus. This time is sometimes referred to as the *latency period*, during which no antibody response is detectable in the test serum. During the latency period, T-cell and B-cell response is occurring, and the first appearance of specific antibody constitutes the beginning of the primary response. Most of the antibodies produced in the beginning of the primary response are immunoglobulin M (IgM), although they are later replaced by immunoglobulin G (IgG) antibodies (Fig. 3–1).[11] After elimination of the antigenic stimulus and the subsequent decline of antibody response, memory T and B cells are stored in organs of the immune system. When the same antigen is encountered again, these memory cells are responsible for the rapid pro-

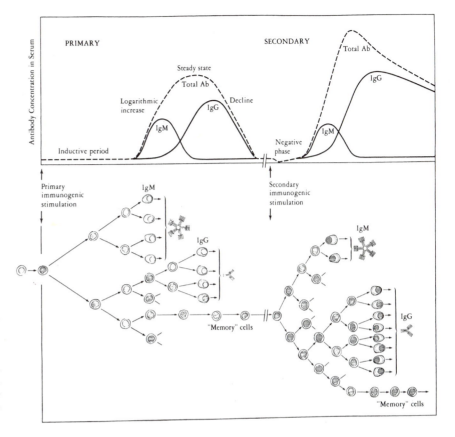

**Figure 3–1.** Schematic representation of primary and secondary antibody responses. Note the enhanced antibody production and expanded antibody-producing cell population during the secondary antibody response. (From Herscowitz, HB: Immunophysiology. In Bellanti, JA (ed): Immunology III. WB Saunders, Philadelphia, 1985, p 117, with permission.)

duction, higher intensity, and longer duration of secondary responses. Secondary responses are characterized by the presence of large amounts of IgG antibodies. IgM antibodies, also formed at the beginning of the response, rapidly decline as they are replaced by IgG antibodies (see Fig. 3–1). Secondary response antibodies have a higher avidity for antigen, are produced at significantly lower doses of antigen than antibodies formed during the primary response, and usually are formed more quickly, in 1 to 2 days. An Rh-negative individual, for example, may require a dose of at least 200 to 300 mL of Rh-positive red cells before mounting a primary response. A secondary exposure to Rh-positive cells, however, may require as little as 0.1 mL of Rh-positive red cells to induce a rapid antibody response.[11]

### Advanced Concepts

#### Cells and Organs of the Immune System: Cell Maturation/Membrane Markers

Macrophages, T lymphocytes, B lymphocytes, and NK cells interact directly from cell to cell or indirectly by mediators through a complex system of cell markers and receptors. In laboratory testing, these cell surface molecules, which specify leukocyte definition and function, are designated as clusters of differentiation (CD), groups that are recognized by various monoclonal antibodies.[12] Many mediator substances such as cytokines, immunoglobulins, and proteins of the complement, kinin, clotting, and fibrinolytic systems represent cellular products that have effects on organ systems, cells, and other substances.[13,14]

Cells of the immune system are arranged in primary lymphoid organs such as the thymus and bone marrow, and secondary lymphoid organs such as lymph nodes and spleen (Table 3–4). In the primary organs, cells differentiate and mature into immunocompetent cells; in the secondary organs, cells associate and communicate with each other and interact with antigens. Immune cells originate from pluripotential stem cells through two main lineages: myeloid and lymphoid. The myeloid cells consist of phagocytic cells, such as monocytes and polymorphonuclear granulocytes, as well as other APCs, such as dendritic cells. The lymphoid cells include the various subpopulations of T cells, B cells, and NK cells.[10]

Myeloid precursors, which give rise to the cells of the mononuclear phagocytic system (MPS), originate in the bone marrow and differentiate into circulating blood monocytes, which can be transformed into macrophages in the tissues. The primary function of the MPS is phagocytosis and processing of antigen to prepare it for further immune outcomes mediated by lymphocytes.[10] Phagocytic cells can be very effective in directly killing bacteria, fungi, and tumor cells.[15] Mononuclear phagocytes also serve as APCs, which present processed antigen to lymphocytes. Mono-

**Table 3–4.** Lymphoid Organs Associated with the Acquired Immune System

| Primary Lymphoid Organs | Secondary Lymphoid Organs |
|---|---|
| • Thymus<br>• Bone marrow | • Lymph nodes<br>• Spleen<br>• Mucosa-associated tissues |
| Site of maturation for T and B cells | Site of cell function for mature T and B cells |
| Lymphocytes differentiate from stem cells, then migrate to secondary lymphoid organs | Cells interact with each other, accessory cells, and antigens |

nuclear phagocytes interact with other immune cells and antigens through a complex system of cellular receptors. When phagocytic cells function in antigen recognition and binding of antibody or of complement-coated (opsonized) antigen, or both, the principal receptors involved are those for the Fc portion of IgG and the CR1 receptor for the complement component C3b.[16] When the monocytes and macrophages function as APCs, they express the Ia antigens, the class II MHC antigens. Dendritic cells, however, although they express the Ia marker, lack the Fc receptor and some of the other distinctive monocyte-macrophage markers.[17]

Polymorphonuclear granulocytes originate in the bone marrow and account for approximately 70 percent of the circulating leukocytes. These cells are further classified as neutrophils, eosinophils, and basophils, based on the staining characteristics of their cytoplasmic granules. The main role of these cells is phagocytosis of microorganisms as they function primarily in acute inflammatory responses with antibody and complement.[18] All granulocytes possess receptors for the Fc portion of IgG (CD16) and complement receptors C5a, CR1(CD35), and CR3(CD11b). Additionally, eosinophils possess low-affinity Fc receptors for IgE. Basophils and mast cells (tissue basophils) possess high-affinity Fc immunoglobulin E (IgE) receptors.

Lymphocytic cells generated in the thymus or bone marrow travel through the circulatory system to the lymph nodes and spleen. Lymphocytes account for approximately 20 percent of circulating leukocytes. In the primary organs, these cells acquire receptors that equip them to meet antigenic confrontations and to differentiate between self and nonself antigens. In the secondary organs, immune cells are provided with an interactive environment in which immune response information is exchanged and specific actions are initiated.[10]

As previously discussed, the two primary classifications of lymphocytes are T cells and B cells. Although these cells may be similar in appearance, they may be distinguished by the presence of distinctive cell markers. The T cell has a T-cell antigen receptor (TCR) usually identified with the CD3 complex. The TCR associates in cell-to-cell contact and interacts with both antigenic determinants and MHC proteins.[19] The CD2 marker, which has the unique ability to bind with

sheep erythrocytes, is also a distinctive molecule found on T cells. $T_H$ cells have the CD4 marker and recognize antigen together with the MHC class II molecules. $T_C$ cells possess CD8 markers and interact with MHC class I molecules.

B cells are generally defined by the presence of Ig on their surface, although they also possess MHC class II antigens; complement receptors, CD35 and CD21; Fc receptors for IgG; and also CD19, CD20, and CD22 markers, which are commonly used to identify B cells. Immunoglobulin may act as an antigen receptor for binding simple structural antigens or those antigens having multiple repeating determinants (T-cell-independent antigens, not requiring the intervention of T-cell help). When T-cell-dependent antigens (structurally complex substances) are encountered, B cells require the intervention of T cells to assist in the production of antibody. When B cells become activated, they develop into plasma cells, which produce and secrete large quantities of soluble Ig into tissue or serum.[20]

Natural killer cells are sometimes referred to as third-population cells (TPCs) because, although they originate in the bone marrow, they have a distinct developmental line apart from those of T and B lymphocytes.[10] Natural killer cells do not have surface Ig or secrete Ig; they do not have an antigen receptor like the TCR found on T lymphocytes. These cells possess CD56 and CD16 markers and do not require the presence of an MHC marker in order to respond to an antigen. The cells are capable of lysing virally infected cells and tumor cells. By possessing receptors for the Fc portion of an Ig molecule, NK cells may bind and lyse antibody-coated cells in a process known as antibody-dependent cellular cytotoxicity (ADCC).[21]

### Cytokines

Cytokines are polypeptides that act as biologic mediators of immune and tissue cells. Cytokines are divided into lymphokines, which are produced by lymphocytes, and monokines, which are produced by monocytes and macrophages. Cytokines modulate the host response to antigens by regulating growth, mobility, and differentiation of leukocytes.[22] One cytokine may function alone to mediate one effect; several cytokines may have increased or decreased quantitative effects; or other cytokines may act in a synergistic man-

*granulocytes*
CD16
CD35
CD11b

*T-cells*
CD3 complex
TCR

CD2 — Sheep erythrocyte binding ability ?          Complement receptors:
                                                                CD21+35

ner, in which one cytokine requires the presence of a second cytokine to produce an effect.[23]

As a result of the various modes of action of cytokines, significant overlay in function may occur. Interleukins (ILs), colony-stimulating factors (CSFs), interferons (INFs), and tumor necrosis factors (TNFs) compose the major classifications of cytokines. Cytokines act by binding to target cell receptors. The number of receptors per cell dramatically increases as the cell is transformed from a resting state to a response state. The initial sign for this transformation may be the binding of antigen or other cytokines to the cell receptor. Interleukin-2 (IL-2), for example, requires this initial signal to be the antigen presented by an APC to a T cell. The production and response of receptor expression for IL-2, therefore, is maximized by an antigen-activated T cell.[17] After binding, both the receptor and the cytokine are internalized by the cell to induce the target cell to produce various biologic responses such as cell growth and differentiation, as well as chemoattractive, antiviral, antiproliferative, and immunomodulating activities for other immune cells (see Table 3–3).[22]

### Genetic Control of the Immune System

The ability to make an immune response to any given antigen varies between individuals. Experiments with guinea pigs testing familial patterns of susceptibility to infection have demonstrated that resistance and susceptibility are inherited characteristics.[24] Individuals may or may not develop antibodies after blood transfusions containing various nonself antigens. Those who have a genetic tendency to develop antibodies are considered *responders*. The terms *high responders* and *low responders* also describe individual responses to antigen challenges.

T cells and B cells have antigen-receptor molecules, which consist of two polypeptide chains. These proteins are synthesized by two genes located on two different chromosomes. Both T- and B-cell antigen receptor protein genes are found on chromosome 14 but at separate loci. The second loci for B cells may be on chromosome 2 or chromosome 22. The second T-cell loci is found on chromosome 7.[25] The enormous diversity of the immune response cannot be explained by one gene coding for every immunoglobin or T-cell receptor. It has been found that antibody genes can move and rearrange themselves. The *germ line DNA* is located at a locus in the unmodified gene of an inherited chromosome and is identical to all other body cells. During early development of the lymphocyte, when differentiation is taking place, the germ line DNA has the capability to move to another position on the chromosome. The germ line DNA demonstrates immense repetition. The mechanism of rearrangement during differentiation also brings together sets of genes that are transcribed and translated into complete protein arrangements. Diversity in antibody specificity is achieved by this rearrangement in different combinations and random assortment of available amino acid sequences. When DNA rearrangement has occurred, the antigenic specificity of that particular cell is fixed. Unnecessary and unused genetic material is then eliminated.[26]

As previously discussed, after antigenic stimulation, one B cell forms an antibody of only one single specificity. During the lifetime of the cell, it can switch to make a different class of antibody while retaining the same antigenic specificity. Class or isotype switching involves further DNA rearrangement in mature B cells. Class switching is dependent on antigenic stimulation and the presence of cytokines released by T cells.[26]

The MHC is the region of the genome that encodes those proteins known as the HLAs. The MHC is very influential in immune recognition and regulation of antigen presentation in cell-to-cell interactions, as well as being significant in certain disease associations, transplantation, and paternity testing.[27,28]

Human leukocyte antigen molecules are categorized into three classes: class I, class II, and class III. Class I molecules are found on all nucleated cells. For antigen to be recognized by a cytotoxic (CD8) T cell, it must be recognized within the context of a class I molecule (Figs. 3–2 and 3–3). After recognition, the cytotoxic cell destroys the target cell bearing the antigen.[27] Class II molecules are found on immunocompetent cells such as B lymphocytes, APCs, and activated T cells.[29] A class II molecule on an APC is essential for presenting processed

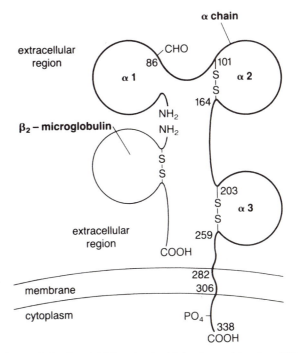

**Figure 3–2.** Class I HLA molecule. Molecule consists of an MW 44,000 polymorphic transmembrane glycoprotein, termed the α *chain,* which bears the antigenic determinant, in noncovalent association with an MW 12,000 nonpolymorphic protein termed β$_2$ *microglobulin.* The α chain has three extracellular domains termed α$_1$, α$_2$, and α$_3$. NH$_2$ = amino terminus; COOH = carboxy terminus; CHO = carbohydrate side chain; -SS- = disulfide bond; PO$_4$ = phosphate radical. (From Swartz,[20] p 47, with permission.)

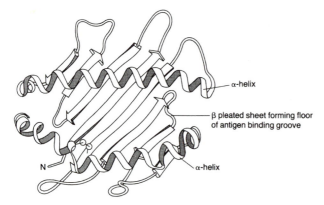

**Figure 3–3.** Top view of a crystalline structure of a class I HLA molecule. The molecule is shown as the T-cell receptor would see it. The antigen-binding site formed by the α helices (ribbonlike structures) and β pleated strands (broad arrows) is shown. N indicates the amino terminus. (From Swartz,[20] p 48, with permission.)

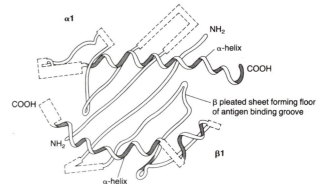

**Figure 3–5.** Top view of a crystalline structure of a class II HLA molecule. The molecule is shown as the T-cell receptor would see it. The antigen-binding site formed by the α chain α1 domain and β chain β1 domain consists of the β pleated sheet platform (thin strands) supporting two α helices (ribbonlike structures) and is very similar to that of the class I molecule (see Fig. 3–3). (From Swartz,[20] p 50, with permission.)

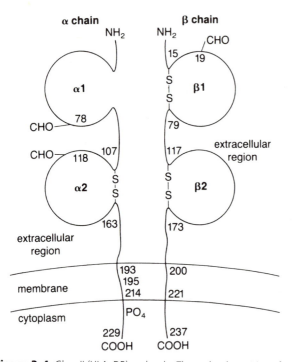

**Figure 3–4.** Class II (HLA–DR) molecule. The molecule consists of an MW 34,000 glycoprotein (the α chain) in a noncovalent association with an MW 29,000 glycoprotein (the β chain). (From Swartz,[20] p 49, with permission.)

antigen to a $T_H$ (CD4) cell (Figs. 3–4 and 3–5). Class III molecules encode components such as C2, C4, and factor B (see discussion of complement system).[27]

## Synopsis

Nearly all immunogens, especially those that elicit the formation of blood group antibodies, need to be processed by an APC to initiate the immune response. After an immunogen, such as an incompatible red blood cell, has entered the bloodstream, it travels to the spleen or liver, where it encounters an APC. The APC processes the foreign antigen in such a way as to present it to a T cell in the context of a class II MHC marker. T cells recognize antigens through the CD3/TCR complex.[19] The TCR contacts portions of both MHC marker and the processed antigen peptide. This binding is assisted by the CD4 marker (for $T_H$ cells) or CD8 marker (for $T_C$ cells). During and after antigen processing, cytokines are generated by source cells, APCs. Their receptors are expressed on recipient lymphocytes; for example, interleukin-1 (IL-1) is secreted by macrophages to activate lymphocytes by promoting the proliferation of T lymphocytes and enhancing production of IL-2 receptors on other T cells.[30] Interleukin-2, a growth factor for other T cells, enhances the activity of $T_C$ cells and NK cells. Stimulated $T_H$ cells are also capable of producing interleukin-4 (IL-4) and interleukin-5 (IL-5) to promote the growth, proliferation, and differentiation of B cells in a T-cell–dependent mechanism for antibody production. B cells are also capable of processing captured antigen through internalization of surface Ig, but this T-cell–independent mechanism is used only for very structurally simple molecules and does not produce immunologic memory. This mechanism is usually not involved in the formation of blood group antibodies. B cells that have been properly stimulated differentiate into antibody-producing plasma cells. B cells also activate other B cells by secretion of cytokines such as interleukin-6 (IL-6).[21] A foreign blood group antigen may initially elicit the production of IgM, but its production may terminate, and IgG may then be produced with the same specificity as IgM. Most immune blood group antibodies are $IgG_1$ and $IgG_3$.[31]

### Immune Suppression

Regulatory and suppressive mechanisms must be present in the normal immune response to control the reaction at all levels of activity. Cytokines react to restrict immune activities through the techniques of competition, mutual suppression, and interaction in cycles regulated by positive and negative feedback routines. In addition, products of the kinin, complement, and lipoxygenase and cyclo-oxygenase pathways, as well as neuroendocrine hormonal peptides such as endorphins and corticosteroids, regulate cytokine activities. Expression of cell membrane receptors also affects the activities of mediator substances.[32] Transforming growth factor (TGF) beta, for example, down-regulates the expression of IL-2 receptors. Interleukin-4 inhibits monocyte function by regulating monocyte adhesion through functional expression of adhesion structures, not necessarily through changes in the surface expression of cytokine receptors.[33]

CD8-positive T cells are generally considered to be the functional set of T cells that suppress immune responses through modulating cytotoxic T cells and antigen-specific T-cell proliferation. These suppressor cells, however, are produced in response to a CD4 subset of helper cells called suppressor-inducer cells.[34] Both subsets are antigen-specific and may act to slow down immune response through an idiotypic transducing effect, similar to the effect of anti-idiotypic antibodies, which suppress specific antibody response. The suppressor cells may also release a soluble suppressor factor that acts on APCs, $T_H$ cells, and B cells.[34,35]

## CHARACTERISTICS OF IMMUNOGLOBULINS

Immunoglobulins are protein molecules produced in response to an immunogen or antigen. Immunoglobulins have specific antibody activity for the antigen that initially invoked their development.[36] As mentioned previously, immunoglobulins are found on the surface of B cells. B cells, on immune stimulation, mature into antibody-producing plasma cells. Immunoglobulins make up approximately 20 percent of the total plasma proteins that are disseminated in body fluids.[36] Although the main function of immunoglob-

ulins is the binding of antigen, these molecules have other biologic functions, such as facilitating phagocytosis, neutralizing toxic substances, fixing complement, and killing microbes.[37]

Immunoglobulins have been classified as IgA, IgD, IgE, IgG, and IgM, corresponding to the chemical structure of the heavy chain of the molecule. In addition to the differences in heavy chain structure, immunoglobulin classes also vary in other features such as serum concentration, molecular weight, biologic activity, percentage of carbohydrate content, and plasma half-life, as illustrated in Table 3–5. The immunoglobulin found in greatest concentration in serum is IgG, which composes approximately 80 percent of the total serum immunoglobulin; 13 percent is IgA (IgA, however, is the major immunoglobulin found in body secretions such as saliva); 6 percent is IgM; 1 percent is IgD; and IgE is present only in trace amounts.[38]

### Immunoglobulin Structure

All classes and subclasses of immunoglobulins have a common chemical structural configuration (Fig. 3–6). The basic immunoglobulin unit is composed of four polypeptide chains: two identical light chains (molecular weights of approximately 22,500 daltons [D]) and two identical heavy chains (molecular weight from approximately 50,000 to 75,000 D). Both light and heavy chains are held together by covalent disulfide bonds. The heavy chains are interconnected by disulfide linkages in the hinge region of the molecule. Light and heavy chains are held together in a similar manner. The immunoglobulin classes are named according to the structure of their heavy chains, and the five types of heavy chains are designated alpha (IgA), delta (IgD), epsilon (IgE), gamma (IgG), and mu (IgM). Only two types of light chains, kappa and lambda, are found in all classes of immunoglobulins.[38]

The immunoglobulin molecule has two terminal regions, the carboxyl (-COOH) and amino (-NH$_2$) terminal regions. The carboxyl region of the heavy chain has a comparatively constant amino acid sequence for any antibody class. This area of the heavy chain com-

**Table 3–5.** Characteristics of Serum Immunoglobulins

| Characteristic | IgA | IgD | IgE | IgG | IgM |
|---|---|---|---|---|---|
| Heavy chain type | Alpha | Delta | Epsilon | Gamma | Mu |
| Sedimentation coefficient(s) | 7–15* | 7 | 8 | 6.7 | 19 |
| Molecular weight (D) | 160–500 | 180 | 196 | 150 | 900 |
| Biologic half-life (d) | 5.8 | 2.8 | 2.3 | 21 | 5.1 |
| Carbohydrate content (%) | 7.5–9.0 | 10–13 | 11–12 | 2.2–3.5 | 7–14 |
| Placental transfer | No | No | No | Yes | No |
| Complement fixation (classic pathway) | − | − | − | + | +++ |
| Agglutination in saline | + | − | − | ± | ++++ |
| Heavy chain allotypes | A$_m$ | None | None | G$_m$ | None |
| Proportion of total immunoglobulin (%) | 13 | 1 | 0.002 | 80 | 6 |

*May occur in monomeric or polymeric structural forms.
D = daltons; d = days; − = absent; ± = weak reactivity; + = slight reactivity; +++ = strong reactivity; ++++ = very strong reactivity.

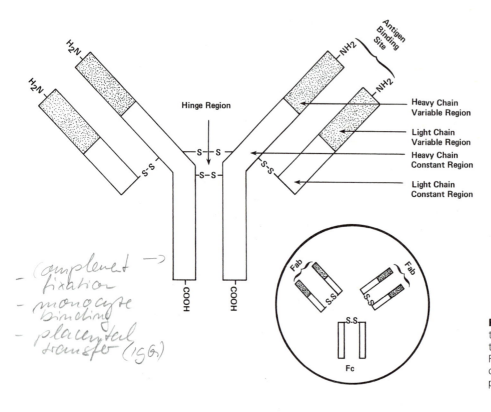

Hinge Region

Heavy Chain
Variable Region

Light Chain
Variable Region

Heavy Chain
Constant Region

Light Chain
Constant Region

Antigen
Binding
Site

**Figure 3–6.** Schematic representation of basic immunoglobulin structure. The inset shows formation of Fab and Fc fragments after enzymatic cleavage of the IgG molecule by papain.

- Complement
  fixation ⟶
- monocyte
  binding
- placental
  transfer (IgG)

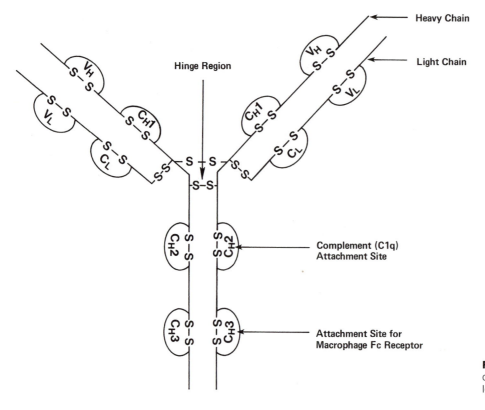

Hinge Region

Heavy Chain

Light Chain

Complement (C1q)
Attachment Site

Attachment Site for
Macrophage Fc Receptor

**Figure 3–7.** Schematic illustration of the domain structure within the IgG molecule.

prises the constant region. The light chain also has a constant region. Enzyme cleavage by papain splits the antibody molecule at the hinge region to give three fragments, one crystallizable (Fc) fragment and two fragment-antigen-binding (Fab) fragments. The Fc fragment encompasses the portion of the immunoglobulin molecule from the carboxyl region to the hinge region. The Fc region is responsible for complement fixation, monocyte binding, and placental transfer (IgG only). The amino terminal regions are known as the variable regions of the light and heavy chains because they are structured according to the variation in antibody specificity against diverse antigens encountered in the immune response. The Fab fragments encompass the portions of the immunoglobulin from the hinge region to the amino terminal. The Fab portion is the region responsible for binding antigen[38] (see Fig. 3–6).

Domains constitute regions of the light and heavy chains that are folded into compact globular loops (Fig. 3–7). Domains are held together by intrachain covalent disulfide bonds. V specifies the variable region, and C, the constant region. One domain ($V_L$) is the variable region and one domain ($C_L$) is in the constant region of each light chain. One variable domain ($V_H$) is also on each heavy chain. The immunoglobulin class determines the number of domains on the constant regions of each heavy chain. There are, therefore, three constant domains: $C_H1$ to $C_H3$, on the heavy chains of IgA, IgD, and IgG; and there are four constant domains, $C_H1$ to $C_H4$, on the heavy chains of IgE and IgM. Antigen-

binding and idiotypic regions (which distinguish one V domain from all other V domains) are located within the three-dimensional structures formed by the $V_L$ and $V_H$ domains. Heavy chain domains are associated with some of the biologic properties of immunoglobulins, especially those of IgG and IgM. Complement fixation, for example, is identified with the $C_H2$ domain. The $C_H3$ domain serves as an attachment site for the Fc receptor of monocytes and macrophages.[38]

## Immunoglobulins Significant for Blood Banking

IgG and IgM are the immunoglobulins having the most significance for blood bankers. Most clinically significant antibodies are IgG, which react at body temperature, 37°C; clinically significant antibodies, therefore, are capable of destroying transfused antigen-positive red cells. IgM antibodies are found as naturally occurring antibodies in the ABO system. Other blood groups such as Lewis, Ii, P, and MNS may also produce IgM antibodies. The primary blood banking testing problem encountered with IgM antibodies is that they may interfere with the detection of clinically significant IgG antibodies by masking their reactivity. Because IgM exists in both a monomeric and a polymeric form with a pentameric configuration containing a J (or joining) chain, IgM can be dissociated through the cleavage of covalent bonds interconnecting the monomeric subunits and the J chain (Fig. 3–8). The blood banker may use 2-mercaptoethanol (2-ME) or dithiothreitol (DTT)

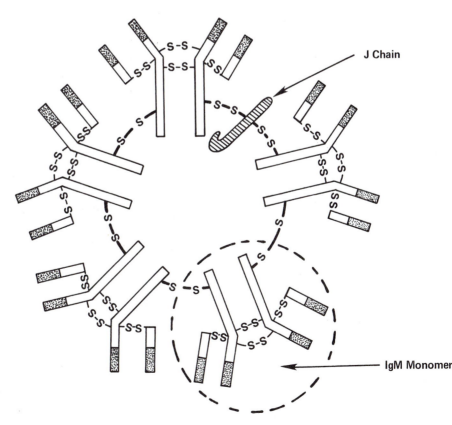

**Figure 3–8.** Schematic representation of the pentameric configuration of the IgM immunoglobulin.

to accomplish the dissociation of the IgM molecule. By the use of these reagents, a mixture of IgM and IgG antibodies can be distinguished because only IgM antibodies are removed by the use of such compounds.[38]

IgG antibodies are significant in the study of immunohematology because they denote the class of immunoglobulins formed in response to the transfusion of incompatible blood products. IgG antibodies are important in hemolytic disease of the newborn (HDN). Maternal IgG immunoglobulins are formed in response to incompatible fetal red cells. Four different subclasses exist for IgG: $IgG_1$, $IgG_2$, $IgG_3$, and $IgG_4$. Small differences in chemical structure within the constant regions of the gamma heavy chains designate the various subclasses. The number of disulfide bonds between the two heavy chains in the hinge region of the molecule constitutes one of the main differences between subclasses. Subclasses also exhibit variations in electrophoretic mobility and biologic properties such as the ability to fix complement and cross the placenta[38] (Table 3–6).

IgG blood group antibodies of a single specificity may show immunoglobulins of all four subclasses or predominantly or exclusively one IgG subclass. Antibodies to the Rh system antigens, for example, are mostly of the $IgG_1$ and $IgG_3$ subclasses. Anti-K (Kell), and anti-Fy (Duffy) antibodies, however, are usually of the $IgG_1$ subclass. Anti-Jk (Kidd) antibodies are mainly $IgG_3$. The purpose for the existence of biologic differences in subclass expression is unknown, but variations in immunologic responsiveness may possibly have underlying clinical significance, especially in HDN.[38] Severe HDN has been most often associated with $IgG_1$ antibodies.[39]

IgA, similar to IgM, exists in two main forms, a monomer and polymer form, with two immunoglobulin molecules in the polymer form joined by a J chain. Serum IgA is found in both monomeric and polymeric forms. Secretory IgA, usually found in the polymer form, also acquires a glycoprotein secretory component as it passes through epithelial cell walls of mucosal tissues and appears in saliva, tears, bronchial secretions, prostatic fluid, vaginal secretions, and the mucous secretions of the small intestine.[40]

IgA is important in the study of immunohematology for several reasons. Approximately one-third of anti-A and anti-B antibodies are of the IgA class (the other two-thirds are IgM and IgG)[41] (Fig. 3–9). Anti-IgA antibodies sometimes form following the transfusion of plasma products to patients who are deficient in IgA. (See Chapter 18 for a discussion of anaphylactic shock in an IgA-deficient individual transfused with a plasma product.) Another reason for the importance of IgA is that secretory IgA antibodies may be found in patients who show autoimmune hemolysis because of multiple antibodies bound to the surface of red cells. IgA antibodies show an augmentation effect of IgG-induced red cell hemolysis.[42]

IgE is normally found only in monomeric form in very small concentrations in serum, composing only about 0.004 percent of total immunoglobulins. The Fc portion of the molecule attaches to basophils and mast cells. When an allergen binds to the Fab portion of the molecule and cross-links with a second molecule on the cell surface, it triggers cellular release of biochemical mediators such as histamine, which is responsible for the manifestation of symptoms associated with the allergic reaction.

Transfusion reactions such as urticaria may occur because of the presence of IgE antibodies. Patients who have repeated allergic reactions to blood products may be given antihistamines to counteract the response when receiving blood products.[43]

IgD, present in only trace amounts (0.2 percent) in serum, has functions that probably relate primarily to the maturation of B cells into antibody-producing plasma cells. IgD may possibly perform some immunoregulatory roles during B-cell differentiation.[44]

## Immunoglobulin Variations

Immunoglobulin structures have genetic variability similar to inherited blood group differences. Three main types of antibody variation exist: isotype, allo-

**Table 3.6.** Biologic Properties of IgG Subclasses

| Characteristic | $IgG_1$ | $IgG_2$ | $IgG_3$ | $IgG_4$ |
|---|---|---|---|---|
| Proportion of total serum IgG (%) | 65–70 | 23–28 | 4–7 | 3–4 |
| Complement fixation (classic pathway) | ++ | + | +++ | − |
| Binding to macrophage Fc receptors | +++ | ++ | +++ | ± |
| Ability to cross placenta | + | ± | + | + |
| Dominant antibody activities: | | | | |
|   Anti-Rh | ++ | − | + | ± |
|   Anti–factor VII | − | − | − | + |
|   Antidextran | − | + | − | − |
|   Anti-Kell | + | − | − | − |
|   Anti-Duffy | + | − | − | − |
|   Antiplatelet | − | − | + | − |
| Biologic half-life (days) | 21 | 21 | 7–8 | 21 |

− = absent; ± = weak (or unusual) reactivity; + = slight (or usual) reactivity; ++ = moderate (or more common) reactivity; +++ = strong reactivity.

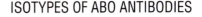

## ISOTYPES OF ABO ANTIBODIES

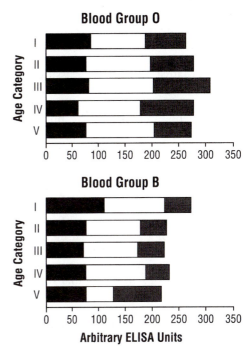

**Figure 3–9.** Distribution of anti-A IgM, IgG, and IgA antibodies by age categories, IgM (black), IgG (white), IgA (gray), expressed as arbitrary ELISA units. Age categories: I = 20–30 years; II = 31–40 years; III = 41–50 years; IV = 51–60 years; V = 61–67 years. (Adapted with permission from TRANSFUSION, published by The American Association of Blood Banks. Rieben et al,[41] p 613.)

type, and idiotype. Isotypic variation refers to variants present in all members of a species (e.g., the different immunoglobulin heavy and light chains and subclasses). All humans, therefore, have the same immunoglobulin classes and subclasses. Allotypic variation is present primarily in the constant region; not all variants occur in all members of a species. Idiotypic variation happens only in the variable region and is specific for each antibody molecule.[45]

Allotypic determinants have been defined as located on the $C_L$ domains of kappa light chains ($K_m$ markers), on the constant domains of $IgA_2$ ($A_{2m}$ markers), and on the constant domains of IgG ($G_m$ markers). Three $K_m$, two $A_m$, and 28 $G_m$ markers have been described. $G_m$ markers specifically have been typed in paternity cases and population genetics studies. Inheritance of certain $G_m$ phenotypes may even define an individual's ability to mount an antibody response of a given immunoglobulin subclass. Certain disease associations, especially autoimmune diseases, have been shown with some $G_m$ phenotypes. The genes that define allotype expression, therefore, may play an additional biologic role similar to that of other immune response (Ir) genes found within the HLA system.[46]

Pregnant women may become immunized to paternal allotypic determinants on fetal immunoglobulins.[47] Alloimmunization may also occur in patients who have received multiple transfusions of blood, plasma, or gamma globulin. Antibodies against $A_{2m}$ allotypes have been implicated in some transfusion reactions, especially in patients who may have an IgA deficiency. Patients with rheumatoid arthritis may spontaneously develop antibodies in the absence of a known sensitizing stimulus.[46]

### Immunoglobulin Fc Receptors on Effector Cells

Mononuclear phagocytes, macrophages, and monocytes are equipped with receptors for the attachment of IgG immunoglobulin. These receptors bind to the $C_H3$ domain in the Fc portion of the IgG molecule. Only the $IgG_1$ and $IgG_3$ subclasses are capable of cytophilic attachment to the Fc receptors. Incompatible red cells, therefore, that are coated with IgG antibody adhere to monocytes and macrophages. Phagocytosis of the antibody-coated cells will be promoted. Other cells with Fc receptors include neutrophils, NK cells (CD16), and mature B cells.[47,48]

## COMPLEMENT SYSTEM

The complement system denotes a group of approximately 25 serum and cell membrane proteins that have a variety of functions within the immune response. One role of the complement system is direct lysis of cells, bacteria, and enveloped viruses. Another capability of complement is the mediation of opsonization, whereby foreign substances are coated with complement to facilitate phagocytosis. A third function of the complement system is the production of split products, which are peptide fragments capable of directing certain inflammatory and immune response operations such as increased vascular permeability, smooth muscle contraction, phagocytic chemotaxis, migration, and adherence.[49,50]

Complement components circulate in inactive form (exception, factor D) and are sequentially activated through two main pathways, the classic pathway and the alternative pathway. The classic pathway is activated by the binding of antigen with antibody of the IgM class or $IgG_1$, $IgG_2$, or $IgG_3$ subclasses. Complement components are sequentially numbered C1 through C9, in order of their discovery, not necessarily their activation sequence. The alternative pathway is activated by polysaccharides and lipopolysaccharides, which may be found on the surfaces of certain target cells such as bacteria, fungi, parasites, and tumor cells. Four serum proteins are unique for the alternative pathway and are designated by letters: factor B, factor D, properdin (factor P), and initiating factor (IF). Divalent cations such as $Ca^{2+}$ and $Mg^{2+}$ are required in the activation process of some components. Complement components or complexes that have been stimulated and that have enzymatic activity are designated by a bar placed over the appropriate number or letter; for example, C4b2a or factor D. The complement system also contains regulatory or inhibitory proteins such as C1 inhibitor (C1INH), factor H, factor I, C4-binding protein (C4BP), anaphylatoxin inactivator, membrane attack complex (MAC) inhibitor, and C3 nephritic factor (NF).[51,52]

## Classic Complement Pathway

The cascading activation of the classic complement pathway is initiated by the binding of C1 to the Fc fragment of an IgM or IgG subclass. The C1 component is composed of three C1 subunits: C1q, C1r, and C1s. The generation of C1s activates C4 and C2, forming a bimolecular complex. This activated complex, C4b2a, is a powerful cleaving esterase enzyme, which uses C3 as a natural substrate. By-products that result from the activation of the classic sequence include C4b and C3b. Human red cells have CR1 receptors for C4b and C3b, and some of the cleavage products will attach to the cell membrane. Later these fragments are further degraded to C4d and C3d through the action of C4BP, factor H (which binds C3b), and factor I (which degrades both C4b and C3b)[52] (Fig. 3–10).

## Alternative Complement Pathway

Factor $\overline{D}$ is analogous to $\overline{C1s}$ in the classic pathway, factor B is analogous to C2, and the cleavage product C3b is analogous to C4. Activation of the alternative pathway requires that a C3b molecule be bound to the surface of a target cell. Small amounts of C3b are generated continuously owing to the spontaneous hydrolytic cleavage of the C3 molecule. When C3b encounters normal cells, it is rapidly eliminated through the combined inactivating interactions of factors H and

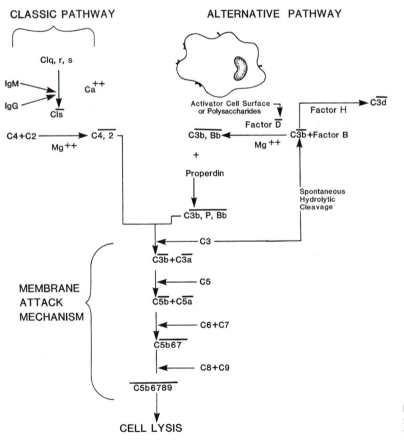

**Figure 3–10.** Schematic diagram illustrating the sequential activation of the complement system via the classic and alternative pathways.

I. The accumulation of C3b on cell surfaces is associated with attachment of C3b to factor B. The complex of C3b and factor B (analogous to C4b2a) is then acted on by factor D. As a result of this action, factor B is cleaved, yielding a cleavage product known as Bb. The C3bBb complex is stabilized by the presence of properdin (P), yielding C3bPBb. This complex acts as an esterase that cleaves C3 into additional C3b. C3b, therefore, acts as a positive feedback mechanism for driving the alternative pathway that bypasses the C142 sequence of the classic pathway (see Fig. 3–10).[52]

## Membrane Attack Complex

The terminal components of the complement sequence compose the MAC. In the classic pathway the MAC is initiated by the enzymatic activity of C4b2a3b on C5. In the alternative pathway C3bBbP has the ability to cleave C5. After C5 is split into C5a and C5b by either the classic or the alternative pathway, C5b continues the complement cascade in initiating the membrane attachment of C6, C7, and C8. After the attachment of C9 to the C5b678 complex, a small transmembrane channel is formed, destroying the integrity of the cell membrane. Osmotic lysis eventually causes total cell destruction.[52,53]

## Binding of Complement by Red Cell Antibodies

Red cell antibody and complement can bring about the destruction of red cells. The effective activation of the classic pathway by C1q necessitates the binding of one C1 molecule to two adjacent immunoglobulin Fc regions. A pentameric IgM molecule provides two Fc regions side by side, thereby binding complement. A monomeric IgG molecule, however, binds C1q less efficiently, and two IgG molecules are unlikely to align themselves side by side to bind complement. As many as 800 IgG anti-A molecules may need to attach to one adult $A_1$ red cell to bind a single C1 molecule.[38] Rh IgG antibodies usually do not bind complement because of the scarcity of Rh antigens on red cell surfaces, although there may be exceptions.[54] An interesting example of an efficient IgG hemolysin is found in patients with paroxysmal cold hemoglobinuria, who have antibodies directed against P blood group determinants. Antibodies to the Lewis blood group system are generally IgM, and they activate complement, on rare occasions causing hemolytic transfusion reactions.[55] With the exception of the ABO system, however, only a few antibodies activate the complement sequence that leads to complement-mediated intravascular hemolysis. Extravascular hemolysis most often occurs as a result of antibody coating of red cells, but the split products of complement activation facilitate the activity of the reticuloendothelial system and cause anaphylatoxic effects.[56] Cells of the mononuclear phagocyte system, monocytes, macrophages, and the cells lining the hepatic and splenic sinusoids also play an important role in the clearance of antibody-coated red cells. These phagocytic cells are equipped with two biologically important types of surface receptors: complement receptors for C3b (CR1) and immunoglobulin Fc receptors (Fig. 3–11). Transfused

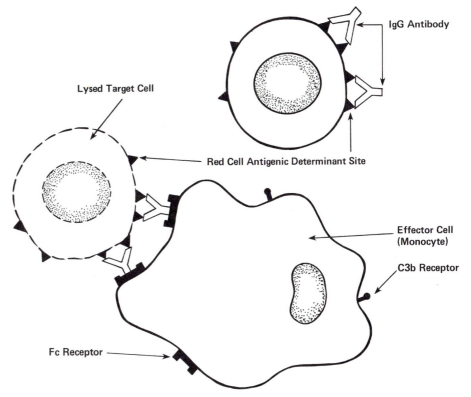

IgG Antibody

Red Cell Antigenic Determinant Site

Lysed Target Cell

Effector Cell (Monocyte)

C3b Receptor

Fc Receptor

**Figure 3–11.** Schematic representation of the mechanism of antibody-dependent cell-mediated cytotoxicity (ADCC). Note the role of effector cell surface receptors for the Fc fragment of IgG.

red cells coated with C3b alone, with antibody, are sequestrated only transiently in the reticuloendothelial organs and otherwise survive normally. Monocytes and macrophages do not have IgM receptors; therefore, IgM-coated red cells are not eliminated through Fc receptor-mediated phagocytosis. If erythrocytes are coated with IgG and complement, however, they will be cleared rapidly from circulation.[52]

Interestingly, the CR1 (C3b/C4b, CD35) receptor on red cells, which is important in immune adherence (attachment of immune complexes to erythrocytes, significant in the metabolism of immune complexes), is also a blood group antigen, Knops/McCoy, which generates high-titer low-avidity (HTLA) antibodies in immunized transfusion recipients.[57,58]

### Blood Samples Required for Testing

Some blood banking tests require the use of serum to ensure that adequate amounts of viable complement are available for fixation by blood group antibodies. An anticoagulated sample, for example, would not be conducive to complement activation because anticoagulants bind $Ca^{2+}$ or $Mg^{2+}$, or both, and inhibit complement activity. Adding 2 mg of $Na_2H_2$ ethylenediaminetetraacetic acid (EDTA) to 1 mL of serum will totally obstruct complement activation. Heparin inhibits the cleavage of C4.[45] Using serum instead of plasma for most blood bank procedures ensures that viable complement is accessible for use in all methods; therefore, serum should be used for all antibody screening and compatibility testing. Serum should be removed as soon as possible from a clotted blood sample. If testing cannot proceed immediately after separation of serum and red cells, then serum should be removed and placed at 4°C for no longer than 48 hours. For longer periods of time, serum should be frozen at –50°C or lower to retain complement activity.

The lytic potential of complement may be abolished by heating serum at 56°C for 30 minutes. C1 and C2 are destroyed and C4 is damaged by this treatment. Factor B is inactivated by heating at 50°C for 20 minutes.[59]

Serum under normal circumstances has some natural complement inhibition. An inhibitor is present that blocks the action of activated Cl by binding to and removing C1s and C1r from the activated complex of C1qrs.[59]

The complement system may become activated during storage of preserved red cell products. In citrate-phosphate-dextrose-adenine (CPDA-1)-preserved red cells, for example, activation of C3 may be caused by activation of the alternate pathway of the complement system by contact of plasma with plastic surfaces.[60] This action may cause some hemolysis in the red cell product.

## CHARACTERISTICS OF ANTIGENS

The immune response is initiated by the presentation of a provocation that takes the form of an *immunogen* or an *antigen*. The difference between an immunogen and an antigen is associated with the body's reactivity to an immune stimulus. Even though "immunogen" and "antigen" are often used as equivalent terms, immunogen actually refers to any substance that can induce an immune response, whereas antigen implies the ability of an immunogenic substance to react with the products, such as antibodies, which result from an immune response.[61] The term "antigen" is more commonly used among blood bankers because their primary testing concern is the detection of antibodies to blood group antigens.

The immune reaction to an immunogen or antigen is determined by host response as well as several characteristics of the foreign substance. Properties such as size, complexity, conformation, charge, accessibility, solubility, digestibility, and chemical composition influence the amount and type of immune response (Table 3–7). A molecule having a small molecular weight (MW), less than 10,000 d, for example, is called a *hapten* and usually does not elicit an immune response by itself. When coupled with a carrier protein having a larger size than MW 10,000 d, however, the hapten can invoke a reaction.[61]

Chemical complexity is another property with implications for the type and extent of immune response generated upon exposure to a foreign substance. The more complex molecules generally produce a greater response. Antibody or cellular response is usually very specific for antigen conformation (e.g., linear versus globular molecules). Antibody response is also formed to the net charge of a molecule, whether it is to positive, negative, or neutral antigenic determinants. The accessibility of determinant groupings influences the immune response and subsequent antibody formation.

Insoluble substances are less likely to elicit an immune response. A molecule may be a protein, lipoprotein, polysaccharide, lipopolysaccharide, glycoprotein, polypeptide, or nucleic acid; the response is generated according to the composition of the stimulus. Red cell antigens, for example, may be proteins (such as the Rh, M, and N blood group substances) or glycolipids (such as the ABH, Lewis, Ii, and P blood group substances). Human, leukocyte antigens are glycoproteins. Because of structural, conformational, and molecular differences, not all blood group substances are equally immunogenic in vivo (Table 3–8). Fifty to seventy percent of Rh-negative recipients of Rh-positive blood would be

**Table 3–7.** Characteristics of Antigens: Properties That Influence Immune Response

Size
Complexity
Conformation
Charge
Accessibility
Solubility
Digestibility
Chemical composition

**Table 3.8.** Relative Immunogenicity of Different Blood Group Antigens

| Blood Group Antigen | Blood Group System | Immunogenicity (%)* |
|---|---|---|
| D (Rh$_o$) | Rh | 50.00 |
| K | Kell | 5.00 |
| c (hr') | Rh | 2.05 |
| E (rh") | Rh | 1.69 |
| k | Kell | 1.50 |
| e (hr") | Rh | 0.56 |
| Fy$^a$ | Duffy | 0.23 |
| C (rh') | Rh | 0.11 |
| Jk$^a$ | Kidd | 0.07 |
| S | MNSs | 0.04 |
| Jk$^b$ | Kidd | 0.03 |
| s | MNSs | 0.03 |

**Source:** Adapted from Williams, WJ, et al (eds): Hematology. McGraw-Hill, New York, 1983, p 1491.
*Percentage of transfusion recipients lacking the blood group antigen (in the first column) who are likely to be sensitized to a single transfusion of red cells containing that antigen.

expected to form antibodies if exposed to the D antigen; however, only approximately 5 percent of K-negative individuals are likely to develop antibodies to the K antigen after being transfused with K antigen–positive blood. Varying immunogenicity for different blood group antigens has practical significance for blood bankers because red cells from donors need to be routinely typed only for ABO and D antigen groupings. Other blood group antigens, from a statistical standpoint, are unlikely to elicit an immune response in a recipient.[62]

## CHARACTERISTICS OF BLOOD GROUP ANTIBODIES

### Polyclonal and Monoclonal Antibodies

As previously discussed, an antigen consists of numerous antigenic determinants or epitopes. Each B cell recognizes an individual epitope as nonself and is stimulated to produce antibody with specificity against that single epitope. Therefore, multiple epitopes on the antigen induce the proliferation of a variety of B-cell clones, resulting in heterogeneous, or *polyclonal*, serum antibodies manufactured in response to a single antigen. In vivo, the polyclonal nature of antibodies improves localization, phagocytosis, and complement-mediated lysis in the antigen-antibody defense mechanism. However, this diversity is not optimal when working with in vitro reagents produced by animals or humans. Because of the natural differences in immune response, polyclonal serums vary in antibody concentration from person to person and animal to animal. Individual sera also differ in the serologic properties of the antibody molecules they contain, the epitopes they recognize, and the presence of additional nonspecific or crossreacting antibodies.[63,64] Individual B cells can be isolated

from a polyclonal population and propagated in cell culture. The supernatant from the cell culture contains antibody of a single epitope specificity, resulting in a *monoclonal* antibody suspension. Monoclonal antibodies are highly specific, well characterized, and uniformly reactive. Refer to the sections on the effect of monoclonal versus polyclonal reagents and on monoclonal and polyclonal gammopathies later in this chapter.

### Naturally Occurring and Immune Antibodies

Red cell antibodies are considered *naturally occurring* when they are found in the serum of individuals who have never been exposed to red cell antigens by transfusion, injection, or pregnancy. Theoretically, these antibodies are produced in response to substances in the environment that are antigenically identical with or similar to red cell antigens. The common occurrence of naturally occurring antibodies suggests that their antigens are widely found in nature—that is, in animals, bacteria, and pollen. Most naturally occurring antibodies are IgM cold agglutinins, which react best at room temperature or below, activate complement, and when active at 37°C may be hemolytic. Common naturally occurring antibodies react with the ABH, Hh, Ii, Lewis, MN, and P blood group systems. Some naturally occurring antibodies that may be found in normal serum are manufactured without a known environmental stimulus.[65]

Red cell antibodies are considered immune when found in serum of individuals who have been exposed to red cell antigens by transfusion, injection, or pregnancy. These antibodies are not generally found in nature, and their molecular makeup is unique to human red cells. Most immune red cell antibodies are IgG warm sensitizing antibodies that react best at 37°C and require the use of antihuman globulin for detection. The most common immune antibodies include those that react with the Rh, Kell, Duffy, Kidd, and Ss blood group systems.[66]

### Unexpected Antibodies

Based on individual's blood type, naturally occurring anti-A and anti-B antibodies are routinely present in human serum. These antibodies are the most significant blood group antibodies and are a useful tool in the confirmation of blood typing. In normal, healthy individuals, anti-A and anti-B antibodies are generally the only red cell antibodies expected to be found in a serum sample. Except in unusual circumstances, these antibodies are easily detected by reverse grouping cells using a direct agglutination technique. (Refer to Chapter 5, The ABO Blood Group System, for a more detailed discussion.)

All other antibodies directed against red cell antigens are considered unexpected. The reactivity of unexpected antibodies is unpredictable; they may be either IgM or IgG; they may hemolyze, agglutinate, or sensitize red blood cells; or they may require enhancing agents for detection. The clinical significance of red cell antibodies is different, depending on the nature of specificity. Because of the polymorphism of the human population, a diversity of red cell antigens exists, requiring a variety of immunologic techniques for their detection and identification. In vitro detection of unexpected antibodies involves the use of antibody screening procedures, which include testing of unknown serum mixed with known reagent cells at various phases of time, temperature, incubation, and media to optimize antigen-antibody reactivity. Routine blood bank testing requires testing of samples for both expected and unexpected antibodies. Refer to Detection of Red Cell Antigen-Antibody Reactions and to Chapter 11, Antibody Detection and Identification, for a more detailed discussion on methods.

### Alloantibodies and Autoantibodies

Antigens that initiate the immune cascade result in the formation of either alloantibodies or autoantibodies. Alloantibodies are produced after exposure to genetically different, or nonself, antigens of the same species. The implication for blood banking is that transfused components carrying nonself antigens are susceptible to immune attack by alloantibodies. Autoantibodies are antibodies produced in response to self-antigens. Cold or warm autoantibodies that react specifically or nonspecifically with blood cell antigens may present both clinical problems for the patient and testing problems for the blood banker.

## CHARACTERISTICS OF ANTIGEN-ANTIBODY REACTIONS

After the immune system has been stimulated and has produced antibody, many properties of antigen and antibody reactions influence the final response outcome. Intermolecular binding forces and antibody affinity, avidity, and specificity determine the extent of the reaction and resultant removal of the antigen. The antigen-binding site of the antibody molecule is uniquely designed to recognize a homologous antigen because of the structural arrangement of amino acid sequences in the variable regions of the light and heavy chains (see Immunoglobulin Structure). The extent of the reciprocal relationship or "fit" between the antigen-binding site of the immunoglobulin molecule and its corresponding antigen is somewhat controlled by the properties of antigen and antibody reactions.

### Intermolecular Binding Forces

Intermolecular binding forces such as hydrogen bonding, electrostatic forces, Van der Waals forces, and hydrophobic bonds do not involve the formation of covalent chemical bonds between antigens and their corresponding antibodies.[67] Antibody affinity is often defined as the strength of a single antigen-antibody

bond produced by the summation of these attractive and repulsive forces. *Avidity* is the term often used to express the binding of a multivalent antigen with antisera produced in an immunized individual. Avidity, therefore, is a measure of the functional affinity of an antiserum for the whole antigen.[67] High-titer low-avidity antibodies may be annoying for blood bankers in that they exhibit low antigen-binding capacity but still show reactivity at high serum dilutions.[68]

### Antibody Specificity

Reaction strengths of antigens and antibodies are often quantified by affinity or avidity; however, the specificity of an antiserum is related to its relative avidity for antigen. Antibody specificity can be further classified as a specific reaction, cross-reaction, or no reaction. A specific reaction implies reaction between similar determinants. A cross-reaction results when some determinants of one antigen are shared by another antigen. No reaction occurs when there are no shared determinants (Fig. 3–12).[67]

The forces of intermolecular binding that ultimately influence affinity, avidity, and specificity can often be manipulated by using various blood bank reagents and methods to enhance the reactivity of certain red cell antigens and antibodies (see Factors That Influence Agglutination Reactions).

### Host Factors

The properties of antigens are not the only factors in determining the immunogenicity of blood group substances; host factors also play a key role in ascertaining an individual's ability to mount an immune response. The immune response can be influenced by such elements as nutritional status, hormones, genetic makeup, age, race, exercise level, and the occurrence of disease or injury. Severe malnutrition can lead to a 50 percent reduction in CD4-positive T cells and result in antibody responses of lower affinity. Hormone receptors are found on immunologic cells and both enhance and suppress immune response. Immune response can be genetically influenced by the genes of the MHC. Ir genes help con-

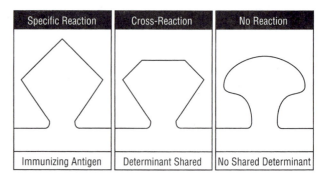

**Figure 3–12.** Types of antigen-antibody reactions: specific reaction, cross-reaction, and no reaction.

trol the type and extent of T-cell and B-cell response to individual antigens. Aging has an influence on immune response; it is generally believed that immune function decreases as age increases.[69] For blood bankers, a decrease in antibody levels in older individuals may result in false-negative reactions. Race may be a factor in the susceptibility and nonsusceptibility to certain diseases. The majority of black individuals who do not inherit the Duffy blood system antigens (Fy[a] or Fy[b]) are resistant to malarial invasion with *Plasmodium knowlesi* and *P. vivax.* The absence of these antigens may make these individuals ideal donors for those who have developed Duffy system antibodies, because most persons who manufacture anti-Fy[a] commonly have the Fy(a − b +) phenotype.

Strenuous exercise, traumatic injury, and the presence of certain diseases are other factors that may have an immunosuppressive effect on the immune response.[69] Blood bankers may observe the consequences of these conditions by detecting negative or weak serum test results, especially on reverse ABO groupings (Table 3–9).[70]

## Tolerance and Immune Unresponsiveness

The concept of tolerance, or failure of the immune system to mount an immune response to an antigen, has important implications for blood bankers. Tolerance may be naturally or experimentally induced in an individual. Exposure to an antigen during fetal life may produce tolerance to that antigen. An example of this type of tolerance is found in the chimera, an individual who receives an in utero cross-transfusion of ABO-incompatible blood from a dizygotic (nonidentical) twin.[62,70,71] The chimera will never produce antibodies against the ABO group of the twin. Forward and reverse ABO grouping of such an individual may appear as a testing discrepancy to the blood banker.

Another blood banking implication involves the deliberate induction of immune unresponsiveness for Rh-positive cells in Rh-negative individuals. When an Rh-negative woman gives birth to an Rh-positive infant, she is exposed to Rh-positive red cells. From 50 to 70 percent of Rh-negative mothers develop anti-D antibodies upon first exposure to Rh-positive cells. The formation of these antibodies can be prevented by the administration of IgG Rh-immune globulin (RHIG) within 48 to 72 hours after the birth of the infant. Interestingly, 25 to 30 percent of Rh-negative individuals

**Table 3–9.** Host Factors: Properties of the Host That Influence Immune Response

| |
|---|
| Nutritional status |
| Hormones |
| Genetics |
| Age |
| Race |
| Exercise level |
| Disease |
| Injury |

are nonresponders and do not produce anti-D antibodies, even when subjected to repeated exposure to Rh-positive cells.

## DETECTION OF RED CELL ANTIGEN-ANTIBODY REACTIONS

### Traditional Laboratory Methods

In vitro testing for the detection of antigens or antibodies may be accomplished by a variety of immunologic techniques. Such techniques as hemoagglutination, precipitation, agglutination inhibition, and hemolysis are the most commonly used methods to detect the presence of blood group antigens or antibodies. Techniques such as radioimmunoassay (RIA), enzyme-linked immunosorbent assay (ELISA) or enzyme immunoassay (EIA), and immunofluorescence, which quantitate antigen or antibody with the use of a radioisotope, enzyme, or fluorescent label, may be used in automated or semiautomated blood banking instrumentation for detecting blood group antigens or antibodies but are rarely used in routine serologic testing of blood products.[72]

In blood bank testing, agglutination reactions are the major manifestation of the blood group antigen-antibody response. Typing for ABO, Rh, and other blood group antigens is accomplished by agglutination reactions. Agglutination can be shown to develop in two stages. In stage 1, known as sensitization, antibody binding occurs. Antigenic determinants on the red cell membrane combine with the antigen-combining site (Fab region) on the variable regions of the immunoglobulin heavy and light chains. Antigen and antibody are held together by noncovalent bonds, and no visible agglutination is seen at this stage. In stage 2, a lattice structure composed of multiple antigen-antibody bridges between antibodies and red cell antigens is formed. Visible agglutination is present during this stage.[73]

The development of a perceptible, insoluble antigen-antibody complex resulting from the mixing of equivalent amounts of soluble antigen and antibody is known as a *precipitation reaction.* The visible clumping depends on multiple binding sites on antibody and antigen. The generation of antigen-antibody complexes results in a lattice formation.

Agglutination inhibition is a method in which a positive reaction is the opposite of what is normally observed in agglutination. Agglutination, which usually occurs as a manifestation of an antigen-antibody reaction, is inhibited when an antigen-antibody reaction has previously occurred in a test system and, therefore, prevents agglutination. A blood bank test illustrating this method is the *secretory study.* To determine whether soluble ABO substances are present in body fluids, saliva containing soluble ABO antigens is mixed with known ABO antisera and allowed to incubate. The antigen and appropriate antisera combine if the soluble ABO antigen is present in the saliva. If binding occurs, no free antibody is present to agglutinate reagent red cells. No agglutination, therefore, indicates that soluble antigen is present and the individual being tested is a secretor; if agglutination occurs, then no soluble antigen is present, the reagent antisera and red cells were available to react with each other, and the individual is a nonsecretor.

Hemolysis represents a positive result and indicates that an antigen-antibody reaction has occurred in which complement has been fixed, and red cell lysis occurs. The Lewis blood group antibodies, anti-Le$^a$ and anti-Le$^b$, may be regarded as clinically significant if hemolysis occurs as a result of an antigen, antibody, and complement reaction.

Radioimmunoassay, ELISA or EIA, and immunofluorescence are immunologic techniques based on quantitating antigen or antibody by the use of a radioisotope, enzyme, or fluorescent label. These techniques measure the initial interaction of the binding of antigen with antibody. Most of these techniques employ reagents that use either antigen or antibody, which is bound in a solid or liquid phase, in a variety of reaction systems ranging from plastic tubes or plates to microscopic particles. These methods also use a separation system to isolate bound and free fractions and a detection system to measure the amount of antigen-antibody interaction. The values of unknown samples are then calculated from the values of standards of known concentration.

## Factors That Influence Agglutination Reactions

Many factors influencing reactivity apply to all antigen-antibody reactions, but the main emphasis here is on agglutination reactions. The agglutination reaction is influenced by the concentration of both antigen and antibody as well as other factors such as pH, temperature, ionic strength, surface charge, antibody class, red cell antigen dosage, and the use of various enhancement media, antihuman globulin reagents, and enzymes.

### Centrifugation

High-speed centrifugation is the simplest and most common technique to enhance agglutination. Centrifugation subjects sensitized red cells to high gravitational forces overcoming the natural repulsive effect of red cells to one another. (See discussion of zeta potential in the section on Effect of Enhancement Media and Potentiators.) Having red cells in closer physical proximity allows for an increase in antigen-antibody bridging (lattice formation) and results in enhanced agglutination.[74]

### Effect of Antigen-Antibody Ratio

Under ideal reactive conditions, an equivalent amount of antigen and antibody bind in optimal proportions. An excess of either antigen or antibody, however, may lead to unbound immunoglobulin (prozone effect) or a surplus of antigen-binding sites (postzone effect) (Fig. 3–13). In either situation, the lattice formation and subsequent agglutination may not occur in the test system, leading to the assumption of false-negative results.[73] To correct the problem of excessive antibody, the serum may be diluted, with each serial dilution of serum tested against red cells. To correct the problem of excessive antigen, the serum-to-cell ratio in the test system may be increased, which tends to increase the number of antibodies available to bind with each red cell.[75] Test systems, therefore, can be manipulated to overcome the effects of excessive antigen or antibody.

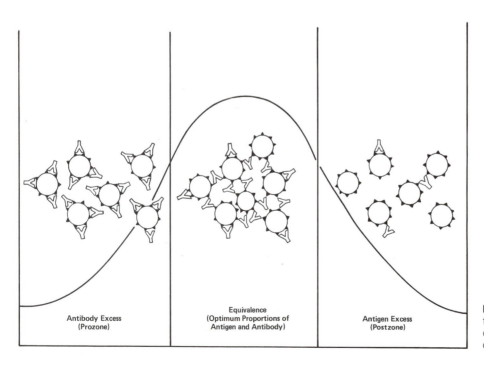

| Antibody Excess (Prozone) | Equivalence (Optimum Proportions of Antigen and Antibody) | Antigen Excess (Postzone) |

**Figure 3–13.** Schematic representation of the effects of varying concentrations of antigen and antibody on lattice formation.

Dosage effect, another reason for lack of antigen sites on red cells, occurs as a result of the inheritance of genotypes, which gives rise to heterozygous expression of red cell antigens. M+ cells from an individual having the genotype *MM*, for example, has more M antigen sites than M+ cells from an individual having the *MN* genotypes. The Rh system is another blood group system that contains certain antigens that show the dosage effect.[76,77] The C, c, E, and e antigens show dosage effect depending on the inheritance of the homozygous versus the heterozygous expression of the genotype for these antigens. *DCe/DCe*, for example, may show a 3+ agglutination with specific antisera for C and e; *DCe/DcE*, however, may show only a 1+ reaction.[64]

### Effect of pH

Agglutination reactions are also affected by pH. The ideal pH of a test system is between 6.5 and 7.5. Exceptions to this range include some examples of anti-M and some antibodies of the Pr(Sp₁) group, which show stronger reactivity below pH 6.5.[75]

### Effect of Temperature

Different types of antibodies may exhibit optimal reactivity at different temperatures. IgM antibodies, for example, usually react optimally at or below 22°C. IgG antibodies usually require 37°C temperatures.[61] By manipulating the temperature range, blood bankers are able to enhance detection of clinically significant antibodies (Fig. 3–14).[73]

### Effect of Immunoglobulin Type

IgM antibodies are generally capable of agglutinating red cells suspended in 0.85 percent saline medium.

**Types of Antibodies Reaction Phases**

| | | |
|---|---|---|
| Immediate Spin Phase | A, B, H<br>I<br>M, N<br>Leᵃ, Leᵇ<br>P1 | IgM |
| Antiglobulin Phase (37°C) | D, C, E<br>c,e<br>K, Fy, Jk<br>S, s<br>Leᵃ, Leᵇ | IgG |

**Figure 3–14.** Types of antibodies and reaction phases. (From Kutt, et al,[66] p 10, with permission.)

The IgM antibody is approximately 750 times as efficient as IgG in agglutination reactions.[78] The IgM molecule easily bridges the distance between two red cells because it is 160 Å larger than an IgG molecule.[75] Another factor that contributes to the difference in reactivity between the IgM and IgG molecules is the number of antigen-combining sites on each type of immunoglobulin. Theoretically, the IgM has the potential to bind 10 antigens; however, in reality this rarely happens owing to the size and spacing of antigens in relation to the size and configuration of the IgM molecule. When the IgM molecule attaches to two red cells, for example, probably two or three antigen-combining sites attach to each red cell.[75] An IgG molecule, however, has only two binding sites per molecule, which implies that an IgG molecule would have to bind two red cells with only one binding site on each cell.[75] Of course, agglutination reactions involve more than one immunoglobulin molecule, but this example may be multiplied many times in order to represent its relevance in the agglutination reaction (Fig. 3–15).

Examples of IgM antibodies that have importance in blood banking include those against the ABH, Ii, MN, Lewis (Leᵃ, Leᵇ), Lutheran (Luᵃ), and P blood group antigens. IgG antibodies are those directed as Ss, Kell (Kk, Jsᵃ, Jsᵇ, Kpᵃ, Kpᵇ), Rh (DCEce), Lutheran (Luᵇ), Duffy (Fyᵃ, Fyᵇ), and Kidd (Jkᵃ, Jkᵇ) (see Figure 3–14).

Because of the basic differences in the nature of reactivity between IgM and IgG antibodies, various serologic systems must be used to detect optimally both classes of clinically significant antibodies. An overview of serologic systems traditionally used for antibody detection in the blood bank laboratory may be seen in Table 3–10.

### Effect of Enhancement Media and Potentiators

As stated previously, agglutination reactions for IgM antibodies and their corresponding red cell antigens are easily accomplished in saline medium. Detection of IgM antibodies, however, may not have the same clinical significance as the detection of most IgG antibodies because IgG antibodies, which react at body temperature, 37°C, are the type generally responsible for hemolytic transfusion reactions and hemolytic disease of the newborn. To discover the presence of IgG antibodies, the blood banker normally uses a variety of enhancement techniques (Table 3–11).

Several enhancement media are aimed at reducing the zeta potential of the red cell membrane. The net negative charge surrounding red cells is part of the force that repels red cells from each other. The zeta potential is an expression of the difference in electrostatic potential at the surface of the red cell and the ionic cloud of positive cations that are attracted to the negative charges on the surface (see Figure 3–15).[73,75] Reducing the zeta potential, therefore, should have the desired effect of allowing red cell agglutination by IgG molecules.

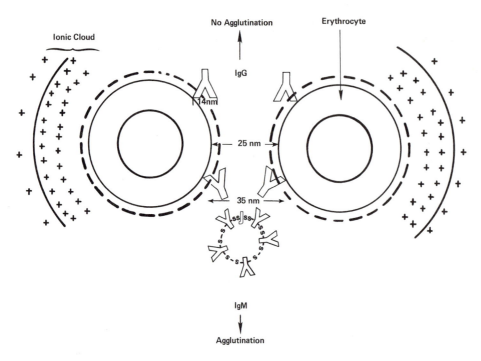

**Figure 3–15.** Schematic representation of the ionic cloud concept and its relevance to hemagglutination induced by IgM and IgG antibodies. Compare the size of the IgG antibody with the IgM molecule. The size of the IgG molecule is not large enough to span the distance between two adjacent red cells.

**Table 3–10.** Serologic Systems Used in Traditional Laboratory Methods for Red Cell Antibody Detection

| Reaction Phase | Ig Class Commonly Detected | Purpose and Mechanism of Reaction | Tests That Use Serologic System | Type of Antibodies Commonly Detected |
|---|---|---|---|---|
| Immediate spin | IgM | IgM antibodies react best at cold temperatures. IgM is an agglutinating antibody that has the ability to easily bridge the distance between red cells. | ABO reverse testing Cross-match Antibody screening/ identification Autocontrol | Expected ABO alloantibodies Unexpected cold-reacting alloantibodies or auto-antibodies |
| 37°C incubation | IgG | IgG antibodies react best at warm temperatures. No visible agglutination commonly seen. IgG is sensitizing antibody with fewer antigen binding sites than IgM and cannot undergo the second stage of agglutination, lattice formation. Complement may be bound during reactivity, which may or may not result in visible hemolysis. | Antibody screening/ identification Cross-match (if needed) Autocontrol | |
| Antiglobulin test (AGT) | IgG | Antihuman globulin (AHG) has specificity for the Fc portion of the heavy chain of the human IgG molecule and/or complement components. AHG acts as a bridge cross-linking red cells sensitized with IgG antibody or complement. | Antibody screening/ identification Cross-match (if needed) Autocontrol Direct antiglobulin test (DAT) | Unexpected warm-reacting alloantibodies or auto-antibodies |

**Table 3–11.** Potentiators

| Reagent | Action | Procedure | Type of Antibody ID |
|---|---|---|---|
| Saline | | 4–22°C (IgM) immediate spin (IS) up to 60 min; 37°C (IgG) for 45–60 min | Primarily IgM; IgG if incubated at 37°C |
| AHG | Cross-links sensitized cells, resulting in visible agglutination | 1. DAT: AHG added directly to washed red cells 2. IAT: serum + screen cells; incubation at 37°C for time determined by additive used; cell washing before addition of AHG | 1. Polyspecific: anti-IgG + anti-complement 2. IgG monospecific: anti-IgG only |
| 22% Albumin* | Causes agglutination by adjusting zeta potential between red cells | Incubation at 37°C for 15–60 min; cell washing prior to indirect anti-globulin test (IAT) | IgG |
| LISS* | Low ionic strength environment causes red cells to take up antibody more rapidly | Incubation at 37°C for 5–15 min; cell washing before IAT | IgG |
| PEG* | Increases test sensitivity; Aggregates red blood cells causing closer proximity of red cells to one another assisting in antibody cross-linking | Incubation at 37°C for 10–30 min; cell washing before IAT NOTE: The test mixture cannot be centrifuged and examined reliably for direct agglutination after 37°C incubation. | IgG |
| Enzymes | Reduces red cell surface charge; Destroys or depresses some red cell antigens; enhances other red cell antigens | 1. One-step: enzymes added directly to serum/red cell mixture 2. Two-step: red cells pretreated with enzymes before addition of serum | Destroys $Fy^a$, $Fy^b$, MNS; enhances reactivity to Rh, Kidd, $P_1$, Lewis, and I antibodies |

*All additives should be added after the IS phase immediately before 37°C incubation.
LISS = low ionic strength solutions; PEG = polyethylene glycol.

**Protein Media.** Various colloidal diluents such as albumin, polyethylene glycol (PEG), polybrene, polyvinylpyrrolidone (PVP), and protamine are used to enhance the agglutination of red cells coated with IgG molecules. These substances may accomplish this enhancement by increasing the dielectric constant (a measure of electrical conductivity), which consequently reduces the zeta potential of the red cell.[73]

**Low Ionic Strength Solution Media.** Low ionic strength solution (LISS) media decrease the ionic strength of a reaction medium and, thus, reduce the zeta potential. With a reduction in zeta potential, there is an increased attraction between positively charged antibody molecules and negatively charged red cells. Low ionic strength solution media generally contain 0.2 percent sodium chloride, and they are often used because they result in an increased rate of antibody uptake during sensitization, with an incubation period of 5 to 15 minutes instead of 30 to 60 minutes, which may be required when using a protein potentiator such as albumin.[73,75,77]

**Polyethylene Glycol and Polybrene.** Polyethylene glycol and polybrene are macromolecule additives used within a LISS to bring sensitized red cells closer to each other in order to assist antibody cross-linking and enhancement of agglutination reactions. Use of these reagents offers some distinct advantages. Polybrene can detect ABO incompatibility as well as clinically significant IgG alloantibodies. The use of PEG produces very specific reactions with reduction in false-positive or nonspecific reactions. Polyethylene glycol is consid-ered to be more effective than albumin, LISS, or manual polybrene for detection of weak antibodies.[74] These reagents have been used in both automated and manual testing systems.

**Enzymes.** The reactions of certain blood group antigens and antibodies are selectively enhanced or suppressed by the use of certain enzymes. Some of the enzymes used in detection and identification of blood group antibodies include ficin (from figs), papain (from papaya), trypsin (from pig stomach), and bromelin (from pineapple). Several theories have been proposed to explain the action of enzymes. One theory proposes that the treatment of red cells with enzymes results in the release of sialic acid from the membrane, subsequent decrease in the negative charges of the red cells, and a reduction of the zeta potential.[73,76] Another theory states that enzyme treatment removes hydrophilic glycoproteins from the membrane of red cells, causing the membrane to become more hydrophobic, thereby allowing the red cells to come closer together. Also, because of removal of glycoproteins from the membrane, antibody molecules may no longer be sterically obstructed from reacting with red cell antigens on the membrane surface.[76] The use of enzymes provides enhanced antibody reactivity to Rh, Kidd, $P_1$, Lewis, and I antigens and destroys or depresses reactivity to red cell antigens $Fy^a$, $Fy^b$, M, N, and S.[77]

**Antihuman Globulin Reagents.** The antihuman globulin (AHG) test is designed to detect red cells coated with antibody or complement, or both. One type of reagent, polyspecific AHG, is used to detect red cells that have been sensitized with IgG antibody or complement components C3b or C3d. Monospecific AHG reagent is used to detect red cells sensitized only with IgG antibody or only with complement.[77] Some AHG reagents are manufactured by injecting animals, usually goats or rabbits, with human globulin. The animals make an antibody response to the foreign human globulin and produce antihuman antibodies to the human globulin components. For the manufacture of polyspecific AHG, both gamma (IgG) and beta (C3b and C3d) globulin components are processed. For monospecific AHG, animals are injected only with IgG and produce antibodies directed against the gamma heavy chain. Monoclonal AHG reagents are also available. Monoclonals are produced by hybridoma technology (see Monoclonal Versus Polyclonal Reagents).

Antihuman globulin reagents act by cross-linking red cells already sensitized with antibody or complement, or both, thus bridging the gap among red cells. The agglutination reaction, therefore, is enhanced by the use of AHG reagents (see Tables 3–10 and 3–11). Refer to Chapter 4 (The Antiglobulin Test) for a more detailed discussion.

### Chemical Reduction of IgG and IgM Molecules

Blood bankers may sometimes discover mixtures of antibodies or the presence of autoantibodies in testing situations in which they must remove or enhance the reactivity of either IgG or IgM antibodies. Dithiothreitol (DTT) and 2 mercaptoethanol (2 ME) are sulfhydryl compounds that break the disulfide bonds of the J chain of the IgM molecule but leave the IgG molecule intact.[79] ZZAP reagent, consisting of a thiol reagent plus a proteolytic enzyme, causes the dissociation of IgG molecules from the surface of sensitized red cells and alters the surface antigens of the red cell.[80]

Chemical reduction of the disulfide bond of the IgG molecule is also used to produce chemically modified reagents that react with red cells in saline.[73,74] Sulfhydryl compounds reduce the disulfide bonds in the hinge region of the IgG molecule, rendering the Fab portions more flexible in facilitating agglutination reactions.[81]

### Monoclonal Versus Polyclonal Reagents

Traditional polyclonal antisera reagents to detect red cell antigens have been produced by immunizing donors and then collecting serum containing antibodies. Antihuman globulin reagents have traditionally been made by injecting animals with human globulin components and then collecting the antihuman antibodies (see Antihuman Globulin Reagents, p 61). Polyclonal reagents, therefore, are directed against multiple epitopes or antigen-binding sites found on the original antigen used to stimulate antibody production in the host animal. Monoclonal reagents, however, are made by hybridoma technology whereby spleen lymphocytes from immunized mice are fused with rapidly pro-

liferating myeloma cells. These hybrid cells, after extensive screening and testing, are selected and cultured to produce lines of immortal cell clones that manufacture a specific antibody directed against only a single epitope. Monoclonal reagents have some distinct advantages over polyclonal reagents. Because monoclonal reagents are produced from immortal clones, no batch variation exists, and high titers of antibodies can be produced. Monoclonal reagents react very specifically and often have higher affinities. For these reasons, monoclonal reagents are not subject to cross-reactivity and interference from nonspecific reactions and may even react strongly with very small quantities of antigen as may be found in subgroups (e.g., subgroups of A).[82,83] Disadvantages of monoclonal antisera include overspecificity, the fact that complement may not be fixed in the antigen-antibody reaction, and problems with sensitivity.[82,84] Some of the disadvantages of monoclonal reagents may be overcome by using blends of different monoclonal reagents or by using polyclonal reagents and monoclonal reagents together.[85] Monoclonal antisera have been used for typing red cell antigens, for AHG testing, and also for phenotyping lymphocyte antigens and HLA typing.

### Nontraditional Laboratory Methods

#### Immunofluorescence Flow Cytometric Techniques

Antibody binding can be visualized by tagging the antibody with a fluorescent dye. Fluorescent testing uses fluorescent dyes such as fluorochrome as markers in immunologic reactions. The fluorescent compound is bound to an antibody molecule. Fluorescence occurs when the compound absorbs light at one wavelength and emits light at a longer wavelength. A red blood cell coated with fluorescent-labeled antibody emits a brightly fluorescent color. The color depends on the fluorochrome dye used.

Both direct and indirect procedures may be used with immunofluorescent antibodies. With direct procedures the specific antibody, called the primary antibody, is directly conjugated with the fluorescent dye and identifies the specific antigen when bound. Indirect procedures involve the use of antihuman serum tagged with fluorescent dye, which is added to an untagged primary antibody bound to a red cell antigen.

The principle of flow cytometry is based on the scattering of light as cells flow in single file through a laser beam. The components of this automated system include a laser for cell illumination, photodetectors for signal detection, and a computer-based management system.[86] Fluorescence is used as an indicator system for the detection of antibody-antigen reactions comparable to hemagglutination. Immunofluorescent antibodies have been used in flow cytometry to quantify fetomaternal hemorrhage, identify transfused cells and follow their survival in recipients, to measure low levels of cell-bound IgG, and to distinguish homozygous from heterozygous expression of blood group antigens.[87] Immunofluorescence flow cytometric techniques are also used in HLA cross-match techniques for transplantation. Refer to Chapter 23 in this text for a detailed discussion.

### Solid-Phase Adherence Test

Solid-phase adherence techniques may be used to detect and to identify both antigens and antibodies. These tests rely on adherence rather than on hemagglutination as an indicator system of antigen-antibody reactions. Polystyrene, polypropylene, or polyvinyl microplate wells may be coated with either antibody or monolayers of cellular material.[88] Solid-phase testing is based on protein or cellular adherence onto a plastic surface by simple passive adsorption. To assist in adsorption, the microplates are chemically pretreated with glutaraldehyde, L-lysine, or a potent serum-specific antibody.[89]

The direct testing procedure consists of reagent antibody of known specificity fixed to the microplate well with the addition of unknown red cells. If an antigen-antibody reaction occurs, the red cells adhere to the sides of the well and the reaction is considered positive. If no antigen-antibody reaction occurs, no adherence occurs and the red cells are free to fall to the bottom of the well. The direct test may be used for red cell typing for specific antigens. The indirect test uses red cells of known antigenic composition bound onto pretreated microplate wells. The test serum is added, incubated, and washed free of unbound serum proteins. IgG-coated indicator cells are then added. As with the direct test, a positive reaction is demonstrated if the IgG-coated cells adhere to the sides of the well, and a negative reaction is determined if the indicator cells settle to the bottom.

### Gel Test

The gel test involves the use of a dextran acrylamide gel contained in a microtube. The microtube is made up of an upper reaction chamber and a gel column with a tapered bottom.[90] The upper reaction chamber is used to test cells, serum (if needed), or both. On centrifugation, the inert gel particles act as a filter to trap red cell agglutinates of different sizes at different levels of the microtube gel column. Larger agglutinates remain at the top of the microtubes with relatively smaller agglutinates filtered out toward lower portions of the column. Unagglutinated cells are driven by centrifugal force to the bottom of the microtube. Neutral gels, specific gels, and antiglobulin gels are available.[90] The gel technique may be used for cell antigen detection and identification, serum antibody detection and identification, and cross-matching.[91]

### Red Cell Affinity-Column Test

The affinity-column test uses immunoreactive gel within a microtube consisting of a mixture of protein G and protein A covalently bonded to beaded agarose gels suspended in a viscous buffer solution. Both protein G and protein A bind specifically to the Fc portion of the IgG molecule. Protein G binds to all four subclasses of human IgG, and protein A to the subclasses IgG1, IgG2, and IgG4, but not to IgG3. Protein G and protein A reactions are comparable to reactions seen with antihuman serum (AHG) and are used in place of AHG in this test system. Serum and cells for testing are mixed and incubated in an area above the gel column. The higher specific gravity of the gel prevents test sample from entering the reaction gel column. On centrifugation, the test mixture passes through the viscous buffer solution, and red cells coated with IgG antibodies adhere to the immunoreactive protein/gel bead. Strong positive reactions produce a band of red cells at the top of the immunoreactive gel column. Other positive reactions produce a band of red cells at the top of the gel column and a button of red cells at the bottom. The thickness of this band of red cells at the top of the gel column is indicative of the strength of the antigen-antibody reactions. Negative reactions result in all the red cells passing through the column and forming a button at the bottom. This IgG binding ability of protein G and protein A gels has been used in red cell affinity chromatography for the detection of IgG antibodies.[92]

## IMMUNE-MEDIATED DISEASES IMPORTANT IN BLOOD BANK TESTING

### Immunodeficiency

Defects in antibody-mediated immunity, cell-mediated immunity, phagocytosis, complement, or other mediator substances may result in immunodeficiency diseases. Immunodeficiencies may be congenital or acquired, may occur secondary to an embryologic abnormality or enzymatic defect, or may be of unknown origin (Table 3–12).[93] Blood bankers need a general knowledge of immunodeficiencies because these disorders may present laboratory and transfusion problems. An individual with a low immunoglobulin level, for example, may have a weak or negative test result for expected serum antibodies in reverse ABO grouping.[94]

### Hypersensitivity

Many immune-mediated diseases with implications for blood banking can be classified as hypersensitivity reactions. Hypersensitivity is an inflammatory response to a foreign antigen and may involve antibody-mediated and cell-mediated reactions or only a cell-mediated reaction. The terms *hypersensitivity* and *allergy* are often used interchangeably, and allergic diseases are often classified according to the mechanisms involved in the response.[95] The Gell and Coombs classification is useful to distinguish between disorders that may be involved with transfusion of blood products and those

**Table 3–12.** Classification of Immunodeficiency Disorders

---

*Antibody (B cell) Immunodeficiency Disorders*
X-linked hypogammaglobulinemia (congenital hypogammaglobulinemia)
Transient hypogammaglobulinemia of infancy
Common, variable, unclassifiable immunodeficiency (acquired by hypogammaglobulinemia)
Immunodeficiency with hyper-IgM
Selective IgA deficiency
Selective IgM deficiency
Selective deficiency of IgG subclasses
Secondary B cell immunodeficiency associated with drugs, protein-losing states
X-linked lymphoproliferative disease

*Cellular (T cell) Immunodeficiency Disorders*
Congenital thymic aplasia (DiGeorge syndrome)
Chronic mucocutaneous candidiasis (with or without endocrinopathy)
T cell deficiency associated with purine nucleoside phosphorylase deficiency
T cell deficiency associated with absent membrane glycoprotein
T cell deficiency associated with absent class I or II MHC antigens or both (base lymphocyte syndrome)

*Combined Antibody-mediated (B cell) and Cell-mediated (T cell) Immunodeficiency Disorders*
Severe combined immunodeficiency disease (autosomal recessive, X-linked, sporadic)
Cellular immunodeficiency with abnormal immunoglobulin synthesis (Nezelof syndrome)
Immunodeficiency with ataxia-telangiectasia
Immunodeficiency with eczema and thrombocytopenia (Wiskott-Aldrich syndrome)
Immunodeficiency with thymoma
Immunodeficiency with short-limbed dwarfism
Immunodeficiency with adenosine deaminase deficiency
Immunodeficiency with nucleoside phosphorylase deficiency
Biotin-dependent multiple carboxylase deficiency
Graft-versus-host disease
Acquired immunodeficiency syndrome

*Phagocytic Dysfunction*
Chronic granulomatous disease
Glucose-6-phosphate dehydrogenase deficiency
Myeloperoxidase deficiency
Chédiak-Higashi syndrome
Job's syndrome
Tuftsin deficiency
Lazy leukocyte syndrome
Elevated IgE, defective chemotaxis, and recurrent infections

---

**Source:** Ammann,[93] p 319, with permission.

that may influence laboratory testing. A type I reaction, also known as anaphylactic or immediate hypersensitivity, involves mast cells or basophils with surface IgE antibody that cross-links allergen and causes release of histamine and other mediators responsible for the allergic reactions associated with the manifestation of the disease. IgA-deficient individuals, for example, who receive plasma products containing IgA may have an anaphylactic reaction to those products. Urticarial reactions may also result from transfusion and may be a response to a substance in donor plasma, such as drugs or certain food allergens.[96,97]

A type II reaction involves IgG or IgM antibody and complement, phagocytic cells, and proteolytic enzymes. Hemolytic disease of the newborn, transfusion reactions caused by blood group antibodies, and autoimmune hemolytic reactions are examples of type II reactions (see Autoimmune Disease and Hemolytic Disease of the Newborn).

Type III reactions also involve IgG and IgM antibodies, complement, and phagocytic cells. The main feature of this type of tissue-damaging reaction is the formation of immune complexes: aggregations of antibody, antigen, polymorphonuclear neutrophils (PMNs), and complement. Drug-induced antibodies, such as those to penicillin, may form complexes and eventually lead to hemolytic reactions.[98]

The type IV reaction is a T-cell-mediated response involving only T cells and their related cytokines. Antibody and complement are not involved in this reaction.[99] Graft-versus-host reaction is the primary clinical example of a type IV reaction that has significance for blood bankers. Transfusion of viable lymphocytes to an immune-suppressed recipient may result in the attack of those transfused lymphocytes against the recipient.

## Monoclonal and Polyclonal Gammopathies

Plasma cell neoplasms result in proliferation of abnormal immunoglobulin that is a product of a single clone of B cells (as monoclonal gammopathies) or of multiple clones (as in polyclonal gammopathies).[100] The proliferation may be of a specific antibody class or only of a light or heavy chain. The increased amounts of immunoglobulin lead to increased viscosity of serum. This situation may present special testing problems for blood bankers. The increased concentrations of serum proteins cause nonspecific aggregation of RBCs. Rouleaux, or stacking of red cells like coins, may result from serum of individuals who have disorders such as multiple myeloma.[101] In some testing situations, special procedures such as saline replacement may be needed to distinguish true cell agglutination from nonspecific aggregation caused by the presence of increased concentrations of abnormal immunoglobulins.

## Autoimmune Disease

Autoantibodies are antibodies produced against an individual's own cells and tissues. Many theories have been proposed to explain why this breakdown occurs in the normal immune response and why pathologic conditions develop. Cross-reactivity of the immune response between body tissues and foreign antigens, disturbance of the anti-idiotypic network, loss of self-tolerance, and aberrant presentation of antigen through MHC markers are among the theories for development of autoimmunity.[102] From a laboratory testing perspective, the autoimmune conditions that have the most significance for blood bankers are the autoimmune hemolytic anemias. These diseases may produce antibodies that cause red cell destruction and resultant anemia and also cause difficulties in red cell antigen testing because of antibody- or complement-coated red cells. A direct antiglobulin test (DAT) using polyspecific antihuman serum with both anti-IgG and anti-C3d is used to detect coated cells. Special procedures such as elutions or chemical treatment to remove antibody may be needed to prepare cells for antigen typing. Unbound serum autoantibodies may interfere with alloantibody detection and compatibility testing. In this situation, procedures such as adsorptions or chemical treatment to denature immunoglobulins may need to be performed to remove autoantibodies from serum and cells so that they do not interfere with the testing for clinically significant antibodies.

## Hemolytic Disease of the Newborn

Immunoglobulins that can cross the placenta are responsible for conferring maternal immunity upon the fetus. In most situations this process is important to protect the fetus and, after birth, the newborn infant until approximately 6 months of age, at which time infants begin to produce their own antibodies. Hemolytic disease of the newborn (HDN) occurs when maternal antibody is directed toward foreign antigen on fetal red cells. If the mother is exposed to fetal red cells as a result of fetomaternal transfer of red cells during pregnancy or childbirth, then she will mount an immune response against those red cell antigens. Memory cells of this encounter will be stored in lymphatic organs. A subsequent pregnancy with a second exposure to the same red cell antigens will result in the production of fetal red cell antigen-specific antibodies. $IgG_1$, $IgG_3$, and $IgG_4$ are capable of crossing the placenta and attaching to fetal red cells.[103] Severe HDN, often requiring exchange transfusion, has been associated with $IgG_1$ antibodies more frequently than with antibodies of other subgroups, such as $IgG_3$.[39] Transplacental antibodies may be focused on antigens A and B of the ABO system, antigens of the Rh system, or other blood group antigens such as those in the Kell system.

## SUMMARY

The immune response consists of an intricate system of many factors including tissues, organs, cells, and biologic mediators that act to defend an organism against intrusion by a foreign substance. The response functions under the genetic control of the HLA system to recognize and to react to an immune stimulus. Immunoglobulins have special significance for blood bankers because blood bank testing is focused primarily on the prevention, detection, and identification of blood group antibodies. The complement system is important because of its interaction with the antibody response and the in vivo and in vitro effects of complement activation and resultant red cell destruction. Blood bankers need to know the antigen characteristics and host factors that have an impact on the immune response to enable them to evaluate and to solve testing problems. An immunologic viewpoint is essential to understand the factors that affect agglutination reactions between red cells and red cell antibodies, especially in test media selection and testing conditions. Finally, to comprehend the consequences of certain immune-mediated disease conditions and their influences on blood bank testing, the blood banker should possess a basic knowledge of these disorders.

# SUMMARY CHART: IMPORTANT POINTS TO REMEMBER (MT/MLT)

n The role of the immune system is:
  • Protection from foreign substances
  • Destruction of the host's own abnormal cells
n The basic mechanism used by the immune system is:
  • Recognition of foreign or abnormal cells
  • Response by destruction and/or elimination
n The acquired immune system demonstrates:
  • Diversity: individual lymphocytes in the overall population possess membrane molecules of unique configuration different from the shape of comparable molecules on other cells in the same population
  • Recognition: lymphocytes possess the capability to differentiate self molecules from nonself molecules
  • Specificity: ability of antibody to recognize and to bind only to the uniquely shaped molecular structure of the antigen
  • Memory: ability to remember the infectious antigen and to enhance the immune response
n There are two populations of lymphocytes: T lymphocytes and B lymphocytes.
  • T lymphocytes: distinguished from B cells by their ability to bind sheep erythrocytes (called the CD2 marker). The definitive T-cell marker is the T-cell antigen receptor (TCR) usually identified with the CD3 complex. T cells require antigen-presenting cells (APCs) to respond to antigens. There are two subpopulations of T lymphocytes distinguished by other major CD markers.
    —$T_H$: T helper cells:
      —carry the CD4 marker
      —are necessary to induce T or B lymphocytes to begin an immune response
      —release lymphokines which help regulate the immune response
      —recognize specific antigens in association with MHC class II molecules
    —$T_C$: T cytotoxic cells:
      —carry the CD8 marker
      —are able to kill specific target cells without the help of antibody
      —recognize specific antigens in association with MHC class I molecules
  • B lymphocytes: make up about 5 to 15% of circulating lymphoid pool and are characterized by their surface immunoglobulins. The surface markers are manufactured by the B cells themselves and are inserted into their surface membrane, where they act as specific antigen receptors.
    —Differentiate into plasma cells to secrete humoral antibody
    —Require the help of T lymphocytes for optimal antibody production and for immunologic memory
      —A single B cell produces a clone that manufactures antibody of a single specificity
n The primary immune response occurs after the first exposure to a foreign antigen. The secondary response or anamnestic response is seen after a secondary exposure with the same specific antigen.
n Complement consists of a group of serum proteins that activate each other in a sequential order to form products that are involved in immune adherence phagocytosis and cell lysis. Complement can be activated through two pathways:
  • The classical pathway initiated by antigen-antibody complexes requires C1q for activation.
  • The alternative pathway activated by the cell walls of some bacteria, fungi, parasites, and tumor cells requires $C\overline{3b}$, serum factors B, D, properdin, and initiating factor.
n There are 5 classes of immunoglobulins, which have a basic four-chain protein structure, consisting of two identical light (L) and two identical heavy (H) chains. Disulfide bonds link each light chain to a heavy chain, and the two heavy chains are linked to each other.
  • Sequence differences between antibody molecules may be isotypic, allotypic, or idiotypic.
  • The N-terminal domains of both H and L chains are the variable (V) regions that make up the combining site of the antibody and vary according to the specificity of the antibody.
n The immune reaction is determined by host response as well as characteristics of the foreign substance. Factors such as size, complexity, conformation, charge, assessability, and chemical composition influence the amount and type of immune response. Blood group antigens may be proteins, glycolipids, or glycoproteins. Not all blood group substances are equally immunogenic in vivo.
n Blood group antibodies may be characterized by such factors as epitope diversity (monoclonal or polyclonal), mode of sensitization (naturally occurring or immune), expected or unexpected presence in routine serum samples, class (IgM or IgG), activity (warm or cold reactive, agglutinating or sensitizing), clinical significance, specificity including alloantibody or autoantibody specificity and chemical reactivity (influence of enzymes, activity with variations in pH, activity with DTT or 2-ME reagents, etc.).
n Red cell antigen-antibody reactions are most commonly detected by hemagglutination procedures. Hemagglutination occurs in two stages: sensitization and lattice formation. A number of traditional and nontraditional methods may be used to detect and identify serum antibodies and red cell antigenic composition.

## REVIEW QUESTIONS

1. Characteristics of the acquired immune system include:
   A. Immediately available defense mechanism
   B. The inflammatory response
   C. Production of antibody
   D. Mechanism does not alter on repeated exposure to the same foreign antigen

2. Substances that help in the regulation and duration of the immune response are called:
   A. Haptens
   B. Opsonins
   C. Cytokines
   D. Lysozymes

3. Which cell is identified primarily by the presence of immunoglobulin on its surface?
   A. $T_H$ cell
   B. NK cell
   C. B cell
   D. Macrophage

4. Which cell functions primarily in antigen processing and presentation?
   A. $T_C$ cell
   B. Macrophage
   C. Plasma cell
   D. NK cell

5. Which of the following is a signal for the expression of IL-2 receptors on a $T_H$ cell?
   A. Antigen internalized by a B cell in a T-independent process
   B. Presentation of antigen by a monocyte to a $T_H$ cell
   C. Binding of immunoglobulin on surface of a macrophage
   D. Cross-linking of antigen on surface of a mast cell

6. Which class(es) of HLA marker(s) is (are) important in immune recognition of antigen in cell-to-cell interactions?
   A. Class II
   B. Class I
   C. Class III
   D. Class I and Class II

7. Which immunoglobulin class would be most important in the study of immune-mediated transfusion reactions due to the presence of alloantibodies?
   A. IgA
   B. IgM
   C. IgE
   D. IgG

8. Which immunoglobulins can activate the classic pathway of the complement systems?
   A. IgA and IgM
   B. IgG (all subgroups) and IgA
   C. IgG1, IgG2, IgG3, and IgM
   D. IgE and IgD

9. Which complement factor is common to both classic and alternative pathways?
   A. Factor B
   B. Factor C3
   C. Factor C1
   D. Factor C4

10. Which of the following patient samples for blood bank testing is *most likely* to contain complement?
    A. EDTA-anticoagulated sample
    B. Heparin-anticoagulated sample
    C. Serum sample stored at 4°C for 72 hours
    D. Serum sample drawn 2 hours ago

11. Which of the following statements is true concerning the formation of antibodies to blood group antigens?
    A. All blood group antigens are equally immunogenic.
    B. Only ABO and Rh blood group antigens are immunogenic.
    C. Antibodies may form to any foreign blood group antigen, but usually only ABO and Rh antibodies form in clinically significant numbers.
    D. Any blood group antigen may elicit an immune response, but only 50 percent of blood recipients will respond with antibody formation.

12. Antibody idiotype is determined by the:
    A. Constant region of heavy chain
    B. Constant region of light chain
    C. Constant regions of heavy and light chains
    D. Variable regions of heavy and light chains

13. Which antibody is produced rapidly and in highest amounts during secondary response?
    A. IgG
    B. IgM
    C. IgA
    D. Both IgM and IgG are produced rapidly and in equal amounts.

14. Which of the following is *most likely* to account for the failure of a visible red cell antigen-antibody reaction?
    A. Homozygous expression of antigen on red cell
    B. pH of 7.1
    C. Incubation at 37°C for suspected IgG antibody
    D. Excess antibody (prozone effect)

15. What is the main advantage of LISS media over other types of enhancement media?
    A. Has rapid antibody uptake
    B. Has increased saturation of antibody molecules
    C. May be used for either manual or automated systems
    D. Selectively enhances or suppresses certain blood group antigen-antibody reactions

16. What is the action of AHG reagent?
    A. Reduces the zeta potential of the red cell, allowing closer approach of red cells
    B. Cross-links red cells that have become sensitized with antibody or complement
    C. Renders the red cell membrane more hydrophobic, allowing red cells to come closer together
    D. Releases sialic acid from the red cell membrane, thereby decreasing negative charges between cells

17. Monoclonal antibodies:
    A. Have specificity for a single epitope
    B. May be manufactured using hybridoma technology
    C. Develop from a single B-cell clone
    D. All of the above

18. A blood cell product is irradiated to prevent the transfusion of viable lymphocytes to an immunocompromised patient. What type of reaction is prevented by this action?
    A. Type I, anaphylactic shock
    B. Type II, transfusion reaction
    C. Type III, immune complex formation
    D. Type IV, graft-versus-host reaction

19. From a blood bank testing perspective, what is the main problem with a patient having an autoimmune hemolytic anemia?
    A. Large amounts of excess protein may coat red cells.
    B. Autoantibodies are formed rapidly and to many blood group determinants.
    C. Autoantibodies may interfere with the detection of clinically significant alloantibodies.
    D. Rouleaux of red cells make antigen typing difficult.

20. Which IgG subclass is most efficient at crossing the placenta?
    A. IgG1
    B. IgG2
    C. IgG3
    D. IgG4

## ANSWERS TO REVIEW QUESTIONS

1. C (p 41)
2. C (p 39)
3. C (p 41)
4. B (p 43)
5. B (p 45)
6. A (pp 45–46)
7. D (p 50)
8. C (p 52)
9. B (pp 52–53)
10. D (p 54)
11. C (pp 55, 57)
12. D (p 51)
13. A (pp 42–43)
14. D (p 58)
15. A (p 61)
16. B (p 62)
17. D (p 62)
18. D (p 64)
19. C (p 65)
20. A (p 50)

## REFERENCES

1. Male, D, and Roitt, I: Introduction to the immune system. In Roitt, I, Brostoff, J, and Male, D (eds): Immunology, ed 4. Mosby, London, 1996, p. 1.2.
2. Kuby, J: Immunology. W. H. Freeman and Co, New York, 1992, p 50.
3. Benjamini, E, Sunshine, G, and Leskowitz, S: Immunology: A Short Course, ed 3. Wiley-Liss, New York, 1996, p 24.
4. Male, D, and Roitt, I: Introduction to the immune system. In Roitt, I, Brostoff, J, and Male, D: Immunology, ed 4. Mosby, London, 1996, p 1.6.
5. Turgeon, ML: Fundamentals of Immunohematology, ed 2. Williams & Wilkins, Philadelphia, 1995, p 5.
6. Kuby, J: Immunology. W. H. Freeman and Co, New York, 1992, p 9.
7. Rook, G: Cell mediated immune reactions. In Roitt, I, Brostoff, J, and Male, D: Immunology, ed 4. Mosby, London, 1996, p 9.1.
8. Benjamini, E, Sunshine, G, and Leskowitz, S: Immunology: A Short Course, ed 3. Wiley-Liss, New York, 1996, p 199.
9. Benjamini, E, Sunshine, G, and Leskowitz, S: Immunology: A Short Course, ed 3. Wiley-Liss, New York, 1996, p 156.
10. Lydyard, P, and Grossi, C: Cells involved in the immune response. In Roitt, I, Brostoff, J, and Male, D: Immunology, ed 4. Mosby, London, 1996, pp 2.1–2.18.
11. Goodman, JW: The immune response. In Stites, DP, and Terr, AI: Basic and Clinical Immunology, ed 7. Appleton & Lange, Norwalk, CT, 1991, pp 40–41.
12. Kamani, NR, and Douglas, SD: Structure and development of the immune system. In Stites, DP, and Terr, AI: Basic and Clinical Immunology, ed 7. Appleton & Lange, Norwalk, CT, 1991, p 16.
13. Goodman, JW: The immune response. In Stites, DP, and Terr, AI: Basic and Clinical Immunology, ed 7. Appleton & Lange, Norwalk, CT, 1991, p 34.
14. Male, D, and Roitt, I: Introduction to the immune system. In Roitt, I, Brostoff, J, and Male, D: Immunology, ed 4. Mosby, London, 1996, pp 1.1–1.3.
15. Kamani, NR, and Douglas, SD: Structure and development of the immune system. In Stites, DP, and Terr, AI: Basic and Clinical Immunology, ed 7. Appleton & Lange, Norwalk, CT, 1991, p 24.
16. Waytes, AT, et al: Preligation of CR1 enhances IgG-dependent phagocytosis by cultured human monocytes. J Immunol 146:2694, 1991.
17. Kamani, NR, and Douglas, SD: Structure and development of the immune system. In Stites, DP, and Terr, AI: Basic and Clinical Immunology, ed 7. Appleton & Lange, Norwalk, CT, 1991, p 21.

18. Lydyard, P, and Grossi, C: Cells involved in the immune response. In Roitt, I, Brostoff, J, and Male, D: Immunology, ed 4. Mosby, London, 1996, pp 2.14–2.18.
19. Goverman, J, and Parnes, JR: The T cell receptor. In Stites, DP, and Terr, AI: Basic and Clinical Immunology, ed 7. Appleton & Lange, Norwalk, CT, 1991, pp 73–77.
20. Lanier, L: Cells of the immune response: Lymphocytes and mononuclear phagocytes. In Stites, DP, and Terr, AI: Basic and Clinical Immunology, ed 7. Appleton & Lange, Norwalk, CT, 1991, p 65.
21. Lanier, L: Cells of the immune response: Lymphocytes and mononuclear phagocytes. In Stites, DP, and Terr, AI: Basic and Clinical Immunology, ed 7. Appleton & Lange, Norwalk, CT, 1991, p 68–70.
22. Oppenheim, JJ, Ruscetti, FW, and Faltynek, C: Cytokines. In Stites, DP, and Terr, AI: Basic and Clinical Immunology, ed 7. Appleton & Lange, Norwalk, CT, 1991, pp 78–79.
23. Feldman, M: Cell cooperation in the antibody response. In Roitt, I, Brostoff, J, and Male, D: Immunology, ed 4. Mosby, London, 1996, pp 8.8–8.11.
24. Cooke, A: Regulation of the immune response. In Roitt, I, Brostoff, J, and Male, D: Immunology, ed 4. Mosby, London, 1996, pp 2.14–2.18.
25. Vengelen-Tyler, V: AABB Technical Manual, ed 12. American Association of Blood Banks, Arlington, VA, 1996, p 189.
26. Benjamini, E, Sunshine, G, and Leskowitz, S: Immunology: A Short Course, ed 3. Wiley-Liss, New York, 1996, pp 93–106.
27. Bryant, NJ: Laboratory Immunology and Serology, ed 3. WB Saunders, Philadelphia, 1992, pp 68–69.
28. Owen, M: T-cell receptors and MHC molecules. In Roitt, I, Brostoff, J, and Male, D: Immunology, ed 4. Mosby, London, 1996, p 5.3.
29. Swam, BD: The human major histocompatibility human leukocyte antigen (HLA) complex. In Stites, DP, and Terr, AI: Basic and Clinical Immunology, ed 7. Appleton & Lange, Norwalk, CT, 1991, p 49.
30. Oppenheim, JJ, Ruscetti, FW, and Faltynek, C: Cytokines. In Stites, DP, and Terr, AI: Basic and Clinical Immunology, ed 7. Appleton & Lange, Norwalk, CT, 1991, p 84.
31. Issitt, PD, and Anstee, DJ: Applied Blood Group Serology, ed 4. Montgomery Scientific, Durham, NC, 1998, p 11.
32. Oppenheim, JJ, Ruscetti, FW, and Faltynek, C: Cytokines. In Stites, DP, and Terr, AI: Basic and Clinical Immunology, ed 7. Appleton & Lange, Norwalk, CT, 1991, p 99.
33. Elliott, MJ, et al: Inhibition of human monocyte adhesion by interleukin 4. Blood 77:2739, 1991.
34. Roitt, I: Essential Immunology, ed 7. Blackwell Scientific, Oxford, 1991, pp 155–157.
35. Goodman, JW: The immune response. In Stites, DP, and Terr, AI: Basic and Clinical Immunology, ed 7. Appleton & Lange, Norwalk, CT, 1991, pp 35–44.
36. Goodman, JW: Immunoglobulin structure and function. In Stites, DP, and Terr, AI: Basic and Clinical Immunology, ed 7. Appleton & Lange, Norwalk, CT, 1991, p 109.
37. Bryant, NJ: Laboratory Immunology and Serology, ed 3. WB Saunders, Philadelphia, 1992, p 72.
38. Goodman, JW: Immunoglobulin structure and function. In Stites, DP, and Terr, AL: Basic and Clinical Immunology, ed 7. Appleton & Lange, Norwalk, CT, 1991, pp 109–118.
39. Nance, SJ, Arndt, PA, and Garratty, G: Correlation of IgG subclass with the severity of hemolytic disease of the newborn. Transfusion 30:381, 1990.
40. Goodman, JW: Immunoglobulin structure and function. In Stites, DP, and Terr, AI: Basic and Clinical Immunology, ed 7. Appleton & Lange, Norwalk, CT, 1991, p 117.
41. Rieben, R, et al: Antibodies to histo-blood group substances A and B: Agglutination titers, Ig class, and IgG subclasses in healthy persons of different age categories. Transfusion 31:607, 1991.
42. Sokol, RJ, et al: Red cell autoantibodies, multiple immunoglobulin classes, and autoimmune hemolysis. Transfusion 30:714, 1990.
43. Vengelen-Tyler, V: AABB Technical Manual, ed 12. American Association of Blood Banks, Arlington, VA, 1996, pp 548–549.
44. Kerr, WG, Hendershot, LM, and Burrows, PD: Regulation of IgM and IgD expression in human B-lineage cells. J Immunol 146:3314, 1991.
45. Hay, F: The generation of diversity. In Roitt, I, Brostoff, J, and Male, D: Immunology, ed 4. Mosby, St. Louis, 1996, p 6.3.
46. Zaleski, MB, et al: Allotopy of Immunoglobulins, Immunogenetics. Pitman, Marshfield, MA, 1983, p 171.
47. Goodman, JW: Immunoglobulin structure and function. In Stites, DP, and Terr, Al: Basic and Clinical Immunology, ed 7. Appleton & Lange, Norwalk, CT, 1991, p 115.
48. Mollison, PL: Red cell antigens and antibodies and their interactions. In Blood Transfusion in Clinical Medicine, ed 9. Blackwell Scientific, London, 1993, pp 132–134.
49. Frank, MM: Complement and kinin. In Stites, DP, and Terr, AI: Basic and Clinical Immunology, ed 7. Appleton & Lange, Norwalk, CT, 1991, p 161.
50. Walport, M: Complement. In Roitt, I, Brostoff, J, and Male, D: Immunology, ed 4. Mosby, St Louis, 1996, p 13.12.
51. Bryant, NJ: Laboratory Immunology and Serology, ed 3. WB Saunders, Philadelphia, 1992, p 47.
52. Frank, MM: Complement and kinin. In Stites, DP, and Terr, AI: Basic and Clinical Immunology, ed 7. Appleton & Lange, Norwalk, CT, 1991, pp 167–169.
53. Frank, MM: Complement and kinin. In Stites, DP, and Terr, AI: Basic and Clinical Immunology, ed 7. Appleton & Lange, Norwalk, CT, 1991, p 166.
54. Wiler, M: The Rh blood group system. In Harmening, D: Modern Blood Banking and Transfusion Practices, ed 3. FA Davis, Philadelphia, 1994, p 126.
55. Mollison, PL: ABO, Lewis, li, and P groups. In Blood Transfusion in Clinical Medicine, ed 9. Blackwell Scientific Oxford, 1993, pp 183–184.
56. Larison, PJ, and Cook, LO: Adverse effects of blood transfusion. In Harmening, D: Modern Blood Banking and Transfusion Practices, ed 2. FA Davis, Philadelphia, 1994, p 354.
57. Moulds, JM, et al: The C3b/C4b receptor is recognized by the Knops, McCoy, Swain-Langley, and York blood group antisera. J Exp Med 173:1159, 1991.
58. Rao, N, et al: Identification of human erythrocyte blood group antigens on the C3b/C4b receptor. J Immunol 146:3502, 1991.
59. Bryant, NJ: Laboratory Immunology and Serology, ed 3. WB Saunders, Philadelphia, 1992, p 55.
60. Schleuning, M, et al: Complement activation during storage of blood under normal blood bank conditions: Effects of proteinase inhibitors and leukocyte depletion. Blood 79:3071, 1992.
61. Goodman, JW: Immunogenicity and antigenic specificity. In Stites, DP, and Terr, AI: Basic and Clinical Immunology, ed 7. Appleton & Lange, Norwalk, CT, 1991, p 101.
62. Issitt, PD: Applied Blood Group Serology, ed 3. Montgomery Scientific, Miami, 1985, p 224.
63. Kuby, J: Immunology. WH Freeman & Co, New York, 1992, p 141.
64. Vengelen-Tyler, V: AABB Technical Manual, ed 12. American Association of Blood Banks, Arlington, VA, 1996, p 204.
65. Mollison, PL: ABO, Lewis, li, and P groups. In Blood Transfusion in Clinical Medicine, ed 9. Blackwell Scientific, London, 1993, pp 100–102.
66. Mollison, PL: ABO, Lewis, li, and P groups. In Blood Transfusion in Clinical Medicine, ed 9. Blackwell Scientific, Oxford, 1993, pp 110–113.
67. Roitt, I: Essential Immunology, ed 8. Blackwell Scientific, Oxford, 1994, pp 85–92.
68. Turgeon, ML: Fundamentals of Immunohematology. Williams & Wilkins, Philadelphia, 1995, pp 135, 137, 156.
69. Roitt, I: Essential Immunology, ed 8. Blackwell Scientific, Oxford, 1994, pp 212–213.
70. Vengelen-Tyler, V: AABB Technical Manual, ed 12. American Association of Blood Banks, Arlington, VA, 1996, p 539–540.
71. Miller, J: Immunological tolerance. In Roitt, I, Brostoff, J, and Male, D: Immunology, ed 4. Mosby, London, 1996, p 12.1.
72. Vengelen-Tyler, V: AABB Technical Manual, ed 12. American Association of Blood Banks, Arlington, VA, 1996, pp 224–225.

73. Vengelen-Tyler, V: AABB Technical Manual, ed 12. American Association of Blood Banks, Arlington, VA, 1996, pp 214–216.

74. Turgeon, ML: Fundamentals of Immunohematology. Williams & Wilkins, Baltimore, 1995, p 73.

75. Issitt, PD, and Anstee, DJ: Applied Blood Group Serology, ed 3. Montgomery Scientific, Durham, NC, 1998, pp 34–35.

76. Issitt, PD, and Anstee, DJ: Applied Blood Group Serology, ed 3. Montgomery Scientific, Durham, NC, 1998, p 37.

77. Kurt, SM, et al: Rh Blood Group System Antigens, Antibodies, Nomenclature, and Testing. Ortho Diagnostic Systems, Raritan, NJ, 1990, pp 13–14.

78. Stites, DP, and Rodgers, RP: Clinical laboratory methods for detection of antigens and antibodies. In Stites, DP, and Terr, AI: Basic and Clinical Immunology, ed 7. Appleton & Lange, Norwalk, CT, 1991, p 253.

79. Mollison, PL: ABO, Lewis, li, and P groups. In Blood Transfusion in Clinical Medicine, ed 9. Blackwell Scientific, London, 1993, pp 99–100.

80. Vengelen-Tyler, VV: AABB Technical Manual, ed 12, American Association of Blood Banks, Arlington, VA, 1996, pp 666–667.

81. Issitt, PD, and Anstee, DJ: Applied Blood Group Serology, ed 3. Montgomery Scientific, Durham, NC, 1998, p 68.

82. Hybridomas and Monoclonal Antibodies. Bioeducational Pub, Rochester, NY, 1982, p 19.

83. Lau, P, et al: Group A variants defined with a monoclonal anti-A reagent. Transfusion 30:142, 1990.

84. Turgeon, ML: Fundamentals of Immunohematology. Williams & Wilkins, Baltimore, 1995, pp 68–69.

85. Vengelen-Tyler, V: AABB Technical Manual, ed 12. American Association of Blood Banks, Arlington, VA, 1996, pp 204–205.

86. Stevens, CD: Clinical Immunology and Serology. FA Davis, Philadelphia, 1996, p 37.

87. Vengelen-Tyler, V: AABB Technical Manual, ed 12. American Association of Blood Banks, Arlington, VA, 1996, p 224.

88. Turgeon, ML: Fundamentals of Immunohematology. Williams & Wilkins, Baltimore, 1995, p 397.

89. Vengelen-Tyler, V: AABB Technical Manual, ed 12. American Association of Blood Banks, Arlington, VA, 1996, p 225.

90. Turgeon, ML: Fundamentals of Immunohematology. Williams & Wilkins, Baltimore, 1995, p 396.

91. Vengelen-Tyler, V: AABB Technical Manual, ed 12. American Association of Blood Banks, Arlington, VA, 1996, p 227.

92. Frame, T: Personal communication, August, 1997.

93. Ammann, AJ: Mechanisms of immunodeficiency. In Stites, DP, and Terr, AI: Basic and Clinical Immunology, ed 7. Appleton & Lange, Norwalk, CT, 1991, p 319.

94. Vengelen-Tyler, V: AABB Technical Manual, ed 12. American Association of Blood Banks, Arlington, VA, 1996, p 241.

95. Terr, AI: Mechanisms of hypersensitivity. In Stites, DP, and Terr, AI: Basic and Clinical Immunology, ed 7. Appleton & Lange, Norwalk, CT, 1991, p 367.

96. Vengelen-Tyler, V: AABB Technical Manual, ed 12. American Association of Blood Banks, Arlington, VA, 1996, pp 548–549.

97. Turgeon, ML: Fundamentals of Immunohematology. Williams & Wilkins, Baltimore, 1995, p 286.

98. Roitt, I: Essential Immunology, ed 8. Blackwell Scientific, Oxford, 1994, p 325–326.

99. Bryant, NJ: Laboratory Immunology and Serology, ed 3. WB Saunders, Philadelphia, 1992, p 78.

100. Parker, JW, and Lukes, RJ: Neoplasms of the immune system. In Stites, DP, and Terr, AI: Basic and Clinical Immunology, ed 7. Appleton & Lange, Norwalk, CT, 1991, p 617.

101. Vengelen-Tyler, V: AABB Technical Manual, ed 12. American Association of Blood Banks, Arlington, VA, 1996, p 636.

102. Steinberg, AD: Mechanisms of disordered immune regulation. In Stites, DP, and Terr, AI: Basic and Clinical Immunology, ed 7. Appleton & Lange, Norwalk, CT, 1991, p 432–437.

103. Goodman, JW: Immunoglobulin structure and function. In Stites, DP, and Terr, AI: Basic and Clinical Immunology, ed 7. Appleton & Lange, Norwalk, CT, 1991, p 117.

## BIBLIOGRAPHY

Benjamini, E, Sunshine, G, and Leskowitz, S: Immunology: A Short Course, ed 3. Wiley-Liss, New York, 1996.

Bryant, NJ: Laboratory Immunology and Serology, ed 3. WB Saunders, Philadelphia, 1992.

Elliott, MJ, et al: Inhibition of human monocyte adhesion by interleukin 4. Blood 77:2739, 1991.

Hybridomas and Monoclonal Antibodies. Bioeducational Pub, Rochester, NY, 1982.

Issitt, PD, and Anstee, DJ: Applied Blood Group Serology, ed 3. Montgomery Scientific, Durham, NC, 1998.

Kerr, WG, Hendershot, LM, and Burrows, PD: Regulation of IgM and IgD expression in human B-lineage cells. J Immunol 146:3314, 1991.

Kuby, J: Immunology. WH Freeman & Co, New York, 1992.

Kutt, SM, et al: Rh Blood Group System Antigens, Antibodies, Nomenclature and Testing. Ortho Diagnostic Systems, Raritan, NJ, 1990.

Lau, P, et al: Group A variants defined with a monoclonal anti-A reagent. Transfusion 30:142, 1990.

Mollison, PL: Blood Transfusion in Clinical Medicine, ed 9. Blackwell Scientific, London, 1993.

Moulds, JM, et al: The C3b/C4b receptor is recognized by the Knops, McCoy, Swain-Langley, and York blood group antisera. J Exp Med 173:1159, 1991.

Nance, SJ, Arndt, PA, and Garratty, G: Correlation of IgG subclass with the severity of hemolytic disease of the newborn. Transfusion 30:381, 1990.

Rao, N, et al: Identification of human erythrocyte blood group antigens on the C3b/C4b receptor. J Immunol 146:3502, 1991.

Rieben, R, et al: Antibodies to histo-blood group substances A and B: Agglutination titers, Ig class, and IgG subclasses in healthy persons of different age categories. Transfusion 31:607, 1991.

Roitt, I: Essential Immunology, ed 8. Blackwell Scientific, Oxford, 1994.

Roitt, I, Brostoff, J, and Male, D: Immunology, ed 4. Mosby, London, 1996.

Schleuning, M, et al: Complement activation during storage of blood under normal blood bank conditions: Effects of proteinase inhibitors and leukocyte depletion. Blood 79:3071, 1992.

Sokol, RJ, et al: Red cell autoantibodies, multiple immunoglobulin classes, and autoimmune hemolysis. Transfusion 30:714, 1990.

Stevens, CD: Clinical Immunology and Serology. FA Davis, Philadelphia, 1996.

Stites, DP, and Terr, AI: Basic and Clinical Immunology, ed 7. Appleton & Lange, Norwalk, CT, 1991.

Turgeon, ML: Fundamentals of Immunohematology. Williams & Wilkins, Baltimore, 1995.

Vengelen-Tyler, V: AABB Technical Manual, ed 12. American Association of Blood Banks, Arlington, VA, 1996.

Waytes, AT, et al: Preligation of CR1 enhances IgG-dependent phagocytosis by cultured human monocytes. J Immunol 146:2694, 1991.

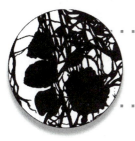

# CHAPTER 4

# THE ANTIGLOBULIN TEST

Peggy Perkins Simpson, MS, MT (ASCP)
and Pamela Ellis Hall, MA, MT (ASCP) SBB

**OBJECTIVES:**

*On completion of this chapter, the learner should be able to:*

1 State the principle of the antiglobulin test.

2 Differentiate monoclonal from polyclonal and monospecific from polyspecific antihuman globulin (AHG) reagents.

3 Describe the preparation of monoclonal and polyclonal AHG reagents.

4 Explain the antibody requirements for AHG reagents.

5 Discuss the use of polyspecific versus monospecific AHG in the indirect antiglobulin test (IAT).

6 Discuss the advantages and disadvantages of anti-complement activity in polyspecific AHG.

7 Compare and contrast the indirect antiglobulin test and the direct antiglobulin test (DAT). Include an explanation of (1) principle, (2) applications, and (3) red cell sensitization.

8 List the reasons for the procedural steps in the DAT and IAT.

9 Interpret the results of a DAT panel.

10 List the factors that affect the antiglobulin test.

11 List the sources of error associated with the performance of the antiglobulin test.

12 Discuss new techniques for antiglobulin testing.

## INTRODUCTION

The antiglobulin test (also called Coombs' test) is based on the principle that antihuman globulins (AHGs) obtained from immunized nonhuman species bind to human globulins such as IgG or complement, either free in serum or attached to antigens on red blood cells (RBCs or red cells).

There are two major types of blood group antibodies, IgM and IgG. Because of their large pentamer structure, IgM antibodies bind to corresponding antigen and directly agglutinate RBCs suspended in saline. IgG antibodies are termed *nonagglutinating* because their monomer structure is too small to agglutinate sensitized RBCs directly. The addition of AHG containing anti-IgG to RBCs sensitized with IgG antibodies allows the hemagglutination of these sensitized cells. Some blood group antibodies have the ability to bind complement to the RBC membrane. Antiglobulin tests detect IgG and/or complement-sensitized RBCs.

## HISTORY OF THE ANTIGLOBULIN TEST

Before the discovery of the antiglobulin test, only IgM antibodies had been detected. The introduction of the antiglobulin test permitted the detection of nonagglutinating IgG antibodies and led to the discovery and characterization of many new blood group systems.

In 1945, Coombs and associates[1] described the use of the antiglobulin test for the detection of weak and nonagglutinating Rh antibodies in serum. In 1946, Coombs and coworkers[2] described the use of AHG to detect in vivo sensitization of the red cells of babies suffering from hemolytic disease of the newborn (HDN). Although the test was initially of great value in the investigation of Rh hemolytic disease of the newborn, it was not long before its versatility for the detection of other IgG blood group antibodies became evident. The first of the Kell blood group system antibodies[3] and its associated antigen were reported only weeks after Coombs had described the test.

Although Coombs and associates[1] were instrumental in introducing the antiglobulin test to blood group serology, the principle of the test had in fact been described by Moreschi[4] in 1908. Moreschi's studies involved the use of rabbit antigoat serum to agglutinate rabbit red cells, which were sensitized with low nonagglutinating doses of goat antirabbit red cell serum.

Coombs's procedure involved the injection of human serum into rabbits to produce antihuman serum. After absorption to remove heterospecific antibodies and dilution to avoid prozone, the antihuman globulin serum still retained sufficient antibody activity to permit cross-linking of adjacent red cells sensitized with IgG antibodies. The cross-linking of sensitized RBCs by AHG produced hemagglutination, indicating that the RBCs had been sensitized by an antibody that had reacted with an antigen present on the cell surface.

The antiglobulin test can be used to detect RBCs sensitized with IgG alloantibodies, IgG autoantibodies, or complement components. Sensitization can occur either in vivo or in vitro. The use of AHG to detect in vitro sensitization of red blood cells is a two-stage technique referred to as the indirect antiglobulin test (IAT). In vivo sensitization is detected by a one-stage procedure, the direct antiglobulin test (DAT). The IAT and DAT still remain the most common procedures performed in blood group serology.

## ANTIHUMAN GLOBULIN REAGENTS

Several AHG reagents have been defined by the Food and Drug Administration (FDA) Center for Biologics Evaluation and Research (CBER). These are listed in Table 4–1 and are discussed in the following paragraphs. Antihuman globulin reagents may be polyspecific or monospecific.

### Polyspecific Antihuman Globulin

Polyspecific AHG contains antibody to human IgG and to the C3d component of human complement. Other anti-complement antibodies such as anti-C3b,

**Table 4–1.** Antihuman Globulin Reagents

| Reagent | Definition |
| --- | --- |
| *Polyspecific* | |
| 1. Rabbit polyclonal | Contains anti-IgG and anti-C3d (may contain other anti-complement and other anti-immunoglobulin antibodies). |
| 2. Rabbit/murine monoclonal blend | Contains a blend of rabbit polyclonal antihuman IgG and murine monoclonal anti-C3b and -C3d. |
| 3. Murine monoclonal | Contains murine monoclonal anti-IgG, anti-C3b, and anti-C3d. |
| *Monospecific Anti-IgG* | |
| 1. Rabbit polyclonal | Contains anti-IgG with no anti-complement activity (not necessarily gamma-chain specific). |
| 2. IgG heavy-chain specific | Contains only antibodies reactive against human gamma chains. |
| 3. Monoclonal IgG | Contains murine monoclonal anti-IgG. |
| *Anti-Complement* | |
| Rabbit polyclonal<br>1. Anti-C3d and anti-C3b<br>2. Anti-C3d, anti-C4b, anti-C4d | Contains only antibodies reactive against the designated complement component(s), with no anti-immunoglobulin activity. |
| Murine Monoclonal<br>1. Anti-C3d<br>2. Anti-C3b, anti-C3d | Contains only antibodies reactive against the designated complement component, with no anti-immunoglobulin activity. |

**Source:** Modified from Tyler, V (ed): Technical Manual, ed 12. American Association of Blood Banks, Bethesda, MD, 1996.

anti-C4b, or anti-C4d may also be present. Commercially prepared polyspecific AHG contains little, if any, activity against IgA and IgM heavy chains. However, the polyspecific mixture may contain antibody activity to kappa and lambda light chains common to all immunoglobulin classes, thus reacting with IgA or IgM molecules.[5]

## Monospecific Antihuman Globulin

Monospecific AHG reagents contain only one antibody specificity: either anti-IgG or antibody to specific complement components such as C3b or C3d. Licensed monospecific AHG reagents in common use are anti-IgG and anti-C3b-C3d.[5]

### Anti-IgG

Reagents labeled "anti-IgG" contain no anti-complement activity. Anti-IgG reagents contain antibodies specific for the Fc fragment of the gamma heavy chain of the IgG molecule. If not labeled "gamma heavy-chain specific," anti-IgG may contain anti-light-chain specificity and therefore react with cells sensitized with IgM and IgA as well as with IgG.[5]

### Anti-Complement

Anti-complement reagents such as anti-C3b-C3d reagents are reactive against the designated complement components only and contain no activity against human immunoglobulins.[5]

## PREPARATION OF ANTIHUMAN GLOBULIN

The classic method of AHG production involves injecting human serum or purified globulin into laboratory animals, such as rabbits. The human globulin behaves as foreign antigen, the rabbit's immune response is triggered, and an antibody to human globulin is produced. For example, human IgG injected into a rabbit results in anti-IgG production; human complement components injected into a rabbit result in anti-complement. This type of response produces a polyclonal antiglobulin serum. Polyclonal antibodies are a mixture of antibodies from different plasma cell clones. The resulting polyclonal antibodies recognize different antigenic determinants (epitopes), or the same portion of the antigen but with different affinities. Hybridoma technology can be used to produce monoclonal antiglobulin serum. Monoclonal antibodies are derived from one clone of plasma cells and recognize a single epitope.

## Preparation of Polyspecific Antihuman Globulin

### Polyclonal Antihuman Globulin Production

Polyclonal AHG is usually prepared in rabbits, although when large volumes of antibody are required, sheep or goats may be used. In contrast with the early production methods, in which a crude globulin fraction of serum was used as the immunogen, modern production commences with the purification of the immunogen from a large pool of normal sera.

Conventional polyspecific antiglobulin reagents are produced by immunizing one colony of rabbits with human immunoglobulin (IgG) antigen and another colony with human C3 antigen. Because of the heterogeneity of IgG molecules, the use of serum from many donors to prepare the pooled IgG antigen used to immunize the rabbits and the pooling of anti-IgG from many immunized rabbits are essential in producing reagents for routine use that are capable of detecting the many different IgG antibodies. This is an advantage of using anti-IgG of polyclonal origin for antiglobulin serum.[6]

Both colonies of animals are hyperimmunized to produce high-titer, high-avidity IgG antibodies. Blood specimens are drawn from the immunized animals, and if the antibody potency and specificity meet predetermined specifications, the animals are bled for a production batch of reagent. Separate blends of the anti-IgG and anti-complement antibodies are made, and each pool is then absorbed with A1, B, and O cells to remove heterospecific antibodies. The total antibody content of each pool is determined, and the potency of the pools is analyzed to calculate the optimum antibody dilution for use. Block titrations for anti-IgG pools are performed by reacting dilutions of each antibody against cells sensitized with different amounts of IgG. This is a critical step in the manufacturing process because excess antibody, especially with anti-IgG, may lead to prozoning and hence false-negative test results.

Because it is not possible to coat cells with measured amounts of complement, the potency of anti-C3 pools is measured using at least two examples each of a C3b- and C3d-coated cell. Both anti-C3b (C3c) and anti-C3d are present in the polyclonal anti-C3 pool. The level of anti-C3d is particularly critical in keeping false-positive tests to a minimum and yet detecting clinically significant amounts of red cell–bound C3d. Additionally, if the dilution of the anti-C3 pool is determined on the basis of the amount of anti-C3d present, the level of anti-C3b (C3c) varies. The inability to determine the potency of anti-C3b and anti-C3d individually is one of the difficulties with polyclonal reagents that can be avoided with monoclonal products.[6] Once the required performance characteristics of the trial blend are obtained, a production blend of the separate anti-IgG and anti-complement pools is made.

### Monoclonal Antihuman Globulin Production

The monoclonal antibody technique devised by Kohler and Milstein[7] has been used to produce AHG and has proved particularly useful in producing high-titer antibodies with well-defined specificities to IgG and to the fragments of C3.[8-10]

Monoclonal antibody production begins with the immunization of laboratory animals, usually mice, with purified human globulin. After a suitable immune response, mouse spleen cells containing antibody-secreting lymphocytes are fused with myeloma cells.

The resulting "hybridomas" are screened for antibodies with the required specificity and affinity. The antibody-secreting clones may then be propagated in tissue culture or by inoculation into mice, in which case the antibody is collected as ascites. Because the clonal line produces a single antibody, there is no need for absorption to remove heterospecific antibodies. All antibody molecules produced by a clone of hybridoma cells are identical in terms of antibody structure and antigen specificity. This has advantages and disadvantages in AHG production. Once an antibody-secreting clone of cells has been established, antibody with the same specificity and reaction characteristics will be available indefinitely. This allows the production of a consistently pure and uncontaminated AHG reagent. The disadvantage of monoclonal antibodies is that all antibodies produced by a clone of cells recognize a single epitope present on an antigen. For antigens composed of multiple epitopes such as IgG, several different monoclonal antibodies reacting with different epitopes may need to be blended, or a monoclonal antibody specificity for an epitope on all variants of a particular antigen may need to be selected to ensure that all different expressions of the antigen are detected. Monoclonal antibodies to human complement components anti-C3b and anti-C3d may be blended with polyclonal anti-IgG from rabbits to achieve potent reagents that give fewer false-positive reactions as a result of anti-complement than conventional polyclonal antiglobulin reagents prepared from a blend of rabbit anti-IgG and rabbit anti-complement.[6] Gamma Biologicals manufactures AHG reagents from an entirely monoclonal source. The anti-IgG component is produced by exposing mice to RBCs coated with IgG. The resulting monoclonal anti-IgG reacts with the $C_H3$ region of the gamma chain of IgG subclasses 1, 2, and 3. The antibody does not react with human antibodies of subclass $IgG_4$, but these are not considered to be clinically significant. Blending the monoclonal anti-IgG with a monoclonal anti-C3b and monoclonal anti-C3d results in a polyspecific AHG reagent. The preparation of polyclonal and monoclonal AHG is diagrammed in Figure 4–1. Before the AHG is available for purchase, manufacturers must subject their reagents to an evaluation procedure, and the results must be submitted to the FDA for approval. Whether produced by the polyclonal or monoclonal technique, the final polyspecific product is one that contains both anti-IgG and anti-complement activity at the correct potency for immediate use. The reagent also contains buffers, stabilizers, and bacteriostatic agents and may be dyed green for identification purposes.

### Preparation of Monospecific Antihuman Globulin

Monospecific AHG is prepared by a production process similar to that described for polyspecific AHG; however, it contains only one antibody specificity. Monospecific anti-IgG is usually of polyclonal origin; however, monoclonal anti-IgG has been effectively pre-

**Conventional Method**

Hybridoma Technology

Polyclonal Antihuman Globulin

Monoclonal Antihuman Globulin

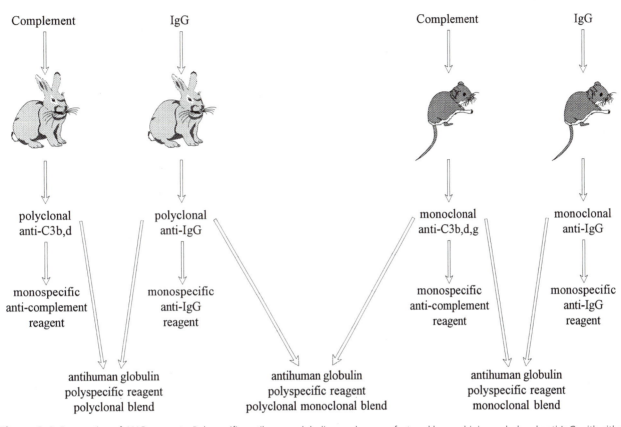

**Figure 4–1.** Preparation of AHG reagents. Polyspecific antihuman globulin may be manufactured by combining polyclonal anti-IgG with either polyclonal or monoclonal anticomplement components. A monoclonal blend may be manufactured by blending monoclonal anti-C3b, monoclonal anti-C3d, and monoclonal anti-IgG. Monospecific antihuman globulin reagents can be manufactured by conventional or hybridoma technology.

pared by hybridoma technology. Monospecific anti-complement reagents are often a blend of monoclonal anti-C3b and monoclonal anti-C3d.

## ANTIBODIES REQUIRED IN ANTIHUMAN GLOBULIN

### Anti-IgG

Antihuman globulin must contain antibody activity to nonagglutinating blood group antibodies. The vast majority of these antibodies are a mixture of $IgG_1$ and $IgG_3$ subclass. Rarely, nonagglutinating IgM antibodies may be found; however, they have always been shown to fix complement and may be detected by anti-complement.[11] IgA antibodies with Rh specificity have been reported; however, IgG antibody activity has always been present as well. The only RBC alloantibodies that have been reported as being solely IgA have been examples of anti-Pr,[12] and those antibodies were

agglutinating. IgA autoantibodies have been reported, although very rarely.[13] Therefore, anti-IgG activity must be present in the AHG reagent. Anti-IgM and anti-IgA activity may be present, but neither is essential. The presence of anti–light-chain activity allows detection of all immunoglobulin classes.

### Anti-Complement

Some antibodies "fix" complement components to the RBC membrane after complexing of the antibody with its corresponding antigen. These membrane-bound complement components can be detected by the anti-complement activity in AHG.

Early AHG reagents were prepared using a crude globulin fraction as the immunogen. In 1947, Coombs and Mourant demonstrated that the antibody activity that detected Rh antibodies was associated with the anti–gamma globulin fraction in the reagent. The first indication that there might be another antibody activity present that had an influence on the final reaction was presented by Dacie in 1951.[14] He observed that different reaction patterns were obtained when dilutions of AHG were used to test cells sensitized with "warm" as compared with "cold" antibodies. In 1957, Dacie and coworkers[15] published data showing that the reactivity of AHG to cells sensitized with "warm" antibodies resulted from anti–gamma globulin activity, whereas anti–nongamma globulin activity was responsible for the activity of cells sensitized by "cold" antibodies. The nongamma globulin component was shown to be beta globulin and had specificity for complement. Later studies[16,17] revealed that the complement activity was a result of C3 and C4.

During the 1960s many reports were published indicating the need for anti-complement activity in AHG to allow the detection of antibodies by the indirect test.[18–21] Many of the specificities mentioned in these reports were ones that are now generally considered to be of little clinical significance (e.g., anti-Le[a], anti-P[1], and anti-H). However, one specificity that was consistently mentioned and that is considered clinically significant was anti-Jk[a]. Evidence was also presented showing that the presence of anti-complement activity would enhance the reactions of clinically significant antibodies (e.g., anti-Fy[a] and anti-K).[18]

## USE OF POLYSPECIFIC VERSUS MONOSPECIFIC ANTIHUMAN GLOBULIN IN THE INDIRECT ANTIGLOBULIN TEST

As previously stated, polyspecific AHG contains both anti-IgG activity and anti-C3 activity. There is considerable debate among immunotransfusionists over the use of monospecific anti-IgG versus polyspecific AHG for routine antibody detection and pretransfusion testing. Because most clinically significant antibodies detected during antibody screening are IgG, the most important function of polyspecific AHG is the detection of IgG antibodies.

There have been numerous reports of clinically significant red cell alloantibodies that were not detectable with monospecific anti-IgG but were detected with the anti-complement component of AHG.[22] Unfortunately, polyspecific AHG has also been associated with unwanted positive reactions that are not caused by clinically significant antibodies. To investigate these variables, Petz and coworkers[23] examined 39,436 sera comparing monospecific anti-IgG with polyspecific AHG. They also compared the albumin technique with low ionic strength solutions (LISS)-suspended RBCs. Four Jk[a] antibodies were detected with polyspecific but not with monospecific anti-IgG using albumin or LISS-suspended RBCs. An additional anti-Jk[a] was detected only with polyspecific AHG when using LISS, but not with albumin. Also, five antibodies of anti-Kell, anti-Jk[a], and Fy[a] specificities were detected when using LISS, but not albumin, with both polyspecific AHG and anti-

IgG. Their results concluded that some clinically significant antibodies are detected with the anti-complement component of AHG, but not with anti-IgG. This is especially true for anti-Jk[a], a complement-binding IgG antibody often associated with delayed hemolytic transfusion reactions.

Petz and others[22] also determined the number of false-positive reactions obtained when using polyspecific AHG versus anti-IgG with LISS and albumin. False-positive reactions were defined as those caused by antibodies with no definable specificity or antibodies considered to be clinically insignificant because of optimum reactivity at cold temperatures (anti-I, anti-H, anti-P[1], anti-M). Ninety-three percent of the unwanted positive reactions were shown to be caused by C3 on the cells. The authors emphasize that, if the first step in evaluating a weakly positive AHG reaction is to repeat using the prewarmed technique, about 60 percent of the false-positive weak reactions become negative.

In a 3-year study, Howard and associates[24] found eight patients whose antibodies were detected primarily or solely by AHG containing anti-complement activity. Seven of these antibodies had anti-Jk[a] or anti-Jk[b] specificity. Some of them could be detected using homozygous Jk[a] or Jk[b] cells and an AHG containing only anti-IgG activity. Two of the anti-Jk[a] antibodies were associated with delayed hemolytic transfusion reactions. The complement-only Kidd antibodies represented 23 percent of all Kidd antibodies detected during the study. The authors concluded that they would continue to use polyspecific AHG reagent for routine compatibility testing.

In summary, one must balance the advantage of detecting clinically significant complement-only antibodies with the disadvantages resulting from using antiglobulin serum containing anti-complement activity.[22] A decision on the use of the AHG reagent for indirect tests is the prerogative of the individual blood bank. Many blood banks have adopted the use of monospecific anti-IgG for routine pretransfusion testing, citing cost-containment measures necessitated by the high number of repeats versus the rarity of complement-only detected antibodies such as anti-Jk[a].

## ANTIHUMAN GLOBULIN REAGENTS AND THE DIRECT ANTIGLOBULIN TEST

The direct antiglobulin test (DAT) detects in vivo sensitization of RBCs with IgG and/or complement components. During complement activation, C3 and C4 are split into two components. C3b and C4b bind to the RBC membrane, whereas C3a and C4a pass into the fluid phase. Further degradation of membrane-bound C3b and C4b occurs by removal of C3c and C4c, to leave C3d and C4d firmly attached to the RBC membrane.[25–27] The final degradation step has been shown to occur in vivo[28] and, in fact, is a common occurrence in both warm and cold autoimmune hemolytic anemias. Engelfriet and others[29] have also shown that

degradation of C3b to C3d can occur in vitro, providing that the incubation period is greater than 1 hour. In 1976, Garratty and Petz[30] confirmed the need for anti-C3d activity in AHG for use in the DAT. They also confirmed Engelfriet's observation that, given sufficient time, cell-bound C3b could be degraded to C3d in vitro.

The detection of C3d on the RBC membrane is important in the investigation of both warm and cold autoimmune hemolytic anemia. Many cases of warm autoimmune hemolytic anemia are associated with both IgG and C3d coating the RBCs. In cold autoimmune hemolytic anemia, C3d may be the only globulin detectable on the RBC. Characterization of autoimmune hemolytic anemias requires the detection of the specific globulin sensitizing the RBCs in vivo, usually IgG or C3d, or both. In the investigation of autoimmune hemolytic anemia, a DAT is performed initially with polyspecific AHG. If globulins are detected on the RBC membrane, follow-up testing with monospecific AHG (anti-IgG, anti-C3d) is performed to identify the coating proteins.

## PRINCIPLES OF THE ANTIGLOBULIN TEST

The antiglobulin test is based on the following simple principles:[31]

1. Antibody molecules and complement components are globulins.
2. Injecting an animal with human globulin stimu-

lates the animal to produce antibody to the foreign protein (i.e., AHG). Serologic tests employ a variety of AHG reagents reactive with various human globulins, including anti-IgG, antibody to the C3d component of human complement, and polyspecific reagents that contain both anti-IgG and anti-C3d activity.

3. Antihuman globulin reacts with human globulin molecules, either bound to RBCs or free in serum.
4. Washed RBCs coated with human globulin are agglutinated by AHG.

The complete procedures for the direct and indirect antihuman globulin tests can be found in the procedural appendix at the end of this chapter. **Color Plate 1** summarizes the methodology of both tests. Figure 4–2 illustrates in vitro sensitization detected in the indirect antiglobulin test (IAT) and in vivo sensitization detected by the DAT.

## DIRECT ANTIGLOBULIN TEST

### Principle and Application of the Direct Antiglobulin Test

The DAT detects in vivo sensitization of RBCs with IgG and/or complement components. Clinical conditions that can result in in vivo coating of red cells with antibody and/or complement are (1) hemolytic disease of the newborn (HDN), (2) hemolytic transfusion reaction (HTR), and (3) autoimmune and drug-

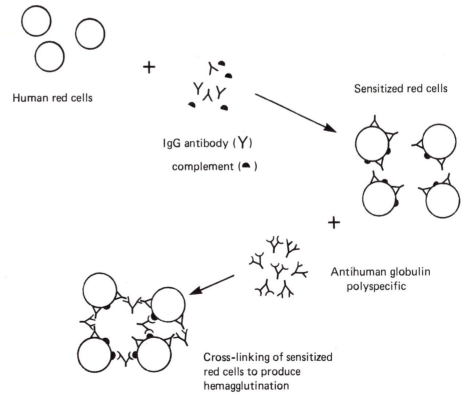

**Figure 4–2.** Antihuman globulin test. The indirect test is employed to determine in vitro sensitization of red cells, whereas the direct test is used to detect in vivo sensitization. Polyspecific antihuman globulin contains anti-IgG and anti-complement activity.

Human red cells

+

IgG antibody (Y)

complement (●)

Sensitized red cells

+

Antihuman globulin polyspecific

Cross-linking of sensitized red cells to produce hemagglutination

**Table 4–2.** Direct Antiglobulin Test

| Principle: Detects In Vivo RBC Sensitization | |
| --- | --- |
| **Application** | **In Vivo Sensitization** |
| HDN | Maternal antibody coating fetal RBCs |
| HTR | Recipient antibody coating donor RBCs |
| AIHA | Autoantibody coating individual's RBCs |

HDN = hemolytic disease of the newborn; HTR = hemolytic transfusion reaction; AIHA = autoimmune hemolytic anemia.

induced hemolytic anemias (AIHA). Table 4–2 lists the clinical application and in vivo sensitization detected for each situation.

## Direct Antiglobulin Test Panel

Initial direct antiglobulin testing includes testing one drop of a 3 to 5 percent suspension of washed RBCs with polyspecific (anti-IgG, anti-C3d) reagent. Positive results are followed by a DAT panel using monospecific anti-IgG and anti-C3d to determine the specific type of protein sensitizing the cell. In warm autoimmune hemolytic anemia, including drug-induced hemolytic anemia, the RBCs may be coated with IgG or C3d, or both. Patterns of reactivity and the type of protein sensitization in autoimmune hemolytic anemia are summarized in Table 4–3. In a transfusion reaction workup, the DAT may demonstrate IgG or C3d, or both, depending on the nature and specificity of the recipient's antibody. In the investigation of HDN, testing for complement proteins is not necessary inasmuch as the protein sensitizing the newborn RBCs is presumed to be maternal IgG.

## Evaluation of a Positive Direct Antiglobulin Test

Clinical consideration should dictate the extent to which a positive DAT is evaluated.[31] Interpreting the significance of a positive DAT requires knowledge of the patient's diagnosis, drug therapy, and recent transfusion history. A positive DAT may occur without clin-

**Table 4–3.** DAT Panel: Patterns of Reactivity in Autoimmune Hemolytic Anemia*

| Anti-IgG | Anti-C3d | Type of AIHA |
| --- | --- | --- |
| + | + | WAIHA (67%) |
| + | − | WAIHA (20%) |
| − | + | CHD, PCH, WAIHA (13%) |

**Source:** Modified from Walker, RH (ed): Technical Manual, ed 10. American Association of Blood Banks, Arlington, VA, 1990.

*The direct antiglobulin test with monospecific antiglobulin reagents is helpful in classifying AIHAs. Other procedures and studies are necessary to diagnose and characterize which form of autoimmune disease is present (see Chapter 21).

WAIHA = warm autoimmune hemolytic anemia; CHD = cold hemagglutinin disease; PCH = paroxysmal cold hemoglobinuria.

ical manifestations of immune-mediated hemolysis. Table 4–4 describes the in vivo phenomena that may be associated with a positive DAT.

The American Association of Blood Banks (AABB) *Technical Manual*[31] states that "results of serological tests are not diagnostic; their significance can only be assessed in relationship to the patient's clinical condition." Answering the following questions before investigating a positive DAT for patients other than neonates will help determine what further testing is appropriate:

1. Is there evidence of in vivo hemolysis?
2. Has the patient been transfused recently?
3. Does the patient's serum contain unexpected antibodies?
4. Is the patient receiving any drugs?
5. Has the patient received blood products or components containing ABO-incompatible plasma?
6. Is the patient receiving antilymphocyte globulin (ALG) or antithymocyte globulin (ATG)?

## INDIRECT ANTIGLOBULIN TEST

### Principle and Application of the Indirect Antiglobulin Test

The IAT is performed to determine in vitro sensitization of red cells and is used in the following situations:

1. Detection of incomplete (nonagglutinating) antibodies to potential donor red cells (compatibility testing) or to screening cells (antibody screen) in serum
2. Identification of antibody specificity using a panel of red cells with known antigen profiles
3. Determination of red cell phenotype using known antisera (e.g., Kell typing, weak D testing)
4. Titration of incomplete antibodies

Table 4–5 lists the IATs and the in vitro sensitization detected for each application.

For in vitro antigen-antibody reactions, the IAT tasks are listed and explained:

| Task | Why |
| --- | --- |
| 1. Incubate RBCs with antisera. | 1. Allows time for antibody molecule attachment to RBC antigen |
| 2. Perform at least three saline washings. | 2. Removes free globulin molecules |
| 3. Add antiglobulin reagent. | 3. Forms RBC agglutinates (RBC antigen + antibody + anti-IgG) |
| 4. Centrifuge. | 4. Accelerates agglutination by bringing cells closer together |
| 5. Examine for agglutination. | 5. Interprets test as positive or negative |

**Table 4–4.** In Vivo Phenomena Associated with a Positive DAT

| | | |
|---|---|---|
| Transfusion | 1. Recipient alloantibody and donor antigen | Alloantibodies in the recipient of a recent transfusion that react with antigen on donor RBC. |
| | 2. Donor antibody and recipient antigen | Antibodies present in donor plasma that react with antigen on a transfusion recipient's RBCs. |
| Drug induced | 1. Drug adsorption | Penicillin adsorbed to RBCs in vivo. Antipenicillin reacts with the penicillin bound to the RBCs. Penicillin-coated RBCs become coated with IgG. |
| | 2. Immune complex adsorption mechanism | Drug and specific antibody form complexes that attach nonspecifically to RBCs and initiate complement activation on the RBC surface. |
| | 3. Membrane modification | RBCs coated with cephalothin (Keflin) adsorb albumin, IgA, IgG, IgM, and α and β (i.e., complement) globulins. The DAT is reactive with anti-IgG and anti-C3d. |
| | 4. Autoimmunity | Following α-methyldopa therapy, autoantibodies are formed, which react with intrinsic RBC antigens. DAT is reactive with anti-IgG. |

| | Type (DAT Reactivity) | |
|---|---|---|
| Autoimmune hemolytic anemia | 1. WAIHA (IgG and/or C3) | Autoantibody reacts with patient's RBCs in vivo. |
| | 2. CHD (C3) | Cold-reactive IgM autoagglutinin binds to RBCs in peripheral circulation (temp 32°C). IgM binds complement, as RBCs return to warmer parts of circulation, IgM dissociates, leaving RBCs coated only with complement. |
| | 3. PCH (IgG) ⊂ ₃ ? | The IgG autoantibody reacts with RBCs in colder parts of body, causes complement to be bound irreversibly to RBCs, and then elutes at warmer temperature. |
| Hemolytic disease of newborn | 1. Maternal alloantibody crosses placenta (IgG) | Maternal (IgG) alloantibody, specific for fetal antigen, coats fetal RBCs. DAT is reactive with anti-IgG. |
| Miscellaneous | 1. Administration of equine preparations of anti-lymphocyte globulin and antithymocyte globulin | Heterophile antibodies that are present in ALG or ATG coat recipient's RBCs. |
| | 2. Administration of high-dose IV gamma globulin | Non–antibody-mediated binding of immunoglobulin to RBCs in patients with hypergammaglobulinemia |

**Source:** Modified from Walker, RH (ed): Technical Manual, ed 10. American Association of Blood Banks, Arlington, VA, 1990.
AIHA = autoimmune hemolytic anemia; CHD = cold hemagglutinin disease; PCH = paroxysmal cold hemoglobinuria.

**Table 4–5.** Indirect Antiglobulin Test

**Principle: Detects in Vitro Sensitization**

| Application | Tests | In Vitro Sensitization |
|---|---|---|
| Antibody detection | Compatibility testing | Recipient antibody reacting with donor cells |
| | Antibody screening | Antibody reacting with screening cells |
| Antibody identification | Antibody panel | Antibody reacting with panel cells |
| Antibody titration | Rh antibody titer | Antibody and selected Rh cells |
| Red cell phenotype | RBC antigen detection (Ex: weak D, K, Fy) | Specific antisera + RBCs to detect antigen. |

6. Grade agglutination reactions.
7. Add antibody-coated RBCs to negative reactions.

6. Determines the strength of reaction
7. Checks for neutralization of antisera by free globulin molecules (the Coombs control cells are D-positive red blood cells that are coated with anti-D)

The DAT does not require the incubation phase because of the antigen-antibody complexes formed in vivo.

## FACTORS AFFECTING THE ANTIGLOBULIN TEST

The antiglobulin test may be able to detect between 150 and 500 IgG molecules per red cell.[32,33] In a study performed by Merry and associates,[32] complete agglutination occurred once a cell had been sensitized with approximately 1000 molecules of IgG. Similar results were obtained for both direct and indirect antihuman globulin tests. The test, therefore, is a poor indicator of the amount of antibody actually sensitizing red cells, inasmuch as there is a very narrow dose-response curve between the number of antibody molecules on the cells and the degree of hemagglutination. In a study using monoclonal antibodies to C3 fragments, Merry and coworkers[34] found that the antiglobulin test had sensitivity for C3 similar to that for IgG.

For the IAT there must be between 100 and 200 IgG or C3 molecules on the cell to obtain a positive reaction. The number of IgG molecules that sensitize a red cell and the rate at which sensitization occurs can be influenced by several factors, outlined as follows:

1. **Ratio of serum to cells.** Increasing the ratio of serum to cells increases the sensitivity of the test system. Generally, a minimum ratio of 40:1 should be aimed for, and this can be achieved by using 2 drops of serum and 1 drop of a 5 percent volume of solute per volume of solution (v/v) suspension of cells.[35] When using cells suspended in saline, it is often advantageous to increase the ratio of serum to cells in an effort to detect weak antibodies (e.g., 4 drops of serum with 1 drop of a 3 percent [v/v] cell suspension will give a ratio of 133:1).

2. **Reaction medium.** *Albumin:* The macromolecules of albumin allow antibody-coated cells to come into closer contact with each other so that aggregation occurs. In 1965, Stroup and MacIlroy[36] reported on the increased sensitivity of the IAT if albumin was incorporated into the reaction medium. Their reaction mixture, consisting of 2 drops of serum, 2 drops of 22 percent (w/v) bovine albumin, and 1 drop of 3 to 5 percent (v/v) cells was shown to provide the same sensitivity at 30 minutes of incubation as a 60-minute saline test. The use of albumin does not seem to provide any advantage over LISS techniques and does add to the cost of the test.[37] Petz and coworkers[23] also showed that an albumin technique may miss a number of clinically significant antibodies.

   *Low ionic strength solutions:* Low ionic strength solutions (LISS) enhance antibody uptake and allow incubation times to be decreased. Some low ionic strength solutions also contain macromolecular substances. The LISS technique introduced by Low and Messeter[38] has critical requirements with respect to the serum-to-cell ratio. Moore and Mollison[39] showed that optimum reaction conditions were obtained using 2 drops of serum and 2 drops of a 3 percent (v/v) suspension of cells in LISS. Increasing the serum-to-cell ratio increased the ionic strength of the reaction mixture, leading to a decrease in sensitivity, thus counteracting the shortened incubation time of the test. A LISS medium may be achieved by either suspending RBCs in LISS or using a LISS additive reagent.

   *Polyethylene glycol:* Polyethylene glycol (PEG) is used as an additive to increase antibody uptake. Its action is to remove water, thereby effectively concentrating antibody. Anti-IgG is the AHG reagent of choice with PEG testing to avoid false-positive reactions.[5] Because PEG may cause aggregation of RBCs, readings for agglutination following 37°C incubation in the IAT is omitted. Several investigators[40] compared the performance of PEG as an enhancement media with that of LISS. Findings indicated that PEG increases the detection of clinically significant antibodies while decreasing detection of clinically insignificant antibodies. Barrett and associates[41] report that since PEG has been used for pretransfusion antibody screening, 6353 red cell components have been transfused without any reported acute or delayed HTRs.

3. **Temperature.** The rate of reaction for the vast majority of IgG antibodies is optimal at 37°C; therefore, this is the usual incubation temperature for the indirect antihuman globulin test. This is also the optimum temperature for complement activation.

4. **Incubation time.** For cells suspended in saline, incubation times may vary between 30 and 120 minutes. The vast majority of clinically significant antibodies can be detected after 30 minutes of incubation, and extended incubation times are usually not necessary. If a LISS technique is being used,[38,39] incubation times may be shortened to 10 to 15 minutes. With these shortened incubation times, it is essential that tubes be incubated at a temperature of 37°C. Extended incubation (i.e., up to 40 minutes) in the LISS technique has been shown to cause antibody to elute from the red cells, causing a decrease in the sensitivity of the test.[42] However, this could not be confirmed by Voak and coworkers.[43]

5. **Washing of cells.** When both the DAT and IAT are performed, RBCs must be saline-washed a minimum of three times before the addition of AHG reagent. Washing the RBCs removes free unbound serum globulins. Inadequate washing may result in a false-negative reaction because of neutralization of the AHG reagent by residual unbound serum globulins.

   Washing should be performed in as short a time as possible to minimize the elution of low-affinity antibodies. The cell pellet should be completely resuspended before adding the next saline wash. All saline should be discarded completely after the final wash because residual saline dilutes the AHG reagent and therefore decreases the sensitivity of the test.

   Centrifugation at each wash should be sufficient to provide a firm cell pellet and therefore minimize the possible loss of cells with each discard of saline. Washing may be performed using an automatic cell washer.[44]

6. **Saline for washing.** Ideally, the saline used for washing should be fresh or alternatively buffered to a pH of 7.2 to 7.4. Saline stored for long periods in plastic containers has been shown to decrease in pH, which may increase the rate of anti-

body elution during the washing process.[45] Changes in pH may have important implications when monoclonal AHG is used, inasmuch as monoclonal antibodies have been shown to have narrow pH ranges for optimum reactivity. Significant levels of bacterial contamination in saline has been reported,[46] and this can contribute to false-positive results.

7. **Addition of antihuman globulin.** Antihuman globulin should be added to the washed cells immediately after washing to minimize the chance of antibody eluting from the cell and subsequently neutralizing the AHG reagent. The volume of AHG added should be as indicated by the manufacturers. However, Voak and associates[47] have shown that adding two volumes of AHG may overcome washing problems when low levels of serum contamination remain. These authors indicated that the neutralization of AHG is a problem only with free IgG left in serum following inadequate saline washings and not with residual serum complement components. The complement fragments free in serum are not the same as the complement fragments bound to RBCs, and therefore residual serum does not contain C3b and C3d to neutralize the anti-C3b and anti-C3d in AHG reagent.

8. **Centrifugation for reading.** Centrifugation of the cell pellet for reading of hemagglutination along with the method used for resuspending the cells is a crucial step in the technique. The CBER-recommended method for the evaluation of AHG uses 1000 relative centrifugal force (RCF) for 20 seconds, although the technique described in this chapter suggests 500 RCF for 15 to 20 seconds. The use of higher RCFs yields more sensitive results; however, depending on how the pellet is resuspended, it may give weak false-positive results because of inadequate resuspension or alternatively may give a negative result if resuspension is too vigorous. The optimum centrifugation conditions should be determined for each centrifuge.

## SOURCES OF ERROR

Some of the more common sources of error associated with the performance of the AHG test have been outlined in the previous section. Table 4–6 lists reasons for false-negative and false-positive AHG reactions. An anticoagulant such as EDTA should be used to collect blood samples for the DAT to avoid the in vitro complement attachment associated with refrigerated clotted specimens.

All negative antiglobulin test reactions must be checked by the addition of IgG-sensitized cells. Adding IgG-coated RBCs to negative test reactions should demonstrate hemagglutination of these RBCs with the anti-IgG in the AHG reagent. If no hemagglutination follows the addition of IgG-coated RBCs, the test result is invalid and the test must be repeated. The most common technical errors that result in failure to demonstrate hemagglutination after the addition of IgG-coated RBCs are inadequate washing, nonreactive AHG reagent, and failure to add AHG reagent.

**Table 4–6.** Sources of Error in the Antihuman Globulin Technique

### False-Positive Results

1. Improper specimen (refrigerated, clotted specimen) may cause in vitro complement attachment
2. Autoagglutinable cells
3. Bacterial contamination of cells or saline used in washing
4. Cells with a positive direct antihuman globulin test used for the indirect antiglobulin test
5. Saline contaminated by heavy metals or colloidal silica
6. Dirty glassware
7. Overcentrifugation and overreading
8. Polyagglutinable cells
9. Preservative-dependent antibody in LISS reagents
10. Contaminating antibodies in the antihuman globulin reagent

### False-Negative Results

1. Inadequate or improper washing of cells
2. Antihuman globulin reagent nonreactive because of deterioration of neutralization
3. Antihuman globulin reagent not added
4. Serum not added in the indirect test
5. Serum nonreactive because of deterioration of complement
6. Inadequate incubation conditions in the indirect test
7. Cell suspension either too weak or too heavy
8. Undercentrifuged or overcentrifuged
9. Poor reading technique

**Source:** Rosenfield, RE, et al: Solid phase serology for the study of human erythrocytic antigen-antibody reactions. Proc Fifteenth Congr Int Soc Blood Trans, Paris, 1976, p 27.

## MODIFIED AND AUTOMATED ANTIGLOBULIN TEST TECHNIQUES

Modifications to the antiglobulin test technique (LISS, PEG, and albumin) have been mentioned; however, some other modifications may be used in special circumstances. Unger[48] reported on the use of enzymes to pretreat cells before performing the indirect antihuman globulin test. With this technique he was able to detect very low titers of Rh antibodies. The technique was also shown to be useful in detecting anti-Jk[a].[49]

In their 1961 paper, Polley and Mollison[18] reported on the use of a two-stage ethylenediaminetetraacetic acid (EDTA) technique to detect complement-fixing antibodies. This technique is particularly suitable for the detection of many Jk[a] and Le[a] antibodies, especially when investigating "aged" serum samples.

In 1980, Lalezari and Jiang[50] reported on the adaptation of the automated low ionic polybrene (LIP) technique for use as a manual procedure. The technique relies on low ionic conditions to rapidly sensitize cells with antibody. Polybrene, a potent rouleaux-forming reagent, is added to allow the sensitized cells to approach each other to permit cross-linking by the attached antibody. A high ionic strength solution is then added to reverse the rouleaux; however, if agglutination is present, it will remain. The test can be carried through to an AHG technique if required. If this is performed, a monospecific anti-IgG reagent must be used because the low ionic conditions cause considerable amounts of C4 and C3 to coat the cells and would give false-positive reactions if a polyspecific reagent were used.

Antiglobulin tests may be performed in reaction vessels other than test tubes. The capillary tube technique, originally introduced by Chown and Lewis[51] for Rh blood grouping, was adapted by them in 1957[52] for the antiglobulin test. Postoway and Garratty[53] have reported on the use of the capillary tube technique in the determination of IgG subclasses using specific subclass-typing antisera.

The antiglobulin test has also been performed using microplates. Crawford and colleagues[54] used microplates for a number of different grouping procedures, including the IAT. Microplate technology is increasingly used in blood group serology, and many techniques are being adapted for it. Redman and associates[55] have adapted the LIP technique for use in microplates. Although their report does not include the use of an AHG phase, this additional step could easily be included.

Solid-phase technology may be used for the performance of antiglobulin tests. Several different techniques have been reported using either test tubes[56] or microplates.[57,58] With the availability of microplate readers, this modification lends itself to the introduction of partial automation.

Immucor Incorporated manufactures a solid-phase system for the detection and identification of alloantibodies. Group O reagent RBC membranes are bound to the surfaces of polystyrene microtitration strip wells. IgG antibodies from patient or donor sera are bound to the membrane antigens. After incubation, unbound immunoglobulins are rinsed from the wells; then a suspension of anti-IgG–coated indicator RBCs is added to the wells. Centrifugation brings the indicator RBCs in contact with antibodies bound to the reagent red cell membranes. If the test result is negative, a pellet of indicator RBCs forms in the bottom of the wells. A positive test causes adherence of the indicator RBCs, forming anti-IgG–IgG complexes and a second immobilized RBC layer.

The gel test is a new process to detect RBC antigen-antibody reactions. In this method, RBCs are centrifuged through a gel contained in a special microtube. The gel acts as a trap; free unagglutinated RBCs form pellets in the bottom of the tube, whereas agglutinated RBCs are trapped in the tube for hours. Therefore, negative reactions appear as pellets in the bottom of the microtube, and positive reactions are fixed in the gel.

There are three different types of gel tests: neutral, specific, and antiglobulin. A neutral gel does not contain any specific reagent and acts only by its property of trapping agglutinates. The main applications of neutral gel tests are antibody screening and identification with enzyme-treated or untreated RBCs and reverse ABO typing. Specific gel tests use a specific reagent incorporated into the gel and are useful for antigen determination. The low ionic antiglobulin test (GLIAT) is a valuable application of the gel test and may be used for the IAT or the DAT. Antihuman globulin reagent is incorporated into the gel. For example, in an indirect antiglobulin gel test, 50 μL of a 0.8 percent RBC suspension is pipetted onto a gel containing AHG, serum is added, and the tube is centrifuged after a period of incubation. At the beginning of centrifugation, the RBCs tend to pass through the gel, but the medium in which they are suspended remains above. This results in separation between the RBCs and the medium without a washing phase. Red blood cells come in contact with AHG in the upper part of the gel, and the positive and negative reactions are separated. The detection of unexpected antibodies by GLIAT compares favorably with conventional AHG methods and provides a safe, reliable, and easy-to-read AHG test.[59]

The changes in blood bank technology, along with the changes in emphasis on the importance of crossmatching versus antibody screening, will probably further modify the role of the antiglobulin test over the coming years. At present, however, it still remains the most important test in the blood bank for the detection of clinically significant antibodies to red cells and for the detection of immune hemolysis.

## CASE STUDIES

### CASE 1

A 50-year-old woman is admitted to the hospital for cardiac surgery. Six units of blood are ordered. The patient is blood type O, D positive. The pretransfusion antibody screen is negative, and the abbreviated immediate spin cross-match is compatible. The patient is given 4 units of O, D-positive blood in transfusion. Ten days after transfusion, the patient is slightly jaundiced, develops malaise and weakness, and voids dark urine. The results from a transfusion-reaction investigation, before and after laboratory testing, are as follows:

Prelaboratory and postlaboratory testing:

| Test | Pretransfusion Sample | Posttransfusion Sample |
|---|---|---|
| Serum haptoglobin | — | Decreased |
| Urine hemoglobin | Negative | 4+ |
| Hematocrit | 35% | 30% |
| Antibody screen | Negative | Negative |
| DAT | — | 2+ |
| Reticulocyte count | — | 7.2% |
| Indirect bilirubin | 0.7 mg/dL | 3.0 mg/dL |

No clerical errors are detected.

**Questions:**

1. Give an explanation for the positive DAT on the posttransfusion sample.

2. What antiglobulin testing is indicated on the posttransfusion sample?

3. Why is the posttransfusion antibody screen negative?

**Answers:**

1. The positive DAT on the posttransfusion sample is the result of an alloantibody present in the patient's serum reacting with recently transfused donor RBC antigen. It was not detected in the pretransfusion sample because of a low titer. The titer increased when the corresponding donor antigen caused an anamnestic response.

2. A DAT panel using monospecific anti-IgG and anti-C3d should be performed to confirm the presence of IgG alloantibody coating the recently transfused donor RBCs. Once the presence of IgG alloantibody is confirmed, an elution must be performed on the posttransfusion specimen to remove alloantibody from the recently transfused donor RBCs. Because the DAT is positive and the antibody screen is negative, this confirms the presence of antibody-coated transfused cells. An antibody identification panel on the eluate confirms the identity of the alloantibody.

3. All of the antibody present is reacting with the recently transfused donor RBC antigens. There is no free antibody in the serum for detection by the antibody screen.

## CASE 2

During preadmission testing on a 45-year-old man, a positive DAT is demonstrated. A DAT panel is performed to characterize the type of protein sensitizing the red blood cells.

| | DAT Panel | | |
|---|---|---|---|
| | Polyspecific Antihuman Serum | Anti-IgG | Anti-C3d |
| Patient's RBCs | + | − | + |

**Questions:**

1. Interpret the DAT panel by indicating what type of protein is sensitizing the RBCs.

2. Name two reasons for this type of protein sensitization.

3. Before investigating a positive DAT, what questions will help determine further appropriate testing?

**Answers:**

1. Complement is sensitizing the RBCs.

2. Cold agglutinins and drugs associated with the immune complex mechanism activate complement.

3. p 78, Questions 1–6.

---

**SUMMARY CHART: IMPORTANT POINTS TO REMEMBER (MT/MLT)**

- The antiglobulin test is used to detect red cells sensitized by IgG alloantibodies, IgG autoantibodies, and/or complement components.
- Antihuman globulin (AHG) reagents containing anti-IgG are needed for the detection of IgG antibodies because the IgG monomeric structure is too small to directly agglutinate sensitized red cells.
- Polyspecific AHG sera contain antibodies to human IgG and the C3d component of human complement.
- Monospecific AHG sera contain only one antibody specificity: either anti-IgG or antibody to anti-C3b-C3d.
- Classic AHG sera (polyclonal) are prepared by injecting human globulins into rabbits, and an immune stimulus triggers production of antibody to human serum.
- Hybridoma technology is used to produce monoclonal antiglobulin serum.

- The direct antiglobulin test (DAT) detects in vivo sensitization of RBCs with IgG and/or complement components. Clinical conditions that can result in a positive DAT include hemolytic disease of the newborn (HDN), hemolytic transfusion reactions (HTR), and autoimmune and drug-induced hemolytic anemia (AIHA).
- The indirect antiglobulin test (IAT) detects in vitro sensitization of RBCs and can be applied to compatibility testing, antibody screen, antibody identification, RBC phenotyping, and titration studies.
- A positive DAT is followed by a DAT panel using monospecific anti-IgG and anti-C3d to determine the specific type of protein sensitizing the red cell.
- EDTA should be used to collect blood samples for the DAT to avoid in vitro complement attachment associated with refrigerated clotted specimens.

## REVIEW QUESTIONS

1. A principle of the antiglobulin test is:
   A. IgG and C3d are required for red cell sensitization.
   B. Human globulin is eluted from RBCs during saline washings.
   C. Injection of human globulin into an animal engenders passive immunity.
   D. AHG reacts with human globulin molecules bound to RBCs or free in serum.

2. Polyspecific AHG reagent contains:
   A. Anti-IgG
   B. Anti-IgG and anti-IgM
   C. Anti-IgG and anti-C3d
   D. Anti-C3d

3. Monoclonal anti-C3d is:
   A. Derived from one clone of plasma cells
   B. Derived from multiple clones of plasma cells
   C. Derived from immunization of rabbits
   D. Reactive with C3b and C3d

4. Which of the following is a clinically significant antibody whose detection may be dependent on anticomplement activity in polyspecific AHG?
   A. Anti-Jk$^a$
   B. Anti-Le$^a$
   C. Anti-P$_1$
   D. Anti-H

5. After the addition of IgG-coated RBCs to a negative AHG reaction during an antibody screen, a negative result is observed. Which of the following is a correct interpretation?

A. The antibody screen is negative.
B. The antibody screen needs to be repeated.
C. The saline washings were adequate.
D. Reactive AHG reagent was added.

6. Red blood cells must be washed in saline at least three times before the addition of AHG reagent to:
   A. Wash away any hemolyzed cells
   B. Remove traces of free serum globulins
   C. Neutralize any excess AHG reagent
   D. Increase the antibody binding to antigen

7. An in vitro phenomenon associated with a positive IAT is:
   A. Maternal antibody coating fetal RBCs
   B. Patient antibody coating patient RBCs
   C. Recipient antibody coating transfused donor RBCs
   D. Identification of alloantibody specificity using panel of reagent RBCs

8. False-positive DAT results are most often associated with:
   A. Use of refrigerated, clotted blood sample in which complement components coat RBCs in vitro
   B. A recipient of a recent transfusion manifesting an immune response to recently transfused RBCs
   C. Presence of heterophile antibodies from administration of globulin
   D. A positive autocontrol caused by polyagglutination

9. Cold hemagglutinin disease is associated with which of the following DAT patterns of reactivity?

|     | Anti-IgG | Anti-C3d | Anti-IgG/C3d |
|-----|----------|----------|--------------|
| A.  | –        | –        | +            |
| B.  | +        | +        | +            |
| C.  | –        | +        | +            |
| D.  | +        | –        | +            |

10. A patient is group O, D negative and is given 3 units of O, D-negative blood by transfusion on June 1. Two additional units of RBCs are ordered on June 10. During pretransfusion testing for the additional units, a weakly positive autocontrol is demonstrated, and the antibody screen is negative. The results on a DAT panel on the pretransfusion specimen (June 1) and posttransfusion EDTA specimen (June 10) are:

|                | Polyspecific antihuman serum | anti-IgG | anti-C3d | Control |
|----------------|------------------------------|----------|----------|---------|
| Pretransfusion  | –                            | –        | –        | –       |
| Posttransfusion | +                            | +        | –        | –       |

Which of the following is the most likely interpretation of these results?
A. An alloantibody formed in response to recently transfused donor RBCs not detectable in patient serum because of in vivo attachment to the recipient RBCs
B. In vivo attachment to recently transfused donor RBCs
C. Autoantibody attached to recipient RBCs
D. Anamnestic response in which stimulated alloantibody production is not detectable in antibody screen because of in vivo attachment to recently transfused donor RBCs

11. DAT panel results on three patients are as follows:

|           | Polyspecific AHG | Anti-IgG | Anti-C3d |
|-----------|------------------|----------|----------|
| Patient 1 | +                | +        | +        |
| Patient 2 | +                | –        | +        |
| Patient 3 | +                | +        | –        |

A correct interpretation of the type of protein coating each patient's RBCs corresponds to:

|    | Patient 1         | Patient 2  | Patient 3  |
|----|-------------------|------------|------------|
| A. | IgG only          | C3d only   | IgG only   |
| B. | Both IgG and C3d  | C3d only   | IgG only   |
| C. | Both IgG and C3d  | IgG only   | C3d only   |
| D. | Both IgG and C3d  | IgG only   | IgG only   |

12. Polyethylene glycol (PEG) enhances antigen-antibody reactions by:
A. Decreasing zeta potential
B. Concentrating antibody by removal of water
C. Increasing antibody affinity for antigen
D. Increasing antibody specificity for antigen

13. Solid-phase antibody screening is based on:
A. Adherence
B. Agglutination
C. Hemolysis
D. Precipitation

14. A positive DAT may be found in which of the following situations?
A. A weak D-positive patient
B. A patient with anti-K
C. Hemolytic disease of the newborn
D. An incompatible crossmatch

## ANSWERS TO REVIEW QUESTIONS

1. D (p 72)
2. C (p 72)
3. A (p 73)
4. A (p 76)
5. B (p 81)
6. B (p 80)
7. D (p 79, Table 4–5)
8. A (p 81, Table 4–6)
9. C (p 78, Table 4–3)
10. D (p 79, Table 4–4)
11. B (p 78)
12. B (p 80)
13. A (p 82)
14. C (p 77)

## REFERENCES

1. Coombs, RAA, et al: A new test for the detection of weak and "incomplete" Rh agglutinins. Br J Exp Pathol 26:255, 1945.
2. Coombs, RRA, et al: In vivo isosentisation of red cells in babies with haemolytic disease. Lancet i:264, 1946.
3. Race, RR, and Sanger, R: Blood Groups in Man, ed 6. Blackwell Scientific, Oxford, 1975, p 283.
4. Moreschi, C: Neue Tatsachen über die Blutkorperchen Agglutinationen. Zentralbl Bakteriol 46:49, 1908.
5. Tyler, V (ed): Technical Manual, ed 12. American Association of Blood Banks, Bethesda, MD, 1996.
6. Issitt, C: Monoclonal Antiglobulin Reagents. Dade International Online, 1997. http://www.dadeinternational.com/hemo/papers/monoanti.htm.
7. Kohler, G, and Milstein, C: Continuous cultures of fused cells secreting antibody of predefined specificity. Nature 256:495, 1975.
8. Lachman, PJ, et al: Use of monoclonal antibodies to characterize the fragments of C3 that are found on erythrocytes. Vox Sang 45:367, 1983.
9. Holt, PDJ, et al: NBTS/BRIC 8: A monoclonal anti-C3d antibody. Transfusion 25:267, 1985.
10. Voak, D, et al: Monoclonal antibodies—C3 serology. Biotest Bull 1:339, 1983.
11. Mollison, PL: Blood Transfusion in Clinical Medicine, ed 7. Blackwell Scientific, Oxford, 1983, p 502.

12. Garratty, G, et al: An IgA high titre cold agglutinin with an unusual blood group specificity within the Pr complex. Vox Sang 25:32, 1973.
13. Petz, LD, and Garratty, G: Acquired immune hemolytic anemias. Churchill Livingstone, New York, 1980, p 193.
14. Dacie, JF: Differences in the behaviour of sensitized red cells to agglutination by antiglobulin sera. Lancet ii:954, 1951.
15. Dacie, JV, et al: "Incomplete" cold antibodies: Role of complement in sensitization to antiglobulin serum by potentially haemolytic antibodies. Br J Haematol 3:77, 1957.
16. Harboe, M, et al: Identification of the component of complement participating in the antiglobulin reaction. Immunology 6:412, 1963.
17. Jenkins, GC, et al: Role of C4 in the antiglobulin reaction. Nature 186:482, 1960.
18. Polley, MJ, and Mollison, PL: The role of complement in the detection of blood group antibodies: Special reference to the antiglobulin test. Transfusion 1:9, 1961.
19. Polley, MJ, et al: The role of 19S gamma-globulin blood group antibodies in the antiglobulin reaction. Br J Haematol 8:149, 1962.
20. Stratton, F, et al: The preparation and uses of antiglobulin reagents with special reference to complement fixing blood group antibodies. Transfusion 2:135, 1962.
21. Stratton, F, et al: Value of gel fixation on Sephadex G-200 in the analysis of blood group antibodies. J Clin Pathol 21:708, 1968.
22. Petz, LD, et al: Clinical Practice of Transfusion Medicine, ed 3. Churchill Livingstone, New York, 1996, p 207.
23. Petz, LD, et al: Compatibility testing. Transfusion 21:633, 1981.
24. Howard, JE, et al: Clinical significance of the anti-complement component of antiglobulin antisera. Transfusion 22:269, 1982.
25. Lachman, PJ, and Muller-Eberhard, HJ: The demonstration in human serum of "conglutinogen-activating-factor" and its effect on the third component of complement. J Immunol 100:691, 1968.
26. Muller-Eberhard, HJ: Chemistry and reaction mechanisms of complement. Adv Immunol 8:1, 1968.
27. Cooper, NR: Isolation and analysis of mechanisms of action of an inactivator of C4b in normal human serum. J Exp Med 141:890, 1975.
28. Brown, DL, et al: The in vivo behaviour of complement-coated red cells: Studies in C6-deficient, Ce-depleted and normal rabbits. Clin Exp Immunol 7:401, 1970.
29. Engelfriet, CP, et al: Autoimmune haemolytic anemias: 111 preparation and examination of specific antisera against complement components and products, and their use in serological studies. Clin Exp Immunol 6:721, 1970.
30. Garratty, G, and Petz, LD: The significance of red cell bound complement components in development of standards and quality assurance for the anti-complement components of antiglobulin sera. Transfusion 16:297, 1976.
31. Walker, RH (ed): Technical Manual, ed 10. American Association of Blood Banks, Arlington, VA, 1990.
32. Merry, AH, et al: Quantitation of IgG on erythrocytes: Correlation of numbers of IgG molecules per cell with the strength of the direct and indirect antiglobulin tests. Vox Sang 47:73, 1984.
33. Petz, LD, and Garratty, G: Acquired immune hemolytic anemias. Churchill Livingstone, New York, 1980, p 307.
34. Merry, AH, et al: The quantification of C3 fragments on erythrocytes: Estimation of C3 fragments on normal cells, acquired haemolytic anaemia cases and correlation with agglutination of sensitized cells. Clin Lab Haematol 5:387, 1983.
35. Voak, D, et al: Improved antiglobulin tests to detect different antibodies: Detection of anti-Kell by LISS. Med Lab Sci 39:363, 1982.
36. Stroup, M, and MacIlroy, M: Evaluation of the albumin antiglobulin technic in antibody detection. Transfusion 5:184, 1965.
37. Mollison, PL: Blood Transfusion in Clinical Medicine, ed 7. Blackwell Scientific, Oxford, 1983, p 519.
38. Low, B, and Messeter, L: Antiglobulin test in low-ionic strength salt solution for rapid antibody screening and cross-matching. Vox Sang 26:53, 1974.

39. Moore, HC, and Mollison, PL: Use of a low-ionic strength medium in manual tests for antibody detection. Transfusion 16:291, 1976.
40. Shirley, R, et al: Polyethylene glycol versus low-ionic strength solution in pretransfusion testing: A blinded comparison study. Transfusion 34:5, 1994.
41. Barrett, V, et al: Analysis of the routine use of polyethylene glycol (PEG) as an enhancement medium. Immunohematology 11:1, 1995.
42. Jorgensen, J, et al: The influence of ionic strength, albumin and incubation time on the sensitivity of indirect Coombs' test. Vox Sang 36:186, 1980.
43. Voak, D, et al: Low-ionic strength media for rapid antibody detection: Optimum conditions and quality control. Med Lab Sci 37:107, 1980.
44. Voak, D, et al: Quality control of antihuman globulin tests: Use of replicate tests to improve performance. Biotest Bull 3:41, 1986.
45. Bruce, M, et al: A serious source of error in antiglobulin testing. Transfusion 26:177, 1986.
46. Green, C, et al: Quality assurance of physiological saline used for blood grouping. Med Lab Sci 43:364, 1968.
47. Voak, D, et al: Antihuman globulin reagent specification: The European and ISBT/ICSH view. Biotest Bull 3:7, 1986.
48. Unger, LJ: A method for detecting $Rh_o$ antibodies in extremely low titre. J Lab Clin Med 37:825, 1951.
49. van der Hart, M, and van Loghem, JJ: A further example of anti-Jk$^a$, Vox Sang 3:72, 1953.
50. Lalezari, P, and Jiang, RF: The manual polybrene test: A simple and rapid procedure for detection of red cell antibodies. Transfusion 20:206, 1980.
51. Chown, B, and Lewis, M: The slanted capillary method of rhesus blood grouping. J Clin Pathol 4:464, 1951.
52. Chown, B, and Lewis, M: The Knell antigen in American Indians, with a note about anti-Knell sera. Am J Phys Anthropol 15:149, 1957.
53. Postoway, N, and Garratty, G: Standardization of IgG subclass antiserums for use with sensitized red cells. Transfusion 23:398, 1983.
54. Crawford, MN, et al: Microplate system for routine use in blood bank laboratories. Transfusion 10:258, 1970.
55. Redman, M, et al: Typing of red cells on microplates by low-ionic polybrene technique. Med Lab Sci 43:393, 1986.
56. Rosenfield, RE, et al: Solid phase serology for the study of human erythrocytic antigen-antibody reactions. Proc 15th Congr Int Soc Blood Trans, Paris, 1976, p 27.
57. Moore, HH: Automated reading of red cell antibody identification tests by a solid phase antiglobulin technique. Transfusion 24:218, 1984.
58. Plapp, FV, et al: A solid phase antibody screen. Am J Clin Pathol 82:719, 1984.
59. Lapierre, Y, et al: The gel test: A new way to detect red cell antigen-antibody reactions. Transfusion 30:2, 1990.

## BIBLIOGRAPHY

Beck, ML, and Marsh, WL: Letter to the editor: Complement and the antiglobulin test. Transfusion 17:529, 1977.
Black, D, and Kay, J: Influence of tube type on the antiglobulin test. Med Lab Sci 43:169, 1986.
Freedman, J, et al: Further observations on the preparation of antiglobulin reagents reacting with C3d and C4d on red cells. Vox Sang 33:21, 1977.
Freedman, J, and Mollison, PL: Preparation of red cells coated with C4 and C3 subcomponents and production of anti-C4d and anti-C3d. Vox Sang 31:241, 1976.
Federal Register 42:41920, 1977.
Federal Register 50:5579, 1985.
Garratty, G, and Petz, LD: An evaluation of commercial antiglobulin sera with particular reference to their anticomplement properties. Transfusion 11:79, 1971.
Giles, C, and Engelfriet, CP: Working party on the standardization of antiglobulin reagents of the expert panel of serology. Vox Sang 38:178, 1980.

Graham, HA, et al: A new approach to prepare cells for the Coombs test. Transfusion 22:408, 1982.

Issitt, PD, et al: Evaluation of commercial antiglobulin sera over a two-year period. Part 1. Anti-beta 1A, anti-alpha 2D, and anti-beta 1E levels. Transfusion 14:93, 1974.

Judd, WJ, et al: Paraben-associated autoanti-Jk$^a$ antibodies: Three examples detected using commercially prepared low-ionic strength saline containing parabens. Transfusion 22:31, 1982.

Petz, LD: Complement in immunohaematology and in neurologic disorders. In International Symposium on the Nature and Significance of Complement Activation. Ortho Research Institute of Medical Science, Raritan, NJ, 1976, p 87.

Plapp, FV, et al: Solid phase red cell adherence tests in blood banking. In Smit Bigings, C Th, Das, PC, and Greenwalt, TJ: Future Development in Blood Banking. Martinus Nijhoff, Boston, 1986, p 177.

# PROCEDURAL APPENDIX

## MANUAL ANTIGLOBULIN TEST TECHNIQUES

### I. Direct Antiglobulin Test

#### A. Procedure

1. Label two 10 or 12 × 75 mm glass test tubes. Test and control, respectively, and add 1 drop of a 3 percent v/v suspension of test cells to each.
2. Wash the cells a minimum of three times with saline and *ensure that all saline is completely decanted after the last wash.*
3. To the tube labeled "test," add 1 to 2 drops of antihuman globulin as recommended by the manufacturer and mix.
4. To the control tube add 1 to 2 drops of 3 percent w/v bovine albumin in saline and mix.
5. Centrifuge both tubes at 500 rcf for 15 to 20 seconds.
6. Following centrifugation, completely resuspend the cell pellet by gently tipping and rolling the tube. Read and score agglutination macroscopically with the aid of a background light source and low-power magnification.
7. Incubate the tubes for another 5 minutes at room temperature and repeat steps 5 and 6. Most manufacturers now recommend this additional step because it has been shown that some negative or even weak reactions may increase in strength. These reactions have been attributed to the presence of C3d and, to a lesser extent, IgA on the cell surface. Conversely, the reaction with some cells may weaken after the extra incubation; this has been attributed to either detachment of IgG antibody or, alternatively, prozoning when excess anti-IgG has been added.

#### B. Controls

To all negative tubes add 1 drop of control cells weakly sensitized with IgG, mix the cells, and repeat steps 5 and 6. A mixed-field weakly positive reaction should now be obtained, indicating that the antihuman globulin had been added to the tube and that it was still reactive. All negative results could therefore be considered valid. If a negative result was obtained after addition of the control cells, it would indicate that the antihuman globulin had not been added or that, if added, it was nonreactive. This could occur if:

1. The reagent had deteriorated in storage.
2. The reagent had been contaminated by serum and the antibody activity neutralized.
3. The cells had been insufficiently washed and residual serum or plasma had neutralized the antihuman globulin reagent when added to the tube.

Control cells weakly sensitized with complement should be used with monospecific anti-C3d reagent to validate negative results.

The control tube containing cells and 3 percent w/v bovine albumin should give a negative result. If the result is positive, it indicates that the cells are autoagglutinable and that the test cannot be properly interpreted.

For reasons previously outlined, the cells used for direct antiglobulin tests should be collected into either EDTA or citrates containing anticoagulant to minimize the possibility of the in vitro attachment of complement components.

### II. Indirect Antiglobulin Test

#### A. Procedure

1. Into a labeled glass 10 or 12 × 75 mm test tube, place 2 to 4 drops of test serum and 1 drop of a washed 3 percent v/v suspension of red cells.

2. Mix the cell suspension and incubate for 30 minutes in a 37°C water bath.
3. Centrifuge the tube at 500 rcf for 15 to 20 seconds.
4. After centrifugation, completely resuspend the cell pellet by gently tapping and rolling the tube. Read and score agglutination macroscopically with the aid of a background light source and low-power magnification.
5. Wash the cells at least three times with saline and *ensure that all saline is completely decanted following the final wash.*
6. Add 1 to 3 drops of antihuman globulin as recommended by the manufacturer and mix.
7. Repeat steps 3 and 4.

### B. Controls

To all negative tubes, add 1 drop of control cells weakly sensitized with IgG, mix the cells, and repeat steps 3 and 4. Negative results can be considered valid if a weakly positive mixed-field reaction is obtained after addition of the control cells. If this reaction is not obtained, the test should be repeated.

When phenotyping red cells using an antihuman globulin–reactive typing serum, it is important to follow the antisera manufacturer's recommendations for the use of the reagent.

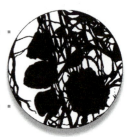

# THE ABO BLOOD GROUP SYSTEM

Denise M. Harmening, PhD, MT(ASCP), CLS(NCA)
and Deborah Firestone, MA, MT(ASCP)SBB
with case history by William Bernard, MT(ASCP)SBB
St. John's Hospital Transfusion Services
Springfield, IL

## OBJECTIVES

*On completion of this chapter, the learner should be able to:*

1 Describe the reciprocal relationship between ABO antigens and antibodies for blood types O, A, B, and AB.

2 Identify the frequencies of the four major blood types in the White, Black, Mexican, and Asian populations.

3 Explain the effect of age on the production of ABO isoagglutinins.

4 Describe the immunoglobulin classes of ABO antibodies in group O, A, and B individuals.

5 Predict the ABO phenotypes and genotypes of offspring from various ABO matings.

6 Explain the formation of H, A, and B antigens on the red cells from precursor substance to immunodominant sugars.

7 Describe the formation of H, A, and B soluble substances.

8 Explain the principle of the hemagglutination inhibition assay for the determination of secretor status.

9 Describe the qualitative and quantitative differences between the $A_1$ and $A_2$ phenotypes.

10 Describe the reactivity of *Ulex europaeus* with the various ABO groups.

11 Describe the characteristics of the weak subgroups of A ($A_3$, $A_x$, $A_{end}$, $A_m$, $A_y$, $A_{el}$).

12 Describe the characteristics of the "Bombay" and "para-Bombay" phenotypes.

13 Explain the effects of disease on the expression of ABH antigens and antibodies.

14 Interpret the results from an ABO typing and resolve any discrepancies if present.

## HISTORICAL PERSPECTIVE

Karl Landsteiner truly opened the doors of blood banking with his discovery of the first human blood group system, ABO. This marked the beginning of the concept of individual uniqueness defined by the red cell antigens present on the red cell membrane. The ABO system still remains the most important of all blood groups in transfusion practice. Transfusion of an incorrect ABO type can result in the death of a patient.

In 1901, Landsteiner drew blood from himself and five associates, separated the cells and serum, and then mixed each cell sample with each serum. He was inadvertently the first individual to perform the forward and reverse grouping. Forward grouping is defined as using known sources of reagent antisera (anti-A, anti-

B) to detect antigens on an individual's red cells (Table 5-1 and Fig. 5-1). Reverse grouping is defined as using reagent cells with known $A_1$ and B antigens and testing the serum of the patient for ABO group antibodies (Table 5-2 and Fig. 5-2).

Groups A, B, and O were the first blood groups described by Landsteiner. He found that serum from group B individuals agglutinated group A red blood cells and, therefore, that an antibody to A antigens was present in group B serum. Conversely, serum from group A individuals agglutinated group B red cells, and, therefore, an antibody to B antigens was present in group A serum. Serum from group O individuals agglutinated both A and B cells, indicating the presence of antibodies to both A and B in group O serum (see Table 5-2 and Fig. 5-2).

In 1902, Landsteiner's associates, Sturle and von Descatello, discovered the fourth ABO blood group, AB. As can be seen from Table 5-2, serum from group AB individuals does not agglutinate group A or group B cells, indicating the absence of antibodies to both A and B.

The frequency of these blood groups in the white population is as follows: group O, 45 percent; group A, 41 percent; group B, 10 percent; and group AB, 4 percent.[1] Therefore, O and A are the most common blood group types, and blood group AB is the rarest. However, frequencies of ABO groups differ in a few selected populations and ethnic groups (Table 5-3).[1-4] For example, group B is found twice as frequently in Blacks and Asians as in Whites, and subgroup $A_2$ is rarely found in Asians.

Landsteiner concluded from the reactions he observed that in the ABO blood group system, individuals have "naturally occurring" antibodies in their serum directed against the missing ABO antigen on the surface of their RBCs. This term "naturally occurring" is really a misnomer, inasmuch as substantial evidence suggests that anti-A and anti-B are stimulated by substances that are ubiquitous in nature. Bacteria have been shown to be chemically similar to human ABO antigens and may serve as a source of stimulation of antibody formation. Springer and coworkers[5] have demonstrated that leghorn chickens kept in a germ-free environment from birth lacked ABO antibodies, whereas, in comparison, control chickens raised under normal conditions had ABO antibodies. Various seeds from pollinating plants are also chemically similar to

**Table 5–1.** ABO Forward Grouping

| Patient's Red Cells | Reaction with Anti-A | Reaction with Anti-B | Interpretation of Blood Group |
|---|---|---|---|
| 1 | Negative | Negative | O |
| 2 | + | Negative | A |
| 3 | Negative | + | B |
| 4 | + | + | AB |

+ = visual agglutination

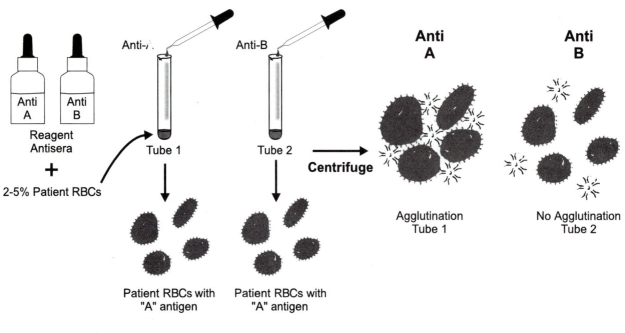

Patient RBCs with          Patient RBCs with
"A" antigen                "A" antigen

## Interpretation:  Group A

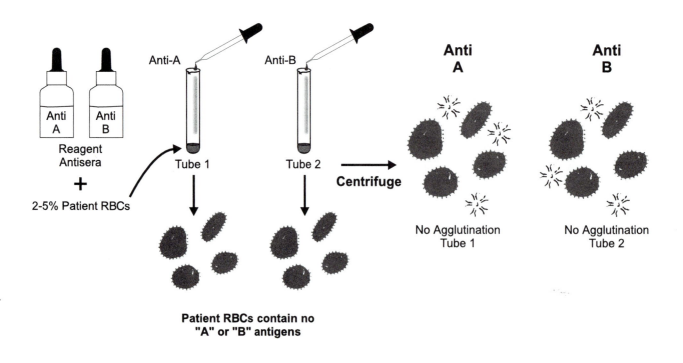

Patient RBCs contain no
"A" or "B" antigens

## Interpretation:  Group O

**Figure 5–1.** Forward grouping: group A individual, group O individual.

**Table 5–2.** ABO Reverse Grouping

| Patient's Serum | Reaction with Reagent A₁ Cells | Reaction with Reagent B Cells | Interpretation of Blood Group |
|---|---|---|---|
| 1 | + | + | O |
| 2 | Negative | + | A |
| 3 | + | Negative | B |
| 4 | Negative | Negative | AB |

+ = visual agglutination

human ABO antigens—so much so that they can be used as a source of antisera (e.g., the reagent anti-A₁ lectin; see ABO Subgroups, later in this chapter).

Whether the source of stimulation to ABO antigens the individual lacks is pollen particles, bacteria, or other substances present in nature, the fact remains that there is a general processing of that particular antigen. This results in a consistent immune response reflected in antibody production. The production of ABO antibodies is initiated at birth, but titers are generally too low for detection until the individual is 3 to 6 months of age. As a result, it is logical to perform only forward grouping on cord blood from newborn infants. The antibody production peaks at 5 to 10 years of age and then declines progressively with advanced age. Patients older than 65 years of age usually have low titers, so that antibodies may be undetectable in the reverse grouping. The ABO blood group system is unique in that all normal, healthy individuals consistently have present in their serum antibodies to antigens they lack on their red cells. The other defined blood group systems do not regularly have in their serum "naturally occurring" antibodies to antigens they lack on their RBCs. Most other blood group systems require the introduction of foreign red cells by transfusion or pregnancy. Some blood groups, however, can occasionally have antibodies present that are not related to the introduction of foreign red cells. These antibodies are usually of the IgM type and are not consistently present in everyone's serum. Performance of a reverse grouping is, therefore, unique to the ABO blood group system. Testing of ABO is relatively easy; therefore, the regular occurrence of anti-A and/or anti-B in persons lacking the corresponding antigen(s) serves as a confirmation of results in the forward grouping. Complete absence of anti-A and anti-B is very rare in healthy individuals (except AB subjects); it occurs in less than 0.01 percent of the random population.[6]

The natural presence of ABO antibodies, however, creates a treacherous situation as far as blood transfusion and some organ transplants are concerned. If group B red cells are given to a group A patient whose serum contains anti-B, the donor's red cells will be destroyed almost immediately, being lysed at a rate of approximately 1 mL of red cells per minute. This produces a very severe—if not fatal—transfusion reaction in the patient. In some situations when ABO incompatible organs are transplanted, there may be an immediate rejection phenomenon.[7] Therefore, both for-

ward and reverse grouping must be performed on all patients' samples, noting the correct reciprocal relationship of antigens and antibodies in a given blood group type (Table 5–4). As a result, group O is referred to as the *universal donor*, and group AB as the *universal recipient*.

## ABO ANTIBODIES

ABO antibodies are generally IgM. Characteristically, IgM antibodies are cold-reacting antibodies that bind complement and do not cross the placenta. (For a review of other characteristic properties of IgM antibodies, see Chap. 3).

In any given serum from a group A and/or B individual, anti-B and/or anti-A may be IgM only, a mixture of IgM and IgG, a mixture of IgM and IgA, or a mixture of all three immunoglobulins.[8] However, the majority of anti-A from a group B individual and anti-B from a group A individual contains predominantly IgM antibody, with minor amounts of IgG or IgA present, if detectable at all. The "immune" form of anti-A or anti-B can be produced by individuals exposed to foreign red cell stimulation, by either transfusion or pregnancy.

Serum from group O individuals contains not only anti-A and anti-B but also anti-A,B. Anti-A,B antibody activity, originally thought to be just a mixture of anti-A and anti-B, cannot be separated into a pure specificity when adsorbed with either A or B cells. Activity toward both A and B cells still remains with anti-A,B even after repeated adsorptions with A or B cells. For example, anti-A,B adsorbed with A cells and then eluted will still react with both A and B cells.[9,10] Anti-A,B, therefore, possesses serologic activity not found in mixtures of anti-A plus anti-B.

Anti-A,B from group O individuals has been reported to be a mixture of IgG and IgM, or IgG, IgM, and IgA. Anti-A,B crosses the placenta more frequently than anti-A or anti-B, confirming the presence of IgG. The "immune" form of anti-A,B can be produced by O individuals exposed to A or B red cells by either transfusion or pregnancy. These anti-A,B "immune" antibodies are predominantly IgG. IgG anti-A and anti-B antibodies develop far more commonly in group O individuals than in A or B individuals. Knowledge of the amount of IgG anti-A, anti-B, or anti-A,B in a woman's serum sometimes allows prediction or diagnosis of hemolytic disease of the newborn caused by ABO incompatibility (see Chap. 20).

There is a wide variation in the titers of ABO isoagglutinins in a random population. Generally, anti-A from a group O individual has a higher titer than anti-A from a group B individual, and anti-A from a group B individual usually has a higher titer than anti-B from a group A individual. Anti-A,B from group O individuals has a higher titer of anti-B and anti-A than that found in group A and B individuals, respectively. This makes A,B antiserum a convenient reagent to use to detect weak ABO antigens.

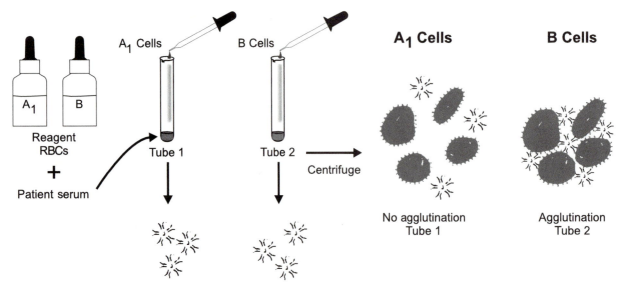

Interpretation:  **Group A**

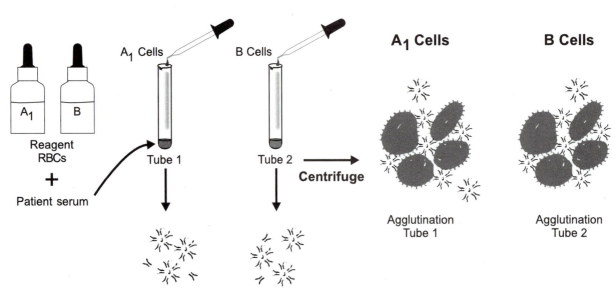

Interpretation:  **Group O**

**Figure 5–2.** Reverse grouping: group A individual, group O individual.

**Table 5–3.** ABO Phenotype Frequencies in U.S. Populations

| Phenotype | White (%) | Black (%) | Mexican (%) | Asian (%) |
|-----------|-----------|-----------|-------------|-----------|
| O | 45 | 49 | 56 | 43 |
| $A_1$ | 33 | 19 | 22 | 27 |
| $A_2$ | 8 | 8 | 6 | Rare |
| B | 10 | 19 | 13 | 25 |
| $A_1B$ | 3 | 3 | 4 | 5 |
| $A_2B$ | 1 | 1 | Rare | Rare |

## INHERITANCE OF THE ABO BLOOD GROUPS

The theory for the inheritance of the ABO blood groups was first described by Bernstein in 1924. He demonstrated that each individual inherits one ABO gene from each parent and that these two genes determine which ABO antigens are present on the red cell membrane. One position, or locus, on each chromosome 9 is occupied by an A, B, or O gene. The O gene is considered an amorph, inasmuch as no detectable antigen is produced in response to the inheritance of this gene. The designations A and B refer to phenotypes, whereas *AA, BO,* and *OO* denote genotypes. In the case of an O individual, both phenotype and genotype are the same, because that individual would have to be homozygous for the O gene. An individual who has the phenotype A (or B) can have the genotype *AA* or *AO* (or *BB* or *BO*). The phenotype and genotype are the same in an AB individual because of the inheritance of both the A and B gene. Table 5–5 lists possible ABO phenotypes and genotypes from various matings. The inheritance of ABO antigens, therefore, follows simple mendelian genetics. ABO, like most other blood group systems, is codominant in expression. (For a review of genetics, refer to Chap. 2.)

### Formation of A, B, and H Antigens

The ABO genes do not actually code for the production of ABH antigens but, rather, produce specific glycosyltransferases that add sugars to a basic precursor substance on the RBC (see Fig. 5–3). A "donor" nucleotide derivative supplies the sugar that confers ABH specificity (Table 5–6). The formation of ABH antigens results from the interaction of ABO genes with several other separate, independent blood group systems. For example, the action of the H gene, which is inherited independently from the ABO genes, is intimately related to the formation of the ABH antigens. A, B, and H antigens are formed from the same basic precursor material, which is itself a genetic product. The basic material has a glycoprotein or glycolipid backbone (depending on whether an ABH red cell antigen or soluble substance is being produced) to which sugars are attached in response to specific enzyme tranferases elicited by an inherited gene. The ABH glycolipid antigens are built upon a common carbohydrate residue, which represents a paragloboside (**Color Plate** 3 and Fig. 5–4).

The precursor substance on erythrocytes is referred to as type 2. This means that the terminal galactose on the precursor substance is attached to the *N*-acetylglucosamine in a beta $-1 \rightarrow 4$ linkage (**Color Plate 6** and Fig. 5–5). A type 1 precursor substance, which will be discussed later, refers to a beta $1 \rightarrow 3$ linkage between galactose and *N*-acetylglucosamine.

### Interaction of Hh and ABO Genes

Inheritance of at least one H gene (genotype *HH* or *Hh*) elicits the production of an enzyme, α-2-L-fucosyltransferase, which transfers the sugar L-fucose from the GDP-Fuc (guanosine-diphosphate L-fucose) donor nucleotide to the terminal galactose of the precursor chain. The H gene, now known as the FUT 1 gene,[11] is present in greater than 99.99 percent of the random population. The allele of H, "h," is quite rare, and the genotype, *hh*, is extremely rare. This *hh* genotype, called the *Bombay phenotype,* lacks normal expression of the ABH antigens because α-2-L-fucosyltransferase is not produced. Even though Bombay (*hh*) individuals may inherit ABO genes, normal expression, as reflected in the formation of A, B, or H antigens, does not occur. (A discussion of the Bombay phenotype can be found later in this chapter.)

The H substance must be formed for the other sugars to be attached in response to an inherited A and/or B gene. Therefore, the Bombay phenotype is devoid of antigens of the ABO system. However, all individuals possess the H gene, in which H substance is formed first, with the subsequent attachment of other sugars,

**Table 5–4.** Summary of Forward and Reverse Groupings

| Patient | Patient's Cells Tested with | | Interpretation: Forward Group | Patient's Serum Tested with | | Interpretation: Reverse Group |
|---------|--------|--------|---------------------------------|----------|---------|---------------------------------|
| | Anti-A | Anti-B | | $A_1$ Cells | B Cells | |
| 1 | Negative | Negative | O | + | + | O |
| 2 | + | Negative | A | Negative | + | A |
| 3 | Negative | + | B | + | Negative | B |
| 4 | + | + | AB | Negative | Negative | AB |

**Table 5–5.** ABO Groups of the Offspring from the Various Possible ABO Matings

| Mating Phenotypes | Mating Genotypes | Offspring Possible Phenotypes (and Genotypes) |
|---|---|---|
| A × A | AA × AA | A (AA) |
| | AA × AO | A (AA or AO) |
| | AO × AO | A (AA or AO) or O (OO) |
| B × B | BB × BB | B (BB) |
| | BB × BO | B (BB or BO) |
| | BO × BO | B (BB or BO) or O (OO) |
| AB × AB | AB × AB | AB (AB) or A (AA) or B (BB) |
| O × O | OO × OO | O (OO) |
| A × B | AA × BB | AB (AB) |
| | AO × BB | AB (AB) or B (BO) |
| | AA × BO | AB (AB) or A (AO) |
| | AO × BO | AB (AB) or A (AO) or B (BO) or O (OO) |
| A × O | AA × OO | A (AO) |
| | AO × OO | A (AO) or O (OO) |
| A × AB | AA × AB | AB (AB) or A (AA) |
| | AO × AB | AB (AB) or A (AA or AO) or B (BO) |
| B × O | BB × OO | B (BO) |
| | BO × OO | B (BO) or O (OO) |
| B × AB | BB × AB | AB (AB) or B (BB) |
| | BO × AB | AB (AB) or B (BB or BO) or A (AO) |
| AB × O | AB × OO | A (AO) or B (BO) |

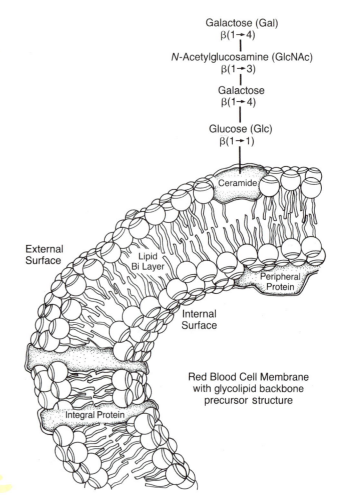

Galactose (Gal)
β(1→4)
|
N-Acetylglucosamine (GlcNAc)
β(1→3)
|
Galactose
β(1→4)
|
Glucose (Glc)
β(1→1)

**Figure 5–3.** Red blood cell precursor structure: lacto-N-neotetraosylceramide (a type-2 chain paragloboside).

depending on whether an A and/or B gene is inherited. The sugars that occupy the terminal positions of this precursor chain and confer blood group specificity are called the immunodominant sugars. Therefore, L-fucose is the sugar responsible for H specificity (blood group O) (**Color Plate 4** and Fig. 5–6).

The A allele codes for the production of α-3-N-acetylgalactosaminyltransferase, which transfers an N-acetyl-D-galactosamine (GalNAc) sugar from the UDP-GalNAc (uridine diphosphate-N-acetyl-D-galactose) donor nucleotide to the H substance. This sugar is responsible for A specificity (blood group A) (**Color Plate 5** and Fig. 5–7). The A-specific immunodominant sugar is linked to a type 2 chain glycolipid precursor that now contains H substance through the action of the H gene. Only type 2 paragloboside chains are found in the erythrocyte membrane being synthesized by the red cell precursors.

The A gene tends to elicit higher concentrations of transferase than the B gene. This leads to the conversion of practically all of the H antigen on the red cell to A antigen sites. As many as 810,000 to 1,170,000 antigen sites exist on an $A_1$ adult red cell in response to inherited genes.

The B allele codes for the production of α-3-D-galactosyltransferase, which transfers a D-galactose (Gal) sugar from the UDP-Gal (uridine diphosphate galactose) donor nucleotide to the H substance. This sugar is responsible for B specificity (blood group B) (**Color Plate 7** and Fig. 5–8). Anywhere from 610,000 to

**Table 5–6.** Donor Nucleotides and Immundominant Sugars Responsible for H, A, and B Antigen Specificities

| Gene | Glycosyltransferase | Nucleotide (Sugar Donor) | Immunodominant Sugar | Antigen |
|---|---|---|---|---|
| H | α-2-L-fucosyltransferase | GDP-Fuc | L-fucose | H |
| A | α-3-N-acetylgalactosaminyltransferase | UDP-GalNAc | N-acetyl-D-galactosamine | A |
| B | α-3-D-galactosyltransferase | UDP-Gal | D-galactose | B |

GDP-Fuc = guanosine-diphosphate L-fucose; UDP-GalNAc = uridine diphosphate-N-acetyl-D-galactose; UDP-Gal = uridine diphosphate galactose

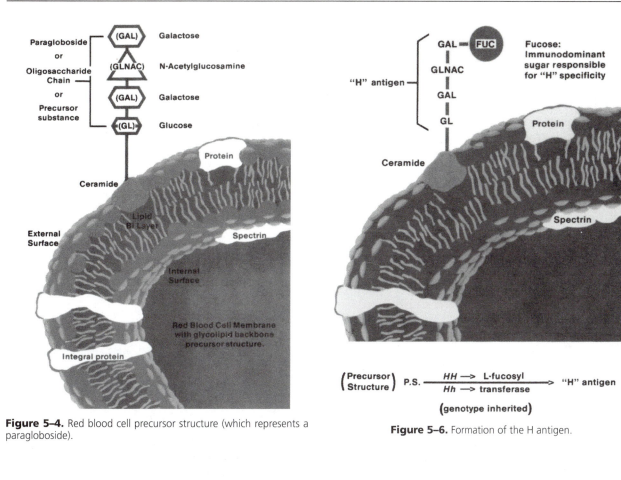

Paragloboside or Oligosaccharide Chain or Precursor substance

(GAL) — Galactose
(GLNAC) — N-Acetylglucosamine
(GAL) — Galactose
(GL) — Glucose

Protein
Ceramide
Lipid Bi Layer
External Surface
Spectrin
Internal Surface
Red Blood Cell Membrane with glycolipid backbone precursor structure.
Integral protein

**Figure 5–4.** Red blood cell precursor structure (which represents a paragloboside).

GAL — FUC
GLNAC
"H" antigen
GAL
GL

Fucose: Immunodominant sugar responsible for "H" specificity

Protein
Ceramide
Spectrin

$$\left(\begin{array}{c}\text{Precursor}\\\text{Structure}\end{array}\right) \text{P.S.} \xrightarrow[\displaystyle Hh \longrightarrow \text{ transferase}]{\displaystyle HH \longrightarrow \text{L-fucosyl}} \text{"H" antigen}$$

(genotype inherited)

**Figure 5–6.** Formation of the H antigen.

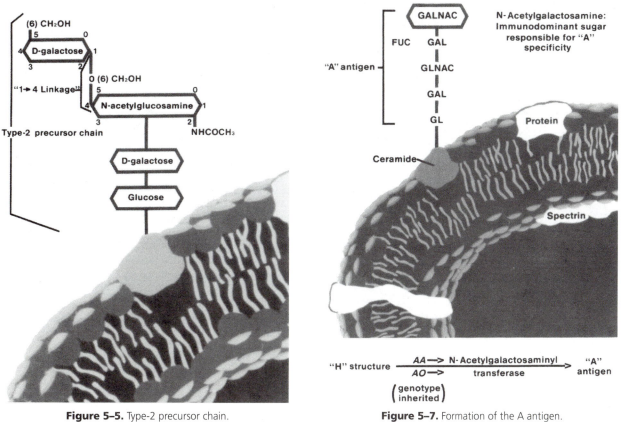

(6) CH₂OH
5        O
4  D-galactose  1
3        2
"1→4 Linkage"
O (6) CH₂OH
5        O
4  N-acetylglucosamine  1
3        2
NHCOCH₃
Type-2 precursor chain
D-galactose
Glucose

**Figure 5–5.** Type-2 precursor chain.

GALNAC
FUC   GAL
"A" antigen
GLNAC
GAL
GL

N-Acetylgalactosamine: Immunodominant sugar responsible for "A" specificity

Protein
Ceramide
Spectrin

$$\text{"H" structure} \xrightarrow[\displaystyle AO \longrightarrow]{\displaystyle AA \longrightarrow \text{N-Acetylgalactosaminyl transferase}} \text{"A" antigen}$$

$$\left(\begin{array}{c}\text{genotype}\\\text{inherited}\end{array}\right)$$

**Figure 5–7.** Formation of the A antigen.

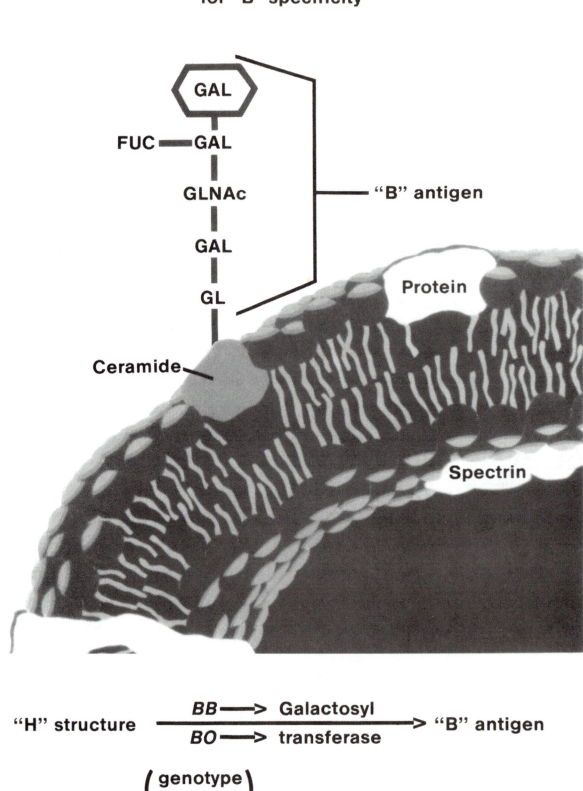

**D-Galactose:** Immunodominant sugar responsible for "B" specificity

"H" structure $\xrightarrow{\quad BB \longrightarrow Galactosyl \quad}$ "B" antigen
$\quad\quad\quad BO \longrightarrow transferase$

$\begin{pmatrix} \text{genotype} \\ \text{inherited} \end{pmatrix}$

**Figure 5–8.** Formation of the B antigen.

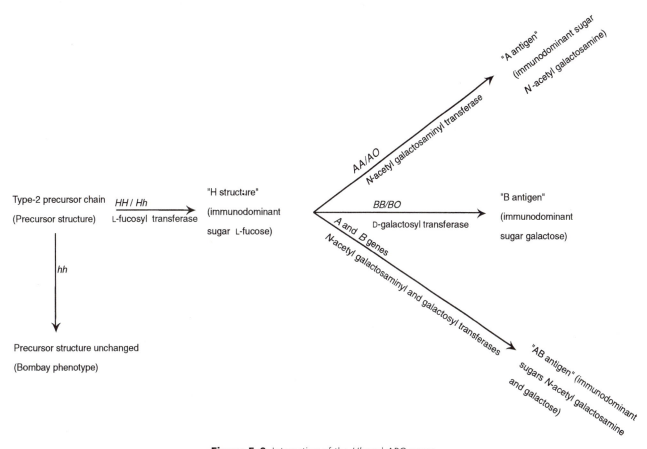

**Figure 5–9.** Interaction of the *Hh* and *ABO* genes.

830,000 B antigen sites exist on a B adult red cell in response to the conversion of the H antigen by the glycosyltransferase elicited by the B gene.

When both A and B genes are inherited, the B enzyme ($\alpha$-3-D-galactosyltransferase) seems to compete more efficiently for the H structure, and the A enzyme ($\alpha$-3-N-acetylgalactosaminyltransferase) is not as successful. Therefore, the average number of A antigens on an AB adult cell is approximately 600,000 sites, compared with an average of 720,000 B antigen sites.

The O allele at the ABO locus, which is sometimes referred to as an amorph, does not elicit the production of a catalytically active polypeptide, and therefore the H substance remains unmodified.[12] As a result, the O blood group has the highest concentration of H antigen. Interaction of the *Hh* and ABO genes is reviewed in Figure 5–9.

Studies at the molecular level using complementary DNA clones have revealed that the difference in the specificities of the A and B transferases may correspond to a difference in four amino acids between the A and B enzymes.[13] A and B alleles that result in subgroups may have additional point mutations that produce transferases that differ in their ability to convert H antigen to A or B antigen.[14] In addition, O genes were identified as having a single base deletion near the N terminus when compared with A genes. This deletion of a single DNA base pair creates a premature stop codon (three adjacent bases) resulting in an O-transferase, which is functionally inactive and incapable of modifying the H antigen. It is unlikely, therefore, that O individuals would express a protein that is immunologically related to that produced by either A or B transferases.[13] The O allele that results from a single nucleotide deletion causing a frame shift is known as O[1] variant and comprises 96 percent of all O alleles. An O[2] variant allele, in which inactivation arises from other mutations causing amino acid changes, makes up 4 percent of all O alleles. It has been suggested that other O variants will occur from inactivation of an A or B gene due to other mechanisms such as promoter inactivation and altered exon expression.[15]

The ABH antigens develop as early as the thirty-seventh day of fetal life but do not increase much in strength during the gestational period. Typically, ABH reactivity of the newborn erythrocyte is not as strong as that of the adult cell. The red cells of the newborn have been estimated to carry anywhere from 25 to 50 percent of the number of antigenic sites found on the adult red cell. In addition to age, the phenotypic expression of ABH antigens may vary with race, genetic interaction, and disease states. The genetic interaction of the ABO blood group system with the Lewis, Ii, and P blood groups is reflected in the synthesis of all these antigens by the sequential addition of sugar residues to a common precursor substance previously described for ABO (Fig. 5–10).

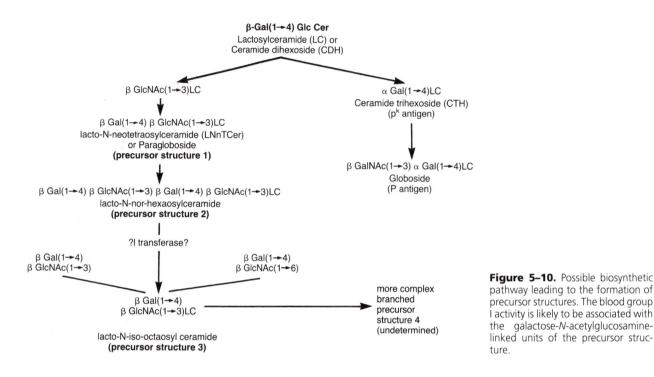

**Figure 5–10.** Possible biosynthetic pathway leading to the formation of precursor structures. The blood group I activity is likely to be associated with the galactose-*N*-acetylglucosamine-linked units of the precursor structure.

### Formation of A, B, and H Soluble Antigens

ABH antigens are present in all organs of the human body and thus are sometimes referred to as histoblood group antigens rather than blood group antigens.[7] ABH-soluble antigens can be synthesized and secreted by tissue cells. Therefore, ABH blood group–specific substances can be found in all the body secretions, and their presence is dependent on the ABO genes inherited as well as the inheritance of another set of genes (secretor genes) that regulate their formation. Approximately 78 percent of the random U.S. population has inherited the Se gene, possessing the genotype *SeSe* or *Sese.* This genotype is given the name *secretor.* The secreted A, B, and/or H antigens are glycoproteins, as opposed to glycolipids, on red blood cell surfaces. People who inherit the *sese* genotype are termed *nonsecretors.* The secretor gene (FUT 2) codes for the production of α-2-L-fucosyltransferase, which is expressed in tissues related to exocrine secretions (as opposed to the product of the H gene, which is expressed in mesodermal tissues such as red blood cells).[7,15] This transferase utilizes type 1 precursors to form type I H determinants, which are the major carriers of the ABH molecules in secretions.[12] The Se gene does not, however, affect the formation of A, B, or H antigens on the red cell and does not control the presence of A, B, or H transferases in hematopoietic tissue. In fact, A or B transferase enzymes, unlike A or B glycoprotein substances or antigens, are found in the secretions of $A_1$ or B individuals regardless of their secretor status. However, it is the presence of the Se-gene-specified α-2-L-fucosyltransferase that determines whether ABH-soluble substances will be secreted (**Color Plate 8** and Fig. 5–11).

### Distinction of A, B, and H Antigens and A, B, and H Soluble Substances

The formation of soluble A, B, and H substances is the same as that described for the formation of A, B, and H antigens on the red cells, except for a few minor distinctions:

1. The secreted substances are glycoproteins; the red cell antigens are glycolipids.
2. The first sugar in the common carbohydrate residue of the precursor substance is *N*-acetylgalactosamine for the glycoprotein secretions, and glucose for the red cell antigens. (review **Color Plates 3, 4, and 8** and Figures 5–4, 5–6, and 5–11).
3. Glycoproteins in secretions are primarily synthesized on type 1 precursor chains.[12] In the case of red cell ABH glycolipid antigens, only type 2 precursor chains are involved. Note that type 1 chain refers to a beta-1→3 linkage in which the number one carbon of the galactose is attached to the number three carbon of the *N*-acetylglucosamine sugar of the precursor substance, as opposed to a beta-1→4 linkage previously described for a type 2 chain.
4. α-2-L-fucosyltransferase produced by the *H* gene (FUT 1) is expressed mainly in the RBC lineage, whereas α-2-L-fucosyltransferase produced by the Se gene (FUT 2) is expressed in secretory tissues.

Tests for ABH secretion may establish the true ABO group of an individual whose red cell antigens are poorly developed. The demonstration of the A, B, and H substances in saliva is evidence for the inheritance of an A gene, a B gene, an H gene, and an Se gene. The term *secretor* refers only to secretion of A, B, or H soluble

**Genotype:** *Se  se*
     *AB*
     *HH*

**water-soluble secretions produced by tissue cells**

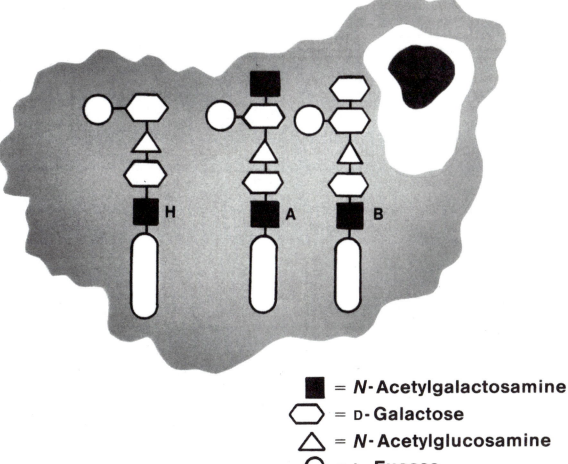

■ = *N*-Acetylgalactosamine
⬡ = D-Galactose
△ = *N*-Acetylglucosamine
○ = L-Fucose
⬭ = Protein backbone

**Figure 5–11.** Secretor ABH glycoprotein substances.

antigens in body fluids. The glycoprotein-soluble substances (or antigens) normally found in the saliva of secretors are listed in Table 5–7. The procedure for determination of secretor status can be found in the Procedural Appendix at the end of this chapter. Table 5–8 summarizes the body fluids in which ABH-soluble substances can be found.

## ABO SUBGROUPS

### A Subgroups

#### Basic Concepts

In 1911 von Dungern described two different A antigens based on reactions between group A RBCs and anti-A and anti-$A_1$ antisera. Group A red cells that react with both anti-A and anti-$A_1$ are classified as $A_1$ whereas those that react with anti-A and not anti-$A_1$ are classified as $A_2$ (Table 5–9).

Classification into $A_1$ and $A_2$ phenotypes accounts for 99 percent of all group A individuals. The cells of approximately 80 percent of all group A individuals are $A_1$, and the remaining 20 percent are $A_2$ or weaker subgroups. The difference between $A_1$ and $A_2$ is both quantitative and qualitative.

The production of both types of antigens is a result of an inherited gene at the ABO locus (Table 5–10). Inheritance of an $A_1$ gene elicits production of high concentrations of the enzyme $\alpha$-3-$N$-acetylgalactosaminyltransferase, which converts almost all of the H precursor structure to $A_1$ antigens on the red cells. $A_1$ is a very potent gene that creates from 810,000 to 1,170,000 $A_1$ antigen sites on the adult red cell. Inheritance of an $A_2$ gene results in the production of only 240,000 to

**Table 5–7.** ABH Substances in the Saliva of Secretors (SeSe or Sese)*

| ABO Group | Substances in Saliva | | |
|---|---|---|---|
| | A | B | H |
| O | None | None | ↑↑ |
| A | ↑↑ | None | ↑ |
| B | None | ↑↑ | ↑ |
| AB | ↑↑ | ↑↑ | ↑ |

*Nonsecretors (sese) have no ABH substances in saliva.
↑↑ and ↑, respectively, represent the concentration of ABH substances in saliva.

**Table 5–8.** Fluids in Which A, B, and H Substances Can Be Detected in Secretors

| | |
|---|---|
| Saliva | Milk |
| Tears | Amniotic fluid |
| Urine | Pathologic fluids: pleural, peritoneal, pericardial, |
| Digestive juices | ovarian cyst |
| Bile | |

**Table 5–9.** $A_1$ versus $A_2$ Phenotypes

| Blood Group | Reactions of Patient's Red Cells with | |
|---|---|---|
| | Anti-A (from B Sera) | Anti-$A_1$ Lectin |
| $A_1$ | + | + |
| $A_2$ | + | Negative |

**Table 5–10.** Additional ABO Genotypes, Phenotypes, and Frequencies

| Genotype | Phenotype | U.S. Frequencies | |
|---|---|---|---|
| | | Whites | Blacks |
| $A_1A_1$ | | | |
| $A_1A_2$ | $A_1$ | 33% | 19% |
| $A_1O$ | | | |
| $A_2A_2$ | $A_2$ | 7% | 5% |
| $A_2O$ | | | |
| $A_1B$ | $A_1B$ | 2% | 2% |
| $A_2B$ | $A_2B$ | 1% | 2% |

290,000 $A_2$ antigen sites on the adult $A_2$ red cell. The immunodominant sugar on both $A_1$ and $A_2$ RBCs is $N$-acetyl-$D$-galactosamine. These quantitative differences have been reflected not only in the number of antigen sites but also in the concentration of $\alpha$-3-$N$-acetyl-galactosaminyltransferase. Studies on the transferases from $A_1$ and $A_2$ individuals have demonstrated greater activity in the sera of $A_1$ individuals than in $A_2$ individuals as evidenced by their ability to convert group O cells to A cells.[16,17] Qualitative differences also exist, inasmuch as 1 to 8 percent of $A_2$ individuals produce anti-$A_1$ in their serum, and 25 percent of $A_2B$ individuals produce anti-$A_1$. In fact, some investigators have demonstrated that anti-$A_1$ can be found in the sera of all $A_2B$ individuals if sensitive enough techniques are utilized. Therefore, some subtle qualitative differences between $A_1$ and $A_2$ antigens must exist, even though the same immunodominant sugar is attached by the same transferase in each case. There must be some change in the antigenic structure, because the $A_2$ and $A_2B$ individuals cannot recognize the $A_1$ antigen as being part of their own red cell makeup and are immunologically stimulated to produce a specific $A_1$ antibody that does not cross-react with $A_2$ red cells.

It is generally presented, however, that $A_1$ has two antigens, A and $A_1$, whereas $A_2$ has only one, A antigen (**Color Plate 9A** and Fig. 5–12). However, to simplify the concept, one can think of $A_1$ as having only $A_1$ antigen sites and $A_2$ as having only A antigen sites. Serum from group B individuals contains two antibodies, anti-A and anti-$A_1$; therefore, this antibody mixture reacts with both $A_1$ and $A_2$ red cells. If serum from a group B individual is adsorbed with $A_2$ cells, the serum left after the cells and attached anti-A are removed by

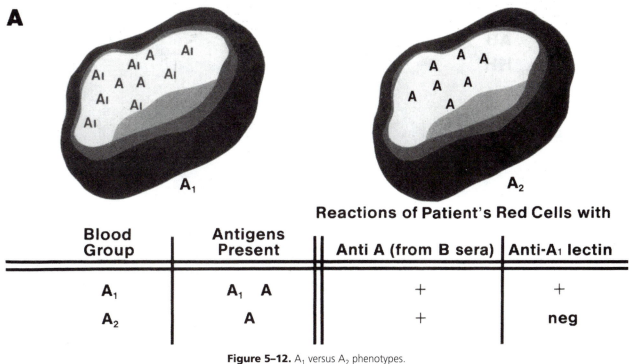

| Blood Group | Antigens Present | Reactions of Patient's Red Cells with | |
|---|---|---|---|
| | | Anti A (from B sera) | Anti-A₁ lectin |
| $A_1$ | $A_1$   A | + | + |
| $A_2$ | A | + | neg |

**Figure 5–12.** $A_1$ versus $A_2$ phenotypes.

centrifugation is referred to as *absorbed serum* (anti-$A_1$). This absorbed serum will react only with $A_1$ antigen sites. The seeds of the plant *Dolichos biflorus* serve as another source of anti-$A_1$, which is known as anti-$A_1$ lectin. Lectins are seed extracts that agglutinate human cells with some degree of specificity. This reagent agglutinates $A_1$ (or $A_1$B) cells but does not agglutinate $A_2$ (or $A_2$B cells) (**Color Plate 9B** and Fig. 5–13). Regardless of which conceptual presentation is used, the fact remains that group A red cells can be subdivided by the results of tests with anti-A (from B donor sera), and anti-$A_1$ (adsorbed serum or lectin). The characteristics of the $A_1$ and $A_2$ phenotypes are presented in Table 5–11.

Most group A infants appear to be $A_2$ at birth, inasmuch as ABH antigens are not fully developed on the red cells at this time. However, no difficulty is usually encountered in grouping cord red cells, inasmuch as most reagents contain potent anti-A and anti-A,B. Most cord $A_2$ cells will eventually group as $A_1$ after a given amount of time for development (usually a few months).

Group AB red cells also can be similarly classified into subgroups. To include these subgroups into the genetic pathways of the biosynthesis of ABH antigens, we must again start with the basic precursor substance. In the diagram in Figure 5–14, one can see that the H gene is necessary for the formation of the A, B, and H antigens. H antigen is found in greatest concentration on the red cells of group O individuals. Group $A_1$ individuals will not possess a great deal of H antigen because, in the presence of the $A_1$ gene, the pressure of the $A_1$ gene; almost all of the H antigen is converted to $A_1$ anti-

gen by placing the large *N*-acetyl-D-galactosamine sugar on the H substance. Because of the presence of so many $A_1$ antigens, the H antigen on $A_1$ and $A_1$B red cells may be hidden and therefore may not be available to react with anti-H antisera. In the presence of an $A_2$ gene, only some of the H antigen is converted to A antigens, and the remaining H antigen is detectable on the cell. Weak subgroups of the A antigen will often have a reciprocal relationship between the amount of H antigen on the RBC and the amount of A antigens formed (i.e., more A antigen formed, less H antigen expressed on the RBC). The H antigen on the RBCs of $A_1$ and $A_1$B individuals is so well hidden by *N*-acetyl-D-galactosamine that anti-H is occasionally found in the serum. This anti-H is a "naturally occurring" IgM cold agglutinin that reacts best below room temperature. As can be expected, this antibody is formed in response to a natural substance and reacts most strongly with cells of group O individuals (which have the greatest amount of H substance on their RBCs) and weakly with the RBCs of $A_1$B individuals (which contain small amounts of H substance). It is an insignificant antibody in terms of transfusion purposes, because it has no reactivity at 37°C, body temperature. However, high-titered anti-H may react at room temperature and present a problem in compatibility testing) (see Chap. 12). It can also be detected during antibody screening procedures, inasmuch as the reagent screening cells used are group O (see Chap. 11). However, because 80 percent of group A and AB donors are $A_1$ and $A_1$B, respectively, these blood types would probably be selected for the appropriate patient and thus be compatible with anti-H, if present, in the patient's serum.

**B**

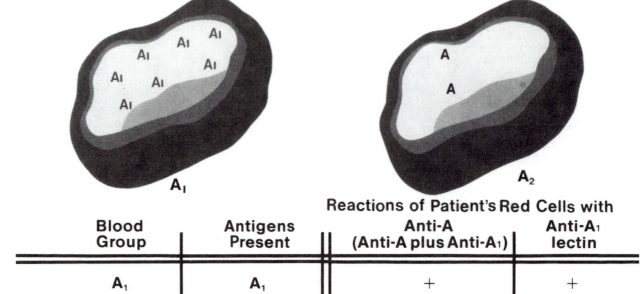

**Figure 5–13.** A$_1$ versus A$_2$ phenotypes (alternative conceptual presentation).

| Blood Group | Antigens Present | Reactions of Patient's Red Cells with | |
| :---: | :---: | :---: | :---: |
| | | Anti-A (Anti-A plus Anti-A$_1$) | Anti-A$_1$ lectin |
| A$_1$ | A$_1$ | + | + |
| A$_2$ | A | + | neg |

**Table 5–11.** Characteristics of A$_1$ and A$_2$ Phenotypes

| Phenotypes | Testing of Red Cells | | | | Naturally Occurring Antibodies in Serum | | Substances Present in Saliva of Secretors | Presence of a Transferase in Serum | Number of Antigen Sites per Red Cell $\times 10^3$ |
| :---: | :---: | :---: | :---: | :---: | :---: | :---: | :---: | :---: | :---: |
| | Anti-A | Anti-B | Anti-A,B | Anti-A$_1$ | Common | Unexpected | | | |
| A$_1$ | ++++ | 0 | ++++ | ++++ | Anti-B | None | A,H | Pos (pH = 6) | 810–1170 |
| A$_2$ | ++++ | 0 | ++++ | 0 | Anti-B | Anti-A$_1$ (1–8% of cases) | A,H | Pos (pH = 7) | 240–290 |

Anti-H lectin from the extract of *Ulex europaeus* closely parallels the reactions of human anti-H. Both antisera agglutinate red blood cells of group O and A$_2$ and react very weakly or not at all with groups A$_1$ and A$_1$B. Group B cells give reactions of variable strength (Fig. 5–15). Apparently the difference in the accessibility of the L-fucose sugar that determines H specificity contributes to the reactivity of anti-H among the various red cell ABO groups.

### Advanced Concepts

The discussion thus far has presented a basic overview of the two major ABO subgroups, A$_1$ and A$_2$. A more plausible, yet more detailed theory of ABO subgroups has been proposed by the identification of four different forms of H antigens, two of which are unbranched straight chains (H$_1$, H$_2$) and two of which are complex branched chains (H$_3$, H$_4$) (**Color** Plate 10 and Fig. 5–16). H$_1$ through H$_4$ correspond to the precursor structures on which the A enzyme can act to convert H antigen to blood group A active glycolipids. Although the chains differ in length and complexity of branching, the terminal sugars giving rise to their antigenic specificity are identical. Studies on the chemical and physical characteristics of the A$_1$ and A$_2$ enzyme transferases have demonstrated that these two enzymes are different qualitatively.[17,18] Straight chain H$_1$ and H$_2$ glycolipids can be converted to A$^a$ and A$^b$ antigens, respectively, by both A$_1$ and A$_2$ enzymes, with the A$_2$ enzyme being less efficient. The more complex branched H$_3$ and H$_4$ structures can be converted to A$^c$ and A$^d$ antigens by A$_1$ enzyme and only very poorly by A$_2$ enzyme. As a result, more unconverted H antigens (specifically H$_3$ and H$_4$) are available on group A$_2$ red cells, and only A$^a$ and A$^b$ A determinants are formed from H$_1$ and H$_2$ structures. In the red cells of some A$_2$ individuals, A$^c$ is extremely

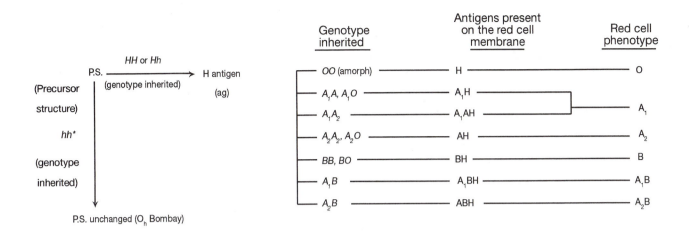

* Bombay individuals may inherit ABO genes (e.g., genotype *OO*, *A₁O*, *A₁A₂*,*A₁B*), but red blood cells are devoid of ABO antigen.

**Figure 5–14.** Summary of the genetic pathway for the biosynthesis of the ABH antigens.

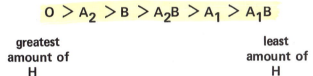

greatest
amount of
H

least
amount of
H

**Figure 5–15.** Reactivity of anti-H antisera or anti-H lectin with ABO blood groups.

low and $A^d$ is completely lacking (Table 5–12). It is feasible to expect that these are the individuals in whom one would find anti-A₁ in the serum. This anti-A₁ antibody could really be an antibody to $A^c$ and $A^d$ determinants, which these A₂ individuals lack. Also, in 22 to 35 percent of A₂B individuals, anti-A₁ can be found in the serum. Inasmuch as the B enzyme transferase is usually more efficient than the A enzyme in converting H structures to the appropriate antigen, A₂ enzymes would probably fail completely when paired with a B enzyme. As a result, A₂B individuals would be far more likely to lack $A^c$ and $A^d$ components, with subsequent production of anti-$A^c$ and anti-$A^d$ (anti-A₁).

As stated previously, most group A infants appear to be A₂ at birth, with subsequent development to A₁ a few months later. Newborn infants have been found to have a deficiency of the branched H₃ and H₄ antigens and, therefore, also the $A^c$ and $A^d$ antigens, possibly accounting for the A₂ phenotype. Adult cells contain a higher concentration of branched H₃ and H₄ structures and, therefore, $A^c$ and $A^d$ determinants of the A antigen in A₁ individuals.

## Weak A Subgroups

### Basic Concepts

Group A phenotypes demonstrating weaker serologic reactivity than A₂ are designated weak subgroups. These subgroups of A make up 1 percent of those encountered in the laboratory and therefore are mainly of academic interest. Reactivity with anti-H, as well as anti-A and anti-A,B, may be used to classify the weaker subgroups of A. In addition, the presence or absence of anti-A₁ in the serum as well as secretor studies and adsorption-elution tests can be utilized to subdivide A individuals into A₃, Aₓ, A_end, and so on (Table 5–13).

Occasionally weak subgroups of A may present practical problems if, for example, an Aₓ donor is mistyped as group O. This is potentially dangerous because the group O patient possesses anti-A,B, which agglutinates and lyses Aₓ red cells. Occasional problems also arise when A₂ or A₂B individuals demonstrate anti-A₁ in their serum. Because anti-A₁ is a naturally occurring IgM cold antibody, it is unlikely to cause a transfusion reaction, but it will be detected in the compatibility testing as well as in reverse grouping.

### Advanced Concepts

It is proposed that the majority of these weak A phenotypes result from expression of an alternate weak allele present at the ABO locus. Some very rare subgroups are hypothesized to be the result of modifying genes that regulate expression of ABO genes. Weak subgroup A alleles, when paired with an O gene, exhibit a dominant mode of inheritance, except in subgroup A_y,

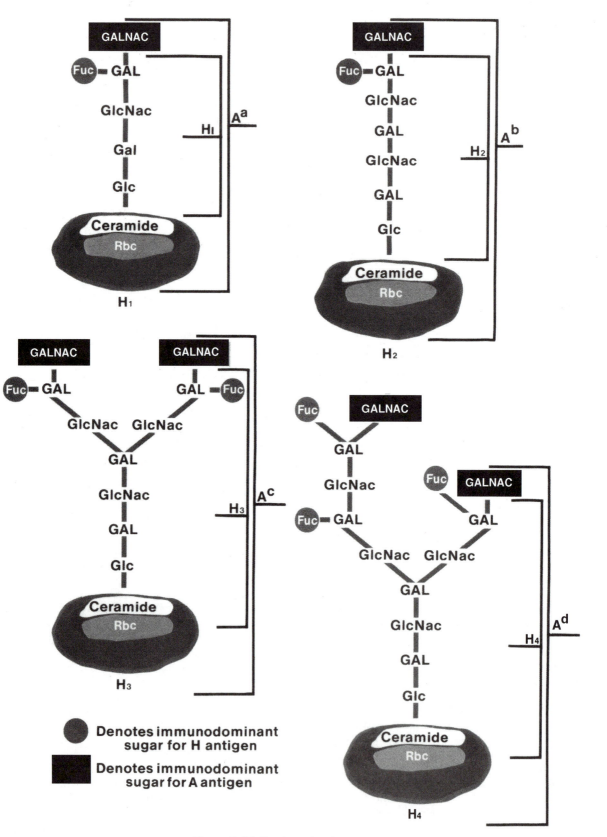

**Figure 5–16.** H-active antigenic structures.

**Table 5–12.** Structural Characteristics of $A_1$ and $A_2$ Red Cells

---

$A_2$ red cells: predominantly $A^a$ and $A^b$ and unconverted $H_3$ and $H_4$ antigen sites
$A_1$ red cells: $A^a$, $A^b$, $A^c$, and $A^d$ determinants and no unconverted $H_3$ and $H_4$ antigen sites

---

which is inherited in a recessive manner.[19] The rare phenotype $A_y$ apparently does not represent an alternate allele, because it is inherited in a recessive fashion and can be observed only in siblings. This observation suggests inheritance of a double dose of a recessive regulatory gene segregating independently of the ABO locus, which modifies expression of the inherited A gene.[18] Glycosyltransferase studies of gene products of these alternate alleles at the A locus have demonstrated evidence of heterogeneous enzymes in $A_3$ and $A_m$ subgroups and absence of transferase activity in the $A_{end}$ and $A_{el}$ subgroups.[20] It should be noted that there are still some reported A variants that do not fit into any of the weak subgroups described, alluding to existence of new alternate alleles or regulation by modifier genes.[18]

Weak A phenotypes can be serologically differentiated using the following techniques:

1. Forward grouping of A and H antigens with anti-A, anti-A,B, and anti-H
2. Serum grouping of ABO isoagglutinins and the presence of anti-$A_1$
3. Adsorption-elution tests with anti-A
4. Saliva studies to detect the presence of A and H substances

Additional special procedures such as serum glycosyltransferase studies for detection of A enzyme can be performed for differentiation of weak subgroups. Absence of a disease process should be confirmed before subgroup investigation, because ABH antigens are altered in various malignancies and other hematologic disorders. (A discussion of ABH Antigens/Antibodies in Disease can be found later in this chapter).

Weak A subgroups can be distinguished as $A_3$, $A_x$, $A_{end}$, $A_m$, $A_y$, and $A_{el}$, using the serologic techniques mentioned previously (see Table 5–13). The characteristics of each weak A subgroup are now presented.

**$A_3$.** $A_3$ red cells characteristically demonstrate a mixed-field pattern of agglutination with anti-A and anti-A,B reagents.[21] The estimated number of A antigen sites is approximately 30,000 per red cell.[18] Weak $\alpha$-3-N-acetylgalactosaminyltransferase activity is detectable in the serum. However, there appears to be a heterogeneity in the $A_3$ glycosyltransferases isolated from various $A_3$ phenotypes. Individuals tested were divided into three groups.[20] Group one consisted of $A_3$ phenotypes with low levels of detectable serum A enzyme, which had an optimal pH of approximately 7.0. Group two consisted of $A_3$ individuals with no detectable A enzyme. Group three consisted of an $A_3$ phenotype demonstrating a serum A enzyme level at 50 percent of the control level, and an optimal pH activity of 6.0. Additionally, serum from this $A_3$ individual in group three was capable of converting O red cells into A red cells.[20] $A_3$ enzyme is a product of an allele at the ABO locus inherited in a dominant manner. Anti-$A_1$ may be present in serum of $A_3$ individuals, and A substance is detected in the saliva of $A_3$ secretors.

**$A_x$.** $A_x$ red cells characteristically are not agglutinated by anti-A reagent but demonstrate weak agglutination with anti-A,B.[21] The estimated number of A antigen sites is approximately 4000 per red cell.[19] A very weak A enzyme has been detected in the serum of this subgroup, which represents the gene product of an alternate allele inherited in a dominant mode at the ABO locus.[20] In some rare exceptions, this mode of inheritance has been questioned. $A_x$ individuals almost always produce anti-$A_1$ in their serum. Routine secretor studies detect the presence of only H substance in $A_x$ secretors. However, $A_x$ secretors contain A substance detectable only by agglutination/inhibition studies using $A_x$ red cells as indicators.[19] Caution should be used in interpreting results of secretor studies using $A_x$ indicator cells and anti-A, because not all $A_x$ cells are agglutinated by anti-A.

**Table 5–13.** Characteristics of Weak ABO Phenotypes

| Phenotypes | Testing of Red Cells | | | | Naturally Occurring Antibodies in Serum | | Substances Present in Saliva of Secretors | Presence of A Transferase in Serum | Number of Antigen Sites per Red Cell $\times 10^3$ |
|---|---|---|---|---|---|---|---|---|---|
| | Anti-A | Anti-B | Anti-A,B | Anti-H | Common | Unexpected | | | |
| $A_3$ | ++mf | 0 | ++mf | +++ | Anti-B | Sometimes anti-$A_1$ | A, H | Weak pos | 30 |
| $A_x$ | wk/0 | 0 | ++ | ++++ | Anti-B | Almost always anti-$A_1$ | H | Very weak pos | 4 |
| $A_{end}$ | wk mf | 0 | wk mf | ++++ | Anti-B | Sometimes anti-$A_1$ | H | Neg | See text |
| $A_m$* | 0 | 0 | 0 | ++++ | Anti-B | No anti-$A_1$ | A, H | Pos (two types) | 0.2–1.9 |
| $A_y$* | 0 | 0 | 0 | ++++ | Anti-B | No anti-$A_1$ | A, H | Weak Pos | — |
| $A_{el}$* | 0 | 0 | 0 | ++++ | Anti-B | Usually anti-$A_1$ Sometimes anti-A also | H | Neg | 0.1–1.4 |

*A specificity demonstrated only by absorption/elution procedures.
mf = mixed-field agglutination; wk = weak; 0 = negative.

**A_end.** $A_{end}$ red cells characteristically demonstrate weak mixed-field agglutination with anti-A and anti-A,B, but only a very small percentage of the red cells ($\leq 10$ percent) agglutinate.[21] The estimated number of A antigen sites on the few agglutinable red cells is approximately 3500, whereas no detectable A antigens are demonstrated on red cells that do not agglutinate.[19] No A glycosyltransferase is detectable in the serum of $A_{end}$ individuals.[20] The $A_{end}$ phenotype is the expression of an A allele inherited in a dominant mode at the ABO locus. Secretor studies detect the presence of only H substance in the saliva of $A_{end}$ secretors. The phenotypes of $A_{finn}$ and $A_{bantu}$ are considered by some investigators to represent variants of the $A_{end}$ subgroup.[19]

**A_m.** $A_m$ red cells are characteristically unagglutinated by anti-A or anti-A,B. A strongly positive adsorption/elution of anti-A confirms the presence of A antigen sites. The estimated number of A antigen sites varies from 200 to 1900 per red cell in $A_m$ individuals.[19] An A enzyme of either the $A_1$ or $A_2$ type previously described is detectable in the serum of $A_m$ subgroups.[22] This $A_m$ enzyme is a product of an alternate allele at the ABO locus that is inherited in a dominant manner and results in the $A_m$ phenotype. These individuals usually do not produce anti-$A_1$ in their sera. A substance in normal quantities is easily detected in the saliva of $A_m$ secretors.

**A_y.** $A_y$ red cells are unagglutinated by anti-A or anti-A,B. Adsorption and elution of anti-A is the method used to confirm the presence of A antigens. Activity of eluates from $A_y$ red cells is characteristically weaker than that of eluates from $A_m$ red cells. Weak A glycosyltransferase is detectable in the serum of $A_y$ individuals, and saliva secretor studies demonstrate H and A substance, with A substance present in below normal quantities.[20] $A_y$ individuals usually do not produce anti-$A_1$. The $A_y$ phenotype can be observed in siblings, implicating a recessive mode of inheritance. This phenotype does not represent expression of an alternate allele at the ABO locus but suggests the action of a separate independent genetic system, designated Yy, regulating expression of the A gene. It is hypothesized that inheritance of a double dose of the recessive regulatory gene ($yy$) results in suppression of the A gene, leading to formation of the $A_y$ phenotype.[19]

**A_el.** $A_{el}$ red cells typically are unagglutinated by anti-A or anti-A,B. Often, adsorption and elution of anti-A is positive when monospecific anti-IgG antisera is used in indirect antiglobulin testing. No detectable A enzyme activity can be demonstrated in the serum of $A_{el}$ individuals by glycosyltransferase studies.[20] The $A_{el}$ phenotype is an expression of an alternate A allele at the ABO locus inherited in a dominant manner when paired with an O gene. $A_{el}$ individuals usually produce an anti-$A_1$ that is reactive with $A_1$ cells and sometimes produce anti-A, which agglutinates $A_2$ red cells.[19] Secretor studies demonstrate the presence of only H substance in the saliva of $A_{el}$ secretors.

A general flowchart for the process of elimination and identification of various subgroups is presented in Figure 5–17, with the assumption that the patient's medical history (e.g., recent transfusion, disease states) has been investigated and excluded as a source of discrepancy.

## B Subgroups

### Advanced Concepts

The *B* gene codes for an $\alpha$-3-D-galactosyltransferase, which transfers a galactose sugar to the H antigen previously formed. Isoelectric focusing of group B serum has demonstrated two B enzyme activities, one with an isoelectric point (pI) equal to 4.8 to 5.2 and the other with a pI of 8.2 to 8.8.[23] Activity of both enzymes in

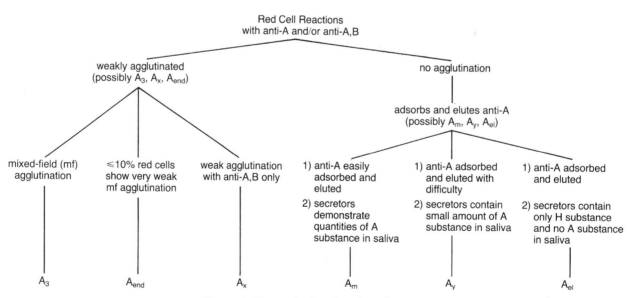

**Figure 5–17.** Investigation of weak A subgroups.

serum is optimum at pH 6.5 and requires the presence of the metallic cofactor $Mn^{2+}$. Both B-glycosyltransferases are specific for the same nucleotide sugar donor (UDP-Gal) and transfer the same immunodominant sugar, D-galactose, to confer B specificity. As a result of the four types of H substrate available to B-glycosyltransferases, four types of B antigenic structures are possible, as previously described for the A blood groups. These B antigens are designated $B_I$, $B_{II}$, $B_{III}$, and $B_{IV}$ with the addition of D-galactose to the respective H glycolipid variant.[24] Only $B_I$ and $B_{II}$ glycolipid variants have been isolated and characterized. $B_{III}$ and $B_{IV}$ structures remain to be isolated and characterized from red blood cells but are considered to be branched structures inasmuch as they are built upon $H_3$ and $H_4$ glycolipids.[24]

## Weak B Subgroups

### Basic Concepts

Subgroups of B are very rare and are less frequent than A subgroups. Red cells demonstrating serologic activity that is weaker than normal are designated weak B phenotypes or B subgroups and include $B_3$, $B_x$, $B_m$, and $B_{el}$ phenotypes[19] (Table 5–14). There are no B subgroups reported that are equivalent to $A_{end}$ or $A_y$. A classification system similar to A subgroups has been used because of common serologic characteristics. Subgroups of B are usually recognized by variations in the strength of the reaction using anti-B and anti-A,B.

### Advanced Concepts

Inheritance of B subgroups, similar to that of the majority of A subgroups, is considered to be a result of alternate alleles at the B locus. Criteria used for differentiation of weak B phenotypes include the following:

1. Strength/type of agglutination with anti-B, anti-A,B, and anti-H
2. Presence or absence of ABO isoagglutinins in the serum
3. Adsorption-elution studies with anti-B
4. Presence of B substance in saliva

These serologic techniques can be used to characterize B subgroups in the following manner.

**$B_3$.** A mixed-field pattern and rapid agglutination are the typical reaction of the $B_3$ phenotype with anti-B reagent.[21] B glycosyltransferase is present in the serum of these individuals, but enzyme activity varies from 10 to 100 percent of control levels.[19] This variability suggests heterogeneity of B enzyme in $B_3$ individuals, which is characteristic also for the subgroup $A_3$. Anti-B is absent in the serum of $B_3$ phenotypes, but B substance is present in normal amounts in the saliva of secretors. The $B_3$ subgroup is the most frequent weak B phenotype.[19]

**$B_x$.** $B_x$ red cells typically demonstrate weak agglutination with anti-B antisera without mixed-field agglutination, although some examples of red cells may not agglutinate at all.[18] Similar to the $A_x$ phenotype, $B_x$ erythrocytes agglutinate stronger with anti-A,B than with anti-B.[21] B glycosyltransferase has not been detected in the serum of $B_x$ phenotypes, but a weakly reactive anti-B usually is produced.[19] $B_x$ red cells readily adsorb and elute anti-B. Secretor studies demonstrate large amounts of H substance, but B substance is undetectable using group B indicator red cells. When $B_x$ indicator red cells are used, a weak B substance can be detected in secretor studies.[19]

**$B_m$.** $B_m$ red cells characteristically are unagglutinated by anti-B or anti-A,B. The $B_m$ red cells easily adsorb and elute anti-B. B glycosyltransferase is present in the serum of $B_m$ phenotypes but is usually lower in activity and varies from individual to individual.[25]

Reduced activity of B enzyme in hematopoietic tissue is clearly the defect causing the formation of the $B_m$ subgroup, inasmuch as normal B plasma incubated with $B_m$ red cells and UDP-galactose transforms them into a normal group B phenotype. Anti-B is not characteristically present in the serum of $B_m$ individuals. Normal quantities of H and B substance are found in the saliva of $B_m$ secretors.

The $B_m$ phenotype is usually the result of inheritance of a rare allele at the ABO locus, although the subgroup $B_m$ may be the product of an interacting modifying gene linked closely to the ABO locus.[25] This modifier gene may depress expression of the B gene, resulting in

**Table 5–14.** Characteristics of B Phenotypes

| Phenotypes | Testing of Red Cells | | | | Naturally Occurring Antibodies in Serum | | Substances Present in Saliva of Secretors | Presence of a B Transferase in Serum |
|---|---|---|---|---|---|---|---|---|
| | Anti-A | Anti-B | Anti-A,B | Anti-H | Common | Unexpected | | |
| B | 0 | ++++ | ++++ | ++ | Anti-A | None | B, H | Pos (normal amount) |
| $B_3$ | 0 | mf++ | ++mf | +++ | Anti-A | None | B, H | Wk pos |
| $B_x$ | 0 | wk/0 | + | +++ | Anti-A | Weak anti-B | H | Neg |
| $B_m$* | 0 | 0 | 0 | +++ | Anti-A | None | B, H | Wk pos |
| $B_{el}$* | 0 | 0 | 0 | +++ | Anti-A | Sometimes a weak anti-B | H | Neg |

*B specificity demonstrated only by absorption/elution procedures.
mf = mixed-field; wk = weak; 0 = negative.

decreased B enzyme activity.[25] The $B_m$ subgroup is reported to be more frequent in Japan.[19]

**$B_{el}$.** $B_{el}$ red cells are unagglutinated by anti-B or anti-A,B. This extremely rare phenotype must be determined by adsorption and elution of anti-B. No B glycosyltransferase has been identified in the serum of B individuals. A weak anti-B may be present in the serum of this subgroup. Only H substance is demonstrated in saliva of $B_{el}$ secretors.

Other weak B phenotypes have been reported that do not possess the appropriate characteristics for classification into one of the groups previously discussed.[26] These may represent new classifications and new representations of ABO polymorphism.

## THE BOMBAY PHENOTYPES ($O_h$)

### Basic Concepts

The H gene appears to be necessary for the formation of A and B antigens (see Figure 5–14). It is very common; 99.99 percent of all individuals have an *HH* or *Hh* genotype. The h allele is very rare and does not produce the α-2-L-fucosyltransferase necessary for formation of the H structure. The genotype *hh* or $H_{null}$ is extremely rare and is known as the Bombay phenotype, or $O_h$.

Bombay cells cannot be converted to group A or B by the specific transferases. This supports the concept that the H structure serves as the acceptor molecule or precursor substance for the product of the A or B gene-specified transferases. The Bombay phenotype was first reported by Bhende in 1952 in Bombay, India. More than 130 Bombay phenotypes have now been reported in various parts of the world. These red cells are devoid of normal ABH antigens. The Bombay red cells fail to react with anti-A, anti-B, and anti-H. Bombay serum contains anti-A, anti-B, anti-A,B, and anti-H. Unlike the anti-H found occasionally in the serum of $A_1$ and $A_1B$ individuals, the Bombay anti-H can often be potent and reacts strongly at 37°C. It is an IgM antibody that can bind complement and cause red cell lysis. Because the H antigen is common to all ABO blood groups, Bombay blood is incompatible with that of all ABO donors. In routine forward grouping, using anti-A and anti-B, the Bombay would phenotype as an O

blood group. However, the red cells of the Bombay phenotype ($O_h$) do not react with the anti-H lectin (*U. europaeus*), unlike those of the normal group O individual, which react strongly with anti-H lectin. Transfusing normal group O blood (with the highest concentration of H antigen) to a Bombay recipient would cause immediate cell lysis by the anti-H in the serum. Therefore, only blood from another Bombay individual will be compatible and can be transfused to a Bombay recipient. Table 5–15 lists the general characteristics of Bombay phenotypes. Inheritance of the genotype *hh* usually occurs in children of consanguineous marriages. When family studies demonstrate which ABO genes are inherited in the Bombay phenotype, the genes are written as superscripts ($O_h^A$, $O_h^B$, $O_h^{AB}$). The serum of Bombay individuals who are genetically A and/or B contains the specific A and/or B transferases, demonstrated by the ability of the Bombay serum to convert group O cells to A or B.

### Advanced Concepts

The Bombay phenotype has now been classified into different categories.

#### Category 1: Classical Bombay

These cells lack H antigen (genotype *hh*) and react stronger with examples of anti-I. This phenomenon gives credence to the theory that I antigen is a precursor to H antigen and A and B antigens. ABH substance is absent in saliva. If a person inherited normal A and/or B genes, the respective enzymes could be detected and the person would be designated $O_h^A$, $O_h^B$, $O_h^{AB}$.

#### Category 2: Para-Bombay

Red cells of these individuals express weak forms of A and B, which are primarily detected by adsorption and elution studies. If a person is genetically A or B, the respective enzymes can be detected, but no H enzyme is detectable, even though it has been shown that there is limited production of H antigen on the RBC.[11,27] It is postulated that homozygous inheritance of a mutant FUT 1 gene codes for the production of low levels of H transferase activity. The small amount of H substance on the RBC is completely used by the A and/or B trans-

---

**Table 5–15.** General Characteristics of Bombay $O_h$ ($H_{null}$) Phenotypes

1. Absence of H, A, and B antigens; no agglutination with anti-A, anti-B, or anti-H lectin
2. Presence of anti-A, anti-B, anti-A,B and a potent wide thermal range of anti-H in the serum
3. A, B, H nonsecretor (no A, B, or H substances present in saliva)
4. Absence of α-2-L-fucosyltransferase (H enzyme) in serum and H antigen on red cells
5. Presence of A or B enzymes in serum
6. Strong reactivity with anti-I reagents (possibly owing to an increase in number of I receptors)
7. A recessive mode of inheritance (identical phenotypes in children but not in parents)
8. Red cells of the Bombay phenotype ($O_h$) will not react with the anti-H lectin (*Ulex europaeus*)
9. Red cells of the Bombay phenotype ($O_h$) are compatible *only* with the serum from another Bombay individual

ferase present. This results in small quantities of A and/or B antigen being present on the RBC with no detectable H antigen. ABH substance is absent in the saliva. The anti-H present in the serum is weaker in reactivity than the anti-H found in the classical Bombay phenotype, although it may be active at 37°C.[11] These individuals are designated $A_h$, $B_h$, or $AB_h$.[11,28]

Two other categories of H-deficient phenotypes are described in the literature as Bombay-like secretors. It appears that this H-deficient phenotype can arise through both autosomal-dominant and autosomal-recessive modes of inheritance. In the dominant form of this phenotype, weak expressions of A, B, and H antigens can be detected on the RBCs along with their corresponding enzymes. Normal levels of ABH substances are present in the saliva. The recessive form of the phenotype fails to express A, B, and H antigens on the RBC, yet normal ABH substances are present in secretions. Table 5–16 summarizes the various Bombay classifications.

## ABH ANTIGENS/ANTIBODIES IN DISEASE

Associations between ABH antigens and practically any disorder known to man can be found throughout medical literature. Even more profound are the associations of blood group specificity and such things as a more pronounced "hangover" in A blood groups, criminality in group B blood groups, and good teeth in group O individuals. There are also several papers correlating blood groups with personality traits. It is no surprise that many scientists refer to these associations as a part of blood group mythology. However, more relevant associations between blood groups and disease are important to the blood banker in terms of blood group serology.

Various disease states seem to alter red cell antigens and result in progressively weaker reactions or additional acquired "pseudoantigens" during forward grouping. Leukemia, chromosome 9 translocations, and any disease inducing stress hematopoiesis (e.g., thalassemia)[29] have been shown to depress antigen strength. Often the cells appear to be a mixed-field agglutination (tiny agglutinates in a sea of unagglutinated cells). These weakened A or B antigens may demonstrate the type of serologic reactions shown in Table 5–17.

The weakening of the antigen tends to follow the course of the disease. The antigen strength will increase again as the patient enters into remission. The isoagglutinins (anti-A, anti-B, or anti-A,B) may also be weak or absent in those leukemias demonstrating hypogammaglobulinemia, such as chronic lymphocytic leukemia (CLL). Various lymphomas, such as the malignant (non-Hodgkin's) variety, may yield weak isoagglutinins owing to moderate decreases in the gamma globulin fraction. Also, immunodeficiency diseases, such as congenital agammaglobulinemia, also yield weak or absent isoagglutinins. If this problem is suspected, a simple serum protein electrophoresis will confirm or rule out this condition. Hodgkin's disease

**Table 5–16.** Characteristics Reported or Postulated for Categories of H-Deficient Phenotypes (Bombays)

| Classification | Proposed Genes Inherited | Glycosyltransferase[¶] | Red Cell Antigens: A, B, and H Detected | A, B, and H Soluble Substances in Secretions | Antibodies in Serum |
|---|---|---|---|---|---|
| 1. Classical Bombay $O_h$, $O_h^B$, $O_h^A$, $O_h^{AB}$ | hh sese | None or A and/or B[†] in serum or red cell stroma | None detectable | None detectable | Anti-A, anti-B, anti-H |
| 2. Para-Bombay $A_h$, $B_h$, $AB_h$ | A and/or B[†] hh[*] sese | A and/or B[†] in serum and red cell stroma | Weak A/B[†] Residual H when A or B immuno-dominant sugar is removed with appropriate enzymes | None detectable | Anti-A/anti-B[†] Weak anti-IH or anti-H |
| 3. $O_m^h$ or $O_{Hm}$ Bombay | Se | A and/or B[†] in serum/red cells | None | H substance (normal amounts) | Weak IH or anti-H[‡] |
| 4. $H_m$ Bombay[§] $H_m$, $A_{Hm}$, $B_{Hm}$, $AB_{Hm}$ | Se | H in serum and red cell stroma (normal activity); A and/or B[†] in serum and red cell stroma (normal activity) | Weak A/B[†] and H | H substance A/B[†] (all normal amounts) | Anti-A/anti-B[†] Anti-A/anti-B[†] |

* = Weak variant present at the Hh locus.
† = Dependent on ABO genotype.
‡ = Majority of cases.
§ = One family reported.
¶ = Refer to Figure 5–9.

**Table 5–17.** Serologic Reactions Typical of Leukemia

| Patient Phenotype | Forward Grouping Reaction of Patient Cells with | | | Reverse Grouping Reaction of Patient Serum with | |
| --- | --- | --- | --- | --- | --- |
| | Anti-A | Anti-B | Anti-A,B | A₁ Cells | B Cells |
| A | + mf | Neg | ++ mf | Neg | +++ |
| B | Neg | ±/+ | + | ++++ | Neg |
| | | | Patient diagnosis: leukemia | | |

mf = mixed field.

has also been reported to weaken or depress ABH red cell antigens, resulting in variable reactions during forward grouping similar to those found in leukemia.

The very young and elderly populations also have weak expression of the ABO isoagglutinins. In the elderly patient, the production of immunoglobulin is depressed. In the infant patient, the production of ABO isoagglutinins is not detectable until 3 to 6 months of age. Also, A antigen production is not fully complete at birth, and newborn cells appear as subgroup A₂. Discrepancies in the reverse grouping are thus observed even in the absence of a disease state.

Individuals with intestinal obstruction, carcinoma of the colon or rectum, or other disorders of the lower intestinal tract may have increased permeability of the intestinal wall, which allows passage of the bacterial polysaccharides from *Escherichia coli* serotype O₈₆ into the patient's circulation. This results in the "acquired B" phenomenon in group A₁ individuals. The patient's group A red cells absorb the B-like polysaccharide, which reacts with anti-B.

A lack of detectable ABO antigens can occur in patients with carcinoma of the stomach or pancreas. The patient's red cell antigens have not been changed, but the serum contains excessive amounts of blood group–specific soluble substances (BGSS) that neutralize the antisera used in the forward grouping.

All these disease states previously mentioned result in discrepancies between the forward and reverse groupings, indicating that the patient's red cell group is not what it seems. All ABO discrepancies must be resolved before blood is released for that patient. In some cases secretor studies may help confirm the patient's true ABO group.

## ABO DISCREPANCIES

ABO discrepancies occur when the expected two positive and two negative reactions are not observed and are usually technical in nature. Some of the more common causes of technical errors leading to ABO discrepancies in the forward and reverse groupings are listed in Table 5–18. ABO discrepancies can usually be resolved by repeating the test on the same sample using a saline suspension of red blood cells if the initial test was performed using RBCs suspended in serum or

**Table 5–18.** Common Sources of Technical Errors Resulting in ABO Discrepancies

1. Inadequate identification of blood specimens, test tubes, or slides
2. Cell suspension either too heavy or too light
3. Clerical errors
4. A mix-up in samples
5. Missed observation of hemolysis
6. Failure to add reagents
7. Failure to follow manufacturer's instructions
8. Uncalibrated centrifuge
9. Contaminated reagents
10. Warming during centrifugation

plasma. It is important to make sure that any and all technical factors that may have given rise to the ABO discrepancy have been reviewed and corrected and to acquire essential information regarding the patient's age, diagnosis, transfusion history, medications, immunoglobulin levels (if determined), and history of pregnancy. If the discrepancy persists, a new sample can be procured from the patient and the test can be repeated. ABO discrepancies may be arbitrarily divided into four major categories.

### Group I Discrepancies

Group I discrepancies are between forward and reverse groupings because of weakly reacting or missing antibodies. These discrepancies are more common than those in the other groups listed. When a reaction in the reverse grouping is weak or missing, a group I discrepancy should be suspected because, normally, forward and reverse grouping reactions are very strong (4+). The reason for the missing or weak isoagglutinins is that the patient has depressed antibody production or cannot produce the ABO antibodies. Some of the more common populations with discrepancies in this group are:

- Newborns
- Elderly patients
- Patients with leukemias demonstrating hypogammaglobulinemia (e.g., CLL)
- Patients with lymphomas demonstrating hypogammaglobulinemia (e.g., malignant lymphomas)
- Patients using immunosuppressive drugs that yield hypogammaglobulinemia

**Table 5–19.** Example of ABO Discrepancy Seen with Weak or Missing Antibodies

| | Forward Grouping Reaction of Patient's Cells with | | | Reverse Grouping Reaction of Patient's Serum with | |
| --- | --- | --- | --- | --- | --- |
| | Anti-A | Anti-B | Anti-A,B | A₁ Cells | B Cells |
| Patient | Neg | +++ | ++++ | Neg | Neg |
| | Patient's probable group: B (elderly patient) | | | | |

- Patients with congenital agammaglobulinemia
- Patients with immunodeficiency diseases
- Patients with bone marrow transplantations (patients develop hypogammaglobulinemia from therapy and start producing a different red cell population from the transplanted bone marrow)

### Resolution of Common Group I Discrepancies

The best way to resolve this discrepancy is to enhance the reverse group reaction by incubating the patient serum with reagent A₁ and B cells at room temperature for approximately 15 to 30 minutes. If there is still no reaction, the serum-cell mixtures can be incubated at 4°C for 15 to 30 minutes. An auto-control and an O cell control must always be tested concurrently with the reverse typing when trying to solve the discrepancy, because the lower temperature of testing will most likely enhance the reactivity of other commonly occurring cold agglutinins, such as anti-I, that react with all adult red blood cells. Table 5–19 shows a type of discrepancy that may be seen with weak or missing antibodies.

### Rare Group I Discrepancies

Chimerism, as illustrated in Figure 5–18, is a rare cause of a weak or missing ABO isoagglutinin. *Chimerism* is defined as the presence of two cell populations in a single individual. Detecting a separate cell population may be easy or difficult, depending on what percentage of cells of the minor population is present. Reactions from chimerism are typically mixed field. True chimerism is rarely found and occurs in twins, in whom two cell populations will exist through the life of the individual. In utero exchange of blood occurs because of vascular anastomosis. As a result, two cell populations

emerge, both of which are recognized as self, and the individuals do not make anti-A or anti-B. Therefore, no detectable isoagglutinins are present in the reverse grouping. If the patient or donor has no history of a twin, then the chimera may be due to dispermy (two sperm fertilizing one egg) and indicates mosaicism. More commonly, artificial chimeras occur, which yield mixed cell populations as a result of: (1) blood transfusions (e.g., group O cells given to an A or B patient); (2) transplanted bone marrows; (3) exchange transfusions; and (4) fetal-maternal bleeding.

### Group II Discrepancies

These discrepancies are between forward and reverse groupings because of weakly reacting or missing antigens. This group of discrepancies is probably the least frequently encountered. Some of the causes of discrepancies in this group include:

Subgroups of A and/or subgroups of B may be present (see the section on ABO subgroups)

Leukemias may yield weakened A or B antigens (see Table 5–17)

Hodgkin's disease has been reported in some cases to mimic the depression of antigens found in leukemia

Excess amounts of blood group–specific soluble substances (BGSS) present in the plasma in association with certain diseases, such as carcinoma of the stomach and pancreas

"Acquired B" phenomenon is most often associated with intestinal obstruction or malignancy of the stomach or intestine (Table 5–20)

Antibodies to low-incidence antigens in reagent anti-A or anti-B (Table 5–21)

### Resolution of Group II Discrepancies

The reaction of weakly reactive antigens with their respective antisera can be enhanced by incubating the test mixture at room temperature for up to 30 minutes to increase the association of antibody with antigen. If negative, reduce the temperature to 4°C. Include group O and autologous cells as controls. Red blood cells can also be pretreated with enzymes and retested with reagent antisera.

Excess amounts of BGSS will neutralize the reagent anti-A or anti-B, leaving no unbound antibody to react

| | Anti-A | Anti-B | Anti-A,B | A₁ | B | | |
| --- | --- | --- | --- | --- | --- | --- | --- |
| Pt. 1 | 0 | 2+MF | 2+MF | 4+ | 0 | Twin 1 | 70% B |
| | | | | | | | 30% 0 |
| Pt. 2 | 0 | +Wk | +Wk | 4+ | 0 | Twin 2 | 30% B |
| | | | | | | | 70% 0 |

**Figure 5–18.** Patients 1 and 2 are examples of chimera twins.

**Table 5–20.** Example of ABO Discrepancy Caused by an Acquired B Antigen

| | Forward Grouping Reaction of Patient's Cells with | | | Reverse Grouping Reaction of Patient's Serum with | |
| --- | --- | --- | --- | --- | --- |
| | Anti-A | Anti-B | Anti-A,B | A₁ Cells | B Cells |
| Patient | ++++ | ++ | ++++ | Neg | ++++ |
| | | | Patient's probable group: A | | |

**Table 5–21.** Example of ABO Discrepancy Caused by Low-Incidence Antibodies in the Reagent Antisera

| | Forward Grouping Reaction of Patient's Cells with | | | Reverse Grouping Reaction of Patient's Serum with | |
| --- | --- | --- | --- | --- | --- |
| | Anti-A | Anti-B | Anti-A,B | A₁ Cells | B Cells |
| Patient | ++++ | + | ++++ | Neg | ++++ |
| | | | Patient's probable group: A | | |

with the patient cells. This yields a false-negative or weak reaction in the forward grouping. Washing the patient cells free of the BGSS with saline should alleviate the problem, resulting in correlating forward and reverse groupings.

The acquired B antigen arises when bacterial enzymes modify the immunodominant blood group A sugar (N-acetyl-D-galactosamine) into D-galactosamine, which is sufficiently similar to the immunodominant blood group B sugar (D-galactose) to cross-react with anti-B antisera. This pseudo-B antigen is formed at the expense of the A₁ antigen and disappears after recovery.[30] The reaction of the appropriate antiserum with these acquired antigens demonstrates a weak reaction, often yielding a mixed-field appearance. There has been an increased incidence in the detection of acquired B in the clinical laboratory as a result of the use of monoclonal anti-B reagents containing ES4 clone, with the strongest reactions associated with those reagents that have a higher pH value.[30] Testing the patient's serum or plasma against autologous red blood cells gives a negative reaction because the anti-B in the serum does not agglutinate autologous RBCs with the acquired B antigen. The acquired-B antigen is also not agglutinated when reacted with anti-B that has a pH greater than 8.5 or less than 6.0.[31] Secretor studies can be performed when trying to characterize the acquired-B phenomenon. If the patient is in fact a secretor, only A substance is secreted in the acquired-B phenomenon. *Bandeiraea simplicifolia II* (BSII) strongly agglutinates acquired-B cells that have been enzyme pretreated.[31] The discovery of the molecular genetics of glycosyltransferases provides an additional approach to the diagnosis of acquired-B status. Because these individuals are genetically blood group A, the B transferase activity will be absent.[32]

Treating RBCs with acetic anhydride reacetylates the surface molecules, then markedly decreases the reactivity of the cells when tested against anti-B. The reactivity of normal B cells is not affected by treatment with acetic anhydride.[14]

It is impossible for manufacturers to screen reagent antisera against all known red cell antigens. It has been reported (although rarely) that this additional antibody in the reagent antisera has reacted with the corresponding low-incidence antigen present on the patient's red cell. This gives an unexpected reaction of the patient's cells with anti-A or anti-B, or both, mimicking the presence of a weak antigen. The best way to resolve this discrepancy is by repeating the forward type, using antisera with a different lot number. If the cause of the discrepancy is a low-incidence antibody in the reagent antisera reacting with a low-incidence antigen on the patient's cells, the chances are that the antibody will not be present in a different lot number of reagent.

## Group III Discrepancies

These discrepancies are between forward and reverse groupings caused by protein or plasma abnormalities and result in rouleaux formation (Table 5–22), or pseudoagglutination, attributable to:

Elevated levels of globulin from certain disease states, such as multiple myeloma, Waldenström's macroglobulinemia, other plasma cell dyscrasias, and certain moderately advanced cases of Hodgkin's lymphomas

Elevated levels of fibrinogen

Plasma expanders, such as dextran and polyvinylpyrrolidone (PVP)

Wharton's jelly

**Table 5–22.** Example of ABO Discrepancy Caused by Rouleaux Formation

| | Forward Grouping Reaction of Patient's Cells with | | | Reverse Grouping Reaction of Patient's Serum with | |
| --- | --- | --- | --- | --- | --- |
| | Anti-A | Anti-B | Anti-A,B | A₁ Cells | B Cells |
| Patient | ++++ | ++ | ++++ | ++ | ++++ |
| | | | Patient's probable group: A | | |

## Resolution of Group III Discrepancies

Rouleaux, or a stacking of erythrocytes that adhere in a coinlike fashion, giving the appearance of agglutination, can be observed on microscopic examination (**Color Plate 2**). Cell grouping can usually be accomplished by washing the patient's red cells several times with saline. Performing a saline dilution or saline replacement technique will free the cells in the case of rouleaux formation in the reverse type. In true agglutination, red cell clumping will still remain after the addition of saline.

Washing cord cells six to eight times should alleviate spontaneous rouleaux due to Wharton's jelly, which is a viscous mucopolysaccharide material present on cord bloods. Even though it is rather illogical to perform reverse groupings on cord samples, a small minority of hospitals still routinely carry out this procedure. Therefore, the student should be aware that washing the cord cells with saline will result in an accurate forward grouping. However, the reverse grouping may still not correlate with the forward grouping because the antibodies detected are usually of maternal origin.

## Group IV Discrepancies

These discrepancies are between forward and reverse groupings owing to miscellaneous problems and have the following causes:

- Polyagglutination
- Cold reactive antibodies (allo and auto)
- Warm autoantibodies
- Unexpected ABO isoagglutinins
- Antibodies other than anti-A and anti-B may react to form antigen-antibody complexes that may then adsorb onto patient's red cells (e.g., some individuals have antibodies against acriflavine, the yellow dye used in some commercial anti-B reagents; the acriflavin–anti–acriflavin complex attaches to the patient's red cells, causing agglutination in the forward type)
- RBCs with the cis "AB phenotype" (a rare occurrence) express a weakly reactive A antigen (analogous to A₂ cells) and a weak B antigen.[31] Weak anti-B (present in the serum of most "cis-AB" individuals) leads to an ABO discrepancy in the reverse grouping

## Resolution of Group IV Discrepancies

Polyagglutination (red cells agglutinating with all human sera) can occur as a result of genetic inheritance or bacterial infection (see Chap. 22). An example of polyagglutination is T polyagglutination, in which exposure of a hidden erythrocyte antigen (T antigen) occurs in patients with bacterial or viral infections. Bacterial contamination in vitro or in vivo produces an enzyme that alters and exposes the hidden antigen on red blood cells, leading to *T activation*. All normal human serum contains anti-T, which reacts with this now exposed hidden T antigen. The strength of the reaction depends upon how much anti-T antibody is in the serum. An example of the type of discrepancy in the forward and reverse groupings caused by T activation is shown in Table 5–23. Anti-T does not present a problem for using monoclonal antibody typing reagents.[31]

If the polyagglutination is suspected, lectin studies should be performed. This consists of testing the patient cells with a series of lectins. Commercial lectin kits are available. Based on the reactions obtained, the type of polyagglutination can be determined. For further information, see Chapter 22. *Tn activation*, although rarely encountered, is another type of polyagglutinability. This condition is permanent, not transient, and is not associated with bacterial or viral infections. Acquired A antigen phenomenon has been reported in Tn activation (see Chap. 22).

Potent cold autoantibodies can cause spontaneous agglutination of the patient's cells. These cells often yield a positive direct Coombs' or antiglobulin test (see Chap. 21). If the antibody in the serum reacts with all adult cells, for example, anti-I (see I Blood Group System in Chapter 8), the reagent A and B cells used in the reverse grouping also agglutinate. The type of discrepancy in the forward and reverse groupings caused by cold autoantibodies is shown in Table 5–24.

To resolve this discrepancy, the patient's red blood cells could be incubated at 37°C for a short period of time, then washed with 37°C saline three times and retyped. If this is not successful in resolving the forward type, the patient's RBCs can be treated with dithiothreitol (DTT) to disperse IgM-related agglutination. As for the serum, the reagent RBCs and serum or plasma can be warmed to 37°C, then mixed, tested, and read at 37°C. The test can be converted to the antihuman globulin phase if necessary. Weakly reactive anti-A and/or

**Table 5–23.** Example of ABO Discrepancy Caused by T Activation

| | Forward Grouping* Reaction of Patient's Cells with | | | Reverse Grouping Reaction of Patient's Serum with | |
| --- | --- | --- | --- | --- | --- |
| | Anti-A | Anti-B | Anti-A,B | A₁ Cells | B Cells |
| Patient | ++ | + | ++++ | ++++ | ++++ |
| | | | Patient's probable group: O | | |

*Note: polyclonal antisera used.

**Table 5–24.** Example of ABO Discrepancy Caused by Cold Autoantibodies

| | Forward Grouping Reaction of Patient's Cells with | | | Reverse Grouping Reaction of Patient's Serum with | |
| --- | --- | --- | --- | --- | --- |
| | Anti-A | Anti-B | Anti-A,B | A₁ Cells | B Cells |
| Patient | ++ | ++++ | ++++ | ++++ | +++ |
| | | | Patient's probable group: B | | |

**Table 5–25.** Example of ABO Discrepancy Caused by Warm Autoantibodies or Transfusion Reactions Yielding Antibody-coated Red Cells

| | Forward Grouping Reaction of Patient's Cells with | | | Reverse Grouping Reaction of Patient's Serum with | |
| --- | --- | --- | --- | --- | --- |
| | Anti-A | Anti-B | Anti-A,B | A₁ Cells | B Cells |
| Patient | + | + | + | ++++ | ++++ |
| | | | Patient's probable group: O | | |

anti-B may not react outside their optimum thermal range. If the reverse typing is negative (and a positive result was expected), an autoabsorption could be performed to remove the autoantibody from the serum, and the absorbed serum can then be used to repeat the reverse typing.

Patients with warm autoimmune hemolytic anemia or those on drugs such as alpha methyldopa may have red cells coated with sufficient antibody to promote spontaneous agglutination. Also, transfusion reactions resulting in antibody production caused by transfused foreign red cell antigens can result in antibody-coated red cells that produce a positive direct Coombs' test. This may promote a mixed-field or weak agglutination in the forward grouping, resulting in an ABO discrepancy. These warm-reacting antibodies, which are coating the patient's red cells, yield weaker reactions at room temperature during ABO testing than at 37°C. The type of discrepancy in the forward and reverse groupings caused by warm autoantibodies or transfusion reactions yielding antibody-coated red cells is shown in Table 5–25.

When a technologist suspects that warm autoantibodies are causing false-positive reactions in the forward grouping, he or she can treat the cells in a manner that removes the bound immunoglobulin. Subjecting the

RBCs to a gentle heat elution at 45°C may remove sufficient antibody that the RBCs can be reliably typed with anti-A and anti-B.

Unexpected ABO isoagglutinins in the patient's serum react at room temperature with the corresponding antigen present on the reagent cells. Examples of this type of ABO discrepancy include A₂ and A₂B individuals who can produce "naturally occurring" anti-A₁, or A₁ and A₁B individuals who may produce "naturally occurring" anti-H. (For review, refer to previous sections on ABO subgroups.) Reverse grouping can be repeated using at least three examples of A₁, A₂, B cells, O cells, and an autologous control (patient's serum mixed with patient's red cells). The specificity of the antibody can be determined by examining the pattern of reactivity (e.g., if antibody agglutinates only A₁ cells, it can most likely be identified as anti-A₁).

Unexpected alloantibodies in the patient's serum other than ABO isoagglutinins (e.g., anti-M) may cause a discrepancy in the reverse grouping. Reverse grouping cells possess other antigens in addition to A and B, and it is possible that other unexpected antibodies present in the patient's serum will react with these cells (Table 5–26). In this situation, a panel should be performed with the patient's serum. Once the unexpected alloan-

**Table 5–26.** Example of ABO Discrepancy Caused by Unexpected Alloantibodies in Patient's Serum

| | Forward Grouping Reaction of Patient's Cells with | | | Reverse Grouping Reaction of Patient's Serum with | |
|---|---|---|---|---|---|
| | **Anti-A** | **Anti-B** | **Anti-A,B** | **A₁ Cells** | **B Cells** |
| Patient | ++++ | ++++ | ++++ | + | + |

Patient's probable group: AB

**Table 5–27.** Example of ABO Discrepancy Caused by a Red Cell–adsorbed, Soluble, Antigen-Antibody Complex

| | Forward Grouping Reaction of Patient's Cells with | | | Reverse Grouping Reaction of Patient's Serum with | |
|---|---|---|---|---|---|
| | **Anti-A** | **Anti-B** | **Anti-A,B** | **A₁ Cells** | **B Cells** |
| Patient | Neg | +++ | Neg | ++++ | ++++ |

Patient's probable group: O

tibody(ies) is(are) identified, $A_1$ and B cells negative for the corresponding antigen can be used in the reverse typing, or once again, the reverse typing can be repeated at 37°C if the ABO isoagglutinins react at this temperature and there is no interference from the unexpected alloantibody.

Some individuals have antibodies against acriflavin in their serum. The patient's antibody combines with the dye and attaches to the patient's red cells, resulting in agglutination in the forward grouping. The type of discrepancy in the forward grouping caused by this red cell–adsorbed, soluble, antigen-antibody complex is shown in Table 5–27. Washing the patient's cells three times with saline and then retyping them should resolve this discrepancy.

Cis-AB refers to the inheritance of both AB genes from one parent carried on one chromosome and an O gene inherited from the other parent. This results in the offspring inheriting three ABO genes instead of two (Fig. 5–19). The designation cis-AB is used to distinguish this mode of inheritance from the more usual AB phenotype in which the alleles are located on different chromosomes. Usually the B antigen yields a weaker reaction with the anti-B from random donors, with mixed-field agglutination typical of subgroup $B_3$ reported in several cases. The serum of most cis-AB individuals contains a weak anti-B, which reacts with all ordinary B red cells, yet not with cis-AB red cells. A and B transferase levels are lower than those found in ordinary group AB sera.[31] Some investigators have suggested that the B antigen in the cis-AB represents only a piece of the normal B antigen. Cis-AB blood can be classified into four categories: $A_2B_3$, $A_1B_3$, $A_2B$, and $A_2B_x$. Various hypotheses have been offered to explain the cis-AB phenotype. Many favor a crossing over of a portion of a gene resulting in unequal expression by the recombinant. However, the banding pattern of the distal end of the long arm of chromosome 9 represent-

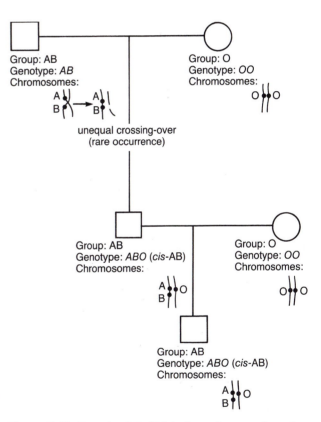

**Figure 5–19.** Example of cis-AB inheritance to unequal crossing-over. □ = male; ○ = female. (From Harmening-Pittiglio,[33] p 7 with permission.)

ing the ABO locus is normal. There have been other examples of cis-ABs that do not fit the above scenario. In these examples, there was a mutation at the ABO locus and an enzyme was produced that was capable of transferring both A-specific and B-specific sugars to the precursor molecule.[33]

**Table 5–28.** ABO Discrepancies between Forward and Reverse Grouping*

| | Forward Grouping | | | Reverse Grouping | | | | | |
|---|---|---|---|---|---|---|---|---|---|
| Patient | Anti-A | Anti-B | Anti-A,B | A₁ Cells | B Cells | O Cells | Auto-control | Possible Causes | Resolution Steps |
| 1 | Neg | Neg | Neg | Neg | Neg | Neg | Neg | Group O newborn or elderly patient; patient may have hypo-gammaglobulinemia or agammaglobulinemia, or may be taking immunosuppressive drugs | Check age and diagnosis of patient and immunoglobulin levels if possible; incubate at RT for 30 min or at 4°C for 15 min; include group 0 and autologous cells at 4°C |
| 2 | 4+ | Neg | 4+ | 1+ | 4+ | Neg | Neg | Subgroup of A; probable A₂ with anti-A₁ | Use anti-A₁ lectin, test serum against additional A₁, A₂, and O cells |
| 3 | 4+ | 4+ | 4+ | 2+ | 2+ | 2+ | 2+ | (1) Rouleaux (multiple myeloma patient; any patient with reversed albumin-to-globulin ratio or patients given plasma expanders) | (1) Wash red cells; use saline dilution or saline replacement technique |
| | | | | | | | | (2) Cold autoantibody (probable group AB with an auto anti-I) | (2) Perform cold panel and autoabsorb or rabbit erythrocyte stroma (REST) absorb (see Chapter 11) or reverse type at 37°C |
| | | | | | | | | (3) Cold autoantibody with underlying cold or RT reacting alloantibody (probable group AB with an auto anti-I and a high-frequency cold antibody, (e.g., anti-P₁, anti-M, anti-Leᵇ) | (3) Perform cold panel autoabsorb or REST, and run panel on absorbed serum; select reverse cells lacking antigen for identified alloantibody; repeat reverse group on absorbed serum to determine true ABO group or at 37°C |
| 4 | 4+ | 4+ | 4+ | 1+ | Neg | Neg | Neg | Subgroup of AB; probable A₂B with anti-A₁ | Use anti-A₁ lectin |
| 5 | 4+ | Neg | 4+ | Neg | 4+ | 3+ | Neg | A₁ with potent anti-H | Confirm A₁ group with anti-A₁ lectin; test additional A₂, O, and A₁ cells and an Oₕ if available |
| 6 | Neg | Neg | Neg | 4+ | 4+ | 4+ | Neg | Oₕ Bombay | Test with anti-H lectin; test Oₕ cells if available; send to reference laboratory for confirmation |
| 7 | Neg | Neg | 2+ | 2+ | 4+ | Neg | Neg | Subgroup of A; probable Aₓ with anti-A₁ | Perform saliva studies or absorption/elution |
| 8 | 4+ | 2+ | 4+ | Neg | 4+ | Neg | Neg | Group A with an "acquired B" antigen | Check history of patient for lower gastrointestinal problem or septicemia; use modified BS-1 lectin if available, or acidify anti-B typing reagent to pH 6.0 by adding 1 or 2 drops of 1N HCl to 1 mL of anti-B anti-sera, and measure with a pH meter (this acidified anti-B antisera would agglutinate only true B antigens, *not* acquired B antigens), test serum against autologous cells |
| 9 | 4+ | 4+ | 4+ | 2+ | Neg | 2+ | Neg | Group AB with alloantibody | Perform antibody screen and panel |
| 10 | Neg | 4+ | 4+ | 4+ | 1+ | 1+ | 1+ | Group B with cold auto-antibody | Enzyme-treat red cells and perform autoabsorption or REST absorption at 4°C or perform prewarmed testing |

*Absorptions should not be performed on patients' cells that have been transfused within the last 3 months.
REST = rabbit erythrocyte stroma; RT = room temperature.
Note: absorption with rabbit stroma decreases reactivity of serum with B cells.

Some examples of serologic reactions involving ABO discrepancies have been provided with answers for review and self-evaluation (Table 5–28). Also, the procedure for determination of secretor status is provided at the end of this chapter. Finally, you have been briefly introduced to ABO, the first and "simplest" blood group system known!

## CASE HISTORY

### William Bernard, MT(ASCP)SBB

### Introduction

The previous discussion of weak subgroups of A, and undoubtedly of B as well, is interesting, but of mainly historical interest. The various subgroups were defined over a period of years using human-source polyclonal reagents. These reagents are no longer available. Today in the United States, the only reagents available commercially are monoclonal reagents. These reagents show subtle differences from the traditional reagents. In most cases these differences are rare and cause few problems in practice. The major difference is that subgroups, such as $A_x$ and $A_{el}$, give positive reactions with monoclonal anti-A reagent and so are not recognized. The only traditional subgroup that can be recognized with modern reagents is $A_1$, and this is only because of the presence of anti-$A_1$ lectin. These changes are not necessarily bad, but one needs to be aware that they exist.

Monoclonal reagents are not all the same, as shown in Table 5–29. Each manufacturer supplies reagents, which are composed of antibody produced by one or more clones. Each of these reagents offers subtle quirks on oc-

**Table 5–29.** Commercially Available Monoclonal Antisera (FDA-approved)

| | REAGENTS | | | | | |
|---|---|---|---|---|---|---|
| | Anti-A | | Anti-B | | Anti-A,B | |
| Company Name | Type of Antibody | Designated Clone | Type of Antibody | Designated Clone | Type of Antibody | Designated Clone |
| Ortho | IgM IgM | MHO4 3D3 | IgM IgM IgM | NB10.5A5 NB10.3B4 NB1.19 | IgM IgM IgM IgM | MHO4 3D3 NB10.5A5 NB1.19 |
| Gamma | IgM | BIRMA 1 | IgM | GAMA11O | IgM IgM IgM | BIRMA 1 ES4 ES15 |
| Immucor | IgM IgM | BIRMA 1 F98 7C6 | IgM IgM IgM | ES4 F84 3D6 F97 2D6 | IgM IgM IgM IgM IgM IgM IgM IgM | BIRMA 1 BIRMA 1 ES4 ES15 F98 7C6 F84 3D6 F97 2D6 F125 7B6 |
| BCA (Biopool, Int.) | IgM | BIRMA 1 | IgM | ES4 | IgM IgM IgM | BIRMA 1 ES4 ES15 |

**Table 5–30.** Advantages and Disadvantages of Monoclonal Antibodies

| Advantages | Disadvantages |
|---|---|
| • Unlimited production, availability, and supply of antibody with batch-to-batch consistency (via hybridoma technology) <br> • Higher titers and therefore stronger reactions (i.e., weak subgroups more readily detected) <br> • Human/animal source materials eliminated <br> • Antibodies are IgM, which give direct agglutination, resulting in shorter time to perform the test <br> • Fewer false-positives as a result of potentiators with these reagents <br> • Contain no contaminating antibodies such as Bg, low incidence, or polyagglutinins <br> • May be used to type DAT– –positive cells | • Specificity may be relative (i.e., all monoclonal reagents from different companies are *not* the same) <br> • Epitope may be shared by several antigens <br> • Single epitope antibodies may not react with all antigen-positive cells <br> • Should not be used for adsorption/elution studies <br> • Unexpected reactions may occur |

casion. All of them meet FDA specifications and can be used. However, one must be aware that they are not the same. Instructions provided by the manufacturer must be followed exactly. In addition, any notes or precautions included in the manufacturer's product insert need to be reviewed. When changing from one reagent to another, even with the same manufacturer, things will not necessarily be the same as before. Table 5–30 lists the advantages and disadvantages of monoclonal antibodies.

The following case may illustrate the situation a transfusion service may have to address after the introduction of the use of monoclonal reagents in the laboratory.

## CASE STUDY

A 74-year-old woman was admitted for total hip replacement. Three units of red cells were requested before surgery. The results obtained when typing the patient's admission blood sample are shown:

| | Anti-A | Anti-B | A₁ Cells | B Cells |
|---|---|---|---|---|
| Patient sample | +4 | 0 | 0 | +3 |

The patient received 2 units of red cells during surgery. No adverse reaction was noted. Seven days after the first surgery, the transfusion service again received a request to have blood available for surgery, this time for a bowel resection. A new specimen was obtained and showed the following results:

| | Anti-A | Anti-B | A₁ Cells | B Cells |
|---|---|---|---|---|
| Patient sample | +4 | +2 | 0 | +3 |

**Questions**

1. What is the cause of the change in results obtained?

2. What technique can be used to determine the patient's blood type?

3. Does this have any clinical effect on the patient?

Further investigation determined that the patient was rather obese and had a pre-existing umbilical hernia. During recovery from the hip replacement surgery, a portion of the patient's bowel became strangulated in this hernia. The second surgery was to remove this section of necrotic bowel.

The anti-B reagent used was obtained from the ES4 clone. As originally formulated, this reagent reacted well with red cells showing the acquired-B phenomenon. Use of this reagent acidified to pH 6.0 gave the expected negative reaction with the patient's second red cell sample.

The problem for the transfusion service was that textbooks described acquired B as occurring only very rarely and then showing only very weak agglutination. The monoclonal reagent would react well with red cells showing this change. What was also unknown was the rapidity with which the change could apparently occur. This change is of no particular significance in itself but can result in serious consequences if the patient is incorrectly determined to be group AB and subsequently transfused with AB red cells. The patient was given an additional unit of group A red cells by transfusion without problem.

---

## SUMMARY CHART: IMPORTANT POINTS TO REMEMBER (MT/MLT)

- ABO frequencies: group O, 45%; group A, 41%; group B, 10%; group AB, 4%
- ABO blood group system has "naturally occurring" antibodies that are primarily IgM
- ABO genes, like most other blood groups, are inherited in a codominant manner
- ABH-soluble antigens are secreted by tissue cells and are found in all body secretions. The antigens secreted depend on the person's ABO group
- ABO reverse grouping is omitted from cord blood testing on newborns because their antibody titers are generally too low for detection
- ABO red cell antigens are glycolipids; ABO-secreted substances are glycoproteins
- L-fucose is the immunodominant sugar responsible for H specificity
- $N$-acetylgalactosamine in the immunodominant sugar responsible for A specificity
- D-galactose is the immunodominant sugar responsible for B specificity
- The $hh$ genotype is known as the Bombay phenotype, or $O_h$, and lacks normal expression of the ABH antigens
- Group O persons contain the greatest amount of H substance; group $A_1B$ persons contain the least amount of H substance
- Approximately 80% of persons inherit the A gene phenotype as $A_1$; the remaining 20% phenotype, as $A_2$ or weaker subgroups
- Approximately 1 to 8% of $A_2$ persons produce anti-$A_1$ in their serum
- Glycoproteins in secretions are formed on type 1 precursor chains
- The ABH glycolipid antigens on red cells are formed on type 2 precursor chains
- Forward and reverse grouping normally yield strong (4+) reaction
- Group A persons contain anti-B in their serum; group B persons contain anti-A in their serum; group AB persons contains neither anti-A or anti-B in their serum; group O persons contain both anti-A and anti-B in their serum
- Approximately 78% of the random population inherit the $Se$ gene and are termed $secretors$; the remaining 22% inherit the $se$ gene and are termed $nonsecretors$
- The $Se$ gene codes for the production of L-fucosyltransferase

## REVIEW QUESTIONS

1. An ABO type on a patient gives the following reactions:

| REACTION OF PATIENT'S CELLS WITH | | | REACTION OF PATIENT'S SERUM WITH | |
|---|---|---|---|---|
| Anti-A | Anti-B | Anti-A,B | $A_1$ cells | B cells |
| 4+ | 4+ | 4+ | neg | neg |

What is the patient's blood type?
A. O
B. A
C. B
D. AB

2. The major immunoglobulin class of anti-B in a group A individual is:
A. IgM
B. IgG
C. IgA
D. All of the above

3. What are the possible ABO phenotypes of the offspring from the mating of a group A to a group B individual?
A. O, A, B
B. A, B

C. A, B, AB
D. O, A, B, AB

4. The immunodominant sugar responsible for blood group A specificity is:
A. L-fucose
B. $N$-acetyl-D-galactosamine
C. D-galactose
D. Uridine diphosphate-$N$-acetyl-D-galactose

5. What ABH substances would be found in the saliva of a group B secretor?
A. H
B. H and A
C. H and B
D. H, A, and B

6. An ABO type on a patient gives the following reactions:

| REACTION OF PATIENT'S CELLS WITH | | | | REACTION OF PATIENT'S SERUM WITH | |
|---|---|---|---|---|---|
| Anti-A | Anti-B | Anti-A,B | Anti-$A_1$ | $A_1$ cells | B cells |
| 4+ | neg | 4+ | neg | 2+ | 4+ |

The reactions above may be because:
A. Patient is $A_1$ with acquired B
B. Patient is $A_1B$ with anti-$A_1$
C. Patient is $A_2$ with anti-$A_1$

D. Patient has increased concentrations of protein in the serum

7. Which of the following ABO blood groups contains the least amount of H substance?
   A. $A_1B$
   B. $A_2$
   C. B
   D. O

8. You are working on a specimen in the laboratory that you believe to be a "Bombay phenotype." Which of the following reactions would you expect to see?
   A. Patient's cells + *Ulex europaeus* = no agglutination
   B. Patient's cells + *Ulex europaeus* = agglutination
   C. Patient's serum + group O donor RBCs = no agglutination
   D. Patient's serum + $A_1$ and B cells = no agglutination

9. An example of a technical error that can result in an ABO discrepancy is:
   A. Acquired-B phenomenon
   B. Missing isoagglutinins
   C. Cell suspensions either too heavy or too light
   D. Acriflavin antibodies

10. An ABO type on a patient gives the following reactions:

| REACTION OF PATIENT'S CELLS WITH | | | REACTION OF PATIENT'S SERUM WITH | | | |
|---|---|---|---|---|---|---|
| Anti-A | Anti-B | Anti-A,B | $A_1$ cells | B cells | O cells | Auto-control |
| 4+ | neg | 4+ | 2+ | 4+ | 2+ | neg |

To resolve this discrepancy, you would:
   A. Check the age and immunoglobulin levels of the patient
   B. Perform antibody screen and panel
   C. Perform cold panel and auto-absorb serum
   D. Wash red cells and use saline replacement

## ANSWERS TO REVIEW QUESTIONS

1. D (p 91)
2. A (p 93)
3. D (pp 95, 96 (Table 5–5))
4. B (p 96)
5. C (pp 100, 102 (Table 5–7))
6. C (p 102)
7. A (p 103)
8. A (p 110)
9. C (p 112 (Table 5–18))
10. B (p 116)

## REFERENCES

1. Mourant, AE, et al: The Distribution of the Human Blood Groups and Other Biochemical Polymorphisms, ed 2. Oxford University Press, Oxford, 1976.
2. Reed, TE: Distributions and tests of independence of seven blood group systems in a large multiracial sample from California. Am J Hum Genet 20:142, 1968.
3. Wiener, AS: Problems and pitfalls in blood grouping tests for non-parentage: Distribution of the blood groups. Am J Clin Pathol 51:9, 1969.
4. Schreffler, DC, et al: Studies on Genetic Selection in a Completely Ascertained US Caucasian Population. I. Frequencies, Age, and Sex Effects and Phenotype Associations for 12 Blood Group Systems. Tecumseh, Michigan: Population 10,000. West European Ancestry. American Society of Human Genetics, 1971.
5. Springer, FG, et al: Origin of anti-human blood group B agglutinins in white leghorn chicks. J Exp Med 110:221, 1959.
6. Dobson, A, and Ikin, E: The ABO blood groups in the United Kingdom: Frequencies based on a very large sample. J Pathol Bacteriol 58:221, 1946.
7. Oriol, R: ABO, Hh, Lewis and secretion: Serology, genetics and tissue distribution. In Cartron, JP, and Rouger, P (eds): Blood Cell Biochemistry, Vol 6: Molecular Basis of Major Human Blood Group Antigens, Plenum, New York, 1995, pp 37–73.
8. Kunkel, HG, and Rockey, JH: B2$_A$ and other immunoglobulins in isolated anti-A antibodies. Proc Soc Exp Biol Med 113:278, 1963.
9. Landsteiner, K, and Witt, DH: Observations on the human blood groups: Irregular reactions. Isoagglutinin in sera of group 4. The fact $A_1$. J Immunol 2:221, 1926.
10. Dodd, BE, et al: The cross-reacting antibodies of group O sera: Immunological studies and a possible explanation of the observed facts. Immunology 12:39, 1967.
11. Mak, KH, et al: Serologic characteristics of H-deficient phenotypes among Chinese in Hong Kong. Transfusion 36:994–999, 1986.
12. Lowe, JB: Biochemistry and biosynthesis of ABH and Lewis antigens: Characterization of blood group–specific glycosyltransferases. In Cartron, JP, and Rouger, P (eds): Blood Cell Biochemistry, Vol 6: Molecular Basis of Major Human Blood Group Antigens. Plenum, New York, 1995, pp 75–115.
13. Yamato, F, Clausen, H, and White, T: Molecular genetic basis of the histo-blood group ABO system. Nature 345:229, 1990.
14. Vengelen-Tyler V (ed): Technical Manual. American Association of Blood Banks, Bethesda, MD, 1996.
15. Olsson, ML, and Chester, MA. Frequent occurrence of a variant $O^1$ gene at the blood group ABO locus. Vox Sang 70:26–30, 1996.
16. Schachter, H, et al: A quantitative difference in the activity of blood group A specific *N*-acetylgalactosaminyl-transferase in serum from $A_1$ and $A_2$ human subjects. Biochem Biophys Res Commun 45:1011, 1971.
17. Schachter, H, et al: Qualitative differences in the alpha-*N*-acetyl-galactosaminyl transferases produced by human $A_1$ and $A_2$ genes. Proc Natl Acad Sci USA 7:220, 1973.
18. Tilley, CA, et al: Human blood group A- and H-specified glycosyltransferase levels in the sera of newborn infants and their mothers. Vox Sang 34:8, 1978.
19. Beattie, KM: Perspectives on some usual and unusual ABO phenotypes. In Bell CA (ed): A seminar on antigens on blood cells and body fluids. American Association of Blood Banks, Washington, DC, 1980, pp 97–149.
20. Cartron, JP, et al: Study of the α-*N*-acetyl-galactosaminyltransferase of sera and red cell membranes of human A subgroups. J Immunogenet 5:107–116, 1978.
21. Lopez, M, et al: Activity of IgG and IgM ABO antibodies against some weak A ($A_3$, $A_x$, $A_{end}$) and weak B ($B_3$, $B_x$) red cells. Vox Sang 37:281–285, 1979.
22. Cartron, JP, et al: Assay of α-N-acetylgalactosaminyltransferase in human sera: Further evidence for several types of $A_m$ individuals. Vox Sang 28:347–365, 1975.
23. Topping, MD, and Watkins, WM: Isoelectric points of the human

blood group $A_1$, $A_2$ and B gene-associated glycosyltransferases in ovarian cysts fluids and serum. Biochem Biophys Res Commun 64:89–96, 1975.

24. Hakomori, SI: Blood group ABH and Ii antigens of human erythrocytes: Chemistry, polymorphism and their developmental change. Semin Hematol 18:39–62, 1981.

25. Koscielak, J, Pacuszka, T, and Dzierzkowa-Borodej, W: Activity of B-gene-specified galactosyltransferase in individuals with Bm phenotypes. Vox Sang 30:58–67, 1976.

26. Boose, GM, Issitt, C, and Issitt, PD: Weak B antigen in family. Transfusion 18:570–571, 1978.

27. Watkins, WM: Changes in the specificity of blood-group mucopolysaccharides induced by enzymes from *Trichomonas foetus*. Immunology 5:245–266, 1962.

28. Salmon, C, et al: H deficient phenotypes: A proposed practical classification Bombay $A_h$, $H_2$, $H_m$. Blood Transfus Immunohaematol 23:233–248, 1980.

29. Reed, ME, and Lomas-Frances, C: The blood group antigen facts group. Academic Press, New York, 1997, pp 3–26.

30. Judd, WJ, and Annesley, TM: The acquired-B phenomenon. Transfus Med Rev 10:111–117, 1996.

31. Mallory, D: Immunohematology Methods and Procedures. American Red Cross, Rockville, MD, 1993.

32. Fischer, GF, Fae, I, and Dub, E: Analysis of the gene polymorphism of ABO blood group specific transferases helps diagnosis of acquired B status. Vox Sang 62:113, 1992.

33. Harmening-Pittiglio, D: Genetics and biochemistry of A, B, H and Lewis antigens. In Wallace, ME, and Gibbs, FL (eds): Blood Group Systems: ABH and Lewis. American Association of Blood Banks, Arlington, VA, 1986.

## BIBLIOGRAPHY

Abe, K, Levery, SB, and Hakomori, S: The antibody specific to type 1 chain blood group A determinant. J Immunol 132(4):1951, 1984.

Adatia, A, et al: Comparison of the absorption of allo-anti-B by red cells and by a synthetic immunoabsorbent using the autoanalyzer. Rev Fr Transfus Immunohematol 26(6):585, 1983.

Anderson, DE, and Haas, C: Blood type A and familial breast cancer. Cancer 54(9):1845, 1984.

Atichartakarn, V, et al: Autoimmune hemolytic anemia due to anti B autoantibody. Vox Sang 49(4):301, 1985.

Baechtel, FS: Secreted blood group substances: Distributions in semen and stabilities in dried semen stains. J Forensic Sci 30(4):1119, 1985.

Bakacs, T, Ringwald, G, and Jokuti, I: Direct ADCC lysis of O, Rh-positive (R 1 R2) erythrocytes by lymphocytes of individuals sensitized against antigen D. Immunol Lett 4(1):53, 1982.

Beattie, KM, et al: Two chimeras detected during routine grouping test by Autoanalyzer. Transfusion 17:681, 1977.

Beattie, KM, et al: Blood group chimerism as a clue to generalized tissue mosaicism. Transfusion 4:77, 1964.

Bensinger, WI, Buckner, CD, and Clift, RA: Whole blood immunoadsorption of anti-A or anti-B antibodies. Vox Sang 48(6):357, 1985.

Bensinger, WI, et al: Immune adsorption of anti-A and anti-B antibodies. Prog Clin Biol Res 88:295, 1982.

Bernoco, M, et al: Detection of combined ABH and Lewis glycosphingolipids in sera of H-deficient donors. Vox Sang 49(1):58:1985.

Bolton, S, and Thorpe, JW: Enzyme-linked immunoabsorbent assay for A and B water soluble blood group substances. J Forensic Sci 31(1):27, 1986.

Boose, GM, Issitt, C, and Issitt, P: Weak B antigen in a family. Transfusion 18:570, 1978.

Bracey, AW, and Van-Buren, C: Immune anti-A1 in A2 recipients of kidneys from group O donors. Transfusion 26(3):282, 1986.

Brand, A, et al: ABH antibodies causing platelet transfusion refractoriness. Transfusion 26(5):463, 1986.

Breimer, ME, and Karlsson, KA: Chemical and immunological identification of glycolipid-based blood group ABH and Lewis antigens in human and kidney. Biochem Biophys Acta 755(2):170, 1983.

Brouwers, HA, et al: Sensitive methods for determining subclasses of IgG anti-A and anti-B in sera of blood-group O women with a blood-group-A or B child. Br J Haematol 66(2):267, 1987.

Cartron, J, et al: Study of the alpha-N-acetylgalactosaminyl-transferase in sera and red cell membranes of human A subgroups. J Immunogenet 5:107, 1978.

Cartron, J, et al: Assay of alpha-N-acetylgalactosaminyl-transferases in human sera: Further evidence for several types of $A_m$ individuals. Vox Sang 28:347, 1975.

Cartron, J, et al: "Weak A" phenotypes: Relationship between red cell agglutinability and antigen site density. Immunology 27:723, 1974.

Cheng, MS: Two similar cases of weak agglutination with anti-B reagent. Laboratory Medicine 12:506, 1981.

Clausen, H, Holmes, E, and Hakomori, S: Novel blood group H glycolipid antigens exclusively expressed in blood group A and AB erythrocytes (type 3 chain H). II. Differential conversion of different H substrates by A1 and A2 enzymes, and type 3 chain H expression in relation to secretor status. J Biol Chem 261(3):1388, 1986.

Clausen, H, et al: Further characterization of type 2 and type 3 chain blood group A glycosphingolipids from human erythrocyte membranes. Biochemistry 25(22):7075, 1986.

Clausen, H, et al: Blood group A glycolipid (Ax) with globo-series structure which is specific for blood group A1 erythrocytes: One of chemical bases for A1 and A2 distinction. Biochem Biophys Res Commun 124(2):523, 1984.

Cohen, F, and Zuelzer, WW: Interrelationship of the various subgroups of the blood group A: Study with immunofluorescence. Transfusion 5:223, 1965.

Dodd, BE, and Lincoln, PJ: Serological studies of the H activity of $O_h$ red cells with various anti-H reagents. Vox Sang 35:168, 1978.

Dodd, BE, and Wood, NJ: Elution of group-specific substance A from RBC of various subgroups of A and its effect on the agglutination of AX RBC. Vox Sang 43(5):248, 1982.

Dunstan, RA: Status of major red cell blood group antigens on neutrophils, lymphocytes and monocytes. Br J Haematol 62(2):301, 1986.

Economidou, J, Hughes-Jones, N, and Gardner, B: Quantitative measurements concerning A and B antigen sites. Vox Sang 12:321, 1967.

Feng, CS, et al: Variant of type B blood in an El Salvador family: Expression of a variant B gene enhanced by the presence of an A2 gene. Transfusion 24(3):264, 1984.

Finne, J: Identification of the blood group ABH-active glycoprotein components of human erythrocyte membrane. Eur J Biochem 104:181, 1980.

Fukuda, MN, and Hakomori, S: Structures of branched blood group A-active glycosphingolipids in human erythrocytes and polymorphism of A- and H-glycolipids in A1 and A2 subgroups. J Biol Chem 257(1):446, 1982.

Furukawa, K, Mattes, MJ and Lloyd, KO: A1 and A2 erythrocytes can be distinguished by reagents that do not detect structural differences between the two cell types. J Immunol 135(6):4090, 1985.

Gardas, A, and Koscielak, J: A, B and H blood group specificities in glycoprotein and glycolipid fractions of human erythrocyte membrane: Absence of blood group active glyco-proteins in the membrane of non-secretors. Vox Sang 20:137, 1971.

Gart, JJ, and Nam, JM: A score test for the possible presence of recessive alleles in generalized ABO-like genetic systems. Biometrics 40(4):887, 1984.

Gemke, RJ, et al: ABO and Rhesus phenotyping of fetal erythrocytes in the first trimester of pregnancy. Br J Haematol 64(4):689, 1986.

Greenwell, P, et al: Fucosyltransferase activities in human lymphocytes and granulocytes: Blood group H gene-specified alpha-2-L-fucosyltransferase is a discriminatory marker of peripheral blood lymphocytes. FEBS Lett 164(2):314, 1983.

Hakomori, S, Stellner, K, and Watanabe, K: Four antigen variants of blood group A glycolipid: Examples of highly complex, branched chain glycolipid of animal cell membrane. Biochem Biophys Res Commun 49:1061, 1972.

Handa, V, et al: The $O_h$ (Bombay group) phenotype. J Indian Med Assoc 82(12):446, 1984.

Hanfland, P: Characterization of B and H blood group active glycosphingolipids from human B erythrocyte membranes. Chem Phys Lipids 15:105, 1975.

Herron, R, et al: A specific antibody for cells with acquired B antigen. Transfusion 22(6):525, 1982.

Hirschfeld, J: Conceptual framework shifts in immunogenetics. I. A new look at cis AB antigens in the ABO system. Vox Sang 33:286, 1977.

Hummell, K, et al: Inheritance of cis-AB in three generations (family Lam). Vox Sang 33:290, 1977.

Kannagi, R, Levery, SB, and Hakomori, S: Blood group H antigen with globo-series structure. Isolation and characterization from human blood group O erythrocytes. FEBS Lett 175(2):397, 1984.

Knowles, RW, et al: Monoclonal anti-type 2 H: An antibody detecting a precursor of the A and B blood group antigens. J Immunogenet 9(2):69, 1982.

Kogure, T, and Furukawa, K: Enzymatic conversion of human group O red cells into group B-active cells by alpha-$N$-galactosyltransferase of sera and salivas from group B and its variant types. J Immunogenet 3:147, 1976.

Koscielak, J, et al: Structures of fucose containing glycolipids with H and B blood group activity and of sialic acid and glucosamine containing glycolipid of human erythrocyte membrane. Eur J Biochem 37:214, 1973.

Koscielak, J, et al: Weak A phenotypes possibly caused by mutation. Vox Sang 50(3):187, 1986.

Le-Pendu, J, et al: Alpha-2-L-fucosyl-transferase activity in sera of individuals with H-deficient red cells and normal H antigen in secretions. Vox Sang 44(6):360, 1983.

Levine, P, et al: $A_h$, an incomplete suppression of A resembling $O_h$. Vox Sang 6:561, 1961.

Lin-Chu, M, et al: The para-Bombay phenotype in Chinese persons. Transfusion 27(5):388, 1987.

Lopez, M, et al: Activity of IgG and IgM ABO antibodies against some weak A ($A_3$, $A_x$, $A_{end}$) and weak B ($B_3$, $B_x$) red cells. Vox Sang 37:281, 1979.

Madsen, G, and Heisto, H: A Korean family showing inheritance of A and B on the same chromosome. Vox Sang 14:211, 1968.

Makela, O, Ruoslahti, E, and Ehnholm, C: Subtypes of human ABO blood groups and subtype-specific antibodies. J Immunol 3:763, 1969.

Marsh, WL, et al: Inherited mosaicism affecting the blood groups. Transfusion 15:589, 1975.

Mohn, JF, et al: An inherited blood group A variant in the Finnish population. I. Basic characteristics. Vox Sang 25:193, 1973.

Mollison, PL, Engelfriet, CP, and Contreras, M. Blood Transfusion in Clinical Medicine. Blackwell Scientific, London, 1993.

Moores, PP, et al: Some observations on "Bombay" bloods, with comments on evidence for the existence of two different $O_h$ phenotypes. Transfusion 15:237, 1975.

Oriol, R, Le Pendu, J, and Mollicone, R. Genetics of ABO, H, Lewis, X and related antigens. Vox Sang 51:161–171, 1986.

Pacuszka, T, et al: Biochemical serological and family studies in individuals with cis AB phenotypes. Vox Sang 29:292, 1975.

Poretz, RD, and Watkins, WM: Galactosyltransferases in human submaxillary glands and stomach mucosa associated with the biosynthesis of blood group specific glycoproteins. Eur J Biochem 25:455, 1972.

Race, C, and Watkins, WM: The action of the blood group B gene-specified alpha-galactosyltransferase from human serum and stomach mucosal extracts on group O and "Bombay" $O_h$ erythrocytes. Vox Sang 23:385, 1972.

Race, RR, and Sanger, R: Blood Groups in Man, ed 6. Blackwell Scientific, Oxford, 1975, pp 522–524, 531–535.

Rawson, AJ, and Abelson, N: Studies in blood group antibodies. III. Observations on the physiochemical properties of isohemagglutinins and isohemolysins. J Immunol 85:636, 1960.

Reed, ME, and Lomas-Francis, C: The Blood Group Antigen Facts Book. Academic Press, New York, 1997, pp 3–26.

Reed, TE, and Moore, BPL: A new variant of blood group A. Vox Sang 9:363, 1964.

Renkonen, KO: Blood-group-specific haemagglutinins in seed extracts. Vox Sang 45(5):397, 1983.

Roath, S, et al: Transient acquired blood group B antigen associated with diverticular bowel disease. Acta Haematol (Basel) 77(3):188, 1987.

Romano, EL, Mollison, PL, and Linares, J: Number of B sites generated on group O red cells from adults and newborn infants. Vox Sang 34:14, 1978.

Romans, DG, Tilley, CA, and Dorrington, KJ: Monogamous bivalency of IgG antibodies. I. Deficiency of branched ABHI-active oligosaccharide chains on red cells of infants causes the weak antiglobulin reactions in hemolytic disease of the newborn due to ABO incompatibility. J Immunol 124:2807, 1980.

Rubinstein, P, et al: A dominant suppressor of A and B. Vox Sang 25:377, 1973.

Rudmann, SV: Textbook of Blood Banking and Transfusion Medicine. WB Saunders, Philadelphia, 1995.

Sabo, B, et al: The cis AB phenotype in three generations of one family: Serological enzymatic and cytogenetic studies. J Immunogenet 5:87, 1978.

Salmon, C, et al: Quantitative and thermodynamic studies of erythrocytic ABO antigens. Transfusion 16:580, 1976.

Sathe, MS, Gorakshakar, AC, and Bhatia, HM: Blood group specific transferases in Bombay ($O_h$) Para-Bombay and weaker A and B variants. Indian J Med Res 81:53, 1985.

Schenkel-Brunner, H: Blood-group-ABH antigens of human erythrocytes. Eur J Biochem 104:529, 1980.

Schenkel-Brunner, H, Chester, MA, and Watkins, WM: Alpha-L-fucosyl-transferases in human serum from donors of different ABO, secretor and Lewis blood group phenotypes. Eur J Biochem 30:269, 1972.

Schenkel-Brunner, H, Prohaska, R, and Tuppy, H: Action of glycosyltransferases upon "Bombay" ($O_h$) erythrocytes: Conversion to cells showing blood group H and A specificities. Eur J Biochem 56:591, 1975.

Schenkel-Brunner, H, and Tuppy, H: Enzymatic conversion of human O into A erythrocytes and of B into AB erythrocytes. Nature 223:1272, 1969.

Schenkel-Brunner, H, and Tuppy, H: Enzymatic conversion of human blood group O erythrocytes into $A_2$ and $A_1$ cells by alpha-$N$-acetyl-D-galacto-saminyltransferases of blood group A individuals. Eur J Biochem 34:125, 1973.

Schmidt, P, et al: A hemolytic transfusion reaction due to the transfusion of $A_x$ blood. J Lab Clin Med 54:38, 1959.

Seyfried, H, Waleska, I, and Werblinska, B: Unusual inheritance of ABO group in a family with weak B antigens. Vox Sang 3:268, 1964.

Smalley, CE, and Tucker, EM: Blood group A antigen site distribution and immunoglobulin binding in relation to red cell age. Br J Haematol 54(2):209, 1983.

Solomon, J, Waggoner, R, and Leyshon, CW: A quantitative immunogenetic study of gene suppression involving $A_1$ and H antigens of the erythrocyte without affecting secreted blood group substances: The ABH phenotypes $A_h$ and $O_h$. Blood 25:470, 1965.

Stayboldt, C, Rearden, A, and Lane, TA: B antigen acquired by normal A1 red cells exposed to a patient's serum. Transfusion 27(1):41, 1987.

Sturgeon, P, Moore, BPL, and Weiner, W: Notations for two weak A variants: $A_{end}$ and $A_{el}$. Vox Sang 9:214, 1964.

Takasaki, S, and Kobata, A: Chemical characterization and distribution of ABO blood group active glycoprotein in human erythrocyte membrane. J Biol Chem 251:3610, 1976.

Takasaki, S, Yamashita, K, and Kobata, A: The sugar chain structures of ABO blood group active glycoproteins obtained from human erythrocyte membrane. J Biol Chem 253:6086, 1978.

Topping, MD, and Watkins, WM: Isoelectric points of the human blood group $A_1$, $A_2$ and B gene-associated glycosyltransferases in ovarian cyst fluids and serum. Biochem Biophys Res Commun 34:89, 1975.

Tuppy, H, and Schenkel-Brunner, H: Occurrence and assay of alpha-H-acetyl-galactosaminyltransferase in the gastric mucosa of humans belonging to blood group A. Vox Sang 17:139, 1969.

Viitala, J, Finne, J, and Krusius, T: Blood group A and H determinants in polyglycosyl peptides of A1 and A2 erythrocytes. Eur J Biochem 126(2):401, 1982.

Watanabe, K, Laine, RA, and Hakomori, S: On neutral fucoglycolipids having long branched carbohydrate chains: H-active I-active glycosphingolipids of human erythrocyte membranes. Biochemistry 14:2725, 1975.

Watkins, WM: Glycoproteins: Their composition, structure and function. In Gottschalk, A (ed): Glycoproteins, ed 2. Elsevier, Amsterdam, 1972, pp 830–891.

Watkins, WM: Blood group substances: Their nature and genetics. In Surgenor, D (ed): The Red Blood Cell. Academic Press, New York, 1974, p 303.

Westerveld, A, et al: Assignment of the $AK_1$: Np: ABO linkage group to human chromosome 9. Proc Natl Acad Sci 73:895, 1976.

Wheeler, DA, et al: Serologic and biochemical studies of a previously unclassified blood type B variant. 63(3):711, 1984.

Wiener, AS, and Cioffi, AF: A group B analogue of subgroup A3. Am J Clin Pathol 58:693, 1972.

Wiener, AS, and Socha, WW: Macro and microdifferences in blood group antigens and antibodies. Int Arch Allergy Appl Immunol 47:946, 1974.

Wittemore, NB, et al: Solubilized glycoprotein from human erythrocyte membranes possessing blood group A, B and H activity. Vox Sang 17:289, 1969.

Wrobel, DM, et al: "True" genotypes of chimeric twins revealed by blood group gene products in plasma. Vox Sang 27:395, 1974.

Wu, AM, et al: Immunochemical studies on blood groups: The internal structure and immunological properties of water-soluble human blood group A substance studied by Smith degradation, liberation, and fractionation of oligosaccharides and reaction with lectins. Arch Biochem Biophys 215(2):390, 1982.

Yamaguchi, H: A review of cis AB blood. Jinrui Idengaku Zasshi 18:1, 1973.

Yamaguchi, H, Okubo, Y, and Hazama, F: Another Japanese $A_2B_3$ blood group family with the propositus having O group father. Proc Jpn Acad 42:517, 1966.

Yamaguchi, H, Okubo, Y, and Tanaka, M: Cis AB bloods found in Japanese families. Jinrui Idengaku Zasshi 15:198, 1970.

Yokoyama, M, Stacey, SM, and Dunsford, I: $B_x$: A new subgroup of the blood group B. Vox Sang 2:348, 1957.

Yoshida, A, et al: An enzyme basis for blood type A intermediate status. Am J Hum Genet 34(6):919, 1982.

Yoshida, A, et al: A case of weak blood group B expression (Bm) associated with abnormal blood group galactosyltransferase. Blood 59(2):323, 1982.

Yoshida, A, Yamaguchi, YF, and Dave, V: Immunologic homology of human blood group glycosyltransferases and genetic background of blood group (ABO) determination. Blood 54:344, 1979.

# PROCEDURAL APPENDIX

## DETERMINATION OF THE SECRETOR PROPERTY

### Principle

Certain blood group substances occur in soluble form in a large proportion (78 percent) of individuals in secretions such as saliva and gastric juice (see Table 5–8). These individuals are termed "secretors" (they possess the Se gene) and secrete ABH-soluble antigens. These water-soluble blood group substances are readily detected in very minute quantities because they have the property of reacting with their corresponding antibodies and thereby neutralizing or inhibiting the capacity of the antibody to agglutinate erythrocytes possessing the corresponding antigen. The reaction is termed *hemagglutination inhibition* and provides a means of assaying the relative activity or potency of these water-soluble blood group substances.

### Materials

paraffin wax
saliva
human polyclonal anti-A and anti-B serum
anti-H lectin from *Ulex europaeus*
test tubes
pipettes
saline
2 to 5 percent washed group A, B, and O cells

### Procedure

1. Chew a piece of paraffin wax to stimulate secretion of saliva.
2. Collect about 2 to 3 mL of saliva in a test tube.
3. Place stoppered tube of saliva in a boiling water bath for 10 minutes. This inactivates enzymes that might otherwise destroy blood group substances.
4. Centrifuge at $1000 \times g$ for 10 minutes.
5. Collect clear supernatant into a clean tube.
6. Dilute saliva 1:2 or 1:4 (undilute saliva contains nonspecific glycoproteins that can inhibit antisera and lead to incorrect results).
7. Add one drop of diluted antiserum to an appropriately labeled tube (anti-A, anti-B, anti-H). For dilution, titrate anti-H, anti-A, and anti-B, testing against appropriate cells at immediate spin. Select the dilution giving 2+ agglutination and prepare a sufficient quantity to complete the test.
8. Add one drop of supernatant saliva to each tube. Mix and incubate at room temperature for 8 to 10 minutes.
9. Add one drop of the appropriate indicator cells (A, B, or O cells) to the properly labeled tube.
10. Mix and incubate at room temperature for 30 to 60 minutes.
11. Centrifuge.
12. Observe for macroscopic agglutination.

## Control

1. One drop of saline is used in place of dilute saliva. Test in parallel with the saliva.
2. Test saliva from a known secretor and a nonsecretor in parallel with test saliva.

## INTERPRETATIONS

1. Nonsecretor: Agglutination of red cells by antiserum-saliva mixture; control tube positive.
2. Secretor: No agglutination of red cells by antiserum and saliva mixture; control tube positive. The antiserum has been neutralized by the soluble blood group substances or antigens in the saliva, which react with their corresponding antibody. Therefore, no free antibody is available to react with the antigens on the reagent red cells used in the testing. This negative reaction is a positive test for the presence of ABH-soluble antigens and indicates that the individual is a secretor.

### ABH Substances in Saliva

| | ABH Substances in Saliva | | |
|---|---|---|---|
| ABO Group | A | B | H |
| *Secretors* | | | |
| A | Much | None | Some |
| B | None | Much | Some |
| O | None | None | Much |
| AB | Much | Much | Some |
| *Nonsecretors* | | | |
| A, B, O, and AB | None | None | None |

# CHAPTER 6

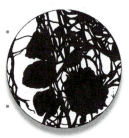

# THE Rh BLOOD GROUP SYSTEM

Merilyn Wiler, MA Ed, MT(ASCP)SBB

## OBJECTIVES

*On completion of this chapter, the learner should be able to:*

**1** Explain the derivation of the term Rh.

**2** Differentiate Rh from LW.

**3** Compare and contrast the Fisher-Race and Wiener theories of Rh inheritance.

**4** Translate the five major Rh antigens, genotypes, and haplotypes from one nomenclature to another, including Fisher-Race, Wiener, Rosenfield, and ISBT nomenclatures.

**5** Define the basic biochemical structure of Rh.

**6** Compare and contrast the genetic pathways for the inherited $Rh_{null}$ and the amorphic $Rh_{null}$.

**7** Describe and differentiate three mechanisms that result in weak D expression on red blood cells.

**8** List three instances in which the weak D status of an individual must be determined.

**9** List and differentiate four types of Rh typing reagents. Give two advantages for each.

**10** Define three characteristics of Rh antibodies.

**11** Describe three symptoms associated with an Rh hemolytic transfusion reaction.

**12** Compare and contrast $Rh_{null}$ and $Rh_{mod}$.

**13** List four Rh antigens (excluding DCcEe), and give two classic characteristics of each.

## INTRODUCTION

The term *Rh* refers not only to a specific red cell antigen but also to a complex blood group system that is currently composed of nearly 50 different antigenic specificities. Although the Rh antibodies were among the first to be described and scientists have spent years unraveling the complexities of the Rh system and its mode of inheritance, the genetic control of the Rh system and the biochemical structure of the Rh antigens still elude scientists.

## HISTORY OF THE Rh SYSTEM

Before 1939, the only significant blood group antigens recognized were those of the ABO system. Transfusion medicine was thus based on matching ABO groups. Despite ABO matching, blood transfusions continued to result in morbidity and mortality.

As the 1930s ended, two significant discoveries were made that would further the safety of blood transfusion and eventually result in defining the most extensive blood group system known. It began when Levine and Stetson[1] described a hemolytic transfusion reaction in an obstetrical patient. After delivery of a stillborn infant, a woman required transfusions. Her husband, who had the same ABO type, was selected as her donor. After transfusion, the recipient demonstrated the classic symptoms of an acute hemolytic transfusion reaction. Subsequently, an antibody was isolated from the mother's serum that reacted both at 37°C and at 20°C with the father's red blood cells. It was postulated that the fetus and the father possessed a common factor that the mother lacked. While the mother carried the fetus, she was exposed to this factor and subsequently built an antibody that reacted against the transfused red cells from the father and resulted in the hemolytic transfusion reaction.

A year later, Landsteiner and Wiener[2] reported on an antibody made by guinea pigs and rabbits when they were transfused with rhesus monkey red cells. This antibody, which agglutinated 85 percent of human red cells, was named "Rh." Another investigation by Levine and coworkers[3] demonstrated that the agglutinin that had caused the hemolytic transfusion reaction and the antibody described by Landsteiner and Wiener appeared to define the same blood group. Many years later it was recognized that the two antibodies were different. However, the name Rh was retained for the human-produced antibody, and the anti-rhesus formed by the animals was renamed anti-LW in honor of those first reporting it (Landsteiner and Wiener).

Further research resulted in defining Rh as a primary cause of hemolytic disease of the newborn (HDN, also called erythroblastosis fetalis) and a significant cause of hemolytic transfusion reactions. Continued investigation[4-7] showed additional blood group factors associated with the original agglutinin. By the mid-1940s five antigens made up the Rh system. Today the Rh blood group system is made up of nearly 50 different specificities.

## NOMENCLATURES OF THE RH SYSTEM

The terminologies used to describe the Rh system are derived from four sets of investigators. Two of the terminologies are based on the postulated genetic mechanisms of the Rh system. The third terminology describes only the presence or absence of a given antigen. The fourth is the result of the combined efforts of the International Society of Blood Transfusion (ISBT) Working Party on Terminology for Red Cell Surface Antigens. The genetic pathways are described in detail after the discussion of the nomenclatures, although reference to the former may be included here.

### Fisher-Race: The DCE Terminology

In the early 1940s, Fisher and Race[8] were investigating the antigens found on human red blood cells, including the newly defined Rh antigen. They postulated that the antigens of the system were produced by three closely linked sets of alleles. This is illustrated in Figure 6–1. Each gene was responsible for producing a product (or antigen) on the red cell surface. Each antigen

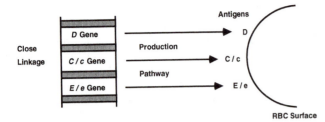

**Figure 6–1.** Fisher-Race concept of Rh (simplified). Each gene produces one product.

**Table 6–1.** Gene Frequency of Rh Antigens

| Gene | Frequency (%) |
|---|---|
| D | 85 |
| d | 15 |
| (absence of D) | |
| C | 70 |
| E | 30 |
| c | 80 |
| e | 98 |

**Table 6–2.** Fisher-Race Phenotypes of the Rh System: Frequencies in the United States

| Gene Combination | Frequency (%) | | | |
|---|---|---|---|---|
| | White | Black | Native American | Asian |
| DCe | 42 | 17 | 44 | 70 |
| dce | 37 | 26 | 11 | 3 |
| DcE | 14 | 11 | 34 | 21 |
| Dce | 4 | 44 | 2 | 3 |
| dCe | 2 | 2 | 2 | 2 |
| dcE | 1 | 0 | 6 | 0 |
| DCE | 0 | 0 | 6 | 1 |
| dCE* | 0 | 0 | 0 | 0 |

**Source:** Widmann,[9] p 130, with permission.
*Frequency less than 1%, but phenotype has been found.

and corresponding gene were given the same letter designation; however, when referring to the gene, the letter is italicized.

Fisher and Race named the antigens of the system D, d, C, c, E, and e. To date, no d antigen has been found, and it is considered an amorph (silent allele) or the absence of D antigen. The phenotype (blood type observed during testing) of a given red cell is defined by the presence of D, C, c, E, and e expression. The gene frequency for each Rh antigen is given in Table 6–1 and the Rh haplotype (the complement of genes inherited from either parent) frequencies are given in Table 6–2. Notice how the frequencies vary with race.

According to the Fisher-Race proposal, each person inherits a set of *Rh* genes from each parent (i.e., one *D*

or *d*, one *C* or *c*, and one *E* or *e*). This is detailed in Figure 6–1. Because *Rh* genes are codominant, each inherited gene expresses its corresponding antigen on the red cell. The combination of maternal and paternal haplotypes determines one's genotype (the *Rh* genes inherited from each parent) and dictates one's phenotype (the antigens expressed on the red cell that can be detected serologically). An individual's Rh phenotype is reported as DCE rather than CDE because Fisher postulated that the *C/c* locus lies between *D/d* and *E/e* loci. This information is based on frequencies of the various gene combinations.

It is essential to remember that d does not represent an antigen but simply represents the absence of the D antigen. C, c, E, and e represent actual antigens recognized by specific antibodies. For many students the Fisher-Race nomenclature represents the easiest way to think about the five major Rh system antigens, but it has shortcomings in that many of the newer Rh antigens are not assigned names using the Fisher-Race nomenclature.

In very rare instances, an individual may fail to express any allelic antigen at one or both Rh loci; that is, a person may express neither C or c, E or e, nor CcEe. The genotype for the Rh-positive person exhibiting a deletion phenotype such as these is written −*De* or −*DE*, *CD*− or *cD*−, or −*D*−, last respectively. The last is sometimes referred to as a double deletion. The person expressing no Rh antigens on the red cell is said to be Rh$_{null}$, and the phenotype may be written as ---/---. Weakened expression of all Rh antigens of an individual has also been reported. These individuals are said to have the Rh$_{mod}$ phenotype, and there is no unique way of indicating this using the Fisher-Race terminology.

## Wiener: The Rh-Hr Terminology

In his early work defining the Rh antigens, Wiener[10] believed that the gene responsible for defining Rh actually produced an agglutinogen that contained a series of blood factors. According to Rh-Hr terminology, this *Rh* gene produces at least three factors within an agglutinogen (Fig. 6–2). The agglutinogen may be considered the phenotypic expression of the haplotype. Each factor is an antigen recognized by an antibody. Antibodies can recognize single or multiple factors (antigens).

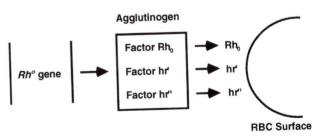

**Figure 6–2.** Wiener's agglutinogen theory. Antibody will recognize each factor within the agglutinogen.

**Table 6–3.** Rh-Hr Terminology of Wiener

| Gene | Agglutinogen | Blood Factors | Shorthand Designation | Fisher-Race Antigens |
|------|-------------|---------------|----------------------|---------------------|
| $Rh^0$ | $Rh_0$ | $Rh_0hr'hr''$ | $R_0$ | Dce |
| $Rh^1$ | $Rh_1$ | $Rh_0rh'hr''$ | $R_1$ | DCe |
| $Rh^2$ | $Rh_2$ | $Rh_0hr'rh''$ | $R_2$ | DcE |
| $Rh^z$ | $Rh_z$ | $Rh_0rh'rh''$ | $R_z$ | DCE |
| $rh$ | rh | $hr'hr''$ | r | dce |
| $rh'$ | rh' | $rh'hr''$ | r' | dCe |
| $rh''$ | rh'' | $hr'rh''$ | r'' | dcE |
| $rh^y$ | $rh_y$ | $rh'rh''$ | $r^y$ | dCE |

Table 6–3 lists the major agglutinogens and their respective factors, along with the shorthand term that has come to represent each agglutinogen. The Wiener terminology is complex and unwieldy; nevertheless, it is used by many blood bankers interchangeably with the other nomenclatures.

Fisher-Race nomenclature may be converted to Wiener nomenclature and vice versa. It is important to remember that an agglutinogen in the Wiener nomenclature actually represents the presence of a single haplotype capable of expressing three different antigens (see Table 6–3). When describing an agglutinogen, the uppercase R denotes the presence of the original factor, the D antigen. The lowercase r indicates the absence of the D antigen. The presence of uppercase C is indicated by a one (1) or single prime ('). Lowercase c is implied when there is no 1 or ' indicated. That is, $R_1$ is the same as $DC\,e$; r' denotes $dCe$; and $R_0$ is equivalent to $Dce$. The presence of E is indicated by the Arabic numeral two (2) or double prime ("). Lowercase e is implied when there is no 2 or " indicated. That is, $R_2$ is the same as $DcE$; r" denotes $dcE$; and r is equivalent to $dce$. When both C and E are uppercase, the letter z or y is used. $R_z$ denotes $CDE$, whereas $r^y$ represents $CdE$. Italics and superscripts are used when describing the *Rh* genes in the

Wiener nomenclature. Standard type is used to describe the gene product or agglutinogen. Subscripts are used with the uppercase R and superscripts with the lowercase r. The phenotypes of $Rh_{null}$ and $Rh_{mod}$ are written as stated. The genotype for the $Rh_{null}$ that arises from an amorphic gene at both Rh loci is written as $\bar{\bar{rr}}$ and pronounced "little r double bar."

When referring to the Rh antigens (or factors) in Wiener nomenclature, the single prime (') refers to either C or c and the double prime (") to either E or e. If the r precedes the h (i.e., rh' or rh"), we are referring to C or E antigens, respectively. When the h precedes the r, we are referring to either c (hr') or e (hr") antigen. $Rh_0$ is equivalent to D. In the Wiener nomenclature, there is no designation for the absence of D antigen. By using these designations, the worker should be able to recognize immediately which factors are present on the red cells described. However, it is difficult to use the Wiener nomenclature to describe adequately additional alleles within an agglutinogen. Because of this, many of the more recently described antigens of the *Rh* system have not been given Rh-Hr designations.

## Rosenfield and Coworkers: Alpha/Numeric Terminology

As the Rh blood group system expanded, it became more difficult to assign names to new antigens using existing terminologies. In the early 1960s Rosenfield and associates[11] proposed a system that assigns a number to each antigen of the Rh system in order of its discovery or recognized relationship to the Rh system (Table 6–4). This system has no genetic basis, but simply demonstrates the presence or absence of the antigen on the red cell. A minus sign preceding a number designates absence of the antigen. If an antigen has not been typed for, its number will not appear in the sequence. An advantage of this nomenclature is that the red cell phenotype is thus succinctly described.

**Table 6–4.** Common Rh Types by Three Nomenclatures

| | Genotype | | | Frequency (%) |
|---|---|---|---|---|
| | **Wiener** | **Fisher-Race** | **Rosenfield** | **(approx., White)** |
| Common genotypes | $R^1r$ | DCe/dce | Rh:1,2,−3,4,5 | 33 |
| | $R^1R^1$ | DCe/DCe | Rh:1,2,−3,−4,5 | 18 |
| | rr | dce/dce | Rh:−1,−2,−3,4,5 | 15 |
| | $R^1R^2$ | DCe/DcE | Rh:1,2,3,4,5 | 11 |
| | $R^2r$ | DcE/dce | Rh:1,−2,3,4,5 | 9 |
| | $R^2R^2$ | DcE/DcE | Rh:1,−2,3,4,−5 | 2 |
| Rarer genotypes | r'r | dCe/dce | Rh:−1,2,−3,4,5 | 1 |
| | r'r' | dCe/dCe | Rh:−1,2,−3,−4,5 | 0.01 |
| | r"r | dcE/dce | Rh:−1,−2,3,4,5 | 1 |
| | r"r" | dcE/dcE | Rh:−1,−2,3,4,−5 | 0.03 |
| | $R^0r$ | Dce/dce | Rh:1,−2,−3,4,5 | 2 |
| | $R^0R^0$ | Dce/Dce | Rh:1,−2,−3,4,5 | 0.1 |
| | $r^yr$ | dCE/dce | Rh:−1,2,3,4,5 | rare |

**Source:** Handbook of Clinical Laboratory Science. CRC Press, Boca Raton, FL, 1977, p 342, with permission.

For the five major antigens, D is assigned Rh1, C is Rh2, E is Rh3, c is Rh4, and e is Rh5. For red cells that type D + C + E + c negative, e negative, the Rosenfield designation is Rh: 1, 2, 3, −4, −5. If the sample was not tested for e, the designation would be Rh:1, 2, 3, −4. All Rh system antigens have been assigned a number.

The numeric system is well suited to electronic data processing. Its use expedites data entry and retrieval. Its primary limiting factor is that there is a similar nomenclature for numerous other blood groups such as Kell, Duffy, Kidd, Lutheran, Scianna, and more. K:1,2 refers to the K and k antigens of the Kell blood group system. Therefore, when using the Rosenfield nomenclature in the computer, one must use both the alpha (Rh:, K:) and the numeric (1, 2, −3, etc.) to denote a phenotype.

## International Society of Blood Transfusion: Numeric Terminology

As the world of blood transfusion began to cooperate and share data, it became apparent that there was a need for a universal language. The ISBT formed the Working Party on Terminology for Red Cell Surface Antigens. Its mandate was to establish a uniform nomenclature that is both eye and machine readable and is in keeping with the genetic basis of blood groups.[12] The ISBT adopted a six-digit number for each authenticated blood group specificity. The first three numbers represent the system and the remaining three the antigenic specificity. The number 004 was assigned to the Rh blood group system, and then each antigen assigned to the Rh system was given a unique number to complete the six-digit computer number. Table 6–5 provides a complete listing of these numbers.

When referring to individual antigens, an alphanumeric designation similar to the Rosenfield nomenclature may be used. The alphabetic names formerly used (e.g., Rh, Kell) were left unchanged but were converted to all uppercase letters (i.e., RH, KELL). Therefore, D is RH1, C is RH2, and so forth. (Note: There is no space between the RH and the assigned number.)

The phenotype designation includes the alphabetical symbol that denotes the blood group, followed by a colon and then the specificity numbers of the antigens defined. A minus sign preceding the number indicates that the antigen was tested for but was not present. The phenotype D+ C− E+ c+ e+ or DccEe or $R_2r$ would be written RH:1,−2,3,4,5.

When referring to a gene, an allele, or a haplotype, the symbols are italicized, followed by a space or asterisk, and then the numbers of the specificities are separated by commas. $R^1$ or DCe would be RH1,2,5.

## Summary: Rh Terminologies

Blood bankers must be familiar with the Fisher-Race, Wiener, Rosenfield, and ISBT nomenclatures and must be able to translate among them when reading about, writing about, or discussing the Rh system. Tables 6–4 and 6–6 summarize the data presented in

**Table 6–5.** The Antigens of the Rh Blood Group System in Four Nomenclatures

| Numeric | Fisher-Race | Weiner | ISBT Number | Other Names or Comment |
|---------|-------------|--------|-------------|------------------------|
| Rh1 | D | $Rh_0$ | 004001 | |
| Rh2 | C | rh' | 004002 | |
| Rh3 | E | rh" | 004003 | |
| Rh4 | c | hr' | 004004 | |
| Rh5 | e | hr" | 004005 | |
| Rh6 | ce | hr | 004006 | f |
| Rh7 | Ce | $rh_i$ | 004007 | |
| Rh8 | $C^w$ | $rh^{w1}$ | 004008 | |
| Rh9 | $C^x$ | $rh^x$ | 004009 | |
| Rh10 | $ce^s$ | $hr^v$ | 004010 | V |
| Rh11 | $E^w$ | $rh^{w2}$ | 004011 | |
| Rh12 | G | $rh^G$ | 004012 | |
| Rh13 | | $Rh^A$ | 004013 | |
| Rh14 | | $Rh^B$ | 004014 | |
| Rh15 | | $Rh^C$ | 004015 | |
| Rh16 | | $Rh^D$ | 004016 | |
| Rh17 | | $Hr_0$ | 004017 | |
| Rh18 | | Hr | 004018 | |
| Rh19 | | $hr^S$ | 004019 | |
| Rh20 | $e^s$ | | 004020 | VS |
| Rh21 | $C^G$ | | 004021 | |
| Rh22 | CE | rh | 004022 | Jarvis |
| Rh23 | $D^W$ | | 004023 | Wiel |
| Rh24 | $E^T$ | | 004024 | |
| Rh25*/† | | | 004025 | |
| Rh26 | c-like | | 004026 | Deal |
| Rh27 | cE | $rh_{ii}$ | 004027 | |
| Rh28 | | $hr^H$ | 004028 | Hernandez |
| Rh29 | | | 004029 | total Rh |
| Rh30 | $D^{cor}$ | | 004030 | $Go^a$ |
| Rh31 | | $hr^B$ | 004031 | |
| Rh32 | | $\overline{R}^N$ | 004032 | Troll |
| Rh33 | | $R_0^{Har}$ | 004033 | Hill |
| Rh34 | | $Hr^B$ | 004034 | Bastiaan |
| Rh35 | | | 004035 | 1114 |
| Rh36 | | | 004036 | $Be^a$ (Berrens) |
| Rh37 | | | 004037 | Evans |
| Rh38† | | | 004038 | Duclos |
| Rh39 | C-like | | 004039 | |
| Rh40 | Tar | | 004040 | Targett |
| Rh41 | Ce-like | | 004041 | |
| Rh42 | $Ce^s$ | $rh_i^S$ | 004042 | Thornton |
| Rh43 | | | 004043 | Crawford |
| Rh44 | | | 004044 | Nou |
| Rh45 | | | 004045 | Riv |
| Rh46 | "Allelic" | to $\overline{R}^N$ | 004046 | Sec |
| Rh47 | | | 004047 | Dav |
| Rh48 | | | 004048 | JAL |
| Rh49 | | | 004049 | Stem |
| Rh50 | | | 004050 | FPTT |
| Rh51 | | | 004051 | |

*Rh25 was formerly assigned to the LW antigen. LW is now known as $LW^a$ and is no longer considered a member of the Rh system.
†Obsolete names: Rh25 formerly LW, Rh38 formerly Duclos.

this section. These tables also include probable genotypes based on the antigens found in selected red blood cell populations.

Table 6–6 correlates Rh phenotypes with the most probable genotype in a designated population. It is important to remember that results of typing do not de-

**Table 6–6.** Eighteen Possible Reaction Patterns with Five Antisera*

| D | C | E | c | e | Whites (%) | Blacks (%) | Whites | Blacks | Other Possibilities (Both Groups) |
|---|---|---|---|---|---|---|---|---|---|
| + | + | − | + | + | 35 | 26 | DCe/dce | DCe/Dce | dCe/Dce |
| + | + | − | − | + | 19 | 3 | DCe/DCe | DCe/DCe | DCe/dCe |
| + | + | + | + | + | 13 | 4 | DCe/DcE | DCe/DcE | DCe/dcE dCe/DcE, DCE/dce DCE/Dce or dCE/Dce |
| + | − | + | + | + | 12 | 16 | DcE/dce | DcE/Dce | dcE/Dce |
| + | − | + | + | − | 2 | 1 | DcE/DcE | DcE/DcE | DcE/dcE |
| + | − | − | + | + | 2 | 42 | Dce/dce | Dce/Dce or Dce/dce | — |
| − | − | − | + | + | 15 | 7 | dce/dce | dce/dce | — |
| − | + | − | + | + | 1 | 1 | dCe/dce | dCe/dce | — |
| − | − | + | + | + | 1 | rare | dcE/ dce | dcE/dce | — |
| − | + | + | + | + | Each of these phenotypes occurs with a frequency of less than 0.2% in both racial groups. | | dCe/dcE | dCE/dce | |
| − | + | − | − | + | | | dCe/dCe | — | |
| − | − | + | + | − | | | dcE/dcE | — | |
| + | + | + | − | + | | | DCE/DCe | DCE/dCe | |
| + | + | + | + | − | | | DCE/DcE | DCE/dcE | |
| + | + | + | − | − | | | DCE/DCE | DCE/dCE | |
| − | + | + | − | + | | | dCE/dCe | — | |
| − | + | + | + | − | | | dCE/dcE | — | |
| − | + | + | − | − | | | dCE/dCE | — | |

*Percentages are rounded off.

fine genotype, only phenotype. Other genotypes that can occur with the given test results are also listed, but they are not commonly seen.

Determining probable genotypes is useful for parentage studies as well as for population studies. Probable genotypes also may be useful in predicting the potential for hemolytic disease of the newborn (HDN) in offspring of an Rh-negative woman with an Rh antibody.

There are substantial differences in the probable genotypes of various populations. These differences must be remembered when trying to locate compatible blood for recipients with unusual or multiple Rh antibodies.

To further emphasize the interchangeable use of the terminologies for the basic antigens, see Table 6–4, which defines common genotypes using the Fisher-Race, Wiener, and Rosenfield nomenclatures. The frequencies listed are for those found in the white population.

## PROPOSED GENETIC PATHWAYS

### Biochemistry of the Rh Antigens

Before any discussion of genetic pathways can occur, it is necessary to understand the result of gene action. The final result of gene action in red blood cell groups is the production of a biochemical structure; in the Rh system it is a nonglycosylated protein. This means that there are no carbohydrates attached to the protein. The Rh antigens are transmembrane polypeptides

and are an integral part of the red cell membrane.[13] The gene products of RHD and RHCE are remarkably similar in that both encode for proteins composed of 417 amino acids that traverse the cell membrane 12 times and that their sequence differs by only 44 base pair.[14] The gene products of RHCE, RHCe, RHce, and RHcE are even more similar. C and c differ from one another in four amino acid positions, and one amino acid differentiates E from e (Fig. 6–3). Only small loops of the Rh proteins are exposed on the surface of the red cell and provide the conformational requirements for the serologic differences between the Rh blood types.

As part of the research on the biochemistry of the Rh antigens, investigations have been performed to determine the quantity of antigen sites on red blood cells of various Rh phenotypes. In comparison with ABO and

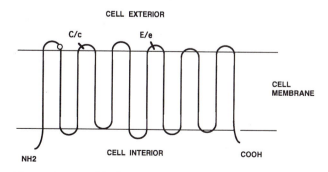

**Figure 6–3.** Model of Rh polypeptide. O denotes where the sequence of D diverges from C/c or E/e. The C/c and E/e respectively denote the region responsible for the serologic difference between C/c and E/e.

**Table 6–7.** Number of D Antigen Sites of Cells with Various Phenotypes

| Rh Phenotype | Number of D Antigen Sites |
|---|---|
| $R_1r$ | 9,900–14,600 |
| $R_0r$ | 12,000–20,000 |
| $R_2r$ | 14,000–16,600 |
| $R_1R_1$ | 14,500–19,300 |
| $R_1R_2$ | 23,000–31,000 |
| $R_2R_2$ | 15,800–33,300 |
| D–– | 110,000–202,000 |

Kell (K) blood groups, $A_1$ cells possess approximately $1.0 \times 10^6$ A antigens, whereas homozygous Kell cells have 6000 K sites. The number of D antigen sites were measured on a variety of Rh phenotypes by Hughes-Jones and coworkers, and the results are summarized in Table 6–7.[15] The greatest number of D antigen sites are on cells of the rare Rh phenotype D––. (D–– cells carry only D antigen and completely lack Cc and Ee.) However, of the commonly encountered Rh genotypes, $R^2R^2$ cells possess the largest number of D antigen sites.

## Mechanisms of Antigen Production

Many theories have been proposed to explain genetically the results of serologic and biochemical studies in the Rh system. Two theories of Rh genetic control were initially postulated. Wiener postulated that a single gene produced a single product that contained separately recognizable factors (see Figure 6–2). In contrast, Fisher and Race proposed that the Rh locus contains three distinct genes that control the production of their respective antigens (see Figure 6–1).

It is currently accepted that only two closely linked genes control the expression of Rh; one gene codes for the presence or absence of *D* and the second gene for either *Ce, cE, ce,* or *CE*[15,16] (Fig. 6–4).

It has been demonstrated through linkage studies that the Rh locus is located on chromosome 1, along with the genes for elliptocytosis, 6-phosphogluconate dehydrogenase (PGD), phosphoglucomutase (PGM), and phosphopyruvate hydratase (PPH).[17]

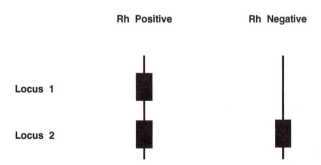

**Figure 6–4.** Rh Inheritance: Two loci theory. Locus 1 codes for the presence or absence of *D/d*. Locus 2 codes for the presence of *Ce, cE, ce, or CE.*

The Rh antigens are inherited as codominant alleles. Offspring inherit one Rh haplotype from each parent. Figure 6–5 is an example of a normal Rh inheritance pattern.

It has been postulated that the genes contained at the Rh locus are very closely linked, so much so that crossing over is an extremely rare event. The frequencies of the various Rh gene complexes strongly support this theory. If the genes were not closely linked, all of the gene complex frequencies would be similar.

One mechanism of Rh antigen production first proposed by Race uses the concept of precursor substances as the building blocks for Rh antigens. Different sets of genes sequentially affect the final expression of the Rh antigens in a given individual. This concept has been used to describe the formation of many other common blood group antigens. When only a few alleles exist, it appears to be an adequate explanation. With the complexity of the Rh system, modification of this proposal is required.

The modification illustrated in Figure 6–6 is based on serologic data gathered during the 1960s.[18] Variation within the $Rh_{null}$ phenotype (phenotype that demonstrates no Rh antigens on the red cell surface) and the discovery that the Rh genes are not linked to the LW genes are better explained by Giblett's interpretation. According to Giblett,[19] precursor substance 1 is acted upon by one of several genes at the Xr locus. Un-

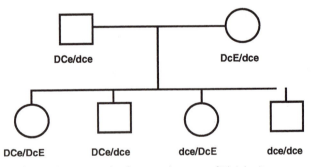

**Figure 6–5.** Example of a normal pattern of Rh inheritance.

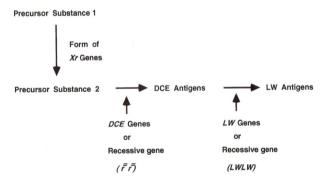

**Figure 6–6.** Giblett's modification of Race's Rh genetic pathway. Alternative forms of *Xr* gene: $X^1r$, $X^0r$, or $X^Qr$. Inheriting $X^1r$ in either the homozygous or heterozygous form results in expected conversion of precursor 1 to precursor 2. Inheriting homozygous $X^0r X^0r$ results in the amorphic $Rh_{null}$. Inheriting homozygous $X^Qr X^Qr$ results in $Rh_{mod}$ expression.

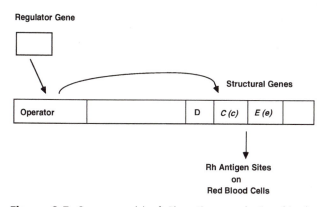

**Figure 6–7.** Operon model of Rh antigen production (simple operon).

der normal circumstances precursor 1 is converted to precursor 2 in the presence of the $X^1r$ gene. (The $X^1r$ may be either homozygous or heterozygous.) In the presence of DCE genes, precursor 2 is converted to DCE antigens. The LW gene(s) then act to express the LW antigens. When the LW/LW genotype (the amorphic genotype) is present, the cells express no LW antigens and type as $LW^{a-b-}$.

When homozygous $X^0r/X^0r$ genes are inherited at the Xr loci, precursor 1 is not converted to precursor 2. Even though the individual has normal CDE and $LW^a$ or $LW^b$ genes and can transfer these genes to offspring, neither the CDE nor LW antigens will be expressed on this individual's red blood cells. When no Rh antigens are expressed on the red cell, the cells are said to be $Rh_{null}$. Because the $X^0r/X^0r$ genes are inherited independently from the Rh genes, this type of $Rh_{null}$ is called the regulator or inhibitor type $Rh_{null}$. Because these individuals carry no Rh antigens on their red cells, they are capable of making antibody to any or all of the Rh antigens.

When homozygous $X^Qr X^Qr$ genes are inherited at the Xr loci, only a limited amount of precursor 1 is converted to precursor 2. This results in a weakened expression of all Rh antigens on the red cell. People with the $Rh_{mod}$ phenotype do not make antibody to the Rh antigens that they possess.

When the $X^1r$ gene is inherited in combination with the rr genes, the individual is said to have the amorphic $Rh_{null}$ phenotype. Precursor 1 is converted to precursor 2; however, the rr genes at the DCE loci do not alter precursor 2. This results in no DCE antigens or LW antigens being produced.

As the understanding of genetics grew, the way of looking at blood group inheritance also changed. The 1973 paper by Rosenfield and colleagues[20] is a comprehensive description of the operon model. This model postulates that an operator gene directs production of a messenger, which in turn directs a structural gene to produce a polypeptide chain (the antigen itself). Furthermore, there may be a regulator gene at another locus that can influence the sequence described. This may result in either altered genetic products or in no production of genetic products. Compatible with this model is the oc-

currence of mutations, which can result in varied expression of products from the Rh locus. The model is diagrammatically interpreted in Figure 6–7. Rosenfield defines a conjugated operon that further explains the unique gene products associated with the Rh system.

As work in the field of genetics and blood groups advances, it may be possible to define the actual pathway of antigen production. As new data become available, new concepts and hypotheses may evolve from current theories and proposals.

## VARIATIONS OF THE $Rh_0$ (D) ANTIGEN

### Weak D

When Rh-positive red cell samples are typed for the D antigen, they are expected to react strongly (macroscopically) with anti-D reagents. However, with certain red cells the testing must be carried through the antiglobulin phase of the tube testing to demonstrate the presence of the D antigen. Red cells carrying the weaker D antigen have historically been referred to as having the Du type. Three different mechanisms have been described that can explain the weakened expression of the D antigen.

### Genetic Weak D

The first mechanism results from inheritance of D genes that code for a weakened expression of the D antigen.[21] The D antigens expressed appear to be complete, but few in number. Inheritance of these genes can be tracked vertically from one generation to the next and are seen most frequently in blacks. The genetic weak D is rarely found in whites.

### C Trans

The second mechanism that may result in weakened expression of the D antigen is described as a position effect or gene interaction effect.[22] In individuals showing the gene interaction weak D, the allele carrying D is trans (or in the opposite haplotype) to the allele carrying C, for example, Dce/dCe. The Rh antigen on the red cell is normal, but the steric arrangement of the C antigen in relationship to the D antigen appears to interfere with the expression of the D antigen. This interference with D expression does not occur when the C gene is inherited in the cis position to D, such as DCe/dce. It is not possible to distinguish the genetic weak D from the position effect weak D serologically. Family studies are necessary to distinguish which type of weakened D antigen is being demonstrated. Practically speaking, this is unnecessary because the D antigen is structurally complete. These individuals can receive D-positive red cells with no adverse effects.

### D Mosaic or Partial D

The third instance in which the D antigen expression can be weakened is when one or more parts of the D antigen is missing. Cells with a mosaic D antigen usually type weaker than expected or may not react at all when routine procedures are used with most commercial anti-D reagents.

In the early 1950s several reports[23,24] described individuals who were typed D-positive but manufactured an anti-D that reacted with all D-positive samples except their own. The formation of alloanti-D by D-positive individuals required explanation.

Wiener and Unger[25] postulated that the D antigen is made of antigenic subparts, genetically determined, that could be absent in rare instances. If an individual lacked one (or more) pieces or epitopes of the total D antigen, alloantibody can be made to the missing fraction(s) if exposed to red cells that possess the complete D antigen. This theory has become well accepted.

Tippett and Sanger[26] worked with red blood cells and sera of D-mosaic individuals to classify these antigens. Their work, which was based on the reactivity of anti-D sera from D-positive people, with red cells from D-positive people who also made anti-D, has led to a method of categorizing the mosaic D. Seven categories were recognized, designated by Roman numerals I through VII. Category I is now obsolete, and a few of the categories have been subdivided further.

With the advent of monoclonal antibodies and the depletion and deterioration of the available anti-D made by persons with partial D genotype, Tippett and coworkers[27] have pursued the classification of partial D antigens using monoclonal anti-D (MAb-D). Table 6–8 presents a summary of the partial D categories. Also, the molecular basis of most partial D antigens has been determined.

Although understanding the difference between the genetic weak D, weak D caused by C trans, and the mosaic or partial D helps explain why some persons with the weak D phenotype develop anti-D and others do not, no differentiation in weak status is made in the routine blood bank. The donors and patients are classified simply as Rh-positive or Rh-negative. It is important, however, to remember that the anti-D made by D-mosaic individuals can cause hemolytic disease of the newborn (HDN) or transfusion reactions, or both. Once anti-D is identified, Rh-negative blood should be used for transfusion. The identification of a person with a D-mosaic gene routinely occurs after the person begins producing anti-D. This discovery should prompt collection of additional samples to be sent to a reference laboratory for $Rh_0(D)$ classification.

## DETERMINATION OF D STATUS

Determining the D status of a red cell sample is essential when testing donor bloods. Blood for transfusion is considered Rh-positive if either the D or the weak D test is positive. Any donor blood sample that is typed $Rh_0(D)$-negative by the slide or rapid tube method must be tested further by an indirect antihuman globulin technique (Color Plate 11). If both tests are negative, the donor sample is considered Rh-negative. If the donor sample tests positive in any phase of $Rh_0(D)$ testing, the sample is considered Rh-positive.

For transfusion recipients, the application of the test for weak D is controversial. Because blood recipients with the C trans weak D and those with the genetic weak D clearly have the complete D antigen and cannot manufacture alloanti-D, Rh-positive blood may be transfused. The very rare D-mosaic individuals can form alloanti-D when exposed to D-positive red cells. However, many workers believe that the number of individuals homozygous for the D-mosaic gene is so small, the risk of sensitizing a D-mosaic individual so low, and the supply of Rh-negative blood so precious that an intended blood recipient who types weak D positive should be given Rh-positive blood. Policy regarding transfusion of weak D recipients is established individually within each transfusion service. Regulatory agencies do not require routine testing for weak D in blood recipients unless the intended recipient has, or in the past has had, anti-D in his or her serum.

**Table 6–8.** Epitope Profiles of Partial D Antigens

| | Reactions with Monoclonal Anti-D Antibodies | | | | | | | |
|---|---|---|---|---|---|---|---|---|
| Cells | epD1 | epD2 | epD3 | epD4 | epD5 | epD6/7 | epD8 | epD9 |
| I | + | : | + | 0 | + | + | + | 0 |
| IIIa | + | + | + | + | + | + | + | + |
| IIIb | + | + | + | + | + | + | + | + |
| IIIc | + | + | + | + | + | + | + | + |
| IVa | 0 | 0 | 0 | + | + | + | + | 0 |
| IVb | 0 | 0 | 0 | 0 | + | + | + | + |
| Va | 0 | + | + | + | 0 | + | + | + |
| VI | 0 | 0 | + | + | 0 | 0 | 0 | + |
| VII | + | + | + | + | + | + | 0 | + |
| DFR | : | : | + | + | : | : | 0 | + |
| DBT | 0 | 0 | 0 | 0 | 0 | : | + | 0 |
| $R_0^{Har}$ | 0 | 0 | 0 | 0 | : | : | 0 | 0 |

+ = positive reaction; 0 = negative reaction; : = positive with some antibodies and negative with other antibodies.

Determining the $Rh_0(D)$ status (including weak D status) of obstetric patients is critical. All Rh-negative, weak D-negative obstetric patients are candidates for Rh immune globulin (RhIG) (a drug injected to prevent Rh-negative individuals who are exposed to Rh-positive red cells from developing anti-D). Likewise, when the mother is Rh-negative and the newborn is typed Rh-negative, the weak D status of the newborn must be determined to assess the likelihood of maternal sensitization and the need for Rh immune globulin prophylaxis for the mother.

There are instances when an accurate Rh type cannot be determined through routine testing. If a newborn's cells are coated with maternal IgG anti-D in utero, very few D antigen sites are available to react with reagent anti-D (termed "blocking phenomena"). Elution of the sensitizing antibody (removing the antibody) and identifying it as anti-D will verify that the infant's red cells are D-positive. Other complex Rh typing difficulties arise in persons suffering from warm autoimmune hemolytic anemia. Many of the antibodies produced in this disorder are directed against the patient's own red cells and react as though they were Rh-specific. Resolution of these anomalies is beyond the scope of this chapter and frequently requires referral to reference laboratories for resolution or confirmation.

## DETECTION OF Rh ANTIBODIES AND ANTIGENS

### Rh Antibodies

Although the Rh system was first recognized by saline tests used to detect IgM antibodies, most Rh antibodies are IgG immunoglobulins and react optimally at 37°C or after antiglobulin testing. Rh antibodies are usually produced following exposure of the individual's immune system to foreign red cells, through either transfusion or pregnancy. Rh antigens are highly immunogenic; the D antigen is the most potent.[28] A comparison of the immunogenicity of the common Rh antigens is described in Figure 6–8. Exposure to less than 1 mL of Rh-positive red cells can stimulate antibody production in an Rh-negative person.

$IgG_1$, $IgG_2$, $IgG_3$, and $IgG_4$ subclasses of Rh antibodies have been reported. $IgG_1$ and $IgG_3$ are of the greatest clinical significance because the reticuloendothelial system rapidly clears red cells coated with $IgG_1$ and $IgG_3$ from the circulation. IgA Rh antibodies have also been reported but are not routinely tested for in the blood bank.[26]

As with most blood group antigen sensitization, IgM Rh antibodies are formed initially, followed by a transition to IgG. Rh antibodies often persist in the circula-

tion for years. An individual with low-titer Rh antibody may experience an anamnestic (secondary) antibody response if exposed to the same sensitizing antigen. Therefore, in the clinical setting, accuracy of D typing is essential, as is the careful checking of patient history to determine whether an Rh antibody has been identified previously. Most commonly found Rh antibodies are considered clinically significant. Therefore, antigen-negative blood must be provided to any patient with a history of Rh antibody sensitization, whether the antibody is currently demonstrable or not.

Rh antibodies do not bind complement. For complement to be fixed (or the complement cascade activated), two IgG immunoglobulins must attach to a red cell in close proximity. Rh antigens (to which the antibody would attach) are not situated on the red cell surface this closely. Therefore, when an Rh antibody coats the red cells, intravascular, complement-mediated hemolysis must occur. Red cell destruction resulting from antibodies is primarily extravascular.

Because Rh antibodies are primarily IgG and can traverse the placenta, and because Rh antigens are well developed early in fetal life, Rh antibodies formed by Rh-negative pregnant women do cross the placenta and may coat fetal red cells that carry the corresponding antigen. This results in the fetal cells testing positive by the direct antiglobulin test and in HDN, if the coated fetal cells are removed prematurely from the fetal circulation (see Chap. 20). Until the discovery of Rh-immune globulin, anti-D was the most frequent cause of HDN.

### Rh Antigen Typing Reagents

The reagents used to type for D and for the other Rh antigens may be derived from a variety of sources. The reagents may be high-protein-based, or low-protein-based, saline-based, chemically modified, monoclonal, or blends of monoclonals.

Saline reactive reagents, which contain IgM immunoglobulin, were the first typing reagents available to test for the D antigen. Saline anti-D has the advantage of being low-protein-based and can be used to test cells that are coated with IgG antibody. The primary disadvantages of saline typing reagents are their limited availability, cost of production, and lengthy incubation time. Because saline anti-D is an IgM immunoglobulin, it cannot be used for weak D typing.

In the 1940s high-protein anti-D reagents were developed. Human plasma containing high-titer D-specific antibody is used as the raw material. Potentiators of bovine albumin and macromolecular additives such as dextran or polyvinylpyrrolidone are added to the source material to optimize reactivity in the standard slide and rapid tube tests.[29] These reagents are commonly referred to as high-protein reagents. The presence of potentiators and the higher protein concentration, however, increase the likelihood of false-positive reactions. To assess the validity of the high-protein Rh typing results, a control reagent was

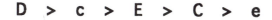

**D > c > E > C > e**

**Figure 6–8.** Immunogenicity of common Rh antigens. (For a detailed discussion, refer to Mollison[28].)

manufactured and had to be tested in parallel with each Rh test. If the control reacted, the test result was invalid and had to be repeated using a different technique or reagent anti-D. The major advantages of high-protein anti-D reagents are reduced incubation time and the ability to perform weak D testing and slide typing with the same reagent.

In the late 1970s, scientists chemically modified the IgG anti-D molecule by breaking the disulfide bonds that maintain the antibody's rigid shape.[30] This allows the antibody to relax and to span the distance between red cells in a low-protein medium. The chemically modified reagents can be used for both slide and tube testing and do not require a separate, manufactured Rh control as long as the samples type as A, B, or O. When samples test AB Rh-positive or when the Rh test is performed by itself, a separate saline control must be used to ensure that the observed reactions are true agglutination and not a result of spontaneous agglutination. Fewer false-positive test reactions are obtained because of the lower-protein suspending medium. Because of its lower-protein base and ready availability, the chemically modified anti-D replaced the need for saline anti-D reagents.

Monoclonal antibody reagents have become available recently. These reagents are derived from single clones of antibody-producing cells. The antibody-producing cells are hybridized with myeloma cells to increase their reproduction rate and thereby to maximize their antibody-producing capabilities. Because the D antigen appears to be a mosaic and the monoclonal Rh antibodies have a narrow specificity, monoclonal anti-D reagents are usually a combination of monoclonal anti-Ds from several different clones to ensure reactivity with a broad spectrum of Rh-positive red cells. Some companies also blend anti-IgM and anti-IgG anti-D to maximize visualization of reactions at immediate spin testing and to allow indirect antiglobulin testing for weak D with the same reagent. The monoclonal blends can be used for slide, tube, microwell, and most automated Rh testing. Because these reagents are not human derived, they lack all potential for transmitting infectious disease.

As with all commercial typing reagents, Rh antigen typing must be performed with strict adherence to manufacturer's directions, use of proper controls, and accurate interpretation of test and control results. Table 6–9 summarizes several common causes of false Rh typing results and suggests corrective actions that may be taken to obtain an accurate Rh type.

## CLINICAL CONSIDERATIONS

### Transfusion Reactions

Rh antigens are highly immunogenic. The D antigen is the most immunogenic antigen outside the ABO system. When anti-D is detected, a careful medical history will reveal red cell exposure through pregnancy or transfusion of products containing red cells. Circulating antibody appears within 120 days of a primary exposure and within 2 to 7 days after a secondary exposure.

Rh-mediated hemolytic transfusion reactions, whether caused by primary sensitization or secondary immunization, usually result in extravascular destruction of immunoglobulin-coated red cells. The transfusion recipient may have an unexplained fever, a mild bilirubin elevation, and decrease in hemoglobin and haptoglobin. The direct antihuman globulin test is usually positive, and the antibody screen may or may

**Table 6–9.** False Reactions with Rh Typing Reagents

| False-Positives | | False-Negatives | |
|---|---|---|---|
| Likely Cause | Corrective Action | Likely Cause | Corrective Action |
| 1. Cell suspension too heavy | 1. Adjust suspension, retype | 1. Immunoglobulin-coated cells (in vivo) | 1. Use saline-active typing reagent |
| 2. Cold agglutinins | 2. Wash with warm saline, retype | 2. Saline-suspended cells (slide) | 2. Use unwashed cells |
| 3. Test incubated too long or drying (slide) | 3. Follow manufacturer's instructions precisely | 3. Failure to follow manufacturer's directions precisely | 3. Review directions; repeat test |
| 4. Rouleaux | 4. Use saline-washed cells, retype | 4. Omission of reagent manufacturer's directions | 4. Always add reagent first and check before adding cells |
| 5. Fibrin interference | 5. Use saline-washed cells, retype | 5. Resuspension too vigorous | 5. Resuspend all tube tests gently |
| 6. Contaminating low-incidence antibody in reagent | 6. Try another manufacturer's reagent or use a known serum antibody | 6. Incorrect reagent selected | 6. Read vial label carefully; repeat |
| 7. Polyagglutination | 7. See chapter on polyagglutination | 7. Variant antigen | 7. Refer sample for further investigation |
| 8. Bacterial contamination of reagent vial | 8. Open new vial of reagent, retype | 8. Reagent deterioration | 8. Open new vial |
| 9. Incorrect reagent selected | 9. Repeat test; read vial label carefully | | |

not demonstrate circulating antibody. When the direct antiglobulin test indicates that the recipient's red cells are coated with IgG, elution studies may be helpful in defining the offending antibody specificity. If antibody is detected in either the serum or eluate, subsequent transfusions should lack the implicated antigen. It is not unusual for a person with a single Rh antibody to produce additional Rh antibodies if further stimulated.[28]

### Hemolytic Disease of the Newborn

Hemolytic disease of the newborn (HDN) is briefly described here because of the historic significance of the discovery of the Rh system in elucidating its cause. As stated previously, anti-D was discovered in a woman after delivery of a stillborn fetus. The mother required transfusion. The father's blood was transfused and the mother subsequently experienced a severe hemolytic transfusion reaction. Levine and Stetson[1] postulated that the antibody causing the transfusion reaction also crossed the placenta and destroyed the red blood cells of the fetus, causing its death. The offending antibody was subsequently identified as anti-D.[3]

Hemolytic disease of the newborn caused by Rh antibodies is often severe because the antigens are well developed on fetal cells and Rh antibodies are primarily IgG, which readily cross the placenta.

After years of research, a method was developed to prevent susceptible (Rh$_0$D-negative) mothers from forming anti-D, thus preventing Rh$_0$(D) HDN. Rh-immune globulin, a purified preparation of anti-D, is given to a D-negative woman during pregnancy and following delivery of a D-positive fetus.[31] Rh-immune globulin is effective only in preventing anti-D HDN. No effort is being made at this time to develop immune globulin products for other Rh antigens (e.g., C, c, E, e). When present, Rh HDN may be severe and may require aggressive treatment. Refer to Chapter 20 for a more detailed discussion of HDN—its etiology, serology, and treatment.

### Rh$_{null}$ SYNDROME Rh$_{mod}$

The rare individual who lacks all Rh antigens is said to have the Rh$_{null}$ syndrome and demonstrates a mild compensated hemolytic anemia,[32] reticulocytosis, stomatocytosis, a slight-to-moderate decrease in hemoglobin and hematocrit, an increase in hemoglobin F, a decrease in serum haptoglobin, and possibly an elevated bilirubin. The severity of the syndrome is highly variable from individual to individual even within one family. When transfusion of individuals with Rh$_{null}$ syndrome is necessary, only Rh$_{null}$ blood can be given.

Individuals of the Rh$_{mod}$ phenotype exhibit features similar to those with the Rh$_{null}$ syndrome; however, the clinical symptoms are usually less severe and rarely clinically remarkable.[33] Rh$_{null}$ and Rh$_{mod}$ red cells exhibit other blood group antigens; however, S, s, and U

antigen expression may be depressed.[34] Rh$_{null}$ red cells are negative for FY5.

## UNUSUAL PHENOTYPES AND RARE ALLELES

Some of the less frequently encountered Rh antigens are discussed briefly in the following paragraphs. Refer to other reference textbooks for in-depth discussions.[13,17]

### C$^w$

The C$^w$ was originally considered an allele at the C/c locus.[35] Later studies showed that it can be expressed in combination with both C and c and in the absence of either allele. Although C$^w$ is usually found in combination with C, its exact origin is not clear. C$^w$ is found in about 2 percent of whites and is very rare in blacks. Anti-C$^w$ has been identified in individuals without known exposure to foreign red cells as well as after transfusion or pregnancy. Anti-C$^w$ may show dosage (i.e., reacting more strongly with cells from individuals who are homozygous for C$^w$). Because of the low incidence of the C$^w$, C$^w$ antigen negative blood is readily available.

### f (ce)

The f antigen is expressed on the red cell when both c and e are present on the same haplotype or are in the cis position, and it has been called a *compound* antigen.[36] However, f is a single entity. Phenotypically, the following samples appear the same when tested with the five major Rh antisera: *Dce/DCE* and *DcE/DCe*. However, when tested with anti-f, only the former reacts. Anti-f has been reported to cause HDN and transfusion reactions.

### rh$_i$ (Ce)

Like anti-f, anti-rh$_i$ is present when C and e are in the cis configuration, has been called a compound antigen, and is a single entity.[36] A sample with the phenotype D + C + E + c + e + can be either *DcE/DCe* or *Dce/DCE*. Anti-rh$_i$ reacts only with *Dce/DCe* red cells.

### G

G is an antigen that is present on most D-positive and all C-positive red blood cells. In the test tube anti-G reacts as though it were a combination of anti-C plus anti-D.[37] G was originally described in an rr person who received Dccee red blood cells. Subsequently the recipient produced an antibody that appeared to be anti-D + C, which should be impossible because the C antigen was not on the transfused red cells. Further investigation showed that the antibody was directed toward D + G.

## Rh:13, Rh:14, Rh:15, Rh:16

Rh:13, Rh:14, Rh:15, Rh:16 defines four different parts of the D mosaic, as it was originally described. Although these parts are included in the D-mosaic categories II to VII as defined by Tippett and Sanger,[26,27,38] they are not directly comparable.

## $Hr_0$, Rh:17

$Hr_0$ is an antigen present on all red blood cells with the "common" Rh phenotypes (e.g., $R_1R_1$, $R_2R_2$, rr).[39] When red cells phenotype as D--, the most potent antibody they make is often one directed against $Hr_0$.

## Rh:23, Rh:30, Rh:40

Rh:23, Rh:30, and Rh:40 are all low-frequency antigens associated with a specific category of D mosaic. Rh:23 (also known as Wiel and $D^w$) is an antigenic marker for category Va D mosaic,[40] Rh:30 (also known as $Go^a$ or $D^{cor}$) is a marker for category IVa D-mosaic,[41] and Rh:40 (also known as Tar or Targett) is a marker for category VII.[42]

## Rh:33

The low-incidence antigen Rh:33 is associated with a rare variant of the $R^0(Dce)$ gene called $R_0{}^{Har}$.[43] $R_0{}^{Har}$ gene codes for normal amounts of c, reduced amounts of e, reduced f, reduced $Hr_0$, and reduced amounts of D antigen. The D reactions are frequently so weak that the cells are frequently mistakenly typed as Rh negative. To denote the weakened expression of an antigen in Fisher-Race nomenclature the letter is placed in parentheses. The $R_0{}^{Har}$ gene expresses (D)c(e) and has been found in whites.

## Rh:32

Rh:32 is a low-frequency antigen associated with a variant of the $R^1[D(C)(e)]$ gene which is called $\bar{\bar{R}}^N$.[44] The C antigen and e antigen are expressed weakly. The D antigen expression is exaggerated or exalted. This gene has been found primarily in blacks.

## e Variants

It appears, especially in the black population, that the e antigen may exhibit the same mosaic quality described for D. Because of these variations, e typings can be unreliable.[17,45]

Among the variants at the e locus are $hr^s$, $hr^B$, and $VS(e^s)$, with a variant $R^0$ or r gene making e plus one or the other of these pieces. Such variants are usually recognized when they make antibodies that behave as anti-e even though their red cells type as e-positive with routine Rh typing reagents.

## V, VS

The $V(ce^s)$ antigen is found in about 30 percent of randomly selected American blacks. In selected indi-viduals it serologically appears to be the counterpart of f because it is present when c is cis with $e^s$.[46] The $VS(e^s)$ antigen is also relatively common in blacks, reacting with all V-positive red cells and additionally with r's red cells.[47] Although the relationship of V to VS remains somewhat less than clear, both are markers associated with the black population.

## Deletions

There are very uncommon phenotypes that demonstrate no Cc and/or Ee reactivity. Many examples lacking all Cc or Ee often have an unusually strong D antigen expression, frequently called an exalted D. The deletion phenotype is indicated by the use of a dash (–), as in the following examples: DC–, Dc–, D–E, D––. The antibody made by D– –people is called anti-Rh 17 or anti-$Hr_0$.

A variation has been recognized within the deletion D––, called D••. The D antigen in the D•• is stronger than that in DC–, D-E, Dc–, or D-e samples but weaker than that of D–– samples. A low-incidence antigen called Evans (Rh:37) accompanies the Rh structure of D•• cells.[48]

Deleted complexes are of particular interest and concern in parentage testing. The absence of antigens can make interpretation of parentage testing results difficult. Transfusion of individuals with a deletion or D•• phenotype is difficult if multiple antibodies are present; blood of a similar phenotype would be required.

## THE LW ANTIGEN

A discussion of the LW antigen begins at the time when Rh antigens were first recognized. The antibody produced by injecting rhesus monkey red cells into guinea pigs and rabbits was identified as having the same specificity as the antibody Levine and Stetson[1] described earlier. The antibody was given the name anti-Rh, for anti-rhesus, and the blood group system was established. Many years later it was recognized that the two antibodies were not identical; the anti-rhesus described by Landsteiner and Wiener[2] was renamed anti-LW in their honor.

Phenotypically, there is a similarity between the Rh and LW systems. Anti-LW reacts strongly with most D-

**Table 6–10.** LW Phenotypes and Genotypes

| Phenotype | Genotype |
|---|---|
| LW(a+b−) | $LW^a LW^a$ or $LW^a LW$ |
| LW(a+b+) | $LW^a LW^b$ |
| LW(a−b+) | $LW^b LW^b$ or $LW^b LW$ |
| LW(a−b−) | $LW LW$ |

**Source:** Sistonen and Tippett[50], p 252, with permission.)
Note: $Rh_{null}$ individuals are phenotypically LW(a− b−) because of the genetic mechanism causing the $Rh_{null}$ status. The LW genotype of $Rh_{null}$ may be determined by family studies.

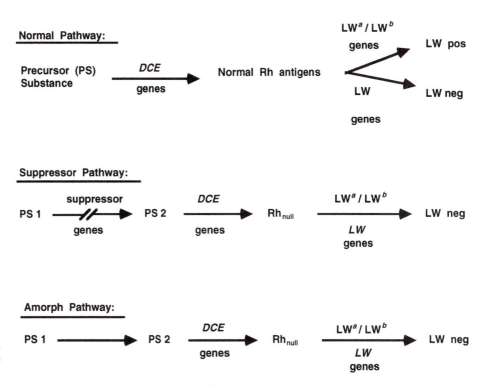

**Figure 6–9.** Genetic pathways relating Rh and LW antigens. Rh antigen precursor substance must be available for LW to be made.

positive red cells, weakly (sometimes not at all) with Rh-negative red cells, and never with $Rh_{null}$ cells. The independent segregation of *LW* from the *Rh* blood group genes was established by a family study on a D-positive, LW-negative woman; other family studies support this point.[44,49]

The nomenclature describing the various expressions of the LW antigen has evolved over time.[50] An excellent description of this is found in other reference texts.[45]

There are three alleles at the LW locus: $LW^a$ $LW^b$, and *LW* (a silent allele). Persons lacking LW antigen altogether are *LW/LW* and express no LW on the red cells. Table 6–10 is a summary of LW phenotypes and genotypes. $LW^a$ is very common, and $LW^b$ somewhat less common. The relationship of LW antigen production to the Rh antigens is summarized in Figure 6–9. Under normal circumstances precursor substance is acted upon by the *Rh* genes to produce normal Rh antigens. The *LW* genes then exert their influence to express LW antigen on the red cell surface.

When the $Rh_{null}$ suppressor genes ($X^orX^or$) are present, the *Rh* and *LW* genes are not expressed on the red cell; however, the *Rh* and *LW* genes are normal and, when passed to offspring with the $X^1r$ gene, will be expressed normally. The amorphic $Rh_{null}$ individual inherits the $\bar{r}\bar{r}$ genes, which do not express Rh antigens; therefore, *LW* genes cannot be expressed.

Anti-LW usually reacts more strongly with D-positive red cells than with D-negative adult red cells. A weak anti-LW may react only with D-positive red cells, and enhancement techniques may be required to demonstrate its reactivity with D-negative cells. Anti-LW reacts equally well with cord cells regardless of D typing.[17] This is an important characteristic to remember when trying to differentiate anti-LW from anti-D. Also, anti-LW more frequently appears as an autoantibody, which does not present clinical problems. Autoanti-LW is occasionally seen in autoimmune hemolytic anemia.

Because of the complexity of the Rh blood group system, a tremendous amount of literature exists. The inquisitive reader can continue to piece together the puzzle by consulting the sources included in the references.

---

## SUMMARY CHART: IMPORTANT POINTS TO REMEMBER (MT/MLT)

- The Rh antibody was so named on the basis of antibody production by guinea pigs and rabbits when transfused with rhesus monkey red cells.
- Rh is a primary cause of hemolytic disease of the newborn (HDN, erythroblastosis fetalis) and a significant cause of hemolytic transfusion reactions.
- Fisher-Race DCE terminology is based on the theory that antigens of the system were produced by three closely linked sets of alleles, and each gene was responsible for producing a product (or antigen) on the red cell surface.
- A person who expresses no Rh antigens on the red cell is said to be $Rh_{null}$, and the phenotype may be written as ---/---.
- In the Wiener Rh-Hr nomenclature, it is postulated that the gene responsible for defining Rh actually produced an agglutinogen that contained a series of blood factors, in which each factor is an antigen recognized by an antibody.
- In the Rosenfield alpha/numeric terminology a number is assigned to each antigen of the Rh system in order of its discovery (Rh1 = D, Rh2 = C, Rh3 = E, Rh4 = c, Rh5 = e).

- Rh antigens are characterized as nonglycosylated proteins in the red cell membrane.
- The most common genotype in whites is $R^1r$ (35%); the most common genotype in blacks is $R^0r$ (42%).
- The Rh antigens are inherited as codominant alleles.
- A D-mosaic individual is characterized as lacking one or more pieces or epitopes of the total D antigen and may produce alloantibody to the missing fraction if exposed to complete D red cells.
- Blood for transfusion is considered Rh-positive if either the D or weak D test is positive; if both the D and weak D tests are negative, blood for transfusion is considered Rh-negative.
- Most Rh antibodies are IgG immunoglobulins and react optimally at 37°C or following antiglobulin testing; exposure to less than 1 mL of Rh-positive red cells can stimulate antibody production in an Rh-negative person.
- Rh-mediated hemolytic transfusion reactions usually result in extravascular hemolysis.
- Rh antibodies are IgG and can cross the placenta to coat fetal (Rh-positive) red cells.

## REVIEW QUESTIONS

1. The Rh system was first recognized in a case report about:
   A. A hemolytic transfusion reaction
   B. Hemolytic disease of the newborn
   C. Circulatory overload
   D. Autoimmune hemolytic anemia

2. What antigen is found in 85 percent of the white population and is always significant for transfusion purposes?
   A. d
   B. c
   C. D
   D. E
   E. e

3. Weaker-than-expected reactions with anti-D typing reagents are categorized as:
   A. $Rh_{mod}$
   B. Partial D
   C. DAT positive
   D. $D^w$

4. Cells carrying a weak D antigen require the use of what test to demonstrate its presence?
   A. Indirect antiglobulin test
   B. Direct antiglobulin test
   C. Microplate test
   D. Warm auto-absorption test

5. Rh antigens are inherited as:
   A. Autosomal recessive alleles
   B. Sex-linked genes
   C. Codominant alleles
   D. X-linked

6. Rh antigens are:
   A. Glycophorins
   B. Simple sugars
   C. Proteins
   D. Lipids

7. Rh antibodies react best at what temperature (°C)?
   A. 22
   B. 18
   C. 15
   D. 37

8. Rh antibodies are primarily of which immunoglobulin class?
   A. IgA
   B. IgM
   C. IgG
   D. IgD
   E. IgE

9. Rh antibodies have been associated with which of the following clinical conditions?
   A. Erythroblastosis fetalis
   B. Thrombocytopenia
   C. Hemolytic transfusion reactions

D. Hemophilia A
E. Both A and C

10. Rh$_{null}$ cells lack:
    A. Lewis antigens
    B. Normal oxygen-carrying capacity
    C. Rh antigens
    D. MNSs antigens

11. The antigen system closely associated phenotypically with Rh is known as:
    A. McCoy
    B. Lutheran
    C. Duffy
    D. LW

12. Anti-LW will not react with which of the following?
    A. Rh-positive red cells
    B. Rh-negative red cells
    C. Rh$_{null}$ red cells
    D. Rh:33 red cells

13. Convert the following genotypes from Wiener nomenclature to Fisher-Race and Rosenfield nomenclatures and list the antigens present in each haplotype.
    A. $R_1r$
    B. $R_2R_0$
    C. $R_zR_1$
    D. $r^yr$

14. The Rh phenotype that has the strongest expression of D is:
    A. $R_1r$
    B. $R_1R_2$
    C. $R_2r$
    D. $R_2R_2$
    E. D--

## ANSWERS TO REVIEW QUESTIONS

1. A (p 129)
2. C (p 130, Table 6–1)
3. B (p 136)
4. A (p 135)
5. C (p 134)
6. C (p 133)
7. D (p 137)
8. C (p 137)
9. E (pp 138–139)
10. C (p 139)
11. D (p 140)
12. C (p 141)
13. $R_1r$    DCe/cde    Rh:1,2,−3,4,5
    $R_2R_0$    DcE/cDe    Rh:1,−2,3,4,5
    $R_zR_1$    DCE/DCe    Rh:1,2,3,−4,5
    $r^yr$    CE/cde    Rh:−1,2,3,4,5
    (see Table 6–3, p 131)
14. E (p 140)

## REFERENCES

1. Levine, P, and Stetson, RE: An unusual case of intragroup agglutination. JAMA 113:126, 1939.
2. Landsteiner, K, and Wiener, AS: An agglutinable factor in human blood recognized by immune sera for rhesus blood. Proc Soc Exp Biol (NY) 43:223, 1940.
3. Levine, P, et al: The role of isoimmunization in the pathogenesis of erythroblastosis fetalis. Am J Obstet Gynecol 42:925, 1941.
4. Race, RR, et al: Recognition of a further common Rh genotype in man. Nature 153:52, 1944.
5. Mourant, AE: A new rhesus antibody. Nature 155:542, 1945.
6. Stratton, F: A new Rh allelomorph. Nature 158:25, 1946.
7. Levine, P: On Hr factor and Rh genetic theory. Science 102:1, 1945.
8. Race, RR: The Rh genotypes and Fisher's theory. Blood 3 (Suppl 2): 27, 1948.
9. Widmann, FK (ed): Technical Manual of the American Association of Blood Banks, ed 9. American Association of Blood Banks, Arlington, VA, 1985.
10. Wiener, AS: Genetic theory of the Rh blood types. Proc Soc Exp Biol (NY) 54:316, 1943.
11. Rosenfield, RE, et al: A review of Rh serology and presentation of a new terminology.
12. Lewis, M (Chair): Blood group terminology 1990. Vox Sang 58:152, 1990.
13. Issitt, PD: Serology and Genetics of the Rh Blood Group System. Montgomery Scientific Publications, Cincinnati, 1985.
14. Vengelen-Tyler, V (ed): Technical Manual, ed 12. American Association of Blood Banks, Bethesda, MD, 1996.
15. Hughes-Jones, NC, Gardner, B, and Lincoln, PJ: Observations of the number of available c, D, and E antigen sites on red cells. Vox Sang 21:210, 1971.
16. Tippett, PA: A speculative model for the Rh blood groups. Ann Hum Genet 50:241, 1986.
17. Race, RR, and Sanger, R: Blood Groups in Man, ed 6. Blackwell Scientific, Oxford, 1975.
18. Race, RR: Modern concepts of the blood group systems. Ann NY Acad Sci 127:844, 1965.
19. Giblett, ER: Genetic Markers in Human Blood. Blackwell Scientific, Oxford, 1969.
20. Rosenfield, RE, Allen, FH, Jr, and Rubinstein, P: Genetic model for the Rh blood group systems. Proc Nat Acad Sci 70(5):1303, 1973.
21. Race, RR, Sanger, R, and Lawler, SD: The Rh antigen D$^u$. Ann Eugen Lond 14:171, 1948.
22. Capellini, R, Dunn, LC, and Turri, M: An interaction between alleles at the Rh locus in man which weakens the reactivity of the Rh$_0$ factor (D$^0$). Proc Nat Acad Sci 41:283, 1955.
23. Shapiro, M: The ABO, MN, P and Rh blood group systems in South African Bantu: A genetic study. South Afr Med J 25:187, 1951.
24. Argall, CI, Ball, JM, and Trentelman, E: Presence of anti-D antibody in the serum of D$^u$ patient. J Clin Lab Med 41:895, 1953.
25. Wiener, AS, and Unger, LJ: Rh factors related to the Rh$_0$ factor as a source of clinical problems. JAMA 169:696, 1959.
26. Tippett, P, and Sanger, R: Observations on subdivisions of the Rh antigen D. Vox Sang 7:9, 1962.
27. Tippett, P, Lomas-Francis, C, and Wallace, M. The Rh antigen D: Partial D antigens and associated low incidence antigens. Vox Sang 70:123–131, 1996.
28. Mollison, PL: Blood Transfusion in Clinical Medicine, ed 6. Blackwell Scientific Publications, Oxford, 1988.

29. Diamond, LK, and Denton, RC: Rh agglutination in various media with particular reference to the value of albumin. J Clin Lab Med 30:821, 1945.

30. Romans, DG, et al: Conversion of incomplete antibodies to direct agglutinins by mild reduction. Proc Nat Acad Sci USA 74:2531, 1977.

31. Queenan, JT: Modern Management of the Rh Problem, ed 2. Harper & Row, New York, 1977.

32. Schmidt, PJ, and Vos, GH: Multiple phenotypic abnormalities associated with $Rh_{null}$ (—/—). Vox Sang 13:18, 1967.

33. Chown, B, et al: An unlinked modifier of Rh blood groups: Effects when heterozygous and when homozygous. Am J Hum Gen 24:623, 1972.

34. Schmidt, PJ, et al: Aberrant U blood group accompany $Rh_{null}$. Transfusion 7:33, 1967.

35. Callendar, ST, and Race, RR: A serological and genetic study of multiple antibodies formed in response to blood transfusion by a patient with lupus erythematosus diffuses. Ann Eugen Lond 13:102, 1946.

36. Rosenfield, RE, and Haber, GV: An Rh blood factor, $Rh_1$ (Ce) and its relationship to hr (ce). Am J Hum Genet 10:474, 1958.

37. Allen, FH, and Tippett, PA: A new Rh blood type which reveals the Rh antigen G. Vox Sang 3:321, 1958.

38. Wiener, AS, and Unger, LJ: Further observations on the blood factors $Rh^A$, $Rh^B$, $Rh^C$, $Rh^D$. Transfusion 2:230, 1962.

39. Allen, FH, Jr, and Corcoran PA. Proc 11th Ann Mtg. AABB, Cincinnati, Abstract, 1958.

40. Chown, B, et al. The Rh antigen $D^w$ (Wiel). Transfusion 4:169, 1964.

41. Lewis, M, et al. Blood group antigen $Go^a$ and the Rh system. Transfusion 7:440, 1967.

42. Lewis, M, et al: Assignment of the red cell antigen Targett (Rh 40) to the Rh blood group systems. Am J Hum Genet 31:630, 1979.

43. Giles, CM, et al: An Rh gene complex which results in a "new" antigen detectable by a specific antibody, anti-Rh 33. Vox Sang 21:289, 1971.

44. Rosenfield, RE, et al: Problems in Rh typing as revealed by a single Negro family. Am J Hum Genet 12:147, 1960.

45. Issitt, PD: Applied Blood Group Serology, ed 3. Montgomery Scientific Publication, Miami, 1985.

46. DeNatale, A, et al: A "new" Rh antigen, common in Negroes, rare in white people. JAMA 159:247, 1955.

47. Sanger, R, et al: An Rh antibody specific for V and $R^s$. Nature (Lond) 186:171, 1960.

48. Contreras, M, et al: The Rh antigen Evans. Vox Sang 34:208, 1978.

49. Vos, GH, et al: A sample of blood with no detectable Rh antigens. Lancet i:14, 1961.

50. Sistonen, P, and Tippett, P: A "new" all allele giving further insight into the LW blood group system. Vox Sang 42:252, 1982.

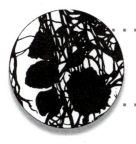

# CHAPTER 7

# THE LEWIS SYSTEM

Denise M. Harmening, PhD, MT (ASCP), CLS (NCA)
and Mitra Taghizadeh, MS, MT (ASCP)

*Areas of concentration for MT and MLT students

## OBJECTIVES

*On completion of this chapter, the learner should be able to:*

1 Describe the formation and secretion of Lewis antigens and their adsorption onto the red cells.

2 Discuss the inheritance of the Lewis genes and their interactions with the other blood group genes.

3 List substances present in secretions and the Lewis phenotypes based on a given genotype.

4 Define the role of secretor genes in formation of Lewis antigens.

5 List the Lewis phenotypes and their frequencies in the white and black populations.

6 Indicate the process of development of the Lewis antigens after birth.

7 Describe the changes in the Lewis phenotypes during pregnancy.

8 List the characteristics of the Lewis antigens.

9 List the characteristics of the Lewis antibodies.

10 Discuss the significance of Lewis antibodies.

11 Discuss the biologic significance of the Lewis antigens.

The Lewis blood group system is unique in that it is believed to be the only system that is not manufactured by the red blood cell. Lewis antigens are not synthesized by the red cell and incorporated into the red cell membrane structure. Instead, these antigens are manufactured by tissue cells and secreted into body fluids. Therefore, the Lewis system has been referred to as a system rather than as a blood group because Lewis antigens are found primarily in the secretions and the plasma. These antigens are then adsorbed onto the red cell membrane from plasma, but they are not really an integral part of the membrane structure. Because Lewis-soluble antigens are manufactured by tissue cells, antigen production depends not only on the inheritance of Lewis genes but also on the inheritance of the secretor gene. Genetic interaction also exists between the Lewis and ABO genes because the amount of Lewis antigen detectable on the red cell is influenced by the ABO genes inherited.

This chapter has been divided into basic concepts and advanced concepts. Students at MT and MLT levels should focus on understanding the topics marked by asterisks in the chapter outline. Other advanced concepts are included for advanced learning.

## INHERITANCE

Similar to ABO genes, the Lewis gene (*Le*) does not actually code for the production of Lewis antigens but, rather, produces a specific glycosyltransferase, L-fucosyltransferase. This enzyme adds L-fucose to the basic

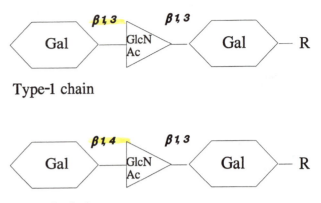

**Figure 7–1.** Structure of type-1 and type-2 chains. Gal = D-galactose; GlcNAc = *N*-acetyl-D-glucosamine; R = other biochemical residues.

precursor substance. The *Le* gene is located on the short arm of chromosome 19 linked to the C3 complement locus,[1] and far from *Se* and *H* genes, which are closely linked on the long arm of the same chromosome.[2] In whites, 90 percent of the population possesses *Le* gene. This gene codes for a specific glycosyltransferase, α-4-L-fucosyltransferase, which transfers L-fucose to type 1 chain oligosaccharide on glycoprotein or glycolipid structures. Type 1 chain refers to the beta linkage of the number 1 carbon of galactose to the number 3 carbon of *N*-acetylglucosamine (GlcNAc) residue of the precursor structure (Fig. 7–1). The inheritance of the *Le* gene acts in competition with ABO genes, adding L-fucose to the GlcNAc sugar of the common precursor structure manufactured by tissue cells (Fig. 7–2 and **Color Plate 12**). The structure formed is known as Le$^a$-soluble antigen. It is then secreted and adsorbed onto the red cell, lymphocytes, and platelet membranes from plasma.[2] In the addition of L-fucose to type 1 chain catalyzed by Lewis enzyme, the number 1 carbon of L-fucose is attached to the number 4 carbon of GlcNAc. This transfer reaction can occur only in type 1 precursor structures. Addition of L-fucose cannot occur with type 2 precursor structures because in type 2 structures number 4 carbon of GlcNAc is already linked to galactose (see Fig. 7–1).

## BASIC CONCEPTS: THE LEWIS (LE) PHENOTYPES

### The Lewis (a+b−) Phenotype: Nonsecretors (LE1-007.001)

Le$^a$ substance is secreted regardless of the secretor status. The term *secretor* refers only to the presence of water-soluble ABH antigen substances in the body fluids, which are influenced by the independently inherited secretor genes *Se* and *se*. (For a review of secretors, refer to Chap. 5.) Therefore, an individual can be a nonsecretor (*sese*) of ABH and still secrete Le$^a$ into the

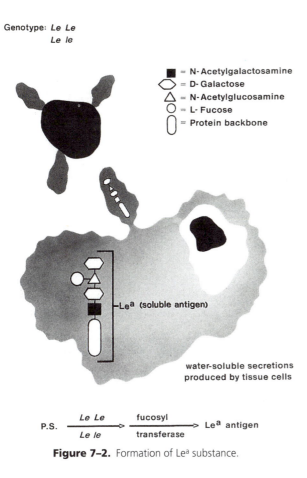

Genotype: *Le Le*
           *Le le*

■ = N- Acetylgalactosamine
◇ = D- Galactose
△ = N- Acetylglucosamine
○ = L- Fucose
▯ = Protein backbone

—Le^a (soluble antigen)

water-soluble secretions
produced by tissue cells

P.S. $\xrightarrow{\dfrac{Le\ Le}{Le\ le}}$ $\xrightarrow[\text{transferase}]{\text{fucosyl}}$ Le^a antigen

**Figure 7–2.** Formation of Le^a substance.

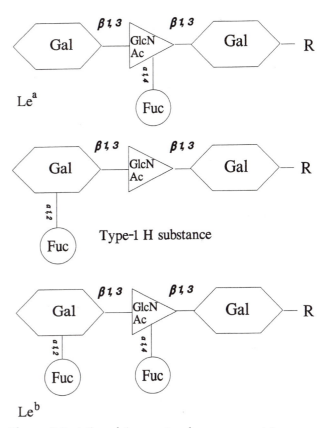

Le^a

Type-1 H substance

Le^b

**Figure 7–3.** Action of Le gene transferase enzyme. Le^a = gene codes for L-fucosyl transferase, which adds L-fucose (FUC) to the carbon number 4 of *N*-acetyl glucosamine of type-1 precursor structure. Type-1 H substance = *Se* gene codes for L-fucosyl transferase, which adds L-fucose to the carbon number 2 of terminal galactose. Le^b = in the presence of Le, Se, a second fucose is added to the carbon number 4 of the subterminal *N*-acetyl glucosamine of type-1 H substance. Gal = D-galactose; G1cNAc = *N*-acetyl-D-glucosamine; FUC = L-fucose; R = other biochemical residues.

body fluids, producing the phenotype Lewis a-positive b-negative on the red blood cells. This is written Le (a+b−). All Le (a+b−) individuals are nonsecretors of ABH substances.[3] Lewis enzyme has been detected in saliva, milk, submaxillary glands, gastric mucosa, and kidney and cyst fluids.[4] Lewis fucosyltransferase has not been detected in plasma or in red cell stroma. Lewis antigens produced in saliva and other secretions are glycoproteins, but Lewis cell-bound antigens absorbed from plasma onto the red cell membranes are glycolipids. Formation of Le^a from type 1 precursor structure is depicted in Figures 7–3 and 7–4.

### The Lewis (a−b+) Phenotype: Secretors (LE2-007.002)

The genetically independent *Sese*, ABO, *Hh*, and Lewis genes are intimately associated in the formation of the Le^b antigen. Le^a and Le^b are not alleles. The phenotype Le (a−b+) is the result of the genetic interaction of *Lele* and *Sese* genes. Le^b antigen represents the product of genetic interaction between *Le(FUT3)* and *Se(FUT2)* genes. Recently it was suggested that the *Se* gene does not control the expression of the *H* gene. Lewis and secretor genes are two independent genes that code for different but related α-2-L-fucosyltransferases.[2,5] The inheritance of the *Se* gene codes for the enzyme α-2-L-fucosyltransferase, which adds L-fucose

to type 1 precursor substance and thus forms type 1 H. The inheritance of the *Le* gene codes for the addition of another L-fucose that is added to the subterminal *N*-acetylglucosamine and thus forms Le^b antigen (see Figures 7–3 and 7–4). Some precursor chains are not acted on by the Se fucosyltransferase, but may accept L-fucose from the Lewis fucosyltranferase forming Le^a (Fig. 7–5 and **Color Plate 12**). Therefore, both Le^a-soluble and Le^b-soluble antigens can be found in the secretions. However, only Le^b adsorbs onto the red cell from plasma. This is probably because higher concentrations of Le^b in plasma allow Le^b-soluble antigen to compete more successfully for sites of adsorption onto the red cell membrane. As a result, the red cells of these individuals always phenotype as Le(a−b+), even though both Le^a- and Le^b-soluble antigens are present in the secretions and plasma. In secretors, biochemical studies indicate that Le and Se fucosyltransferases compete for type 1 chain precursor.[6] Se glycosyltransferase catalyzes synthesis of H on type 1 chain precursor structures. The respective amounts of Le^a and type 1 H substances formed in

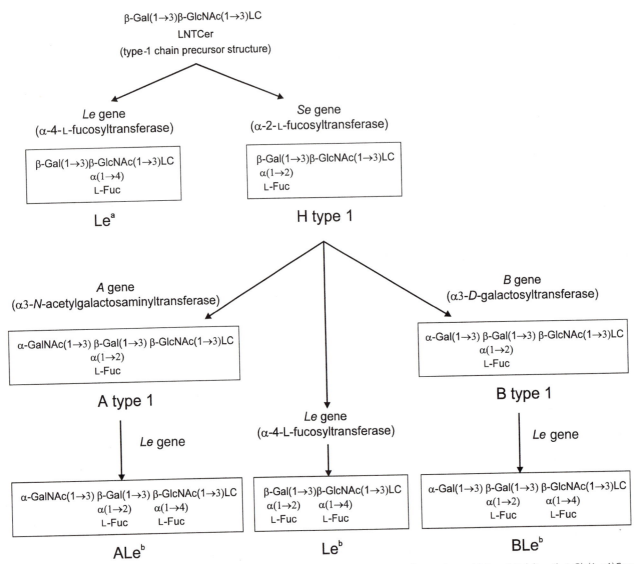

**Figure 7–4.** Formation of Lewis antigens (le$^a$, le$^b$, Ale$^b$, Ble$^b$) adsorbed from plasma. LC (lactosylceramide) = β-Gal (1→4) β-Glc(1→1)Cer; LNTCer = lacto-N-tetraosylceramide; Gal = galactose; GlcNAc = N-acetylglucosamine; Fuc = fucose; GalNAc = N-acetylgalactosamine.

secretions are determined by the ratio of these two fucosyltransferases. In nonsecretors (*sese*), only Le$^a$ antigens are formed in secretions, inasmuch as no Se enzyme is present in secretory cells. As a result, all type 1 chain precursor glycoproteins are available for the Le enzyme α-4-L-fucosyltransferase. The *H* gene functions in adding L-fucose to D-galactose of type 2 chain on the red cell membrane paragloboside structure, forming the H antigen as described for formation of ABH antigens (see Chap. 5). Therefore, only Le$^a$ antigen is secreted by the tissue cells and subsequently adsorbed onto the erythrocyte from plasma yielding the phenotype Le(a+b−). Lewis antigens have also been detected on the surface of platelets and lymphocytes, regardless of the secretor status, but not on the surface of granulocytes or monocytes.[2,7,8]

## The Lewis (a−b−) Phenotype: Secretors or Nonsecretors

A third type of red cell phenotype is the Lewis a-negative b-negative written Le(a−b−) (Fig. 7–6). Recently it was suggested that the lack of the Lewis antigens on the red cells of this group is not caused by the absence of the Lewis gene (*FUT3*), but rather by the specific point mutations in the *Le* gene. These mutations give rise to a nonfunctional or partially active Lewis transferase (Le$^w$) causing the negative expression of the Lewis antigen on the red cells.[5,9] According to this finding, the Lewis antigen is absent only on the red cells tested serologically with the Lewis antisera; however, the Lewis antigen (<5 percent compared with that made by the Lewis-positive individuals)[2] is present in

Genotype: *Le*
*Se*

water-soluble secretions
produced by tissue cells

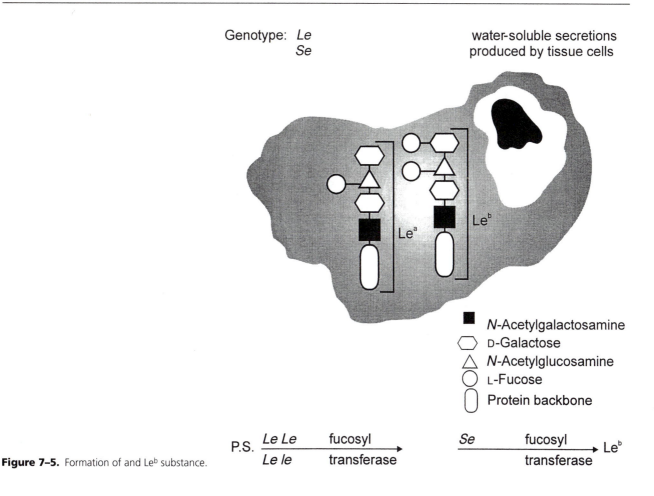

■ *N*-Acetylgalactosamine
⬡ D-Galactose
△ *N*-Acetylglucosamine
○ L-Fucose
⬭ Protein backbone

P.S. $\dfrac{Le\ Le}{Le\ le}$ $\xrightarrow[\text{transferase}]{\text{fucosyl}}$ $Se$ $\xrightarrow[\text{transferase}]{\text{fucosyl}}$ Le$^b$

**Figure 7–5.** Formation of and Le$^b$ substance.

the tissues and secretions of the Le(a−b−) secretors.[5,9] The main substances found in the secretions of the Le(a−b−) individuals depend on the secretor status and the ABO genotype of the person. The Le(a−b−) nonsecretors express type 1 precursor, whereas the Le(a−b−) secretors express H type 1 substances plus ABH antigens associated with the related ABO genes inherited.

The *lele* genotype is much more common in blacks than in whites. The frequencies of these Lewis red cell phenotypes in the white population are as follows: Le(a−b+), 72 percent; Le(a+b−), 22 percent; and Le(a−b−), 6 percent. In the black population the frequencies are Le(a−b+), 55 percent; Le(a+b−), 23 percent; and Le(a−b−), 22 percent (Table 7–1). All Le(a−b+) individuals are ABH secretors and also secrete Le$^a$ and Le$^b$. All Le(a+b−) individuals are ABH nonsecretors, yet all secrete Le$^a$. It is no surprise, then, that the frequencies of these Lewis phenotypes parallel the frequency of the secretor gene. Approximately 78 to 80 percent of whites are secretors, and 20 percent are nonsecretors. In terms of Le(a−b−) individuals, 80 percent are ABH secretors and 20 percent ABH nonsecretors. The antigen expressed by Le(a−b−) secretors is type 1 H (Le$^d$) substance, whereas the antigen expressed by Le(a−b−) nonsecretors is type 1 precursor substance (Le$^c$)[2] (see Figures 7–1, 7–3, and 7–6).

## ADVANCED CONCEPTS: BIOCHEMISTRY OF LEWIS ANTIGENS

The Lewis antigens or substances found in the secretions are glycoproteins, as are the ABH substances from secretors. The glycoproteins are composed of 80 percent carbohydrates and 15 percent amino acids.[10] In plasma, Lewis antigens are glycolipids (glycosphingolipids). These antigens are carried by lipoproteins present in plasma that adhere to red cell membranes, forming glycosylceramides. All of the Lewis antigens found on red cells have been absorbed from plasma. The exact site for the synthesis of Lewis glycolipids in the plasma is not known; however, it has been postulated that they may originate mainly from the intestinal tract epithelial cells. Other exocrine organs such as the liver, kidney, and pancreas also contribute to the plasma glycolipids.[2,5,11] About one-third of the total Lewis glycolipids in blood are bound to the red cells, and the rest are in plasma.[2] Using plasma as a source of Lewis glycosphingolipids, Le(a−b−) red cells incubated with Le$^a$-positive or Le$^b$-positive plasma can be converted to Le(a+b−) or Le(a−b+), depending on the substance present in the plasma. With saliva as a source of Lewis substances, Le(a−b−) red cells cannot be converted into Lewis-positive phe-

Genes inherited

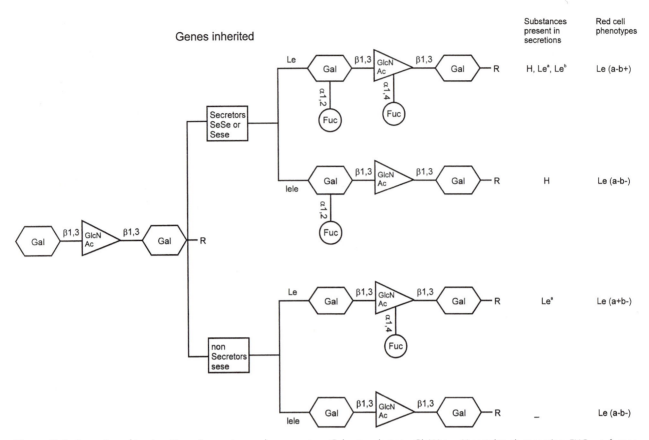

**Figure 7–6.** Formation of Lewis antigens in secretors and nonsecretors. Gal = D-galactose; GlcNAc = N-acetyl-D-glucosamine; FUC = L-fucose; R = other biochemical residues.

**Table 7–1.** Phenotypes and Frequencies in the Lewis System

| | Adult Phenotype Frequency (%) | |
|---|---|---|
| Phenotype | Whites | Blacks |
| Le(a+b−) | 22 | 23 |
| Le(a−b+) | 72 | 55 |
| Le(a−b−) | 6 | 22 |

**Table 7.2.** Substances Present in Secretions and Antigens Present on Red Cells, Depending on the Lewis, Hh, and ABH Genes Inherited

| Gene Inherited | Substances Present in Secretions | Red Cell Phenotype |
|---|---|---|
| *Le, Se*, A/B/H | Le$^a$, Le$^b$, A, B, H | A, B, H, Le(a−b+) |
| *lele, Se*, A/B/H | A, B, H | A, B, H, Le(a−b−) |
| *Le, sese*, A/B/H | Le$^a$ | A, B, H, Le(a+b−) |
| *lele, sese*, A/B/H | — | A, B, H, Le(a−b−) |
| *Le, sese, hh*, A/B | Le$^a$ | O$_h$, Le(a+b−) |
| *Le, Se, hh*, A/B | Le$^a$, Le$^b$, A, B, H | A, B, Le(a−b+)* |

* = Para-Bombay phenotype.

notypes because Lewis substances in saliva, being glycoproteins, are not adsorbed onto the red cell membranes. The Lewis specificity similar to ABH antigens resides in the carbohydrate portion of the molecule. Both Le$^a$ and Le$^b$ are formed by the addition of a fucose molecule to the precursor structure of a type 1 chain in secretions (see Figures 7–2, 7–5, **Color Plates 12, 13**). In addition, A or B enzymes in secretor individuals can form A or B antigens in secretions by adding the appropriate sugar residue to type 1 or type 2 H substances. The substances present in secretions and antigens present on red cells, depending upon *Lele, Sese,* and ABO genes inherited, are listed in Table 7–2. The Lewis gene–specified fucosyltransferase com-

petes with A and B gene–specified enzymes for the same type 1 H substrate. As a result, individuals who inherit *Le* and *Se* genes have more Lewis and fewer A or B plasma glycolipids than *Se, lele* individuals. Le$^a$ and Le$^b$ antigens, once formed in secretions, can no longer be used as substrates for H and A or B enzymes, owing to chain termination signaled by the Lewis transferase. As a result, presence or absence of *Le* gene affects the concentration of H, A, and B type 1 chain substances found in secretions. *Le* gene does not affect synthesis of type 2 chain H, A, and B-soluble antigens

**Table 7–3.** Characteristics of Lewis, A, B, and H Substances Found in Secretions

| | Lewis Substances in Secretion | ABH Substances in Secretion |
|---|---|---|
| Genetic control | *Le* gene (Le$^a$ formation is not dependent or controlled by *Se* gene) | *Se* gene |
| Glycosyltransferase | α-4-L-fucosyltransferase (Le) | α-4-L-fucosyltransferase (H) <br> α-3-*N*-acetylgalactosaminyltransferase (A) <br> α-3-D-galactosyltransferase (B) |
| Substrate precursor structure | Type 1 chains | Type 1 or type 2 chains |
| Factors affecting formation | 1. Once formed, Le$^a$ and Le$^b$ are no longer substrates for H or AB enzymes, respectively. <br><br> 2. Lewis and H fucosyltransferases compete for type 1 chain precursor structure. <br><br> 3. Lewis and AB enzymes compete for type 1 H substance. | 1. Type 2 chain, A, B, and H substance formation is unaffected by the presence of the Lewis enzyme. <br> 2. A or B type 1 substances can act as substrates for Lewis enzyme forming ALe$^b$ or BLe$^b$ "compound" antigenic glycoproteins. <br> 3. Formation of type 1 chain, A, B, and H substances is competitively inhibited by the presence of Lewis enzyme. |

found in secretions. Antigens of all other blood group systems are built on type 2 precursor chains found on the red cell membrane because these determinants are manufactured by the red cell. Characteristics of Lewis and ABH substances found in secretions are compared in Table 7–3.

## DEVELOPMENT AND CHANGES OF LEWIS ANTIGENS AFTER BIRTH

Depending on the genes inherited, Le$^a$ and Le$^b$ glycoproteins as well as ABH substances will be present in the saliva of newborn infants. In plasma there are no detectable Lewis glycosphingolipids at birth.[12] Therefore, cord blood and red cells from newborn infants phenotype as Le(a−b−). It is the low level of plasma Lewis antigens that accounts for this fact, because the plasma of newborn infants has been demonstrated to be incapable of transforming Le(a−b−) adult cells into Lewis-positive phenotype. However, Le(a−b−) erythrocytes from infants can be transformed into Le(a+b−) phenotype at incubation with plasma from an Le(a+b−) adult.[13] When the genotypes *Le* and *sese* are inherited, Lewis antigens (Le$^a$ and Le$^b$) are not detectable on cord red cells, but these infants do secrete Le$^a$ substance in their saliva. Lewis glycosphingolipids become detectable in plasma after approximately 10 days of life. In individuals who inherit *Le* and *Se* genes, a transformation can be followed from Le(a−b−) phenotype at birth to Le(a+b −) after 10 days, to Le(a+b+), and finally to Le(a−b+), the true Lewis phenotype after 6 to 7 years.[14,15] In contrast, individuals who inherit *Le* and *sese* genes phenotype as Le(a−b−) at birth and transform to Le(a+b−) after 10 days. The Le(a+b−) phenotype persists throughout life. Individuals with *lele*

genes phenotype as Le(a−b−) at birth and for the rest of their lives.

## CHANGES IN LEWIS PHENOTYPE

A decrease in expression of Lewis antigens has been demonstrated on red cells from many pregnant women, resulting in Le(a−b−) phenotypes during gestation.[16] The mechanism causing production of this phenotype during pregnancy is uncertain. It has been suggested that physiologic changes in the composition of blood that affect distribution of Lewis glycolipid between plasma and red cells are responsible for this phenomenon. Of the total Lewis glycolipids in whole blood, approximately one-third of Le$^b$ is associated with red cells, and the rest is bound to plasma lipoproteins.[16] Other investigators have proposed that the large increase in the ratio of plasma lipoproteins to red cell mass that occurs during pregnancy is responsible for Le(a−b−) phenotypes.[17] In this instance, a greater amount of Le$^b$ glycolipids would be bound to plasma lipoproteins instead of adsorbing onto the red cells.[14] Lack of expression of Lewis antigens (Le$^a$ and Le$^b$) has been demonstrated on the red cells of patients with cancer, alcoholic cirrhosis, and viral and parasitic infections. This transformation of Lewis-positive phenotypes to Lewis-negative phenotypes is caused by abnormal lipid metabolism, changes in triglycerides and high-density proteins,[2] and/or other neoplastic changes occurring in cancer patients.[18,19] Other factors involved in the expression of the Lewis phenotype may be genetic, such as a single-point mutation caused by leucine to arginine substitution in the Lewis fucosyltransferase.[2] This mutation causes decrease in adsorption of Lewis antigen onto red cells from plasma, resulting in Le(a−b−) phenotype in individuals who

**Table 7–4.** Lewis Antigens

Poorly developed at birth
Reversibly adsorbed onto red cells from plasma
Not found on cord blood or newborn red cells Le(a−b−)
Lewis glycolipids detectable in plasma after approximately 10 days of life
Transformation of Lewis phenotype after birth seen in individuals who inherit *Le* and *Se* genes: Le(a−b−) to Le(a+b−) to Le(a+b+) to Le(a−b+) (the true phenotype)
Decrease in expression demonstrated in red cells from many pregnant women, resulting in Le(a−b−) phenotype during gestation
Do not show dosage in serologic reactions

**Table 7–5.** Lewis Antibodies

Usually naturally occurring
Predominantly IgM
May cause in vivo hemolysis of red cells
Sometimes reacts at 37°C and Coombs phase more weakly than at room temperature
Enhanced by enzymes
Readily neutralized by Lewis blood group substances
Rarely causes in vitro hemolysis; however, in vivo posttransfusion hemolysis reported in cases in which Lewis Ab strongly reacts in Coombs phase

have Le$^a$ and Le$^b$ in their saliva.[2] A summary of Lewis antigen characteristics can be found in Table 7–4.

## LEWIS ANTIBODIES

### Basic Concepts

Antibodies to the Lewis blood group antigen (anti-Le$^a$ and anti-Le$^b$) are frequently detected in antibody screening procedures. Lewis antibodies are generally produced by Le(a−b−) persons. Lewis antibodies are considered naturally occurring because they are present without previous exposure to the antigen-positive red cells. They are generally immunoglobulin M (IgM) in nature and do not cross the placenta to cause hemolytic disease of the newborn (HDN). However, because they are IgM antibodies, these hemolysins can activate complement and therefore can occasionally cause in vivo and in vitro hemolysis. An interesting aspect of Lewis antibodies is that they occur quite frequently in the sera of pregnant women.[20] Lewis antibodies are more reactive with enzyme-treated cells than with untreated cells and more reactive with group O cells than with group A or B cells. Anti-Le$^a$ and anti-Le$^b$ may occur together and can be neutralized by the Lewis substances present in plasma or saliva.

#### Anti-Le$^a$

Anti-Le$^a$ is the most commonly encountered antibody of the Lewis system produced in 20 percent of individuals with Le(a−b−) phenotypes. The antibody is often of IgM class; however, some may have IgG components or may be entirely IgG.[21] The IgG form of anti-Le$^a$ does not bind to the red cells as efficiently as the IgM form does and thereby is not generally detected in routine blood bank procedures. However, IgG anti-Le$^a$ has been detected on red cells using enzyme-linked immunosorbent assay (ELISA).[21] The IgG Lewis antibodies can be formed after massive transfusions of Lewis-positive antigens in individuals whose serum lacked Lewis antibodies before receiving Lewis-positive red cell transfusion.[20,22] The IgM form of Le$^a$ antibody binds complement and therefore can cause in vivo and

**Table 7–6.** Serologic Characteristics of Anti-Le$^a$ and Anti-Le$^b$ Antibodies in Vitro

| | Anti-Le$^a$ | Anti-Le$^b$ |
|---|---|---|
| Saline 4–22°C | Most | Most |
| Albumin 37°C | Few | Few |
| AHG | Many | Few |
| Enzymes | Many | Few |
| Hemolysis | Some | Occasional |

in vitro hemolysis. The antibody reactivity is enhanced by enzyme-treated red cells. The Le$^a$ antibody is frequently detected with saline-suspended cells at room temperature. However, it sometimes reacts at 37°C and Coombs phase and therefore can cause hemolytic transfusion reactions.[14] Anti-Le$^a$ is easily neutralized with plasma or saliva that contains Le$^a$ substance. Persons who are Le(a−b+) do not make anti-Le$^a$ because (1) the Le$^a$ antigen structure is contained within Le$^b$ antigen epitope, and (2) Le(a−b+) persons have Le$^a$ substance present in their plasma and saliva.[2,14] Caution must be used, however, because the agglutinates can be dispersed easily if the red blood cells are not resuspended gently.

#### Anti-Le$^b$

Anti-Le$^b$ is not as common or generally as strong as anti-Le$^a$. Although it is usually an IgM agglutinin, it does not fix complement as readily as anti-Le$^a$. Anti-Le$^b$ is usually produced by an Le(a−b−) individual; only occasionally will an Le(a+b−) individual produce an anti-Le$^b$. Like anti-Le$^a$, anti-Le$^b$ is neutralized by plasma or saliva containing Le$^b$ substance. A summary of Lewis antibodies and their serologic characteristics can be found in Tables 7–5 and 7–6, respectively.

### Advanced Concepts

#### Anti-Le$^b$

An interesting aspect of anti-Le$^b$ is that it can be classified into two categories: anti-Le$^{bH}$ and anti-Le$^{bL}$. Anti-Le$^{bH}$ reacts best when both the Le$^b$ and the H antigens are present on the red cell, such as group O and A$_2$ cells.

**Table 7–7.** Lewis Antigen on the Red Cells and Possible Antibodies Produced in the Plasma

| Red Cell Phenotype | Possible Antibodies Produced |
| --- | --- |
| Le(a+b−) | Anti-Le$^b$ |
| Le(a−b+) | — |
| Le(a−b−) | Anti-Le$^a$, Anti-Le$^b$ |
| Le$^x$ | — |

Anti-Le$^{bH}$ is probably an antibody to a compound antigen. It is important to remember that in phenotyping red cells, especially $A_1$ and $A_1B$ cells, the antiserum being used is not anti-Le$^{bH}$. Anti-Le$^{bL}$ is the Le$^b$ antibody that recognizes any Le$^b$ antigen regardless of the ABO type. Anti-Le$^{bH}$ can be neutralized by either H or combined H and Le$^b$ substance. Anti-Le$^{bL}$ is the antibody of choice for phenotyping red cells.

Neither anti-Le$^{bH}$ nor anti-Le$^{bL}$ is frequently implicated in hemolytic transfusion reactions, and the lack of reports in the literature suggests that anti-Le$^b$ in general has no clinical significance.[20] Formation of possible Lewis antibodies in different red cell phenotypes is summarized in Table 7–7.

### Anti-Le$^x$

Anti-Le$^x$ agglutinates all Le(a+b−) and Le(a−b+) red cells and is formed by all individuals who are phenotyped as Le(a−b−). Anti-Le$^x$ also agglutinates approximately 90 percent of all white cord blood initially phenotyping as Le(a−b−). In 1981, Schenkel-Brunner and Hanfland[23] defined the binding site of Le$^x$ antibodies by immunoadsorption studies. The binding site of Le$^x$ antibodies was found to be the smaller disaccharide structure of fucose-$\alpha(1{\rightarrow}4)$GlcNAc-R.[12,23] The reactivity of Le$^x$ determinant as defined by these authors is inhibited by the Le$^a$ glycolipid similar to the inhibition of normal anti-Le$^a$ because the specificities of both antibodies are determined by a fucose-$\alpha(1{\rightarrow}4)$GLcNAc linkage, which is present in both Le$^x$ determinant and Le$^a$ antigens as a product of the Lewis $\alpha$-4-L-fucosyltransferase.

Le(a−b−x+) cord cells do not react with anti-Le$^a$ or anti-Le$^b$. This may be a result of the hidden nature of the Le$^x$ determinant, which is covered by the addition of many more carbohydrates to the disaccharide chain. A somewhat similar analogy can be made with the A, B, and H antibodies and antigens, in that H-positive O cells, analogous to Lewis (a−b−x+) cells, do not react anti-A or anti-B, but anti-H (analogous to anti-Le$^x$) does agglutinate selected B and A cells. The fact that the reactivity of anti-Le$^x$ cannot be separated using Le(a+b−) or cord red cells indicates that this antibody is detecting a Lewis precursor antigen present in the biochemical structure of Le$^a$ and Le$^b$.[2,14,24]

The x determinant recognized by anti-x should not be confused with the Le$^x$(X) structure, which is a type 2 isomer of Le$^a$.[2] (Fig. 7–7).

## CLINICAL SIGNIFICANCE OF LEWIS ANTIBODIES

Although some cases of hemolytic transfusion reactions caused by anti-Le$^a$ have been reported and there have been cases of in vivo red cell destruction due to anti-Le$^b$, Lewis antibodies are generally considered insignificant in blood transfusion practices. This is because:

1. Lewis antibodies can be neutralized by the Lewis substances present in the plasma and can thereby be decreased in quantity.
2. The Lewis antigens dissociate from the red cells as readily as they bind to the red cells. In other words, the Lewis-positive donor red cells can become Lewis-negative red cells following transfusion into an individual with a Lewis-negative phenotype. These antigens released into the plasma can further neutralize any Lewis antibodies present in the recipient plasma.
3. Lewis antibodies are generally IgM and therefore cannot cross the placenta and cause HDN. In addition, Lewis antigens are not fully developed at birth (Table 7–8).

For these reasons, the presence of Lewis antibodies in a patient's serum does not require transfusions of Lewis-negative red cells, as long as pretransfusion tests performed at 37°C and Coombs phase are compatible and there is no evidence of in vitro hemolysis. The Lewis antibodies reactive at 37°C and antihuman globulin phase, however, should not be ignored because these antibodies can cause in vivo red cell destruction.

## ADVANCED CONCEPTS: OTHER LEWIS ANTIGENS

### The Lewis (a+b+) Phenotype: Partial Secretors

It is postulated that a weak variant of the secretory gene (Se) referred to as Se$^w$ is responsible for the expression of Le(a+b+) phenotype. The Se$^w$ allele is rare or absent in whites and should not be confused with the occasional expression of Le$^a$ antigen in Le(a−b+) individuals. Le(a+b+) phenotype is referred to as *partial secretory phenotype* and is frequently found in Polynesians, Australians, and Asians.[5] Individuals with Se$^w$ gene have a reduced amount of ABH substances in their secretions because of the competition of Le and Se transferases for type 1 precursors. In non–group O individuals there is even more competition for H type 1 by the A and B glycosyltransferase, and therefore less Le$^b$ is formed.[25] Lewis(a+b+) phenotype has been reported more in group O than in non–group O individuals. Detection of Le(a+b+) phenotype is also dependent on the potency and type of the antisera used.[2,5]

It is worth noting that the Se$^w$ allele has been cloned, and it is suggested that the weak expression of secretor

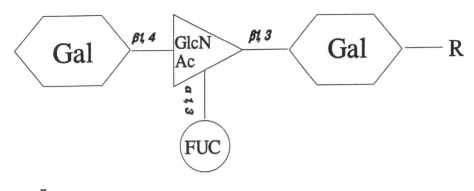

Le$^x$

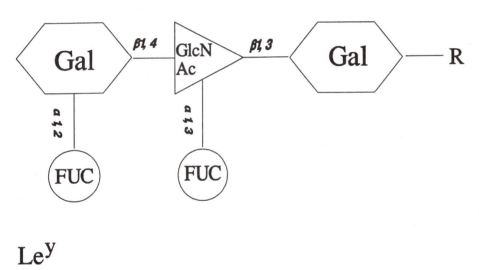

Le$^y$

**Figure 7–7.** Structure of Le$^x$ and Le$^y$ from type-2 chains. Gal = D-galactose; G1cNAc = *N*-acetyl-D-glucosamine; R = other biochemical residues.

**Table 7–8.** Factors Contributing to Clinical Insignificance of Lewis Antibodies

Neutralization of Lewis antibodies by Lewis substances present in the plasma
Loss of red cell Lewis antigen(s) into the plasma
Lack of reactivity at 37°C and antihuman globulin phase
Generally IgM in nature and incapable of crossing placenta
Lewis antigens poorly developed in newborn infants

transferase (*Se$^w$*) is caused by point mutations in the coding region of FUT2.[5] In addition, the frequency of the nonsecretor gene (*se*) has been found to be uncommon in Polynesians.[3]

### Le$^c$ and Le$^d$ (Type 1 Precursor and Type 1 H Structure)

Le$^d$ antigen was first described by Potapov,[26] who reported an antibody in the serum that reacted with red cells from Le(a−b−) ABH-secretor individuals. In his

report, he predicted another hypothetic antibody, anti-Le$^c$, which would detect the Lewis antigen on red cells of Lewis (a−b−) ABH nonsecretors. In 1972, Gunson and Latham reported such an antibody that defined the Le$^c$ antigen.[27]

Le$^c$ and Le$^d$ type 1 chain structures also have been proposed by Graham[28] and Hanfland[29] and their co-workers, who obtained anti-Le$^c$ and anti-Le$^d$ antibodies following immunization of goats with human saliva. In their investigation, anti-Le$^d$ was strongly inhibited by a fucose containing saccharide of the type 1 H chain structure. These investigators suggest that neither Le$^c$ nor Le$^d$ antigens are associated with the Lewis system. Le$^c$ represents type 1 precursor structure, and Le$^d$ is type 1 H structure (Fig. 7–8). More recent findings suggest that there are two types of Le$^c$ substances referred to as single Le$^c$ and branched Le$^c$.[2,30,31]

Le$^c$ present in saliva, plasma, and the red cells is a combination of a branched structure and unbranched forms.[2,31] The branched structures are the main glycolipids on the red cells in Le(a−b−) nonsecretors and cause agglutination using polyclonal antibodies. The

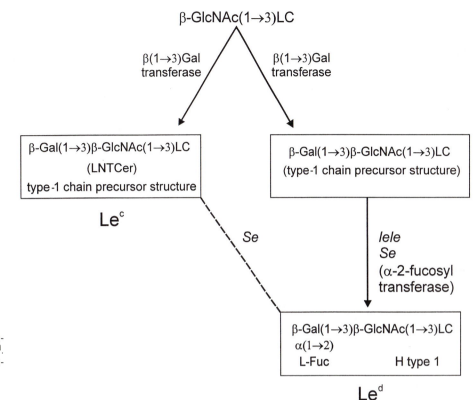

$\beta$-GlcNAc(1$\rightarrow$3)LC

$\beta$(1$\rightarrow$3)Gal transferase     $\beta$(1$\rightarrow$3)Gal transferase

$\beta$-Gal(1$\rightarrow$3)$\beta$-GlcNAc(1$\rightarrow$3)LC
(LNTCer)
type-1 chain precursor structure

Le$^c$

$\beta$-Gal(1$\rightarrow$3)$\beta$-GlcNAc(1$\rightarrow$3)LC
(type-1 chain precursor structure)

*Se*

*lele*
*Se*
($\alpha$-2-fucosyl transferase)

$\beta$-Gal(1$\rightarrow$3)$\beta$-GlcNAc(1$\rightarrow$3)LC
$\alpha$(1$\rightarrow$2)
L-Fuc       H type 1

Le$^d$

**Figure 7–8.** A hypothetical pathway. Formation of Le$^c$ and Le$^d$. Based on the work of Graham, Hanfland, and associates.[28,29]

branched structures are either absent or poorly detected on Le(a−b−) cord cells because of the lack of specificity of anti-Le$^c$ antibodies for the cord cells. Le$^c$ in its unbranched single form (lactotetraosylceramide) does not cause agglutination of the red cells with polyclonal antibodies. Single Le$^c$ is the precursor to Le$^a$ and Le$^d$ (type 1 H). Le$^d$ is formed by the action of the Se transferase on type 1 precursor substance (Le$^c$).[2]

Formation of Lewis antigens in secretions and through their adsorption onto red cells depends on the genetic makeup of the individual (Table 7–9). The Le$^c$ and Le$^d$ antigens are found in Lewis-negative individuals (*lele*) who have phenotypes of Le(a−b−). Le$^c$ antigen is found only in Le(a−b−) individuals who are ABH nonsecretors. Le$^d$ antigen is found only in Le(a−b−) individuals who are ABH secretors. In view of these findings, perhaps Lewis phenotype would be correctly written as Le(a−b−c+d−) and Le(a−b−c−d+), similar to the new phenotypes previously described. Le$^c$ is analogous to Le$^a$; they are biochemically very similar and secreted only by ABH nonsecretors (*sese*). Similarly, Le$^c$ is adsorbed onto the red cell only after exposure to the plasma or secretion containing the soluble antigen. This close similarity between Le$^a$ and Le$^c$ accounts for the observation that the Le(a−b−) individuals who produced anti-Le$^a$ are all ABH secretors with an Le(a−b−c−d+) phenotype.

The presence of Le$^c$ in Le(a−b−) ABH nonsecretors probably prevents the formation of anti-Le$^a$, inasmuch as Le$^c$ and Le$^a$ are biochemically very similar. Saliva from these Le(a−b−c+d−) ABH nonsecretors has been found to contain Le$^c$-soluble antigens.

Le$^d$ antigen is analogous to the Le$^b$ antigen and is found only in Le(a−b−) secretors; its correct phenotype is Le(a−b−c−d+). Le$^d$ is also thought to be biochemically similar to Le$^b$. The Le$^c$-soluble and Le$^d$-soluble antigens subsequently adsorb (as all Lewis antigens do) to the red cell membrane after exposure to the plasma containing the soluble antigen.

In the rare Bombay phenotype O$_h$ (see Chap. 5), individuals cannot synthesize the H, A, B antigens on their red cells because they lack the H structure necessary for formation of these antigens (see Figures 7–2, 7–5; **Color Plates 12, 13**). As a result, all O$_h$ individuals have a phenotype of either Le(a+b−), if the Lewis gene (*Le*) is inherited, or Le(a−b−), if the Lewis genotype is *lele* (Fig. 7–9). A more specific phenotype for the O$_h$ individual of the Lewis genetic makeup (*lele*) would be Le(a−b−c+d−) because all O$_h$ individuals are nonsecretors of all ABH substances, yet are capable of secreting Le$^c$ substances in the saliva.

In equally rare para-Bombay individuals, at least one functional *Se* gene is present in addition to two null alleles at the H locus. These individuals have A, B, and H antigens in their secretions, with a weak AB antigen on their red cells. The weak antigen on their red cells may be adsorbed from plasma or may be due to the presence of an alternative gene at the H locus.[14,24] The indicated alternative gene gives rise to a small amount of H antigen, all of which is transformed into the A and B antigens.

To make the Lewis system even more complicated and intriguing, interaction among *ABO, H, Se,* and *Le* genes results not only in the formation of the Le$^a$ and Le$^b$ substances but also in the compound antigen prod-

**Table 7–9.** Review of the Genetic Interaction among Lewis, *Hh,* Secretor, and ABH Genes

| Hypothetic Genotype | Substances Present in Saliva | Red Cell Phenotype |
|---|---|---|
| *LeLe HH SeSe AA* | A, H, Le$^a$, Le$^b$ | A Le(a−b+) |
| *lele Hh Sese AO* | A, H | A Le(a−b−) |
| Lele Hh sese AO | *Le$^a$* | A Le(a+b−) |
| *lele HH sese AO* | Le$^c$ | A Le(a−b−) |
| *lele HH sese AB* | Le$^c$ | AB Le(a−b−) |
| LeLe HH, Sese, AB | A, B, H, Le$^a$, Le$^b$ | AB Le(a−b+) |
| *lele Hh SeSe AB* | A, B, H, Le$^c$, Le$^d$ | AB Le(a−b−) |
| Lele Hh sese AB | Le$^a$ | AB Le(a+b−) |
| Lele HH SeSe OO | H, Le$^a$, Le$^b$ | O Le(a−b+) |
| *lele Hh SeSe OO* | H, Le$^c$, Le$^d$ | O Le(a−b−) |
| LeLe HH sese OO | Le$^a$ | O Le(a+b−) |
| *lele Hh sese OO* | Le$^c$ | O Le(a−b−) |
| *lele hh Sese AB*\* | A, B, H | AB Le(a−b−)\* |
| *LeLe hh SeSe AB*\* | Le$^a$, Le$^b$, A, B, H | AB Le(a+b−)\* |
| Lele hh sese AB | Le$^a$ | O$_h$ Le(a+b−) |
| lele hh sese AB | Le$^c$ | O$_h$ Le(a−b−) |

\*Para-Bombay phenotype.

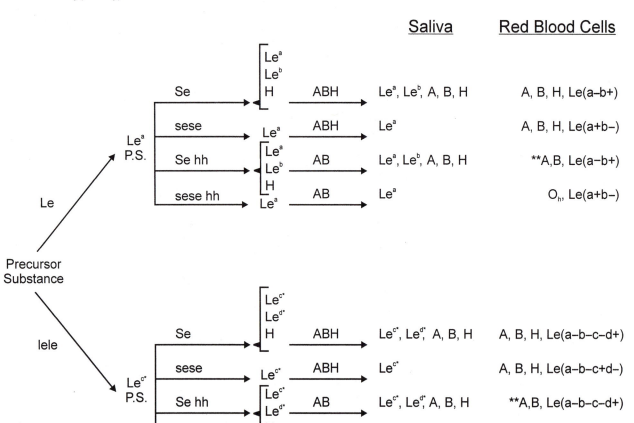

\* Provisional pathway for Le$^c$ and Le$^d$ antigens

\*\* Para-Bombay Phenotype

**Figure 7–9.** Genetic pathway for the production of the A, B, H, Le$^a$, and Le$^b$ blood group substances.

ucts ALe[b] and BLe[b]. This has been confirmed because an anti-A[1] Le[b] antibody has been described in the Lewis system. The compound antibody reacts only with red cells that possess both the A[1] and the Le[b] antigenic determinants and is felt to be the result of genetic interaction among the *A[1]*, *Le*, *H*, and *Se* genes.[32] For a review of the genetic interaction that occurs between the *Le*, *H*, *Se*, and *ABO* genes, which results in the various substances found in secretions as well as red cell phenotypes, the reader should study Table 7–9, which gives various hypothetical genotypes.

### Le[x] and Le[y]

Le[x](X) is referred to as a type 2 isomer of Le[a],[2,5,13] which is formed by the addition of fucose-α (1→3) GlcNAc linkage on type 2 chain (see Figure 7–7). This Le[x] is the same antigenic structure called stage-specific embryonic antigen-1 (SSEA-1),[1] which is different from Le[x] as a binding site for the anti-Le[x] discussed previously. Le[y](Y) is defined as a type 2 isomer of Le[b] and is made by addition of fucose-α (1→3) GlcNAc linkage on type 2 H substance (see Figure 7–7).

Other Lewis-related type 2 structures are ALe[x] (AX), ALe[y] (AY), and BLe[y] (BY). ALe[y] and BLe[y] are important markers of the cell membrane.[2,5]

Lewis and secretor fucosyltransferases can use type 1 and type 2 precursor substances to form type 1 and type 2 antigens; however, type 2 antigens are primarily made by other α-3-fucosyltransferases, such as FUT4, FUT5, FUT6, and FUT7.[2] In addition, *Se* and *H* genes can both act on the type 2 precursors to form H type 2 and related structures. However, the H type 2 and related structures found in the secretions are formed by the effect of the *Se* gene on type 2 precursor.[5] Table 7–10 summarizes the Lewis antigens made from type 1 and type 2 precursor substances.

### BIOLOGIC SIGNIFICANCE OF LEWIS SYSTEM

Although the Lewis system is not considered a significant system in transfusion medicine, it has significance at the tissue level for the establishment of a biologic relationship between blood group antigens and the diseases.[2,5]

The biologic role of the Lewis system in disease is intricate because of the complexity of the Lewis structure,

**Table 7–10.** Type 1 and Type 2 Antigens

| Type 1 | Type 2 |
|---|---|
| Le[c] | Type 2 precursor |
| Le[d] | H type 2 |
| Le[a] | Le[x] |
| Le[b] | Le[y] |
| A type 1 | A type 2 |
| ALe[b] | A Le[y] |

causing diversity of the cell surface markers. However, it is clearly known that the Lewis system is associated with factors causing certain diseases, such as peptic ulcers, ischemic heart disease, cancer, and kidney transplant rejection. In addition, Lewis antigens have receptors to interact with microorganisms expressing a particular lectin. For example, Le[b] has receptors for *Helicobacter pylori*.[5,33,34] Furthermore, lack of *Le* and *Se* genes in Le(a−b−) phenotype is associated with pathologic conditions. Le[x] and Le[y] are associated with gastrointestinal, colorectal, and lung cancers.[14] Le[x] antigen is a marker for Reed-Sternberg cells of Hodgkin's disease.[14]

It has also been postulated that the presence of Lewis antibodies in Lewis-negative individuals is associated with a higher renal allograft rejection than in Lewis-positive people.[5] Anti-Le[a] has been reported to be associated with renal failure in Lewis-negative bone marrow transplant patients. Some Lewis antibodies occur in patients with cancer, such as anti-ALe[d] in patients with cancer of the stomach, anti-Le[c] in patients with bronchogenic carcinoma, anti-Le[bH] in patients with metastatic carcinoma of the bladder, and auto-anti-Le[a] in Le(a−b+) individuals with carcinoma of esophagus. The presence of some Lewis antibodies is found to be beneficial to patients; for example, anti-Le[c] is responsible for the regression of the patient's tumor, and mono-clonal antibodies to type 1 Lewis substance has antitumor effect both in vivo and in vitro.[2] The biologic significance of the Lewis system needs more research because of controversial findings in some areas.

### SUMMARY

Traditionally, six antigens have been associated with the Lewis system: Le[a], Le[b], Le[c], Le[d], Le[x], and Le[y]. All these antigens can be detected in secretions and on red cells (after adsorption from plasma). The Lewis system represents a tissue group, inasmuch as Lewis antigens are not synthesized by red cells but rather are adsorbed from plasma. In secretions, these antigens exist as glycoproteins. In plasma and on red cells, they are glycolipids. The structure of the Le[a] and Le[b] glycosphingolipids from human plasma and red cells has been defined biochemically. Le[a] represents a lacto-*N*-fucopentaosyl[5] ceramide, depicted here:

β-Gal(1→3) β-GlcNAc(1→3) β-Gal(1→4)) β-Glc(1→1)Cer
|
α(1→4)
|
Fuc

Type 1 chain

Le[b] represents a lacto-*N*-difucohexaosyl (1) ceramide, depicted here:

β-Gal(1→3) β-GlcNAC(1→3) β-Gal(1→4)β-Glc(1→1) Cer
|     |
α(1→2)   α(1→4)
|     |
Fuc     Fuc

Type 1 chain

Le$^c$ is found in the Lewis-negative (*lele*) nonsecretors, Le$^d$ in *lele* secretors. The biochemical structure of Le$^c$ and Le$^d$ are type 1 precursor and type 1 H substance, respectively (see Figure 7–8). Le$^c$ as a compound structure (type 1 and type 2) has also been demonstrated. Le$^x$ antigen is defined as type 2 isomer of Le$^a$, and Le$^y$ antigen is defined as type 2 isomer of Le$^b$.

## CASE STUDY

A 35-year-old woman was seen by her obstetrician for a prenatal care examination. A blood test for prenatal type and screen showed the following:

| ABO-Rh Typing | | | | | |
|---|---|---|---|---|---|
| Anti-A | Anti-B | Anti-D | Rh Control | A$_1$ Cell | B Cell |
| 0 | 4+ | 4+ | 0 | 4+ | 0 |

| Antibody Screen | | | |
|---|---|---|---|
| | IS | 37°C | Antihuman Globulin |
| I | R$_1$R$_1$ | | |
| I | R$_1$R$_1$ 1+ | 1+ | 1+ |
| II | R$_2$R$_2$ 1+ | 1+ | 0 |

The results of a 10–red cell panel indicate that anti-Le$^a$ and anti-Le$^b$ are present in the patient's serum. The anti-Le$^b$ reactivity is seen only at IS and 37°C, with the 37°C reactivity most likely a carryover from the IS reading. Therefore, anti-Le$^b$ is not clinically significant because it does not react at antihuman globulin.

The anti-Le$^a$ reactivity is present at all phases—IS, 37°C, and antihuman globulin. A prewarmed antibody screen should be performed before considering the anti-Le$^a$ to be clinically significant. The majority of the anti-Le$^a$ antibodies are nonreactive at antihuman globulin using the prewarmed technique.

The results in this case illustrate that:

1. Lewis antibodies are present in the serum of pregnant women.

2. The antibodies are insignificant or are not associated with HDN, or both, because newborn infants lack the Lewis antigens and IgM antibodies do not cross the placenta.

---

## SUMMARY CHART: IMPORTANT POINTS TO REMEMBER (MT/MLT)

n Lewis blood group antigens are not synthesized by the red cells. These antigens are made by tissue cells, secreted into body fluids and plasma, and adsorbed onto the red cell membrane.

n Lewis antigens present in secretions are glycoproteins; Lewis cell–bound antigens absorbed from plasma onto red cell membranes are glycolipids.

n The *Le* gene codes for L-fucosyltransferase, which adds L-fucose to the type 1 chain

n *Le* gene is needed for the expression of Le$^a$ substance, and *Le* and *Se* genes are needed to form Le$^b$ substance.

n Le$^a$ antigen is formed by the addition of L-fucose to the number 4 carbon of *N*-acetylglucosamine of type 1 precursor structure.

n All Le(a+b−) persons are ABH nonsecretors and have only Le$^a$ substance in secretions.

n Le$^b$ antigen is formed when a second L-fucose is added to the number 4 carbon of the subterminal *N*-acetyl-D-glucosamine of type 1 H.

n All Le(a−b+) persons are ABH secretors and have both Le$^a$ and Le$^b$ substances in secretions.

n The most common Lewis phenotype in both whites and blacks is Le(a−b+).

n The *lele* genotype is more common among blacks than in whites and will phenotype as Le(a−b−).

n Lewis antigens are poorly expressed at birth.

n Lewis antigens do not demonstrate dosage in serologic reactions.

n Lewis antibodies are generally IgM (naturally occurring); antibodies are capable of binding complement and are enhanced by enzymes; Lewis substance in secretions can neutralize Lewis antibodies.

n Lewis antibodies are frequently encountered in pregnant women.

n Lewis antibodies are not considered significant in transfusion medicine.

---

## REVIEW QUESTIONS

1. Where are the Lewis antigens produced?
   A. Platelets
   B. Red blood cells
   C. White blood cells
   D. Tissue cells
   E. All of the above

2. Biochemically, Lewis antigens are classified as what in secretions?
   A. Glycoproteins
   B. Glycolipids
   C. Polyproteins
   D. Glycophorins

3. Biochemically, Lewis antigens are classified as what

in plasma and on red cells? (Use answer choices for Question 2.)

4. Which of the following characteristics best describes Lewis antibodies?
   A. IgM, naturally occurring, causes HDN
   B. IgM, naturally occurring, does not cause HDN
   C. IgG, in vitro hemolysis, causes hemolytic transfusion reactions
   D. IgG, in vitro hemolysis, does not cause hemolytic transfusion reactions

5. The *Le* gene codes for a specific glycosyltransferase that transfers an L-fucose to the *N*-acetylglucosamine on:
   A. Type 1 precursor chain
   B. Type 2 precursor chain
   C. Types 1 and 2 precursor chain
   D. Either type 1 or type 2 in any one individual but not in both

6. Secretions of a person with the genes *B*, *Se*, and *Le* contain which of the following?
   A. B substance, H substance, Le$^a$ and Le$^b$ substances
   B. B substance, Le$^a$ substance
   C. H substance, Le$^a$ and Le$^b$ substances
   D. H substance, Le$^a$ substance

7. Secretions of a person with the genes *B*, *sese*, and *Le* contain which of the following?
   A. B substance, Le$^a$ substance
   B. H substance, Le$^a$ substance
   C. H substance, Le$^a$ and Le$^b$ substance
   D. Le$^a$ substance

8. An individual with genes *A*, *H*, *Se*, and *lele* has which of the following phenotypes?
   A. ABH, Le(a−b−)
   B. ABH, Le(a+b−)
   C. AH, Le(a−b−)
   D. AH, Le(a+b−)

9. Transformation to Le$^b$ phenotype after birth may be as follows:
   A. Le(a−b−) to Le(a+b+) to Le(a−b+)
   B. Le(a+b−) to Le(a−b−) to Le(a−b+)
   C. Le(a−b+) to Le(a+b+) to Le(a−b+)
   D. Le(a+b+) to Le(a+b+) to Le(a−b+)

10. In what way do the Lewis antigens change during pregnancy?
    A. Le$^a$ antigen increases only
    B. Le$^b$ antigen increases only
    C. Le$^a$ and Le$^b$ both increase
    D. Le$^a$ and Le$^b$ both decrease

11. Le$^c$ and Le$^d$ antigens are found in individuals with the phenotype of:
    A. Le(a−b−)
    B. Le(a+b−)
    C. Le(a−b+)
    D. Le(a+b−)

12. Anti-Le$^x$ agglutinates which of the following antigens?
    A. All Le(a+b−) red cells
    B. All Le(a−b+) red cells
    C. All Le(a−b−) red cells
    D. Two of the above

13. The Lewis phenotype that is most commonly associated with *H. pylori* infection is:
    A. Le(a+b−)
    B. Le(a−b+)
    C. Le(a−b−)
    D. Le(a−x+)

## ANSWERS TO REVIEW QUESTIONS

1. D (p 146)
2. A (p 147)
3. B (p 147)
4. B (p 152)
5. A (p 146)
6. A (p 150, Table 7–2)
7. D (p 150, Table 7–2)
8. C (p 150, Table 7–2)
9. A (p 511)
10. D (p 151)
11. A (p 154)
12. D (p 153)
13. B (p 157)

## REFERENCES

1. Oriol, R, et al: Genetics of ABO, H, Lewis, X and related antigens. Vox Sang 51:161, 1986.
2. Henry, S, et al: Lewis histo-blood group system and associated secretory phenotypes. Vox Sang 69:166, 1995.
3. Henry, S, et al: A second nonsecretor allele of the blood group α(1,2) fucosyltransferase gene (FUT2). Vox Sang 70:21, 1996.
4. Salmon, C, et al: The human blood groups. Masson Pub, New York, 1984, p 162.
5. Henry, SM: Immunohematology: Journal of blood group serology and education. American Red Cross 13(2):51, 1996.
6. Watkins, WM, et al: Regulation of expression of carbohydrate blood group antigens. Biochimie 70:1597, 1988.
7. Dunstan, RA: Status of major red cell blood group antigens on neutrophils, lymphocytes, and monocytes. Br J Haematol 62:301, 1986.
8. Dunstan, RA: The expression of ABH antigens during in vitro megakaryocyte maturation: Origin of heterogeneity of antigen density. Br J Haematol 62:587, 1986.
9. Elmgren, A, et al: DNA sequencing and screening for point mutations in the human Lewis (*FUT3*) gene enables molecular genotyping of the human Lewis blood group system. Vox Sang 70:97, 1996.
10. Watkins, WM: Blood group substances: In the ABO system the genes control the arrangement of sugar residues that determines blood group specificity. Science 152:172, 1966.

11. Hauser, R: Le^a and Le^b tissue glycosphingolipids. Transfusion 53:577, 1995.

12. Wendell, RF: Clinical Immunohematology: Basic Concept and Clinical Applications. Blackwell Scientific, Oxford, England, 1990, pp 187–199.

13. Hanfland, P, and Graham, HA: Immunochemistry of the Lewis blood-group system: Partial characterization of Le^a, Le^b, and H-type 1 (Le^dH) blood group active glycosphingolipids from human plasma. Arch Biochem Biophys 210:383, 1981.

14. Petz, LD, et al: Clinical Practice of Transfusion Medicine, ed 3. Churchill Livingstone, New York, 1995, pp 81–89.

15. Walker, RH: Technical Manual, ed 12. American Association of Blood Banks, Bethesda, MD, 1996, pp 246–248.

16. Churchill, WH, and Kutz, SR: Transfusion Medicine. Blackwell Scientific, Oxford, England, 1988, p 57.

17. Hammar, L, et al: Lewis phenotype of erythrocytes and Le^b active glycolipid in serum of pregnant women. Vox Sang 40:27, 1981.

18. Langkilde, NC, et al: Letter to the Editor. Lancet I:926, 1990.

19. Idikio, HA, and Manickavel V: Lewis blood group antigens (a and b) in human breast tissues: Loss of Lewis-b in breast cancer cells and correlation with tumor grade. Cancer 68(6): 1303, 1991.

20. Mollison, PL, et al: Blood Transfusion in Clinical Medicine, ed 9. Blackwell Scientific, Oxford, England 1993, pp 175–198.

21. Cowles, JW, et al: The fine specificity of Lewis blood group antibodies: Evidence for maturation of immune response. Vox Sang 56:107, 1989.

22. Cheng, MS, and Lukomskyj, L: Lewis antibody following a massive blood transfusion. Vox Sang 57:155, 1989.

23. Schenkel-Brunner, H, and Hanfland, P: Immunochemistry of the Lewis blood group system. III. Studies on the molecular basis of the Le^x property. Vox Sang 40:358, 1981.

24. Bryant, NJ: An Introduction to Immunohematology, ed 3. WB Saunders, Philadelphia, 1994, pp 110–111, 129–136.

25. Turgeon, ML: Fundamentals of Immunohematology: Theory and Technique, ed 2. Williams & Wilkins, Philadelphia, 1995, pp 120–124.

26. Potapov, MI: Detection of the antigen of the Lewis system, characteristic of the erythrocytes of the secretor group Le(a−b−). Probl Hematol Blood Transfus (USSR) 1970, pp 11:45.

27. Clamagirand-Milet, C, et al: Isoelefocusing pattern of 2-L, 3-L and 4-L-fucosyltransferases from human milk and serum. FEBS Lett 126:123, 1981.

28. Graham, HA, et al: Genetic and immunochemical relationships between soluble and cell-bound antigens of the Lewis system. In Mohn, JF, et al (eds): Human Blood Groups. Proc Fifth Intern Conv Immunology. Karger, Basel, 1977, 257–267.

29. Hanfland, P, et al: Immunochemistry of the Lewis blood-group system. FEBS Lett 142:77, 1982.

30. Hanfland, P, et al: Immunochemistry of the Lewis blood-group system: Isolation and structures of Lewis-c active and related glycosphingolipids from the plasma of blood group O Le(a−b−) nonsecretors. Arch Biochem Biophys 246:655, 1986.

31. Oriol, R: Genetic control of the fucosylation of ABH precursor chains: Evidence for new epistatic interactions in different cells and tissues. J Immunogenet 17:235, 1990.

32. Seaman, MJ, et al: Siedler: An antibody which reacts with A, (Le(a−b−) red cells. Vox Sang 15:25, 1968.

33. Reid, ME, and Lomas-Francis, C: The Blood Group Antigen Facts Book. Academic Press, San Diego, 1997, pp 210–215.

34. Silberstein, LE: Molecular and Functional Aspects of Blood Group Antigens. American Association of Blood Banks, Bethesda, MD, 1995, pp 52, 181–182.

## BIBLIOGRAPHY

Abhyankar, S, et al: Positive cord blood "DAT" due to anti-Le^a: Absence of hemolytic disease of the newborn. Am J Pediatr Hematol Oncol 11(2):185, 1989.

Bernoco, M, et al: Detection of combined ABH and Lewis glycosphingolipids in sera of deficient donors. Vox Sang 49(1):58, 1985.

Boorman, KE, et al: Blood Group Serology, ed 6. Churchill Livingstone, New York, 1988, pp 69–80.

Boren, T, et al: Attachment of *Helicobacter pylori* to human gastric epithelium mediated by blood group antigens. Science 262:1892, 1993.

Caillard, T, et al: Failure of expression of alpha-3-fucosyltransferase in human serum is coincident with the absence of the X (or Le(x)) antigen in the kidney but not on leukocytes. Exp Clin Immunogenet 5(1):15, 1988.

Clausen, H, and Hakomori, S: ABH and related histo-blood group antigens: Immunochemical differences in carrier isotypes and their distribution. Vox Sang 56:1, 1989.

Cowels, JW, et al: Comparison of monoclonal antisera with conventional antisera for Lewis blood group antigen determination. Vox Sang 52(1–2): 83, 1987.

Hanfland, P, et al: Immunochemistry of the Lewis blood group system: Isolation and structures of Lewis-c active and related glycosphingolipids from the plasma of blood group Le(a−b−) nonsecretors. Arch Biochem Biophys 246(2):655, 1986.

Issitt, PD, and Anstee, DJ: Applied Blood Group Serology, ed 4. Montgomery Scientific, Durham, NC, 1998, pp 247–271.

Le-Pendu, J, et al: Expression of ABH and X (Le^x) antigens in various cells. Biochimie 70(11):1613, 1988.

Mollicone, R, et al: Acceptor specificity and tissue distribution of three human alpha-3-fucosyltransferase. Eur J Biochem 191(1):169, 1990.

Mollison, PL, et al: Blood Transfusion in Clinical Medicine, ed 9. Blackwell Scientific, Oxford, England, 1993, pp 175–198.

Oriol, R: Genetic regulation of the expression of ABH and Lewis antigens in tissues. APMIS Suppl 27:28, 1992.

Rossi, EC, et al: Principles of Transfusion Medicine. Williams & Wilkins, Baltimore, 1992, p 70.

Shulman, IA: Problem Solving in Immunohematology, ed 4. ASCP Press, Chicago, 1992, pp 62–64.

Turgeon, ML: Fundamentals of Immunohematology: Theory and Technique. Lea & Febiger, Philadelphia, 1989, pp 137–159.

Ura, Y, et al: Quantitative dot blot analyses of blood group related antigens in paired normal and malignant human breast tissues. Int J of Cancer 50(1):57, 1992.

Walker, RH: Technical Manual, ed 12. American Association of Blood Banks, Bethesda, MD, 1996, pp 246–248.

Watkins, WM, et al: Regulation of expression of carbohydrate blood group antigens. Biochimie 70(11):1597, 1988.

Whitlock, SA: The Clinical Laboratory Manual Series: Immunohematology. Delmar, Albany, NY, 1997, pp 79–80.

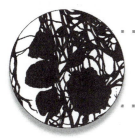

CHAPTER **8**

# OTHER MAJOR BLOOD GROUP SYSTEMS

Loni Calhoun, MT(ASCP)SBB

**Introduction**
Terminology
Evaluating Antigen Biochemistry

**The MNSs (002) Blood Group System**
Basic Concepts
- MN antigens
- Ss antigens
- Anti-M
- Anti-N
- Anti-S and anti-s

Advanced Concepts
- Biochemistry
- Genetics
- M and N lectins
- Null phenotypes
- The Miltenberger series
- Other antibodies in the MNSs system
- Autoantibodies
- Disease associations

**The P (003) and P$^k$ (209) Blood Group Systems**
Basic Concepts
- The P$_1$ antigen
- Anti-P$_1$

Advanced Concepts
- Biochemistry
- Genetics
- Other sources of P$_1$ antigen and antibody
- Anti-PP$_1$P$^k$
- Anti-P
- Anti-P$^k$
- Antibodies to compound antigens
- Luke (LKE) antigen and antibody
- The p antigen and antibody
- Disease associations

**The I (207) Blood Group Collection**
Basic Concepts
- The Ii antigens
- Anti-I
- Anti-i

Advanced Concepts
- Biochemistry and genetics
- Other sources of Ii antigen
- The I$^T$ antigen and antibody
- The specificities I$^D$, I$^F$, I$^S$
- Antibodies to compound antigens
- Disease associations

**The Kell (006) Blood Group System**
Basic Concepts
- K and k antigens
- Kp$^a$, Kp$^b$, Kp$^c$, and VLAN antigens
- Js$^a$ and Js$^b$ antigens
- Anti-K
- Antibodies to Kp$^a$, Js$^a$, and other low-frequency Kell antigens
- Antibodies to k, Kp$^b$, Js$^b$, and other high-frequency Kell antigens

Advanced Concepts
- Biochemistry
- Genetics
- The Kx antigen
- The K$_0$ phenotype
- Other Kell antigens
- The McLeod phenotype
- Altered expressions of Kell antigens
- Autoantibodies

**The Duffy (008) Blood Group System**
Basic Concepts
- Fy$^a$ and Fy$^b$ antigens
- Anti-Fy$^a$ and anti-Fy$^b$

Advanced Concepts
- Biochemistry
- Genetics
- The Fy$^x$ gene
- Fy3 antigen and antibody
- Fy4 antigen and antibody
- Fy5 antigen and antibody
- Fy6 antigen and antibody
- Fy3 and Fy5 antibody characteristics
- The Duffy-malaria association

**The Kidd (009) Blood Group System**
Basic Concepts
- Jk$^a$ and Jk$^b$ antigens
- Anti-Jk$^a$ and anti-Jk$^b$

Advanced Concepts
- Biochemistry
- Genetics
- Jk(a−b−) phenotype
- Anti-Jk3
- Autoantibodies
- Disease associations

**The Lutheran (005) Blood Group System**
Basic Concepts
- Lu$^a$ and Lu$^b$ antigens
- Anti-Lu$^a$
- Anti-Lu$^b$

Advanced Concepts
- Biochemistry
- Genetics
- Lu(a−b−) phenotypes
- Anti-Lu3
- Lu6/Lu9 and Lu8/Lu14
- Au$^a$ (Lu18) and Au$^b$ (Lu19)
- Other Lutheran antigens

## OBJECTIVES

*On completion of this chapter, the learner should be able to:*

### ANTIGEN CHARACTERISTICS

1  List the antigen frequencies for the common antigens K, M, S, s, Fy$^a$ Fy$^b$, Jk$^a$, Jk$^b$, and P$_1$.

2  Define Kp$^a$, Js$^a$, and Lu$^a$ as low-frequency antigens and Kp$^b$, Js$^b$, Lu$^b$, and I as high-frequency antigens.

3  Associate the antigen phenotypes S−s−U−, Js(a+), and Fy(a−b−) with blacks.

4  Define the null phenotypes En(a−), U−, M$^k$, p, K$_0$, Fy(a−b−) Jk(a−b−), and Lu(a−b−) and describe their role in problem solving.

5  Compare both dominant and recessive forms of the Lu(a−b−) and Jk(a−b−) phenotypes.

6  Describe the reciprocal relationship of I antigen to i antigen.

7  Associate I, P$_1$, and Lutheran antigens as being poorly expressed on cord cells.

8  Define the association of MN with glycophorin A and Ss with glycophorin B.

### ANTIBODY CHARACTERISTICS

9  Define M, N, I, and P$_1$ antibodies as non–red-cell–induced ("naturally occurring"), cold-reacting agglutinins that are usually clinically insignificant.

10  Describe K, k, S, s, Fy$^a$, Fy$^b$, Jk$^a$, and Jk$^b$ antibodies as usually induced by exposure to foreign red cells ("immune"), antiglobulin-reactive antibodies that are clinically insignificant.

11  Differentiate the antibody specificities that commonly show dosage (M/N, S/s, K/k, Jk$^a$/Jk$^b$) from those that show dosage less frequently (Fy$^a$/Fy$^b$ and Lu$^a$/Lu$^b$).

12  Differentiate antigens that are denatured by routine blood bank enzymes (M, N, S, s, Fy$^a$, Fy$^b$) from antigens whose reactivity with antibody is enhanced (Ii, P$_1$, Jk$^a$, Jk$^b$).

13  List the antibodies in the Kell and Lutheran blood group systems that do not react with 2-aminoethylisothiouronium–treated red cells and those antibodies in the Kell, MNSs, and Duffy systems that do not react with ZZAP-treated red cells.

### CLINICAL SIGNIFICANCE AND DISEASE ASSOCIATION

14  Identify or correlate the common 37°C antihuman globulin–reactive antibodies K, k, S, s, Fy$^a$, Fy$^b$, Jk$^a$, and Jk$^b$ with transfusion reactions and hemolytic disease of the newborn.

15  Describe the Kidd antibodies as a common cause of delayed hemolytic transfusion reactions.

16  Describe the association of autoanti-I with *Mycoplasma pneumoniae* infections and autoanti-i with infectious mononucleosis.

17  Describe the common characteristics of the McLeod phenotype, including very weak Kell antigen expression, acanthocytosis, and late onset of muscular dystrophy–like syndrome.

18  Describe the association of the Fy(a−b−) phenotype with *Plasmodium vivax* resistance.

19  Identify Jk(a−b−) red cells with a resistance to lysis normally in 2M urea, a common diluting fluid used for automated platelet counters.

20  Define those autoantibodies that sometimes have specificity to antigens in certain blood group systems and describe why the strength of the corresponding antigen sometimes weakens during this time.

## INTRODUCTION

This chapter contains more information than blood bank technologists or technicians need to know to work capably at the bench. It is hoped that the extra details will challenge them to learn more and will serve as a reference when the antigens and antibodies are encountered in real-life situations.

Antigen and antibody characteristics are summarized on the front and back cover of this book so that students can easily access pertinent information when performing antibody identification. Students should review the objectives, read the material, and then refer to the antigen-antibody characteristic chart to see how much they really know.

### Terminology

A blood group system is a group of antigens produced by alleles at a single gene locus or at loci so closely linked that crossing over does not occur or is very rare.[1] With a few notable exceptions, most blood group genes are located on the autosomal chromosomes and are inherited in straightforward mendelian fashion.

Most blood group alleles are codominant and express a corresponding antigen. For example, a person who inherits alleles *K* and *k* carries both K and k antigens on his or her red cells. Some genes code for complex structures that carry more than one antigen (e.g., the glycophorin B structure, which carries S or s antigen, also carries 'N' and U specificity).

Silent or amorphic alleles that make no apparent antigen exist, but they are rare. When paired chromosomes carry the same silent allele, a null phenotype results. Red cells with null phenotypes can be very help-ful when evaluating antibodies to unknown high-frequency antigens. For example, an antibody reacting with all test cells except those with the phenotype Lu(a−b−) may be directed against the antigens in the Lutheran system or an antigen phenotypically related to the Lutheran system.

Some blood group systems have regulator or modi-fying genes, which alter antigen expression. These are not necessarily located at the same locus as the blood group genes they affect and may segregate indepen-dently. One such modifying gene is *In(Lu)*, which in-hibits or suppresses the expression of all the antigens in the Lutheran blood group system as well as many other antigens, including $P_1$ and i. It is a rare dominant gene inherited independently of the genes coding for Lutheran, P, and Ii antigens.

Although gene and antigen names seem confusing at first, certain conventions are followed when writing al-leles, antigens, and phenotypes.[1] Some examples are given in Table 8–1. Genes are underlined or written in italics, and their allele number or letter is always superscript. Antigen names are not italicized and are most easily learned by everyday use. Phenotype des-ignation depends on the antigen nomenclature and whether letters or numbers are used. These are also best learned through use.

Antibodies are described by their antigen notation with the prefix "anti-." To help standardize blood group system and antigen names, the International So-ciety of Blood Transfusion (ISBT) Working Party of Ter-minology for Red Cell Surface Antigens has devised a numeric system based on nomenclature first proposed in 1980.[2] Each known system is given a number and letter designation, and each antigen within the system is numbered sequentially in order of discovery. For ex-ample, the Kell blood group system is 006 or KEL; the K antigen is 006.001 or KEL1.

One must remember that serologic tests determine only red cell phenotype, not genotype. Genotype is de-termined usually by family studies. Genetic studies and statistical analyses of inheritance data are required be-fore an antigen is assigned to a blood group system.

## Evaluating Antigen Biochemistry

Although blood bank personnel use routine sero-logic tests to detect red cell antigens, researchers use more sophisticated techniques to analyze their bio-chemistry and structure. Because these methods con-tribute so greatly to our knowledge of antigen function and expression, students should understand the prin-ciples behind some of the basic research tools.

Red cell proteins can be studied by staining intact membranes from osmotically lysed "ghost" red cells, but more often the membranes are dissociated first into lipid and protein components. Lipids are separated with organic solvents, loosely bound proteins are solu-bilized by changing pH or ionic strength or by using chelating agents, and tightly bound proteins are solu-bilized with detergents such as sodium dodecyl sulfate (SDS).

Solubilized proteins can be separated from one an-other using polyacrylamide gel electrophoresis (PAGE), wherein protein migration depends on mole-cular size and charge. When SDS and PAGE are used to-gether, the negative charge of the detergent overpowers the charge of the protein, and separation occurs by size alone. By comparing relative electrophoresis mobilities with SDS-PAGE, the relative molecular mass of a pro-tein, is determined. This value relates to, but is not quite the same as, the actual molecular weight of the protein or the molecular weight calculated from amino acid sequencing studies.

After proteins are separated, the electrophoretic bands can be stained with Coomassie blue R 250, which stains protein, or periodic acid–Schiff stain (PAS), which stains carbohydrates. Bands detected with PAS represent glycoprotein. Common membrane proteins identified with SDS-PAGE and Coomassie blue/PAS stains are summarized elsewhere.[1,3]

Membrane proteins can also be separated according to their biologic activity by passing them through affin-ity chromatography columns. The support media in a column can be coupled with specific antibodies, lectins, membrane receptors, or special enzymes. Only high-affinity proteins bind; others can be washed away. Once isolated, the bound protein can be eluted and its amino acid sequence determined.

The carbohydrates attached to proteins and lipids can also be studied. Glycopeptide linkages, the attachment of sugars to proteins, are categorized as *N*-glycosidic (*N*-acetylglucosamine [GlcNAc] attached to asparagine [Asn]) or *O*-glycosidic (sugars, usually *N*-acetylgalac-tosamine [GalNAc] or galactose [Gal], attached to ser-ine [Ser] or threonine [Thr]). The sugars with a carbo-

**Table 8–1.** Examples of Correct Blood Group Terminology

| Gene | Antigen | Other Names | Phenotype Antigen Positive | Phenotype Antigen Negative | Blood Group Antibody | Blood Group System |
|------|---------|-------------|----------------------------|----------------------------|----------------------|---------------------|
| *K* | K | K1,006.001 | K+ | K− | Anti-K | Kell or KEL |
| *Jkᵃ* | Jkᵃ | JK1,009.001 | Jk(a+) | Jk(a−) | Anti-Jkᵃ | Kidd or JK |
| *P¹ᵏ* | P¹ | P1,003.001 | $P_1$+ | $P_1$− | Anti-$P_1$ | P |
| *Lu⁴* | Lu⁴ | LU4,005.004 | Lu:4 | Lu:−4 | Anti-Lu⁴ | Lutheran or LU |

hydrate chain itself are studied by sequentially removing them with specific glycosidase enzymes.

Deoxyribonucleic acid (DNA) technology has also enhanced our knowledge of red cell antigens.[4, 5] When isolated from cells or obtained by the reverse transcription of mRNA, DNA can be amplified by polymerase chain reaction and cloned and sequenced for amino acid configuration and tertiary structure.

## THE MNSs (002) BLOOD GROUP SYSTEM

Following the discovery of the ABO blood group system, Landsteiner and Levine began immunizing rabbits with human red cells, hoping to find new antigen specificities. Among the antibodies recovered from these rabbit sera were anti-M and anti-N, both of which were reported in 1927.[6,7] Data from family studies suggested that the genes coding for M and N were alleles to one another. Thus, MN became a blood group system.

In 1947, after the implementation of the antiglobulin test, Walsh and Montgomery[8] discovered S, a distinct antigen genetically linked to MN. Its antithetical partner, s, was found in 1951,[9] and the MN system became MNSs, a two-loci system. The phenotypic frequencies of MN and Ss are listed in Table 8–2.

In 1953, an antibody to a high-frequency antigen, U, was reported by Weiner.[10] The observation by Greenwalt and associates[11] that all U− red cells were also S−s− resulted in the inclusion of U into the system.

Forty antigens have now been included in the MNSs system, making it almost equal to Rh in size and complexity (Table 8–3). Many of these antigens are associated with variant MNSs structures: Some behave as low-frequency antithetical antigens to M, N, S, or s; others behave as satellite antigens inherited concomitantly with M, N, S, and s. Still others represent high-frequency antigens or epitopes found elsewhere on the common MN or Ss glycoproteins.

To recognize its early discovery, the MNSs system has been assigned the ISBT numeric designation 002, second after ABO.

**Table 8–2.** Frequency of MNSs Phenotypes and Key Facts*

| Phenotype | Whites (%) | Blacks (%) |
|---|---|---|
| M+N− | 28 | 26 |
| M+N+ | 50 | 44 |
| M−N+ | 22 | 30 |
| S+s− | 11 | 3 |
| S+s+ | 44 | 28 |
| S−s+ | 45 | 69 |
| S−s−U− | 0 | <1 |

*Antigens: Well developed at birth.
Antibodies: Anti-MN: Clinically insignificant; some examples are pH/glucose dependent. Anti-Ss: Clinically significant. Reactivity is destroyed by enzymes. Usually show dosage.

## Basic Concepts

### MN Antigens

The M and N antigens are found on a well-characterized glycoprotein called MN-sialoglycoprotein (MN-SGP), α-sialoglycoprotein, or glycophorin A (GPA). The antigens are defined by the first and fifth amino acid (aa) on this structure (see Biochemistry section and Figure 8–1), but antibody reactivity may also encompass adjacent carbohydrate chains, which are rich in sialic acid.

There are about $10^6$ copies of GPA per red cell.[12] The antigens exhibit dosage. For example, red cells from people who are homozygous MM carry a double dose of the M antigen and react more strongly with anti-M than do red cells from heterozygous MN individuals who carry only a single dose of M.

The antigens can be detected as early as 9 weeks' gestational age, and they are well developed at birth. This makes them very useful in paternity exclusion cases involving newborns or the very young (when only well-developed antigens can be reliably typed).

Because MN antigens are at the outer end of GPA, they are easily destroyed or removed by the routine blood bank enzymes ficin, papain, and bromelain and by the less common enzymes trypsin and pronase. The antigens are also destroyed by ZZAP, a solution of dithiothreitol (DTT) and papain, but they are not affected by DTT alone, S-(2-aminoethyl) isothiuronium bromide (AET), α-chymotrypsin, chloroquine, or acid treatment. Treating red cells with neuraminidase, which cleaves sialic acid (also known as neuraminic acid or NeuNAc), abolishes reactivity with only some examples of antibody. M and N antibodies are heterogeneous; some may recognize only specific amino acids, but others recognize both amino acids and carbohydrate chains.

M and N are primarily red cell antigens. Although older data suggested that M antigen may be present on lymphocytes, M and N were not detected on lymphocytes, monocytes, or granulocytes by immunofluorescence flow cytometry, nor have they been detected on platelets. MN antigens have been detected on renal capillary endothelium and epithelium.[13] This is especially interesting because a strain of *Escherichia coli* associated with urinary tract infection has been identified as having recognition sites for the $NH_2$ terminal end of MN-SGP.[14]

### Ss Antigens

Ss antigens are located on a smaller glycoprotein that is very similar to MN, called Ss-sialoglycoprotein (Ss-SGP), δ-SGP, or glycophorin B (GPB) (see Biochemistry and Figure 8–1). The aa at position 29 on GPB is critical to antigen expression—S has methionine, whereas s has threonine. The epitope may also include the glutamic acid residue at position 28 and the glycosidic chain attached to threonine at position 25.[15] Ss-SGP complexes with Rh protein, which helps Ss-SGP stabilize or incorporate into the red cell membrane.[4] $Rh_{null}$ red cells have greatly reduced Ss expression.

**Table 8–3.** Summary of MNSs Antigens

| ISBT Number | Common Name | Alternate Name | Frequency (%) | Year Discovered | Biochemistry* |
|---|---|---|---|---|---|
| *I. Common Antigens Encoded by GPA or GPB* | | | | | |
| 1 | M | — | 78 | 1927 | GPAM aa1-5:Ser-Ser*-Thr*-Thr*-Gly |
| 2 | N | — | 72 | 1927 | GPAN aa1-5:Leu-Ser*-Thr*-Thr*-Glu |
| 3 | S | — | 55 | 1947 | GPBS aa29:Met |
| 4 | s | — | 89 | 1951 | GPBs aa29:Thr |
| *II. Low-Frequency Antigens Encoded by GPA, GPB, or Hybrids* | | | | | |
| 6 | He | Henshaw | 0.8 | 1951 | GPBAB aa1-5 |
| 7 | Mi<sup>a</sup> | Miltenberger | <1 | 1951 | GPA aa24-34 |
| 8 | M<sup>c</sup> | — | <0.1 | 1953 | GPABA aa1-5 |
| 9 | Vw | Verweyst | <1 | 1954 | GPABA aa28:Met |
| 10 | Mur | Murrell | <0.1 | 1961 | GPBAB aa34-41 |
| 11 | M<sup>g</sup> | Gilfeather | <0.01 | 1958 | GPABA aa1-5:Leu-Ser*-Thr-Asn-Glu |
| 12 | V<sup>r</sup> | Verdegaal | <0.1 | 1958 | — |
| 13 | M<sup>e</sup> | — | <1 | 1961 | GPA or B aa5:Gly |
| 14 | Mt<sup>a</sup> | Martin | 0.25 | 1962 | (Ns association) |
| 15 | St<sup>a</sup> | Stones | <0.1 | 1962 | GPBA or AA aa23-31 |
| 16 | Ri<sup>a</sup> | Ridley | <0.1 | 1962 | (Ns association) |
| 17 | Cl<sup>a</sup> | Caldwell | <0.1 | 1963 | (Ms association) |
| 18 | Ny<sup>a</sup> | Nyberg | <0.1 | 1964 | (Ns association) |
| 19 | Hut | Hutchinson | <0.1 | 1966 | GPABA aa28:Lys |
| 20 | Hil | Hill | <0.1 | 1966 | GPAB<sup>s</sup> or BAB<sup>s</sup> aa54-67 |
| 21 | M<sup>v</sup> | Armstrong | <0.6 | 1966/1980 | GPB |
| 22 | Far | Kamhuber | <0.1 | 1977 | — |
| 23 | s<sup>D</sup> | Dreyer | <0.01 | 1981 | GPB |
| 24 | Mit | Mitchell | 0.12 | 1980 | — |
| 25 | Dantu | — | <0.1 | 1981/1984 | GPB<sup>s</sup>A aa37-42 |
| 26 | Hop | — | <0.1 | 1982 | GPBAB or ABA aa45-54 |
| 27 | Nob | — | <0.1 | 1982 | GPABB aa49-53 |
| 29 | EnKt | — | <0.1 | 1985 | GPA aa49-52 |
| 31 | Or | Orriss | (Low) | 1987 | GPA variant? |
| 32 | DANE | — | (Low) | 1991 | GPABA |
| 33 | TSEN | — | (Low) | 1992 | GPAB<sup>s</sup> or BAB aa54-67 |
| 34 | MINY | — | (Low) | 1992 | GPAB or BAB aa54-67 |
| 35 | MUT | — | (Low) | 1995 | GPABA or BAB aa28:Lys |
| 36 | SAT | — | (Low) | 1994 | GPA4B5 exons aa69-74 |
| 37 | ERIK | — | (Low) | 1993 | GPA aa59:Lys |
| 38 | Os<sup>a</sup> | — | (Low) | 1983 | GPA? |
| *III. High-Frequency Antigens Encoded by GPA or GPB* | | | | | |
| 5 | U | — | >99.9 | 1953 | GPB aa33-39 |
| 28 | En<sup>a</sup> | — | >99.9 | 1969 | GPA aa26-56 |
| 30 | "N" | — | >99.9 | 1978 | GPB aa1-5 |
| 39 | ENEP | — | >99.9 | 1995 | GPB aa65:Ala |
| 40 | ENEH | — | >99.9 | 1992 | GPB aa28:Thr |

**Source:** Carton, JP, and Rouger, P (eds): Blood Cell Biochemistry, Vol 6: Molecular Basis of Human Blood Group Antigens. Plenum, New York, 1995; Reid, MD, and Lomas-Francis, C: The Blood Group Antigen Facts Book. Academic Press, New York, 1997.
* = attachment site for alkali-labile oligosaccharides
Ser = Serine
Thr = Threonine
Gly = Glycine
Asn = Asparagine
Leu = Leucine
Glu = Glutamic Acid
Met = Methionine
Ala = Alanine

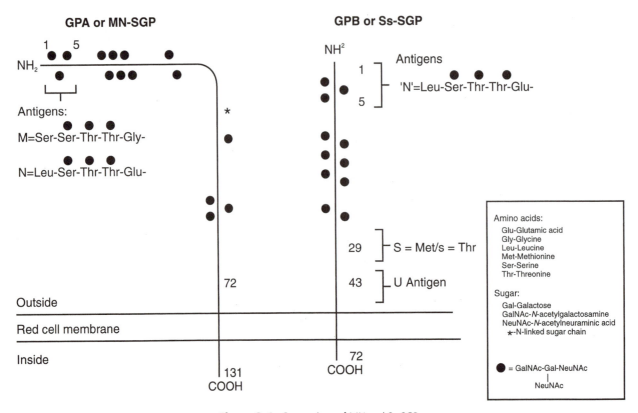

**Figure 8–1.** Comparison of MN and Ss-SGP.

There are about $2 \times 10^5$ copies of Ss-SGP/red cell,[12] but not all these may be available for antibody attachment. Masouredis and others[16] found only 12,000 available s sites on ss red cells. Data also suggest that red cells from SS people carry more copies of GPB than ss people.[15] Like MN, Ss antigens exhibit dosage. They also are well developed at birth and appear on red cells at an early gestational age (12 weeks).

The Ss antigens are less easily degraded by enzymes because the antigens are located farther down the glycoprotein, and enzyme-sensitive sites are less accessible. Ficin, papain, bromelain, pronase, and chymotrypsin can destroy Ss activity, but the amount of degradation may depend on the strength of the enzyme solution, length of treatment, and enzyme-to-cell ratio. Trypsin does not destroy Ss activity; neither does DTT, AET, chloroquine, or acid treatment. Weak concentrations (0.0005 to 0.005 percent) of sodium hypochlorite, or common household bleach, selectively destroy S reactivity by oxidizing the methionine amino acid at position 29.[17] Such bleach-treated cells can be useful in identifying antibodies found in combination with anti-S.

Like MN, Ss are considered red cell antigens. They are not found on platelets, lymphocytes, monocytes, and granulocytes.[5]

### Anti-M

Most examples of anti-M are naturally occurring, cold-reactive saline agglutinins. Although we may think of them as IgM, 50 to 80 percent are IgG or have an IgG component.[1] They usually do not bind complement, regardless of their immunoglobulin class, and they do not react with enzyme-treated red cells. The frequency of finding saline-reactive anti-M in routine blood donors is 1 in 2500 to 5000.[5] It appears to be more common in children than adults, and is particularly common in patients with burns.[12]

Because of antigen dosage, M antibodies may react better with M+N− red cells (genotype *MM*) than with M+N+ red cells (genotype *MN*). Very weak anti-M may not react with M+N+ red cells at all, making panel identification difficult. Antibody reactivity can be enhanced by increasing the serum-to-cell ratio or incubation time, or both, by decreasing incubation temperature or by adding a potentiating medium such as albumin or low-ionic-strength solution (LISS).

Some examples of anti-M are pH-dependent, reacting best at pH 6.5. These antibodies may be detected in plasma, which is slightly acidic from the anticoagulant, but not in unacidified serum. It is suggested that their antibody-binding site includes the histidine residue at position 9 on GPA, because its steric orientation is known to vary with pH.[1]

Other examples of anti-M react only with red cells exposed to glucose solutions. Such antibodies react with M+ reagent red cells or donor cells stored in preservative solutions containing glucose but do not react with freshly collected M+ cells. The significance of both pH-dependent and glucose-dependent antibodies in transfusion is questionable.

As long as anti-M does not react at 37°C, it is not clinically significant in transfusion. It is sufficient to provide units that are crossmatch compatible at 37°C and the antiglobulin phase without typing for M antigen. Sometimes compatible units carry the M antigen; for example, M+N+ red cells, which do not react with weak anti-M. Only rarely do such units stimulate a change in the antibody's thermal range.

Anti-M rarely causes hemolytic transfusion reactions, decreased cell survival, or hemolytic disease of the newborn (HDN). However, when 37°C reactive IgG anti-M is found in a pregnant woman, her physician should be forewarned; some HDN cases have been severe.[1]

### Anti-N

The serologic characteristics of anti-N are similar to those of anti-M: It is a cold-reactive IgM or IgG saline agglutinin that does not bind complement or react with enzyme-treated red cells. It demonstrates dosage, reacting better with M−N+ (*NN*) red cells than with M+N+ (*MN*) red blood cells (RBCs). Rare examples are glucose-dependent (see above).[18]

Also like anti-M, anti-N is not clinically significant unless it reacts at 37°C. It has been implicated only with rare cases of HDN.

Anti-N is rarer than anti-M because the terminal end of GPB carries the same amino acid sequence and sugars as the N antigen on GPA. This N-like structure, called 'N', may prevent N- individuals from recognizing N as a foreign antigen. In a series of 86,000 patients, only 2 examples of anti-N were seen.[5] The most potent antibodies are found in rare individuals who type M+N−S−s− and lack N and 'N'.

Anti-N is also seen in renal patients, regardless of their MN type, who are dialyzed on equipment sterilized with formaldehyde. Dialysis-associated anti-N reacts with any N+ or N− red cell treated with formaldehyde and is called anti-N$^f$. Formaldehyde may alter the MN antigen so that it is recognized as foreign. The antibody titer decreases when dialysis treatment and exposure to formaldehyde stop. Because anti-N$^f$ does not react at 37°C, it is clinically insignificant in transfusion. However, it has been associated with the rejection of a chilled transplanted kidney.[19]

### Anti-S and Anti-s

Most examples of anti-S and anti-s are IgG, reactive at 37°C and the antiglobulin test phase. A few express optimal reactivity at colder temperatures. If anti-S or anti-s specificity is suspected, incubating tests at room temperature or 4°C and performing a "cold" antiglobulin test may help in its identification.

The antibodies may or may not react with enzyme-treated red cells, depending on the degree of treatment. Treated red cells should be tested for S or s antigen expression with known antisera before enzyme reactions are interpreted. Although seen less often than anti-M, S or s antibodies are more likely to be clinically significant. They may bind complement, and they have been implicated with severe hemolytic transfusion reaction with hemoglobinuria. They have also caused HDN.

Units selected for transfusion must be antigen-negative and crossmatch compatible. Because only 11 percent of whites and 3 percent of blacks are s−, it can be difficult providing blood for a patient with anti-s. S− units are much easier to find (45 percent of whites and 69 percent of blacks are S−), but antibodies to low-frequency antigens are commonly found in sera containing anti-S, and these can cause unexplained incompatible crossmatches.

### Advanced Concepts

#### Biochemistry

Glycophorin A has a molecular weight of 36 kd and contains 131 aa.[20] The hydrophilic NH$_2$ terminal end, which lies outside the red cell membrane, has 72 aa residues, 15 *O*-glycosidically linked oligosaccharide chains (GalNAc-serine/threonine), and 1 *N*-glycosidic chain (sugar-asparagine). The portion that traverses the membrane is hydrophobic and contains 23 aa.[12] The hydrophilic COOH end of the peptide chain, which contains 36 aa and no carbohydrates, lies inside the membrane and interacts weakly with the membrane cytoskeleton. MN antigens differ in their aa residue at positions 1 and 5 (see Figure 8–1): M has a serine and glycine at these positions, whereas N has leucine and glutamic acid.

The Ss-SGP or GPB has a molecular weight of 20 kd and contains 72 aa and 11 *O*-linked oligosaccharide chains.[20] It has an outer glycosylated portion of 43 aa and a hydrophobic portion of 24 aa that traverses the red cell membrane. The small remaining "tail" may become embedded in the lipid layer or may rest at the surface of the cytoplasmic compartment.

Because the first 26 aa on GPA are identical to those on GPB, cells truly negative for N were not found, and researchers thought perhaps N was a precursor to M. We now call the *N*-like structure on GPB 'N' and recognize that it can react with some anti-N. Other similarities between GPA and GPB exist: GPB residues 27 to 35 and 46 to 71 are almost identical to GPA residues 59 to 67 and 75 to 100, respectively. However, the middle portion of GPB has no counterpart on GPA, and GPB carries no *N*-linked carbohydrate chain on aa26.

Most *O*-linked carbohydrate structures on GPA and GPB are branched tetrasaccharides containing one GalNAc, one Gal, and two NeuNAc (sialic acid). Heterogeneity does occur within these chains—they can lack a sugar or have sugar substitutions—but their significant feature is NeuNAc, which helps give the red cell its negative charge. About 70 percent of a red cell's NeuNAc is carried on GPA, and about 16 percent is carried by GPB.[15]

Other antigens within the MNSs system have been evaluated biochemically (see Table 8–3). Some have altered GPA because of aa substitutions and/or changes in carbohydrate chains. Others appear to be variants of GPB. Still others are hybrids of both GPA and GPB, probably arising from gene crossover during meiosis. Such hybrid structures can have the outer $NH_2$ portion of GPA attached to the inner COOH end of GPB or vice versa. This results in changes in glycosylation, changes in molecular weight, loss of high-frequency antigens, the appearance of novel low-frequency antigens, and alterations in the expression of MNSs antigens.[12,15]

Both GPA and GPB can exist in dimeric form in the red cell membrane. Whereas GPB appears to complex with Rh protein, GPA associates with protein band 3. The area of association between GPA or GPB with these other structures may give rise to additional antigen specificities.

The heterogeneity of GPA and GPB leads to speculation about their physiologic function. Red cells that lack GPA and/or GPB are not associated with disease or decreased survival. Perhaps these glycoproteins and their negative charge prevent red cells from adhering to each other or to vessel walls. Perhaps the water attracted to their carbohydrates helps protect red cells from damage during circulation.[1] They may also play a role in the translocation of band 3 protein (an anion transporter) to the surface of the red cell membrane.[2]

### Genetics

The genes *GYPA* and *GYPB*, which code for GPA and GPB, represent two closely linked loci on chromosome 4 (4p28-q31). The known alleles for *GPA (M/N)* and *GPB (S/s)* are codominant. Because of their many similarities and primate antigen studies, some suggest that *GPB* arose from a duplication of an ancestral *GPA* gene and that the other alleles arose by further mutations.[1,20] The most common gene complex is *Ns*, followed by *Ms, MS,* then *NS*.

*GYPA* is organized into seven exons (portions that are translated into functional protein—the unused portions or introns are spliced out): A1 encodes for a leader protein that helps insert the structure into the membrane during formation; A2 encodes the first 26 aa; A3 has inverted repeat sequences known to be sites for DNA recombination; A4 encoded the remaining extracellular portion; A5, the transmembrane protein; A6 and A7, the cytoplasmic portion. A7 also contains the stop code.[20]

*GYPB* has a similar size and arrangement to *GYPA* but only five exons: B1 and B2, which are nearly identical to A1 and A2, encode a leader protein and aa 1 through 26; B3 is analogous to A4, encoding the portion of the molecule that carries Ss; B4, similar to A5, encodes a larger transmembrane portion because of a mutation that affects an mRNA splice site; B5 encodes the cytoplasmic portion and final stop code. There is no counterpart to A3 because of another splice site mutation, nor is there an A6 or A7 counterpart.

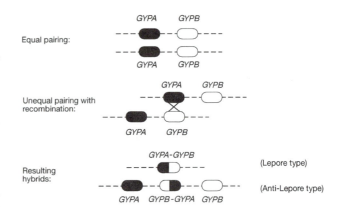

**Figure 8–2.** How unequal pairing and recombination during meiosis can lead to *GYPA–GYPB* hybrids.

Once the genetic complexity of *GYPA* and *GYPB* is understood, it is easy to account for the variant alleles. There may be point mutations, deletions, and unequal pairing during meiosis with subsequent recombination (Fig. 8–2), resulting in hybrids. A *GYPA-GYPB* hybrid (called Lepore type for a similar hemoglobin hybrid) encodes only altered structures that contain the beginning $NH_2$ end of GPA and the COOH end of GPB. A *GYPB-GYPA* hybrid (called anti-Lepore type) encodes normal GPA, normal GPB, and a hybrid structure that contains the $NH_2$ end of GPB and the COOH end of GPA.[2,20]

### M and N Lectins

A number of plant lectins have proved useful in studying GPA biochemistry, some with practical application.[1,21] Those having N reactivity include *Bauhinia variegata, B. candicans, B. bonatiana, B. purpura,* and *Vicia graminea. Vicia graminea* lectin is not commonly used. It reaches with the O-linked tetrasaccharides near the $NH_2$ end of both M-SGP and N-SGP, but when properly diluted it will appear to react only with N-SGP and so makes an appropriate typing reagent.[1]

Anti-M reactivity has been found in seeds from the plants *Iberis amara, I. umbellate, I. semperivens,* and the Japanese turnip. *Maclura aurantiaca,* made from the Osage orange, reacts with the tetrasaccharides on both M-SGP and N-SGP and has been used to screen for rare red cells lacking MN-SGP.[21]

When antigen typing red cells with lectins, one must keep in mind that only specific carbohydrate structures are recognized by these reagents. Results may not parallel those obtained with human antibody or other lectins, especially when altered or variant SGPs are tested.

### Null Phenotypes

**U Negative Phenotype.** The U (for *universal*) antigen is located on GPB very close to the red cell membrane between aa 33 and 39, and its expression may be influenced by nearby membrane structures, possibly the Rh glycoprotein.[12] This high-frequency antigen is found in all individuals except about 1 percent of American blacks (and 1 to 35 percent of African blacks),[20] who lack GPB because of a partial or complete deletion of *GYPB*. They usually type S−s−U− and make anti-U in response to transfusion or pregnancy.

Some examples of anti-U react with apparent U− red cells, although weakly, by absorption and elution.[15] Such cells are said to be U variant. It is thought that "true" U− individuals lack *GPB*, whereas U variants may lack only a portion of *GPB* or have a mutation that results in a quantitative and qualitative alteration in expression. There is a strong correlation between the antigen He and U variant expression.[2] Red cells that lack Rh protein on the red cell membrane have less GPB, hence Rh$_{null}$ and Rh$_{mod}$ individuals may also appear U−. Nevertheless, U is present and can be confirmed with absorption-elution studies.

Because U antibodies are heterogeneous, U− units selected for transfusion must be crossmatched using the patient's antibody. Simply knowing the unit types U− does not guarantee compatibility, nor does an antiglobulin crossmatch if expression is very weak. Some patients may tolerate U variant units; others may not. If the patient is U− and N−, the antibody may actually have N and U specificity, making the search for compatible blood even more difficult.

**En$^a$ Negative Phenotype.** In 1969, Darnborough and associates[22] and Furuhjelm and coworkers[23] described an antibody to the same high-frequency antigen, called En$^a$ (for *envelope*), which reacted with all cells except those of the propositi. Both En(a−) individuals appeared to be M−N− with reduced NeuNAc on their red cells, but both had normal Ss expression.

Although the gene responsible for this phenotype has been termed *En*, it is now known that the Finnish En(a−) individuals lacked GPA because of a complete or nearly complete deletion of *GYPA*, whereas the English En(a−) individuals had a Lepore type *GYPA-GYPB* hybrid gene that encodes a small amount of M, designated 'M', and S.

Most En(a−) adults produce anti-En$^a$, which defines portions of GPA unrelated to M or N, but not all antibodies detect the same portion. Anti-En$^a$ TS recognizes a trypsin-sensitive (TS) area on GPA between aa 20 and 39. Anti-En$^a$ FS reacts with a ficin-sensitive (FS) area between aa 46 and 56, and anti-En$^a$ FR reacts with a ficin-resistant (FR) area around aa 62 to 72.[2]

**M$^k$ Phenotype.** The rare silent gene *M$^k$* was identified in 1964 by Metaxas and Metaxas-Buhler[24] in the heterozygous state when they studied an M−N+ (*NM$^k$*) mother who had an M+N− (*MM$^k$*) child. The red cells of these rare individuals expressed half the amount of normal MN and Ss on SDS-PAGE analysis. In 1979, Tokunaga and associates[25] reported finding two related homozygous MkMk blood donors in Japan. These null individuals typed M−N−S−s−U− but had a normal hematologic picture. More individuals have since been identified, and it is now known that the *M$^k$* gene represents a single, near-complete deletion of both *GYPA* and *GYPB*.[20] The *M$^k$M$^k$* genotype is associated with increased glycosylation and, consequently, increased relative mass of red cell membrane bands 3 and 4.1 but a decreased size in the glucose transporter.

### The Miltenberger Series

The Miltenberger series was developed to explain the relationship of several low-frequency antigens in the MNS blood group system. They appeared to be related to one another because red cells containing one of these antigens often had more than one, which would be statistically unlikely if they were genetically independent.

After the first five antigens were defined, Cleghorn performed a series of cross tests with their respective antibodies and separated the red cells into five phenotypes: Mi$^I$, Mi$^{II}$, Mi$^{III}$, M$^{IV}$, and Mi$^V$.[26] These phenotypes have been redefined and expanded to 11 with the discovery of additional antigens (Table 8–4).[2,4]

**Table 8–4.** The Miltenberger Series

| Current Class | Proposed # Terminology | Antigens | | | | | | | | | | Biochemistry* | |
|---|---|---|---|---|---|---|---|---|---|---|---|---|---|
| | | Vw | Mur | Hil | Hut | Hop | Nob | DANE | MUT | TSEN | MINY | | |
| Mi.I | GP.Vw | + | 0 | 0 | 0 | 0 | 0 | 0 | 0 | 0 | 0 | GP ABA | aa28 Thr→Ser |
| Mi.II | GP.Hut | 0 | 0 | 0 | + | 0 | 0 | 0 | + | 0 | 0 | GP ABA | aa28 Thr→Lys |
| Mi.III | GP.Mur | 0 | + | + | 0 | 0 | 0 | 0 | + | 0 | + | GP BAB | |
| Mi.IV | GP.Hop | 0 | + | 0 | 0 | 0 | 0 | 0 | + | + | + | GP BAB | |
| Mi.V | GP.Hil | 0 | 0 | + | 0 | 0 | 0 | 0 | 0 | 0 | + | GP AB | |
| Mi.VI | GP.Bun | 0 | + | + | 0 | + | 0 | 0 | + | 0 | + | GP BAB | |
| Mi.VII | GP.Nob | 0 | 0 | 0 | 0 | 0 | + | 0 | 0 | 0 | 0 | GP ABA | aa49 Arg→Thr aa52 Thr→Ser |
| Mi.VIII | GP.Joh | 0 | 0 | 0 | 0 | + | + | 0 | 0 | NT | 0 | GP ABA | |
| Mi.IX | GP.Dane | 0 | + | 0 | 0 | 0 | 0 | + | 0 | 0 | 0 | GP ABA | |
| Mi.X | GP.HF | 0 | 0 | + | 0 | 0 | 0 | 0 | + | 0 | + | GP BAB | |
| Mi.XI | GP.JL | 0 | 0 | 0 | 0 | 0 | 0 | 0 | NT | + | + | GP AB$^s$ | |

**Source:** Reid, MD, and Lomas-Francis, C: The Blood Group Antigen Facts Book. Academic Press, New York, 1997.
NT = not tested.

Biochemical and molecular studies have simplified our understanding of the Miltenberger series. Each phenotype represents a distinct variant GPA or hybrid molecule. Tippett and colleagues[27] proposed that the Miltenberger terminology be dropped in favor of one that recognized the glycoprotein variant and the name of the first propositus. Many other variant MN glycoproteins associated with the Miltenberger phenotypes are described elsewhere.[2,4,27]

### Other Antibodies in the MNSs System

Antibodies to antigens other than M, N, S, and s are rarely encountered and can usually be grouped into two categories: those directed against low-frequency antigens and those directed against high-frequency antigens.

Antibodies to high-frequency antigens are easily detected with antibody screening cells. Antibodies to low-frequency antigens are rarely detected by the antibody screen but are seen as an unexpected incompatible crossmatch or an unexplained case of HDN. Few hospital blood banks have the test cells available to identify the specificity, but enzyme reactivity and MNSs antigen typings may offer clues.

It is common practice with these antibodies to transfuse units that are crossmatch-compatible at 37°C and in the antiglobulin phase—an easy task if the antigen frequency is low but quite difficult if it is high. Typing sera for other MNSs specificities are not generally available, so the antigen status of compatible red cells can seldom be confirmed.

### Autoantibodies

Autoantibodies to M and N have been reported.[1] Autoantibodies to U and En[a] are more common and may be associated with warm-type autoimmune hemolytic anemia.

Not all examples of anti-M in M+ individuals or anti-N in N+ individuals are autoantibodies. Many fail to react with the patient's own cells. It may be that these individuals have altered GPA and that their antibody is specific for a portion of the common antigen they lack.

### Disease Associations

As already mentioned, GPA may serve as the receptor by which certain pyelonephritogenic strains of *E. coli* gain entry to the urinary tract.

The malaria parasite *Plasmodium falciparum* may use sites associated with the glycophorins, or the NeuNAc attached to glycophorins, or both, for cell invasion. In an attempt to identify the receptor, its invasion rate into cells with normal and rare phenotypes has been studied. Reduced invasion is seen with En(a−) cells, U− cells, $M^kM^k$ cells, Tn and Cad cells (which have altered oligosaccharides on glycophorins), Ge− cells, and normal cells treated with neuraminidase and trypsin.[28] The extent to which GPA and GPB are involved is unclear,

but it appears that NeuNAc on *O*-linked oligosaccharides is critical to the invasion process.

## THE P (003) AND P^k (209) BLOOD GROUP SYSTEMS

The P blood group system was introduced in 1927 by Landsteiner and Levine.[7] In their search for new antigens, they injected rabbits with human red cells and produced an antibody, initially called anti-P, that divided human red cells into two groups: P+ and P−.

In 1959, Levine and associates[29] described anti-Tj[a] (now known as anti-PP$_1$P[k]), an antibody to a high-frequency antigen that Sanger[30] later related to the P system. Because it defined an antigen common to P+ and P− cells and was made by an apparent P null individual, the original antigen and phenotypes were renamed. Anti-P became anti-P$_1$; the P+ phenotype became P$_1$; the P− phenotype became P$_2$; and the rare P null individual became known as p.

The P blood group became more complex in 1959, when Matson and coworkers[31] described the P[k] phenotype. These rare individuals lack an antigen, P, which is common to all red cells except those with the phenotype p or P[k]. In its place is another high-frequency antigen, P[k], one not commonly seen on red cells but one that is well expressed on all fibroblasts except those from p individuals. The puzzling association of P and P[k] was not truly understood until the biosynthetic pathway became known.

This knowledge has prompted the ISBT to divide the antigens into both a blood group system and an associated antigen "collection." The antigen P$_1$ is assigned to the P blood group system (designated P1 or 003) and given the number 003.001. The antigens P, P[k], and Luke are assigned to the globoside collection of antigens (209) and are given the numbers 209.001, 209.002, and 209.003; p antigen has not yet been assigned. To simplify terminology for the reader, this section will refer to all the antigens as P system antigens.

The antigens and phenotypes associated with the P system are summarized in Table 8–5. The P$_1$ and P$_2$ phenotypes are analogous to A$_1$ and A$_2$ in the ABO system. The antibodies generally fall into two categories: clinically insignificant or potently hemolytic.

### Basic Concepts

The P system antigens are biochemically related to the carbohydrate chains that make up the ABH and I antigens. P$_1$, P, or P[k] may be found on red cells, platelets, leukocytes, tissue fibroblasts, smooth muscle of the digestive tract, and uroepithelial cells; P and P[k] have also been found in plasma as glycosphingolipids. The antigens have not been identified in secretions.[5] Red cells carry approximately $14 \times 10^6$ copies of globoside, the P and P[k] structure, per adult red cell and about $5 \times 10^5$ copies of P$_1$.[12] The antigen P[k] is also known as CD77.

**Table 8–5.** P System Phenotypes, Antigens, and Antibodies

| Phenotype | Detectable Antigens* | Possible Antibodies† | Frequency | |
|---|---|---|---|---|
| | | | Whites | Blacks |
| $P_1$ | $P_1$, P | — | 79% | 94% |
| $P_2$ | P | Anti-$P_1$ | 21% | 6% |
| p | — | Anti-PP$_1$P$^k$ | Rare | Rare |
| $P_1{}^k$ | $P_1$, P$^k$ | Anti-P | Very rare | Very rare |
| $P_2{}^k$ | P$^k$ | Anti-P, Anti-$P_1$ | Most rare | Most rare |

*Antigens: $P_1$ poorly developed at birth; combined frequency of rare phenotypes 10:1,000,000.
†Antibodies: Anti-$P_1$; Usually clinically insignificant. Anti-PP$_1$P$^k$. Hemolytic; associated with early abortion. Anti-P: Hemolytic; associated Donath-Landsteiner antibody and early abortion. Reactivity enhanced by enzymes.

## The $P_1$ Antigen

The expression of $P_1$ changes during fetal development. The antigen is found on fetal red cells as early as 12 weeks, but it weakens with gestational age: Ikin and colleagues[32] found that young fetuses were more frequently and more strongly $P_1$+ than older fetuses. The antigen is poorly expressed at birth and may take up to 7 years to be fully expressed.[33]

Antigen strength in adults varies from one individual to another, a fact first noted by Landsteiner and Levine,[7] who found that some $P_1$+ people were $P_1$ strong and others were $P_1$ weak. These differences appear to be quantitative, not qualitative, and may either be genetically controlled or represent homozygous versus heterozygous inheritance of the gene making $P_1$. The strength of $P_1$ also can vary with race. Blacks have a stronger expression of $P_1$ than whites. The rare dominant gene *In(Lu)*, discussed in the Lutheran section, inhibits the expression of $P_1$ so that $P_1$ individuals who inherit it may serologically type as $P_1$-negative.

The $P_1$ antigen deteriorates rapidly on storage. When old cells are typed or used as controls for typing reagents, or when older cells are used to detect anti-$P_1$ in serum, false-negative reactions may result.

## Anti-$P_1$

Anti-$P_1$ is a common, naturally occurring IgM antibody in the sera of $P_2$ individuals. It is usually a weak, cold-reactive saline agglutinin not seen in routine testing. Stronger examples react at room temperature or bind complement, which is detected in the antiglobulin test when polyspecific reagents are used. Antibody activity can be neutralized or inhibited with soluble $P_1$ substance or bypassed using prewarmed test methods.

Because $P_1$ antigen expression on red cells varies and deteriorates during storage, antibodies may react only with cells having the strongest expression and give inconclusive patterns of reactivity when panel identification is performed. Laboratory staff members can incu-

bate tests in the cold or pretreat test cells with enzymes to enhance reactions and to confirm specificity, but most repeat the tests using prewarmed methods instead. If activity is no longer seen, the antibody may be considered clinically insignificant, and specificity need not be identified.

Providing units that are crossmatch-compatible at 37°C and the antiglobulin phase, regardless of their $P_1$ status, is an acceptable approach to transfusion. Giving $P_1$+ units under these circumstances does not cause a rise in antibody titer or a change in its thermal range of reactivity.[5]

Rare examples of $P_1$ antibodies that react at 37°C can cause in vivo red cell destruction; both immediate and delayed hemolytic transfusion reactions have been reported.[5] These rare antibodies react well in the antiglobulin phase, bind complement, and may lyse test cells, especially if they are enzyme-treated. Although it is tempting to assume that such antibodies are IgG, many have been identified as IgM; IgG forms are rare. Hemolytic disease of the newborn is not associated with anti-$P_1$, presumably because the antibody is usually IgM in nature and the antigen is so poorly developed on fetal cells.

## Advanced Concepts

### Biochemistry

The antigens of the P system exist as glycosphingolipids and glycoproteins. As with ABH, the antigens are immunodominant sugars added sequentially to a precursor structure. Biochemical analyses have shown that the structures carrying P determinants also carry I and ABH antigens. However, the genes of the P system act first, hence their antigens are closer to the membrane than A, B, H, or I. Also as with ABH, P system antigens are resistant to enzyme, DTT, chloroquine, or acid degradation.

A simplified biosynthetic pathway of the P$^k$, P, and Luke antigens is given in Figure 8–3.[4] Ceramide dihexose (CDH), also called lactosylceramide, is a glycolipid precursor that can be acted upon by several different sugar transferases. The addition of galactose in an α1–4 linkage makes ceramide trihexose (CTH) or P$^k$ antigen. With another sugar addition, the P$^k$ structure becomes globoside, or the P antigen. This explains why the high-frequency antigen P$^k$ is not readily apparent on red cells; the P sugar makes P$^k$ less accessible to react with its antibody. In sheep, globoside becomes the precursor for the Forssman antigen; in humans it is the precursor for the LKE or Luke antigen.

In an alternative biosynthetic pathway, CDH can acquire two more sugars and become paragloboside, a precursor for the $P_1$ antigen (the p antigen, which will be discussed later) and Ii and ABH antigens.[4]

### Genetics

The problem with the biosynthetic pathway was finding a genetic model that fits serologic data. Both

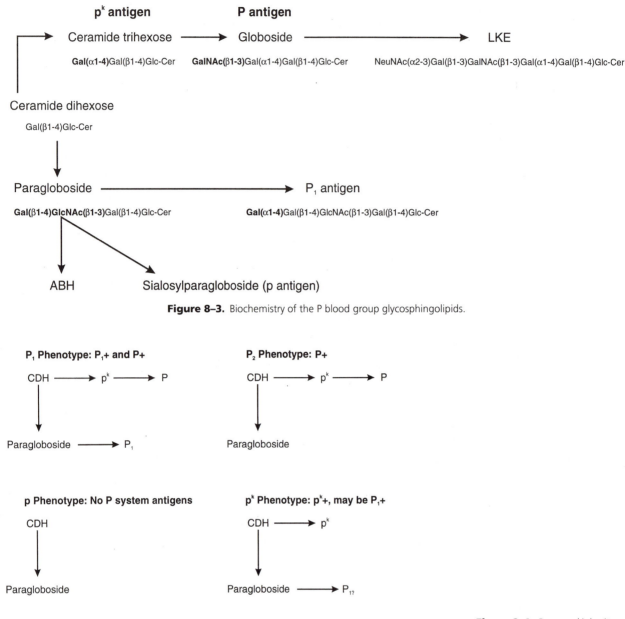

**Figure 8–3.** Biochemistry of the P blood group glycosphingolipids.

**Figure 8–4.** Proposed inheritance P blood group antigens.

CDH = Ceramide Dihexose

two- and three-gene models have been proposed.[34] The current blood system assignment of $P_1$ antigen to a paragloboside system and Pk and P to a globoside system favors a three-gene model: each gene makes a transferase, which adds the appropriate sugar to the appropriate precursor. Each gene may have more than one allele: a common allele that encodes the transferase and a less common one that does not.

The final P phenotype of an individual depends on the alleles inherited at all loci, as illustrated in Figure 8–4. P nulls (p phenotype) make no P system antigens; such individuals are very rare—5.8 in a million. P nulls are slightly more common in Japan, North Sweden, and in an Amish group in Ohio.[1] Individuals

with the $P^k$ phenotype may express $P_1$ antigen, depending on their alleles at the $P$ locus. Data suggest that the gene coding for $P_1$ is located on chromosome 22(q11.2-qter).[12]

## Other Sources of $P_1$ Antigen and Antibody

The discovery of strong anti-$P_1$ in two $P_2$ individuals infected with *Echinococcus granulosus* tapeworms led to the identification of $P_1$ and $P^k$ substance in hydatid cyst fluid.[35] This fluid was subsequently used in many of the studies that identified the biochemical structure of P system antigens.

A $P_1$-like antigen has also been found in the red cells,

plasma, and droppings of pigeons and turtledoves, as well as in the egg white of turtledoves. Exposure to these birds may place $P_2$ bird handlers at risk of making strong, clinically significant anti-$P_1$. The $P_1$ antigen in bird droppings may be attributed to certain gram-negative avian bacteria rather than to the birds themselves.[36]

Strong antibodies to $P_1$ also have been associated with fascioliasis (bovine liver fluke disease), *Clonorchis sinensis*, and *Opisthorchis viverrini* infections. $P_1$ substance has been identified in extracts of *Lumbricoides terrestris* (the common earthworm) and *Ascaris suum*.[2]

Soluble $P_1$ substances have potential use in the blood bank and are commercially available. When it is necessary to confirm antibody specificity or to identify underlying antibodies, these substances can be used to neutralize anti-$P_1$ if prewarmed methods do not eliminate reactivity.

Antibody-like substances, similar to plant lectins, also have been reported. Extracts of salmon and trout roe contain activity for $P_1$, $P^k$, and B antigen. Serum from the snake *Python sebae* contains an anti-P activity detected with enzyme-treated red cells.

## Anti-PP₁Pᵏ

Originally called Tj$^a$, this antibody was first described in the serum of Mrs. Jay, a p individual with adenocarcinoma of the stomach.[29] Her tumor cells carried P system antigens, and the antibody was credited as having cytotoxic properties that may have helped prevent metastatic growth postsurgery (the T in the Tj$^a$ refers to *tumor*).

Anti-PP$_1$P$^k$ is produced by all p individuals early in life without red cell sensitization and reacts with all red cells except those of other P nulls. Unlike systemwide reactive antibodies made by other blood group nulls, most examples are a mixture of separable anti-P, anti-$P_1$, and anti-$P^k$. The antibodies are predominantly IgM, sometimes IgG. They react over a wide thermal range and efficiently bind complement, which makes them potent hemolysins. Anti-PP$_1$P$^k$ has the potential to cause severe hemolytic transfusion reactions and hemolytic disease of the newborn.

The antibody is also associated with spontaneous abortions in early pregnancy. Although the reason for this is not fully known, it has been suggested that having an IgG anti-P component is an important factor.[37] Women with such antibodies and a history of multiple abortions have successfully delivered infants after being plasmapheresed to reduce their antibody level during pregnancy.[38]

Vos and coworkers[39] described an unusual Tj$^a$-like autoantibody in the serum of habitual aborters found transiently only during pregnancy and only in Australia. The antibody did not agglutinate cells or react in an antiglobulin test; it was detected only by its hemolysis. This activity was not complement-dependent, although it was destroyed by heat and may reflect some Australian environmental factor.

## Anti-P

In addition to being an antibody component in p individuals (see above), anti-P is found as a naturally occurring alloantibody in the sera of all $P^k$ individuals. Its reactivity is similar to anti-PP$_1$P$^k$ in that it is usually a potent hemolysin reacting with all cells except the autocontrol and those with a $P_{null}$ phenotype. However, it differs from anti-PP$_1$P$^k$ in that it does not react with cells having the extremely rare $P^k$ phenotype and the individual making the antibody may type $P_1+$.

Alloanti-P is rarely seen in the blood bank, but because it is hemolytic with a wide thermal range of reactivity, it is very significant in transfusion. IgG fractions may occur and have been associated with habitual early abortion.

Anti-P specificity is also associated with the cold reactive IgG autoantibody in patients with paroxysmal cold hemoglobinuria (PCH). This autoimmune disorder is seen transiently in children following viral infections and in tertiary syphilis. Antibody activity is biphasic. It attaches to red cells in the cold and lyses them as they warm. The autoantibody reacts only weakly or not at all in routine test systems. Its true hemolytic nature is best demonstrated by the Donath-Landsteiner test. The etiology and diagnosis of PCH are more fully discussed in Chapter 21.

## Anti-Pᵏ

This antibody has been isolated from some examples of anti-PP$_1$P$^k$ by selective adsorption with $P_1$ cells, and it has been reported in the serum of $P_1$ individuals with biliary cirrhosis and autoimmune hemolytic anemia.[2] A murine monoclonal antibody having $P^k$ specificity now exits. Anti-$P^k$ activity can be inhibited with hydatid cyst fluid.

## Antibodies to Compound Antigens

Considering the biochemical relationship of the P system antigens to ABH and I, it is not surprising that antibodies requiring more than one antigenic determinant have been described, including IP$_1$, iP$_1$, I$^T$P$_1$, and IP. Most examples are cold-reactive agglutinins.

## Luke (LKE) Antigen and Antibody

In 1965, Tippett and associates[40] described an antibody in the serum of a patient with Hodgkin's lymphoma that divided the population into three phenotypes: 84 percent tested Luke+, 14 percent were weakly positive or Luke(w), and 2 percent were Luke−. Although this mendelian dominant gene segregated independently of the P system, it was thought to be phenotypically related because the antibody reacted with all cells except 2 percent of $P_1$ and $P_2$ phenotypes and those having the rare p and $P^k$ phenotypes. All individuals with the p and $P^k$ phenotype are Luke−. Using the original antibody, the Luke(w) phenotype was more commonly found with $P_2$ than $P_1$ and more common with $A_1$ and $A_1B$ than with $A_2$, B, or O phenotypes, although subsequent examples did not parallel these findings.

Only four human antibodies have been described. The original was a saline agglutinin that reacted best at 4°C. Using enzyme methods and additional complement, it became a potent hemolysin. The other examples were much weaker and clinically insignificant.

Luke's association with the P system was clarified, thanks to a murine monoclonal antibody directed against a stage-specific embryonic mouse antigen called SSEA-4. Tippett and associates discovered the similarity between this antigen and Luke, and the antibody was renamed LKE for Luke erythrocyte antigen.[41] Anti-LKE is inhibited by NeuNAc($\alpha$2-3)Gal($\beta$1-3)GalNAc-, the structural equivalent of globoside (P antigen) with galactose and neuraminic acid attached. The rarity of human antibody makes monoclonal anti-LKE a truly important tool.

### The p Antigen and Antibody

In 1972, Engelfriet and associates[42] described a transient antibody in the serum of a $P_1$ individual that reacted best with p red cells, less well with $P_2$, and weakest with $P_1$ cells. Because of this pattern of reactivity, it was called anti-p. The antigen it detects is sialosylparagloboside—that is, paragloboside with NeuNAc (sialic acid) attached. This oligosaccharide is present in great quantity on p cells but is neither a precursor to P system antigens nor genotypically related.

Only a few examples of anti-p have been reported. They react preferentially with p red cells either at 4°C or at the antiglobulin phase. Reactions can be inhibited with sialosylparagloboside. Anti-p reactivity is destroyed with neuraminidase but enhanced with papain.

### Disease Associations

Several diseases with pathologic conditions associated with the P system have been described here: parasitic infections are associated with anti-$P_1$, early abortions with anti-PP$_1$P$^k$ or anti-P, and PCH with anti-P.

The antigens may also be associated with urinary tract infections. Some pyelonephritogenic strains of *Escherichia coli* ascend the urinary tract in ladderlike fashion by adhering to $P_1$ and/or P$^k$ glycolipids on uroepithelial cells. The fimbriae or pili of such organisms have receptor sites for structures involving Gal($\alpha$1-4)Gal($\beta$1-4), the terminal sugars for $P_1$ and P$^k$. This supports the findings of Lomberg and associates,[43] who found more urinary infections in young girls who were $P_1$+ than in those who were $P_1$−. It has also been shown that persons with the p phenotype are not susceptible to acute pyelonephritis associated with *E. coli*. However, specific receptor molecules may vary or be influenced by other factors because Mullholland and coworkers[44] found more infections in a $P_1$− postmenopausal group.

Other globoside associations have been identified with infection. *Streptococcus suis*, which occasionally causes meningitis and septicemia in humans, binds exclusively to P$_k$ antigen. A class of toxins secreted by *Shigella dysenteriae, Vibrio cholerae, V. parahaemolyticus,* and some pathogenic strains of *E. coli* also has binding specificity for a Gal($\alpha$1-4)Gal($\beta$1-4) moiety. In addition, globoside is the receptor of human parvovirus B19.[4]

## THE I (207) BLOOD GROUP COLLECTION

The existence of cold agglutinins in the serum of people with acquired hemolytic anemia has long been recognized. In 1956, Wiener and associates[45] gave a name to one such agglutinin, calling its antigen "I" for *individuality*. The antibody reacted with all but 5 of 22,000 blood specimens tested (i.e., most were I+). The nonreactive I− specimens were thought to be homozygous for a rare gene producing the "i" antigen. Many cold autoagglutinins were found to have I specificity. In 1960, Marsh and Jenkins[46] reported finding anti-i, and the unique relationship between I and i began to unfold.

Because I and i are not discrete antithetical antigens produced by allelic genes, they are classified not as a system but rather as a "collection" of blood group antigens that has been given the numeric designation 207 by the ISBT.[2] I is assigned the number 207.001 and i is assigned 207.002. Both represent common related structures defined by a heterogeneous collection of autoantibodies.

### Basic Concepts

#### The Ii Antigens

The antigens are best introduced by classic serologic facts. Both I and i are high-frequency antigens expressed in a wide range of strengths that are inversely proportional to one another. At birth, infant red cells are rich in i; I is almost undetectable. During the first 18 months of life, the quantity of i slowly decreases as I increases until adult proportions are reached; adult red cells are rich in I and have only trace amount of i antigen.

The number of I copies per adult red cell is about 5 $\times$ 10$^5$, but a wide normal range of reactivity can be observed with both anti-I and anti-i.[5] Data suggest that a red cell's i reactivity is inversely proportional to marrow transit time and red cell age in circulation.

Some people appear not to change their i status after birth. They become the rare i adult, or "I" negative phenotype. Two i adult phenotypes have been reported:[46,47] $i_1$ has the least amount of I antigen and is found in whites; $i_2$ has slightly more I antigen and is associated with blacks. A spectrum of Ii phenotypes and their characteristics are listed in Table 8–6.

**Table 8–6.** Ii Phenotypes and Key Facts*

| Phenotype | I Antigen Content | i Antigen Content | Frequency |
|---|---|---|---|
| I | Strong | Weakest | Common in adults |
| I$_{int}$ | Intermediate | Intermediate | Rare in adults (?heterozygote) |
| i Cord | Weak | Strong | Common in newborn infants |
| i$_2$ | Weaker | Stronger | 1:10,000 black adults |
| i$_1$ | Weakest | Strongest | <1:10,000 white adults |

*Antigens: Infants are born with i antigen. I normally developing by 18 months of age. I activity based on ABH precursor branching.
Antibodies: Anti-I: Common cold reactive autoantibody; associated with *Mycoplasma pneumoniae*. Anti-i: Rare autoantibody; associated with infectious mononucleosis. Reactivity enhanced by enzymes.

## Anti-I

Anti-I is a common autoantibody that can be benign or pathologic.[1,48] Consistently strong reactions with adult cells and weak reactions with cord cells define its classic activity but are no guarantee of its specificity. Cord cells have weak expression of other antigens, and additional testing may be needed to confirm or to rule out these specificities. For example, the high-frequency antibody anti-Yt$^a$ may mimic anti-I but should not cause a positive autocontrol, and anti-I typically does. Common reactivity patterns are in Table 8–7.

Benign anti-I, found in the serum of many normal healthy individuals, is not associated with in vivo red cell destruction. It is usually a weak, naturally occurring, saline-reactive IgM agglutinin that goes undetected in routine testing because it usually reacts only at 4°C. Stronger examples agglutinate test cells at room temperature and/or bind complement, which can be detected in the antiglobulin test if polyspecific reagents are used. Some may react only with the strongest I+ cells and give inconsistent panel reactions.

Although incubating tests in the cold enhances anti-I reactivity and helps confirm its identity, many blood bankers prefer to repeat tests using prewarmed methods. If the weak reactions disappear, they are clinically insignificant and can be ignored. If identification is necessary, albumin and enzyme methods also enhance anti-I reactivity. Using enzymes with slightly acidified serum may even promote hemolysis. Thimerosol-dependent autoanti-I, seen only when the preservative thimerosol is present in the test system, has also been reported.[49]

Pathologic antibodies are more potent IgM agglutinins with higher titers and a broader thermal range of activity, that is, reacting up to 30 or 32°C. When peripheral circulation cools in response to low ambient temperatures, these antibodies attach in vivo and cause autoagglutination and vascular occlusion (Raynaud's phenomenon) or intravascular hemolysis. Refer to the chapter on autoimmune hemolytic anemias for more information.

Strong examples of anti-I can react with adult and cord cells equally well, and antibody specificity may not be apparent unless the serum is diluted or warmed to 37°C. Potent cold autoantibodies can also mask clinically significant underlying alloantibodies and complicate transfusions. Procedures to deal with these problems are discussed in other chapters. When a patient with pathologic autoanti-I must be transfused, use of a blood warmer is advised, especially when fast infusion rates are required. Blood warmers are not needed with weaker benign examples of anti-I or with slow infusion rates.

The production of autoanti-I may be stimulated by microorganisms carrying I-like antigen on their surface. Patients with *Mycoplasma pneumoniae* often develop strong cold agglutinins with I specificity as a cross-reactive response to mycoplasma antigen[50] and can experience a transient episode of acute abrupt hemolysis just as the infection begins to resolve. A *Listeria monocytogenes* organism from a patient with cold autoimmune hemolytic anemia has been reported to absorb anti-I and stimulate its production in rabbits.

Anti-I also exists as an IgM or IgG alloantibody in the serum of most i adults. It has been traditional to transfuse compatible i units to these people, although such practice may be unnecessary, especially when the antibody is clinically insignificant and not reactive at 37°C. Technologists must be aware that strong autoanti-I can mimic alloanti-I: if enough autoantibody attaches to a patient's red cells, blocking the antigenic sites, they may falsely type I-negative.

Anti-I is not associated with HDN because the antigen is poorly expressed on infant red cells.

**Table 8–7.** Typical Reactions of Some Cold Autoantibodies*

| Antibody | A$_1$ Adult | A$_2$ Adult | B Adult | O Adult | O Cord | A Cord | O$_h$ Adult | O$_i$ Adult |
|---|---|---|---|---|---|---|---|---|
| Anti-I | ++++ | ++++ | ++++ | ++++ | 0/+ | 0/+ | ++++ | (0) |
| Anti-i | 0/+ | 0/+ | 0/+ | 0/+ | ++++ | ++++ | 0/+ | ++++ |
| Anti-H | 0/+ | ++ | +++ | ++++ | +++ | 0/+ | (0) | +++ |
| Anti-IH | 0/+ | ++ | +++ | ++++ | 0/+ | 0/+ | (0) | (0) |
| Anti-IA | ++++ | +++ | 0/+ | 0/+ | 0/+ | 0/+ | (0) | (0) |

*Reactions vary with antibody strength; very potent examples may need to be diluted before specificity can be determined.
0 = negative; + = positive.

CHAPTER 8

## Anti-i

Alloanti-i has never been described. Most autoanti-i are IgM and react best with saline-suspended cells at 4°C. Only very strong autoantibodies are detected in routine testing because standard test cells (except cord cells) have poor i expression. See Table 8–6.

Unlike anti-I, autoanti-i is not seen as a common benign antibody in healthy individuals. Potent examples are associated with infectious mononucleosis (Epstein-Barr virus infections) and diseases of the reticuloendothelial system (e.g., reticuloses, myeloid leukemias, and alcoholic cirrhosis). High-titer autoantibodies with a wide thermal range may contribute to hemolysis, but because i expression is generally weak, they seldom cause significant hemolysis. IgG anti-i has also been described and has been associated with HDN.[51]

## Advanced Concepts

### Biochemistry and Genetics

An early association of Ii to ABH was demonstrated by complex antibodies involving both ABH and Ii specificity (see Antibodies to Compound Antigens, further on). It was also known that I activity increased when ABH sugars were removed with specific enzymes and that adults with the Bombay phenotype ($O_h$) had the greatest amount of I antigen on their cells.[52] Thanks to these observations and work by Feizi, Hakomori, Watanabe, and Kabat (reviewed elsewhere[48,53,54]) we now know that Ii antigens are defined by a series of carbohydrates on the inner portion of ABH oligosaccharide chains.

ABH and Ii determinants on the red cell membrane are carried on precursor structures that attach either to proteins or to lipids. See Figure 8–5 for four glycolipid examples. Little i activity is defined by at least two repeating N-acetyllactosamine [Gal($\beta$1-4)GlcNAc($\beta$1-3)] units in linear form. Branched N-acetyllactosamine units [Gal($\beta$1-4)GlcNAc($\beta$1-6)] are associated with I activity. In the examples given, $H_2$ has i activity, $H_3$ has I activity, and $H_1$ carries no Ii activity because it is too short. $H_4$ is heterogeneous and not well characterized

but has both branched and linear regions. Studies on rabbit cells suggest that the linear regions on $H_4$ may contribute to the expression of i on adult red cells.[48]

In summary, fetal, cord, and adult i red cells predominantly carry unbranched chains and have an i phenotype.[54] Normal adult cells have more branched structures and express I antigen. The gene responsible for I antigen most likely codes for the branching enzyme, $\beta$(1-6)glucosaminyl transferase. Hybridization studies indicate that the gene is located on chromosome 9q21.[2]

Family studies show that the adult i phenotype is recessive. Heterozygous children having one I and one i parent have intermediate I expression. One family in India has a reported I−i− phenotype: 15 of 93 family members had greatly reduced I and i, and 6 had partial depression of both. It may be that they have variant Ii structures that cannot react with common forms of anti-I and anti-i.[1]

### Other Sources of Ii Antigen

Ii antigens are found on the membranes of leukocytes and platelets in addition to red cells. Indeed, some potent Ii antibodies have been shown to be lymphocytotoxic. It is quite likely that the antigens exist on other tissue cells, much like ABH, but this is not confirmed.

I and i have also been found in the plasma and serum of adults and newborns and in saliva, human milk, amniotic fluid, urine, and ovarian cyst fluid. The antigens in secretions do not correlate with red cell expression and are thought to develop under separate genetic control. For example, the quantity of I antigen in the saliva of adult i individuals and newborns is quite high.

Technologists occasionally attempt to neutralize potent examples of anti-I with human milk or saliva to identify underlying alloantibodies. Because so few antibodies will neutralize, this technique is not as helpful as it might appear.

The I antigen has been found on the red cells or body fluids of other animal species, including rabbits, sheep, and cattle.[5] The red cells from most adult primates express i antigen and mimic those from newborn or i adults.

| Ii Activity | H Precursor | Structure |
|---|---|---|
| (none) | $H_1$ | Gal($\beta$1-4)GlcNAc($\beta$1-3)Gal($\beta$1-3)Gal($\beta$1-4)Glc-Cer |
| i | $H_2$ | Gal($\beta$1-4)GlcNAc($\beta$1-3)Gal($\beta$1-4)GlcNAc($\beta$1-3)Gal($\beta$1-4)Glc-Cer |
| I | $H_3$ | Gal($\beta$1-4)GlcNAc($\beta$1-3) \ Gal($\beta$1-4)GlcNAc($\beta$1-3)Gal($\beta$1-4)Glc-Cer / Gal($\beta$1-4)GlcNAc($\beta$1-6) |
| I | $H_4$ | (Highly branched, not well characterized) |

**Figure 8–5.** ABO precursor structures having Ii activity.

### The I^T Antigen and Antibody

In 1965, Curtain and colleagues[55] reported a cold agglutinin in Melanesians that did not demonstrate classical I or i specificity. In 1966, Booth and associates[56] confirmed the antibody's high incidence and carefully described its reactivity. It reacted strongly with cord cells, more weakly with normal adult cells, and most weakly with adult i cells. They concluded that it might represent a transition state of i into I and designated the specificity I^T (T for *transition*). Although the association of this antibody to transitional I has since been questioned, its serologic pattern of reactivity is not in dispute.

Anti-I^T is a common, naturally occurring antibody in several populations: The Melanesians, coastal residents of Papua New Guinea, and the Yanomama Indians in Venezuela. Whether or not it is associated with an organism or parasite in these regions is unknown.

The antibody has also been associated with Hodgkin's lymphoma. Garratty and associates[57] investigated over 50 patients with Hodgkin's disease: three of the four patients in this group with evidence of warm autoimmune-mediated hemolysis demonstrated IgG autoanti-I^T. The antibody has also been reported in a patient with non-Hodgkin's lymphoma and in patients with hemolytic anemia, plus a few with no evidence of hemolysis.[1]

### The Specificities I^D, I^F, I^S

In 1971, Marsh and coworkers,[58] thinking that the I antigen might be a mosaic, proposed two subdeterminants based on serologic differences. I^F (fetal) described the I antigen detected on cord cells that remained constant on all cells, including i adults throughout life. I^D (developed) referred to the I antigen not detected on cord cells but which developed later at the expense of i antigen. Anti-I^D appeared as common benign examples of antibody and could be inhibited with human milk. In contrast, anti-I^F was not inhibited and was seen as the pathologic component in hemolytic antibodies.

The term I^S was used to describe the soluble I antigen in secretions (human milk and saliva). The rare anti-I^S reported in 1975 by Dzierzkowski-Borodej and coworkers[59] was completely inhibited by saliva and IgA colostrum and appeared similar to Marsh's inhibitable I^D antibodies.

Understanding the specificities I^T, I^F, I^D, and I^S is difficult until one considers the complex biochemistry of Ii structures. They might represent different heterogeneous portions of ABH oligosaccharides.

### Antibodies to Compound Antigens

Many other I-related antibodies have been described: IA, IB, IAB, IH, iH, IP_1, I^TP_1, IHLe^b, and iHLe^b. Bearing in mind the close relationship of I to the biochemical structures of ABH, Lewis, and P, one should not be surprised to find antibodies that recognize compound antigens. Such antibodies require all involved antigens to react optimally. Table 8–7 summarizes some common specificities with this collection.

### Disease Associations

Well-known associations between strong autoantibodies and disease or microorganisms have already been discussed: anti-I and *M. pneumoniae*, anti-i and infectious mononucleosis, anti-I^T and Hodgkin's lymphoma. Cold autoantibodies have also been reported in influenza infections, but other associations are rare. Isolated cases include Coxsackie virus type A infection, acute cytomegalovirus infection, relapsing fever, malaria, trypanosomiasis, and bacterial infections.[48]

Diseases can also alter the expression of Ii antigen on cells. Conditions associated with increased i antigen on red cells include those which stress the bone marrow or shorten the marrow maturation time: acute leukemias, hypoplastic anemias, megaloblastic anemias, sideroblastic anemias, hemoglobinopathies, chronic hemolytic anemias, even patients phlebotomized too much and too often. Except in some cases of leukemia, the increase in i on red cells is not usually associated with a decrease in I antigen; the expression of I antigen can appear normal or sometimes enhanced. Reactive lymphocytes in infectious mononucleosis are reported to have increased i antigen. Those from patients with chronic lymphocytic leukemia have less i antigen than normal controls.

Chronic dyserythropoietic anemia type II or hereditary erythroblastic multinuclearity with a positive acidified serum test (HEMPAS) is associated with much greater i activity on red cells than control cord cells. HEMPAS cells are very susceptible to lysis with both anti-i and anti-I, and lysis by anti-I appears to be the result of increased antibody uptake and increased sensitivity to complement.[14]

I antigen may be involved in binding immune complexes consisting of drug and drug antibodies. Immune complexes involving rifampin, nitrofurantoin, dexchlorpheniramine, and thiopental have been associated with binding to I antigens on red cells and subsequent complement activation and hemolysis.[4]

In the Japanese, the gene coding for i is linked to an autosomal recessive gene for congenital cataracts.[2]

## THE KELL (006) BLOOD GROUP SYSTEM

The Kell blood group system is an interesting mix of high-frequency and low-frequency antigens. The first one was discovered in 1946 shortly after the introduction of antiglobulin testing.[54] It was defined by an antibody in the serum of a Mrs. Kellacher, which reacted with the red cells of her newborn infant, her older daughter, her husband, and about 9 percent of the random population. The antigen was called K (Kell). In 1949, Levine and coworkers[60] reported its high-frequency antithetical partner k (Cellano).

Kell remained a two-antigen system until Allen and associates[61,62] described the antithetical antigens Kp^a and Kp^b in 1957 and 1958, respectively. Inheritance patterns and statistics confirmed their relation to the Kell system.

Likewise, Js$^a$, described in 1957 by Giblett,[63] and Js$^b$, described by Walker and associates in 1963,[64] were found to be antithetical and related to the Kell system.

The discovery of the null phenotype in 1957,[65] designated K$_0$, helped associate many other antigens with the Kell system. Antibodies that reacted with all red cells except those with the K$_0$ phenotype recognized high-frequency antigens that are phenotypically related. Some were found to be made by closely linked loci to K/k; for others the genetic status was not clear. These were called para-Kell or Kell-like antigens.

More discoveries followed, including the description of the McLeod phenotype by Allen and colleagues in 1961.[66] This phenotype, with its weakened expression of Kell antigens and pathologic syndrome, brought into focus another antigen, Kx, made by a gene on the X chromosome. Research aimed at understanding the association of Kell and Kx has expanded our knowledge of the system's inheritance and biochemistry.

The 25 antigens now included in the Kell blood group system, designated KEL or 006 by the ISBT, are listed in Table 8–8. The associated antigen Kx is part of the XK system, which carries the numeric designation 019.

## Basic Concepts

Kell blood group antigens are found only on red cells. They have not been found on platelets or on lymphocytes, granulocytes, or monocytes using immunofluorescent flow cytometry.

The K antigen can be detected on fetal cells as early as 10 weeks (k at 7 weeks) and is well developed at birth. The total number of K antigen sites per red cell is quite low and shows dosage: Hughes-Jones and Gardner[67] found about 6000 sites on K+k− red cells and only 3500 sites on K+k+ red cells, although others have found up to 18,000 copies per red cell. Despite its lower quantity, K is very immunogenic and reacts well with its antibody.

The antigens are not denatured by routine blood bank enzymes ficin and papain but are destroyed by trypsin and chymotrypsin used in combination.[4] Solutions of dithiothreitol (DTT) and ZZAP (which contains DTT) denature all Kell system antigens but not K$_x$ antigens; 2-aminoethylisothiuronium bromide (AET) destroys all Kell antigens but not K$_x$.[5] Beta-mercaptoethylamine (MEA) and 2-mercaptoethanol (2ME) are known to denature the Kell antigens K, k, Kp$^a$, Kp$^b$, Js$^a$, Js$^b$, and Ku. The frequencies of common Kell phenotypes and key facts are listed in Table 8–9.

## K and k Antigens

These antithetical antigens warrant special attention because they are so immunogenic. K is rated second only to D in immunogenicity. When K− people are transfused with 1 unit of K+ blood, the probability of their developing anti-K may be as high as 10 percent.[67] Fortunately, the frequency of K is low and the chance of receiving a K+ unit is small. If anti-K develops, compatible units are easy to find.

Blood banks are seldom involved with the k antigen. Only two in 1000 individuals lack k and are capable of

**Table 8–8.** Summary of Kell Antigens

| ISBT Number | Common Name | Alternate Name | Frequency (%) | Year Discovered | Comments* |
|---|---|---|---|---|---|
| | | | *I. Antigens Known to Be Encoded by the Kell Gene* | | |
| 1 | K | Kell | 9.0 | 1946 | Antithetical to k, aa193:Met |
| 2 | k | Cellano | 99.8 | 1949 | Antithetical to K, aa193:Thr |
| 3 | Kp$^a$ | Penney | 2W | 1957 | Antithetical to Kp$^b$, aa281:Trp |
| 4 | Kp$^b$ | Rautenberg | >99.9 | 1958 | Antithetical to Kp$^a$, VLAN, aa281:Arg |
| 5 | Ku | Peltz | >99.9 | 1961 | aa128:Arg |
| 6 | Js$^a$ | Sutter | <0.1W/20B | 1958 | Antithetical to Js$^b$, aa597:Pro |
| 7 | Js$^b$ | Matthews | >99.9W/99B | 1963 | Antithetical to Js$^a$, aa597:Leu |
| 10 | Ul$^a$ | Karhula | <3 Finns | 1968 | aa494:Val |
| 11 | — | Cote | >99.9 | 1976 | Antithetical to K17, aa302:Val |
| 12 | — | Bockman | >99.9 | 1973 | Para-Kell |
| 13 | — | Sgro | >99.9 | 1974 | Para-Kell |
| 14 | — | Santini | >99.9 | 1973 | Antithetical to K24, aa180:Arg |
| 16 | — | (k-like) | 99.8 | 1976 | Absent from McLeod cells |
| 17 | Wk$^a$ | Weeks | 0.3 | 1974 | Antithetical to K11, aa302:Ala |
| 18 | — | Marshall | >99.9 | 1975 | Para-Kell |
| 19 | Kx | Sublett | >99.9 | 1979 | Para-Kell |
| 20 | Km | — | >99.9 | 1979 | Absent from K$_0$ McLeod cells |
| 21 | Kp$^c$ | Levay | <0.1 | 1945/1979 | Antithetical to Kp$^a$ and Kp$^b$ |
| 22 | — | Ikar | >99.9 | 1982 | Para-Kell |
| 23 | Cent | Centauro | <0.5 | 1987 | Para-Kell |
| 24 | Callais | Cls | <2.0 | 1985 | Antithetical to K14, aa180:Pro |
| 25 | — | VLAN | (Low) | 1996 | Antithetical to Kp$^b$ |

**Source:** Reid, MD, and Lomas-Francis, C: The Blood Group Antigen Facts Book. Academic Press, New York, 1997.

**Table 8–9.** Frequencies of Common Kell Phenotypes and Key Facts*

| Phenotype | Whites (%) | Blacks (%) |
|---|---|---|
| K−k+ | 91.0 | 96.5 |
| K+k+ | 8.8 | 3.5 |
| K+k− | 0.2 | <0.1 |
| Kp(a+b−) | <0.1 | 0 |
| Kp(a+b+) | 2.3 | Rare |
| Kp(a−b+) | 97.7 | 100 |
| Js(a+b−) | 0 | 1 |
| Js(a+b+) | Rare | 19 |
| Js(a−b+) | 100 | 80 |

*Antigens: Well developed at birth. Expression very weak on McLeod phenotype cells.
Antibodies: Anti-K: Most common antibody after anti-D; reacts less well in low-ionic media. Clinically significant. Reactivity destroyed by AET and DTT. May show dosage.

developing the antibody. The likelihood that these few individuals have received transfusions and become immunized is even less.

### $Kp^a$, $Kp^b$, $Kp^c$, and VLAN Antigens

Alleles $Kp^a$ and $Kp^c$ are low-frequency mutations of their high-frequency partner $Kp^b$. The $Kp^a$ antigen is found in about 2 percent of whites. Its gene is unique because it suppresses the expression of other Kell genes in cis position, including k, $Js^b$, K11, K14, and K18.[68]

The $Kp^c$ antigen is even rarer. In 1979, Yamaguchi and colleagues[69] discovered several siblings from a consanguineous marriage in Japan who typed Kp(a−b−) but otherwise had normal Kell antigens. They concluded that both parents carried a new allele, $Kp^c$, which the children inherited in a homozygous state. Gavin and coworkers[70] then showed that $Kp^c$ and Levay, the first low-frequency antigen ever described, were identical. (Levay was not placed into the system when it was reported because Kell had not yet been discovered!) Recently, the rare antigen VLAN, found in only one family, was reported as a possible fourth allele at this locus.[71]

### $Js^a$ and $Js^b$ Antigens

The $Js^a$ antigen, antithetical to the high-frequency antigen $Js^b$, is found in about 20 percent of blacks but in less than 0.1 percent of whites. It is interesting that the frequency of $Js^a$ in blacks is almost 10 times greater than the frequency of the K antigen in blacks.[5] $Js^a$ and $Js^b$ were linked to the Kell system when it was discovered that $K_o$ red cells were Js(a−b−).

### Anti-K

Outside the ABO and Rh antibodies, anti-K is the most common antibody seen in the blood bank. It is usually an IgG antibody reactive in the antiglobulin phase, but some examples agglutinate saline-suspended cells. About 20 percent bind complement up to C3, but they are seldom lytic. The antibody is made in response to antigen exposure through pregnancy and transfusion, and can persist for many years.

Naturally occurring IgM examples of anti-K are rarer and have been associated with bacterial infections. Marsh and coworkers[71] studied an anti-K in an untransfused 20-day-old infant with an *E. coli* O125:B15 infection whose mother did not make anti-K. The organism was shown to have a somatic K-like antigen that reacted with the infant's antibody, so it was thought to have been the stimulus. The antibody disappeared after recovery. Other organisms implicated with naturally occurring anti-K or known to react with anti-K include mycobacteria, *Enterococcus faecium, Morganella morganii, Campylobacter jejuni*, and *C. coli*.[5,72]

Some examples of anti-K react poorly in low-ionic media such as LISS, LISS-polybrene or LIP, and in some automated systems.[72] The most reliable method of detection is the indirect antiglobulin test, but even this is no guarantee, especially when LIP is used. Routine blood bank albumin or enzyme methods do not affect antibody reactivity, but using DTT, ZZAP, 2ME, MEA, or AET decreases reactivity. The potentiating medium, polyethylene glycol (PEG), may increase reactivity.

Anti-K shows a dosage effect, as do many other Kell antibodies; however, dosage is not always evident. Many factors other than gene zygosity can weaken or otherwise affect antigen expression (see subsequent text).

The K antibody has been implicated in severe hemolytic transfusion reactions. Although some antibodies bind complement, in vivo red cell destruction is usually extravascular via the macrophages in the spleen.

Anti-K is also associated with severe hemolytic disease of the newborn (HDN). Titer does not always accurately predict the severity of disease, inasmuch as stillbirth has been seen with AHG titers as low as 64. When a pregnant woman is identified as making anti-K, it is prudent to type the father for the K antigen, and if K+, monitor the fetus carefully for signs of HDN.[72]

### Antibodies to $Kp^a$, $Js^a$, and Other Low-Frequency Kell Antigens

These antibodies are rare because so few people are exposed to the antigen. Because routine antibody screening cells do not carry low-frequency antigens, the antibodies are most often detected through unexpected incompatible crossmatches or cases of HDN. Not all blood banks have the antigen-positive cells needed to confirm the specificity, but everyone should be able to provide compatible units for transfusion.

The serologic characteristics and clinical significance of these antibodies parallel anti-K except that reports of HDN have been mild. The original anti-$Kp^a$ was "naturally occurring," but most antibodies are "immune."

## Antibodies to k, Kp<sup>b</sup>, Js<sup>b</sup>, and Other High-Frequency Kell Antigens

*Antibodies to k, Kpᵇ, Jsᵇ, and Other High-Frequency Kell Antigens*

Antibodies to high-frequency Kell antigens are rare, because so few people lack the antigen. They also parallel anti-K in serologic characteristics and clinical significance but have been associated with mild cases of HDN.

The antibodies are easy to detect but difficult to work with because most blood banks do not have the antigen-negative panel cells needed to rule out other alloantibodies, nor do they have typing reagents to phenotype the patient's red cells. However, if the antibody does not react with AET-treated red cells, this is a clue that it may be related to Kell, and it provides the technologist with more "rule-outs" for other specificities. Caution is needed when interpreting results because AET denatures other high-frequency antigens, including JMH, Yk<sup>a</sup>, Hy, Kn<sup>a</sup>, McC<sup>a</sup>, and Vel.[1] DTT-treated cells can be used with similar cautions.

Finding compatible units for transfusion can be difficult; siblings and rare donor inventories are the most likely sources. Patients with these kinds of antibody should be encouraged to give autologous units.

## Advanced Concepts

### Biochemistry

Early evidence suggested that Kell antigens involved both protein and carbohydrates. The glycoprotein was finally isolated by sensitizing red cells with Kell antibody, solubilizing the membranes, separating the antibody-antigen complexes, and analyzing them with SDS-PAGE. The same 93-kd protein was isolated using antibodies to K, k, Kp<sup>b</sup>, Ku, Js<sup>b</sup>, K12, K13, K14, K19, K22, and K23, indicating that all these specificities rested on the same structure.

The *Kell* gene was recently cloned, and from its cDNA, the Kell protein was deduced to be a single-pass transmembrane glycoprotein having 732 aa.[20,73] About 47 aa at the *N*-terminus reside in the cell cytoplasm and complex with the internal cell cytoskeleton. A 665-aa segment on the extracellular surface of the cell has six possible *N*-glycosylation sites and 15 cysteine residues. This suggests that the protein is highly folded with disulfide bonds; its folded configuration, as well as critical amino acids and glycosylation, may be essential to antigen specificity and reactivity (Fig. 8–6).

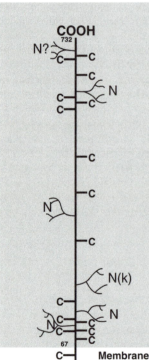

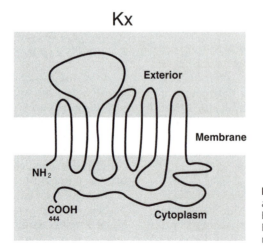

**Figure 8–6.** Proposed structures for Kell and Kx proteins. (From Daniels, G: Human Blood Groups. Blackwell Science Ltd, Osney Mead, Oxford, pp 407 and 412, with permission.)

The structure and amino acid sequence of Kell protein is very similar to a family of zinc-binding endopeptidases. It is possible that Kell protein catalyzes the activation or inactivation of biologically important peptides in the peripheral blood.[2] It appears that the protein complexes with other membrane proteins, including band 4.1, spectrin (a protein similar to actin), and glycophorin C (which carries the Gerbich antigens).

## Genetics

The Kell antigens were said to be encoded by a "gene complex" that had at least 4 "sub-loci." From chimpanzee studies, it was hypothesized that $kKp^bJs^aK^{11}$ was the ancestral complex, with $Js^b$ arising after the human and chimp evolutionary lines separated, making $kKp^bJs^bK^{11}$ the common gene complex in humans.

We now know that the *KEL* gene, with its 19 exons of coding sequence,[4] encodes the entire 732-aa Kell glycoprotein. Specific base pair mutations have been identified, which result in aa substitutions and the antithetical antigens K, $Kp^a$, $Js^a$, and K14, and in many low-frequency antigens. Table 8–8 summarizes known aa differences and their positions on the glycoprotein. Typically, a *KEL* gene variant codes for only one low-frequency antigen. People who test positive for two low-frequency Kell antigens have always been found to carry them on different chromosomes. For example, someone who types Kp(a+) and Js(a+) is genetically $kKp^aJs^b$ on one chromosome and $kKp^bJs^a$ on the other. A rare silent allele to *KEL* called $K^o$ has also been identified. When inherited in a homozygous $K^oK^o$ state, no Kell antigens are expressed.

The *KEL* gene is linked with the Yt blood group and the gene that enables us to taste phenylthiocarbamide. Data suggest that it resides on the long arm of chromosome 7 at position 7q33.

## The Kx Antigen

When Kell antigens are denatured with AET or DTT, the expression of Kx (now called XK1) increases. Because of this inverse relationship, it was initially suggested that Kx might be a precursor or backbone for Kell, or part of a Kell protein complex, and it was initially given the designation K15. However, no evidence between the two antigens has been found to date, and Kx has been placed in its own blood group system, called XK.

Kx activity is found on a 444-aa, 37-kd polypeptide having 16 cysteine residues and 10 hydrophobic membrane spanning domains (see Figure 8–6). Its aa sequence is similar to an $Na^+$-dependent glutamate transporter in rabbits.[2]

The Kx antigen is encoded by the gene *XK*, located on the X chromosome at position Xp21.1.[12] Two alleles are proposed: *XK1*, which codes for Kx antigen, and *XK0*, which does not produce Kx and results in the McLeod phenotype. However, *XK0* may actually represent a small or partial deletion of the X chromosome in this area.[68]

## The $K_o$ Phenotype

$K^o$ is a silent Kell allele or some closely linked gene regulator. Inheriting two $K^o$ genes results in a recessive null phenotype that expresses no Kell antigens, although Kx antigen expression is enhanced. $K_o$ cells have no membrane abnormality and survive normally in circulation. The phenotype is rare; data suggest a frequency of 1:25,000 in whites[68]; only 40 to 50 examples are known.

When $K_o$ individuals are immunized, they can make antibodies to any or all Kell antigens that they lack, including Ku (K5), a "universal" Kell antigen present on all cells except $K_o$ nulls. The true nature of Ku is not known, but it may involve an arginine at aa 128. Its antibody is clearly different from anti-$Js^b$, but sufficient studies are not always done to prove it is not a complex mixture of Kell antibodies.[1]

Because $K_o$ red cells are negative for k, $Kp^b$, $Js^b$, and so forth, they are very useful in investigating complex antibody problems. They can help confirm Kell specificity or rule out other underlying specificities. When $K_o$ cells are not available, they can be made by treating normal cells with AET.

## Other Kell Antigens

**K11 and K17.** In 1971, Guevin and colleagues[74] described anti-Cote (now called anti-K11), which reacted with all red cells tested except those of the propositus, two of her eight siblings, and Kell null cells. Its antigen appeared to be phenotypically related to the Kell system. Three years later, Strange and associates[75] discovered that the low-frequency antigen $Wk^a$ (Weeks) was strongly expressed on K:-11 red cells and definitely traveled with the *KEL1* gene. Once this antithetical relationship was confirmed, $Wk^a$ was given the name K17 to show its placement into the Kell system. K11 has a valine at aa position 302 on the Kell protein, whereas K17 has alanine.

**K14 and K24.** K14, like K11, was a high-frequency antigen phenotypically related to the Kell system. In 1985, its antithetical low-frequency antigen, K24, was described.[76] Anti-K24 reacts best with rare K:-14,24 red cells, moderately well with K:14,24 cells, and not at all with common K:14,−24 or AET-treated K:24 red cells. K14 is associated with arginine at aa position 180 on the Kell glycoprotein, whereas K24 has a proline substitution.

**UI$^a$.** UI$^a$ describes a low-frequency antigen found in about 3 percent of random Finns, 0.46 percent Japanese, and 1 of 12 Chinese.[2] Three informative families helped place UI$^a$ (K10) into the Kell system. A high-frequency antithetical antigen has not yet been described. UI$^a$ reactivity is associated with a valine at aa position 494.

**K12, K13, K18, K19, and K22.** These discrete, very high frequency antigens were phenotypically related to the Kell system because they were not found on $K_o$ red cells and they were weakly expressed on McLeod phenotype red cells. Using MAEIA (monoclonal antibody-specific immobilization of erythrocyte antigens) assays, these antigens and other Kell antigens of low frequency have all been located on the Kell glycoprotein.[5]

**Miscellaneous Kell Antigen Assignments.** The antigens K8 (also called K$^W$) and K9 (KL) are no longer used. K15 is also obsolete: its antigen Kx has been moved to the XK system and given the designation XK1 (ISBT 019.001). The specificities KL, Kx, and Km (K20) are related: a young boy named Claas with both the McLeod phenotype and probable chronic granulomatous disease made an antibody called anti-KL, which was found to be two separable antibodies to Kx and Km.[77] Kx and Km are high-frequency antigens present on all red cells with two exceptions: cells with the McLeod phenotype are Kx−, Km−, and $K_0$ cells are Kx+, Km−. The expression of Kell antigens on red cells with common, McLeod, and $K_0$ phenotypes is summarized in Figure 8–7.

K16 refers to a high-frequency k-like antigen seen on k+ red cells that is expressed differently on McLeod red cells. K23 is assigned to a low-frequency antigen identified in only one family; researchers assigned it to the Kell system when they isolated it on Kell protein.

### The McLeod Phenotype

In 1961, Allen and associates[66] described a young male blood donor who initially appeared to be Kell null but who demonstrated weak expression of k, Kp$^b$, and Js$^b$ with adsorption-elution methods. This unusual phenotype was called McLeod, after the donor.

More than 60 examples of this rare phenotype have now been identified. All who have it are male and all lack Kx (XK1) and Km (K20) on their red cells and have poor expression of Kell antigens. These individuals have a variety of associated clinical anomalies called the McLeod syndrome.[73,78]

Red cells lacking Kx have abnormal morphology. Many are acanthocytic (having irregular shapes and protrusions) and are removed from circulation in the spleen. As a result, people with the McLeod phenotype have a chronic but often well-compensated hemolytic anemia with reticulocytosis, bilirubinemia, splenomegaly, and reduced serum haptoglobin levels.

The red cells have normal enzymes, sodium/potassium/phosphorus transport, intracellular ATP, membrane microviscosity, and phospholipid ratios. However, some have a reduction in total lipid content, and data suggest that the abnormal shape is caused by a lipid deficiency on the inner membrane bilayer.[79] McLeod red cells have enhanced transbilayer mobility of phosphatidylcholine and show increased phosphorylation of protein band 3 and the B band of spectrin. Whether these changes are due to the lack of Kx is not known.

McLeod individuals develop a slow, progressive form of muscular dystrophy between ages 40 and 50, which is associated with areflexia (a lack of deep tendon reflexes), choreiform movements (well-coordinated but involuntary movements), and cardiomegaly leading to cardiomyopathy. They have elevated serum creatinine phosphokinase (CPK) levels of the MM type (cardiac/skeletal muscle) and carbonic anhydrase III levels.

An association between the McLeod phenotype and X-linked chronic granulomatous disease (CGD) was made in 1971, when Giblett and associates[80] reported that the rare McLeod phenotype was common among young boys suffering the equally rare disorder CGD. Chronic granulomatous disease is characterized by the inability of phagocytes to make NADH-oxidase, an enzyme important in generating $H_2O_2$, which is used to kill ingested bacteria.[81] Afflicted children die at an early age from overwhelming infections.

At one time it was suggested that CGD was caused by a lack of Kx on white cells, and several alleles at the XK locus were proposed to explain Kx expression on McLeod red cells and CGD white cells. More recent data have shown that this theory is not valid. The Xk gene appears to reside on the X chromosome near deletions associated with CGD, Duchenne muscular dystrophy, even retinitis pigmentosa, near position Xp21.[79]

The expression of Kx in women who are carriers of the McLeod phenotype (XK1,XK0) follows the Lyon hypothesis. The Lyon hypothesis states that in early embryo development, one X chromosome randomly shuts down in female cells that have two. All cells descending from the resulting cell line express only the allele on the active chromosome. Hence, McLeod carriers

| X-linked gene | + Autosomal Kell gene | = | Red cell antigen expression | | | Phenotype |
|---|---|---|---|---|---|---|
| | | | Kell antigens | Km | Kx | |
| *Xk¹* | + *kKp$^b$Js$^b$K11* | → | k, Kp$^b$, Js$^b$, K11...<br>(normal) | Strong | Weak | Common |
| *Xk¹* | + *K₀* | → | None | None | Strong | $K_0$ |
| *Xk⁰* | + *kKp$^b$Js$^b$K11* | → | k, Kp$^b$, Js$^b$, K11...<br>(trace only) | None | None | McLeod |

**Figure 8–7.** Summary of Kell antigens on red cells having normal, $K_0$, and McLeod phenotypes.

exhibit two red cell populations: one having Kx and normal Kell antigens, the other having the McLeod phenotype and atypical morphology.

### Altered Expressions of Kell Antigens

Weaker-than-normal Kell antigen expression is associated with the McLeod phenotype, the suppression by $Kp^a$ gene (cis-modified effect) on Kell antigens, and a dosage effect seen when $Kp^a$ is paired with $K^o$.

Depressed Kell antigens are also seen on red cells with the K:−13 phenotype and the Gerbich system phenotypes Ge:−1, −2, −3 and Ge:−2, −3, which lack normal β- and γ-sialoglycoproteins and may influence the configuration of Kell antigens.[68]

Marsh and Redman[82] propose the umbrella term $K_{mod}$ to describe other phenotypes with weak Kell expression, including those called Day and Mullins. As a group, these phenotypes have very weak Kell antigens and enhanced Kx expression, and some make nonidentical Ku-like antibodies.

Patients with autoimmune hemolytic anemia, in which the autoantibody is directed against a Kell antigen, may have depressed expression of that antigen. Antigen strength returns to normal when the anemia resolves. This phenomenon appears more common in the Kell system than in others.[1]

Finally, red cells may appear to acquire Kell antigens. McGinnis and associates[83] described a K− patient who acquired a K-like antigen during a *Enterococcus faecium* infection. Cultures containing the disrupted organism converted K− cells to K+, but bacteria-free filtrates did not.

### Autoantibodies

Marsh and associates[84] reported that 1 in 250 autoantibodies do not react with $K_0$ red cells and are therefore related to the Kell system. The actual frequency of these antibodies could be much higher, because their study detected autoantibody with pure Kell specificity, not mixtures of Kell with other autoantibodies.[1] They may be benign or hemolytic.

Most Kell autoantibodies are directed against undefined high-frequency Kell antigens, but identifiable autoantibodies to K, $Kp^b$, and K13 have been reported. Issitt and Anstee have noted a possible association between autoanti-K and head injuries or brain tumors.[1]

Mimicking specificities have been reported, such as when an autoanti-K is eluted from K− red cells. But not all of these antibodies may have true mimicking specificity. In some cases of apparent autoanti-K, there may be concurrent weakened K antigen expression.

## THE DUFFY (008) BLOOD GROUP SYSTEM

The Duffy blood group system was named for Mr. Duffy, a multiply transfused hemophiliac who, in

1950, was found to have the first described example of anti-Fy[a].[85] One year later the antibody defining its antithetical antigen, Fy[b], was described by Ikin and coworkers[86] in the serum of a woman who had had three pregnancies.

In 1955, Sanger and colleagues[87] reported that the majority of blacks tested were Fy(a−b−). The gene responsible for this null condition was called *Fy*. Although *FyFy* appeared to be a common genotype in blacks, especially in Africa, the gene was exceedingly rare in whites. In 1975, Miller and coworkers[88] provided an explanation for this observation: Fy(a−b−) red cells were shown to resist infection by the malaria organism *Plasmodium knowlesi* and, as we now know, by *P. vivax*—an example of natural selection in human beings!

Additional Duffy antibodies have since been recognized. Although they are rarely seen in the blood bank, their antigens—Fy3, Fy4, Fy5, Fy6—have contributed to our understanding of the blood group system, which is designated FY or 008 by the ISBT.

### Basic Concepts

#### Fy[a] and Fy[b] Antigens

The Duffy antigens most important in routine blood bank serology are Fy[a] (FY1 or 008.001) and Fy[b] (FY2 or 008.002). They can be identified on fetal red cells as early as 6 weeks' gestational age and are well developed at birth. Masouredis and associates[16] estimated the number of Fy[a] sites on Fy(a+b−) red cells to be 13,300 per cell; an Fy(a+b+) cell carries only 6900 sites. The antigens have not been found on platelets, lymphocytes, monocytes, or granulocytes, but they have been identified in other body tissues, including brain, colon, endothelium, lung, spleen, thyroid, thymus, and kidney cells.[4]

The frequencies of the common phenotypes in the Fy system are given in Table 8–10. The disparity in distribution in different races is quite notable.

Fy antigens do not store well, even in the frozen state. They tend to elute from red cells stored in a medium with low pH or low ionic strength. This can lead to inhibitory substances in the supernatant fluid, which can weaken the reactivity of an anti-Fy[a] or anti-Fy[b].[5]

**Table 8–10.** Frequency of Duffy Phenotypes and Facts*

| Phenotype | Whites (%) | American Blacks (%) | Chinese (%)[92] |
|-----------|-----------|---------------------|-----------------|
| Fy(a+b−) | 17 | 9 | 90.8 |
| Fy(a+b+) | 49 | 1 | 8.9 |
| Fy(a−b+) | 34 | 22 | 0.3 |
| Fy(a−b−) | Very rare | 68 | 0 |

*Antigens: Well developed at birth. Moderately immunogenic.
Fy(a−b−): Resistant to malaria infection.
Antibodies: Clinically significant. Reactivity destroyed by enzymes.
Dosage not obvious.

They also elute from red cells stored in saline for 2 weeks at pH 7.0. These changes are not seen in red cells stored in licensed anticoagulants or the reagent solutions used by commercial manufacturers.[1]

Fy$^a$ and Fy$^b$ antigens are destroyed by common proteolytic enzymes such as ficin, papain, bromelain, and chymotrypsin, and the IgG cleaving reagent ZZAP. They are also denatured by formaldehyde or by heating to 56°C for 30 minutes. They are not affected by AET or acid treatment, but prolonged exposure to chloroquine diphosphate can weaken Fy$^b$. Neuraminidase may reduce the molecular weight of Fy$^a$ and Fy$^b$, but it does not destroy antigenic activity; neither does purified trypsin.

The ability of bromelain to denature Fy$^a$ and Fy$^b$ antigen puzzled those who detected their antibodies using autoanalyzer methods and bromelain. Rosenfield and coworkers[89] suggested that in such systems the antibody may bind first and protect the antigen from enzyme degradation.

### Anti-Fy$^a$ and Anti-Fy$^b$

Because Duffy antigens are only moderate immunogens, anti-Fy$^a$ occurs three times less frequently than anti-K. Anti-Fy$^b$ is 20 times less common than anti-Fy$^a$ and often occurs in combination with other antibodies. Fy$^a$ appears to be more immunogenic in Fy(a−b+) whites than in Fy(a−b−) blacks: in two series, only 25 of 130 patients with anti-Fy$^a$ were Fy(a−b−) blacks.[5]

The antibodies are usually IgG and react best at the antiglobulin phase. Complement binding is rare: about half bind complement only to C3. A few examples are saline agglutinins; these are sometimes seen following a second stimulation. Antibody activity is enhanced in a low ionic strength medium. Anti-Fy$^a$ and anti-Fy$^b$ do not react with enzyme-treated red cells, a helpful characteristic to know when identifying multiple antibodies in a serum containing anti-Fy$^a$ or −Fy$^b$.

The antibodies may or may not show dosage. This discrepancy occurs because it is difficult to differentiate the genotype of some cells. For example, an Fy(a+b−) red cell may have a double or single dose of Fy$^a$ antigen, depending on whether the donor's genotype is *Fy$^a$Fy$^a$* or *Fy$^a$Fy*. Other antigen typings may offer important clues: cells testing R$_o$, S−s−, V+VS+, Js(a+), or Le(a−b−) are more likely to be from black donors and heterozygous. Dosage is also more likely to be seen with saline agglutinating antibodies and with more sensitive techniques.

Anti-Fy$^a$ and anti-Fy$^b$ have been associated with hemolytic transfusion reactions, although hemolysis is seldom severe. Once the antibody is identified, Fy(a−) or Fy(b−) blood must be given, and finding such units in a random population is not difficult. Duffy antibodies have been implicated in delayed hemolytic transfusion reactions, especially in Fy(a−b−) patients with sickle cell disease who have multiple antibodies. Duffy specificity should be looked for or carefully ruled out in such situations. Anti-Fy$^a$ is associated with HDN

ranging from mild to severe. Anti-Fy$^b$ has the same potential.

Rare autoantibodies with mimicking Fy$^a$ and Fy$^b$ specificity have been reported (e.g., anti-Fy$^b$ that can be adsorbed onto and eluted from Fy(a+b−) red cells). Issitt and Anstee[1] suggest that these may represent alloantibodies with "sloppy" specificity made early in an immune response.

### Advanced Concepts

#### Biochemistry

Enzymes, membrane solubilization methods, SDS-PAGE analysis, immunoblotting, and radiolabeling have all been used to study the biochemistry of Duffy antigens.[90] It appears that Fy activity resides on a protein that has a relative mass of 35 to 45 kd and two potential sites for *N*-glycosylation (Fig. 8–8). The glycoprotein traverses the cell membrane seven or nine times and has aa sequencing homologous to human interleukin-8 receptors on leukocytes.[2] Perhaps the Duffy protein acts as a red cell "clearance receptor" for inflammatory mediators or chemokines.

The aa at position 44 on the Duffy glycoprotein defines Fy$^a$ and Fy$^b$ antigen: Fy$^a$ has glycine, and Fy$^b$ has asparagine. Fy3 activity, as defined by monoclonal antibody, is associated with the third extracellular loop, and Fy6 appears to involve aa 31 through 40.[12]

#### Genetics

In 1968, the Duffy gene was linked to a visible inherited abnormality of chromosome 1, thus becoming the first human gene to be assigned to a specific chromosome.[91] It appears to be located near the centromere on the long arm of the chromosome at position 1q22-23. The *Fy* locus is syntenic to *Rh*, which is located near the tip of the short arm; that is, they are on the same chromosome, but they segregate independently.

Modern biotechnology has helped our understanding of the Duffy phenotypes: base pair mutations result in aa variation and variant gene products. The gene in Fy(a−b−) blacks has been found to be an *Fy$^b$* variant

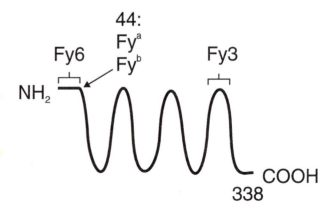

**Figure 8–8.** Proposed structure for the Duffy protein.

with a tryptophane to cysteine substitution at position −46, which disrupts the binding site for mRNA transcription in the red cell.[12] Consequently, Fy(a−b−) blacks do not express Fy$^b$ protein on their red cells but can express it in other tissue. A molecular analysis of Fy(a−b−) whites revealed a 14 base pair deletion in the *Fy* gene, resulting in a reading frame shift and the introduction of a translation stop codon.[2] These individuals carry no Duffy protein on their red cells or on other tissues.

Duffy antigen typings have been performed using the red cells of chimpanzees, gorillas, and old and new world monkeys. The results suggest that *Fy3* developed first, then *Fy$^b$*, but that *Fy$^a$* arose during human evolution.[92]

### The Fy$^x$ Gene

The gene *Fy$^x$* was described in 1965 by Chown and associates[93] as a new allele at the Duffy locus. It does not produce a distinct antigen but, rather, an inherited weak form of Fy$^b$ that reacts with some but not all examples of anti-Fy$^b$. Fy(x+) individuals may type Fy(b−), but their red cells adsorb and elute anti-Fy$^b$. They also have depressed expression of their Fy3 and Fy5 antigen. The red cells from *Fy$^x$Fy$^x$* people also react weakly with anti-Fy5 and anti-Fy6.[92]

Presence of the gene can confuse paternity studies if the weak antigen is not detected. *Fy$^x$* and the silent allele *Fy* or *Fy4* can initially mimic one another. *Fy$^x$* is probably more common than *Fy* in whites, but both are rare.

### Fy3 Antigen and Antibody

In 1971, Albrey and colleagues[94] reported finding anti-Fy3 in the serum of an Fy(a−b−) white Australian female. It reacted with all red cells tested except those of the Fy(a−b−) phenotype. Because it was an inseparable anti-Fy$^a$Fy$^b$, it was thought to react with an antigenic determinant or precursor common to both Fy$^a$ and Fy$^b$ and was called Fy3 (ISBT 008.003). Unlike Fy$^a$ and Fy$^b$, the Fy3 antigen is not destroyed by enzymes. (See the Biochemistry section for its location on the Duffy glycoprotein.)

Anti-Fy3 is made by Fy(a−b−) individuals who truly express no Duffy glycoprotein (see Genetics section above). These Duffy nulls have been found in white, black, and Cree Indian families.[1] Examples of anti-Fy3 produced by nonblacks appear to react with all Duffy positive cells equally well. Those made by blacks are similar but react weakly or not at all with Duffy positive cord cells. Perhaps biotechnology will someday resolve these observed differences.

### Fy4 Antigen and Antibody

All Fy(a−b−) individuals were thought to be homozygous for a silent allele *Fy* until 1973, when Behzad and colleagues[95] discovered anti-Fy4 in the serum of a young Fy(a+b+) black female with sickle cell anemia. The antibody reacted with red cells from all Fy(a−b−) blacks, many Fy(a+b−) and Fy(a+b+) blacks, but not with Fy(a+b+) blacks and not with whites of any Duffy type. It was concluded that most Fy(a−b−) blacks carry an Fy4 antigen, perhaps in place of Fy$^a$, Fy$^b$, and Fy3, and are genetically *Fy$^4$Fy$^4$*. It was suggested that Fy4 offered protection from immunization to Fy$^a$ and Fy$^b$ because so many transfused Fy(a−b−) blacks do not make corresponding antibodies. The Fy4 antigen, like Fy3, is not destroyed by enzymes.

It is now thought unlikely that Fy4 is located on the Duffy glycoprotein.[2] Instead, it may represent a conformational difference in some associated membrane structure that occurs in the absence of Duffy glycoprotein.

### Fy5 Antigen and Antibody

Anti-Fy5 was discovered by Colledge and associates[96] in 1973 in the serum of an Fy(a−b−) black child who later died of leukemia. Initially it was thought to be anti-Fy3 because it reacted with all Fy(a+) or Fy(b+) red cells but not with Fy(a−b−) cells. The antibody differed in that it reacted with the cells from a Fy(a−b−)Fy:−3 white female, but it did not react with Fy(a+) or Fy(b+) Rh$_{null}$ red cells and reacted only weakly with Fy(a+) or Fy(b+) D−− red cells.

The molecular structure of Fy5 (ISBT 008.005) is not known, but it appears to be the result of interaction between Rh and Duffy genes. People who are Fy(a−b−) and/or Rh$_{null}$ do not make Fy5 and are at risk of making the antibody, although few do so. Like Fy3, it is not destroyed by enzymes.

### Fy6 Antigen and Antibody

In 1987, Nichols and coworkers[97] described a murine monoclonal antibody they had prepared that reacted much like anti-Fy3 except that its reactivity was destroyed by ficin, papain, and chymotrypsin. Trypsin enhanced its reactivity. The antibody appeared to define the Duffy receptor used by *P. vivax* to penetrate red cells. It is now known that Fy6 involves aa 31–40 on the Duffy glycoprotein. No human examples of anti-Fy6 have been reported to date.

### Fy3 and Fy5 Antibody Characteristics

Anti-Fy3 or anti-Fy5 are "immune" and IgG and antiglobulin reactive. They react with enzyme-treated red cells, sometimes with enhanced reactivity. Although not all have been so implicated, they have the potential to cause transfusion reactions and HDN.

These antibodies are rarely seen in routine blood banking, and their special patterns of reactivity may not be immediately recognized on standard antibody identification panels. Typing the patient's red cells for Duffy and Rh antigens can provide helpful clues.

## The Duffy-Malaria Association

A correlation between the Duffy antigens and malaria infection has long been suspected. Since 1955, it was known that Africans and black Americans were resistant to infection by *P. vivax* and that these same populations were Fy(a−b−).

Because *P. vivax* could not be grown in culture at that time, Miller and associates[88] conducted in vitro studies with the simian parasite *P. knowlesi*, which could be cultured and would invade human red cells. They confirmed that malaria merozoites invaded only red cells carrying normal Fy$^a$ or Fy$^b$ antigen. When antigen sites were blocked by antibody or denatured with certain enzymes, the cells became resistant to invasion. Because the resistance factors for *P. knowlesi* and *P. vivax* were so parallel in West African populations, it was suggested that Fy$^a$ and Fy$^b$ might also be the invasion receptor for *P. vivax*. In vivo epidemiologic data supported this hypothesis.[98–100]

Close evaluation of the invasion process of *P. knowlesi* suggests that two receptor sites are involved: one for attachment and one for junction.[28,90] Initial attachment occurs regardless of Duffy type and is characterized by the formation of thin filaments between the merozoite and the red cell surface. Junction, the point where the merozoite and red cell membranes actually join, leads to invagination of the red cell membrane and formation of a parasitophorous vacuole (i.e., invasion), which is Duffy antigen–dependent.

Analyses of the Duffy antigens on human and old or new world monkey red cells and their resistance to invasion before and after treatment with various enzymes have led researchers to conclude that Fy6 is the receptor for invasion for *P. vivax* but that Fy3 is a more probable receptor for *P. knowlesi*.[92]

## THE KIDD (009) BLOOD GROUP SYSTEM

The Kidd blood group is the simplest and most straightforward system described in this chapter. In 1951, Allen and coworkers[101] reported finding anti-Jk$^a$ in the serum of a Mrs. Kidd, whose infant had HDN. Its antithetical antigen, Jk$^b$, was found two years later by Plaut and associates.[102] The null phenotype, Jk(a−b−), was described by Pinkerton and associates[103] in 1959. The propositus made an antibody to a high-frequency antigen called Jk3, which was present on any red cell positive for Jk$^a$ or Jk$^b$. No other antigens have been described.

The Kidd system is designated JK or 009 by the ISBT. It has special significance to routine blood banking because of its antibodies, which can be difficult to detect and are a common cause of hemolytic transfusion reactions.

### Basic Concepts

#### Jk$^a$ and Jk$^b$ Antigens

Jk$^a$ (JK1 or 009.001) and Jk$^b$ (JK2 or 009.002) are common red cell antigens. Table 8–11 summarizes the

**Table 8–11.** Frequencies of Kidd Phenotypes and Key Facts*

| Phenotype | Whites (%) | Blacks (%) | Asians (%) |
|---|---|---|---|
| Jk(a+b−) | 28 | 57 | 23 |
| Jk(a+b+) | 49 | 34 | 50 |
| Jk(a−b+) | 23 | 9 | 27 |
| Jk(a−b−) | Exceedingly rare | Exceedingly rare | 0.9–<0.1 |

*Antigens: Well developed at birth. Not very immunogenic. Jk(a−b−): Resistant to urea lysis.
Antibodies: Clinically significant; associated with delayed hemolytic transfusion reactions. Bind complement well. Fade quickly from circulation. Reactivity is enhanced by enzymes. Demonstrate dosage well.

frequencies of the four known phenotypes. There are notable racial differences in antigen frequency: 91 percent blacks, 77 percent whites, but only 50 percent Chinese are Jk(a+); 57 percent blacks and only 28 percent whites are Jk(b−).

Jk$^a$ antigens are detected on fetal red cells as early as 11 weeks, 7 weeks for Jk$^b$. They are well developed at birth, which contributes to the potential for HDN. Red cells from homozygous *Jk$^a$Jk$^a$* individuals express the antigen more strongly than heterozygous *Jk$^a$Jk$^b$* individuals; *Jk$^a$Jk$^a$* red cells carry 14,000 antigen sites per cell.[16]

Kidd antigens are not altered by enzymes, ZZAP, chloroquine diphosphate, AET, DTT, or acid, reagents which readily affect many other blood group antigens. They may not be very accessible on the red cell surface but may well be clustered.[104] This might explain why they do not always react well with their antibody, but antibody that is bound activates complement. They are also not strong immunogens: the risk of making anti-Jk$^a$ after one exposure to Jk(a+) blood appears to be 7 out of 1000.[104]

The antigens are not found on platelets, lymphocytes, monocytes, or granulocytes using sensitive radioimmunoassay or immunofluorescent techniques.[5]

### Anti-Jk$^a$ and Anti-Jk$^b$

Kidd antibodies have a notorious reputation in the blood bank. They show dosage, are often weak, and are found in combination with other antibodies, all of which make them difficult to detect. Their reactivity is not proportional to their clinical significance in transfusion.

Anti-Jk$^a$ is more common than anti-Jk$^b$. Both are IgG (primarily IgG3) and antiglobulin-reactive, although IgM examples have been reported.[5] Antibodies are made in response to pregnancy or transfusion; "naturally occurring" examples have not been reported.

Kidd antibodies bind complement very well. This can be detected in the antiglobulin test using polyspecific reagents; they may also cause in vitro hemolysis. Rare examples are detected only by the complement they bind (i.e., they are nonreactive in antiglobulin tests using anti-IgG reagents). Using polyspecific reagents with both anti-IgG and anti-complement can be helpful in these situations.[1]

Antibody reactivity can also be enhanced by using LISS or PEG (to promote IgG attachment), by using 4 drops of serum instead of 2 (to increase the antibody/antigen ratio), or by using enzymes such as ficin or papain. Enzymes may cleave surrounding proteolytic structures and make the antigen more accessible to react with its antibody; this also promotes hemolysis. Hemolysis may be influenced by antigen dose.

The ability of Kidd antibodies to show dosage can confound inexperienced serologists. An anti-Jk[a] that reacts only with Jk(a+b−) red cells (carrying a double dose of the antigen) can give inconclusive panel results and appear compatible with Jk(a+b+) cells (carrying only a single dose). Readers are urged to rule out Kidd antibodies only with panel cells that have a double dose of antigen (Jk[a+b−]) and to type all crossmatch compatible units with commercial antisera to make sure they are Jk(a−). To ensure that stored antisera can indeed detect weak expressions of the antigen, Jk(a+b+) positive control cells should be tested in parallel.

Kidd antibodies do not store well. When Jk[a] or Jk[b] specificity cannot be confirmed in a serum, which can happen when reference labs test samples sent from hospitals, sample "freshness" and complement activity must be considered. To boost complement levels and to enhance Kidd system antibody reactivity with polyspecific antiglobulin reagents, some investigators add fresh serum[1]; others use a two-stage EDTA method.[105] Identification is easiest when the freshest possible sample is used.

The titer of anti-Jk[a] or anti-Jk[b] quickly declines in vivo. A strong antibody identified today may be undetectable in a few moments. This confirms the need to check blood bank records for previously identified antibodies before a patient is transfused. It is equally important to inform the patient that he or she has such an antibody and to provide a wallet card that notes the specificity in case the patient is transfused elsewhere.

Kidd antibodies are a common cause of hemolytic transfusion reactions, especially of the delayed type. Although intravascular hemolysis has been noted in severe reactions, coated red cells more often are removed extravascularly in the liver. The rate of clearance of incompatible red cells can vary but is usually rapid, so once a delayed reaction is suspected, the patient should be carefully monitored for hemolysis.

Contrary to its hemolytic reputation in transfusion, most Kidd antibodies are associated with relatively infrequent and mild cases of HDN. In a review of 14 cases, only two infants required exchange transfusion, and both of these were before 1969.[106] Perhaps the facts that Kidd antibodies have lower titers and that an affected fetus carries only a single dose of the antigen help protect an infant at risk.

## Advanced Concepts

### Biochemistry

Unraveling the biochemistry of the Kidd protein became a challenge when Heaton and McLoughlin[107] reported in 1982 that Jk(a−b−) red cells resist lysis in 2M urea, a solution commonly used to lyse red cells in a sample before it is used in some automated platelet-counting instruments. Urea crosses the red cell membrane, causing an osmotic imbalance and an influx of water, which rapidly lyses normal cells. With Jk(a−b−) cells, lysis is delayed 15 to 30 minutes. Whether the anomaly lies in the movement of urea or water, or both, was not clear. Data suggested that water movement across the membrane of Jk(a−b−) red cells was also restricted in the presence of urea.[108]

Sinor and colleagues[109] identified the Jk[a] protein as a single band with a relative mass of 45 kd that was not affected by reduction and alkylation and appeared not to be glycosylated. More recently, Olives and associates[110] cloned cDNA and predicted the urea transport and Jk protein to have 391 aa with 10 membrane spanning domains, 2 N-glycosylation sites, and 10 cysteine residues. See Figure 8–9 for a proposed structure. The cysteine residues may explain why treatment with disulfide reagents has an inhibitory effect on urea transport. However, the reagents AET and 2ME do not affect Kidd system antigen reactivity; perhaps the Kidd antigens reside outside the functional site of the transport protein.[4] The specific epitopes for Jk[a] or Jk[b] have not been identified.

No clinical abnormalities have been associated with the Jk(a−b−) phenotype to date. Several unrelated Jk(a−b−) individuals have been found to have normal blood urea nitrogen, creatinine, and serum electrolytes, but studies on two individuals show a marked defect in their ability to concentrate urine.[4] Analysis of Jk(a−b−) red cells using SDS-PAGE shows normal membrane proteins, but using PAGE without SDS (which separates protein by both weight and charge) reveals a unique protein with a relative mass of 67 kd.[111]

### Genetics

The alleles Jk[a] and Jk[b] are mendelian-codominant. Although Jk is called a "silent" allele (because null cells

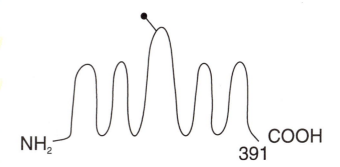

**Figure 8–9.** Proposed structure for Kidd protein.

carry no Kidd antigens), it most likely makes a protein, albeit abnormal, given the results of PAGE analyses with and without SDS. Geitvik and coworkers[112] linked *Jk* to chromosome 18 using a restriction fragment polymorphism. Studies indicate that it is near the centromere at position 18q11–12.

### Jk(a−b−) Phenotype

People with the null phenotype lack Jk$^a$, Jk$^b$, and the common antigen Jk3. Although they are very rare, most have been identified in the Far East and the Pacific Ocean arena (Hawaii, New Zealand, Samoa, Tonga, and Polynesia).[1] The null phenotype has also been reported in several white families and in the Mato Grosso Indians of Brazil. The delayed lysis of Jk(a−b−) red cells in 2M urea has proved an easy way to screen families and/or populations for this rare phenotype.

Family studies show that most Jk(a−b−) nulls are homozygous for the rare "silent" allele *Jk*. Parents of *JkJk* offspring and children of *JkJk* parents type Jk(a+b−) or Jk(a−b+)—never Jk(a+b+)—because they are genetically *Jk$^a$Jk* or *Jk$^b$Jk*. They also demonstrate a single dose of Jk$^a$ or Jk$^b$ antigen in titration studies. Serologists must consider the presence of the *Jk* allele whenever Kidd discrepancies are encountered in paternity studies.

Another genetic explanation for the Jk(a−b−) phenotype was reported by Okubo and associates.[111] They discovered a dominant pattern of inheritance within a Japanese family and proposed the existence of a dominant inhibitor to the Kidd system, *In(Jk)*, analogous to *In(Lu)* in the Lutheran blood group system. Dominant type Jk(a−b−) red cells absorb and elute anti-Jk$^a$ and anti-Jk3, indicating that the antigens are expressed, but only very weakly.

Other evidence for suppression or heterogeneity in the Kidd blood group system has been offered. Arcara and colleagues[113] described a Jk(a−b−) mother who had seven Jk(a+b−) children, five with a double dose of Jk$^a$ on their red cells and two with a single dose. She never made anti-Jk$^a$ or −Jk3, although her Jk(a−b−) brother did. They suggested the brother was truly *JkJk*, whereas she carried a Jk$^a$ gene she could not express. Humphrey and Morel[114] also encountered unexpected titration and dose results when testing Jk$^a$Jk and Jk$^b$Jk individuals. Their red cells appeared to carry single doses of Jk$^a$ and Jk$^b$, but double doses of Jk3, except for an Asian who demonstrated a single dose of both Jk$^a$ and Jk3. How these data fit into a genetic picture is not clear.

### Anti-Jk3

Alloanti-Jk3 is an IgG, antiglobulin-reactive antibody that looks like an inseparable anti-Jk$^a$Jk$^b$. Because panel cells are Jk(a+) or Jk(b+), it reacts with all cells tested except the auto-control. Most blood banks do not have the rare cells needed to confirm its identity; however, they can easily determine its most probable

specificity through antigen typings. The individual making the antibody will type Jk(a−b−). As with other Kidd antibodies, enzymes enhance the reactivity.

Anti-Jk3 is associated with mild HDN and delayed hemolytic transfusion reactions. Compatible units are best found by typing siblings or searching the rare donor files. One example of the antibody has been found in an untransfused male.

### Autoantibodies

Autoantibodies with Kidd specificity (Jk$^a$, Jk$^b$, and Jk3) are rare, but they have been associated with autoimmune hemolytic anemia.[104] Some examples are drug-related: One was found in a patient taking alphamethyldopa (Aldomet);[115] another was chlorpropamide-dependent;[116] that is, it reacted with Jk(a+) red cells only when the drug was present. Because the patient was Jk(a+) and being treated with the drug, a hemolytic anemia developed. This antibody cross-reacted with three other drugs, all containing a urea group: acetohexamide, tolbutamide, and tolazamide.

Examples of benign autoanti-Jk$^a$ have been associated with butyl, ethyl, methyl, and propyl esters of parahydroxybenzoate or paraben.[117] These chemicals are used in some commercially prepared LISS, cosmetics, food preservatives, and pharmaceuticals. The antibodies are seen when paraben-containing LISS is used in antibody detection tests with Jk(a+) cells. These antibodies may arise from viral or bacterial stimulation.

As with other blood groups, Kidd autoantibodies may have mimicking specificity or be associated with depressed antigen expression. One pregnant woman with an apparent compensated anemia was found to have mimicking autoanti-Jk$^b$ and −Jk3; the antibodies could be absorbed by Jk(a+b−) and Jk(a−b−) red cells.[118] In another report, a woman who was Jk(a+b−) transiently typed as Jk(a−b−) and had anti-Jk3.[119]

### Disease Associations

Although Jk$^a$ and Jk$^b$ are thought to be human red cell antigens, three organisms have been associated with Jk$^b$-like specificity. Two, *Enterococcus faecium* and *Micrococcus*, were able to convert Jk(b−) cells to Jk(b+), and one, *Proteus mirabilis*, may have been the stimulus for an autoanti-Jk$^b$.[120]

## THE LUTHERAN (005) BLOOD GROUP SYSTEM

Lutheran antigens have been recognized since 1945, when the first example of anti-Lu$^a$ was discovered in the serum of a patient with lupus erythematosus diffusus, following the transfusion of a unit of blood carrying the corresponding low-frequency antigen.[121] (This patient also made anti-c, anti-N, the first example of anti-C$^W$, and anti-Levay, now known as Kp$^c$!) The new antibody was named Lutheran, a misinterpretation of the donor's name, Luteran. In 1956, Cutbush and Chanarin[122] described anti-Lu^b, which defined the antithetical partner to Lu^a.

The blood group system appeared complete until 1961, when Crawford and coworkers[123] described the first Lu(a−b−) phenotype. Unlike most null phenotypes at the time, this one was inherited in a dominant fashion. In 1963, Darnborough and associates[124] found a more traditional Lu(a−b−) phenotype inherited as a recessive silent allele.

Using rare Lu(a−b−) red cells to test antibodies to unknown high-frequency antigens, some sera showed a phenotypic relationship to Lutheran. That is, they reacted with all red cells tested except those with the Lu(a−b−) phenotype, even though the antibody producers appeared to have normal Lutheran antigens. These specificities were not identical to one another, and they were given the numeric designations Lu4, Lu5, Lu6, and so on to represent their association to the system. Some of these antigens have been found to be products to allelic genes at the Lutheran locus; others have been associated phenotypically. All are summarized in Table 8–12.

The ISBT designation of the Lutheran blood group system is LU or 005.

## Basic Concepts

Blood bankers seldom deal with the serology of the Lutheran blood group system because the antigens have either very high or very low frequency. Either so many people have the antigen, so only a few are capable of making alloantibody, or the antigens are so rare that only a few people are ever exposed. Consequently, the antibodies are infrequently seen. The antigens also have questionable immunogenicity.

### Lu^a and Lu^b Antigens

Lu^a and Lu^b are antigens produced by allelic codominant genes. Common phenotypes are listed in Table 8–13. Most individuals are Lu(b+); only a few are Lu(a+).

Although the antigens have been detected on fetal red cells as early as 10 to 12 weeks of gestation, they are poorly developed at birth and do not reach adult levels until age 15. Using a murine monoclonal antibody with anti-Lu^b activity, the number of Lu^b site per red cells is estimated to be 1630 to 4070 on Lu(a−b+) cells and 845 to 1820 on Lu(a+b+) cells.[125]

The antigens show dosage, with clear differences noted between homozygous and heterozygous members within the same family. However, antigen expression varies greatly from one family to another[2] and is more pronounced with Lu^a than with Lu^b.

Lutheran antigens are thought to be red cell antigens, but Lu^b-like glycoproteins have been found on kidney endothelial cells and liver hepatocytes (especially in fetal livers) using the monoclonal antibody BRIC 108.[126] Other tissues expressing Lutheran activity include the brain, lung, pancreas, placenta, and skeletal muscle.[12] Lutheran antigens have not been detected on platelets, lymphocytes, monocytes, or granulocytes using sensitive radioimmunoassay or immunofluorescent techniques.[5]

### Anti-Lu^a

Most examples are "naturally occurring" saline agglutinins that react better at room temperatures than 37°C. A few react at 37°C by indirect antiglobulin test. Some are capable of binding complement, but in vitro hemolysis has not been reported. Lutheran antibodies are unusual in that they may be IgA, as well as IgM and IgG.[5]

**Table 8–12.** Summary of the Lutheran Antigens

| ISBT Numbers | Common Name | Frequency (%) | Year Discovered | Comments |
|---|---|---|---|---|
| 1 | Lu^a | 8.0 | 1945 | Antithetical to Lu^b |
| 2 | Lu^b | 99.8 | 1956 | Antithetical to Lu^a |
| 3 | Lu^3(Lu^aLu^b) | >99.9 | 1963 | Only nonreactive w/Lu_null cells |
| 4 | Lu^4 | >99.9 | 1971 | Para-Lutheran |
| 5 | Lu^5 | >99.9 | 1972 | Para-Lutheran |
| 6 | Lu^6 | >99.9 | 1972 | Antithetical to Lu9 |
| 7 | Lu^7 | >99.9 | 1972 | Para-Lutheran |
| 8 | Lu^8 | >99.9 | 1972 | Antithetical to Lu14 |
| 9 | Lu^9(Mull) | 2.0 | 1973 | Antithetical to Lu6 |
| 11 | Lu^11 | >99.9 | 1974 | Para-Lutheran |
| 12 | Lu^12(Much) | >99.9 | 1973 | Para-Lutheran |
| 13 | Lu^13(Hughes) | >99.9 | 1983 | Para-Lutheran |
| 14 | Lu^14 | 2.4 | 1977 | Antithetical to Lu8 |
| 16 | Lu^16 | >99.9 | 1980 | Para-Lutheran |
| 17 | Lu^17 | >99.9 | 1979 | Para-Lutheran |
| 18 | Au^a | 80.0 | 1961 | Antithetical to Au^b |
| 19 | Au^b | 50.0 | 1989 | Antithetical to Au^a |
| 20 | Lu^20 | >99.9 | 1992 | Para-Lutheran |

**Table 8–13.** Frequencies of Lutheran Phenotypes and Key Facts*

| Phenotypes | Whites (%) | Blacks (%) |
|---|---|---|
| Lu(a+b−) | 0.15 | 0.1 |
| Lu(a+b+) | 7.5 | 5.2 |
| Lu(a−b+) | 92.35 | 94.7 |
| Lu(a−b−) | Very rare | Very rare |

*Antigens: Poorly developed at birth. Lu(a−b−): Dominant, recessive, and X-linked types.
Antibodies: Questionable clinical significance. May be IgM, IgG, or IgA. Dosage not obvious. Reactivity possibly destroyed by AET.

Anti-Lu$^a$ often goes undetected in routine testing because most reagent cells are Lu(a−). They are more likely encountered as an incompatible crossmatch or during an antibody workup for another specificity. Experienced technologists recognize Lutheran antibodies by their characteristic loose, mixed-field reactivity in a test tube. In capillary testing, their agglutination resembles a pine tree.[127]

Antibody reactivity is not profoundly altered with the common blood bank enzymes ficin and papain, but it can be destroyed with trypsin, chymotrypsin, pronase, and AET. Although anti-Lu$^a$ can show dosage, this may not be apparent because antigen expression is so variable.

Most Lu$^a$ antibodies are clinically insignificant in transfusion. Lu(a+) red cells have been reported to have normal or near-normal survival in a patient making anti-Lu$^a$.[128] Such transfusions do not appear to increase antibody production or change its thermal range of reactivity. In fact, some antibodies have been observed to disappear several months following detection.[127]

Because Lutheran antigens are poorly expressed on cord cells, most cases of HDN associated with anti-Lu$^a$ are mild. Infants may exhibit weakly positive or negative direct antiglobulin tests (DATs) and mild to moderate elevations in bilirubin. Many require no treatment; others respond to simple phototherapy. In one report of mild HDN, the mother's antibody titer rose to 4096.[129]

### Anti-Lu$^b$

Although the first example was a room temperature agglutinin, and IgM and IgA antibodies have been noted, most are IgG (often IgG4) and reactive at 37°C and the antiglobulin phase. They are made in response to pregnancy or transfusion.

Alloanti-Lu$^b$ reacts with all cells tested except the auto-control, and reactions are often weaker with Lu(a+b+) red cells and cord cells. Ficin or papain does not significantly alter reactivity, although AET may. Autologous red cells will test Lu(a+) if the hospital has typing sera available.

Anti-Lu$^b$ has been implicated with shortened survival of transfused cells and posttransfusion jaundice,

but severe or acute hemolysis has not been reported. Chromium survival studies demonstrate a rapid initial clearance of some Lu(b+) red cells but much slower removal of those remaining.[5] Anti-Lu$^b$ may be regarded as clinically significant, but blood should not be withheld in emergency situations just because compatible units cannot be found. Like anti-Lu$^a$, Lu$^b$ antibodies are associated with only mild cases of HDN.

### Advanced Concepts

#### Biochemistry

Using immunoblot methods and a new monoclonal antibody BRIC 108, which had Lu$^b$-like activity, Parsons and associates[130] identified two proteins with molecular weights of 85 and 78 kd. The Lu$^b$ activity of these two glycoproteins depends on at least one N-glycosidically linked oligosaccharide and intrachain disulfide bond. Daniels and Khalid,[131] using human antibodies to Lu$^a$, Lu$^b$, Lu3, Lu4, Lu6, Lu8, and Lu12, showed that all are located on the same membrane components, and these appear identical to those defined by BRIC 108.

Parsons and colleagues[132] have since cloned cDNA encoding the Lutheran protein. The predicted protein contains 597 aa with five potential N-glycosylation sites and multiple O-glycans. It traverses the cell membrane just once and has a cytoplasmic tail of 60 aa (Fig. 8–10). The external portion contains five disulfide bonded domains (three are constant and two are variable) that are related to the "immunoglobulin superfamily" of proteins. This superfamily includes im-

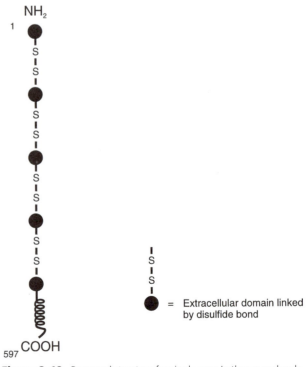

**Figure 8–10.** Proposed structure for single-pass Lutheran molecule.

munoglobulin heavy and light chains, HLA class I and II peptides, T-cell adhesion molecules, CD4 and CD8, immunoglobulin receptors, and the neuronal adhesive molecule N-CAM, among others. Although its biologic role is still uncertain, the Lutheran protein most probably plays some role in adhesion or intracellular signaling.

The specific epitopes for Lutheran antigens have not been identified. However, they are destroyed by trypsin, chymotrypsin, and pronase but are relatively unaffected by ficin, papain, and chloroquine treatment. Red cells treated with 6 percent AER or 200-mM DTT, which break disulfide bonds, fail to react with Lutheran antibodies, although some researchers report otherwise.[126] Perhaps minor variations in treatment explain the discrepant findings, or perhaps there are different specificities of Lu[b], some affected by AET and some not.

### Genetics

The *Lu* gene is located on chromosome 19, along with *H, Se, Le, LW, C3,* and genes coding for Ok[a], apolipoprotein C-II (APO), and myotonic dystrophy. Gene order on the chromosome may be *Ok-Le-C3-LW-APO-Lu-Se-H,*[125,127] with *Lu* residing at position 19q13.2. It is closely linked to *Se* and was the first example of autosomal linkage described in humans.[1]

Because *H, Se,* and *Le* all encode or control fucosyltransferases and Lutheran antigens are associated with glycosylated structures, Daniels[125] suggests that chromosome 19 carries a whole family of glycosyltransferase genes which glycoslyate polypeptides or lipids.

The *Lu* gene, like *Kell,* was thought of as a "gene complex" of at least four subloci, each having two known codominant alleles: *Lu[a]/Lu[b], Lu6/Lu9, Lu8/Lu14,* and *Au[a]/Au[b].* The original *Lu* gene may have encoded a protein carrying many epitopes, including the high-frequency antigens Lu3, Lu[b], Lu6, Lu8, and Au[a]. Subsequent base pair mutations in the gene may explain how the low-frequency antithetical antigens such as Lu[a], Lu9, Lu14, and Au[b] arose.

### Lu(a−b−) Phenotypes

Several genetic explanations for the Lu(a−b−) phenotype have been described. These are summarized in Figure 8–11.

**Dominant In(Lu) Type.** The first Lu(a−b−) family study was reported by the propositus herself.[123] Because the phenotype was seen in successive generations in 50 percent of members in her family and others, and because null individuals passed normal Lutheran genes to their offspring, the expression of Lutheran was thought to be suppressed by a rare dominant regulator gene later called *In(Lu)* for "inhibitor of Lutheran." *In(Lu)* segregates independently from Lutheran. Blood donor screenings have shown the frequency of this type Lutheran null to be 1:3000–5000.[133]

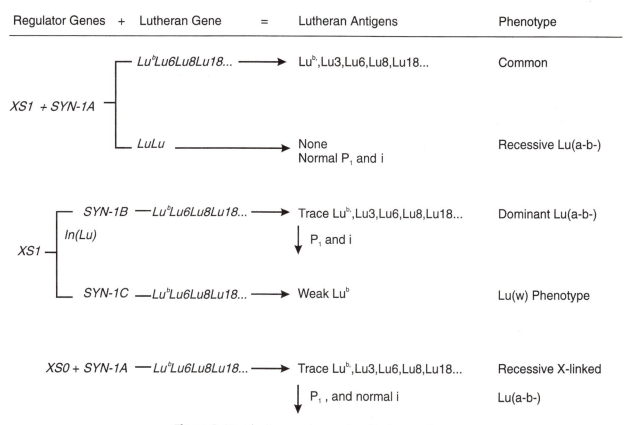

**Figure 8–11.** Inheritance and expression of Lutheran antigens.

Dominant-type Lu(a−b−) red cells carry trace amounts of Lutheran and para-Lutheran antigens as shown by absorption-elution studies. For example, a person who inherits two normal *Lu^b* genes plus *In(Lu)* will type Lu(a−b−) with routine methods but will absorb and elute anti-Lu^b. This trace amount may protect individuals from making alloanti-Lu^b.

Inheriting just one *In(Lu)* gene prevents normal expression of all Lutheran antigens, as well as P_1, i, and Anton/Wj, which are genetically independent. The I antigen appears unaffected. Other unrelated antigens that are suppressed include Cs^a, Yk^a, Kn^a, Sl^a, In^a, and In^b, MER2, epitopes on the common glycoprotein CDw44, concanavalin A receptor, and the receptor for horse antilymphocyte globulin.[126]

Because *In(Lu)* affects the synthesis or expression of so many antigens outside the Lutheran system, Marsh and coworkers[134] have proposed changing its name to *SYN-1*, with *SYN-1A* representing the common allele and *SYN-1B* representing *In(Lu)* (SYN refers to *synthesis*). Although many agree that the name *In(Lu)* is outmoded, they prefer not to change it until the mechanism of the action is better understood. Some propose that *In(Lu)* causes abnormal glycosylation of a common carbohydrate sequence present in many glycoproteins and some glycolipids. It may also alter membrane conformation and affect antigen quantity or its ability to bind with antibody.[126]

*In(Lu)* may also affect red cell shape and metabolism.[126] Udden and others[135] observed abnormal poikilocytosis and acanthocytosis in some *In(Lu)* individuals, although this was variable within families. Red cells from the original *In(Lu)* propositus appear morphologically normal when first collected but become abnormal during storage more quickly than those with normal typings. These red cells also hemolyze more during 4°C storage in modified Alsever's solution. Consequently, *In(Lu)* individuals do not make ideal blood donors. The osmotic fragility of *In(Lu)* red cells is normal, but these cells significantly resist lysis when incubated in plasma at 37°C. *In(Lu)* red cells appear to lose more K^+ than they acquire in Na^+ under these conditions.[126]

**Recessive *LuLu* Type.** In some families, the Lu(a−b−) phenotype is inherited in a recessive fashion, the result of having two rare silent alleles *LuLu* at the Lutheran locus.[124] The parents and offspring of these nulls may type Lu(a−b−), but dosage studies and titers show them to carry a single dose of Lu^b.

Unlike the *In(Lu)* null, recessive Lu(a−b−) people truly lack all Lutheran antigens and can make an inseparable anti-Lu^ab called anti-Lu3. They also have normal antigen expression of P_1, i, and the many other antigens that *In(Lu)* affects. This distinction emphasizes the importance of testing an antibody against recessive Lu(a−b−) red cells before calling its antigen phenotypically related.

**Recessive Sex-linked Inhibitor Type.** In 1986, Norman and associates[136] described an Lu(a−b−) phenotype that fit neither an *In(Lu)* nor an *LuLu* pattern. All Lu(a−b−) family members were male and carried trace amounts of Lu^b detected by absorption-elution. Although P_1 expression was weak, i was well expressed, but I was depressed. The pattern of inheritance suggested an X-borne inhibitor to Lutheran. They proposed calling the locus *XS:XS1* being the common allele and *XS2*, the rare inhibitor that which suppresses in a hemizygous state.

**Lu(w) Phenotype.** Several Lu(a−b+^w) and Lu(a+^wb+^w) individuals with weakened Lutheran antigens have been described. Although not proved, this phenotype, also known as Lu(w), may result from *In(Lu)* with a lesser degree of penetrance or an allele to *In(Lu)* that causes less suppression (*SYN-1C*).

### Anti-Lu3

Anti-Lu3 is a rare antibody that reacts with all red cells except those testing Lu(a−b−). The antibody looks like inseparable anti-Lu^aLu^b and recognizes a common antigen, Lu3, that is present whenever Lu^a or Lu^b are present (much like Jk3's association with Jk^a and Jk^b). It is usually antiglobulin reactive.

This antibody is made only by *LuLu* individuals. Perhaps the very weak expression of Lu3 found on dominant *In(Lu)* and sex-linked *XS2* type nulls protects them from making this antibody. Red cells from dominant and sex-linked type Lutheran nulls can be safely transfused to patients with anti-Lu3.

### Lu6/Lu9 and Lu8/Lu14

In 1972, Lu6[137] and Lu8[138] designations were given to two nonidentical antibodies directed against high-frequency antigens, related to the Lutheran system. The antibodies reacted with all red cells except autologous and Lu(a−b−) cells, but they were made by Lu(a−b+) individuals.

In 1973, Molthan and colleagues[139] described anti-Lu9, an antibody that reacted with 2 percent of random donors and that gave very strong reactions with Lu:−6 red cells. In 1976, Judd and associates[140] reported on anti-Lu14, another antibody to a low-frequency antigen that was strongly expressed on Lu:−8 red cells.

It is now known that these antigens are made by two polymorphic subloci within the Lutheran gene. *Lu6/Lu9* and *Lu8/Lu14* are related to *Lu^a/Lu^b* the way *Kp^a/Kp^b* and *Js^a/Js^b* are related to *K/k*.

### Au^a (Lu18) and Au^b (Lu19)

Au^a (Auberger) was described in 1961 by Salmon and colleagues[141] as an antigen found in 80 percent of whites. In 1989, its antithetical antigen, Au^b, was reported by Frandson and colleagues.[142] Because the antigens were suppressed by *In(Lu)* and *XS2* and were destroyed by trypsin, chymotrypsin, and pronase, they were closely associated with the Lutheran system except that in one family study, they were inherited independently. Serologists considered them just another set of antigens suppressed by Lutheran inhibitors and assigned them to an antigen collection (204) with the designations 204.001 and 204.002.

This has now changed.[143,144] Au$^a$ and Au$^b$ are found on the same glycoprotein expressing Lu$^a$, Lu$^b$, Lu3, Lu4, Lu6, and Lu12 activity and are known to be absent on *LuLu* red cells. The Au(a−) family members associated with the earlier genetic exclusion were retested and found to test Au(a+), so this exclusion was not invalid. Finally, through DNA linkage studies, they were shown to reside on chromosome 19 at position 19q13.2—the Lutheran locus. Au$^a$ and Au$^b$ are now considered a fourth allelic pair within the Lutheran locus and have been redesignated *Lu18* and *Lu19*, respectively.

### Other Lutheran Antigens

Lu4, Lu5, Lu7, Lu12, Lu13, and Lu20 represent discrete, high-frequency antigens phenotypically related to Lutheran. Their antibodies parallel the characteristics of anti-Lu6 and anti-Lu8: they do not react with Lu(a−b−) red cells or autologous cells, which carry otherwise normal Lutheran antigens. They have been included as epitopes on Lutheran glycoproteins through immunoblotting studies.

The high-frequency antigens Lu11, Lu16, and Lu17 are also phenotypically related to Lutheran by virtue of their antibody reactivity (nonreactive with Lu[a−b−] red cells), but confirmation that they are present on Lutheran protein has not been documented, and their inheritance is unknown.

The An/Wj antigen was once associated with the Lutheran system and given the designation Lu15. An/Wj is an interesting high-frequency antigen defined by alloantibodies (anti-Anton) and autoantibodies (anti-Wj). Infants are born An/Wj−, but become An/Wj+ almost within 2 months of birth.[126] The antigen is acquired, not inherited, by all individuals except

**Table 8–14.** Summary of Antibody Characteristics

| Antibody | Reactivity | | | Enzymes | Bind Complement | In Vitro Hemolysis | HTR | HDN | Compatible in U.S. Population (%) | Comments |
|---|---|---|---|---|---|---|---|---|---|---|
| | ≤RT | 37 | AHG | | | | | | | |
| M | Most | Few | Few | Destroy | (Rare)* | No | Few | Mild–severe | 22 | Usually clinically insignificant |
| N | Most | Few | Few | Destroy | (Rare) | No | Rare | Moderate | 28 | |
| S | Some | Some | Most | Variable effect | Some | No | Yes | Mild | 45 W 69 B | |
| s | Few | Few | Most | Variable effect | Few | No | Yes | Mild–severe | 11 W 3 B | |
| U | Rare | Some | Most | No change | (Rare) | No | Yes | Mild–severe | <1 B | |
| P$_1$ | Most | Some | Rare | Enhance | Rare | Rare | Rare | (No) | 21 | Usually clinically insignificant |
| PP$_1$P$^k$ | Most | Some | Some | Enhance | Most | Most | (Yes) | Mild | <0.1 | Potent hemolysins May be associated with early abortions |
| P | Most | Some | Some | Enhance | Most | Some | (Yes) | Mild–severe | <0.1 | |
| I | Most | Few | Few | Enhance | Most | Few | Rare | (No) | See text | Usually autoantibodies clinically insignificant |
| i | Most | Few | Few | Enhance | Most | Few | (?) | Mild | See text | |
| K | Some | Some | Most | No change | Some | No | Yes | Mild–severe | 91 | |
| k | Few | Few | Most | No change | (Some) | No | Yes | Mild | 0.2 | |
| Kp$^a$ | Some | Some | Most | No change | (Some) | No | Yes | Mild | 99.7 | |
| Kp$^b$ | Few | Few | Most | No change | (Some) | No | Yes | Mild | <0.1 | |
| Js$^a$ | Few | Few | Most | No change | (Some) | No | Yes | Moderate | 100 W 80 B | |
| Js$^b$ | (No) | (No) | Most | No change | (Some) | No | Yes | Mild–moderate | 1B | |
| Fy$^a$ | Rare | Rare | Most | Destroy | Some | No | Yes | Mild–severe | 34 W | |
| Fy$^b$ | Rare | Rare | Most | Destroy | Some | No | Yes | (Yes) | 17 W 77 B | |
| Jk$^a$ | Few | Few | Most | Enhance | All | Some | Yes | Mild | 23 | Associated with severe delayed HTR |
| Jk$^b$ | Few | Few | Most | Enhance | All | Some | Yes | Mild | 28 W 57 B | |
| Lu$^a$ | Most | Few | Few | Variable effect | Some | No | (?) | Mild | 92 | IgG$_4$ and IgA antibody classes seen |
| Lu$^b$ | Few | Few | Most | Variable effect | Some | No | Yes | Mild | 0.15 | |

*Comments in parentheses are postulated and not based on reported cases.
B = blacks; HDN = hemolytic disease of the newborn; HTR = hemolytic transfusion reactions; ≤ RT = room temperature or colder; W = whites.

those with the rare *In(Lu)* Lu(a−b−) and An/Wj− phenotypes. Some strains of *Haemophilus influenzae* bind to red cells by the An/Wj antigen, although this does not appear to be the organism's receptor on epithelial cells.[126] When An/Wj was found on *LuLu* cells, its designation was changed to the unassigned high-frequency series 900.030.

Lu10 is another designation no longer used. It was reserved for Singleton, an antigen thought to be the allele of Lu5; the antibody reacted strongly with Lu:−5 red cells. However, five other examples of Lu:−5 cells were later tested and found to be negative with the Singleton serum.[1]

## APPLICATIONS TO ROUTINE BLOOD BANKING

The major blood group systems outside of ABO and Rh become important only after patients develop unexpected antibodies. Then a fundamental knowledge of antibody characteristics, clinical significance, and antigen frequency is needed to help confirm antibody specificity and to select appropriate units for transfusion.

Only a few antibody specificities are commonly seen: M, $P_1$, and I antibodies react at room temperature and are considered clinically insignificant; K, S, s, Fy^a, Fy^b, Jk^a, and Jk^b antibodies react in the antiglobulin phase and are clinically significant. These and selected others are summarized in Table 8–14.

Not all antibody problems are easily solved; panel reactions are sometimes inconclusive. This is when all the esoteric information about the blood groups should be searched for clues. What other antibodies should be considered? What other special techniques or special cells might be used? What information will be gained by antigen typing the patient's cells? If antigen typings are weaker than normal, what is the reason? A systematic review of the blood groups may provide the answer.

Laboratory staff performing paternity tests need to be aware of inheritance patterns and the existence of silent genes, regulators, inhibitors, and modifying situations. Knowing the genetics and biochemistry of the blood group antigens can provide insight into their red cell function and observed disease associations. Perhaps these esoterica will stimulate readers to learn more.

# SUMMARY CHART: IMPORTANT POINTS TO REMEMBER (MT/MLT)

## The I Blood Group System
- I and i antigens appear to have an antithetical relationship.
- Most adult red cells are rich in I and have only trace amounts of i antigen.
- At birth, infant red cells are rich in i; I is almost undetectable; over the next 18 months of development the infant's red cells will convert from i to I antigen.
- Benign anti-I is a weak, "naturally occurring," saline-reactive IgM autoagglutinin detectable only at 4°C.
- Pathologic anti-I is a potent cold autoagglutinin that demonstrates high titer reactivity and reacts over a wide thermal range (0 to 30°C).
- Potent cold autoantibodies can mask clinically significant underlying alloantibodies and complicate transfusions.
- Patients with *Mycoplasma pneumoniae* infections may develop strong cold agglutinins with auto-anti-I specificity.
- Anti-i is an IgM agglutinin and reacts optimally at 4°C; potent examples may be associated with infectious mononucleosis.

## The P Blood Group System
- The P system consists of three antigens, P, $P_1$, and $P^k$, which are biochemically related to the ABH and I antigens.
- $P_1$ antigen expression is variable; $P_1$ antigen is poorly developed at birth.
- Anti-$P_1$ is a common, "naturally occurring" IgM antibody in the sera of $P_2$ individuals; it is usually a weak, cold reactive saline agglutinin seldom detected in routine testing and can be neutralized with soluble $P_1$ substance found in hydatid cyst fluid.
- Anti-$PP_1P^k$ is produced by all p individuals early in life without red cell sensitization and reacts with all red cells except those of other p individuals; antibodies are predominantly IgM, efficiently bind complement, and may demonstrate in vitro hemolysis.
- Anti-P is found as a "naturally occurring" alloantibody in the sera of all $P^k$ individuals.
- Paroxysmal cold hemoglobinuria (PCH) is usually caused by autoantibodies that demonstrate anti-P specificity.
- PCH autoantibodies are IgG biphasic hemolysins demonstrable by the Donath-Landsteiner test.

## The Lutheran Blood Group System
- $Lu^a$ and $Lu^b$ are antigens produced by allelic codominant genes; they are poorly developed at birth.
- Anti-$Lu^a$ may be a "naturally occurring" saline agglutinin that reacts optimally at room temperature.
- Anti-$Lu^b$ is an IgG antibody reactive at the antihuman globulin reagent (AHG) phase; usually produced in response to foreign red cell exposure during pregnancy or transfusion.
- The Lu(a−b−) phenotype is rare and may result from three different genetic backgrounds.

## The MNSs Blood Group System
- Anti-M and anti-N are cold-reactive saline agglutinins that do not bind complement or react with enzyme-treated cells; anti-N has been found in renal patients undergoing dialysis treatment; both anti-M and anti-N may demonstrate dosage.
- Anti-S and anti-s are IgG antibodies, reactive at 37°C and the antiglobulin phase; they may bind complement and have been associated with hemolytic disease of the newborn (HDN) and hemolytic transfusion reactions (HTR).

## The Kell Blood Group System
- The Kell blood group antigens are found only on red cells, are well developed at birth, and are not destroyed by enzymes.
- The K (Kell) antigen is rated second only to D antigen in immunogenicity.
- K2 (previously called Cellano) is a high-frequency antigen.
- Anti-K is usually an IgG antibody reactive in the AHG phase and is made in response to pregnancy or transfusion of red cells; it has been implicated in severe hemolytic transfusion reactions and HDN.
- The McLeod phenotype is described as a rare phenotype with decreased Kell system antigen expression and abnormal red cell morphology, which has been associated with X-linked chronic granulomatous disease (CGD), a rare disorder affecting only males.

## The Duffy Blood Group System
- $Fy^a$ and $Fy^b$ antigens are destroyed by enzymes and ZZAP; they are well developed at birth. The Fy(a−b−) phenotype is prevalent in blacks but virtually nonexistent in whites.
- Fy(a−b−) red cells were shown to resist infection by the malaria organisms *P. knowlesi* and *P. vivax*.
- Anti-$Fy^a$ and anti-$Fy^b$ are usually IgG antibodies and react optimally at the antiglobulin phase of testing; both antibodies have been implicated in delayed hemolytic transfusion reactions and HDN.

## The Kidd Blood Group System
- Anti-$Jk^a$ and anti-$Jk^b$ may demonstrate dosage, are often weak, and are found in combination with other antibodies; both are IgG and antiglobulin reactive.
- Kidd system antibodies bind complement and are made in response to foreign red cell exposure during pregnancy or transfusion.
- Kidd system antibodies are a common cause of delayed hemolytic transfusion reactions.
- Kidd system antibody reactivity is enhanced with enzymes, low ionic strength solution (LISS), and polyethylene glycol (PEG).
- Kidd system antigens are well developed at birth, contributing to the potential for HDN.

# REVIEW QUESTIONS

1. Which of the following best describes MN antigens and antibodies?
   A. Well developed at birth, susceptible to enzymes, generally saline-reactive
   B. Not well developed at birth, susceptible to enzymes, generally saline-reactive
   C. Well developed at birth, not susceptible to enzymes, generally saline-reactive
   D. Well developed at birth, susceptible to enzymes, generally antiglobulin-reactive

2. Which autoantibody specificity is found in patients with paroxysmal cold hemoglobinuria (PCH)?
   A. I
   B. i
   C. P
   D. P$_1$

3. Which of the following is the most common antibody seen in the blood banks after ABO and Rh antibodies?
   A. Anti-Fy$^b$
   B. Anti-k
   C. Anti-Js$^a$
   D. Anti-K

4. Which blood group system is associated with resistance to malaria?
   A. P
   B. Kell
   C. Duffy
   D. Kidd

5. Which antibody does *not* fit with the others with respect to optimum temperature of reactivity?
   A. Anti-S
   B. Anti-P$_1$
   C. Anti-Fy$^a$
   D. Anti-Jk$^b$

6. Which of the following Duffy phenotypes is prevalent in blacks but virtually nonexistent in whites?
   A. Fy(a+b+)
   B. Fy(a−b+)
   C. Fy(a−b−)
   D. Fy(a+b−)

7. Antibody screening cells will *not* routinely detect:
   A. Anti-M
   B. Anti-Kp$^a$
   C. Anti-Fy$^a$
   D. Anti-Lu$^b$

8. About how many donors will need to be antigen-typed to find three Fy(a−) units for crossmatch?
   A. 3
   B. 5
   C. 10
   D. 12

9. Which blood group system is known for showing dosage?
   A. I
   B. P
   C. Kidd
   D. Lutheran

10. Which antibody is most commonly associated with delayed hemolytic transfusion reactions?
    A. Anti-s
    B. Anti-k
    C. Anti-Lu$^a$
    D. Anti-Jk$^a$

11. A patient with a *Mycoplasma pneumoniae* infection will most likely develop a cold autoantibody with specificity to:
    A. I
    B. i
    C. P
    D. P$_1$

12. Which antigen is routinely destroyed by enzymes?
    A. P$_1$
    B. Js$^a$
    C. Fy$^a$
    D. Jk$^a$

## ANSWERS TO REVIEW QUESTIONS

1. A (p 164)
2. C (p 173)
3. D (p 179)
4. C (p 186)
5. B (p 193, Table 8–14)
6. C (p 183, Table 8–10)
7. B (p 179)
8. C (p 193, Table 8–14; also Chap. 11)
9. C (p 186)
10. D (p 187)
11. A (p 175)
12. C (p 184)

## REFERENCES

1. Issitt, PD, and Anstee, DJ: Applied Blood Group Serology, ed 4. Montgomery Scientific, Durham, NC, 1998.
2. Daniels, GL, et al: Blood group terminology. Vox Sang 69:265–279, 1995.
3. Vengelen-Tyler, V, and Judd, WJ (eds): Recent Advances in Blood Group Biochemistry. American Association of Blood Banks, Arlington, VA, 1986.
4. Cartron, JP, and Rouger, P (eds): Blood Cell Biochemistry, Vol 6: Molecular Basis of Human Blood Group Antigens. Plenum, New York, 1995.

5. Mollison, PL, Engelfriet, CP, and Contreras, M: Blood Transfusion in Clinical Medicine. Blackwell Scientific, London, 1997.

6. Landsteiner, K, and Levine, P: A new agglutinable factor differentiating individual human bloods. Proc Soc Exp Biol 24:600, 1927.

7. Landsteiner, K, and Levine, P: Further observations on individual differences of human blood. Proc Soc Exp Biol 24:941, 1927.

8. Walsh, RJ, and Montgomery, C: A new human isoagglutinin subdividing the MN groups. Nature 160:504, 1947.

9. Levine, P, et al: A new blood group factor, s, allelic to S. Proc Soc Exp Biol 78:218, 1951.

10. Wiener, AS, Unger, LJ, and Gordon, EB: Fatal hemolytic transfusion reaction caused by sensitization to a new blood group factor U. JAMA 153:1444, 1953.

11. Greenwalt, TJ, et al: An allele of the S(s) blood group genes. Proc Nat Acad Sci 40:1126, 1954.

12. Reid, MD, and Lomas-Francis, C: The Blood Group Antigen Facts Book. Academic Press, New York, 1997.

13. Hawkins, P, et al: Localization of MN blood group antigens in kidney. Transplant Proc 17:1697, 1985.

14. Vaisanen, V, et al: Blood group M specific haemagglutinin in pyelonephritogenic *Escherichia coli*. Lancet 2:1192, 1982.

15. Rolih, S: Biochemistry of MN antigens. In Unger, PJ, and Laird-Fryer, B (eds): Blood Group Systems: MN and Gerbich. American Association of Blood Banks, Arlington, VA, 1989.

16. Masouredis, SP, et al: Quantitative immunoferritin microasssay of $Fy^a$, $Fy^b$, $Jk^a$, U and $Di^b$ antigen site numbers on human red cells. Blood 56:969, 1980.

17. Rygiel, SA, Issitt, CH, and Fruitstone, MJ: Destruction of the S antigen by sodium hypochlorite. Transfusion 25:274, 1985.

18. Morel, P, et al: Sera exhibiting hemagglutination of N red blood cells stored in media containing glucose (abstract). Transfusion 15:522, 1975.

19. Belzer, FO, Kountz, SL, and Perkins, HA: Red cell cold autogglutinins as a cause of failure of renal transplantation. Transplantation 11:422, 1971.

20. Lutz, P, and Dzik, WH: Molecular biology of red cell blood group genes. Transfusion 32:467, 1992.

21. Holliman, SM: The MN blood group system: Distribution, serology and genetics. In Unger, PJ, and Laird-Fryer, B (eds): Blood Group Systems: MN and Gerbich. American Association of Blood Banks, Arlington, VA, 1989.

22. Darnborough, J, Dunsford, I, and Wallace, JA: The $En^a$ antigen and antibody: A genetical modification of human red cells affecting their blood grouping reactions. Vox Sang 17:241, 1969.

23. Furuhjelm, V, et al: The red cell phenotype En(a−) and anti-$En^a$: Serological and physiochemical aspects. Vox Sang 17:256, 1969.

24. Metaxas, MN, and Metaxas-Buhler, M: $M^k$: An apparently silent allele at the MN locus. Nature 202:1123, 1964.

25. Tokunaga, E, et al: Two apparently healthy Japanese individuals of type $M^kM^k$ have erythrocytes which lack both the blood group MN and Ss-active sialoglycoproteins. J Immungenet 6:383, 1979.

26. Cleghorn, TE: A memorandum on the Miltenberger blood groups. Vox Sang 11:219, 1966.

27. Tippett, P, et al: The Miltenberger subsystem: Is it obsolescent? Transfus Med Rev 4:170, 1966.

28. Hadley, TJ, McGinniss, MH, and Miller, LH: Blood group antigens and invasion of erythrocytes by malarial parasites. In Red Cell Antigens and Antibodies. American Association of Blood Banks, Arlington, VA, 1986.

29. Levine, P, et al: Isoimmunization by a new blood factor in tumor cells. Proc Soc Exp Biol 77:403, 1951.

30. Sanger, R: An association between the P and Jay systems of blood groups. Nature 176:1163, 1955.

31. Matson, GA, et al: A "new" antigen and antibody belonging to the P blood group system. Am J Hum Genet 11:26, 1959.

32. Ikin, EW, et al: $P_1$ antigen in the human foetus. Nature 192:883, 1961.

33. Heiken, A: Observations on the blood group receptor $P_1$ and its development in children. Hereditas 56:83, 1966.

34. Graham, H: An overview of the biochemistry of the Lewis, ABH and P systems. In Bell, CA (ed): A Seminar on Antigens on Blood Cells and Body Fluids. American Association of Blood Banks, Washington, DC, 1980.

35. Cameron, GL, and Staveley, JM: Blood group P substance in hydatid cyst fluids. Nature 179:147, 1957.

36. Roland, FP: $P^1$ blood group and urinary tract infection. Lancet 1:946, 1981.

37. Cantin, G, and Lyonnais, J: Anti-$PP_1P^k$ and early abortion. Transfusion 23:350, 1983.

38. Shirey, RS, et al: Plasmapheresis and successful pregnancy after fourteen miscarriages in the $P_1^k$ with anti-P (abstract). Transfusion 24:427, 1984.

39. Vos, GH, et al: Relationship of a hemolysin resembling anti-$Tj^a$ to threatened abortion in western Australia. Transfusion 4:87, 1964.

40. Tippett, P, et al: An agglutinin associated with the P and the ABO blood group systems. Vox Sang 10:269, 1965.

41. Tippett, P: Contributions of monoclonal antibodies to understanding one new and some old blood group systems. In Garratty, G (ed): Red Cell Antigens and Antibodies. American Association of Blood Banks, Arlington, VA, 1986.

42. Engelfriet, CP, et al: Haemolysins probably recognizing the antigen p. Vox Sang 23:176, 1971.

43. Lomberg, H, et al: $P_1$ blood group and urinary tract infection. Lancet 1:551, 1981.

44. Mulholland, SG, Mooreville, M, and Parson, CL: Urinary tract infections and P blood group antigens. Urology 24:232, 1984.

45. Wiener, AS, et al: Type-specific cold autoantibodies as a cause of acquired hemolytic anemia and hemolytic transfusion reactions: Biologic test with bovine red cells. Ann Intern Med 44:221, 1956.

46. Marsh, WL, and Jenkins, WJ: Anti-i: A new cold antibody. Nature 188:753, 1960.

47. Marsh, WL: Anti-i: A cold antibody defining the Ii relationship in human red cells. Br J Haematol 7:200, 1961.

48. Beck, ML: The I blood group collection. In Moulds, JM, and Woods, LL (eds): Blood Groups: P, I, $Sd^a$ and Pr. American Association of Blood Banks, Arlington, VA, 1991.

49. Shirey, S, Harris, J, and Moore, L: An autoanti-I greatly enhanced in the presence of Thimerosol (abstract). Transfusion 19:642, 1979.

50. Taney, FA, Lee, LT, and Howe, C: Cold hemagglutinin crossreactivity with *Mycoplasma pneumoniae*. Infect Immun 22:29, 1978.

51. Gerbal, A, et al: Sensibilisation des hematies d'un nouveaune par un auto-anticorps anti-i d'origine maternelle nature IgG. Nouv Rev Hematol 11:689, 1971.

52. Moores, PP, et al: Some observations on "Bombay" bloods with comments on evidence for the existence of two different $O_h$ phenotypes. Transfusion 15:237, 1975.

53. Feizi, T: The blood group Ii system: A carbohydrate antigen system defined by naturally monoclonal or oligoclonal autoantibodies of man. Immunology Communications 10:127, 1981.

54. Hakomori, S: Blood group ABH and Ii antigens on human erythrocytes: Chemistry, polymorphism and their developmental change. Semin Hematol 18:39, 1981.

55. Curtain, DD, et al: Cold haemagglutinis: Unusual incidence in Melanesian populations. Br J Haematol 11:247, 1965.

56. Booth, PB, Jenkins, WL, and Marsh WL: Anti-$I^T$: A new antibody of the I blood group system occurring in certain Melanesian sera. Br J Haematol 12:341, 1966.

57. Garratty, G, et al: Autoimmune hemolytic anemia in Hodgkin's disease associated with anti-$I^T$. Transfusion 14:226, 1974.

58. Marsh, WL, Nichols, ME, and Reid, ME: The definition of two I antigen components. Vox Sang 20:209, 1971.

59. Dzierzkowski-Borodej, W, Seyfried, H, and Lisowaka, E: Serological classification of anti-I sera. Vox Sang 28:110, 1975.

60. Levine, P, et al: A new human hereditary blood property (Cellano) present in 99.8 percent of all bloods. Science 109:464, 1949.

61. Allen, FH, and Lewis, SJ: $Kp^a$ (Penney), a new antigen in the Kell blood group system. Vox Sang 2:81, 1957.

62. Allen, FH, Lewis, SJ, and Fudenberg, HH: Studies of anti-Kp^b, a new alloantibody in the Kell blood group system. Vox Sang 3:1, 1958.

63. Giblett, ER: Js, a "new" blood group antigen found in negroes. Nature 181:1221, 1958.

64. Walker, RH, et al: Anti-Js^b, the expected antithetical antibody of the Sutter blood group system. Nature 197:295, 1963.

65. Chown, F, Lewis, M, and Kaita, H: A "new" Kell blood group phenotype. Nature 180:711, 1957.

66. Allen, FH, Krabbe, SM, and Corcoran, PA: A new phenotype (McLeod) in the Kell blood group system. Vox Sang 6:555, 1961.

67. Hughes-Jones, NC, and Gardner, B: The Kell system: Studies with radioactively labelled anti-K. Vox Sang 21:154, 1971.

68. Daniels, G: The Kell blood group system: Genetics. In Laird-Fryer, B, et al (eds): Blood Group Systems: Kell. American Association of Blood Banks, Arlington, VA, 1990.

69. Yamaguchi, H, et al: A "new" allele, Kp^c, at the Kell complex locus. Vox Sang 36:29, 1979.

70. Gavin, J, et al: The red cell antigen once called Levay is the antigen Kp^c of the Kell system. Vox Sang 36:31, 1979.

71. Marsh, WL, et al: Naturally occurring anti-Kell stimulated by E. coli enterocolitis in a 20-day-old child. Transfusion 18:149, 1978.

72. Schultz, MH: Serology and clinical significance of Kell blood group system antibodies. In Laird-Fryer, B, et al (eds): Blood Group System: Kell. American Association of Blood Banks, Arlington, VA, 1990.

73. Marsh, WL, and Redman, CM: The Kell blood group systems: A review. Transfusion 30:158, 1990.

74. Guevin, RM, Taliano, V, and Waldmann, O: The Cote serum, an antibody defining a new variant in the Kell system (abstract). 24th Annual Meeting Abstract Booklet. American Association of Blood Banks, Washington, DC, 1971.

75. Strange, JJ, et al: Wk^a (weeks), a new antigen in the Kell blood group system. Vox Sang 27:81, 1974.

76. Eicher, C, et al: A new low frequency antigen in the Kell system: K24 (Cls) (abstract). Transfusion 25:448, 1985.

77. Van der Hart, M, Szaloky, A, and Van Loghem, JJ: A "new" antibody associated with the Kell blood group system. Vox Sang 15:456, 1968.

78. Marsh, WL: Deleted antigens of the Rhesus and Kell blood groups: Association with cell membrane defects. In Garratty, G (ed): Blood Group Antigens and Disease. American Association of Blood Banks, Arlington, VA, 1983.

79. Rouger, P: Defects of McLeod red blood cells and association with disease. In Laird-Fryer, B, et al (eds): Blood Groups Systems: Kell. American of Blood Banks, Arlington, VA, 1990.

80. Giblett, ER, et al: Kell phenotypes in chronic granulomatous disease: A potential transfusion hazard. Lancet 1:1235, 1971.

81. Marsh, WL, Uretsky, SC, and Douglas, SD: Antigens of the Kell blood group system on neutrophils and monocytes: Their relation to chronic granulomatous disease. J Pediatr 87:1117, 1975.

82. Marsh, WL, and Redman, CM: Recent developments in the Kell blood group system. Transfus Med Rev 1:4, 1987.

83. McGinnis, MH, Maclowry, JD, and Holland, PV: Acquisition of K:1-like antigen during terminal sepsis. Transfusion 24:28, 1984.

84. Marsh, WL, Dinapoli, J, and Øyen, R: Autoimmune hemolytic anemia caused by anti-K13. Vox Sang 36:174, 1979.

85. Cutbush, M, Mollison, PL, and Parkin, DM: A new human blood group. Nature 165:188, 1950.

86. Ikin, EW, et al: Discovery of the expected hemagglutinin, anti-Fy^b. Nature 168:1077, 1951.

87. Sanger, R, Race, RR, and Jack, J: The Duffy blood groups of New York Negroes: The phenotype Fy(a−b−). Br J Haematol 1:370, 1955.

88. Miller, LH, et al: Erythrocyte receptors for (Plasmodium knowlesi) malaria: Duffy blood group determinants. Science 189:561, 1975.

89. Rosenfield, RE, Szymanski, O, and Kochwa, S: Immunochemical studies of the Rh system: III. Quantitative hemagglutination that is relatively independent of source of Rh antigens and antibodies. Cold Spring Harb Symp Quant Biol 29:427, 1964.

90. Valko, DA: The Duffy blood group system: Biochemistry and role in malaria. In Pierce, KR, and Macpherson, CR (eds): Blood Group System: Duffy, Kidd and Lutheran. American Association of Blood Banks, Arlington, VA, 1988.

91. Donahue, RP, et al: Probable assignment of the Duffy blood group locus to chromosome 1 in man. Proc Natl Acad Sci USA 61:949, 1968.

92. Beattie, KM: The Duffy blood group system: Distribution, serology and genetics. In Pierce, SR, and Macpherson, CR (eds): Blood Group Systems: Duffy, Kidd and Lutheran. American Association of Blood Banks, Arlington, VA, 1988.

93. Chown, B, Lewis, M, and Kaita, H: The Duffy blood group system in Caucasians: Evidence for a new allele. Am J Hum Genet 17:384, 1965.

94. Albrey, JA, et al: A new antibody, anti-Fy3, in the Duffy blood group system. Vox Sang 20:29, 1971.

95. Behzad, O, et al: A new anti-erythrocyte antibody in the Duffy system: Anti-FY4. Vox Sang 24:337, 1973.

96. Colledge, KI, Pezzulich, M, and Marsh, WL: Anti-Fy5 an antibody disclosing a probable association between the Rhesus and Duffy blood group genes. Vox Sang 24:193, 1973.

97. Nichols, ME, et al: A new Duffy blood group specificity defined by a murine monoclonal antibody. J Exp Med 166:776, 1987.

98. Mason, SJ, et al: The Duffy blood group determinants: Their role in susceptibility of human and animal erythrocytes to Plasmodium knowlesi malaria. Br J Haematol 36:327, 1977.

99. Miller, LH, et al: The Duffy blood group phenotype in American blacks infected with Plasmodium vivax in Vietnam. Am J Trop Med 27:1069, 1978.

100. Spencer, HC, et al: The Duffy blood group and resistance to Plasmodium vivax in Honduras. Am J Trop Med 27:664, 1978.

101. Allen, FH, Diamond, LK, and Niedziela, B: A new blood group antigen. Nature 167:482, 1951.

102. Plaut, G, et al: A new blood group antibody, anti-Jk^b. Nature 171:431, 1953.

103. Pinkerton, FJ, et al: The phenotype Jk(a−b−) in the Kidd blood group system. Vox Sang 4:155, 1959.

104. Mougey, R: The Kidd blood group system: Serology and genetics. In Pierce, SR, and Macpherson, CR (eds): Blood Group Systems: Duffy, Kidd and Lutheran. American Association of Blood Banks. Arlington, VA, 1988.

105. Polley, MT, and Mollison, PL: The role of complement in the detection of blood group antibodies: Special reference to the antiglobulin test. Transfusion 1:9, 1961.

106. Dorner, I, Moore, JA, and Chaplin, H: Combined maternal erythrocyte autosensitization and materno-fetal Jk^a incompatibility. Transfusion 14:211, 1974.

107. Heaton, DC, and McLoughlin, K: Jk(a−b−) red blood cells resist urea lysis. Transfusion 22:70, 1982.

108. Edwards-Moulds, J: The Kidd blood group system: Drug-related antibodies and biochemistry. In Pierce, SR, and Macpherson, CR (eds): Blood Group System: Duffy, Kidd and Lutheran. American Association of Blood Banks, Arlington, VA, 1988.

109. Sinor, LT, et al: Dot-blot purification of the Kidd blood group antigen (abstr). Transfusion 26:561, 1986.

110. Olives, F, et al: Cloning and functional expression of a urea transporter from human bone marrow cells. J Biol Chem 269:31649–31652, 1994.

111. Okubo, Y, et al: Heterogeneity of the phenotype Jk(a−b−) found in Japanese. Transfusion 26:237, 1986.

112. Geitvik, GA, et al: The Kidd (Jk) blood group locus assigned to chromosome 18 by close linkage to a DNA-RFLP. Hum Genet 77:205, 1987.

113. Arcara, PC, O'Conner, MA, and Dimmette, RM: A family with three Jk(a−b−) members (abstract). Transfusion 9:282, 1969.

114. Humphrey, AJ, and Morel, PA: Heterogeneity within the Kidd system. Transfusion 16:242, 1976.

115. Patten, E, et al: Autoimmune hemolytic anemia with anti-Jk^a specificity in a patient taking Aldomet. Transfusion 17:517, 1977.

116. Sosler, SD, et al: Acute hemolytic anemia due to a chloro-

propamide-dependent autoanti-Jk<sup>a</sup> (abstract). Transfusion 19:641, 1979.

117. Judd, WJ, Steiner, EA, and Cochrane, RK: Paraben-associated autoanti-Jk<sup>a</sup> antibodies. Transfusion 22:31, 1982.

118. Ellisor, SS, et al: Autoantibodies mimicking anti-Jk<sup>b</sup> plus anti-Jk3 associated with autoimmune hemolytic anemia in a primipara who delivered an unaffected infant. Vox Sang 45:53, 1983.

119. Obarski, G, et al: The Jk(a−b−) phenotype, probably occurring as a transient phenomenon (abstract). Transfusion 27:548, 1987.

120. McGinnis, MH: The ubiquitous nature of human blood group antigens as evidenced by bacterial, viral and parasitic infections. In Garraty, G (ed): Blood Group Antigens and Disease. American Association of Blood Banks, Arlington, VA, 1983.

121. Callender, ST, Race, RR, and Paykos, ZV. Hypersensitivity to transfused blood. Br Med J 2:83, 1945.

122. Cutbush, M, and Chanarin, I: The expected blood group antibody, anti-Lu<sup>b</sup>. Nature 178:855, 1956.

123. Crawford, MN, et al: The phenotype Lu(a−b−) together with unconventional Kidd groups in one family. Transfusion 1:228, 1967.

124. Darnborough, J, et al: A "new" antibody anti-Lu<sup>a</sup>Lu<sup>b</sup> and two further examples of the genotype Lu(a−b−). Nature 198:796, 1963.

125. Daniels, G: The Lutheran blood group system: Monoclonal antibodies, biochemistry and the effect of In(Lu). In Pierce, SR, and Macpherson, CR (eds): Blood Group System: Duffy, Kidd and Lutheran. American Association of Blood Banks, Arlington, VA, 1988.

126. Anstee, DJ, et al: Evidence for the occurrence of Lu<sup>b</sup>-active glycoproteins in human erythrocytes, kidney and liver (abstract). International Congress ISBT-BBTS Book of Abstracts, 1988, p 263.

127. Crawford, M: The Lutheran blood group system: Serology and genetics. In Pierce, SR, and Macpherson, CR (eds): Blood Group System: Duffy, Kidd and Lutheran. American Association of Blood Banks, Arlington, VA, 1988.

128. Greendyke, RM, and Chorpenning, FW: Normal survival of incompatible red cells in the presence of anti-Lu<sup>a</sup>. Transfusion 2:52, 1960.

129. Francis, BJ, and Hatcher, DE: Hemolytic disease of the newborn apparently caused by anti-Lu<sup>a</sup>. Transfusion 1:248, 1961.

130. Parson, SF, et al: Evidence that the Lu<sup>b</sup> blood group antigen is located on red cell membrane glycoproteins of 85 and 78 kd. Transfusion 27:61, 1987.

131. Daniels, G, and Khalid, G: Identification, by immunoblotting, of the structures carrying Lutheran and para-Lutheran blood group antigens. Vox Sang 57:137, 1989.

132. Parsons, SF, Mawby, WJ, and Anstee, DJ: Lutheran blood group glycoprotein is a new member of the immunoglobulin superfamily of proteins (abstract). Vox Sang (suppl 2):67:1, 1994.

133. Poole, J: Review: The Lutheran blood group system—1991. Immunohematology 8:1, 1992.

134. Marsh, WL, Johnson, CL, and Mueller, KA: Proposed new notation for the In(Lu) modifying gene. Transfusion 24:371, 1984.

135. Udden, MM, et al: New abnormalities in the morphology, cell surface receptors, and electrolyte metabolism in In(Lu) erythrocytes. Blood 69:52, 1987.

136. Norman, PC, Tippett, P, and Beal, RW: A Lu(a−b−) phenotype caused by an X-linked recessive gene. Vox Sang 51:49, 1986.

137. Marsh, WL: Anti-Lu5, anti-Lu6 and anti-Lu7: Three antibodies defining high frequency antigens related to the Lutheran blood group system. Transfusion 12:27, 1972.

138. MacIlroy, M, McCreary, J, and Stroup, M: Anti-Lu8, an antibody recognizing another Lutheran-related antigen. Vox Sang 23:455, 1972.

139. Molthan, L, et al: Lu9, another new antigen of the Lutheran blood group system. Vox Sang 24:468, 1973.

140. Judd, WJ, et al: Anti-Lu14: A Lutheran antibody defining the product of an allele at the Lu8 blood group locus. Vox Sang 32:214, 1977.

141. Salmon, C, et al: Un nouvel antigene de groupe sanguin erythrocytaire present chez 80% des sujets du race blanche. Nouv Revue Fr Hemat 1:649, 1961.

142. Frandson, S, et al: Anti-Au<sup>b</sup>: The antithetical antibody to anti-Au<sup>a</sup>. Vox Sang 56:54, 1989.

143. Daniels, GL, et al: The red cell antigens Au<sup>a</sup> and Au<sup>b</sup> belong to the Lutheran system. Vox Sang 60:191, 1991.

144. Zelinski, T, et al: Assignment of the Auberger red cell antigen polymorphism to the Lutheran blood group system: Genetic justification. Vox Sang 61:275, 1991.

# CHAPTER 9

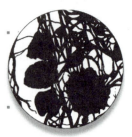

# THE RED CELL SURFACE ANTIGEN TERMINOLOGY AND OTHER BLOOD GROUP SYSTEMS AND ANTIGENS

Deirdre DeSantis, MS, MT(ASCP), SBB, CLS(NCA)

## OBJECTIVES

*On completion of this chapter, the learner should be able to:*

1 Describe the terminology for red cell surface antigens and the four groups into which "authenticated" antigens may be classified.

2 Define the following terms and provide three examples of each: high-incidence antigen, low-incidence antigen.

3 Discuss the notable characteristics of antigens (and corresponding antibodies) in the following blood group systems:

  a Diego (DI) blood group system
  b Cartwright (YT) blood group system
  c XG (XG) blood group system
  d Scianna (SC) blood group system
  e Dombrock (DO) blood group system
  f Colton (CO) blood group system
  g Chido/Rodgers (CH/RG) blood group system
  h Gerbich (GE) blood group system
  i Knops (KN) blood group system

4 Discuss the notable characteristics of the following antigens (and corresponding antibodies) that are classified into a system, collection, series, or the miscellaneous white cell antigen heading.

  a Cromer (CROM) antigens
  b Indian (IN) antigens
  c Cost (Cs$^a$) antigen
  d JMH antigen
  e Vel antigen
  f Sid (Sd$^a$) antigen
  g Bg antigens

## TERMINOLOGY FOR RED CELL SURFACE ANTIGENS

More than 250 red cell surface antigens have been described since the discovery of the ABO system by Landsteiner in 1900. Over this time, numerous nomenclatures and antigenic representations have been introduced, and this has led to inconsistency in terminology. The terminology for red cell surface antigens was initiated to develop a standard numeric system for describing and reporting red cell antigens in a format that is "both eye and computer readable." The first monograph of this numeric system was released in 1990, and a number of amendments have been made.

Through ongoing advances in gene mapping, many blood group antigens have been reclassified, new blood group systems have been created, new antigens have been discovered, and a few antigens have been determined to be obsolete.[1] In keeping with the genetic basis for red cell antigens, the International Society of Blood Transfusion (ISBT) organized a working party to develop a world standard for terminology that would provide a uniform numeric system suitable for electronic data processing equipment.[2] This terminology for red cell surface antigens assigns a six-digit identification number to each "authenticated" blood group antigen. The first three numbers represent the blood group system, collection, or series (e.g., 004 for the RH system), and the last three numbers represent antigen specificity (e.g., 001 for the D antigen). Accordingly, the ISBT number for the D antigen would be 004001. The original (alphabetical) names for the systems and most antigens have not been changed; however, the symbols for each system have been converted to capital letters (e.g., from Rh to RH). An alternative method for identifying antigens in a blood group system according to ISBT would be the system symbol followed by the antigen number (e.g., RH1 for the D antigen). Please refer to Table 9–1 for an abbreviated listing of the blood group systems and the related ISBT terminology and numbers. Phenotypes are designated by the system symbol with a colon followed by the specificity numbers separated by commas. Any negative result (or absent antigen) would be preceded by a minus sign. The phenotype DcEe would be represented in the ISBT system as RH:1, −2, 3, 4, 5. This numeric system is designed as an alternative terminology for computer use and would not be practical for verbal and publication purposes.

All "authenticated" antigens are assigned to a system, a collection, a low-incidence series, or a high-incidence series. To meet the criteria for a blood group system, an antigen must be an inherited character that is controlled by a single gene or by two genes so closely linked that recombination is seldom observed. In addition, "the games must be assigned to a unique chromosomal locus or be inherited discretely from any other gene."[3] The last requirement for membership in a system is the serologic definition of each antigen through testing with the corresponding antibody. At the time of this publication, 23 blood group systems have been established, and 195 antigens have been catalogued into these systems with an ISBT number.[4]

Collections include antigens that demonstrate a biochemical, serologic, or genetic relationship but do not meet the criteria for independent inheritance. Antigens classified as a collection are assigned a 200 number. For instance, the COST collection has been designated as ISBT 205. Refer to Table 9–2 for a listing of the ISBT collections. All remaining red cell antigens that are not associated with a system or a collection are catalogued into the 700 series of low-incidence antigens or the 901 series of high-incidence antigens. Refer to Table 9–3 for an abbreviated listing of high-incidence antigens according to ISBT. High-incidence and low-incidence antigens represent antigens observed in greater than 90 percent or less than 1 percent of most random populations, respectively.

Approximately 260 red cell surface antigens have been described that may or may not represent independent blood group systems. Accordingly, it would be difficult to try to present all of the known red cell surface antigens. Only the more commonly studied blood group systems are addressed briefly, depending on the information currently available. Antigens are grouped into a blood group system, collection, series, or the miscellaneous white cell heading.

## THE DIEGO BLOOD GROUP SYSTEM: DI (ISBT 010)

The Diego system is composed of two sets of independent pairs of antithetical antigens: $Di^a/Di^b$ and $Wr^a/Wr^b$; and three low-incidence antigens: $Wd^a$, $Rb^a$, and WARR. Represented in each antithetical pair are high-incidence $Di^b$ and $Wr^b$ and low-incidence $Di^a$ and $Wr^a$. In 1953, the discovery of anti-$Di^a$ antibody defined the $Di^a$ specificity,[5] and in 1967, the antithetical $Di^b$ antigen was characterized with the newly identified anti-$Di^b$ antibody. The DI antigens are inherited as codominant alleles on chromosome 17. Table 9–1 provides a complete listing of the chromosomal assignments for all ISBT blood group systems. $Di^a$ antigen is described to be a low-incidence antigen (0.01 percent) that is rarely noted in white populations but more commonly noted in individuals of Asian origin. The $Di^a$ antigen has served as a useful tool in anthropologic studies of Mongolian ancestry. South American Indians have been shown to have an incidence of $Di^a$ as high as 36 percent, Chippewa Indians an incidence of 11 percent, Chinese an incidence of 5 percent, and Japanese an incidence of 12 percent.[4,6] $Di^b$ is a high-incidence antigen in white and black populations. The Di (a−b−) phenotype has not been observed. $Di^a$ and $Di^b$ antigens are located on the anion exchange molecule, AE-1,[7] which is an integral transport protein involved in the anion exchange of bicarbonate for chloride in the red blood cell membrane.[8] Of interest, mutations in AE-1 (also known as erythrocyte band 3) may result

**Table 9–1.** Abridged ISBT Terminology for Red Blood Cell Surface Antigens in Blood Group Systems*

| ISBT System Number | System | Symbol | Antigen | ISBT Antigen Number | Chromosomal† Number | Total # of AGs |
|---|---|---|---|---|---|---|
| 001 | ABO | ABO | A | 001 | 9q | 4 |
| | ABO | ABO | B | 002 | | |
| | ABO | ABO | A, B | 003 | | |
| | ABO | ABO | A1 | 004 | | |
| 002 | MNS | MNS | M | 001 | 4q | 39 |
| | MNS | MNS | N | 002 | | |
| | MNS | MNS | S | 003 | | |
| | MNS | MNS | s | 004 | | |
| | MNS | MNS | U | 005 | | |
| 003 | P | P | P1 | 001 | 22q | 1 |
| 004 | Rh | RH | D | 001 | 1p | 52 |
| | Rh | RH | C | 002 | | |
| | Rh | RH | E | 003 | | |
| | Rh | RH | c | 004 | | |
| | Rh | RH | e | 005 | | |
| | Rh | RH | $C^w$ | 008 | | |
| 005 | Lutheran | LU | $Lu^a$ | 001 | 19q | 20 |
| | Lutheran | LU | $Lu^b$ | 002 | | |
| | Lutheran | LU | Lu3 | 003 | | |
| | Lutheran | LU | Lu4 | 004 | | |
| | Lutheran | LU | Lu5 | 005 | | |
| | Lutheran | LU | Lu6 | 006 | | |
| | Lutheran | LU | Lu7 | 007 | | |
| 006 | Kell | KEL | K | 001 | 7q | 25 |
| | Kell | KEL | k | 002 | | |
| | Kell | KEL | $Kp^a$ | 003 | | |
| | Kell | KEL | $Kp^b$ | 004 | | |
| | Kell | KEL | Ku | 005 | | |
| | Kell | KEL | $Js^a$ | 006 | | |
| 007 | Lewis | LE | $Le^a$ | 001 | 19p | 3 |
| | Lewis | LE | $Le^b$ | 002 | | |
| 008 | Duffy | FY | $Fy^a$ | 001 | 1q | 6 |
| | Duffy | FY | $Fy^b$ | 002 | | |
| | Duffy | FY | Fy3 | 003 | | |
| | Duffy | FY | Fy4 | 004 | | |
| | Duffy | FY | Fy5 | 005 | | |
| | Duffy | FY | Fy6 | 006 | | |
| 009 | Kidd | JK | $Jk^a$ | 001 | 18q | 3 |
| | Kidd | JK | $Jk^b$ | 002 | | |
| | Kidd | JK | Jk3 | 003 | | |
| 010 | Diego | DI | $Di^a$ | 001 | 17q | 7 |
| | Diego | DI | $Di^b$ | 002 | | |
| | Diego | DI | $Wr^a$ | 003 | | |
| | Diego | DI | $Wr^b$ | 004 | | |
| 011 | Cartwright | YT | $Yt^a$ | 001 | 7q | 2 |
| | Cartwright | YT | $Yt^b$ | 002 | | |
| 012 | Xg | XG | $Xg^a$ | 001 | Xp | 1 |
| 013 | Scianna | SC | $Sc^a$ | 001 | 1p | 3 |
| | Scianna | SC | $Sc^b$ | 002 | | |
| | Scianna | SC | Sc3 | 003 | | |
| 014 | Dombrock | DO | $Do^a$ | 001 | Not Known | 5 |
| | Dombrock | DO | $Do^b$ | 002 | | |
| | Dombrock | | $Gy^a$ | 003 | | |
| | Dombrock | | Hy | 004 | | |
| | Dombrock | | $Jo^a$ | 005 | | |
| 015 | Colton | CO | $Co^a$ | 001 | 7p | 3 |
| | Colton | CO | $Co^b$ | 002 | | |
| | Colton | CO | Co3 | 003 | | |
| 016 | Landsteiner-Wiener | LW | $Lw^a$ | 001 | 19p | 3 |
| | Landsteiner-Wiener | LW | $Lw^{ab}$ | 002 | | |
| | Landsteiner-Wiener | LW | $LW^b$ | 003 | | |
| 017 | Chido/Rodgers | CH | Ch1 | 001 | 6p | 9 |
| | Chido/Rodgers | CH | Ch2 | 002 | | |
| | Chido/Rodgers | CH | Ch3 | 003 | | |
| | Chido/Rodgers | CH | $Rg^1$ | 011 | | |
| | Chido/Rodgers | CH | $Rg^2$ | 012 | | |
| 018 | H | H | H | 001 | 19q | 1 |

(continued)

**Table 9–1.** Abridged ISBT Terminology for Red Blood Cell Surface Antigens in Blood Group Systems* (*Cont.*)

| ISBT System Number | System | Symbol | Antigen | ISBT Antigen Number | Chromosomal[†] Number | Total # of AGs |
|---|---|---|---|---|---|---|
| 019 | Kx | XK | Kx | 001 | Xp | 1 |
| 020 | Gerbich | GE | Ge2 | 002 | 2q | 7 |
| | Gerbich | GE | Ge3 | 003 | | |
| | Gerbich | GE | Ge4 | 004 | | |
| 021 | CROMER | CROM | Cr$^a$ | 001 | 1q | 10 |
| | CROMER | CROM | Tc$^a$ | 002 | | |
| | CROMER | CROM | Tc$^b$ | 003 | | |
| | CROMER | CROM | Tc$^c$ | 004 | | |
| 022 | Knops | KN | Kn$^a$ | 001 | 1q | 5 |
| | Knops | KN | Kn$^b$ | 002 | | |
| | Knops | KN | McC$^a$ | 003 | | |
| | Knops | KN | Sl$^a$ | 004 | | |
| | Knops | KN | Yk$^a$ | 005 | | |
| 023 | Indian | IN | In$^a$ | 001 | 11p | 2 |
| | Indian | IN | In$^b$ | 002 | | |

*Only the more commonly known antigens are presented. The antigen listing for the following blood group systems is incomplete: MNS, RH, LU, DI, GE, CROM, and KN.
[†]The gene location is designated by the chromosomal number, and the p (short) or q (long) arm.
AGs = antigens.

**Table 9–2.** Antigen Collections According to ISBT

| Collection | | | Antigen | | |
|---|---|---|---|---|---|
| Number | Name | Symbol | Number | Symbol | *Comments* |
| 205 | Cost | COST | 205001 | Cs$^a$ | Cs$^a$: high-frequency antigen with variable expression. Antibodies: IgG, AHG, high titer. Significance: HTR: no; HDN: no. Anti-Cs$^b$ extremely rare |
| | | | 205002 | Cs$^b$ | |
| 207 | Ii | I | 207001 | I | Refer to Chapter 8 |
| | | | 207002 | i | |
| 208 | Er | ER | 208001 | Er$^a$ | Er$^a$ antigen: high frequency. Er$^b$ antigen: low frequency. Antibodies: Er$^a$, IgG, AHG. Significance: HTR: no; HDN: no. Anti-Er$^b$ extremely rare |
| | | | 208002 | Er$^b$ | |
| 209 | | GLOB | 209001 | P | Formerly in P1 system |
| | | | 209002 | p$^k$ | |
| | | | 209003 | LKE | Refer to Chapter 8 |
| 210 | | | 210001 | Le$^c$ | Formerly in Lewis system |
| | | | 210002 | Le$^d$ | Refer to Chapter 7 |

in hereditary spherocytosis,[9] congenital acanthocytosis,[10] and Southeast Asian ovalocytosis.[11]

Both anti-Di$^a$ and anti-Di$^b$ are characterized as red cell–stimulated, IgG antibodies that do not bind complement and are reactive in indirect antiglobulin testing (IAT). Anti-Di$^b$ is reported to show dosage. Although both antibodies have been associated with causing moderate-to-severe transfusion reactions and hemolytic disease of the newborn (HDN), milder forms of HDN are noted with anti-Di$^b$.

The Wright antigens, discovered in 1953,[12] include two allelic antigens: Wr$^a$, a low-incidence antigen occurring in less than 0.01 percent of the random population; and Wr$^b$, a high-incidence antigen occurring in 99.9 percent of the random population. Historically, most red cell surface antigens have been identified and

catalogued according to classical family studies and population statistics. The Wright antigens were first classified as an independent blood group system and later as a collection. The recent work of Bruce and coworkers[13] reveals that the Wr antigens are determined by amino acids Lys-658 or Glu-658 and are housed on the anion transporter AE-1. The Wr antigens, like the Diego antigens, are then linked with anion exchange in the red blood cell membrane.[8] As a result of these findings, the Wright antigens have been reclassified to the Diego blood group system.[1]

Although the antigen Wr$^a$ is extremely rare, the antibody anti-Wr$^a$ has been reported quite frequently. Two types of anti-Wr$^a$ have been observed, a "naturally occurring" IgM and an immune-stimulated IgG. "Naturally occurring" anti-Wr$^a$ is frequently found in the

**Table 9–3.** Notable Antigens in the High-Incidence Series (901)

| Antigen | Name | Ig Class | HDN | HTR | ISBT Number |
|---|---|---|---|---|---|
| Vel | | IgM and few IgG | No | Rare | 901.001 |
| | | | | Severe | |
| | | | | Hemolytic | |
| Comments | • Binds complement — few hemolytic | | | | |
| | • IAT reactivity optimally with enzyme-treated cells | | | | |
| | • Red cell–stimulated | | | | |
| | • Vel(−) incidence: 1 in 4000 with higher frequency in Swedish populations | | | | |
| | • Weak expression on cord cells | | | | |
| Lan | Langereis | IgG1 and IgG3 | mild | Rare | 901.002 |
| | | | | Severe | |
| Comments | • Few bind complement | | | | |
| | • IAT reactivity | | | | |
| | • Red cell–stimulated | | | | |
| At$^a$ | August | IgG | No | Few | 901.003 |
| | | | | Moderate | |
| Comments | • IAT reactivity | | | | |
| | • Red cell–stimulated | | | | |
| | • At ($^a$−) noted in blacks only | | | | |
| JMH | John Milton Hagen | IgG | No | No | 901.007 |
| Comment | • Weak reactivity at IAT | | | | |
| | • Formerly classified as HTLA | | | | |
| | • Autoantibodies in elderly due to reduced antigen expression with age | | | | |
| | • Sensitive to enzyme treatment | | | | |
| Sd$^a$ | Sid | IgM and few IgG | No | Very rare | 901.012 |
| Comments | • RT and IAT reactivity—enhanced by enzymes | | | | |
| | • Red cell–stimulated | | | | |
| | • Variable expression in adults with the most on polyagglutinable Cad cells: super-Sid (Chapter 22) | | | | |
| | • Mixed-field agglutinates, shiny and refractile hemagglutination inhibition with Sd($^a$+) urine which is carried by Tamm Horsfall glycoprotein | | | | |
| | • Depressed antigen expression during pregnancy | | | | |
| | • Weak expression on cord cells | | | | |

serum of individuals who have never been pregnant or received transfusions. Red cell–stimulated anti-Wr$^a$ is typically an IgG$_1$ antibody that is reactive only in IAT testing. The IgG anti-Wr$^a$ is reported to cause mild-to-severe HDN and transfusion reactions.

Only two examples anti-Wr$^b$ alloantibody have been described, so little is known about its clinical significance.[4] Anti-Wr$^b$ may commonly be found as a warm autoantibody in patients with autoimmune hemolytic anemia.

Recent molecular studies have led to the assignment of three low-frequency antigens, Rb$^a$, Wd$^a$, and Warr, to the DI blood group system.[1] All three antigens are found on the third ectoplasmic loop of AE-1.[14] Figure 9–1 provides a molecular representation of the loca-

tion of the DI antigens on the AE-1 transporter protein. Little data are available on the clinical importance of anti-Wd$^a$ and of anti-Rb$^a$. Anti-WARR has been associated with causing mild HDN.

## THE CARTWRIGHT BLOOD GROUP SYSTEM: YT (ISBT 011)

The Cartwright blood group system was discovered 1956 with the observation of Yt$^a$.[15] The YT system is composed of two antigens: Yt$^a$, a high-incidence antigen presenting in 99.8 percent of the general population, and the antithetical partner, Yt$^b$, a low-incidence antigen, presenting in 8 percent of the general popula-

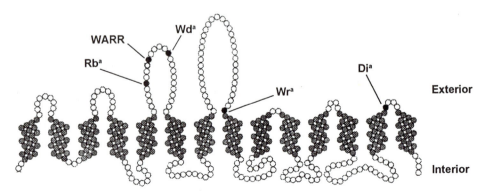

**Figure 9–1.** A molecular illustration of the Diego antigens on the AE-1 transporter molecule.

tion. Three phenotypes have been described, virtually with the same frequencies in both the white and black populations: Yt(a+b−) occurs in 91.9 percent, Yt(a+b+) in 7.8 percent, and Yt(a−b+) in 0.3 percent.[16] The null phenotype Yt(a−b−) has not been observed. The YT antigens have been located on erythrocyte acetylcholinesterase,[17] which is an enzyme involved in neurotransmission.[7]

The Yt[a] antigen is not well developed at birth; therefore, cord bloods are usually Yt[a] negative. Conversely, in adults, the Yt[a] antigen is described as strongly immunogenic, which accounts for the relative frequency in which the anti-Yt[a] antibody is encountered. Interestingly, a case has been reported of a Yt[a] antigen–positive individual presenting with an alloanti-Yt[a], suggesting heterogeneity in antigen expression.[16]

The Yt[b] antigen is well developed at birth but appears to be a poor immunogen. In fact, only a few examples of anti-Yt[b] have been observed in patients who have been frequently transfused and who have produced multiple antibodies.[18]

Both anti-Yt[a] and anti-Yt[b] are IgG antibodies reactive in IAT and are considered to be clinically important because they are predominantly red cell–stimulated. Anti-Yt[a] has been associated with transfusion reactions. No reports have been made of HDN related to the YT antibodies. Studies have shown both Yt[a] and Yt[b] to be inherited as codominant alleles on chromosome 7.

## THE XG BLOOD GROUP SYSTEM: XG (ISBT 012)

The XG blood group was discovered in 1962,[19] and other examples soon followed.[20,21] At present only the Xg[a] antigen has been identified with no known antithetical partner. The blood group is unique in that the gene that encodes for the Xg allele is located on the petite (short) arm of the X chromosome. Many family studies have confirmed the inheritance of the Xg[a] antigen on an X-linked basis; thus, a difference in the frequency of the Xg[a] antigen is noted between the sexes. Approximately 89 percent of the female population expresses Xg[a], whereas 66 percent of the male population expresses Xg[a].

Males are hemizygotes for the XG gene, inasmuch as they carry only one X chromosome. Men, then, may be of genotype *Xg[a]* or *Xg*, whereas women may be *Xg[a]Xg[a]*, *Xg[a]Xg*, or *XgXg*. Thus, the mating of an Xg(a+) man with an Xg(a−) woman would produce all Xg(a+) daughters and Xg(a−) sons.

The infrequently encountered anti-Xg[a] antibodies are predominantly IgG immunoglobulins reactive in the IAT testing and sensitive to enzymes (e.g., bromelain, ficin) but not dithiothreitol (DTT) treatment. These antibodies are described to variably bind complement and react in IAT testing. Most Xg[a] antibodies are the result of red cell stimulation but have not been associated with causing transfusion reactions or HDN. Consequently, Xg[a] antigen does not appear to be an effective immunogen. One example of autoanti-Xg[a] has been reported.[22]

The Xg[a] antigen is carried by a protein with cell adhesion properties that has been demonstrated to have homology with the CD99 molecule.[23] The role of this adhesion molecule in the red cell remains uncertain.

## THE SCIANNA BLOOD GROUP SYSTEM: SC (ISBT 013)

The SC system is composed of the Sc1, Sc2, and Sc3 antigens. Sc1 and Sc2 are antithetical antigens inherited as codominant characters on chromosome 1. Although the antithetical relationship of the Sc1 and Sc2 antigens was not realized until 1967,[24] the Sc1 antigen was first identified as the Sm antigen in 1962[25] and the Sc2 antigen as the rare Bu[a] antigen one year later.[26] The Sc1 is a high-incidence antigen, occurring in approximately 100 percent of the random population. Sc2 is a low-incidence antigen, occurring in less than 1 percent of Northern Europeans.[4] At present the function of the SC antigens remains unknown.

The anti-Sc1 and anti-Sc2 antibodies are rarely observed. Most anti-Sc1 and anti-Sc2 antibodies are IgG, red cell–stimulated, and react in IAT testing. Anti-Sc1 has been described to bind complement, whereas anti-Sc2 has not. Neither anti-Sc1 nor anti-Sc2 has been implicated in transfusion reactions; however, anti-Sc2 has been described in causing mild HDN.[4] A few cases of autoanti-Sc1 have been noted.

The Sc3 antigen is of high frequency and is present on red cells carrying the Sc1 and/or the Sc2 antigens, but it does not appear in the null phenotype Sc(1−2−). Sc3 was identified after anti-Sc3 was observed in two Sc(1−2−) individuals from the Marshall Islands and Papua New Guinea, respectively.[27,28] Later, six other individuals with the Sc null phenotype were found in the same New Guinea village. Anti-Sc3 reacts with all red cells except Sc(1−2−) cells. The antibody does not reveal a discrete specificity in adsorption studies. Anti-Sc3 is characterized as IgG, red cell–stimulated, and reacting in the IAT phase of testing. In regard to clinical importance, the antibody has been linked to causing mild transfusion reactions. No case of HDN has been reported.

## THE DOMBROCK BLOOD GROUP SYSTEM: DO (ISBT 014)

Since the initial discovery of the Dombrock blood group in 1965 with the definition of the Do[a] antigen,[29] four more antigens have been added to the system. The antithetical partner, Do[b], was reported in 1973 when the antibody anti-Do[b] was observed.[30] Most recently, immunochemical and serologic findings have led to the reclassification of the high-incidence antigens Gregory (Gy[a]), Holley (Hy), and Joseph (Jo[a]) to the DO blood group system.[1] In the null phenotype,

Do(a−b−), the Gy$^a$, Hy, and Jo$^a$ antigens are also absent, with all DO antigens being carried by the same membrane glycoprotein.[31] Furthermore, Hy− and Jo($^a$−) red cells express the other DO antigens weakly and are noted exclusively in black populations. The chromosomal location of the DO gene has not been assigned.

Do$^a$ and Do$^b$ are inherited as codominant alleles. The incidence of the Do$^a$ antigen is variable, with 67 percent of whites, 56 percent of blacks and Native Americans, and 24 percent of Japanese carrying the antigen. The Do$^b$ antigen may be observed in nearly 82 percent of whites and 89 percent of blacks. Four phenotypes have been described in the Dombrock system with the following frequencies in whites: Do(a+b−) at 18 percent, Do(a+b+) at 49 percent, and Do(a−b+) at 33 percent. The phenotype Do(a−b−) has infrequently been noted in white and Japanese populations, and, as previously noted, the Gy$^a$, Hy, and Jo$^a$ antigens are also lacking.

Rarely encountered anti-Do$^a$ and anti-Do$^b$ are described as IgG, red cell–stimulated antibodies that react primarily in IAT with polyethylene glycol (PEG) or enzyme enhancement. These DO antibodies are more often observed in combination with other antibodies. Neither anti-Do$^a$ nor anti-Do$^b$ has been associated with clinical HDN; nevertheless, both have been reported to cause acute to delayed transfusion reactions.[32]

Antibodies to Gy$^a$, Hy, and Jo$^a$ have been characterized as IgG, red cell–stimulated, and IAT-reactive. Because antigen expression is weak on cord cells, no cases of clinical HDN have been described. All have been associated with causing moderate transfusion reactions.

## THE COLTON BLOOD GROUP SYSTEM: CO (ISBT 015)

The Colton system is composed of three antigens: Co$^a$, Co$^b$, and Co3 (formerly Co$^{ab}$). Co$^a$ and Co$^b$ are antithetical partners inherited as codominant antigens on chromosome 7. The Colton blood group system was discovered in 1967 when the antibody to the Co$^a$ antigen was described.[33] Co$^b$ was defined in 1970 when the antibody anti-Co$^b$ was observed.[34] Co$^a$, a high-frequency antigen, is present in 99.9 percent of most random populations. Co$^b$ is noted in 10 percent of most random populations. Three phenotypes have been described in the Colton system with the following approximate frequencies: Co(a+b−), 90 percent; Co(a+b+), 9.5 percent; Co(a−b+), 0.5 percent; and Co(a−b−), less than 0.01 percent. Disease associations have linked the Co(a−b−) phenotype with monosomy-7[35] and a rare form of dyserythropoietic anemia.[36] The CO antigens have been located on the transport protein known as channel-forming integral protein (CHIP), which forms the primary erythrocyte water channel and is responsible for water permeability.[8] Moreover, CHIP and the CO antigens are expressed in the tissues of the proximal and descending

tubules and the collecting ducts of the kidney and are believed to account for 80 percent of the reabsorption of water.

Although encountered rarely, both anti-Co$^a$ and anti-Co$^b$ are IgG, red cell–stimulated and reactive in IAT. Anti-Co$^b$ has been shown to bind complement weakly. Both anti-Co$^a$ and anti-Co$^b$ have been associated with acute to delayed transfusion reactions. Unlike the situation with anti-Co$^a$, no reports have implicated anti-Co$^b$ as causing HDN. Of the 12 known examples of anti-Co$^b$, most were noted in individuals with multiple antibodies, with nearly one-half reacting only with bromelain-treated red cells.[37]

The Co3 antigen is of high incidence and is present on red cells carrying the Co$^a$ and/or the Co$^b$ antigens, but it is not expressed in the null phenotype Co(a−b−). Anti-Co3 reacts with all red cells except Co(a−b−) cells. The antibody does not demonstrate a discrete specificity in adsorption studies. Anti-Co3 is characterized as IgG, red cell–stimulated, complement binding, and reacting in the IAT phase of testing. In regard to clinical importance, the antibody has been associated with causing severe HDN. No incidence of transfusion reaction has been reported.

## THE CHIDO/RODGERS BLOOD GROUP SYSTEM: CH/RG (ISBT 017)

The Chido/Rodgers blood group system includes nine antigens, which are subdivided into six Chido antigens, two Rodgers antigens, and the WH antigen. CH1, CH2, CH3, RG1, and RG2 are described as high-incidence antigens, with CH1 being noted in approximately 100 percent and RG1 in 98 percent of all random populations. None of the antigens have been shown to be antithetical. All of CH/RG antigens are poorly expressed on cord cells, adsorbed onto the red cell membrane in individuals with antigen-positive plasma, and sensitive to treatment with ficin, papain, and pronase.[4]

Formerly, the anti-Ch/Rg antibodies were collectively grouped as high-titer, low-avidity (HTLA), along with other antibodies sharing common serologic properties (Table 9–4). High-titer, low-avidity antibodies are characterized as weak and variably reacting IgG antibodies, reacting in the IAT phase of testing. Ag-

**Table 9–4.** Antibodies Formerly Classified as HTLAs owing to Similar Serologic Reactivity

| Antibody | Name | ISBT Class |
|---|---|---|
| Anti-Ch | Chido | Blood Group System: CH/RG |
| Anti-Rg | Rodgers | Blood Group System: CH/RG |
| Anti-Kn | Knops | Blood Group System: KN |
| Anti-McC | McCoy | Blood Group System: KN |
| Anti-Yk$^a$ | York | Blood Group System: KN |
| Anti-Cs$^a$ | Cost | Collection 205: COST |
| Anti-JMH | John Milton Hagen | High-Incidence Series (901) |

glutination strength seldom exceeds 1+, because low avidity (poor binding) and reaction patterns are not always reproducible. These antibodies demonstrate similar weak reactivity at dilutions of 1:64 and higher. Generally they are of the $IgG_4$ subclass[38] and viewed as clinically insignificant. With advances in gene mapping and immunochemical studies, most of the HTLA antigens have been assigned to independent blood group systems or the high-incidence series (901). Consequently, the term HTLA is now regarded to be out of favor.[39]

The Chido antigens were first described in 1967 by Harris when three antibody producers presented with "nebulous" reacting antibodies directed toward a common high-frequency antigen that created problems in compatibility testing.[40] Soon after, Chido specific substance was identified in plasma and serum because of the ability to neutralize anti-Ch antibodies.[41] Anti-Rg was not described until 1976 when a similar but separate antibody demonstrated weak and variable reactivity.[42]

Because of the observation that many serum samples containing anti-Ch and/or anti-Rg antibodies also contained white cell–associated antibodies such as anti-Bg[a], it was postulated that the CH/RG antigens were associated with the human leukocyte antigen (HLA) system. Since this time, the alleles for RG and CH have been located on two closely linked genes known as *C4A* and *C4B* on chromosome 6.[8] In addition, the antigen products have been demonstrated on the C4d fragments of the C4A (Rodgers) and C4B (Chido) glycoproteins of the C4 complement component.[43,44] These findings substantiated the link with the HLA system. The null CH and RG phenotypes, because of C4 deletion, have been associated with a number of autoimmune diseases such as systemic lupus erythematosus,[45] Graves' disease, rheumatoid arthritis, and psoriasis vulgaris.

Anti-Ch/Rg antibodies are usually stimulated in multitransfused individuals lacking one or more of the corresponding antigens. As noted, these antibodies are IgG and weakly reactive in the IAT phase of testing. Antibody producers have routinely been given transfusions of antigen-positive red cells without evidence of increased red cell destruction. However, severe anaphylactic reactions have been reported in a number of antibody-producing patients transfused with large amounts of plasma products.[38] Anti-Ch/Rg antibodies have not been implicated in causing HDN.

The presence of anti-Ch/Rg antibodies often complicates pretransfusion testing and antibody identification because they present with weak and variable serologic patterns that are not reproducible. It is important to identify their presence, inasmuch as they may obscure the detection of more important underlying alloantibodies, such as anti-K, Jk, Fy, Rh, or Vel. Two procedures, antibody screening with C4-coated red cells[46] and plasma inhibition, are routinely used to confirm the identity of suspected anti-Ch/Rg antibodies. Antibody screening with C4-coated red cells is particularly useful for the rapid identification and differentiation of

anti-Ch/Rg antibodies from other antibodies with similar serologic reactivity (see Table 9–4). Plasma inhibition is a valuable tool in compatibility testing and antibody identification procedures in that the anti-Ch/Rg antibodies are removed from the test system, thereby allowing for the detection of possible underlying alloantibodies (see Procedural Appendix at end of chapter). Underlying alloantibodies have been reported in approximately 25 percent of samples being investigated for presenting with "nebulous" reactivity. In addition, anti-Ch and anti-Rg are the only antibodies formerly classified as HTLAs that may be neutralized or inhibited by plasma that is positive for these antigens. Caution must be exercised when using plasma inhibition because other antibodies, namely anti-Le[a] and anti-Le[b], may also be neutralized by plasma or serum containing the corresponding Lewis substance. Plasma inhibition, then, should not be the only method used to identify Ch or Rg antibodies.[39]

## THE GERBICH BLOOD GROUP SYSTEM: GE (ISBT 020)

The Gerbich blood group is a complex system that is composed of three high-incidence antigens (Ge2, Ge3, and Ge4) and four low-incidence antigens (Wb, Ls[a], An[a], and Dh[a]).

The GE antigens were first reported in 1960 when three antibodies were described as reacting with the red cells of all individuals but not with the original three propositi.[47] Soon after, a fourth antibody with similar, but not identical, serologic reactivity was characterized.[48] Accordingly, it was proposed that more than one antibody specificity was represented by these samples. The development of monoclonal GE antibody led to the revision of the GE system in that the Ge2, Ge3, and Ge4 antigens were authenticated and the Ge1 antigen was declared obsolete. Examples of anti-Ge2,[1] anti-Ge3, and anti-Ge4 have been used to define the three GE-negative phenotypes presented in Table 9–5. Two forms of the GE null phenotype have been identified as the Leach types PL and LN, as a result of deletions in exons 3 and 4 and a deletion of nucleotide 134, respectively.[49]

The seven GE antigens are inherited on chromosome 2 and are expressed on altered (because of exon deletion) and unaltered forms of glycophorins C (GPC) and/or D (GPD).[8] GPC and GPD are associated with

**Table 9–5.** Gerbich Negative Phenotypes

| Phenotype | Type | Antibody |
|---|---|---|
| GE: −2, 3, 4 | Yus | Anti-Ge2 |
| GE: −2, −3, 4 | Gerbich | Anti-Ge2 or anti-Ge3 |
| GE: −2, −3, −4 | Leach types: PL LN | Anti-Ge2 or anti-Ge3 |

the red blood cell (RBC) membrane band 4.1, which is integral for maintaining normal erythrocyte shape. Individuals of the Leach phenotype (GE: −2, −3, −4) present with a change in erythrocyte morphology in the form of elliptocytosis.[50]

The incidence of Ge2, Ge3, and Ge4 is cited to be 100 percent in all populations except Melanesians, in whom the incidence of Ge3 is reported to be 50 percent.[4] Antibodies to high-incidence GE antigens are described to be predominantly IgG, red cell–stimulated, variably binding complement, and reacting in the IAT phase of testing. Anti-GE2 and anti-GE3 have also been noted as naturally occurring IgM immunoglobulins and as autoantibodies. Anti-Ge2 and anti-Ge3 are implicated in causing acute to delayed transfusion reactions but not in cases of clinical HDN. No information is available on the clinical significance of anti-Ge4. Likewise, little is known about the pathogenicity of the antibodies to the low-incidence GE antigens; anti-Wb, anti-Ls$^a$, anti-An$^a$, and anti-Dh$^a$.[4] All four are described as predominantly IgG with an IgM component and as not binding complement. Anti-Wb and anti-Ls$^a$ are generally "naturally occurring."

## THE CROMER BLOOD GROUP SYSTEM: CROM (ISBT 021)

The Cromer system is composed of seven high-incidence antigens (Cr$^a$, Tc$^a$, Dr$^a$, Es$^a$, IFC, UMC, and WES$^b$) and three low-incidence antigens (Tc$^b$, Tc$^c$, and WES$^a$). In 1965, the Cr$^a$ antigen was reported by Stroup and McCreay in a black woman after delivery.[51] The CROM antigens are distributed in serum, plasma, urine, platelets, white blood cells, and placental tissue. These antigens are sensitive to chymotrypsin and pronase treatment. In addition, they are poorly expressed on cord cells and depressed during pregnancy. The locus for the CROM antigens is encoded on chromosome 1. All are carried by decay accelerating factor (DAF), which is involved with the regulation of complement activation by accelerating the decay of the C3 and C5 convertases. A null phenotype, INAB, lacks all CROM antigens as well as DAF and has been possibly linked with chronic intestinal conditions. INAB(−) individuals may produce anti-IFC, which is reactive with all samples except INAB red cells.

Anti-CROM antibodies are described as predominantly IgG1, red cell–stimulated, and reactive in IAT testing. Neutralization may be accomplished with concentrated serum, plasma, or urine. The CROM antibodies are rarely observed, with the majority of examples presenting in black individuals. Mild transfusion reactions have been associated with anti-CROM antibodies. Because placental tissue carries DAF, anti-CROM antibodies may be absorbed. This absorption is believed to prevent the passage of antibody into fetal circulation, thereby limiting the occurrence of HDN. To date, no cases of HDN have been reported.

## THE KNOPS BLOOD GROUP SYSTEM: KN (ISBT 022)

The Knops blood group system is composed of five antigens: Kn$^a$ (Knops), Kn$^b$, McC$^a$ (McCoy), Sl$^a$, and Yk$^a$ (York). With the exception of Kn$^b$, all are described as high-incidence antigens in most populations. Kn$^b$ is a low-incidence antigen, noted in 4.5 percent of whites. Of this system, the first antigen to be reported was Kn$^a$ in 1964.[52] Kn$^a$, McC$^a$, Sl$^a$, and Yk$^a$ are expressed poorly on cord cells and depressed in patients presenting with autoimmune disease and the Lu(a−b−) phenotype because of the In(Lu) gene.[53] The antithetical partners McC$^b$ and Sl$^b$ have been reported; however, inadequate evidence is available for their assignment to the ISBT terminology.[54] The alleles for the KN blood group have been located on chromosome 1, with the antigens residing on complement receptor one (CR1). On erythrocytes, CR1 participates in an immune adherence mechanism, whereby the receptor attaches to C3b-marked complexes and delivers them to the liver for removal.[55] Certain autoimmune diseases, such as systemic lupus erythematosus and chronic cold agglutinin disease, have been implicated in depressing the expression of the KN antigens caused by loss of erythrocyte CR1.[56]

The antibodies directed toward the KN blood group antigens were formerly described as having the serologic properties of HTLA antibodies. For more information on HTLA antibodies, refer to the Chido/Rodgers blood group system in this chapter. Advances in gene mapping and immunochemical studies have led to the assignment of Kn$^a$, Kn$^b$, McC$^a$, Sl$^a$, and Yk$^a$ antigens (formerly in the HTLA category) to the KN blood group system. The KN antibodies are characterized as IgG, red cell–stimulated, and reacting weakly and variably at the IAT phase of testing. Reactivity is diminished with trypsin- or chymotrypsin-treated red cells and variable with DTT treatment. The KN antibodies are viewed to be of little clinical importance, inasmuch as none has been associated with causing clinical HDN or HTR.

## THE INDIAN BLOOD GROUP SYSTEM: IN (ISBT 023)

The most recent blood group system, Indian (IN), was discovered in 1973 by Badakere and associates.[57] The IN system is composed of two antithetical antigens, In$^a$ and In$^b$, which are of relatively low and high incidence, respectively. The frequency of In$^a$ is higher in Iranians and Arabs (11 percent), whereas it is much lower in whites, blacks, and Asians (0.1 percent). In$^b$ is noted in 96 percent of whites and 96 percent of Indians.[4] The antigens are inherited as codominant alleles on chromosome 11. Most enzymes denature these antigens. They are poorly expressed on cord cells and depressed during pregnancy. Furthermore, In$^b$ expression may also be depressed in individuals presenting with the Lu(a−b−) phenotype, owing to *In(Lu)* gene. The IN antigens are carried on the hematopoietic isoform of the CD44 marker, which is known for its immune adhesion properties.[8]

IN antibodies are characterized as IgG, red cell–stimulated, and reactive in IAT testing. Unlike the situation with anti-In[b], no reports have linked anti-In[a] with causing HTR. Neither In[a] nor In[b] antibodies have been associated with clinical HDN.

## COLLECTIONS AND NOTABLE ANTIGENS OF THE HIGH-INCIDENCE SERIES

The red cell antigen collections, and a few notable antigens in the high-incidence series, are presented in Tables 9–2 and 9–3. Other texts, such as *Human Blood Groups* by Daniels[58] and *The Blood Group Antigen Facts Book* by Reid and Francis-Lomas,[4] provide additional information on these and other antigens.

## THE MISCELLANEOUS WHITE CELL ANTIGENS: Bg

Three specificities of Bg antigen were first described in 1967 as Bg[a], Bg[b], and Bg[c].[59] The corresponding Bg antibodies are directed toward human leukocyte antigens (HLA). These antigens are categorized into class I and class II antigens. For the purposes of blood banking, only class I antigens will be addressed. Class I antigens are designated as three classes, HLA-A, HLA-B, and HLA-C, which are distributed on all nucleated cells as well as a number of nonnucleated cells. Red cells and platelets are nonnucleated cells that contain nuclei during their developmental stages and carry residual amounts of HLA (Bg) antigen at maturity. Accordingly, weak and obscure Bg reactivity may be observed in serologic testing. The Bg[a] antigen corresponds with HLA-B7, Bg[b] with HLA-B17, and Bg[c] with HLA-A28 (Table 9–6). Inasmuch as the Bg antigens are located

**Table 9–6.** Bg Antigens and HLA

| Bg Antigen | Related HLA Antigen | Comments |
|---|---|---|
| Bg[a] | B-7 | • Formerly known as Bennett-Goodspeed |
| Bg[b] | B-17 | • White cell antigens<br>• Weak and variable IAT reactivity |
| Bg[c] | A-28 | • Clinically benign |

primarily on leukocytes, they are not eligible for assignment to the ISBT terminology for red cell surface antigens.

The Bg antibodies are characterized as IgG and reacting weakly and variably in IAT, with only one or two panel cells that happen to carry higher amounts of Bg antigen. Reactivity is seldom reproducible. Serologically, Bg antibodies are described as "nuisance" antibodies that may be destroyed by treatment with chloroquine or a glycine-HCL/EDTA solution. Because platelets express variable amounts of HLA-A, HLA-B and HLA-C, commercial human platelet concentrate (HPC) is routinely used to adsorb anti-Bg from serum.[60] The absorbed serum is then tested for significant underlying alloantibody without interference.

Serum samples from individuals with multiple transfusions presenting with anti-Bg antibodies also often contain anti-Ch, anti-Rg, or anti-Kn. Bg antibodies have historically been reported as contaminants in commercial reagents, especially antiserums; however, chloroquine is now used for inactivation.[61] In regard to clinical significance, the Bg antibodies are viewed as benign because they have not been implicated with causing HDN or HTR. Interestingly, transient increases in the Bg antigens have been observed in various disease states, such as infectious mononucleosis, leukemia, polycythemia, and hemolytic anemia.[62]

---

## SUMMARY CHART: IMPORTANT POINTS TO REMEMBER (SBB)

- The terminology for red cell surface antigens according to ISBT provides a standard numeric system for naming "authenticated" red cell antigens that is suitable for electronic data processing equipment.
- In the ISBT system, red cell antigens are assigned a six-digit identification number, and the symbols are converted to capital letters. All antigens are catalogued into one of the following four groups:
  - A blood group system if controlled by one discrete gene or by two closely linked genes
  - A collection if shown to share a biochemical, serologic, or genetic relationship
  - The high-incidence series (901) if independently noted in greater than 90 percent of most populations
  - The low-incidence series (700) if independently noted in less than 1 percent of most populations
- The discovery that the Wright antigens are located on the same transport protein (AE-1) as the Diego antigens led to their assignment to the Diego system (DI).
- The low-incidence antigen, $Di^a$, is a useful anthropologic marker for Mongolian ancestry.
- Anti-$Di^a$, anti-$Di^b$, and anti-$Wr^a$ are generally viewed to be clinically significant, inasmuch as all have been described to cause severe HTR and HDN.
- Anti-$Yt^a$ is a fairly common antibody that is associated with mild HTR.
- The $Xg^a$ antigen is found on the petite arm of the X chromosome and is noted with higher frequency in females than in males.
- The Scianna system (SC) is composed of the antithetical Sc1 and Sc2 antigens as well as the high-incidence Sc3 antigen, which is present on all Sc1 and/or Sc2 positive cells.
- The rare null phenotype in the SC system has been observed only in the Marshall Islands and New Guinea.
- In addition to the $Do^a$ and $Do^b$ antigens, the $Gy^a$, Hy, and $Jo^a$ antigens have been assigned to the Dombrock system (DO).
- Antibodies to the DO antigens have occasionally been described to cause moderate HTR.
- The Colton system (CO) is composed of the antithetical $Co^a$ and $Co^b$ antigens as well as the high-frequency Co3 antigen, which is present on all $Co^a$-positive and/or $Co^b$-positive cells.
- The rare antibodies in the CO system have been associated with causing mild HTR and HDN.
- The nine antigens in the Chido/Rodgers system are located on the complement fragments, C4B and C4A, respectively.
- The clinically insignificant CH and RG antibodies present with weak and "nebulous" reactivity at IAT and may be identified by plasma inhibition methods and adsorption with C4-coated cells.
- The eleven Cromer antigens are carried on the decay accelerating factor (DAF) and are distributed in body fluids and on red cells, white cells, platelets, and placental tissue.
- The rare anti-CROM antibodies have been noted only on black individuals and associated with mild HTR.
- In addition to the $Kn^a$ and $Kn^b$ antigens, the $McC^a$, Yk, and $Sl^a$ antigens have been assigned to the Knops system (KN).
- The KN antigens are located on complement receptor 1 (CR1) with expression being depressed by the $In(Lu)$ gene and autoimmune disease.
- The clinically insignificant KN antibodies present with weak and "nebulous" reactivity at IAT.
- The $In^a$ antigen is more prevalent in Arab and Iranian populations, with $In^a$ and $In^b$ antigen expression being depressed by the $In(Lu)$ gene.
- Antibodies directed against the Vel antigen have occasionally been described to cause hemolysis in the test tube and severe hemolytic reactions.
- Anti-$Sd^a$ antibodies present with weak reactivity at IAT, which appears shiny and refractile under the microscope and may be inhibited with Sd-positive urine.
- $Bg^a$, $Bg^b$, and $Bg^c$ white cell antigens correspond with the class I HLA antigens B-7, B-17, and A-28, respectively.
- The clinically insignificant anti-Bg antibodies present with weak and variable reactivity at IAT, which may be destroyed by chloroquine treatment.

## REVIEW QUESTIONS

1. Which blood group system is under control of a gene located on the petite (short) arm of the X chromosome?
   A. GE
   B. DI
   C. YT
   D. XG

2. Which of the following presents with depressed or absent antigen expression due to the $In(Lu)$ regulator gene?
   A. GE and DI
   B. KN and IN
   C. CROM and CH/RG
   D. IN and GE

3. Mutations in the carrier molecule for this blood

group system may result in changes of red blood cell shape in the forms of elliptocytosis, acanthocytosis, or ovalocytosis.
A. DI
B. DO
C. CO
D. SC

4. According to the red blood cell surface antigen terminology by ISBT, all authenticated antigens may be assigned to a blood group system, provided they are:
A. Controlled by a single gene or by two closely linked genes
B. Inherited from multiple regulator genes
C. Shown not to follow mendelian principles
D. Shown to share serologic characteristics with other members of the blood group system

5. The antibody to this red cell antigen in the 901 series demonstrates mixed-field agglutination that appears shiny and refractile under the microscope.
A. Vel
B. JMH
C. Lan
D. Sd$^a$

6. The antibody to this red cell antigen in the 901 series has been associated with causing severe immediate hemolytic transfusion reactions.
A. Anti-JMH
B. Anti-Bg$^a$
C. Anti-Vel
D. Anti-Sd$^a$

7. Which of the following antibodies is directed toward HLA antigens and may be inactivated by chloroquine treatment?
A. Anti-Ch2
B. Anti-Yk$^a$
C. Anti-Bg$^a$
D. Anti-Kn$^b$

8. The most useful methods for rapidly identifying antibodies in the CH/RG blood group system are:
A. Prewarmed technique and titration studies
B. Plasma inhibition and adsorption with C4-coated cells
C. DTT and chloroquine treatment
D. Trypsin and chymotrypsin treatment

9. The following antibodies are generally viewed to be clinically insignificant because they have not been associated with causing increased destruction of red cells, HDN, or hemolytic transfusion reactions.
A. Anti-Do$^a$ and anti-Co$^a$
B. Anti-Ge3 and anti-Wr$^a$
C. Anti-Ch2 and anti-Kn$^a$
D. Anti-Di$^b$ and anti-Yt$^a$

10. Match the system name from column II with the correct antibody in column I.

| Column I | Column II |
|---|---|
| 1. Anti-Ch3 | A. Chido/Rodgers |
| 2. Anti-Yt$^b$ | B. Knops |
| 3. Anti-Di$^a$ | C. XG |
| 4. Anti-Xg$^a$ | D. Scianna |
| 5. Anti-McC$^a$ | E. Cartwright |
| 6. Anti-Sc2 | F. Diego |
| 7. Anti-Co$^b$ | G. Colton |
| 8. Anti-Ge3 | H. Dombrock |
| 9. Anti-Yk$^a$ | I. Gerbich |
| 10. Anti-Wr$^b$ | |

## ANSWERS TO REVIEW QUESTIONS

1. D (p 205)
2. B (p 208)
3. A (pp 201, 203)
4. A (pp 201–203)
5. D (p 204, Table 9–3)
6. C (p 204, Table 9–3)
7. C (p 209)
8. B (p 207)
9. C (pp 207, 208)
10. A = 1 (p 206)
    E = 2 (pp 204–205)
    F = 3 (p 201)
    C = 4 (p 205)
    B = 5 (p 208)
    D = 6 (p 205)
    G = 7 (p 206)
    I = 8 (p 207)
    B = 9 (p 208)
    F = 10 (p 201)

## REFERENCES

1. Daniels, J, et al: Blood group terminology 1995, from the ISBT working party on terminology for red cell surface antigens. Vox Sang 69:265, 1995.
2. Issit, PD, and Moulds, JJ: Blood group terminology suitable for use in electronic data processing equipment. Transfusion 32:7, 1992.
3. Lewis, M, et al: Blood group terminology 1990, from the ISBT working party on terminology for red cell surface antigens. Vox Sang 58, 1990.
4. Reid, M, and Francis-Lomas, C: The Blood Group Antigen Facts Book. Academic Press, New York, 1997.
5. Levine, P, et al: The Diego blood factor. Nature 77, 1956.
6. Layrisse, M, and Arend, T: The Diego blood factor in Chinese and Japanese. Nature 77, 1956.
7. Bruce, LJ, et al: Band 3 Memphis variant II: Altered stilbene disul-

fonate binding and the Diego (Di[a]) blood group antigen are associated with the human erythrocyte band 3 mutation Pro → Leu. J Biol Chem 269, 1994.

8. Silberstein, LS, (ed): Molecular and Functional Aspects of Blood Group Antigens. American Association of Blood Banks. Bethesda, MD, 1995.

9. Jarolim, P, et al: Mutations conserved arginines in the membrane domain of erythroid band 3 lead to a decrease in membrane-associated band 3 and to the phenotype of hereditary spherocytosis. Blood 85, 1995.

10. Bruce, LJ: Band 3HT, a human red-cell variant associated with acanthocytosis and increased anion transport carries the mutation Pro → Leu in the membrane domain of band 3. Biochem J 293, 1993.

11. Schofield, AE, et al: Basis of unique red cell membrane properties in hereditary spherocytosis. J Mol Biol 223, 1992.

12. Holman, CA: A rare new blood group antigen (Wr[a]). Lancet, 2:119, 1953.

13. Bruce, LJ, et al: Changes in the blood group Wright antigens are associated with a mutation at amino acid 658 in human erythrocyte band 3: A site of interaction between band 3 and glycophorin A under certain conditions. Blood 85, 1995.

14. Jarolim, P, et al: Molecular basis of Rb[a], Tr[a], and Wd[a]. Transfusion 37, 1997.

15. Eaton, BR, et al: A new antibody, anti-Yt[a], characterizing a blood group antigen of high incidence. Br J Haematol 2:333, 1956.

16. Mazzi, G, et al: Presence of anti-Yt[a] antibody in a Yt(a+) patient. Vox Sang 66, 1994.

17. Spring, FA, Gardner, B, and Anstee, DJ: Evidence that the antigens of the Yt blood group system are located on human erythrocyte acetylcholinesterase. Blood 80:21, 1992.

18. Giles, CM, et al: A family showing independent segregation of Bu[a] and Yt[b]. Vox Sang 18:265, 1970.

19. Mann, J, et al: A sex-linked blood group. Lancet 1:8, 1962.

20. Cook IA, et al: A second example of anti-Xg[a]. Lancet i:857, 1963.

21. Sausais, L, et al: Characteristic of a third example of Anti-Xg[a] (abstract). Transfusion 4:312, 1964.

22. Yokoyama, M, et al: The first example of autoanti-Xg[a]. Vox Sang 12:198, 1967.

23. Scholossman, SF, et al: CD antigens. Blood 83, 1994.

24. Lewis, M, Chown, B, and Kaita, H: On blood group antigens Bu(a) and Sm. Transfusion 7:92, 1967.

25. Schmidt, PR, Griffitts, JJ, and Northam, FF: A new antibody anti-Sm, reacting with a high incidence antigen. Cited by Race, RR, and Sanger, R, 1962.

26. Anderson, C, et al: An antibody defining a new blood group antigen, Bu[a]. Transfusion 3:30, 1963.

27. McCreary, J, et al: Another minus-minus phenotype: Bu(a−): two examples in one family (abstract). Transfusion 13:350, 1973.

28. Nason, SG, et al: A high incidence antibody (anti-Sc3) in the serum of a SC: −1, −2 patient. Transfusion 20:531–535, 1980.

29. Swanson, JL, et al: A "new" blood group antigen, Do[a]. Nature 206:313, 1965.

30. Molthan, L, et al: Enlargement of the Dombrock blood group system: The finding of anti-Do[b]. Vox Sang 24:382, 1973.

31. Banks, JA, Hemming, M, and Poole, J: Evidence that the Gy[a], Hy and Jo[a] antigens belong to the Dombrock blood group system. Vox Sang 68, 1995.

32. Halverson, G, et al: The first reported case of anti-Do[b] causing an acute hemolytic transfusion reaction. Vox Sang 66, 1994.

33. Heisto, H, et al: Three examples of a red cell antibody, anti-Co[a]. Vox Sang 12:18, 1967.

34. Giles, CM, et al: Identification of the first example of anti-Co[b]. Br J Haematol 19:267, 1970.

35. De la Chapelle, A, et al: Monosomy-7 and the Colton blood groups. Lancet 2:817, 1975.

36. Parsons, SF, et al: A novel form of congenital dyserythropoietic

anemia associated with deficiency of erythroid CD44 and a unique blood group phenotype [In(a−b−), Co(a−b−)]. Blood 83, 1994.

37. Hoffman, JJML, and Overbeeke, MAM: Characteristics of anti-Co[b] in vitro and in vivo: A case study. Immunohematology 1:12, 1996.

38. Westhoff, CM, et al: Severe anaphylactic reactions following transfusions of platelets to a patient with anti-Ch. Transfusion 6:32, 1992.

39. Moulds, JM, and Laird-Fryer, B (eds): Blood Groups: Chido/Rodgers, Knops/McCoy/York and Cromer. American Association of Blood Banks, Bethesda, MD, 1992.

40. Harris, JP, et al: A nebulous antibody responsible for cross-matching difficulties (Chido). Vox Sang 30, 1967.

41. Middleton, J, and Crookston, MC: Chido substance in plasma. Vox Sang 12, 1972.

42. Longster, G, and Giles, CM: A new antibody specificity: Anti-Rg[a] reacting with a red cell and serum antigen. Vox Sang 30, 1976.

43. O'Neil, GJ, et al: Chido and Rodgers blood groups are distinct antigenic components of human complement C4. Nature 273, 1978.

44. Tilley, CA, et al: Localization of Chido and Rodgers determinants to the C4d fragment of human C4. Nature 273, 1978.

45. Moulds, JM: Incidence of Rodgers-negative individuals in systemic lupus erythematosus patients. Immunohematology 4:6, 1990.

46. Judd, JW, et al: The rapid identification of Chido and Rodgers antibodies using C4d-coated red blood cells. Transfusion 21, 1981.

47. Rosenfield, RE, et al: Ge, a very common red cell antigen. Br J Haemat 6, 1960.

48. Barnes, R, and Lewis, TLT: A fourth example of anti-Ge. Lancet 2, 1961.

49. Reid, ME, and Spring, FA: Molecular basis of glycophorin C variants and their associated blood group antigens. Transfus Med 4, 1994.

50. Telen, MJ, et al: Molecular basis for elliptocytosis associated with glycophorin C and D deficiency in the Leach phenotype. Blood 78, 1991.

51. Stroup, M, and McCreay, J: Cr[a], another high frequency blood group factor (abstract). Transfusion 15, 1975.

52. Helgeson, M, et al: Knops-Helgeson (Kn[a]): A high-frequency erythrocyte antigen. Transfusion 10, 1970.

53. Daniels, GL, et al: The effect of In(Lu) on some high frequency antigens. Transfusion 26, 1986.

54. Rolih, S: A review: Antibodies with high titer, low-avidity characteristics. Immunohematology 3:6, 1990.

55. Ahearn, JM, and Fearon, DT: Structure and function of the complement receptor, CR1 (CD35) and CR2 (CD21). Adv Immunol 46, 1989.

56. Ross, GD, et al: Disease-associated loss of erythrocyte complement receptors (CR1, C3b receptors) in patients with systemic lupus erythematosus and other diseases involving autoantibodies and/or complement activation. J Immunol 135, 1985.

57. Badakere, SS, et al: Evidence of a new blood group antigen in the Indian population (a preliminary report). Ind J Med Res 62, 1973.

58. Mollison, PL, et al: Blood Transfusion in Clinical Medicine, ed 9. Blackwell Scientific, Oxford, 1993.

59. Seaman, MJ, et al: The reactions of the Bennett-Goodspeed group of antibodies with 380: The autoanalyzer. Br J Haematol 13:464, 1967.

60. Organon Teknika package insert for Human Platelet Concentrate (HPC), Durham, NC, 1992.

61. Moulds, JM, and Masouredis, S (eds): Monoclonal Antibodies. American Association of Blood Banks, Arlington, VA, 1989.

62. Morton, JA, et al: Changes in red cell Bg antigens in haematological disease. Immunology Communications 9:173, 1980.

# PROCEDURAL APPENDIX

### Plasma Inhibition Studies*

*Materials and Methods*

   Sera (plasmas) and cells: unknown patient serum, indicator cells (screening cells) Chido-Rodgers positive plasma: Ch(a+) Rg(a+) plasma, Ch(a+) Rg(a−) plasma

1. Set up two sets of each of the following mixtures and incubate at room temperature for 15 minutes:
   A. 2 drops unknown serum, 1 drop Ch(a+) Rg(a−) plasma
   B. 2 drops unknown serum, 1 drop Ch(a−) Rg(a+) plasma
   C. 2 drops unknown serum, 1 drop Ch(a+) Rg(a+) plasma
2. Incubate a set of selected screening cells with the foregoing three mixtures for 60 minutes at 37°C. Wash three times with saline and convert to the antihuman globulin test.
3. If multiple alloantibodies are suspected after the previous results are obtained, test a complete genotyped panel of donors with the appropriate mixture.

*Interpretation of Results*

1. If mixture A is reactive with both screening cells and mixtures B and C are nonreactive, the antibody is anti-Rg$^a$ and no other alloantibodies are detected in the unknown serum.
2. If mixture B is reactive and mixtures A and C are nonreactive with the screening cells, the antibody is anti-Ch$^a$ and no other alloantibodies are detected in the unknown serum.
3. If mixture C is reactive and either mixture A or mixture B is nonreactive, it could mean that there is not sufficient quantity of Ch$^a$ or Rg$^a$ substance in the Ch$^a$- or Rg$^a$-positive plasma to inhibit the antibody but that there is enough in mixture A or mixture B plasma to inhibit the antibody.
4. If all three mixtures are nonreactive, the serum antibody is too weak to allow dilution studies.
5. If one screening cell is negative and the other positive with any of the mixtures, then anti-Ch$^a$ and anti-Rg$^a$ and a second or third antibody may be present in the serum. The appropriate mixtures should then be incubated with a panel of selected genotyped cells.

*From Moulds, MK: Serological investigation and clinical significance of high-titered, low-avidity (HTLA) antibodies. Am J Med Tech 10:794, 1981, with permission.

# CHAPTER 10

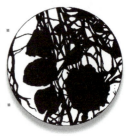

# DONOR SELECTION AND COMPONENT PREPARATION

Patricia A. Wright, BA, MT(ASCP)SBB, and
Virginia C. Hughes, MS, MT(ASCP)

## OBJECTIVES

*On completion of this chapter, the learner should be able to:*

1. Identify the demographic information required from every prospective blood donor to ensure adequate identification.

2. Give the minimum acceptable levels for the following tests, for both allogeneic and autologous donors:
   a. Weight
   b. Temperature
   c. Pulse
   d. Blood pressure
   e. Hemoglobin
   f. Hematocrit

3. Select an acceptable allogeneic blood donor when given the results of the physical examination and medical history.

4. State the medical history information that would be cause for permanent, indefinite deferral.

5. Identify information that would be cause for temporary deferral, and state the length of time for the deferral.

6. List the special medical history and physical examination information required of a pheresis donor.

7. Explain the four major types of autologous blood donation procedures.

8. State the procedure for performing a whole blood donor phlebotomy, including arm preparation, blood collection, and postphlebotomy care instructions for the donor.

9. Recognize a donor reaction; identify the difference between mild, moderate, and severe reactions; and state the recommended treatments for each.

10. List the 10 tests that are required to be performed on all allogeneic blood donor units.

11. List the information that is required to be on the blood unit label.

12. Identify the primary ingredient, storage conditions, shelf life, quality control requirements, and indications for use for each of the following blood components:
   a. Red blood cells
   b. Leukocyte-reduced red blood cells
   c. Washed red blood cells
   d. Frozen, deglycerolized red blood cells
   e. Platelet concentrates (random, single donor)
   f. Single-donor plasma (fresh frozen, frozen within 24 hours, liquid, frozen)
   g. Cryoprecipitate concentrate
   h. Granulocyte concentrate
   i. Factor VIII concentrates
   j. Factor IX concentrates
   k. Rh immunoglobulin
   l. Plasma derivatives (immune serum globulin, plasma protein fraction, normal serum albumin, volume expanders)

## DONOR SELECTION

The process of blood donor selection is designed to provide the blood bank with the answers to two major questions: (1) Will a donation of approximately 450 mL of whole blood at this time be harmful to the donor? (2) Could blood drawn from this donor at this time potentially transmit a disease to the recipient? If the answer to each of these questions is no, the donation can proceed. If the answer to either question is yes, the donor must be deferred either temporarily or indefinitely, depending on the circumstances.

The following are the guidelines established by the blood banking community, which are considered to be the minimum acceptable standards. They are designed to protect both the donor and the public.

### Registration Information and General Requirements

Each donor must be clearly and uniquely identified so that a specific donor can be traced through the entire process and, if necessary, recalled.[1] Please note the top section of the donor card (Fig. 10–1). This demographics section of the donor card is designed to fulfill the identification and recall requirements. The following data are required:

1. **Donor's name.** First name, last name, and middle initial are needed.
2. **Donor's address and phone number.** If the donor works outside the home, it is helpful to have the business address and phone number also.
3. **Gender.**
4. **Date of birth and age.** Prospective donors must be at least 17 years of age. The minimum age limit may be exempted for autologous blood donors. This exception should be determined by the blood bank medical director and then stated in writing in the facility's procedure manual. In some states donors between 17 and 21 years of age may, by law, be considered minors and therefore require parental permission before donation. Check individual state laws. There is no longer an upper age limit for blood donors. Any individual who is in good health and meets all the other donor requirements may donate.
5. **Date of donation.**
6. **Donor's consent.** The donor must provide written, informed consent for the blood bank to take and use his or her blood; the consent must be obtained before the donation. All aspects of the do-

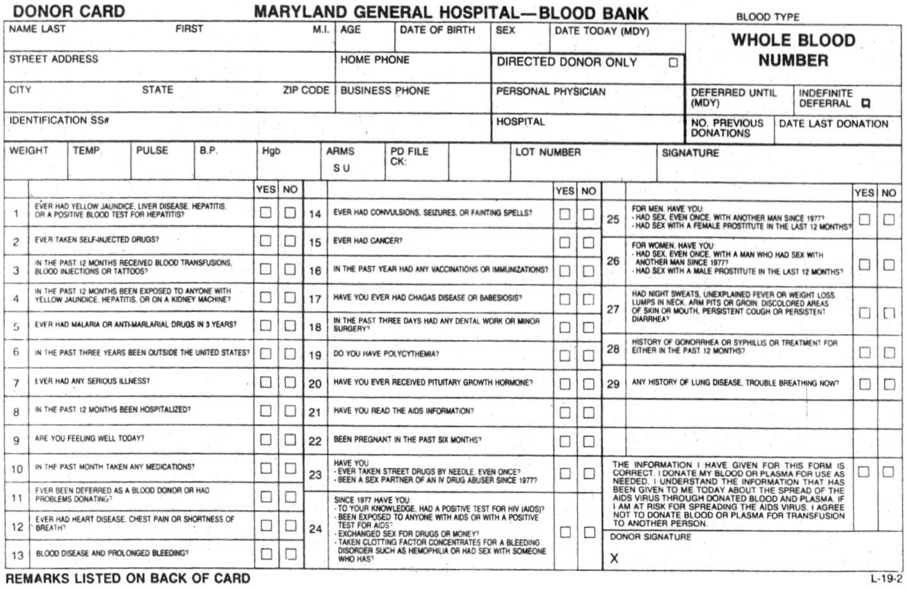

DONOR CARD MARYLAND GENERAL HOSPITAL—BLOOD BANK

BLOOD TYPE

NAME LAST | FIRST | M.I. | AGE | DATE OF BIRTH | SEX | DATE TODAY (MDY) | WHOLE BLOOD NUMBER

STREET ADDRESS | HOME PHONE | DIRECTED DONOR ONLY ☐

CITY | STATE | ZIP CODE | BUSINESS PHONE | PERSONAL PHYSICIAN | DEFERRED UNTIL (MDY) | INDEFINITE DEFERRAL ☐

IDENTIFICATION SS# | HOSPITAL | NO. PREVIOUS DONATIONS | DATE LAST DONATION

WEIGHT | TEMP. | PULSE | B.P. | Hgb | ARMS S U | PD FILE CK: | LOT NUMBER | SIGNATURE

| | | YES | NO | | | YES | NO | | | YES | NO |
|---|---|---|---|---|---|---|---|---|---|---|---|
| 1 | EVER HAD YELLOW JAUNDICE, LIVER DISEASE, HEPATITIS, OR A POSITIVE BLOOD TEST FOR HEPATITIS? | ☐ | ☐ | 14 | EVER HAD CONVULSIONS, SEIZURES, OR FAINTING SPELLS? | ☐ | ☐ | 25 | FOR MEN, HAVE YOU: - HAD SEX, EVEN ONCE, WITH ANOTHER MAN SINCE 1977? - HAD SEX WITH A FEMALE PROSTITUTE IN THE LAST 12 MONTHS? | ☐ | ☐ |
| 2 | EVER TAKEN SELF-INJECTED DRUGS? | ☐ | ☐ | 15 | EVER HAD CANCER? | ☐ | ☐ | 26 | FOR WOMEN, HAVE YOU: - HAD SEX, EVEN ONCE, WITH A MAN WHO HAD SEX WITH ANOTHER MAN SINCE 1977? - HAD SEX WITH A MALE PROSTITUTE IN THE LAST 12 MONTHS? | ☐ | ☐ |
| 3 | IN THE PAST 12 MONTHS RECEIVED BLOOD TRANSFUSIONS, BLOOD INJECTIONS OR TATTOOS? | ☐ | ☐ | 16 | IN THE PAST YEAR HAD ANY VACCINATIONS OR IMMUNIZATIONS? | ☐ | ☐ | | | | |
| 4 | IN THE PAST 12 MONTHS BEEN EXPOSED TO ANYONE WITH YELLOW JAUNDICE, HEPATITIS, OR ON A KIDNEY MACHINE? | ☐ | ☐ | 17 | HAVE YOU EVER HAD CHAGAS DISEASE OR BABESIOSIS? | ☐ | ☐ | 27 | HAD NIGHT SWEATS, UNEXPLAINED FEVER OR WEIGHT LOSS, LUMPS IN NECK, ARM PITS OR GROIN, DISCOLORED AREAS OF SKIN OR MOUTH, PERSISTENT COUGH OR PERSISTENT DIARRHEA? | ☐ | ☐ |
| 5 | EVER HAD MALARIA OR ANTI-MARLARIAL DRUGS IN 3 YEARS? | ☐ | ☐ | 18 | IN THE PAST THREE DAYS HAD ANY DENTAL WORK OR MINOR SURGERY? | ☐ | ☐ | | | | |
| 6 | IN THE PAST THREE YEARS BEEN OUTSIDE THE UNITED STATES? | ☐ | ☐ | 19 | DO YOU HAVE POLYCYTHEMIA? | ☐ | ☐ | 28 | HISTORY OF GONORRHEA OR SYPHILLIS OR TREATMENT FOR EITHER IN THE PAST 12 MONTHS? | ☐ | ☐ |
| 7 | EVER HAD ANY SERIOUS ILLNESS? | ☐ | ☐ | 20 | HAVE YOU EVER RECEIVED PITUITARY GROWTH HORMONE? | ☐ | ☐ | 29 | ANY HISTORY OF LUNG DISEASE, TROUBLE BREATHING NOW? | ☐ | ☐ |
| 8 | IN THE PAST 12 MONTHS BEEN HOSPITALIZED? | ☐ | ☐ | 21 | HAVE YOU READ THE AIDS INFORMATION? | ☐ | ☐ | | | | |
| 9 | ARE YOU FEELING WELL TODAY? | ☐ | ☐ | 22 | BEEN PREGNANT IN THE PAST SIX MONTHS? | ☐ | ☐ | | | | |
| 10 | IN THE PAST MONTH TAKEN ANY MEDICATIONS? | ☐ | ☐ | 23 | HAVE YOU - EVER TAKEN STREET DRUGS BY NEEDLE, EVEN ONCE? - BEEN A SEX PARTNER OF AN IV DRUG ABUSER SINCE 1977? | ☐ | ☐ | | THE INFORMATION I HAVE GIVEN FOR THIS FORM IS CORRECT. I DONATE MY BLOOD OR PLASMA FOR USE AS NEEDED. I UNDERSTAND THE INFORMATION THAT HAS BEEN GIVEN TO ME TODAY ABOUT THE SPREAD OF THE AIDS VIRUS THROUGH DONATED BLOOD AND PLASMA. IF I AM AT RISK FOR SPREADING THE AIDS VIRUS, I AGREE NOT TO DONATE BLOOD OR PLASMA FOR TRANSFUSION TO ANOTHER PERSON. | ☐ | ☐ |
| 11 | EVER BEEN DEFERRED AS A BLOOD DONOR OR HAD PROBLEMS DONATING? | ☐ | ☐ | 24 | SINCE 1977 HAVE YOU: - TO YOUR KNOWLEDGE, HAD A POSITIVE TEST FOR HIV (AIDS)? - BEEN EXPOSED TO ANYONE WITH AIDS OR WITH A POSITIVE TEST FOR AIDS? - EXCHANGED SEX FOR DRUGS OR MONEY? - TAKEN CLOTTING FACTOR CONCENTRATES FOR A BLEEDING DISORDER SUCH AS HEMOPHILIA OR HAD SEX WITH SOMEONE WHO HAS? | ☐ | ☐ | | DONOR SIGNATURE X | | |
| 12 | EVER HAD HEART DISEASE, CHEST PAIN OR SHORTNESS OF BREATH? | ☐ | ☐ | | | | | | | | |
| 13 | BLOOD DISEASE AND PROLONGED BLEEDING? | ☐ | ☐ | | | | | | | | |

REMARKS LISTED ON BACK OF CARD

L-19-2

**Figure 10–1.** Front of the donor history card for allogenic donation. (Courtesy Maryland General Hospital, Baltimore.)

nation procedure must be explained in terms that the donor can understand, including information on significant risks in the procedure and any tests that will be performed on the donated unit. The donor should be given the opportunity to ask questions about the procedure and to refuse consent. Informed consent for a minor must be in accordance with applicable state laws.[2]

Although not required by the American Association of Blood Banks (AABB) standards, the following information may be useful to have as part of the donor record:

7. **Additional identification.** Social security or driver's license number is good because each is a unique number and most donors have one or the other.
8. **Donor's occupation.** Donors with hazardous jobs or activities (e.g., police officers, firefighters, pilots, heavy machinery operators, runners) need to be informed and cautioned concerning safe return to their full range of job activities.
9. **Time of last meal.** It is better that a donor not be fasting at the time of donation. If it has been longer than 4 hours since the last meal, the donor should be given something to eat and drink before the donation.
10. **Race.** It may prove useful later to know the racial origin of the donor when screening for some phenotypes (e.g., Lewis or Duffy negatives).
11. **Intended recipient, replacement credit, donor group.** Many blood donations are designated by the donor for a specific donor group or patient. When this occurs, it is important to obtain the patient or credit information to ensure proper crediting. Even if the donor is rejected or deferred, the information may still be useful or necessary. Any of the following information may be needed: (1) patient name and hospital, (2) patient identification or hospital number, or (3) donor group name.

## Physical Examination

A brief physical examination is required and is primarily designed to ensure the donor's safety. The elements of the examination should rule out or defer any donor whose physical condition is such that a blood donation at this time could be detrimental. It must be done on the day of donation and is generally performed at the time of donation along with the medical history.

1. **General appearance.** The donor should be in good health. If there are signs of alcohol or drug intoxication or obvious symptoms of a cold or other infection or disease, the donor should be deferred.
2. **Weight: 110 lb (50 kg).** The donation of a unit of blood should not exceed approximately 10 percent of the donor's blood volume. This means that for the standard donation of 525 mL, including pilot tubes, the donor should weigh at least 110 lb (50 kg). Blood can be drawn from donors who weigh less than 110 lb, provided the amount of blood collected is proportionately reduced. If less than 300 mL is to be drawn, the amount of anticoagulant in the bag must be reduced accordingly. The following formulas can be used to calculate the amount of anticoagulant to be removed from the primary bag.
   a. Amount of blood to be drawn

$$\frac{\text{Donor's weight (lb)} \times 450 \text{ mL}}{110 \text{ lb}} = \text{Allowable amount(mL)}$$

b. Amount of anticoagulant needed

$$\frac{\text{Allowable amount}}{100} \times 14 = \text{Anticoagulant needed(mL)}$$

c. Amount of anticoagulant to remove

63 mL—anticoagulant (mL) = Anticoagulant to remove(mL)

For institutions that routinely want or need to draw blood from donors weighing less than 110 lb and that have a need for low-volume units of blood, donor bags are available that are designed to draw 150 mL or 250 mL rather than 450 mL.

3. **Temperature: Orally should not exceed (99.5°F 37.5°C).** The purpose of determining the donor's temperature is to eliminate any donor who may have an infection or disease that may be transmissible through the donated blood. Fever is a symptom of infection. There is no low-temperature limit because a low temperature is most frequently caused by cold environmental temperatures and is rarely associated with disease.[3] Care should be taken to ensure that sufficient time has elapsed since eating, drinking, or smoking so that the temperature reading will not be affected.

4. **Pulse: 50 to 100 beats per minute.** The pulse should be checked for at least 30 seconds, and if there is any doubt about the rate or rhythm, assessment should be extended to a full minute. Pulse rates greater than 100 beats per minute must be further evaluated. Increased pulse rates may be caused by physiologic factors such as anxiety, fear, or recent physical exercise. Allow the donor to relax for 10 to 15 minutes, then check the pulse again for a full minute. If it is still elevated, consult the blood bank medical director or defer the donor, or both.

Pulse rates of less than 50 beats per minute may frequently occur in athletes who have a high tolerance to exercise (e.g., marathon runners, professional ball players). A statement indicating the athletic activity and its frequency should be made a part of the permanent donor record. Any irregularities in heart rhythm should be cause for deferral.

5. **Blood pressure: Systolic no greater than 180 mm Hg, diastolic no greater than 100 mm Hg.** Donors with pressure readings higher than these limits must be evaluated by the blood bank medical director before being accepted.

6. **Hematocrit and hemoglobin: 38 percent (12.5 g/dL), venipuncture or fingerstick.** Although determination of either hemoglobin (Hb) or hematocrit (Hct) is acceptable, large donor collection sites will probably prefer the hemoglobin determination using a copper sulfate ($CuSO_4$) method. This method uses the principle that a drop of whole blood, when dropped into a solution of $CuSO_4$, which has a given specific gravity, will maintain its own density for approximately 15 seconds. The density of the drop is directly proportional to the amount of hemoglobin in that drop. If the drop is denser than the specific gravity of the solution, the drop sinks to the bottom; if not, it floats on top. The test solution should have a specific gravity of 1.053. This is not a quantitative test, but it is quick, easy, and quite accurate for screening donors. If a donor fails this procedure or there is a question concerning the results, it is advisable to confirm the results with a microhematocrit. Hemoglobin levels can also be determined using spectrophotometric methods, which are very accurate but more expensive. Several small, portable, easy-to-use hemoglobinometers are available that are well suited for mobile operation use. Smaller donor operations—fewer than 10 to 20 donors per day—may still elect to use a microhematocrit method because at that level it is the cheapest method.

7. **Skin lesions, arm check.** The antecubital area of both arms must be inspected for evidence of habitual drug use or the presence of skin eruptions such as poison ivy, rash, or psoriasis. If there is evidence of self-injected drug use that the donor does not adequately explain, the donor must be indefinitely deferred. There is an extremely high risk of hepatitis and human immunodeficiency virus (HIV) infection in abusers of self-injected drugs. If there is evidence of a rash or infection at the phlebotomy site, the donor must be deferred until the problem has cleared up. This is to help protect both the donor and the donated unit from contamination.

8. **Review of permanent deferral file.** All donors must be checked against a file of indefinitely deferred donors. This check must be performed at some time before the release of the unit from quarantine to distribution.

## Medical History

The medical history is both fact finding and diagnostic. Its purpose is to obtain a profile of the prospective donor's health status to determine his or her suitability for donating blood.[4] The questions are designed to determine whether the donation might be harmful to the donor or whether the blood obtained might transmit disease. The questions should be phrased so that the donor can answer with a simple "yes" or "no" that can be elaborated on if necessary.

The interviewer should be familiar with the questions so that he or she can observe the donor during the interview, be aware of the donor's body postures and facial expressions, and be ready to elaborate on any question if the donor seems not to understand it.

The medical history must be performed on the day of donation and is usually performed at the same time as the physical examination. The interview must be conducted in a somewhat secluded place that has few distractions and permits privacy. It is recognized that the safety of the country's blood supply is critically tied to the quality and effectiveness of the predonation donor medical history. In response to this, the American Association of Blood Banks (AABB) Ad Hoc Committee on Donor History/Interview Process has developed a uniform set of questions that everyone can use and that ensures adherence to both the AABB standards and the Food and Drug Administration (FDA) regulations and recommendations. It is hoped that the use of these questions will help ensure that the donor history is comprehensive, understandable, and dependable to the degree that that is possible[5]:

1. **Have you ever had jaundice, liver disease, hepatitis, or a positive test result for hepatitis? In the past 12 months, have you received blood or had an organ or tissue transplant? In the past 12 months, have you had a tattoo, ear or skin piercing, acupuncture, or an accidental needlestick? In the past 12 months, have you had close contact with a person with jaundice or hepatitis, or have you been given hepatitis B immunoglobulin (HBIg)? Have you ever used a needle, even once, to take any drug (including steroids)?**

All of these questions are considered "hepatitis questions." Laboratory tests are not 100 percent effective in eliminating units of blood that are capable of transmitting viral hepatitis. The medical history cannot completely eliminate the hazard either, but in combination with sensitive testing methods and an emphasis on volunteer donors, the risk has been significantly reduced. (Donors with a history of abuse of self-injected drugs are also at high risk for HIV infection.)

A donor must be indefinitely or permanently deferred if he or she:

a. Gives a history of viral hepatitis after the 11th birthday
b. Currently has or previously has had a confirmed positive test result for hepatitis B surface antigen (HBsAg)
c. Has had more than one reactive test result for hepatitis B core antibody (anti-HBc)
d. Has present or past evidence (either clinical or laboratory) of hepatitis C infection
e. Indicates past or present abuse of self-injected drugs
f. Was the donor of the only unit involved in documented case of posttransfusion hepatitis

A 12-month deferral is given to a potential donor who has had close contact with someone who has hepatitis. "Close contact" is defined as sharing the same household, kitchen, or bathroom facilities. This may include a student living in a dormitory where several cases of hepatitis have occurred or any person who is institutionalized in a prison, psychiatric hospital, or institution for the retarded. It does not routinely apply to hospital personnel performing normal duties, but care should be taken to ensure that hospital workers are aware of and follow infection and body fluid precaution protocols (gloves, gowns, and masks as appropri-

ate). Guidelines for the selection or deferment of personnel working in dialysis centers or units must be defined by the blood bank medical director.

Donors who have received blood transfusions or injections of blood or blood products, an organ or tissue transplant (including skin allografts), a tattoo, ear or other skin piercing, acupuncture, or an accidental needlestick injury should also be deferred from allogeneic donation for 12 months.

There is a 12-month deferral also for any donor who has received HBIg because HBIg is given for exposure to possible infection and it may delay the onset of symptoms of disease. Receipt of hepatitis B vaccine is, however, not a cause for deferral. The vaccine is now generally made from recombinant material and is given prophylactically, not as a result of exposure.

2. **In the past 3 years, have you had malaria or taken antimalarial drugs? In the past 3 years, have you been outside the United States or Canada?**

Malaria parasites reproduce in the red blood cells (RBCs) and can remain in the blood and tissues for years. After the initial infection, some people develop a chronic infection, characterized by periodic relapses.[6] Prospective donors who have had malaria or have been treated for malaria must be deferred for 3 years following therapy or departure from the endemic area, or both. They must remain asymptomatic and not take antimalarial drugs during the 3-year period.

Visitors, immigrants, or refugees from an area considered to be endemic for malaria by the Centers for Disease Control (CDC) Malaria Programs must be deferred for 3 years after departure from the area and must remain asymptomatic and not take antimalarial drugs for that period.

Donors who have traveled to areas considered endemic for malaria are deferred for 12 months after departure from the area, provided that they remain asymptomatic and have not taken antimalarial drugs. It is not necessary to defer a donor who has started antimalarial therapy in preparation for travel but who has not yet been to the endemic area.[7]

3. **In the past 12 months, have you been under a doctor's care or had a major illness or surgery?**

A "yes" answer here requires the interviewer to investigate further. Prospective donors who have recently undergone surgical procedures need to be evaluated to identify those who received blood or blood product (except Rh immune globulin) transfusions at the time. A blood transfusion requires a 12-month deferral owing to the risk of exposure to hepatitis, HIV, or other viral disease. Surgical procedures that are uncomplicated and do not require any blood transfusions are cause for deferral only until healing is complete and the donor has resumed his or her full range of activity.[8]

Any indication that a biopsy was performed should be evaluated further, inasmuch as a large number of patients with acquired immunodeficiency syndrome (AIDS) or AIDS-related complex (ARC) have had lymph node biopsies.[9] If the biopsy findings indicate or suggest either of these diagnoses, the donor must be deferred indefinitely. A person who has been hospitalized for AIDS or AIDS-related diseases must be deferred permanently.

### 4. Are you feeling well and healthy today?

The prospective donor should be in general good health and free from any acute upper respiratory infection or disease. Donors who have active cold or flu symptoms must be deferred until the symptoms are gone. Be aware that many people take over-the-counter medications that mask or eliminate the signs and symptoms of colds and flu. Remember also that some sore throats and nasal stuffiness may be caused by smoking, shouting, environmental pollution, allergies, low humidity, or air conditioning. This question is the only one that requires a "yes" answer. It can be used as a general lead-off question to help relax the donor and to begin the questioning process, or it can be used in the middle of the interview to help ensure that both the donor and the interviewer are alert and listening to the questions and answers.

### 5. Have you ever taken Tegison for psoriasis? In the past 4 weeks, have you taken any pills, medications, or Accutane? In the past 3 days, have you taken aspirin or anything that has aspirin in it?

This question is designed to help identify those donors who are being treated for a serious illness or condition that could defer them as blood donors. In most cases it is not the medication itself that is a cause for deferral but, rather, the underlying condition for which it is prescribed.[10] The blood bank should maintain a list of drugs and medications (generic and brand names) that cause temporary or indefinite deferral. Tegison is potentially teratogenic and AABB standards mandate that donors taking Tegison be deferred indefinitely.[11] Accutane (isotretinoin for acne therapy) is also a potent teratogen that can remain in the blood for several weeks and therefore carries a recommended 4-week deferral. Teratogens in the donor unit could be harmful to an embryo or fetus of a pregnant recipient.[12] The following common medications generally *do not* disqualify a donor: oral contraceptives, mild analgesics, minor tranquilizers, psychic energizers, vitamins, diet pills, hormones, and marijuana (if not currently under the influence). Aspirin and aspirin-containing medications are acceptable, provided that the donor is not being evaluated for a platelet pheresis procedure. Aspirin causes a significant decrease in platelet function for up to 3 days.

### 6. In the past 8 weeks, have you given blood, plasma, or platelets? Have you ever been refused as a blood donor or told not to donate blood? Have you ever given blood under a different name?

The time interval between whole blood donations is 8 weeks (56 days). If a donor has been participating in a pheresis program (plasma, platelets, leukocytes), there must be a 48-hour interval between the last pheresis donation and the anticipated whole blood donation. Pheresis donors will need to wait 8 weeks after a whole blood donation before returning to the pheresis program. The second part of this question is a leading one. If the answer is "yes," further investigation as to why the donor was deferred or told not to donate is required. Regarding the last part of this question, the FDA now requires that donors be asked if they have ever donated under a different name so that a more accurate check of a Donor Deferral Register can be made. It is thought that this will help increase the probability that unsuitable donors will be identified and that units or products from these persons will be removed from the transfusable blood supply.

### 7. Have you ever had chest pain, heart disease, or lung disease?

A history of cardiovascular, coronary, or rheumatic heart disease is usually cause for deferral. In cases in which there is no disability, no limitations of activity, or restrictions imposed by the primary physician, the donor may be acceptable on approval of the blood bank medical director. Active pulmonary tuberculosis (TB) or other active pulmonary disease is cause for deferral. Donors who have had TB that has been successfully treated and that is now inactive are acceptable, as are donors who have a positive skin test (Purified Protein Derivative [PPD]) result but no other signs (on x-ray examination) or symptoms of the disease.

### 8. Have you ever had cancer, a blood disease, or a bleeding problem? Have you ever taken clotting factor concentrates for a bleeding problem such as hemophilia?

A history of cancer, leukemia, or lymphoma is generally a cause for indefinite deferral. Exceptions can be made for some cases, such as basal or squamous cell (skin) cancer, carcinoma in situ of the cervix, and papillary thyroid carcinoma that have been surgically removed and cured. Any donor presenting with a history of any type of cancer should be reviewed by the blood bank medical director before being accepted. A history of leukemia, lymphoma, Kaposi's sarcoma, aplastic anemia, granulocytopenia, sickle cell anemia, thalassemia, any of the hemoglobinopathies, or polycythemia is cause for indefinite deferral. Any history of prolonged or abnormal bleeding following surgery, childbirth, tooth extraction, or cuts and abrasions must also be further evaluated. Persons with a history of abnormal bleeding should be deferred because they may experience excessive bleeding from the venipuncture and because their plasma may lack significant levels of some clotting factors. Persons with a history of hemophilia A or B, von Willebrand's disease, or severe thrombocytopenia, or a history of having ever received clotting factor concentrates, must be permanently deferred from donating blood or blood products.

**9. Have you had convulsions, seizures, or fainting spells?**

A donor with a history of epilepsy or frequent convulsions, other than febrile convulsions in early childhood, is usually deferred because of the possibility of a serious donor reaction. Donors whose seizures are well controlled with or without medication may be accepted. Final decision of acceptability of these donors lies with the blood bank medical director. It should be noted that this question is no longer required by either the AABB or the FDA but is still included on many donor history cards.

**10. In the past 4 weeks, have you had any shots or vaccinations? In the past 12 months, have you been given rabies shots?**

Killed viral, bacterial, rickettsial vaccines, or toxoids are acceptable if the donor is afebrile and symptom free. These include diphtheria, pertussis, typhoid, tetanus, paratyphoid, cholera, hepatitis B, typhus, Rocky Mountain spotted fever, influenza (killed virus), plague, Salk (polio), and rabies (duck embryo or human diploid). Attenuated virus vaccines such as smallpox, Sabin (oral) polio, measles (rubeola), mumps, yellow fever, and influenza (live virus) carry a 2-week deferral. German measles (rubella) vaccine and varicella zoster (chickenpox) carry a 4-week deferral. Rabies vaccine, if given after the bite of a rabid animal, requires a 12-month deferral, as does HBIg. If a prospective donor has received IV immune serum globulin (IVIg), he or she must be evaluated and deferred, if necessary, based on the underlying reason for the immunization.[13]

**11. Have you had a tooth extraction or dental work in the past 3 days? (not a required question)**

Although not required, this question may still be used by many blood banks or blood centers. There may be some risk of bacterial infection following oral surgery, and some procedures require the prophylactic use of antibiotics, which may be cause for a temporary deferral. The final ruling on this question rests with the blood bank medical director.

**12. In the past 6 weeks have you been pregnant, or are you pregnant now?**

A prospective donor should be deferred during pregnancy and for 6 weeks following a third-trimester delivery. Exceptions can be made by the blood bank medical director for autologous donation or if the woman's blood is needed for the exchange transfusion of her infant.

A first-trimester or second-trimester abortion or miscarriage need not be a cause for deferral. If, however, blood is transfused during or following an abortion or delivery, the donor must be deferred for 12 months.

**13. Have you ever been given growth hormone?**

Because of the risk of transmission of Creutzfeldt-Jakob disease (CJD) through infected blood transfu-

sions, a prospective donor who has ever received pituitary growth hormone of human origin must be deferred indefinitely. Recombinant growth hormones (Protropin, Humatrope) do not require deferral, but it must be clear that the donor had received *only* recombinant hormones.[14]

**14. Have you ever had Chagas' disease or babesiosis?**

Any history of Chagas' disease or babesiosis is cause for permanent deferral.

**15. In the past 12 months, have you had a positive test result for syphilis? In the past 12 months, have you had or been treated for syphilis or gonorrhea?**

Prospective donors who have had or been treated for syphilis or gonorrhea are to be deferred for at least 12 months following completion of treatment. Any person with a positive result to a serologic test for syphilis (STS) must be deferred for 12 months. The reason for deferral is not so much a fear of transmission of either syphilis or gonorrhea but that, as they are sexually transmitted diseases, the donor has a higher-than-normal risk of exposure to HIV and hepatitis infections.

**16. Have you ever had night sweats; unexplained fever or weight loss; lumps in the neck, armpits, or groin; discolored areas of the skin or mouth; persistent cough; or persistent diarrhea?**

A donor who has any of the foregoing symptoms must be further evaluated to determine whether or not these symptoms are consistent with AIDS or ARC. Any donor whose symptoms are consistent with the diagnosis of AIDS or ARC (briefly described here) must be indefinitely deferred.

a. Persistent night sweats (repeated sweating at night so that the sheets are wet)
b. Fever of greater than 100.5°F (30.2°C) for more than 10 days
c. Unexplained weight loss of 10 lb or more in less than 2 months
d. Lymphadenopathy (swollen lymph nodes in the neck, armpits, or groin)
e. Discolored areas of the skin (bluish purple areas under the skin typical of Kaposi's sarcoma) or white spots in the mouth or mucous membranes (typical or opportunistic thrush infection), or both
f. Persistent diarrhea that lasts for several days or weeks and returns frequently
g. Persistent cough or shortness of breath
h. Malaise (fatigue, loss of energy)

**17. Do you have AIDS or have you had a positive test result for the AIDS virus? In the past 12 months, have you had sex, even once, with anyone who has AIDS or tested positive for the AIDS virus?**

Donors who have tested positive for the HIV antibody must be indefinitely deferred. Donors who have had sexual contact with a person who had AIDS, ARC, or tested positive for the HIV antibody must also be indefinitely deferred.

**18. In the past 12 months, have you had sex with anyone who has ever used a needle, even once, to take any drug (including steroids)? In the past 12 months, have you ever had sex, even once, with anyone who has ever taken clotting factor concentrates for a bleeding problem such as hemophilia?**

Sexual contact with any person who is at high risk of exposure to HIV infection must be deferred for 12 months from the date of last high-risk sexual contact. The 12-month deferral should provide adequate time for seroconversion to occur if the sexual contact has resulted in the donor's infection with the HIV virus.

**19. At any time since 1977, have you taken money or drugs for sex? In the past 12 months, have you had sex, even once, with anyone who has done so? In the past 12 months, have you given money or drugs to anyone to have sex with you?**

Prostitution is a high-risk behavior. Many drug abusers use prostitution to support their drug habit, and frequent, casual sexual contact with many different partners dramatically increases a person's risk of becoming infected with HIV or the hepatitis virus, or both. Permanent deferral is required for anyone who, since 1977, has traded sex for drugs or money. A 12-month deferral must be given to anyone who, even once, has given someone money or drugs in payment for sex or who has ever had sex with someone he or she knows to have exchanged money or drugs for sex.

**20.** *Male donors:* **Have you had sex with another male, even once, since 1977?**
*Female donors:* **In the past 12 months, have you had sex with a male who has had sex, even once since 1977, with another male?**

These, too, are questions that inquire about a donor's possible participation in high-risk behavior. HIV is very prevalent in the male homosexual population, and sexual contact by men or women with a homosexual or bisexual man is cause for deferral. Permanent deferral is required for any male donor who, since 1977, has had *any* homosexual episode with another male. A 12-month deferral is required of any female donor who has had sex with a bisexual male. As in the previous questions, this 12-month deferral should provide time for seroconversion to take place and be detectable upon routine donor testing.

**21. Are you giving blood in order to be tested for AIDS?**

There are no specific requirements by either the AABB or the FDA to ask this question, but it is a good question to evaluate further a donor's motivation for donating at this time. It is well known publicly that donors' blood is tested for the HIV antibody and that if the result is positive the donor will be notified. It is also known that this test is completely free of charge to the donor. If performed by a private physician, the test is quite expensive. Although many clinics, health departments, and blood centers provide free and anonymous testing, many people still feel threatened by going to such a place for the testing.

**22. Do you understand that if you have the AIDS virus, you can give it to someone else, even though you may feel well and test negative for HIV?**

The FDA recommends that, as part of an effort to educate the general public more fully about AIDS and HIV infection, blood donors need to be informed about the time ("window period") between early infection when a person is able to transmit the virus and the development of the HIV antibody that is detectable in the screening test.[15]

**23. Have you read and understood all the donor information presented to you, and have all your questions been answered?**

The FDA requires that donors be provided with written information about high-risk behaviors, signs and symptoms of disease, the risk of transmitting HIV through blood transfusion, and the importance of self-exclusion. It requires that this information be written in language that the donor can understand and that the interviewer provide an opportunity for the donor to ask questions about anything that he or she does not understand. Figure 10–2 is an example of an information sheet that should be given to every donor each time he or she presents for donation. This example also includes information on other transfusion-transmitted diseases and the tests that will be performed on the donated unit of blood.

**24. The information I have given for this form is correct. I donate my blood or plasma for use as needed. If I am at risk for spreading the AIDS virus, I agree not to donate blood or plasma for transfusion to another person.**

This is the informed consent statement that the donor must read and sign at the completion of the medical history screening. Figure 10–3 is an example of an additional self-exclusion form that every donor should be asked to complete. It is designed to be a confidential form that the donor can complete in private, seal, and return before the donation. The form should not be reviewed until later, usually at the time of donor processing. Many large donor centers use a machine-readable (bar code) sticker that the donor selects and places on the donor card. It provides a mechanism for donors who are at risk but afraid to be deferred at the donor site, to ensure that their donation is not used for transfusion purposes.

MARYLAND GENERAL HOSPITAL

827 Linden Avenue
Baltimore, Maryland 21201
301 225-8000                    AN IMPORTANT MESSAGE TO ALL BLOOD DONORS

  Please read this information sheet carefully before you agree to donate
blood today.  At the completion of the medical history review you will
be asked to sign a statement that says you have read this information
today, that you understand it and that if you are at risk for spreading
the AIDS virus you will not donate blood or plasma for transfusion
to another person.  If any of the information below applies to you, **DO NOT DONATE
BLOOD, BECAUSE IT MIGHT HARM THE PATIENT WHO RECEIVES IT.**

ACQUIRED IMMUNE DEFICIENCY SYNDROME (AIDS)

AIDS is a disease in which the body's normal defense mechanisms against certain
diseases and infections has been broken down.  AIDS can be spread through donated
blood and plasma.  AIDS is associated with the HIV (HTLV-I) virus.  Blood tests
to detect antibody to the AIDS virus are very good, but they are not perfect.
It is possible for a person in the early stage of infection to have a negative
test result. Therefore, people who are at risk for getting AIDS must not donate
blood or plasma.

**You are at risk of getting AIDS and spreading the AIDS virus if:**

- You are a man who has had sex with another man since 1977, **even one time!**
- You have ever taken ("shot up") illegal drugs by needle.
- You have AIDS or one of its signs or symptoms which include:
      *Unexplained weight loss (10 pounds or more in less than 2 months)
      *Night sweats (reoccurring sweating at night which wets the sheets)
      *Blue/purple spots on or under the skin or in the mouth (Kaposi Sarcoma)
      *Long lasting white spots in the mouth (Thrush infection)
      *Swollen lymphnodes (lumps in the neck, arm pits or groin) lasting more
       than a month.
      *Fever of greater than 99 degrees lasting for several days or weeks and/or
       reoccurring frequently
      *Persistant diarrhea (lasting more than a month)
- You have ever had a positive test for AIDS or the AIDS virus (Anti-HIV)
- You are a hemophiliac who has taken clotting factor concentrates since 1977
- You have, since 1977, had sex with any person described above.
- You are a woman or a man who has been a prostitute at any time since 1977.
- You are a man who has had sex with a female prostitute or a woman who has
  had sex with a male prostitute in the past 12 months.

HEPATITIS

If you have ever had hepatitis (a liver disease that can be caused by a virus),
**DO NOT DONATE BLOOD OR PLASMA.**

If you have ever had a positive test for hepatitis (HBsAg, Anti-HCV, Anti-HBc),
**DO NOT DONATE BLOOD OR PLASMA**

SYPHILIS and/or GONORRHEA

If you have or have been treated for syphilis or gonorrhea, in the past 12 months,
**DO NOT DONATE BLOOD OR PLASMA**

(OVER)

**Figure 10–2.** Donor information sheet for viral marker testing. (Courtesy Maryland General Hospital, Baltimore.)

MALARIA

If you have visited or lived in a country where malaria exists, DO NOT DONATE BLOOD FOR 6 MONTHS AFTER YOU LEAVE THAT COUNTRY.

If you are a native of a country where malaria exists, DO NOT DONATE BLOOD FOR 3 YEARS after you have left the area and entered the United States.

If you have had malaria or have taken anti-malarial drugs, DO NOT DONATE BLOOD FOR 3 YEARS after your last attack of malaria and/or after stopping your anti-malarial drug therapy.

IF ANY OF THE ABOVE INFORMATION APPLIES TO YOU, DO NOT DONATE BLOOD OR PLASMA, **EVEN IF YOU FEEL HEALTHY.** YOU MAY LEAVE NOW WITHOUT PROVIDING AN EXPLANATION. IF YOU ARE NOT SURE YOU SHOULD DONATE, PLEASE TALK PRIVATELY WITH THE DONOR ROOM PHLEBOTOMIST.

## Your blood will be tested for hepatitis viruses, syphilis, the AIDS virus (HIV) and certain other viruses.

If the tests for hepatitis show that you probably are a carrier of hepatitis, or if the HIV antibody test shows that you probably have been exposed to the AIDS virus, we will not use your blood or plasma. You will be notified confidentia of the test results and we will put your name and other identifying information on a confidential list of persons who should not donate blood or plasma.

If the results of your hepatitis tests or HIV antibody test are unclear, we will not use your blood or plasma even though you are probably healthy. Your name will be put on a confidential list for special testing the next time you donate blood. You will not however, be informed of these unclear results unless the blood bank medical director decides that the special test results mean that your health might be affected.

**We report positive test results to applicable health departments as required by federal, state and local law.**

WE APPRECIATE THE TIME AND EFFORT INVOLVED IN MAKING A TRIP TO THE BLOOD BANK AND HOPE THAT ALL DONORS WILL RECOGNIZE THE NECESSITY OF THE VOLUNTARY SCREENING PROCEDURES WHICH HAVE BEEN INSTITUTED.

**Figure 10–2. (Continued)**

## Pheresis Donor Selection

The donor selection requirements for a pheresis donor are generally the same as those for a whole blood (WB) donor. Under normal conditions, a pheresis donor must meet all the criteria for a whole blood donor. In addition, the following criteria are specific for the potential pheresis donor and need to be investigated before proceeding with the donation.

### Medical History

1. **A history of donor reactions, particularly to previous pheresis procedures.** Possible adverse reactions to hydroxyethyl starch (HES), steroids, or heparin must be determined and carefully evaluated.

2. **A history of bleeding problems or thrombocytopenia, or both.** This may be critical if a procedure using heparin is to be performed. It is best to defer female donors from heparin procedures during menses.

3. **Allergies to beef or pork.** They are generally a source of heparin.

4. **An indication or history of fluid retention problems.** This may be a significant problem in using HES or steroids, or both, in the pheresis procedure.

5. **An underlying medical condition that may be aggravated by steroids.** These include hypertension, tuberculosis, and diabetes mellitus.

6. **The donor weight.** The size of the bowl used in the procedure (225 mL or 375 mL) will alter the volume of blood that is outside the body (extra-

MARYLAND GENERAL HOSPITAL

827 Linden Avenue
Baltimore, Maryland 21201          DONOR SELF-EXCLUSION FORM
301 225-8000

PLEASE READ AND COMPLETE THIS FORM BEFORE YOU LEAVE THE DONOR ROOM

AIDS can be spread through blood and plasma.  Therefore, blood or plasma
from people at risk for getting AIDS and spreading the AIDS virus must
not be transfused to another person.

YOU ARE AT RISK FOR GETTING AIDS AND SPREADING IT THROUGH YOUR BLOOD AND PLASMA
IF:

- You are a man who has had sex with another man since 1977, <u>even one time.</u>
- You have ever taken illegal drugs by needle.
- You are a native of Haiti, Burundi, Kenya, Rwanda, Tanzania, Uganda or Zaire
  who has entered the United States since 1977.
- You have AIDS or one of the signs or symptoms of AIDS.  (listed on the "An
  Important Message To All Blood Donors" sheet)
- You have ever had a positive test for HIV (HTLV-III) antibody, showing past
  exposure to the AIDS virus.
- You have hemophilia.
- You are or have been the sex partner of any person described above.
- You are a woman or man who is now or has been a prostitute since 1977.
- You have been the heterosexual partner of a male or female prostitute within
  the last twelve (12) months.

If any of the above information applies to you, your blood or plasma <u>MUST NOT
BE TRANSFUSED</u> TO ANOTHER PERSON.  Please take time to think about this important
issue and then mark the correct box below.

SYPHILIS OR GONORRHEA:  <u>DO NOT</u> donate blood for transfusion to another person
if:

- You have or have been treated for syphilis in the last twelve (12) months.
- You have or have been treated for gonorrhea in the last twelve (12) months.


YOU MUST MARK ON OF THE BOXES BELOW IN ORDER FOR YOUR BLOOD TO BE USED.  FAILURE
TO MARK ONE OF THE BOXES WILL REQUIRE THAT YOUR BLOOD BE DISCARDED.

MARK ONLY ONE BOX!    YOUR RESPONSE IS STRICTLY CONFIDENTIAL!



          I believe my blood              My blood should <u>NOT</u>
          is <u>SAFE FOR TRANS-</u>            <u>BE TRANSFUSED</u> to
          <u>FUSION</u> to another            another person.
          person.

After marking the correct box, fold and seal the form so that nobody can see
your answer.  Do not put your name on the form.  Give the sealed form to the
Donor Room nurse.

THANK YOU FOR YOUR INTEREST IN DONATING BLOOD AND FOR HELPING US MAINTAIN A
SAFE BLOOD SUPPLY.

**Figure 10–3.** Donor self-exclusion form. (Courtesy Maryland General Hospital, Baltimore.)

corporeal) and therefore will change the donor's weight requirements. No more than 15 percent of the donor's total blood volume can be extracorporeal. The small bowl requires 110 lb; the large about 150 lb.

7. **Medications.** Use of any medication that might increase the donor's risk or decrease the effectiveness of the product, most particularly aspirin (or aspirin-containing substances), must be evaluated. The donor should be free of aspirin ingestion for 3 to 5 days before platelet pheresis or leukopheresis.

### Physical Examination and Laboratory Tests

As with the medical history, the pheresis donor must meet all the minimum physical examination requirements of a WB donor. Depending on which pheresis procedure is being performed, the following additional laboratory tests must be performed before each donation:

1. Hemoglobin and hematocrit
2. Serum protein
3. Platelet count (not less than 50,000/$\mu$L)
4. White blood cell (WBC) count and differential
5. Partial thromboplastin time (PTT), if using heparin

Perform the following tests after the donation:

1. Hemoglobin and hematocrit
2. Platelet count
3. WBC count

Protein electrophoresis should be performed every 4 months if the donor is a regular, biweekly plasma donor.

### Autologous Donor Selection

An autologous donor is one who is donating blood for his or her own future use. Autologous blood is the safest blood possible for transfusion. There is no risk of disease transmission; alloimmunization to RBCs, platelets, WBCs, or plasma proteins; or transfusion reactions, and the phlebotomy process stimulates the bone marrow to increase cell production. The use of autologous blood decreases the need for allogeneic blood, frequently decreases the total amount of blood needed, and may actually increase the supply of allogeneic blood if the unused autologous units are crossed over into the general inventory.[16] All of this adds up to a big advantage to the donor recipient and a strong reason for blood banks and physicians to encourage its use. There are four types of autologous donations-transfusions. *Predeposit donation* refers to blood that is drawn some time before the anticipated transfusion and stored, usually liquid but occasionally frozen, in the blood bank. *Intraoperative autologous transfusion* occurs when blood is collected during a surgical procedure and usually reinfused immedi-

ately. A third type of autologous donation is the *immediate preoperative hemodilution*. In this procedure, once the patient is in the operating room, 1 to 3 units of WB are collected and the volume is replaced with colloid or crystalloid, or both, thus reducing the patient's hemoglobin level by about 1 to 3 g/dL. The blood remains in the operating room and is used for transfusion during the surgical procedure. The fourth type of autologous donation is *postoperative "salvage,"* in which a drainage tube is placed in the surgical site and postoperative bleeding is salvaged, cleaned, and reinfused.

### Predeposit Donation

Predeposit autologous donation is usually performed for a scheduled elective surgical procedure in which there is a reasonable chance that transfusion will be required. Because the donor will also be the recipient, the donor requirements can be significantly different from those required of an allogeneic WB donor (Fig. 10–4)

**General Requirements**

1. The donor-patient must have a signed written statement from his or her physician requesting the procedure (Fig. 10–5).
2. The physician's request must be reviewed and approved by the blood bank medical director (Fig. 10–6).
3. The donor-patient must give signed, informed consent (Fig. 10–7).

**Donor Criteria**

1. **Age.** Generally no age limits exist, although a child should be old enough to understand what is happening and to be cooperative. Almost any person who is a good candidate for elective surgery can be an autologous donor. The final decision rests with the donor-patient's physician and the blood bank medical director.
2. **Weight.** No strict weight requirements exist. If the donor weighs less than 110 lb (50 kg), a proportionately smaller volume of blood must be drawn. (See the guidelines provided in the discussion of the physical examination, earlier in this chapter, for calculations necessary.) As a rule of thumb, reduce the volume to be drawn by 4 mL for each pound under 110.
3. **Hemoglobin and hematocrit.** The hemoglobin should not be less than 11 g/dL; the hematocrit, not less than 33 percent.
4. **Frequency.** Donations should not be more frequent than every 3 days, and the final donation must be completed at least 3 days before the scheduled surgical procedure. This allows the donor's plasma volume to return to normal before surgery. It is recommended that donors be placed on oral iron therapy if several units are to be drawn or if the units are to be drawn very frequently.

**DONOR CARD**   **MARYLAND GENERAL HOSPITAL—BLOOD BANK**   BLOOD TYPE

| NAME LAST | FIRST | M.I. | AGE | DATE OF BIRTH | SEX | DATE TODAY (MDY) | **WHOLE BLOOD NUMBER** |
| --- | --- | --- | --- | --- | --- | --- | --- |
| STREET ADDRESS | | | HOME PHONE | | AUTOLOGOUS USE ONLY ☐ | | |
| CITY | STATE | ZIP CODE | BUSINESS PHONE | | PERSONAL PHYSICIAN | | DEFERRED UNTIL (MDY) / INDEFINITE DEFERRAL ☐ |
| IDENTIFICATION SS# | | | | HOSPITAL | | | NO. PREVIOUS DONATIONS / DATE LAST DONATION |

| WEIGHT | TEMP. | PULSE | B.P. | Hgb | ARMS S U | TIME START | TIME COMPLETED | LOT NUMBER | SIGNATURE |
| --- | --- | --- | --- | --- | --- | --- | --- | --- | --- |

| | | YES | NO |
| --- | --- | --- | --- |
| 1 | HAVE YOU BEEN PREVIOUSLY REJECTED? IF SO WHY? | ☐ | ☐ |
| 2 | ILLNESS, INFECTIOUS DISEASE RECENTLY (SPECIFICALLY DIARRHEA, NAUSEA, VOMITING, OR ABDOMINAL PAIN WITHIN THE LAST 7 DAYS?) | ☐ | ☐ |
| 3 | CONVULSIONS/FAINTING SPELLS/ABNORMAL BLEEDING? | ☐ | ☐ |
| 4 | MINOR OR DENTAL SURGERY WITHIN THE LAST 3 DAYS? | ☐ | ☐ |
| 5 | MAJOR SURGERY IN THE LAST 12 MONTHS? | ☐ | ☐ |
| 6 | FEELING WELL TODAY? | ☐ | ☐ |
| 7 | RECEIVED BLOOD/BLOOD PRODUCTS IN THE LAST 12 MONTHS? | ☐ | ☐ |
| 8 | HAVE YOU EVER HAD CHEST PAIN, HEART, KIDNEY, LIVER, OR LUNG DISEASE? | ☐ | ☐ |
| 9 | DO YOU HAVE DIABETES? | ☐ | ☐ |
| 10 | ARE YOU ON ANY DRUG THERAPY INCLUDING ANTIBIOTICS? | ☐ | ☐ |
| 11 | HAVE YOU HAD ANY UNEXPLAINED WEIGHT LOSS? | ☐ | ☐ |
| 12 | ARE YOU PREGNANT OR BEEN PREGNANT WITHIN THE LAST 6 MONTHS? | ☐ | ☐ |

| DATE | DONOR NUMBER | Anti A | Anti B | Cells A₁ | Cells B | Anti D | Rh Cont | Du | Check Cell | Du Cont | Check Cell | Interp. | Tech. |
| --- | --- | --- | --- | --- | --- | --- | --- | --- | --- | --- | --- | --- | --- |

LABELING INFO:    I    II    III

Date Drawn:    RT  37°C    RT  37°C    RT  37°C

| DATE | I.S. Sal | 10' LISS | AHG | Check Cell | I.S. Sal | 10' LISS | AHG | Check Cell | I.S. Sal | 10' LISS | AHG | Check Cell |
| --- | --- | --- | --- | --- | --- | --- | --- | --- | --- | --- | --- | --- |

Date Expires:

Labeled By:

REMARKS:

Label Checked By:

THE INFORMATION I HAVE GIVEN FOR THIS FORM IS CORRECT. I DONATE MY BLOOD OR PLASMA FOR USE AS NEEDED. IF I AM AT RISK FOR SPREADING THE AIDS VIRUS, I AGREE NOT TO DONATE BLOOD OR PLASMA FOR TRANSFUSION TO ANOTHER PERSON.    YES ☐  NO ☐   DONOR SIGNATURE   X

L-19 (Rev. 9-92)

**Figure 10–4.** Donor history card for autologous donation. (Courtesy Maryland General Hospital, Baltimore.)

5. **Medical history.** Because the donor will also be the recipient, most medical history questions need not be cause for deferral. Any medical condition that could make the phlebotomy dangerous to the donor-patient (e.g., bacteremia) must be evaluated by the patient's physician and the blood bank medical director (see Fig. 10–4).

## Intraoperative Blood Collection

During a surgical procedure, blood is collected, by aspiration, from the surgical site. It is then processed by centrifugation, washing, and filtering, and is reinfused to the patient during or immediately after surgery.

The procedure can be used in most procedures as long as there is no contamination (sepsis or penetrating bowel wound) of the surgical site or contamination with malignant tumor cells. It has frequently been used in orthopedic, vascular, cardiac, obstetric and gynecologic, and neurosurgical procedures.[17] The procedure tends to be somewhat expensive, so it is advisable to limit the use of this method to situations in which multiple (three or more) units of blood may be needed. Blood collected by this method is not suitable for transfusion to any other patient. It can be stored at room temperature for up to 6 hours and generally does not leave the operating or recovery room. If longer storage is desired, harvested units can be sent to the blood bank to store at 1 to 6°C for up to 24 hours. If this is done, there must be a system in place to identify the unit positively before leaving the operating room and a mechanism, in the blood bank, to prevent accidental release of the blood to the general inventory or the wrong patient. There must be a written protocol for the intraoperative procedure, the blood bank medical director should be involved in establishing the protocol, and the hospital's transfusion committee must approve it.[18]

## Immediate Preoperative Hemodilution

This procedure is used particularly with heart surgery (cardiopulmonary bypass [CPB]) procedures. After the patient is under anesthesia and before the bypass surgery begins, 1 to 3 units of blood are removed and the blood volume is restored using volume expanders (colloid or crystalloid, or both). The patient's hematocrit is typically lowered to about 20 percent. The advantages of this procedure include:

1. Surgical bleeding occurs at a lower hematocrit, and therefore the amount of RBC mass that is lost is less.
2. The donated blood that can be reinfused during or immediately after surgery is very fresh and contains viable platelets, adequate protein levels, and good levels of all the plasma clotting factors.[19]
3. The blood flow through the microcirculation is improved because of the greatly reduced hematocrit.[20]

The collected blood usually does not leave the operating room. It can be stored at room temperature for up to 4 hours, or in the refrigerator (1 to 6°C) for up to 24 hours. As with the intraoperative collection, longer storage should be handled by the blood bank, and all procedures and policies must be in place to ensure proper collection, handling, storage, identification, distribution, and disposition of the blood.

## Postoperative "Shed" Blood Collection

This procedure collects blood from a drainage tube placed in the surgical site. It is particularly useful in collecting "shed" blood from a chest tube following CPB surgery and is frequently used following total knee surgery. The procedure can be used alone or in con-

**MARYLAND GENERAL HOSPITAL**

827 Linden Avenue
Baltimore, Maryland 21201     PHYSICIAN ORDER FORM FOR PREDEPOSIT AUTOLOGOUS TRANSFUSION
410 225-8000

PATIENT NAME: _____

ADDRESS: _____

TELEPHONE: _____ BIRTHDATE: _____ HOSP. # _____

I request that the above-named patient donate _____ units of autologous blood in

advance of his/her surgical procedure _____ scheduled
                                                  (PROCEDURE)

for _____ .
          (DATE)

I have explained this procedure to my patient, including the advantages and disadvantages. In view of my patient's current medical status, I do not foresee any
contraindications to this procedure. I have advised my patient to begin a high
iron diet or prescribed oral iron with the instructions to begin the recommended
iron regime one (1) week prior to the first phlebotomy.

I authorize the release of all unused autologous blood components from this patient
after the post-operative interval specified below. They may be used for transfusion
to other patients or any other use deemed appropriate by the blood bank medical
director. I may extend the holding period by contacting the blood bank at any time
through the end of the originally designated interval. If only autologous red
blood cells are requested, I authorize release of other components immediately
following donation.

_____       _____ , M.D.
      (Date)                        (Requesting Physician's Signature)

------------------------------------------------------------------------
UNLESS OTHERWISE SPECIFIED, THE FOLLOWING CONDITIONS ARE UNDERSTOOD:

| Components reserved for autologous use: | Red Cells (only) | _____ (specify FFP if desired) |
|---|---|---|
| Minimum donor hematocrit: | 34% | |
| | | _____ (specify other) |
| Minimum interval between donations: | 7 days | |
| | | _____ (specify other) |
| Minimum interval between last donation & date of surgery: | 72 hours | |
| | | _____ (specify other) |
| Blood held after surgery: | 72 hours | |
| | | _____ (specify other) |

Oral iron therapy begun: _____     Dose: _____
                              (date)

**Figure 10–5.** Front of the physician's order form for autologous donation. (Courtesy Maryland General Hospital, Baltimore.)

# BLOOD BANK USE ONLY

Medical Director's review and approval          APPROVED:      YES_____   NO_____

COMMENTS: _____

_____

_____

_____

_____


_____          _____
(Signature)                                                      (Date)

**Figure 10–6.** Back of the physician's order form for autologous donation; the blood bank medical director's review for approval. (Courtesy Maryland General Hospital, Baltimore.)

junction with other autologous blood collection procedures. The blood collected by this method must be used within 6 hours of collection.

## WHOLE BLOOD COLLECTION AND PHLEBOTOMY

Once the donor has been registered and has successfully passed the physical examination and medical history requirements, the next step is the actual collection of the donor unit.

1. The personnel performing the phlebotomy procedure must be well trained and under the supervision of a qualified, licensed physician.
2. The blood must be drawn in an aseptic manner, using a sterile, closed system and a single venipuncture.
   a. The phlebotomy site on the donor's arm(s), usually the antecubital area, must be free of any skin lesions or rash, or both, which could cause contamination of the unit or infection to the donor.
   b. The venipuncture site must be thoroughly cleaned and disinfected. A surgical preparation is used to provide maximum protection. Table 10–1 lists two acceptable methods used by most blood banks.
3. A system must be established that will uniquely and positively identify each donor unit, subsequent products prepared, the medical history form, and all pilot tubes. The system may use numbers, letters, or other symbols, or various

combinations thereof. It must, however, provide positive donor identification that is traceable. The numbers (or other identification system) must be applied to the bags, medical history form, and pilot tubes before proceeding with the phlebotomy.

4. Any of the following anticoagulants and additive solutions are considered acceptable by the FDA. Additive solutions (AS) are added to the RBCs after the plasma has been removed:
   a. Acid-citrate-dextrose (ACD)
   b. Heparin
   c. Citrate-phosphate-dextrose (CPD)
   d. Citrate-phosphate-dextrose-adenine (CPDA-1)
   e. CPD plus AS-1 or AS-2, consisting of saline, dextrose, mannitol, and adenine
   f. Citrate-phosphate–double dextrose (CP2D) plus AS, consisting of saline, dextrose, and adenine.
5. The pilot samples to be used for donor processing should be attached firmly to the container before the phlebotomy. They must be filled at the time when the donor unit is being drawn, usually immediately following the collection of the unit, by the same individual who drew the unit.

   Samples (segments) to be used for subsequent compatibility testing must be prepared from the integral tubing (the tubing that runs from the needle to the primary bag) in a manner that allows each segment to be separated without contamination of the unit.
6. Phlebotomy procedure and pilot tube collection. DO NOT LEAVE THE DONOR UNATTENDED AT ANY TIME DURING THE PHLEBOTOMY PROCEDURE.

MARYLAND GENERAL HOSPITAL

827 Linden Avenue
Baltimore, Maryland 21201          PREDEPOSIT AUTOLOGOUS DONOR PROGRAM
301 225-8000

STATEMENT OF CONSENT FOR AUTOLOGOUS DONATION AND TRANSFUSION

A.   The advantages, nature and purpose of autologous donation/transfusion,
     the risks involved and the possibility of complications have been explained
     to me by _____, M.D.  I acknowledge such counseling.

     I understand that:

     1.   The blood drawn from me for later transfusion to me is the safest
          blood for me to receive and that there is virtually no risk of my
          aquiring hepatitis or AIDS from the transfusion of such blood.

     2.   The procedure for donating my own blood is identical to routine blood
          donation.  Each unit (approximately 1 pint) is collected by placing
          a needle into a vein in my arm; blood flows into a sterile plastic
          bag containing an anticoagulant.  After the procedure, the needle
          is removed and pressure and a bandage are applied to my arm to prevent
          bleeding.  Each unit is labeled and stored for my own use during my
          subsequent hospitalization.

     3.   A mild anemia and/or decrease in my blood volume may temporarily result
          from frequent blood donations for autologous transfusion.  Because
          of these possible changes, I should refrain from strenuous athletic
          events and hazardous occupations or endeavors between the time the
          first unit is drawn and the scheduled use of predeposit units.

     4.   I may be asked to take oral iron supplements to replenish the iron
          lost with each donated unit.

     5.   I should contact my personal physician or the blood bank if I feel
          faint, weak, lightheaded, dizzy or otherwise ill.  The blood bank
          is open Monday-Friday from 8:00am - 5:00pm for any questions I may
          have about symptoms related to autologous donation.  The Blood Bank
          phone # is 225-8462.

     6.   The blood which I am donating for autologous purposes may not be used
          to transfuse me if my physician determines that autologous transfusion
          is not medically appropriate.  I also understand that there may be
          situations where additional blood products are required.  In any event,
          I agree to accept homologous (other donor's) blood if my physician
          determines that such transfusion(s) is(are) appropriate.

     7.   If I am physically and mentally able, I must identify my signature
          on the autologous transfusion tag prior to the administration of each
          unit of autologous blood.

     8.   If the scheduled procedure is delayed for any reason, it may be
          necessary to transfuse an older unit back to me and withdraw a fresh
          unit to prevent expiration and discarding of the older unit.

     9.   If the blood is to be transfused at Maryland General Hospital, no
          infectious disease testing will be performed on the donated unit.

                                                                    (OVER)

**Figure 10–7.** Predeposit consent form for autologous donation. (Courtesy Maryland General Hospital, Baltimore.)

10. If I or my physician request that the donated blood be transferred to another facility or hospital, all infectious disease testing required by state and federal law will be performed. These include tests for Hepatitis B surface Antigen (HBsAg), Hepatitis C Virus Antibody (Anti-HCV), Aminoalanine transaminase (ALT), Antibody to the Hepatitis B core antigen (Anti-HBc), Human Immunodeficiency Virus Antibody (Anti-HIV), Human T-lymphotropic Virus Type I Antibody (Anti-HTLV-I).

11. If the tests for infectious deseases show that I am a carrier of hepatitis or have been exposed to the AIDS virus, I will be notified confidentially of the test results and my name and other identifying information will be placed on a confidential list of persons who should not donate blood or plasma for transfusion to other people.

12. If Maryland state laws or federal laws require that these positive test results be reported to state or federal health authorities, this will be done in accordance with such laws.

B. I consent to the withdrawal of blood, by authorized members of the staff of the Maryland General Hospital Blood Bank, for autologous transfusion purposes and further consent to such additional procedures pursuant to autologous transfusion as may be necessary or desirable. Should I not require transfusion of the blood withdrawn for autologous transfusion, during the time frame specified by my physician/surgeon, I further consent to the disposal of my blood in any manner deemed appropriate by the blood bank medical director.

_____ (Date)

Donor/Patient Signature or Authority to Consent if not the Patient's own signature

_____ (Date)

Witness

**Figure 10–7. (Continued)**

a. Make the donor comfortable. Confirm the donor's identification.
b. Select and locate the desired vein. Marking may be necessary if the vein is deep and does not distend visually.
c. Prepare the site and cover.
d. Set up and check the bag and scale unless previously completed.
e. Place a clamp on the tubing between the needle and the primary bag.
f. Give the donor something to squeeze. Instruct the donor to clench the fist a couple of times and then hold it tight.
g. Use a tourniquet or blood pressure cuff (maximum 60 mm Hg) to increase the distention of the vein.
h. Perform the venipuncture. Place the thumb of your free hand below the prepared site and pull the skin taut. With the needle at a 45° angle to the skin, make a quick clean puncture. Once in the skin, reduce the angle of the needle to about 10° to 20°, orient the line of the vein, and make a second push through the vein wall; thread the needle up the vein about one-half inch to aid in securing the needle.
i. Release the clamp on the tubing and check to make sure the flow is fairly rapid and steady.
j. Tape the needle and tubing lightly to the arm.

**Table 10–1.** Arm Preparation Methods

---

### *Method I*

---

1. Scrub the site (2 × 2 inches) for 30 sec using an aqueous iodophor scrub solution (0.7%). Iodophor is a polyvinylpyrrolidone-iodine or poloxamer iodine complex.
2. Apply iodophor complex and let stand for 30 sec. Use a concentric spiral motion, starting in the center and moving outward. Do not go back toward the center. Removal of the iodophor solution is not necessary. The iodine is complexed and will not usually cause skin irritation.
3. Site is now ready for venipuncture. Cover with sterile gauze until ready for needle insertion.

---

### *Method II*

---

1. Scrub vigorously for 30 sec using a 15% aqueous solution of soap ("green soap"). Scrub area should be at least 2 × 2 inches around the intended venipuncture site. The scrub is designed to remove dirt, oils, and loose skin cells.
2. Remove the soap using an alcohol (70%) and acetone (10%) solution (9:1 ratio). Apply solution in the aforementioned concentric, spiral motion. Allow to dry.
3. Apply a tincture of iodine solution (3% iodine in 70% alcohol). Use the same concentric motion as with the alcohol. Allow to dry.
4. Remove the iodine with the alcohol-and-acetone solution as in step 2. The iodine should be removed; it is no longer needed to maintain the cleanliness of the area and, if left on, may cause skin irritation.
5. Site is now ready for venipuncture. Cover with sterile gauze until ready for needle insertion.

---

This will help to prevent accidentally pulling the needle out. Cover with a sterile gauze.

k. Reduce the tourniquet or blood pressure cuff to approximately 40 mm Hg.

l. Continue to monitor the donor for signs of a reaction. Continue to observe the flow rate and periodically mix the blood to ensure contact with the anticoagulant. Mixing is not required if vacuum equipment is being used.

m. When the primary unit has tripped the preset scale, instruct the donor to stop squeezing and clamp off (or tie a knot in) the tubing. The volume-weight conversion for WB is 1.06 g/mL. A unit of WB should weigh between 430 g and 525 g plus the weight of the bag, anticoagulant, and the empty pilot tubes.

n. Collect the pilot tubes before removing the needle from the donor's arm. The most convenient system is one with an in-line needle or in-line pouch; however, this is not mandatory.

o. Release the tourniquet or blood pressure cuff.

p. Permanently clamp or seal the donor tubing close to the needle.

q. Remove the needle from the donor's arm, apply pressure to the site (over the gauze), instruct the donor to raise his or her arm with the elbow straight, and continue pressure to the site. Once the bleeding has stopped (approxi-

mately 2 minutes), have the donor lower his or her arm. Check for bleeding and place a bandage over the site.

r. Strip the tubing to ensure that the blood is completely mixed with the anticoagulant. Allow the tubing to refill, being careful to avoid any bubbles. Seal the tubing in segments at approximately 3-inch intervals, making sure that the lot number is present on each segment. The seal between each segment should be clean and should allow easy separation. These segments will be used for compatibility testing (see step 5).

s. Place the units in storage. All units except those that will be used for platelet production are to be stored at 1 to 6°C or placed into a container for transportation, which will gradually reduce the temperature at 4°C. Those units designed for platelet production are to be stored at 20 to 24°C until the platelets have been removed.

7. Before allowing the donor to leave the area, instruct him or her in postphlebotomy care. The following are some examples of instructions that should be given:

a. Increase fluid intake for the next few hours (may be up to 24 hours). Have something to eat or drink, or both, before leaving the donor area. Remain in the area for at least 10 minutes.

b. Do not drink alcoholic beverages before the next meal.

c. Do not smoke for the next half hour.

d. Leave the bandage on for a few hours.

e. Do not put strong pressure on or try to lift or carry heavy objects with the donating arm for the next few hours.

f. If bleeding occurs from the phlebotomy site, reapply direct pressure until it stops.

g. If you feel dizzy or faint, sit down with your head lowered between your knees or lie down with your feet elevated. If the symptoms continue, return to the blood bank or see your doctor.

h. Refrain from very strenuous activity or hazardous work for a few hours.

## DONOR REACTIONS

Although the majority of donations proceed without any complications, occasionally a donor will have an adverse reaction to the donation. Most reactions are vasovagal reactions. The reactions may result from psychological influences, such as the sight of blood, excitement, fear, or apprehension, or they may be a neurophysiologic response to the actual donation. The reactions can be roughly grouped into three categories based on the degree of severity.

### Mild Reactions

Mild reactions are the most frequently encountered type of reaction, in which the donor exhibits signs of shock but does not lose consciousness. The signs and symptoms of mild reactions include one or more of the following:

1. Nervousness, anxiety
2. Complaints of feeling warm
3. Pallor, sweating
4. Increased or thready pulse (lacking a complete vibration in the beat)
5. Increased respirations leading to hyperventilation
6. Decreased blood pressure
7. Nausea and possibly vomiting

In general, treatment for mild reactions include:

1. Stop the donation; remove the tourniquet and needle from the donor's arm.
2. Have the donor breathe into a paper bag, which will counteract the effects of hyperventilation by increasing the amount of carbon dioxide ($CO_2$) in the air the donor is breathing.
3. Loosen any tight clothing, particularly a necktie or shirt buttoned around the neck.
4. Ensure that the donor has a clear airway.
5. Have the donor pull his or her knees up (with feet on the donor bed) or raise his or her feet (approximately 45 degrees) for a while. The feet may be lowered as the donor recovers.
6. Apply a cold towel to the forehead and neck and use aromatic spirits of ammonia if necessary.
7. Talk to the donor as the treatment is being given to reassure the donor and to reduce his or her stress or anxiety, or both, which may have been the primary causes of the reaction.
8. If the donor does not quickly respond and recover, additional medical help should be summoned.
9. DO NOT LEAVE THE DONOR.

## Moderate Reactions

Moderate reactions are characterized by signs and symptoms similar to those found in mild reactions, plus the fact that the donor loses consciousness. In moderate reactions, the following signs and symptoms, in addition to those listed for mild reactions, may occur:

1. Periods of unconsciousness (which may be repetitive)
2. Decreased pulse rate
3. Rapid, shallow respirations and hyperventilation
4. Continued decrease in blood pressure (hypotension; systolic pressure may drop as low as 60 mm Hg)

The recommended countermeasures for moderate reactions include the following:

1. Proceed with the appropriate measures listed for treatment of mild reactions.
2. Check blood pressure, pulse, and respirations frequently until they return to normal.
3. Administer 95 percent oxygen ($O_2$); 5 percent $CO_2$.

4. Separate the donor from the general donor area by use of screens or move the donor to another room. Sight of a reaction in one donor may trigger reactions in others.

## Severe Reactions

To classify a severe reaction, add convulsions to the previously listed symptoms. Convulsions or seizures can be caused by cerebral ischemia associated with vasovagal syncope (reduced blood flow to the brain owing to the deepening shock symptoms), by marked hyperventilation (severe $CO_2$ depletion can cause convulsions or tetany), or by epilepsy. These severe reactions can be further categorized by the symptoms they produce.

1. Hyperventilation tetany (the earliest stage of convulsions caused by hyperventilation)
   a. The donor has not lost consciousness and may complain of stiffness or tingling in the fingers.
   b. The fingers and thumb may spasm and assume an unnatural position.
   c. The symptoms will progress to deeper, more pronounced convulsions if $CO_2$ intake is not increased.
   The recommended countermeasures include:
   a. Remain calm; do not alarm other donors if possible.
   b. Have the donor rebreathe air from a paper bag.
   c. DO NOT LEAVE THE DONOR. However, help should be summoned inasmuch as the reaction may progress to a more severe state.
2. Mild convulsions
   a. Short lapse of consciousness
   b. Voice fadeout
   c. Slight involuntary movement of the arms and legs
3. Severe convulsions
   a. Rigid body and tightly clenched teeth
   b. Temporary loss of breathing, followed by rasping or stertorous breathing
   c. Slight involuntary movement of the arms and legs
   The recommended countermeasures for both moderate and severe convulsions include:
   a. Gently restrain the donor to prevent injury. It may be necessary to move the donor from the donor couch to the floor.
   b. Summon help immediately. Remain calm and with the donor.
   c. Ensure an adequate airway.
   d. 95 percent $O_2$; 5 percent $CO_2$ may be administered.
   e. Maintain observation of the donor until fully recovered and released by the blood bank physician.

## Cardiac and/or Respiratory Problems

If the donor develops respiratory difficulties or appears to be having cardiac problems, call for medical assistance immediately. If the donor goes into cardiac arrest, administer cardiopulmonary resuscitation (CPR) until medical help arrives.

## Hematomas

Hematomas are not an uncommon complication of the phlebotomy process. They can occur if the needle is not seated properly and there is leakage of blood around the needle entry site into the tissue or if the needle went through the vein and punctured the back wall. If a hematoma develops, remove the tourniquet and the needle. Apply pressure to the venipuncture site and raise the arm for 5 to 10 minutes. Make sure the bleeding has completely stopped, then apply a bandage. If the arm is stiff or sore, a cold (ice) pack can be used over the dressing. Caution the donor that a "black-and-blue" area will develop and, if it is sore or uncomfortable, ice packs can be applied. If the arm becomes painful, the donor should see a doctor or return to the donor center. The discoloration will last a while and will gradually change color from blue-black to purple to red-brown to yellow.

A report of any adverse reaction should be kept on file in the blood bank as a part of the donor record.

## DONOR PROCESSING

All donor units must be processed to some degree before being released for compatibility testing and transfusion. Although there are some minor differences between the AABB standards and the FDA regulations as to which tests are needed, the following criteria will satisfy both organizations' minimum requirements.

All reagents used in donor blood testing and screening must meet or exceed the minimum standards for reactivity established by the FDA. The commercially prepared reagents that are licensed by the FDA must meet these standards, so the blood bank need not be concerned with reagent testing other than routine quality control procedures (see Chap. 13). Each major step of the testing and processing system must be documented and the records maintained so that any unit or component, or both, can be traced. The example given in Figure 10–8 uses a system in which the processing test results are kept as part of the donor record (on the back of the medical history card).

## ABO Grouping

Regulations require that two different tests be used to determine the ABO type of each donor unit. The detection of the antigens present on the red cells is commonly called a "forward or front" type and requires the use of anti-A and anti-B sera. The use of anti-A, B is optional, although still in some use, particularly to confirm the forward type of group O units. The detection of the antibodies present in the plasma or serum is commonly called the "reverse or back" type. Reagent $A_1$ cells and B cells are required; $A_2$ cells are optional.

The results of both tests must be recorded, compared, and found in agreement before the unit can be released. Any discrepancies must be investigated and resolved before releasing the unit, and the results of the investigation must be kept as part of the processing record.

## Rh Typing

The Rh type is determined by the use of anti-$Rh_0$ (D) serum. If the result is positive after the immediate spin phase (D-positive), the unit is labeled Rh-positive. If

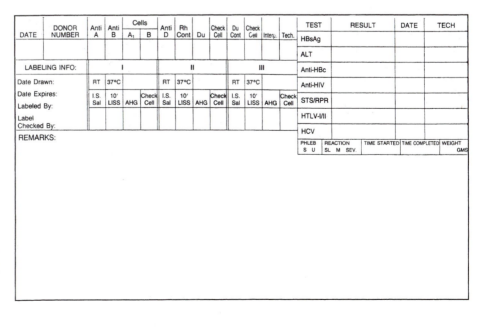

**Figure 10–8.** Form for blood testing for allogeneic donation (back of the donor history card; see Fig. 10–1). (Courtesy Maryland General Hospital, Baltimore.)

the immediate spin phase is negative, an antihuman globulin (AHG) or Coombs phase to detect the D variant (Du) antigen is performed. If the Du test (weak D) is positive, the unit is labeled Rh-positive. If the Du test is negative, the unit is labeled Rh-negative. Large automated blood typing machines are now being used (mostly in large blood centers) that are so sensitive that the Rh type can be accurately determined without the need for the AHG phase.

## Antibody Screen

Although an antibody screen is required only on those donors who give a history of previous pregnancy or transfusion, or both,[21] it is standard practice to perform an antibody screen on all donor units. The procedure must be designed so that the presence of clinically significant antibodies will be detected. Most antibody screening procedures consist of an incubation at 37°C in saline, low ionic strength solution (LISS), or albumin (a new enhancement medium, polyethylene glycol [PEG], is becoming widely used also) and an AHG phase. Because it is widely agreed that antibodies that react only in the cold (less than 37°C) have little or no clinical significance, the use of the immediate spin or a 22°C (room temperature) incubation phase, or both, has generally been dropped. It is acceptable practice to use serum pooled from several donors or pooled screening cells, or both, when performing the antibody screening test on donor units. Donor units in which clinically significant antibodies have been detected should be used for transfusion as RBCs. The plasma must not be used for the preparation of single-donor plasma, liquid or fresh frozen, and should not be used for the production of platelet concentrates or cryoprecipitate.

## Serologic Test for Syphilis

The serologic test for syphilis (STS) is a test that detects previous exposure to syphilis. The rapid plasma reagent (RPR) test is quick, easy to perform, and inexpensive, which makes it good for mass screening of blood donors. However, the test is also prone to false-positive results. Consequently, any positive RPR test result must be confirmed with the more specific, but far more expensive and complicated, fluorescent treponemal antibody absorption (FTA-ABS) test.

Over the years there has been much debate as to the need for an STS. Most have believed that the test is unnecessary because the *Treponema pallidum* spirochete does not survive in citrated blood stored at 1 to 6°C for more than 72 hours, meaning that platelet concentrates are about the only products at risk of transmitting the disease, and there have been no documented cases of transfusion-transmitted syphilis.

The STS is a universally required donor screening test not because there is a concern with transfusion-transmitted syphilis but rather because syphilis is, like hepatitis B, hepatitis C, and HIV, a sexually transmitted disease. A donor who proves to be syphilis-positive is probably at higher risk for exposure to hepatitis and HIV because it implies that safe sexual practices have not been followed.[22]

If the RPR test result is positive, the donor unit is not to be used for transfusion purposes. If the FTA-ABS test result also is positive, the donor needs to be notified.

## Hepatitis B Surface Antigen

The test procedure used must be one approved by the FDA or a documented equivalent method. The methods currently approved are radioimmunoassay (RIA), enzyme-linked immunosorbent assay (ELISA), and reverse passive hemagglutination (RPHA). Of these approved methods the ELISA is by far the most common procedure in use. All of the newer viral marker tests use the ELISA method, and many facilities perform all of the tests on a single instrument.

Any unit found to be positive for HBsAg must not be used for transfusion. (Units drawn for only autologous transfusion can be accepted.)

In an emergency, blood and blood products can be released before HBsAg testing is completed, provided that the test is performed, the results are transmitted to the transfusion service as soon as possible, and the unit is conspicuously labeled or tagged to indicate that testing is not complete. Record of the early release and the subsequent test results must be maintained. If the test result should be positive, the recipient's physician must be notified and a record of that notification must be maintained.[23]

## Hepatitis C Antibody

The hepatitis C virus (HCV) was identified in 1988 and accounts for most, but not all, of what we used to call *non-A, non-B hepatitis*. The test is an ELISA procedure that detects the presence of antibody formed against the hepatitis C virus (anti-HCV). Any donor unit that tests positive for anti-HCV must not be used for transfusion except, as with HBsAg testing, as an autologous transfusion.

The rules for emergency release of a unit, before testing for anti-HCV, are the same as for HBsAg testing.

## Hepatitis Surrogate Testing

In late 1986, surrogate testing for non-A, non-B hepatitis was instituted based on the results of two major studies: one by the National Institutes of Health (NIH) and the other by a multi-institutional cooperative study (Transfusion-Transmitted Virus Study [TTVS]). These studies indicated a significant incidence of elevated ALT levels or anti-HBc, or both, present in donor units implicated in posttransfusion non-A, non-B hepatitis infection.[24] However, in 1995 an NIH consensus panel voted to discontinue the serum ALT test for blood donors because specific anti-HCV testing has eliminated more than 85 percent of posttransfusion hepatitis C infection.[25] Studies have shown that the increased sensitivity with the second generation HCV 2.0 EIA test has supported AABB and NIH in dropping the ALT test as a surrogate marker for blood donors.[26] However, the anti-HBc marker is still mandated in the prevention of posttransfusion hepatitis B.

*Anti-HBc:* This antibody is directed against a "core" or interior protein on the hepatitis B virus. It usually develops before general symptoms of disease are apparent and has been found in donor units that have been implicated in non-A, non-B transfusion-transmitted hepatitis (TTH). Any unit that is repeatedly reactive for anti-HBc should not be used for transfusion.

## Human Immunodeficiency Virus Antibody

All donor units must be screened for the presence of the HIV-1/2 antibody using an EIA procedure approved by the FDA. If the EIA screening test result is positive, the test is repeated. If the repeat test result is negative, the unit can be used for transfusion. If the repeat screening test result is positive, the unit is discarded and a confirmation Western blot test performed. If the Western blot test result is negative or inconclusive, the donor's name is placed in a temporary holding file. The donor need not be notified or deferred from future donations. If the Western blot test result is positive, the donor must be notified, preferably in person, and counseled on what the test results mean. The donor is indefinitely deferred.

HIV-2 has been isolated from several patients with frank AIDS. Although endemic in West Africa, this virus is uncommon in the United States.[27] In 1992, in an effort to ensure the safest blood supply possible, it was required that all donor blood be tested for the presence of both HIV-1 and HIV-2 antibodies (anti-HIV 1/2). In most centers this is done by the use of a new, combined test.

## Human Immunodeficiency Virus (HIV-1 p24) Antigen

This test was introduced in 1996 and was added to the battery of tests because it helps shorten the "window" period between *infection* and the presence of *detectable antibody*. This is a monoclonal test that detects the presence of the p24 antigen in the capsule of the virus. According to a study published in the *New England Journal of Medicine* in December 1995, this test should shorten the window period from 22 to 16 days and reduce the risk of transmission of HIV from 1 in 562,000 to 1 in 825,000 per units of blood screened.[28] The confirmation test for HIV-1 antigen is a neutralization test EIA. The donor should be permanently deferred if the confirmation test is positive. If the neutralization test is negative, the result of the HIV Ag is indeterminant and donors should be temporarily deferred for 8 weeks.[29] If the antigen test is negative after the 8 weeks, donors can be re-entered.

## Human T-Cell Lymphotropic Virus Type I Antibody

This virus is believed to cause adult T-cell leukemia (ATL) and has been associated with a neurologic disorder called HTLV-associated myelopathy (HAM). Because the incubation period for the diseases associated with HTLV-1 infection may be very long and because the results of an American Red Cross study in 1986 to 1987 indicated a possible transfusion-transmitted infection rate of 2800 recipients per year, this virus was added to the growing list of viral markers that must be screened for in all donor blood.[30] HTLV-1 infection is prevalent in Southern Japan and Brazil. Persons can be infected via sexual contact and through breast milk (mother to child). HTLV-II is genetically similar to type I; however, the former is found with higher frequency among intravenous (IV) drug users and in some Native American populations. Donor screening for HTLV is an EIA test that does not discriminate between types I and II. However, as of February 15, 1998, AABB standards in accordance with FDA guidelines will require a separate test for HTLV-II antibodies.[31] Any units that test positive for HTLV must not be used for transfusion unless the unit is labeled as autologous.

## Testing Requirements for Autologous Donors

Units that are donated exclusively for autologous transfusion must be tested for ABO and Rh only if the unit is to be transfused at the same facility that collected it. However, if the unit is to be shipped from the collecting facility to a transfusing facility, the first unit from a specific donor within a 30-day period must be tested for HBsAg, anti-HIV 1/2, HIV-1 Ag, anti-HCV, anti-HBc, STS, and any other test that is required or recommended by the FDA.[32]

If any of the disease marker test results are found to be positive, a "biohazard" label must be attached to the unit. If either the HBsAg or the anti-HIV 1/2 tests are confirmed to be reactive, the unit must not be shipped unless *written* request and consent are obtained from the patient's physician. The patient's physician must also be notified if the anti-HBc, anti-HCV, or STS is found to be repeatedly reactive.

If an autologous donor has met all of the standard requirements for an allogeneic blood donor and the blood bank wishes to use the unit of allogeneic (crossover) transfusion, should it not be needed by the donor, all of the standard tests identified in this section must be performed.

## Labeling

Once all testing is completed, the WB or component(s) must be labeled. The label shall include the following information (Fig. 10–9):

1. Classification of the donor (volunteer, paid, autologous)

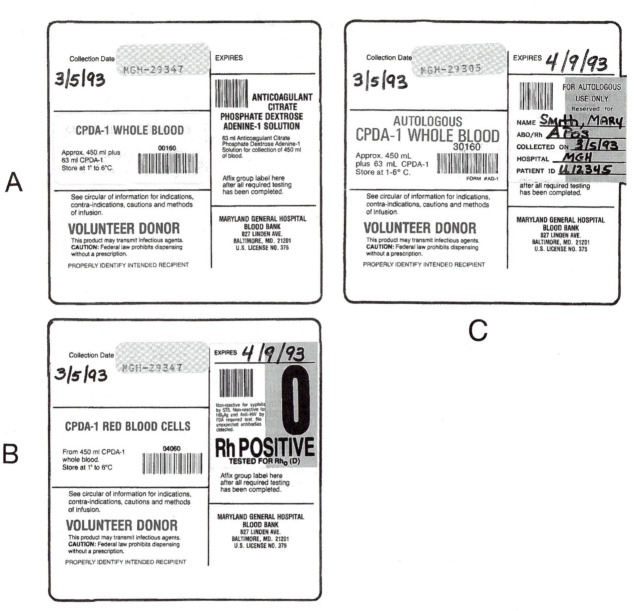

**Figure 10–9.** Donor base labels: (*A*) at time of collection, (*B*) after completion of all testing, and (*C*) for an autologous donor's unit.

2. Name of the component and any modifier(s), if applicable
3. Name of the anticoagulant used (not required for components prepared by hemapheresis or for frozen, deglycerolized, rejuvenated, or washed RBCs)
4. Amount of blood collected or, for platelets, fresh frozen plasma, or low-volume RBCs, volume in the container
5. Donor or WB number (the alphanumeric identification system)
6. Name, address, and registration or license number of the collecting facility
7. Required storage temperature for the specific component
8. ABO group and Rh type of the donor
9. Expiration date (month, day, and year) and, if appropriate, time
10. "See circular of information for indications, contraindications, cautions, and methods of infusion"
11. "Caution: Federal law prohibits dispensing without prescription"
12. "Properly identify intended recipient"
13. "This product may transmit infectious agents"

## Repeat Testing

If the blood-collecting facility is separate from the transfusion facility, the latter is required to perform some repeat testing before issuing the blood or component for transfusion. The tests that must be repeated are:

1. ABO group on all WB and RBC units
2. Rh type on all Rh-negative WB and RBC units (immediate spin phase is required, but Du testing is not required)

These tests are to be performed on a segment sample from the attached integral tubing.

## COMPONENT PREPARATION

Today effective transfusion therapy depends on the availability of many different blood components. These components, used separately or in various combinations, can adequately meet most patient transfusion needs while keeping the risks of transfusion to a minimum.

Component transfusion therapy has the added benefit of using a limited natural resource more effectively by providing needed therapeutic material to several patients from a single donation.

The following section reviews each of the major components in terms of their preparation and general use. Table 10–2 outlines the various components.

### Red Blood Cells

Red blood cells are prepared by removing approximately 80 percent of the plasma from a unit of WB. Regulations require that the final hematocrit of an RBC unit not exceed 80 percent. The average hematocrit is between 65 and 80 percent.

Red blood cells contain the same RBC mass and therefore the same $O_2$-carrying capacity as WB, but with approximately one-half the volume (average volume is 250 to 300 mL). They can be used in any situation that requires increased $O_2$-carrying capacity. RBCs are particularly useful in patients who require the increased RBC mass but may be at risk of circulatory overload (e.g., patients with chronic severe anemia with a compensated [normal] blood volume or those with anemia along with cardiac failure). The advantages of using RBCs rather than WB include:

1. Equal $O_2$ capacity in half the volume
2. Significant reduction in the level of isoagglutinins (anti-A and anti-B), thus facilitating the safe transfusion of group O cells to non–group O recipients
3. Significant reduction in the levels of acid, citrate, and potassium in units prepared just before transfusion. This reduces the risk of acid level, citrate toxicity, and potassium load in patients with cardiac, renal, or liver disease. Units that are prepared at the time of collection have reduced levels of acid and citrate (most of the anticoagulant is removed with the plasma), but potassium, which is released as the RBCs age, will remain a problem.

Red blood cells can be prepared any time during the normal dating period by centrifugation or sedimentation. Between 200 and 250 mL of plasma are usually removed from units collected in CDPA-1. An extra 50 mL of plasma can be removed from units drawn in CPD plus adenine-saline because 150 mL of adenine-saline preservative solution will be added to the cells, returning the hematocrit to about 80 percent. The expiration date of RBCs prepared in a closed system will not change from that of the WB (35 days for CPDA-1 and 42 for CPD plus adenine-saline). Should the unit have to be entered, the expiration date is reduced to 24 hours from the time the unit was entered. Sterile docking-connecting devices are now available that allow entrance to a unit without altering the original expiration date.

The following is a general procedure for RBC production using centrifugation:

1. Weigh and balance each unit.
2. Place the balanced units into the centrifuge. The centrifuge of choice is a swinging bucket type. It produces a better pack and a better plasma cell interface. The refrigerated centrifuges should be checked on each day of use for correct speed and temperature (calibration should be performed every 6 months), and quality control documents should be maintained.
3. Centrifuge for the specified time and speed. Although the average speed is approximately 3600 rpm for about 5 minutes, each centrifuge must be calibrated individually to ensure a quality product. The speed and time change, depending on the plasma product(s) prepared. The AABB *Technical Manual* contains some centrifuge calculation data and procedures.[33]
4. When the centrifuge has come to a complete stop, remove the unit carefully and place on an expressor.
5. Express the plasma into the attached satellite bag. The hematocrit can be estimated by expressing enough plasma to bring the plasma cell interface to the top corner (shoulder) of the bag or by removing a specified weight of plasma. The AABB *Technical Manual* suggests 230 to 256 g (225 to 250 mL).
6. When the desired amount of plasma has been removed, seal the tubing using a dielectric heat sealer or metal clips.
7. Separate the plasma and the RBCs. Store the RBCs at 4°C. The plasma can be stored at 4°C, 22°C, or −30°C, depending on the product desired. Ensure that the satellite bags have the same donor number as the primary bag.

As part of the quality control program, each month hematocrit values must be calculated on a representative number of units (usually 1 to 4 units, depending on the total number prepared). Seventy-five percent of samples tested must meet the approved criteria (80 percent or less).

### RBC Aliquots

Aliquotted red blood cells is the product most often transfused during the neonatal period. Indications for

**Table 10–2.** Summary of Blood Components

| Component | Shelf Life | Storage Temp. | Quality Control | Volume | Indications for Use | Content | Dosage Effect | Transfusion Criteria |
|---|---|---|---|---|---|---|---|---|
| RBCs | CPD—21 d, CPDA-1—35 d, CP2D—21 d, CPD-AS—42 d, Heparin—2 d, CPDA-1—24 h | 1–6°C | Hematocrit must be 80% or less | 250–300 mL | Restore oxygen-carrying capacity in symptomatic anemia | RBCs (65–80%) Plasma (20–35%) Some: Platelets, WBCs | 1 unit RBCs ↑ Hct 3% ↑ Hb 1 g | ABO and Rh/xm |
| Aliquots | | | | Varies | | | | O-neg/CMV– |
| Leukocyte-reduced RBCs | Closed system: same as for RBCs; Open system: 24 h | 1–6°C | $5 \times 10^6$ residual WBC 85% Recovery of RBC | 250–300 mL | Patients who require replacement of RBC mass and reduced exposure to WBC: Febrile reactions | RBCs (85–95%) Plasma (5–20%) Residual WBCs ($<5 \times 10^6$) | Same for RBC | ABO/Rh/xm compatible |
| Washed RBCs | 24 h (open system) | 1–6°C | Plasma removal | 250–300 mL | Patients with a history of plasma protein antibodies, diagnosis of PNH, febrile reactions | RBCs (60–80%) Saline (20–40%) | Same as for RBC | ABO/Rh/crossmatch compatible |
| Frozen, thawed, deglycerolized RBCs | Frozen—10 yr Deglycerolized—24h | Frozen: –65°C or –120°C Deglycerolized—1–6°C | 80% recovery RBC mass <1% residual glycerol <300 mg residual-free hemoglobin | 200–300 mL | Long-term storage of "rare" units and/or autologous units | RBCs (60–80%) Saline with dextrose (20–40%) <1–2% residual WBCs, platelets | Same as for RBC | ABO/Rh/crossmatch compatible antigen profile |
| Platelets Random-donor (Prepared from WB) | 5 d 2 d | 20–24°C 1–6°C | $5.5 \times 10^{10}$ platelets prepared within 6 hr of WB collection pH=6.0 or greater at the end of the storage time | 50–65 mL 30–40 mL | Thrombocytopenia, bleeding, DIC, platelet disorders | Platelets: $5.5 \times 10^{10}$ Plasma: 50–65 mL Residual WBC | Increase platelets 5000–10,000/unit | ABO/Rh compatible (if possible) |
| Aliquots | 4 h (syringe) | 20–24°C | | Varies | Intraventricular bleeding | | | CMV-neg |
| Platelets Single-donor (prepared by pheresis) | 5 d (closed system) 24 h (open system) | 20–24°C | $3.0 \times 10^{11}$ platelets pH ≥ 6.0 or greater at the end of the storage time | 300 mL | To correct thrombocytopenia in patients who demonstrate refractoriness to random-donor platelets (platelet antibodies) | Platelets: $3.0 \times 10^{11}$ Plasma: 300 mL approx. May have significant RBC and WBC | ↑ platelet count: 30–60,000 per unit | ABO and Rh compatible HLA typed (sometimes) Crossmatch compatible (may be required) |
| Single-donor plasma FFP or SPD-24 | Frozen = 1 yr Thawed = 24 h | –18°C 1–6°C | FFP: Prepare within 6 hr of whole blood collection (ACD) SDP-24: Prepare within 24 h of whole blood FFP: 8 h of collection (CPD, CP2D, CPDA-1) | 150–250 mL | Treatment of multiple coagulation factor deficiencies (massive transfusion, trauma, liver disease, DIC, unidentified deficiency) | Plasma, all coagulation factors except platelets 400 mg fibrinogen 1 unit/mL all other factors | Increase factor levels 20–30% per dose of 10–15 mL/kg of body weight | ABO compatible |

| Component | Expiration | Storage Temperature | Preparation | Volume | Indications/Uses | Contents | Dosage | Special Considerations |
|---|---|---|---|---|---|---|---|---|
| Single-donor plasma (SDP) Liquid/frozen | Liquid: up to 5 d beyond whole blood expiration date (26–40 d) Frozen: 5 y | 1–6°C −18°C or colder | Must be frozen within 6 h of transfer to final container | 150–250 mL | Treatment of stable clotting factor deficiencies Source plasma for manufacture into NSA, PPF, ISG | Plasma stable clotting factors only | | ABO compatible |
| Cryoprecipitated antihemophilic factor (Cryo) | Frozen: 1 yr Thawed: 6 h Pooled: 4 h | −18°C or colder 20–24°C | Factor VIII:C (80 IU) Thaw at 37°C | 10–25 mL | Correction of F VIII deficiency (hemophilia A, von Willebrand's) Factor XIII deficiency Fibrinogen deficiency owing to congenital hypofibrinogenemia Some fibrinogen consumption problems Source of "fibrin glue" | Factor VIII:C (80–150 IU) Fibrinogen: (150–250 mg) Factor XIII (20–30% of WB level) vWF (40–70% of WB level) | Plasma volume × % factor level needed = No. units needed ÷ 80 −100 = No. cryoprecipitate bags needed | ABO compatible |
| Granulocyte concentrate | 24 h | 20–24°C | $1.0 \times 10^{10}$ granulocytes Total WBC count with differential | 200–600 mL | Correct severe neutropenia (<500 polymorphonuclear neutrophils/mL) Fever unresponsive to antibiotic therapy for 24–48 h Myeloid hypoplasia of bone marrow with reasonable chance of survival | Granulocytes: $1.0 \times 10^{10}$ WBCs Platelets Plasma RBCs (15% Hct) | | ABO and Rh specific HLA matched (usually) Cross-match compatible |
| Factor VIII concentrate (AHF) | Varies (expiration date listed on each vial) | 1–6°C (lyophilized) | — | 10–30 mL | Treatment of moderate to severe factor VIII deficiencies (hemophilia A) | Factor VIII:C (level stated on label of each vial) Some fibrinogen | See cryoprecipitate for dosage calculations 1 U factor VIII per kilogram body weight should ↑ factor VIII level by 2% | Reconstitute before infusion |
| Factor IX concentrate (prothrombin complex) | Varies (expiration date listed on each vial) | 1–6°C (lyophilized) | — | 20–30 mL | Treatment of factor IX deficiency (hemophilia B, Christmas disease) Treatment of some factor II, VII, X deficiencies | Factors II, VII, IX, X (levels stated on each vial) | See cryoprecipitate for dosage calculations 1 U factor IX per kilogram body weight should ↑ factor IX level by 1.5% | Reconstitute before infusion |
| ISG | 3 yr: Intramuscular injection 1 yr: Intravenous solution | — | — | Varies according to patient size and indications for use | Prophylactic treatment for exposure to certain diseases such as hepatitis, chickenpox | Gamma globulins (intramuscular = 16.5 g/dL) (intravenous = 5 g/dL) Primarily IgG, some IgA, IgM | | Intramuscular or intravenous, depending on product used |

(continued)

**Table 10–2.** Summary of Blood Components (*continued*)

| Component | Shelf Life | Storage Temp. | Quality Control | Volume | Indications for Use | Content | Dosage Effect | Transfusion Criteria |
|---|---|---|---|---|---|---|---|---|
| NSA 5 or 25% | 3 yr<br>5 yr | 20–24°C<br>1–6°C | — | 50 mL or 250 mL | Plasma volume expansion: surgery, trauma, burns, etc. | 96% Albumin<br>4% Globulin | | |
| PPF 5% | 3 yr<br>5 yr | 20–24°C<br>1–6°C | — | 250 mL | Plasma volume expansion | Albumin (80–85%)<br>Globulin (15–20%) | — | — |
| Synthetic volume expanders | Varies | — | — | Varies | Plasma volume expansion (colloid or crystalloid) | Normal saline<br>Ringer's<br>Electrolyte solution<br>Dextran<br>HES | | |
| Rh₀D Ig | 3 yr | 1–6°C | — | 1 mL | Prevention of Rh₀(D) Immunization | Full dose = 300-μg anti-D<br>Mini-dose = 50-μg anti-D<br>IV = 120-μg anti-D | Termination at 12 weeks or more, antepartum dose<br>Termination <12 weeks Amniocentesis | Injection given within 72 h of delivery, abortion, or miscarriage Rh-neg recipient; no evidence of serum anti-D |

transfusion include anemia caused by spontaneous fetomaternal or fetoplacental hemorrhage, twin-twin transfusion, obstetric accidents, and internal hemorrhage. Blood drawn from infants for laboratory testing (iatrogenic anemia) also may warrant a neonatal transfusion if more than 10 percent of the blood volume has been removed.[34] Transfusions for neonates require only small volumes of red cells (10 to 25 mL), so several aliquots may be prepared from a single donor unit.

Initial testing for neonates includes ABO, Rh, and antibody screen for unexpected antibodies, which can be performed on serum or plasma from the infant or mother. Although the procedure in each hospital may vary, it is unnecessary to perform compatibility testing for subsequent transfusions in any one hospitalization, provided that the initial antibody screen is negative and group O or ABO-compatible red cells are transfused. It is not necessary to perform reverse typing on neonates unless they are given non-group-O red cells. If the infant's serum contains an unexpected antibody, the infant must be given red cells lacking the corresponding antigen. The anticoagulant used most often for neonate transfusions is CPDA-1. A transfusion of 10 mL/kg in a unit with a hematocrit of 80 percent should raise the hemoglobin by 3 g/dL. The following is a procedure for preparing red cell aliquots:

1. Select an O-negative, CMV-negative unit, preferably 5 days old or less, but 7 days is acceptable if fresher units are not available.
2. Add 7 mL to the amount requested by the doctor to be transfused. Mix the unit well before aliquotting a volume slightly larger than needed into one of the attached transfer packs of a multipack unit. Heat-seal the tubing between the transfer pack and the main unit. Note: Determine the volume of red cells by weighing the transfer pack on a scale. Tare the empty transfer pack on the scale and weigh enough blood for the aliquot. Example: 50 g of blood should provide enough for a 30 mL aliquot.
3. Label a 30 or 60 mL syringe to indicate the volume contained in the syringe on the product label. Note: The expiration time is 24 hours from the time the transfer pack was entered.
4. Place a hemostat on the tubing between a sterile 20-$\mu$m filter set and the cap on the filter set. Make sure the slide clamp attached to the filter is above the hemostat.
5. Spike the transfer pack with the filter set.
6. Remove the cap from the tubing on the filter set and place it on sterile gauze. Attach the syringe to the filter set tubing.
7. Withdraw the desired amount of blood into the syringe. Close the slide clamp and remove the hemostat. Note: Draw the amount requested for transfusion plus 7 mL to allow for tubing.
8. Remove the syringe from the tubing and replace the caps on both the syringe and the tubing.
9. Place a label on the parent unit indicating that aliquots have been made and specifying how many milliliters have been removed.
10. Store at 1 to 6°C for 24 hours.

## Irradiation

In the past several years the use of irradiated blood products (primarily RBCs and platelets) has risen dramatically. It has long been known that gamma irradiation of blood products would reduce the risk of transfusion-associated graft versus host (TA-GVH) disease in patients receiving allogeneic bone marrow transplants (BMT), and for such patients it is standard practice to irradiate any blood product that is contaminated with donor lymphocytes. More recently it has become clear that other patients are also at risk for TA-GVH disease. The risk appears to be well defined in BMT patients, patients with congenital immunodeficiency syndrome or Hodgkin's disease, for intrauterine transfusions, and for blood transfusions from first-degree family members. Still under investigation, but also felt to carry some degree of risk, are premature newborn infants, solid organ transplant patients, patients with non-Hodgkin's malignancies, and those with solid tumors. To date there has been no reported incidence of TA-GVH disease in AIDS patients.

Most blood product irradiation uses either cesium-137 ($^{137}$Cs) or cobalt-60 ($^{60}$Co) as the source of gamma rays. The American Association of Blood Banks requires that products be given a minimum of 25 Gy, and the range can run as high as 35 Gy.

The shelf life of irradiated RBCs is 28 days from the date of irradiation or original expiration date on unit, whichever comes first.[35] Studies have shown that there is an increase in extracellular potassium following irradiation.[36]

## Leukocyte-reduced Red Blood Cells

Leukocyte-reduced RBCs are products in which the absolute WBC count in the unit is less than $5 \times 10^6$ ($5 \times 10^8$ is acceptable for the prevention of febrile transfusion reactions). The method used must also ensure that at least 85 percent of the original RBC mass is retained. It has been thought for some time that donor leukocytes in blood transfusions are responsible for febrile nonhemolytic (FNH) transfusion reactions and transfusion-related acute lung injury (TRALI). More recently there have been concerns about transfusion-transmitted infectious agents such as cytomegalovirus (CMV), Epstein-Barr virus (EBV), and HTLV-1, all known to be carried primarily in the leukocytes, as well as TA-GVH disease.[37] Many patients, including multiple-transfused, leukemia, aplastic anemia, immunosuppressed, and immunodeficient patients and multiparous women, are potential candidates for leukocyte-reduced blood products. It should be noted that leukocyte-reduced RBCs are not indicated as a measure for preventing posttransfusion GVHD.

Several techniques exist for preparing leukocyte-reduced RBCs. The technique used may depend on the patient's particular need, the equipment available in the blood bank, whether the method can be done in a closed system, and the *cost*. The following is a brief summary of the acceptable techniques.

## Centrifugation

This is one of the easiest and least costly of methods, and it can be done in a closed system, but it is also the least efficient. It reduces the WBC level only by 70 to 80 percent (less than 1 log reduction) and sacrifices as much as 20 percent of the RBC volume.[38] In some instances this technique may not produce a finished product that meets minimum standards for WBC reduction. Today this method has largely been replaced by other, more effective techniques.

## Filtration

Many types of filters are available today that can produce an acceptable leukocyte-reduced product, depending on the purpose for the WBC reduction and the intended recipient.

Microaggregate filters are typically polyester or plastic screen filters with a pore size of 20 to 40 μm.[39] The unit is generally centrifuged before filtration. This increases the size of the microaggregates (e.g., platelets, WBCs), which are then filtered out during the administration of the unit. The effectiveness of the leukocyte reduction can be increased by cooling the unit at 4°C for 3 hours after centrifugation and before filtering. Filters of this type usually give a 1- to 2-log reduction (90 to 99 percent) of leukocytes in the unit ($5 \times 10^8$) and recover most of the original RBC volume.[40] The procedure is easy, quick, and relatively inexpensive. Red blood cell units prepared by this method are quite suitable for patients who have experienced FNH transfusion reactions or for those who are receiving transfusions outside the hospital (e.g., home transfusions), where FNH reactions should be avoided.

Newer leukocyte-reducing filters (third generation) use selective adsorption of leukocytes or leukocytes and platelets. They are made of polyester or cellulose acetate and will produce a 2- to 4-log (more than 99.9 percent) reduction of the WBCs ($<5 \times 10^6$) or platelets, or both.[41] As with the microaggregate filters, there is very little loss of RBC volume, and the procedure is quite easy. These filters provide a leukocyte-reduced product with normal shelf life. Because these filters are so effective in eliminating the leukocytes or platelets, or both, they can be used to help prevent alloimmunization to HLA antigens, CMV transmission-reactivation, and FNH reactions. They are suitable for use with BMT patients, patients receiving intrauterine transfusions, and chemotherapy patients.[42] Bedside filters do not consistently meet the leukocyte reduction standards and are not always suitable for surgical patients because of slow blood flow through the filters.

## Freezing, Deglycerolizing, and Saline Washing

All of these techniques can produce a leukocyte-reduced product. They are not as efficient at removing WBCs as the newer filters (95 to 99 percent reduction), but because they all have a saline-washing step, they remove all of the donor plasma. This makes these products particularly good for patients with plasma protein problems such as paroxysmal nocturnal hemoglobinuria (PNH) or immunoglobulin A (IgA) deficiency with circulating anti-IgA. The disadvantages here are the 24-hour expiration date because of the open system, the special equipment that is necessary, and the overall cost, including the disposable washing sets. Caution must also be used with saline washing alone, because although the plasma removal is acceptable, not all automated systems are approved for leukocyte removal using this technique.

## Frozen, Deglycerolized Red Blood Cells

In the past 15 years, frozen RBCs have come into widespread general use. They provide an RBC product that is almost free of leukocytes, platelets, and plasma. It has an extended shelf life (10 years or more) in the frozen state, which has made long-term storage of rare units possible and autotransfusions more plausible.

Many procedures are used to freeze and to deglycerolize RBCs. The reader should consult the AABB *Technical Manual*, numerous articles in various journals, the American Red Cross blood service directive on RBC freezing and deglycerolizing, and the manufacturer's directions on the use of the equipment. Table 10–3 summarizes key steps of high-glycerol freezing procedures.

## High Glycerol (40 Percent Weight per Volume)

This method increases the cryoprotective power of the glycerol, thus allowing a slow, uncontrolled freezing process. The freezer used is generally a mechanical freezer that provides storage at −65°C. This particular procedure is probably the most widely used method because the equipment involved is fairly simple and the products require less delicate handling. It does, however, require a larger volume of wash solution for deglycerolizing.

## Low Glycerol (20 Percent Weight per Volume)

In this method, the cryoprotection of the glycerol is minimal, and a very rapid, more controlled freezing procedure is required. Liquid nitrogen ($N_2$) is routinely used for this method. The frozen units must be stored at about −120°C, which is the temperature of liquid $N_2$ vapor. Because of the minimal amount of protection by the glycerol, temperature fluctuations during storage can cause RBC destruction.

The quality control procedures necessary for RBC freezing include all of the standard procedures for

**Table 10–3.** Key Steps in Freezing Red Cells Using High Glycerol Concentration

| Preparation | Glycerolization | Deglycerolization |
| --- | --- | --- |
| Weigh red cells<br>Adjust to 260–400 g with 0.9% NaCl<br>Prewarm red cells and glycerol to 25°C | Place red cells on a shaker and add<br>  100 mL glycerol<br>Stop agitation and allow cells to equilibrate<br>  for 5–30 min | Thaw frozen cells at 37°C in a water<br>  bath or dry block<br>Deglycerolize cells using a continuous<br>  flow washer |
| Set glycerol bottles in a water bath<br>  for 15 min at 25–37°C | Let partially glycerolized cells flow into<br>  freezing bag; slowly add remaining glycerol | Apply a deglycerolization label to<br>  transfer pack, ABO, RH, whole blood<br>  unit numbers, expiration date |
| Label the freezing bag with name of<br>  facility, whole blood unit numbers,<br>  ABO, Rh, date collected, date frozen,<br>  cryoprotective agent, expiration date,<br>  and "red blood cells (human) frozen" | Maintain glycerolized cells at 24–32°C until<br>  ready to freeze (should not exceed 4 h) | Dilute unit with hypertonic 12% NaCl<br>  and let equilibrate for 5 min |
| | Freeze at −65°C or colder | Wash with 1.6% NaCl until residual<br>  glycerol is less than 1%<br>Suspend cells in isotonic saline with<br>  0.2% dextrose; store at 1–6°C |

monitoring refrigerators, freezers, water baths, dry thaw baths, and centrifuges. They also include procedures to ensure good RBC recovery (80 percent), good viability (70 percent survival at 24 hours posttransfusion) and adequate glycerol removal (less than 1 percent residual intracellular glycerol). Cells should be frozen within 6 hours of collection unless they have been rejuvenated (24 hours).

1. RBC recovery can be determined easily by estimating the recovered RBC mass (final volume × final hematocrit = RBC mass recovered). Compare with the initial (prefreeze) RBC mass.

2. A posttransfusion survival study should be done when the program is first being set up to ensure the proper use of the equipment and procedure. If the procedure being used is a standard procedure with data already published in the literature, these survival studies are not required.

3. Glycerol must be removed to a level of less than 1 percent residual. The published procedures should accomplish this. It is important, however, to perform this check on each unit before releasing it for transfusion. The procedures are very simple.

   a. Measure the osmolarity of the unit using an osmometer. The osmolarity should be about 420 mOsm (maximum 500 mOsm).

   b. Perform a simulated transfusion. Place one segment (approximately 3 inches) of deglycerolized cells into 7 mL of a 0.7 percent NaCl. Mix, centrifuge, and check for hemolysis. Compare with a standard hemoglobin color comparator. If the hue exceeds the 500 mOsm level, hemolysis is too great and the unit is not transferable. Postdeglycerolized tests include confirmation of ABO, Rh, and a direct antihuman globulin test (DAT).

5. Preglycerolizing tests may include the following:

   a. **DAT.** A unit with a positive DAT result should not be used.

   b. **Sickle test.** Cells that carry the sickle trait do not survive routine freezing and deglycerolizing procedures. It is recommended that cells known to carry the sickle trait not be used routinely in a frozen RBC program. If for some reason the cells must be frozen, there is a special deglycerolizing procedure that may be used.[43] If there is a high percentage of black donors in the area, it may be worthwhile to prescreen units before freezing.

   c. **Accurate and complete records.** Good record keeping must be maintained for all phases of the glycerolizing and deglycerolizing procedures.

## Platelet Concentrate

Platelet concentrates are one of the primary products produced during the routine conversion of WB into concentrated RBCs. They have widespread use for a variety of patients: actively bleeding patients who are thrombocytopenic (less than 50,000/µL) due to decreased production or decreased function; cancer patients, during radiation and chemotherapy, because of an induced thrombocytopenia (less than 20,000/µl); and thrombocytopenic preoperative patients (less than 50,000/µL). Prophylactic platelet transfusions are not usually indicated or recommended in disseminated intravascular coagulation (DIC) or idiopathic thrombocytopenic purpura (ITP). In both cases, there is an induced thrombocytopenia owing to increased destruction. ITP is generally thought to be caused by an autoantibody, and DIC to mass consumption.

Platelet concentrates prepared from WB are generally referred to as random-donor platelets to distinguish them from single-donor platelets produced by pheresis. Random-donor platelet concentrates contain at least $5.5 \times 10^{10}$ platelets, are stored at 20 to 24°C with continuous agitation, contain 50 to 70 mL of plasma (pH > 6), and have a shelf life of 5 days. Single-donor platelet concentrates or "superpack" platelets, as they are sometimes called, are prepared by pheresis (see Chapter 17), contain at least $3.0 \times 10^{11}$ platelets, are stored at 22 to 24°C with agitation, contain approximately 300 mL of plasma, and also have a shelf life of 5 days. Pheresed platelets are generally indicated for patients who are unresponsive or *refractory* to random platelets due to HLA alloimmunization or to limit the platelet exposure from multiple donors.[44]

Whole blood used for the preparation of platelet concentrates must be drawn by a single, nontraumatic venipuncture, and the concentrate must be prepared within 6 hours of collection. The following is a general procedure for preparing random-donor platelets.

1. Maintain the WB at 20 to 24°C before and during platelet preparation.
2. Set the centrifuge temperature at 22°C. The rpm and time must be specifically calculated for each centrifuge. It will generally be a short (2- to 3-minute), light (3200 rpm) spin. This spin should separate most of the RBCs but leave most of the platelets suspended in the plasma.
3. Platelet preparation should be done in a closed, multibag system.
4. Express off the platelet-rich plasma into one of the satellite bags. Enough plasma must remain on the RBC to maintain a 70 to 80 percent hematocrit. The hematocrit estimation methods stated in the RBC procedure can be used here.
5. Seal the tubing between the RBC and the plasma. Disconnect the RBC and store it at 4°C.
6. Recentrifuge the platelet-rich plasma at 22°C using a heavy spin (approximately 3600 rpm for 5 minutes). This will separate the platelets from the plasma.
7. Express the majority of the plasma into the second satellite bag, leaving approximately 50 to 70 mL on the platelets. The volume is important to maintain the pH (above 6.0) during storage.
8. Seal the tubing between the bags and separate. Make segments for both the platelets and the plasma for testing purposes.
9. The plasma can be frozen as fresh frozen plasma (FFP), single-donor plasma frozen within 24 hours (SDP-24), or stored as liquid recovered plasma. Be sure to record the plasma volume on the bag.
10. Allow the platelet concentrate to lie undisturbed for 1 to 2 hours at 20 to 24°C. Be sure the platelet button is covered with the plasma. Platelets should be resuspended. Gentle manipulation can be used if needed.
11. Store on a rotator, allowing constant, gentle agitation.
12. Shelf life is 5 days from the date of collection. If the system is opened, transfusion must be

within 6 hours. The volume, expiration date, and time (if indicated) must be on the label.
13. All of the units for a single dose (typically 6 to 8 units for an adult) can be pooled into a single bag before transfusion. Once pooled, the product must be transfused within 4 hours of pooling. The pooled unit must be given a unique "pool number," which must be on the label.

The quality control procedures must include a platelet count ($5.5 \times 10^{10}$ for random donor, $3.0 \times 10^{11}$ for single donor); pH (6.0 or greater); and volume (must be sufficient to maintain an acceptable pH until the end of the dating period). These procedures are to be performed regularly—usually 1 to 4 units per month, depending on the production volume—at the end of the product's dating period. Seventy-five percent of all units tested must meet or exceed the minimum standards. Temperature monitoring must be performed during each major stage of production and records maintained of all procedures performed.

Platelets, either random donor or single donor, can be irradiated if the patient's diagnosis indicates that it is appropriate. The irradiation requirements are the same as for RBCs (25 to 35 Gy). Irradiation can occur any time during the platelet shelf life and will not affect or change the expiration date.

### Platelet Aliquots

Transfusion of platelet concentrates is indicated for neonates whose count falls below 50,000/μL and who are experiencing bleeding. Factors that may be associated with thrombocytopenia include immaturity of the coagulant system (preterm infant), platelet dysfunction, increased destruction of platelets, dilution effect secondary to massive transfusion or exchange transfusion, or intraventricular hemorrhaging.[45] Either random or apheresed platelets may be transfused and should increase the platelet count by 50,000 to 100,000 given in a dose of 5 to 10 mL/kg. The following procedure is used in the preparation of platelet aliquots for neonates:

1. Select unit to be aliquotted. Either AB or group specific units should be selected. CMV-negative or volume-reduced platelets may be requested by the doctor. For volume-reduced platelets, where infants cannot tolerate large intravenous infusion of plasma, stored platelets are centrifuged and the plasma removed. The platelets remain undisturbed at room temperature for 20 to 60 minutes before being resuspended in residual plasma.
2. Platelets should rotate for at least 30 minutes at room temperature following volume reduction if platelets are shipped from another facility.
3. Remove cap from stopcock apparatus and attach to end of blood set. Use a 170- to 260-μm filter.
4. Remove second cap from stopcock and cap from syringe to be filled and lay it on a piece of sterile gauze. Attach syringe to the stopcock.

5. Close the roller clamps at the spike end of the blood set above the filter and spike the platelet unit.
6. Open the roller clamp on the spike and draw the platelets through the filter and into the syringe. Remove the syringe from the filter set and force the excess air back out of the syringe.
7. Label the syringe with proper labels (see Fig. 10–9). Indicate volume of aliquot on platelet product label.
8. The expiration date is 4 hours from the time the unit was spiked.

## Single-Donor Plasma: Fresh Frozen and Frozen within 24 Hours

Frozen plasma, either FFP or SDP-24, is a frequent by-product of concentrated RBC and platelet concentrate production. It is fresh plasma obtained from a single, uninterrupted, nontraumatic venipuncture. The plasma is then frozen within 8 hours of collection for FFP if the anticoagulant used was CPD, CP2D, or CPDA-1 (6 hours for ACD)[46] or within 24 hours of collection for SDP-24, and stored at −18°C or colder. The product is RBC-free and contains therapeutic levels of all the plasma clotting factors, including factors V and VIII. Fresh frozen plasma contains somewhat higher levels of factors V and VIII, but the levels in SDP-24 are more than adequate, and this product is now being used in some areas instead of FFP. Fresh frozen plasma production is then used for further manufacture into factor VIII concentrate. The shelf life for FFP or SDP-24 is 12 months in the frozen state (−18°C) and 24 hours after thawing, if stored at 1 to 6°C.

The use of SDP-24 or FFP is indicated in patients who are actively bleeding and have multiple clotting factor deficiencies. Examples include massive trauma, surgery, liver disease, DIC, and when a specific disorder cannot be or has not yet been identified.

Specific deficiencies such as factor VIII or fibrinogen are more appropriately treated with cryoprecipitate. Factor II, VII, IX, and X deficiencies would be better treated using the prothrombin complex concentrates.

A single unit of FFP or SDP-24 should contain 150 to 250 mL of plasma, approximately 400 mg of fibrinogen, and about 1 unit of activity per milliliter of each of the stable clotting factors. Fresh frozen plasma also contains the same level (1 unit/mL) of factors V and VIII; SDP-24 contains somewhat less than that level.

If FFP or SDP-24 is to be prepared from WB as part of the production of platelet concentrates, follow the procedure outlined in the platelet concentrate section. At step 9, after the platelet concentrate has been separated from the plasma, proceed in the following manner:

1. Weigh the plasma and determine the volume. Record the volume on the bag.
2. Place the plasma in a protective container and freeze. The plasma must be frozen in such a way that evidence of thawing can be determined. Freezing some sort of indentation into the bag,

which is visible as long as the plasma remains frozen, is an easy way to accomplish this. The container is important because the plastic bag becomes quite brittle when frozen at low temperatures and can be cracked or broken easily.

3. The plasma must be frozen solid within the 8-hour time allotment. The lower the temperature of the freezer and the greater the air circulation around the plasma, the faster the freeze. Freezers at −65°C, blast freezers, packing units between dry ice, or the use of an ice-ethanol or ice-antifreeze bath can be used to speed up the freezing process.[47]
4. Before freezing, be sure that any tubing segments and the transfusion ports ("ears") of the bag are tucked in or placed in such a manner as to prevent or to minimize possible breakage.
5. The label on the frozen plasma must include all of the standard information required. See Code of Federal Regulations, Title:21 CFR 606.121 for specifics. Frozen plasma can also be produced directly from WB, without preparing platelet concentrates. The procedure changes to eliminate the platelet production section, and the general volume of the plasma will be greater.

There are no specific testing procedures required as part of the quality control program. Specific factor levels are not required. Records must be maintained on the production process to ensure that the product was prepared within the time required and that the product was prepared, frozen, and stored at the appropriate temperatures.

## Single-Donor Plasma: Liquid or Frozen

Recovered plasma or single-donor plasma (liquid) and single-donor plasma (frozen) can be prepared directly from the WB or as a byproduct of platelet concentrate or cryoprecipitate production. The products can be used as volume expanders or for treatment of stable clotting factor deficiencies. Because of the availability of hepatitis and HIV-free volume expanders, single-donor plasma is generally not used for that purpose. Most recovered plasma is used for the manufacture of plasma fractionation products such as plasma protein fraction (PPF), normal serum albumin (NSA), and immune serum globulin (ISG).

When produced from WB, recovered ("salvaged") plasma can be removed from the cells any time during the normal dating period and up to 5 days after expiration (26 to 40 days after collection for CPD and CPDA-1, respectively). If SDP (frozen) is being prepared, the plasma is to be stored at −18°C and must be frozen within 6 hours of its transfer to the final container. The shelf life is 5 years in the frozen state. FFP or SDP-24 that has not been used within the 12-month period can be converted to SDP (frozen). Liquid SDP is collected in the same manner, stored at 1 to 6°C, and must be used within 26 to 40 days of whole blood collection.

The production procedure is like that for platelets

and FFP, and quality control measures are limited to production and storage temperatures.

### Cryoprecipitated Antihemophilic Factor

Cryoprecipitate is the cold-precipitated concentration of factor VIII, the antihemophilic factor (AHF). It is prepared from FFP thawed slowly between 1 and 6°C. The product contains most of the factor VIII and part of the fibrinogen from the original plasma. It contains at least 80 units of AHF activity and 150 to 250 mg of fibrinogen. Other significant factors found in cryoprecipitate are factor XIII and von Willebrand factor. Cryoprecipitate has a shelf life of 12 months in the frozen state and must be transfused within 6 hours of thawing or within 4 hours of pooling. Like FFP and SDP-24, cryoprecipitate should be thawed quickly at 37°C. Once thawed, FDA recommends storing at room temperature (22 to 24°C) until transfused. Cryoprecipitate is indicated in the treatment of classic hemophilia (hemophilia A), von Willebrand's disease, and factor XIII deficiency, and as a source of fibrinogen for hypofibrinogenemia. In recent years, cryoprecipitate has also been used to make "fibrin glue," a substance composed of cryoprecipitate (fibrinogen) and topical thrombin. When combined, they produce an adhesive substance that, applied to a surgical site usually via fine spray, can reduce bleeding. It has been most frequently used in cardiac, otologic, and facial cosmetic surgery. The WB donor requirements and preparation requirements for cryoprecipitate are the same as those for platelets and FFP.

1. The venipuncture must be nontraumatic.
2. The WB can be cooled before and during production because platelets are not usually prepared from the units. The volume of plasma required to remain on the RBC and the platelet concentrate will reduce the amount of plasma available for cryoprecipitate production enough to reduce the final AHF activity significantly in the precipitate. At least 200 mL of plasma should be used to ensure that the final product will contain at least 80 AHF units.
3. The plasma must be frozen within 8 hours of collection and within 1 hour from the time freezing was initiated.
4. The second stage of cryoprecipitate preparation begins by allowing the frozen plasma to thaw slowly in the refrigerator at 1 to 6°C. This takes 14 to 16 hours when plasma is thawed in a standard blood bank refrigerator. If a circulating cryoprecipitate thaw bath (4°C water bath) is used, the thawing time is reduced to about 4 hours. The endpoint is when the plasma becomes slushy.
5. Centrifuge the plasma at 4°C for a "hard" spin (typically 3400 to 3600 rpm for 3 to 7 minutes, depending on the centrifuge).
6. Express the supernatant plasma into the attached satellite bag. The cryoprecipitate will be a small white mass in the original plasma bag. Leave only 10 to 15 mL of plasma on the precipitate.
7. Separate and refreeze the cryoprecipitate immedi-

ately. It should be no longer than 1 hour from the time the plasma reaches the slushy stage until the cryoprecipitate is refrozen. A delay in refreezing, or exposure of the unit to elevated temperatures during processing, will significantly decrease the factor VIII activity level in the final product. The centrifuge temperature must be at 4°C, and it is better if the centrifuge cups are well chilled.
8. The final product should be placed in a protective container because of the brittle nature of the plastic bag at freezer temperatures. Store at −18°C or colder for up to 12 months.
9. Labeling requirements are the same as for other products (see Donor Processing).

The quality assurance requirements mandate that the volume and AHF activity of the final product must be tested on at least 4 units monthly.[48] The volume should not exceed 25 mL, and 75 percent of all units tested must show a minimum of 80 IU of AHF activity. Records must be maintained of all quality assurance testing performed.

## Granulocyte Concentrates

Granulocyte concentrates are prepared by cytapheresis (see Chap. 17). Each product should contain $1 \times 10^{10}$ granulocytes if steroids or hydroxyethyl starch (HES), or both, are used. Corticosteroids, usually administered to the donor 12 to 24 hours before pheresis, will increase the number of circulating granulocytes by pulling them from the marginating pool. Hydroxyethyl starch is a sedimenting agent that increases the separation between the WBCs or RBCs, thus facilitating a better recovery of the buffy coat. Granulocyte concentrates contain 200 to 600 mL of plasma and should be stored at 20 to 24°C. The shelf life for this product is 24 hours, but the product should be transfused as soon as possible after preparation. The RBCs in granulocyte concentrates must be ABO-compatible with recipient plasma if concentrates contain more than 2 mL of red blood cells.

Granulocyte concentrates have very limited application and a very narrow success rate. Generally, patients with severe neutropenia (less than 500 polymorphonuclear neutrophils per milliliter), fever that has been unresponsive to antibiotic or other therapy for 24 to 48 hours, and myeloid hypoplasia of the bone marrow and those who have a reasonable chance for survival are candidates for granulocyte transfusions. With improvements in antibiotic therapy and chemotherapy, granulocyte transfusions in adults have become almost nonexistent.[49] They are still used in the treatment of neonatal sepsis.

Recipients of this product are at risk for contracting hepatitis, HIV, and CMV infection.

## Factor VIII Concentrate

This product is used in the treatment of classic hemophilia A bleeding disorders and persons deficient in factor VIII. In addition, persons with von Willebrand's disease have benefited from concentrates containing active vWF, including humate-P and alphanate.

Factor VIII concentrates are still generally manufactured from large volumes of pooled plasma but, because of the very high risk of viral disease transmission with this product, a great deal of effort has gone into developing methods that will inactivate or eliminate virus contamination in the final product. A brief description of the product preparation methods now being used follows.

## Pasteurization

In this method, stabilizers, usually albumin, sucrose, or glycine, are added to the factor VIII concentrate to prevent denaturation. The concentrate is then heated to 60°C for 10 hours, after which the stabilizers are removed and the product lyophilized. The process is effective in producing a product that is safe from HIV-1 and hepatitis infection, but there is a significant loss of factor VIII activity (30 to 40 percent of the original fraction level) in the final product.[50]

## Solvent and Detergent

This method uses a solvent and detergent to disrupt the viral coat chemically, thus inactivating any virus present. The solvents most frequently in use are ethyl ether and tri-(n-butyl) phosphate (TNBP). The detergents are sodium cholate and Tween 80. The concentrate is then purified to remove the solvent and detergent and then lyophilized. Very little of the factor VIII activity is lost (about 10 percent) in this method, and the resulting product is considered safe from viral transmission.[51]

## Monoclonal Purification

Immunoaffinity chromatography is used here. A murine monoclonal antibody directed at the factor VIII or von Willebrand factor (vWF) moiety is bound on a solid-phase substrate and used to absorb selectively the factor VIII:vWF complex.[52] The product is then lyophilized. Large concentrations of very pure factor can be obtained with this method, and products produced in this manner have not yet been known to transmit viral disease.

## Recombinant Products

With the identification and isolation of the gene for human factor VIII, it has become possible to produce factor VIII using recombinant DNA technology. The products made this way have thus far proved to be safe and effective, although also quite expensive.

## Porcine Factor VIII

This product, made from porcine (pig) plasma, has been available for quite some time. It is generally used to treat patients with hemophilia A who have developed inhibitors to human factor VIII. In the past this product has had many adverse side effects, but the newer products, which are better purified, appear to have considerably reduced side effects while still giving good clinical results. Because this is not a product derived from human sources, there is no risk of human virus transmission.[53]

## 1-Deamino-8-D-Arginine Vasopressin

This is actually not a factor VIII product but a synthetic analog of vasopressin. When injected, it will cause the endothelial cells to release intracellular stores of factor VIII and vWF. If this product is to work, the patient's cells must be able to produce some factor levels. It appears to be suitable for treatment of some types of von Willebrand's disease or mild cases of hemophilia A or both types of disorders. 1-Deamino-8-D-arginine vasopressin can be used in combination with epsilon aminocaproic acid, which will help to stabilize clot formation.[54] For most of the foregoing products, the amount of factor VIII activity is indicated on the bottle or vial. They are usually stored at 1 to 6°C and require reconstitution before transfusion.

## Factor IX Concentrate (Prothrombin Complex)

Factor IX concentrates are available in two forms. Prothrombin complex contains significant levels of the vitamin K–dependent clotting factors: II, VII, IX, and X. Like some of the factor VIII products, factor IX concentrate is prepared from large volumes of pooled plasma by adsorbing the factors out using barium sulfate or aluminum hydroxide or by using a cellulose or sephadex column. The concentrate is then lyophilized and virally inactivated. Inactivation is accomplished by various techniques: dry heat at 60 to 70°C for 20 to 150 hours, depending on the particular manufacturer; heat treatment in an organic solvent; or solvent-detergent treatment. All of the products now being made are safe from HIV-1 and HBsAg transmission, but some may not be as good against HCV transmission. The possibility of causing thrombosis, which always was and still is a problem with these products, has led some manufacturers to add heparin to the product for control of this situation. In contrast, the newly developed coagulation factor IX concentrate, developed by monoclonal antibody purification, is less thrombogenic. Only trace amounts of factors II, VII, and X are detected. This product contains 20 to 30 percent of factor IX, compared with 1 to 5 percent for prothrombin complex.[55] These products, like factor VIII products, are stored in the refrigerator and, because they are lyophilized, must be reconstituted before infusing.

This product is used primarily to treat patients with factor IX deficiency (hemophilia B or Christmas disease), but it is also valuable for treatment patients with congenital factor VII and factor X deficiencies.

## Immune Serum Globulin

Immune serum globulin (ISG) is a concentrate of plasma gamma globulins in an aqueous solution. It is prepared from pooled plasma by cold ethanol fractionation. Although the primary serum globulin is IgG, IgA and IgM may also be present.[56]

Plasma found to contain high levels of antibody to special antigens such as hepatitis B or herpes zoster can be used to prepare hyperimmune ISG. Immune serum globulin is now available in both an intramuscular (IMIg) form and an intravenous (IVIg) form. IMIg is used as prophylactic for patients who have been exposed to certain diseases and are at risk of infection. It is also used as replacement therapy for patients with primary immunodeficiencies such as congenital agammaglobulinemia, combined variable immunodeficiency, Wiskott-Aldrich syndrome, and severe combined immunodeficiency. IVIg seems to work better for treating at-risk patients with ITP, for exposure prophylaxis in bone marrow transplant patients, and for patients with AIDs-related thrombocytopenia.[56]

Because of the preparation method for ISG, there appears to be no risk of hepatitis or HIV-1 transmission.

## Normal Serum Albumin

Normal serum albumin (NSA) is prepared from salvaged plasma, pooled and fractionated by a cold alcohol process, then treated with heat inactivation, which removes the risk of hepatitis or HIV infection. It is composed of 96 percent albumin and 4 percent globulin and other proteins.[57] It is available in 25 or 5 percent solutions, stored at 1 to 6°C, and has a shelf life of 5 years. Albumin is used as a colloid volume expander in patients who are hypovolemic and hypoproteinemic.

## Plasma Protein Fraction

Plasma protein fraction is similar to NSA except that the albumin to globulin ratio is lower—83 percent albumin and 17 percent globulin.[57] It is prepared in a 5 percent solution and can be stored at room temperature for 3 years, or 1 to 6°C for 5 years. Like albumin, PPF is used as a volume expander in patients who need volume and protein.

## Synthetic Volume Expanders

These are crystalloids and colloid solutions used as volume expanders alone or in combination with other products. They include normal saline, Ringer's solution, Ringer's lactate, balanced electrolyte solution, dextran (high-molecular-weight or low-molecular-weight), and HES.

## Rh$_0$(D) Immunoglobulin

Rh immunoglobulin (RhIg) is a solution of concentrated anti-Rh$_0$(D), which is manufactured from pooled, hyperimmune plasma. It is used to prevent Rh$_0$(D) immunization of an unsensitized Rh-negative patient after an abortion, miscarriage, or delivery of an Rh-positive baby or after transfusion exposure to Rh-positive cells. It is also routinely given as an antepartum dose at 28 weeks' gestation to reduce the risk of Rh immunization during pregnancy. Like NSA, PPF, and other ISGs, RhIg does not transmit hepatitis, HIV, or the other transfusion-transmitted viruses.

RhIg is available in two concentrations: an intravenous (IV) 300-μg solution, or "full" dose; and an intramuscular 50-μg solution, or "micro" or "mini" dose. Both concentrations come in a 1-mL volume suitable for intramuscular injection. The 300-μg dose is used for abortions, miscarriages, or deliveries that occur at 12 weeks' or more gestation; for antepartum injections; and for transfusion accidents or emergencies resulting in the transfusion of an Rh-positive unit to an Rh-negative patient. The 300-μg dose protects up to 15 mL of D-positive red cells. The 50-μg dose can be used for abortions, miscarriages, or bleeding episodes that occur during the first trimester (less than 12 weeks' gestation). In addition, there is an intravenous 120-μg dose of RhIg that is indicated for termination of pregnancy and amniocentesis.[58]

## Antithrombin III Concentrate

Antithrombin III concentrate is prepared by fractionation of pools of plasma and then heat-treated to reduce the risk of virus transmission. It is used to treat patients who have an inherited deficiency of antithrombin III who are at risk of spontaneous thrombosis. Liquid plasma and FFP are alternative sources of antithrombin.

## SUMMARY CHART: IMPORTANT POINTS TO REMEMBER (MT/MLT)

- A blood donor should weigh at least 110 lb (50 kg).
- The pulse rate of a potential blood donor should be between 50 and 100 beats per minute.
- The hematocrit of a blood donor should be at least 38 percent.
- A donor must be permanently deferred if he or she has had a confirmed positive test for HBsAg.
- The deferral period for persons who have been treated for malaria is 3 years following therapy.
- Persons who have had a blood transfusion are deferred for 12 months owing to risk of exposure to hepatitis, HIV, or other viral diseases.
- Platelet pheresis donors should not have taken aspirin for 3 days before donation because it decreases platelet function.
- The interval between whole blood donation is 8 weeks.
- A person with a history of hemophilia A or B, von Willebrand's disease, or severe thrombocytopenia must be permanently deferred from donating blood.
- Attenuated virus vaccines such as smallpox, measles, mumps, yellow fever, and influenza (live virus) carry a 2-week deferral.
- A blood donor who has tested positive for STS must be deferred for 12 months.
- Donors who have tested positive for the HIV antibody must be indefinitely deferred.
- Predeposit autologous donation refers to blood that is drawn before an anticipated transfusion (e.g., surgery) and stored until used.
- Intraoperative autologous transfusion occurs when blood is collected during a surgical procedure and usually reinfused immediately.
- Immediate preoperative hemodilution takes place in the operating room when 1 to 3 units of whole blood are collected and the patient's volume is replaced with colloid or crystalloid. The blood is reinfused during the surgical procedure.
- Postoperative salvage is an autologous donation in which a drainage tube is placed in the surgical site and postoperative bleeding is salvaged, cleaned, and reinfused.
- The hematocrit for an autologous donation should be at least 33 percent.
- A unit of whole blood should weigh between 430 and 525 g plus the weight of the bag, anticoagulant, and empty pilot tubes.
- All whole blood units should be stored at 1 to 6°C; those units destined for platelet production should be stored at 20 to 24°C until platelets have been removed.
- Donor units must be tested for the presence of STS, anti-HIV-1/2, HIV-antigen, anti-HBc, HBsAg, anti-HCV, anti-CMV, and anti-HTLV-1/2.
- If the blood collection facility is separate from the transfusion facility, then the latter is required to perform a repeat ABO grouping and a repeat $Rh_0(D)$ on all Rh-negative RBC and whole blood units (immediate spin only).
- RBCs are prepared by removing approximately 80 percent of plasma from a unit of whole blood; the final hematocrit must not exceed 80 percent, and the average volume is 250 to 300 mL.
- Irradiated blood products must be given a minimum of 25 Gy, and the expiration date is 28 days from the date of irradiation or the originally assigned outdate on the unit (whichever comes first).
- Leukocyte-reduced RBCs are products in which the absolute WBC count is less than $5 \times 10^6$ and is used to prevent febrile-nonhemolytic reactions and viral transmission (e.g., CMV).
- Random-donor platelets must contain at least $5.5 \times 10^{10}$ platelets, and single-donor platelets must contain $3.0 \times 10^{11}$ platelets, with a shelf life of 5 days.
- Fresh frozen plasma must be prepared within 8 hours of whole blood collection and single-donor plasma within 24 hours of collection; units are stored at −18°C or colder with a shelf-life of 12 months.
- Cryoprecipitate is prepared from FFP and contains at least 80 units of antihemophilic factor and 150 to 250 mg of fibrinogen; the product is indicated for hemophilia A, vWD, factor XIII deficiency, and hypofibrinogenemia.
- RhIg is a solution of concentration anti-$Rh_0(D)$, which is manufactured from pooled hyperimmune plasma. It is used in the prevention of $Rh_0(D)$ immunization of an unsensitized Rh-negative mother after an abortion, miscarriage, or delivery of an Rh-positive infant.

## REVIEW QUESTIONS

1. Which of the following information is not required for WB donors?
   A. Name
   B. Address
   C. Occupation
   D. Sex
   E. Date of birth

2. Which of the following would be cause for temporary deferral?

A. Temperature 99.2°F
B. Pulse 90 beats per minute
C. Blood pressure 110/70 mm Hg
D. Hematocrit 37 percent
E. None of the above; the donor is acceptable

3. Which of the following would be cause for permanent deferral?
   A. History of hepatitis after 10 years of age
   B. Positive hepatitis C test result
   C. Positive HTLV-I antibody
   D. Positive anti-HBc test result
   E. All of the above

4. Immunization for rubella would result in a temporary deferral for:
   A. 4 weeks
   B. 8 weeks
   C. 6 months
   D. 1 year
   E. No deferral required

5. Which of the following donors is acceptable?
   A. Donor who had a first-trimester therapeutic abortion 4 weeks ago
   B. Donor whose husband is a hemophiliac who regularly received cryoprecipitate before 1989
   C. Donor who was treated for gonorrhea 6 months ago
   D. Donor who received HBIg 6 months ago
   E. Donor who had a needlestick injury 10 months ago

6. Which of the following tests is *not* required as part of the donor-processing procedure?
   A. ABO typing
   B. Hct
   C. STS
   D. Anti-HTLV I/II
   E. Malaria

7. Which of the following is the correct shelf life for the component listed?
   A. Deglycerolized RBCs—24 hours
   B. RBCs (CPD plus adenine-saline)—35 days
   C. Platelet concentrate—7 days
   D. FFP—5 years
   E. RBCs (CPDA-1)—21 days

8. Each unit of cryoprecipitate, prepared from WB, should contain approximately how many units of AHF activity?
   A. 40 IU
   B. 80 IU
   C. 120 IU
   D. 160 IU
   E. 180 IU

9. Platelet concentrates prepared by pheresis should contain *how* many platelets per μL?
   A. $5.5 \times 10^{10}$
   B. $6.0 \times 10^{10}$
   C. $3.0 \times 10^{11}$

D. $5.5 \times 10^{11}$
E. $6.0 \times 10^{11}$

10. The required storage temperature for frozen RBCs is:
    A. 4°C
    B. −20°C
    C. −18°C
    D. −30°C
    E. −65°C

11. Platelets prepared from a WB donation require which of the following?
    A. A light spin, then a hard spin
    B. Two light spins
    C. A light spin and two heavy spins
    D. A hard spin, then a light spin
    E. Two heavy spins

12. Once thawed, FFP must be transfused within:
    A. 4 hours
    B. 6 hours
    C. 8 hours
    D. 12 hours
    E. 24 hours

13. The quality control requirements for RBCs require a maximum hematocrit of:
    A. 75 percent
    B. 80 percent
    C. 85 percent
    D. 90 percent
    E. 95 percent

14. AHF concentrates are used to treat:
    A. Thrombocytopenia
    B. Hemophilia B
    C. Hemophilia A
    D. von Willebrand's disease
    E. Hemorrhage secondary to liver disease

15. Prothrombin complex concentrates are used to treat which of the following?
    A. Factor IX deficiency
    B. Factor VIII deficiency
    C. Factor XII deficiency
    D. Factor XIII deficiency
    E. Factor V deficiency

## ANSWERS TO REVIEW QUESTIONS

1. C (p 215)

2. D (p 217)

3. E (p 218)

4. A (p 220)

5. A (p 220)

6. E (pp 233–235)

7. A (pp 238–240, Table 10–2)

8. B (p 246)

9. C (p 244)

10. E (p 242)

11. A (p 244)

12. E (p 245)

13. B (p 237)

14. C (p 246)

15. A (p 247)

## REFERENCES

1. Vengelen-Tyler, VT (ed): Technical Manual, ed 12. American Association of Blood Banks, Bethesda, MD, 1996, p 74.
2. Menitove, JE (ed): Standards for Blood Banks and Transfusion Services, ed 18. Bethesda, MD, 1997, p 10.
3. Cumor, A: Local Health History Criteria. American Red Cross Blood Services, Chesapeake and Potamac Region, Baltimore, MD, 1985, p 42.
4. Menitove, JE, op cit, p 6.
5. Orrell, J (ed): Bulletin #92-4. In News Briefs (Nov/Dec). American Association of Blood Banks, Bethesda, MD, 1992, p 5.
6. Cook, GC: Parasitic Disease in Clinical Practice. Springer-Verlag, New York, 1990, p 1.
7. Jones, FS (ed): Accreditation Requirements Manual, ed 4. American Association of Blood Banks, Bethesda, MD, 1992, p 29.
8. Vengelen-Tyler, V, op cit, p 89.
9. Burke, AP, et al: Systemic lymphadenopathic histology in human immunodeficiency virus-1 seropositive drug addicts without apparent AIDS. Hum Pathol 25(3):248, 1994.
10. Vengelen-Tyler, V, op cit, p 87.
11. Menitove, JE, op cit, p 7.
12. Geiger, JM, et al: Teratogenic risk with etretinate and acrtretin treatment. Dermatology 189(2): 109, 1994.
13. Vengelen-Tyler, V, op cit, p 97.
14. Jones, FS, loc cit.
15. Anonymous: From the CDC and prevention persistent lack of detectable HIV-1 antibody in a person with HIV infection Utah—1995. JAMA 275(12): 903, 1996.
16. Vengelen-Tyler, V, op cit, p 103.
17. Berstsson, A, and Bentson, JP: Autologous transfusion: Preoperative blood collection and blood salvage techniques. Acta Anaesthesiol Scand 40:1041, 1996.
18. Vengelen-Tyler, V, op cit, p 109.
19. Gilcher, RD: Autologous blood. In Garner, RJ, and Silvergleid, AJ: Autologous and Directed Blood Programs. American Association of Blood Banks, Bethesda, MD, 1987, p 3.
20. D'Ambro, M, and Kaplan, D: Alternatives to allogeneic blood use in surgery. Am J Surg 170(6A):49S, 1995.
21. Menitove, JE, op cit, p 18.
22. Assefa, A, et al: Seroprevalence of HIV-1 and syphilis antibodies in blood donors in Gonder, Ethiopia 1989–1993. Journal of AIDS 7(12):1282, 1994.
23. Menitove, JE, op cit, p 46.
24. Stevens, CE, et al: Hepatitis B virus antibody in blood donors and the occurrence of non-A non-B hepatitis in transfusion recipients. Ann Intern Med 101:733, 1984.
25. Anonymous: Infectious disease testing for blood transfusion NIH consensus development panel on infectious disease testing for blood transfusion. JAMA 274:1374, 1995.
26. Cable, R, et al: Limited utility of alanine transferase screening of hepatitis C antibody screened blood donors. Transfusion 37:206, 1997.
27. Paul, SM, et al: Emerging infectious disease: New and resistant strains of HIV. NJ Med 94(6):43, 1997.
28. Lackritz, EM, et al: Estimated risk of transmission of the HIV by screened blood in the US. N Engl J Med 333(26):1722, 1995.
29. FDA Memorandum: Additional recommendations for donor screening for a licensed test for HIV-1 antigen. March 14, 1996, Congressional and Consumer Affairs, Rockville, MD.
30. Busch, MP: Retroviruses and blood transfusion: The lessons learned and the challenge yet ahead. In Nance, SJ (ed): Blood Safety Current Challenges American Association of Blood Banks, Bethesda, MD, 1992, p 17.
31. Menitove, JE, op cit, p 8.
32. Ibid, p 48.
33. Vengelen-Tyler, V, op cit, p 695.
34. Ibid, p 486.
35. Menitove, JE, op cit, p 14.
36. Heaton, TC: Quality of red blood cells. In Vanoss, CJ: Transfusion Immunology and Medicine. Dekker, New York, 1995, p 385.
37. Capon, SM: Blood component preparation and therapy. In Chambers, LA, and Kasprisin, CA (eds): Transfusion Therapy from Donor to Patient. American Association of Blood Banks, Bethesda, MD, 1992, p 18.
38. O'Neill, EM: Red blood cell transfusions. In Kasprisin, CA, and Rzasa, M (eds): Transfusion Therapy: A Practical Approach. American Association of Blood Banks, Bethesda, MD, 1991, p 18.
39. Ibid, p 19.
40. Ibid, p 20.
41. Vengelen-Tyler, V, op cit, p 142.
42. Rossi, EL: Leukoreduced blood components: Laboratory and clinical aspects. In Dzik, NA: Principles of Transfusion Medicine, ed 2. Williams & Wilkins, Baltimore, 1996, p 363.
43. Meryman, HT, and Hornblower, M: Freezing and deglycerolization of sickle trait red blood cells. Transfusion 16:627, 1976.
44. Lane, TA (ed): Blood Transfusion Therapy, ed 5. American Association of Blood Banks, Bethesda, MD, 1996, p 50.
45. Vengelan-Tyler, V, op cit, p 495.
46. Menitove, JE, op cit, p 15.
47. Vengelan-Tyler, V, op cit, p 143.
48. Ibid, p 144.
49. Lane, TA, op cit, p 23.
50. Julius, C: Coagulation products for hemophilia A, hemophilia B, and von Willebrand's disease. In Hackel, E, et al: Transfusion Management of Some Common Heritable Blood Disorders. American Association of Blood Banks, Bethesda, MD, 1992, p 11.
51. Ibid, p 11.
52. Ibid, p 12.
53. Ibid, p 13.
54. Ibid, p 14.
55. Lane, TA, op cit, p 41.
56. Ibid, p 50.
57. Ibid, p 46.
58. Ibid, p 52.

## BIBLIOGRAPHY

American Red Cross Blood Services: Guidelines for the Management of Reactions and Complications Associated with Blood Donors, ARC Form No. 1783. American Red Cross, Washington, DC, 1984.

Baldwin, ML, and Jeffries, LC (eds): Irradiation of Blood Components. American Association of Blood Banks, Bethesda, MD, 1992.

Baldwin, ML, and Kurtz, SR (eds): Transfusion Practice in Cardiac Surgery. American Association of Blood Banks, Bethesda, MD, 1991.

Garner, RJ, and Silvergleid, AJ (eds): Autologous and Directed Blood Programs. American Association of Blood Banks, Bethesda, MD, 1987.

Hackel, E, et al (eds): Transfusion Management of Some Common Heritable Blood Disorders. American Association of Blood Banks, Bethesda, MD, 1992.

Jones, FS (ed): Accreditation Requirements Manual, ed. 4. American Association of Blood Banks, Bethesda, MD, 1992.

Kasprisin, CA, and Rzasa, M (eds): Transfusion Therapy: A Practical Approach. American Association of Blood Banks, Bethesda, MD, 1991.

Katz, AJ (ed): Fundamentals of a Pheresis Program. American Association of Blood Banks, Bethesda, MD, 1979.

Lane, TH (ed): Blood Transfusion Therapy: A Physician's Handbook. American Association of Blood Banks, Bethesda, MD, 1996.

Maffei, LM, and Thurer, RL (eds): Autologous Blood Transfusion: Current Issues. American Association of Blood Banks, Bethesda, MD, 1988.

Menitove, JE (ed): Standards for Blood Banks and Transfusion Services, ed 18. American Association of Blood Banks, Bethesda, MD, 1997.

Milam, JD, et al (eds): Donor Room Procedures. American Association of Blood Banks, Bethesda, MD, 1977.

Mollison, PL: Blood Transfusion in Clinical Medicine, ed 9. Blackwell Scientific, Oxford, 1996.

Nance, ST (ed): Blood Safety: Current Challenges. American Association of Blood Banks, Bethesda, MD, 1992.

Pittiglio, DH, et al: Treating Hemostatic Disorders: A Problem-Oriented Approach. American Association of Blood Banks, Bethesda, MD 1984.

Sandler, SG, and Silvergleid, AJ (eds): Autologous Transfusion. American Association of Blood Banks, Bethesda, MD, 1983.

U.S. Department of Health and Human Services, Food and Drug Administration: The Code of Federal Regulations, 21 CFR 600–799. U.S. Government Printing Office, Washington, DC, 1996.

Vengelen-Tyler, V (ed): Technical Manual, ed 12. American Association of Blood Banks, Bethesda, MD 1996.

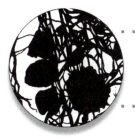

CHAPTER **11**

# DETECTION AND IDENTIFICATION OF ANTIBODIES

Beth Lingenfelter, MS, MT(ASCP)SBB,
Frankie Gillen Gibbs, MS, MT(ASCP)SBB, and
Steven D. Sosler, MS, SBB(ASCP)

## OBJECTIVES

*On completion of this chapter, the learner should be able to:*

1 Define *adsorption, screening cell antigen profile, dosage, eluate, neutralization,* and *unexpected antibody.*

2 Differentiate between the following antibodies: expected and unexpected, red cell immune and non–red cell immune, autoantibodies and alloantibodies, warm and cold.

3 Describe the purpose and limitations of the antibody screening tests.

4 List and discuss characteristics of antibody screening red blood cells.

5 List the benefits and risks for using monospecific anti-IgG over polyspecific antiglobulin reagents for routine antibody screening tests.

6 Outline the procedure used for antibody screening tests and describe the purpose of enhancement reagents and Coombs control red blood cells.

7 Properly interpret results of antibody detection and identification tests.

8 Describe how a patient's medical history is useful in antibody identification.

9 Explain the purpose of the autologous control in antibody screening and identification tests.

10 Correlate knowledge of the serologic characteristics of commonly encountered blood group antibodies with antibody identification studies.

11 Describe the rationale for properly ruling out antibody specificities in identification studies.

12 Explain the criteria for conclusive identification of an antibody.

13 Describe the use of selected cells and antigen typing in antibody identification.

14 Given initial panel results, properly select additional cells needed to complete antibody identification.

15 Select appropriate donor units for transfusion to patients with unexpected antibodies.

16 Calculate the approximate number of random-donor units needed for screening to find a specific number of compatible units for a patient with unexpected antibodies.

17 Describe the principle and list applications for the gel test and solid-phase techniques.

18 List advantages of using a panel of enzyme-pretreated red blood cells in conjunction with an untreated panel and explain why enzyme-pretreated panels cannot be used alone.

19 Describe the effect that chemicals such as proteolytic enzymes, DTT, ZZAP, CDP, and AET have on certain blood group antigens.

20 Describe the principles of and applications for the following techniques: elution adsorption, neutralization, and antibody titers.

21 Briefly describe the principles of the three types of elution techniques described in this chapter.

22 Recognize panel results that indicate the presence of multiple alloantibodies and antibodies to high-frequency and low-frequency antigens and list steps to resolve these antibody problems.

23 Compare and contrast the serologic characteristics of warm and cold autoantibodies.

24 List and describe four techniques used to avoid detection of cold autoantibodies in antibody detection tests.

25 Outline the serologic investigation of warm autoantibodies, including the use of elutions, adsorptions, and ZZAP.

Routine pretransfusion testing consists of ABO and Rh typing, antibody screening, and compatibility testing. The purpose of the antibody screen is to detect red blood cell (RBC) antibodies other than "expected" anti-A or anti-B. These antibodies are called "unexpected" because only 0.3 to 2 percent[1,2] of the general population have positive antibody screens. These unexpected antibodies are usually allo (directed against an RBC antigen that is lacking on the antibody producer's RBCs) but may be auto (directed against an RBC antigen that is on the antibody producer's RBCs). In addition, these unexpected autoantibodies or alloantibodies may be further subclassified by their temperature of reactivity into warm or cold reactive. Unexpected alloantibodies are usually red cell immune (formed by exposure to RBCs via transfusion or pregnancy) but may also be classified as non–red cell immune (sometimes referred to as "naturally occurring"). Once an unexpected antibody is detected, antibody identification studies are performed to determine the antibody's specificity and speculate on its clinical significance. An RBC antibody is significant if it causes shortened survival of antigen-positive RBCs. For example, anti-K is a clinically significant antibody because it binds to K-positive RBCs, resulting in immune destruction or hemolysis.

Blood group antibodies are not always easy to detect and to identify. Some patients, such as those with sickle cell disease, have very high alloimmunization rates,[3] and many of these patients may have multiple alloantibodies, making their identification difficult. Another complication is that many blood group antibodies are labile (42 percent have been reported to disappear over a 5-year period) and may reappear over time.[4] With proper record keeping and if the patient uses the same hospital and physician, this may not be a problem; but if clinically significant antibodies disappear and accurate records of their presence are not available, the patient is a candidate for receiving antigen-positive blood, which is likely to cause a delayed hemolytic transfusion reaction. Another complication is that clinically important alloantibodies are sometimes masked by either warm or cold autoantibodies. This creates unique challenges for the blood banker because resolution is often complicated and time consuming.

Proper detection and identification of RBC antibodies are very important for the selection of appropriate blood for transfusion and in the investigation of hemolytic disease of the newborn (HDN) (see Chap. 20), immune hemolytic anemias (see Chap. 21), and transfusion reactions. This chapter discusses antibody detection and introduces the student to antibody identification studies.

## THE ANTIBODY SCREEN

### Reagent Red Blood Cells

Antibody screening tests involve testing patients' serum or plasma against two or three reagent RBC samples called *screening cells*. Screening cells are commercially prepared group O cell suspensions obtained from individual donors that are phenotyped for the most commonly encountered and clinically important RBC antigens. Group O cells are used so that "naturally occurring," expected anti-A or anti-B will not interfere

with detection of unexpected antibodies. The cells are selected so that the following antigens are present on at least one of the RBC samples: D, C, E, c, e, M, N, S, s, $P_1$, $Le^a$, $Le^b$, K, k, $Fy^a$, $Fy^b$, $Jk^a$, and $Jk^b$. If a set of screening cells did not contain a particular antigen—K, for example—the corresponding antibody would not be detected when serum samples were tested against these cells. An antigen profile listing the antigen makeup of each cell is provided with each lot of screening cells issued from a manufacturer. It is important that the lot number on the screening cells matches the lot number printed on the antigen profile because antigen makeup varies with each lot. Examples of screening cell antigen profiles are illustrated in Figures 11–1 to 11–3.

The "ideal" screening cells have RBCs from individuals who have a homozygous expression of as many antigens as possible. Red blood cells from a homozygous individual have a double dose of an antigen, which results from the inheritance of two genes that code for the same antigen (e.g., Jk [a+b −] RBCs are usually from a $Jk^aJk^a$ donor) and heterozygous expression if the donor has only one copy of the gene (e.g., Jk[a+b+], RBCs are from a $Jk^aJk^b$ donor). Table 11–1 lists examples of some RBC phenotypes and whether they come from homozygous or heterozygous individuals. There is no requirement that screening cells contain RBCs from individuals with homozygous expression of antigens; however, most workers prefer that such RBCs be included in screening cell sets because many antibodies—especially antibodies in the Kidd,

| | Rh | | | | | | | MNS | | | | Lutheran | | P | Lewis | | Kell | | Duffy | | Kidd | | | | | |
|---|---|---|---|---|---|---|---|---|---|---|---|---|---|---|---|---|---|---|---|---|---|---|---|---|---|---|
| CELL | D | C | E | c | e | f | $C^w$ | M | N | S | s | $Lu^a$ | $Lu^b$ | $P_1$ | $Le^a$ | $Le^b$ | K | k | $Fy^a$ | $Fy^b$ | $Jk^a$ | $Jk^b$ | | | | |
| 426509 | + | + | + | + | + | 0 | 0 | 0 | + | + | 0 | 0 | + | + | + | 0 | + | + | 0 | + | 0 | + | | | | |
| 109632 | + | + | + | + | + | 0 | 0 | + | 0 | + | + | 0 | + | 0 | 0 | + | 0 | + | + | + | + | 0 | | | | |

**Figure 11–1.** Antigen profile of pooled screening cell.

| | Rh | | | | | | | MNS | | | | Lutheran | | P | Lewis | | Kell | | Duffy | | Kidd | | | | | |
|---|---|---|---|---|---|---|---|---|---|---|---|---|---|---|---|---|---|---|---|---|---|---|---|---|---|---|
| CELL | D | C | E | c | e | f | $C^w$ | M | N | S | s | $Lu^a$ | $Lu^b$ | $P_1$ | $Le^a$ | $Le^b$ | K | k | $Fy^a$ | $Fy^b$ | $Jk^a$ | $Jk^b$ | | | | |
| 426509 | + | + | + | + | + | 0 | 0 | 0 | + | + | 0 | 0 | + | + | + | 0 | + | + | 0 | + | 0 | + | | | | |
| 109632 | + | + | + | + | + | 0 | 0 | + | 0 | + | + | 0 | + | 0 | 0 | + | 0 | + | + | + | + | 0 | | | | |

**Figure 11–2.** Antigen profile of two-cell antibody-screening cell.

| | Rh | | | | | | | | MNS | | | | Lutheran | | P | Lewis | | Kell | | Duffy | | Kidd | | | | | |
|---|---|---|---|---|---|---|---|---|---|---|---|---|---|---|---|---|---|---|---|---|---|---|---|---|---|---|---|
| CELL | D | C | E | c | e | f | V | $C^w$ | M | N | S | s | $Lu^a$ | $Lu^b$ | $P_1$ | $Le^a$ | $Le^b$ | K | k | $Fy^a$ | $Fy^b$ | $Jk^a$ | $Jk^b$ | | | | |
| R1R1-29 | + | + | 0 | 0 | + | 0 | 0 | 0 | + | 0 | + | 0 | 0 | + | + | + | 0 | 0 | + | + | 0 | + | 0 | | | | |
| R2R2-45 | + | 0 | + | + | 0 | 0 | 0 | 0 | + | + | 0 | + | 0 | + | + | 0 | + | + | + | + | 0 | 0 | + | | | | |
| rr-86 | 0 | 0 | 0 | + | + | + | 0 | 0 | 0 | + | 0 | + | 0 | + | + | + | 0 | 0 | + | 0 | + | + | + | | | | |

**Figure 11–3.** Antigen profile of three-cell structure set.

Duffy, and MNSs blood group systems—show dosage and give stronger reactions when tested against cells from individuals who have RBCs with a homozygous expression of their corresponding antigen.[5,6] As a result of dosage, weakly reacting antibody may not be detected if serum samples are not tested against RBCs with homozygous expression of their corresponding antigen. The most notorious examples of this are anti-Jk[a] and anti-Jk[b]. These antibodies are often hard to detect and are capable of causing severe delayed transfusion reactions when the antibodies are not detected and antigen-positive donor units are transfused (see Chapter 8). Table 11–2 lists some blood group systems that exhibit dosage.

Screening cells are available in three forms: (1) a single vial of no more than two donors pooled together in one vial (see Figure 11–1); (2) two vials, each from a different donor (see Figure 11–2); and (3) three vials representing three different donors (see Figure 11–3). Pooled cells are less sensitive but may be used for the detection of antibodies in donor units. Weakly reactive antibodies may not be detected, but low levels of antibody in the plasma of a donor unit will not harm the recipient.[7] When using pooled reagent screening cells, a mixed-field reaction (both agglutinated and free RBCs in the same serologic reaction) may be observed because half of the RBCs (from one donor) may be antigen-positive, whereas the other half (from the other donor) are antigen-negative. For example, if a serum sample that contains anti-K is tested against a pool of RBCs that contains 50 percent K+ and 50 percent K− RBCs, agglutination will take place with the K+ RBCs, but the K− RBCs will remain as free cells in the reaction.[8] Two-cell or three-cell screening sets are required for detection of antibodies in pretransfusion testing.[9] Detection of very low levels of antibody in a recipient's serum is important because transfusion of antigen-positive RBCs may result in a secondary immune response with rapid production of antibody and subsequent destruction of transfused RBCs.

Serum or plasma may be used for antibody detection and identification procedures, and several prospective

**Table 11–1.** Examples of Some RBC Phenotypes and Whether They Come from Homozygous or Heterozygous Individuals

| | |
|---|---|
| Jk(a−b+) | Homozygous |
| Jk(a+b+) | Heterozygous |
| Fy(a+b−) | Homozygous |
| Fy(a+b+) | Heterozygous |

**Table 11–2.** Some Blood Group Systems That Exhibit Dosage

Rh
Kidd
Duffy
MNSs

comparisons have yielded comparable results among samples that contain alloantibody. Some workers feel that serum is better because complement is present and complement-binding antibodies bind complement to indicator RBCs. This has become less relevant in recent times because standard operating procedure (SOP) in most laboratories calls for the use of anti-IgG antiglobulin sera for indirect antiglobulin tests.

### Enhancement Reagents

Enhancement reagents are solutions added to serum and cell mixtures to promote antigen-antibody binding or agglutination. There is no requirement for the use of enhancement reagents in antibody detection tests; however, SOP in the majority of laboratories requires the use of these reagents because they decrease incubation times and increase the sensitivity of the assays. Enhancement reagents increase the ability to detect lower levels of antibody by changing the RBC/serum environment. As a result, RBCs are able to come closer together in the serologic reaction so that smaller IgG molecules can attach and cross-link RBCs. In addition, a greater number of antibody molecules are able to attach to their respective antigen sites at a faster rate (even if the antibody has a low affinity).[10]

Various enhancement reagents are available, but the most widely used are low ionic strength saline (LISS), PEG (polyethylene glycol), and bovine albumin. Low ionic strength saline and PEG enhance antibody detection tests at the antiglobulin test phase by increasing the quantity and/or rate at which antibodies bind to RBC antigens.[11-13] Antibody binding to RBC antigen is called sensitization and represents the first phase of a hemagglutination reaction (see Chap. 3). Alternatively, bovine albumin is thought to enhance the second phase or actual agglutination of antibody detection tests. The likely mechanism is the reduction of zeta potential (charge), which permits sensitized RBCs to get closer together in solution, resulting in the enhancement of agglutination at the preantiglobulin test phase (usually 37°C).[14]

### Antihuman Globulin Reagents

Antihuman globulin (AHG) is used in immunohematology tests to promote agglutination of RBCs sensitized with immunoglobulin G (IgG) or complement molecules (see Chap. 4). The American Association of Blood Banks (AABB) Standards[9] state that tests for unexpected antibodies (antibody screens) must include an AHG test, but there is no requirement relative to the use of polyspecific or anti-IgG. In some institutions SOP calls for the use of polyspecific AHG as the concluding step in antibody screening, whereas most others have switched to monospecific anti-IgG. There is a twofold rationale for the use of monospecific anti-IgG:

1. Interference from "naturally occurring" cold agglutinins in patients' sera is reduced. Cold agglutinins are clinically insignificant antibodies that

are commonly detected in patient sera. Detection of insignificant antibodies in screening tests is not desirable because it does not benefit the patient and may lead to delays in transfusion while the antibody problem is resolved.

2. Some controversy still surrounds the need for the anti-complement component in AHG. There have been reports of clinically significant antibodies detected only by the anti-complement component of polyspecific AHG.[15,16] However, most workers believe that such antibodies are rare and that the benefits of using monospecific anti-IgG outweigh the risks.

## Coombs Control Red Blood Cells

Coombs control cells are RBCs coated with human IgG antibody. They are usually prepared by incubating D-positive RBCs with potent anti-D. They are used to ensure that AHG tests with negative results are not false negatives because of inactivation of the AHG reagent. When an AHG test result is negative, there should be free AHG reagent in the test tube. When the Coombs control cells are added, the free AHG in the test should cause agglutination of the sensitized RBCs. This positive reaction is mixed-field in nature because half of the RBCs in the mixture lack IgG on their surface (screening cells) and are free cells, whereas half of the RBCs have IgG (Coombs control cells) and are agglutinated.[8]

If the Coombs control cells do not agglutinate, it indicates that the AHG reagent was omitted or neutralized. Such tests are invalid and must be repeated. Neutralization of the AHG reagent is usually the result of inadequate removal of unbound antibodies during the washing procedure. The unbound antibodies bind to the AHG reagent, making it unavailable to cause agglutination of sensitized RBCs.

## Methodology

Antibody screening tests using a test tube method are performed in a variety of ways. American Association of Blood Banks Standards[9] requires that these tests detect clinically significant antibodies and that they include a 37°C incubation and an AHG test. Generally, testing includes the following steps:

1. Appropriately label each tube.
2. Add 2 drops of patient serum to each tube.
3. Add 1 drop of appropriate screening cells to each tube.
4. Centrifuge, then gently resuspend the cell button and read for agglutination or hemolysis. Record results. It should be noted that this step is optional because most significant antibodies are IgG and do not cause agglutination of saline-suspended RBCs.
5. Add 2 drops of enhancement reagent to each tube (may vary with enhancement reagent used).
6. Incubate at 37°C for 15 to 30 minutes, according to the manufacturer's recommendation for the

enhancement reagent being used. During the incubation, antibody in the patient serum will bind to antigens on the reagent RBC. This is called the sensitization phase.

7. Centrifuge, then gently resuspend the cell button and read for agglutination or hemolysis. Record results.
8. Fill all tubes with saline, centrifuge, and discard supernatant. This is called washing, and it removes unbound IgG that neutralizes the AHG reagent.
9. Repeat step 8 two or three times to remove unbound antibody completely.
10. Add 2 drops of AHG to each tube (polyspecific or anti-IgG).
11. Centrifuge, then gently resuspend the cell button and read for agglutination or hemolysis. Tests that are macroscopically negative are usually checked for microscopic agglutination. Record results.
12. Add 1 drop of Coombs control cells (or "check cells") to all negative tests.
13. Centrifuge and read for agglutination. Repeat test if agglutination is not observed.

## Grading Reactions

Agglutination or hemolysis of test RBCs is the visible endpoint of an antigen-antibody interaction. Test results should be evaluated immediately after centrifugation because delays may cause false-negative test results. The first step in evaluating hemagglutination reactions is inspection of the supernatant for signs of hemolysis (red or pink coloration). Next, the RBCs are resuspended by gently shaking or tilting the tube until the cells no longer adhere to the sides. Agglutination is graded during the time that the RBCs are resuspended. In the blood bank, agglutination reactions are routinely graded as negative (no agglutination), weakly positive, and 1+ through 4+ (Color Plate 2). Reactions of 1+ through 4+ may also be described as strong or weak (e.g., $1+^s$, $3+^w$). The degree of the positive reaction generally indicates the amount of antibody participating in the reaction, not its significance. In other words, an anti-D that reacts weakly will have a lower titer than one that reacts 4+, but they are equally significant. Most workers advocate the use of a light source and optical aid (e.g., agglutination viewer) to help standardize and enhance observation of weak reactions.

## Autologous Control

In many laboratories SOP includes an autologous control as part of the antibody screen. The autologous control is performed in parallel with the antibody screen and involves testing the patient's serum against the patient's RBCs. A positive autologous control is an abnormal finding and usually means that the patient has a positive direct antiglobulin test (DAT) and/or free autoantibody in the patient's serum.

The autologous control aids in the interpretation of a positive antibody screen and provides useful information as to whether the antibody is auto or allo in nature. However, the autologous control is not a required test, and there is some controversy concerning its use. Positive autologous controls are associated with autoimmune hemolytic anemia, drug-induced hemolytic anemia (see Chapter 21), and hemolytic transfusion reactions (HTR) (see Chapter 18). Sometimes in a patient experiencing a delayed hemolytic transfusion reaction (DHTR), the autocontrol (DAT) may be positive before free serum alloantibody is available to cause a positive antibody screen.[17] However, positive autologous controls and DAT results are also associated with a variety of benign conditions. For example, increased serum protein or blood urea nitrogen is associated with clinically insignificant positive autologous controls and DATs.[18] In addition, several studies have reported that the use of the autologous control or DAT in routine testing rarely provides significant information.[19] As a result, many laboratories have discontinued the routine use of the autologous control, whereas others have streamlined or restricted evaluation of positive autologous controls.

## Interpretation

Agglutination or hemolysis at any stage of testing is a positive test result, indicating the need for antibody identification studies. However, evaluation of the antibody screen and autologous control results can provide clues and give direction for the identification and resolution of the antibody or antibodies. The investigator should consider the following questions:

### 1. In what phase(s) did the reaction(s) occur?

Antibodies of the IgM class react best at low temperatures and are capable of causing agglutination of saline-suspended RBCs (immediate spin reading). Antibodies of the IgG class react best at the AHG phase. Of the commonly encountered antibodies, anti-N, anti-I, and anti-$P_1$ are frequently IgM, whereas those directed against Rh, Kell, Kidd, and Duffy antigens are usually IgG. Lewis and M antibodies may be IgG, IgM, or a mixture of both.

### 2. Is the autologous control negative or positive?

A positive antibody screen and a negative autologous control indicate that an alloantibody has been detected. A positive autologous control may indicate the presence of autoantibodies or antibodies to medications. If the patient has been recently transfused, the positive autologous control may be caused by alloantibody coating circulating donor RBCs. Evaluation of samples with positive autologous control or DAT results is often complex and may require a lot of time and experience on the part of the investigator.

### 3. Did more than one screening cell sample react, and, if so, did they react at the same strength and phase?

More than one screening cell sample is positive when the patient has multiple antibodies, when the antibodies' corresponding antigen is found on more than one screening cell, or when the patient's serum contains an autoantibody. A single antibody specificity should be suspected when all cells react at the same phase and strength. Multiple antibodies are most likely when cells react at different phases and strengths, and autoantibodies are suspected when the autologous control is positive. Figure 11–4 provides several examples of antibody screen results with possible causes.

### 4. Is hemolysis or mixed-field agglutination present?

Certain antibodies—such as anti-Le$^a$, anti-Le$^b$, anti-$P+P^1+P^k$, and anti-Vel—are known to cause in vitro hemolysis. Mixed-field agglutination is associated with anti-Sd$^a$ and Lutheran antibodies.

### 5. Are the cells truly agglutinated, or is rouleaux present?

Serum from patients with altered albumin-to-globulin ratios (e.g., patients with multiple myeloma) or who have received high-molecular-weight plasma expanders (e.g., dextran) may cause nonspecific aggregation of RBCs, known as rouleaux. Rouleaux is not a significant finding in antibody screening tests, but it is easily confused with antibody-mediated agglutination. Knowledge of the following characteristics of rouleaux helps in differentiation between rouleaux and agglutination:

a. Cells have a "stacked coin" appearance when viewed microscopically (see **Color Plate 2**).
b. Rouleaux is observed in all tests containing the patient's serum, including the autologous control and the reverse ABO typing.
c. Rouleaux does not interfere with the AHG phase of testing because the patient's serum is washed away prior to the addition of the AHG reagent.
d. Unlike agglutination, rouleaux is dispersed by the addition of 1 to 3 drops of saline to the test tube.

## Limitations

Antibody screening tests are designed to detect significant RBC antibodies, but they cannot detect all such antibodies. Antigens with frequencies of less than 10 percent (e.g., C$^w$, Lu$^a$, Kp$^a$) are not usually represented on screening cells, and, as a result, their corresponding antibodies are not detected in routine screening tests. Antibody screening tests may also yield negative results when the titer or concentration of antibody drops below detectable limits. As described in Chapter 3, antibody levels decrease over time when the individual is no longer exposed to the corresponding antigen. If the level of an RBC antibody drops too low, results of antibody screening tests and crossmatches will appear negative and may lead to transfusion of donor units that carry the corresponding antigen. Reexposure to the RBC antigen will elicit a secondary immune response, resulting in a

**RESULTS**

| | | | | |
|---|---|---|---|---|
| cell | IS | 37° | AGT (poly) | 1. Single alloantibody |
| SC I | neg | neg | neg | 2. Two alloantibodies, antigens only present on cell II |
| SC II | neg | neg | 2+ | |
| auto | neg | neg | neg | 3. Probable IgG antibody |

| | | | | |
|---|---|---|---|---|
| cell | IS | 37° | AGT | 1. Multiple antibodies |
| SC I | neg | 1+ | 3+ | 2. Single antibody (dosage) |
| SC II | neg | neg | 1+ | 3. Probably IgG |
| auto | neg | neg | neg | |

| | | | | |
|---|---|---|---|---|
| cell | IS | 37° | AGT | 1. Single or multiple antibodies |
| SC I | 1+ | neg | neg | 2. Probably IgM antibodies |
| SC II | 2+ | neg | neg | |
| auto | neg | neg | neg | |

| | | | | |
|---|---|---|---|---|
| cell | IS | 37° | AGT | 1. Multiple antibodies, warm and cold |
| SC I | 2+ | neg | 1+ | |
| SC II | 3+ | 1+ | 2+ | 2. Potent cold antibody binding complement in AGT |
| auto | neg | neg | neg | |

| | | | | |
|---|---|---|---|---|
| cell | IS | 37° | AGT | 1. Single warm antibody, antigen present on both cells |
| SC I | neg | neg | 1+ | 2. Antibody to high-frequency antigen |
| SC II | neg | neg | 1+ | |
| auto | neg | neg | neg | 3. Complement binding by a cold antibody not detected at IS |

| | | | | |
|---|---|---|---|---|
| cell | IS | 37° | AGT | 1. Warm antibody |
| SC I | neg | neg | 3+ | 2. Transfusion reaction |
| SC II | neg | neg | 3+ | 3. Probable IgG antibody |
| auto | neg | neg | 3+ | |

**Figure 11–4.** Examples of reactions that may be observed in antibody detection tests.

dramatic increase in the antibody titer and possible immunologic destruction of the transfused RBCs. As mentioned earlier, this is called a delayed hemolytic transfusion reaction (DHTR) because it occurs days or weeks after the transfusion. The student should keep in mind that proper performance and interpretation of antibody detection tests minimize the risk of DHTRs.

## ANTIBODY IDENTIFICATION

Antibody identification studies are performed to determine the specificity of the antibody(ies). Once

this is known, one can speculate (based on reports in the literature) on the clinical significance of the antibody(ies). This information is important when selecting donor units for transfusion and for monitoring potential cases of HDN. The majority of patient samples with unexpected RBC antibodies contain single alloantibodies and are relatively simple to identify. Identification studies for samples containing multiple RBC antibodies or autoantibodies may be very complex and require a great deal of time and expertise on the part of the investigator. This section discusses an approach to antibody identification that will resolve the majority of cases and introduces the student to special problems and techniques used to resolve more complex problems.

## Patient History

Information concerning the patient's age, sex, race, diagnosis, transfusion and pregnancy history, medication, and intravenous solutions may provide valuable clues in antibody identification studies, especially with complex cases. The patient's race may be valuable because some antibodies are associated with a particular race. For example, anti-U is associated with persons of African descent because most U-negative individuals are found in this race. Transfusion and pregnancy histories are helpful because patients who have been exposed to "nonself" RBCs via transfusion or pregnancy are more likely to have immune antibodies (i.e., Rh antibodies). "Naturally occurring" antibodies (e.g., anti-M, Le$^b$) should be suspected in patients with no transfusion or pregnancy history. Medications such as intravenous immunoglobulin (IVIG), Rh-immunoglobulin (RhIG), and antilymphocyte globulin (ALG)

may passively transfer antibodies such as anti-A or anti-B, anti-D, and antispecies antibodies, respectively. This will result in the presence of an unexpected serum antibody that is likely to confound the interpretation of antibody identification. The patient's history is especially important when the autologous control or DAT is positive. Certain infections and autoimmune disorders are associated with production of RBC autoantibodies, and some medications are known to cause positive DATs (see Chapter 21). Furthermore, in a recently transfused patient (within 3 months), a positive DAT result may indicate a DHTR. Information regarding recent transfusions is also important when antigen typing the patient's RBCs. Antigen-typing results must be interpreted carefully when the patient has recently received a transfusion because positive reactions may be caused by the presence of donor RBCs in the patient's circulation. Positive reactions caused by donor RBCs usually show mixed-field agglutination, but this depends on how recently the transfusion was received and how much blood was transfused. A sample of a patient history form is shown in Figure 11–5.

PATIENT'S NAME _____

AGE ___ RACE ___ SEX ___ DR'S NAME _____

DIAGNOSIS _____

PREVIOUS TRANSFUSIONS _____ NUMBER OF UNITS _____ DATES _____

PROBLEMS? _____

PREGNANCIES: NUMBER _____ DUE DATE IF CURRENTLY PREGNANT _____

PROBLEMS? _____

MEDICATIONS:
1. _____   5. _____
2. _____   6. _____
3. _____   I.V. Solutions _____
4. _____

IMMEDIATE BLOOD NEEDS? _____

**Figure 11–5.** Patient history form.

## Reagent Red Blood Cells

Antibody identification is performed in the same manner as the antibody screen, except that a panel of reagent RBCs is used in place of screening cells. Panels are expanded versions of the antibody screen, consisting of 8 to 16 group O RBC suspensions. The panel is accompanied by an antigen profile that lists the antigenic makeup of each RBC sample and may also serve as a worksheet to record results (Fig. 11–6). The antigen profile states whether each donor cell tests positive or negative for the following antigens:

D, C, E, c, e, and usually V, VS, f, $C^w$

M, N, S, s

$Fy^a$, $Fy^b$

$Jk^a$, $Jk^b$

K, k, and usually $Kp^a$, $Kp^b$, $Js^a$, $Js^b$

$Lu^a$, $Lu^b$

$Le^a$, $Le^b$

$P_1$

$Xg^a$

Other blood group antigens may be included, and panel cells with rare phenotypes are usually indicated. Rare phenotypes include cells lacking high-frequency antigens (i.e., U, Vel, $Yt^a$) or cells possessing low-frequency antigens (i.e., $Wr^a$, $C^w$, $Co^b$). As with screening cells, it is important to match the lot number appearing on the antigen profile sheet with the lot number on the RBC panel because the pattern of reactions changes with each issue.

The specificity of antibodies in a serum sample is de-termined by comparing the pattern of positive and negative reactions with the antigen profile. In other words, a serum sample containing anti-K should react with cells 3, 4, and 7 when tested against the panel shown in Figure 11–6. The remaining cells (1, 2, 5, 6, 8, and 9) should not react with the serum because they do not carry the K antigen. The presence of other antibodies is ruled out when a serum sample does not react with a cell known to carry the corresponding antigen. In our anti-K example, anti-D is ruled out because RBC sample 2 on the panel is D-positive but does not react with the serum sample. A well-designed panel will identify most commonly encountered antibodies and eliminate or rule out the presence of antibodies that are not present.

## Evaluation of Panel Results

Evaluation of panel results should be carried out in a logical step-by-step method to ensure proper identification and avoid missing antibody specificities that may be masked by other antibodies. A logical approach to antibody identification is outlined here, using a series of questions and the example illustrated in Figure 11–7.

**1. Is the autologous control (last row in panel antigen profile) positive or negative?**

In this case, the autocontrol is negative, indicating that the positive reactions are caused by alloantibody, not by autoantibody. The presence of autoantibodies

| CELL | D | C | E | c | e | f | V | Cw | M | N | S | s | Lua | Lub | P1 | Lea | Leb | K | k | Fya | Fyb | Jka | Jkb | IS | 37°c | IgG |
|---|---|---|---|---|---|---|---|---|---|---|---|---|---|---|---|---|---|---|---|---|---|---|---|---|---|---|
| | | | Rh | | | | | | | MN | S | | Luth | eran | P1 | Lew | is | Ke | ll | Duf | fy | Kid | d | IS | 37°c | IgG |
| 1. r'r-2 | 0 | + | 0 | + | + | + | 0 | 0 | + | + | 0 | + | 0 | + | 0 | 0 | + | 0 | + | + | 0 | + | + | 0 | 0 | 0 |
| 2. R1wR1-1 | + | + | 0 | 0 | + | 0 | 0 | + | + | + | + | 0 | + | + | + | 0 | + | 0 | + | 0 | + | + | 0 | 0 | 0 | 0 |
| 3. R1R1-6 | + | + | 0 | 0 | + | 0 | 0 | 0 | 0 | + | 0 | + | 0 | + | + | + | 0 | + | 0 | + | 0 | + | 0 | 0 | 0 | 2+ |
| 4. R2R2-8 | + | 0 | + | + | 0 | 0 | 0 | 0 | + | + | + | + | 0 | + | + | 0 | + | + | 0 | 0 | + | 0 | + | 0 | 0 | 2+ |
| 5. r"r-3 | 0 | 0 | + | + | + | + | 0 | 0 | + | + | + | 0 | 0 | + | + | 0 | + | 0 | 0 | + | 0 | + | 0 | 0 | 0 | 0 |
| 6. rr-32 | 0 | 0 | 0 | + | + | + | + | 0 | + | 0 | + | 0 | 0 | + | + | 0 | 0 | 0 | + | + | + | + | 0 | 0 | 0 | 0 |
| 7. rr-10 | 0 | 0 | 0 | + | + | + | 0 | 0 | + | + | + | + | 0 | + | 0 | 0 | + | + | 0 | + | + | + | 0 | 0 | 0 | 2+ |
| 8. rr-12 | 0 | 0 | 0 | + | + | + | 0 | 0 | 0 | + | 0 | + | 0 | + | + | 0 | + | 0 | + | + | 0 | 0 | + | 0 | 0 | 0 |
| 9. Ro-4 | + | 0 | 0 | + | + | + | 0 | 0 | + | 0 | 0 | + | 0 | + | 0 | + | 0 | 0 | + | 0 | 0 | 0 | + | 0 | 0 | 0 |
| Cord cell | / | / | / | / | / | / | / | / | / | / | / | / | / | / | / | 0 | 0 | / | / | / | / | / | / | | | |
| Patient | | | | | | | | | | | | | | | | | | | | | | | | | | |

**DIRECT ANTIHUMAN GLOBULIN TEST**

| | |
|---|---|
| Poly | |
| IgG | |
| C3 | |

**Figure 11–6.** Antigen profile of reagent red blood cells used in antibody identification.

| CELL | D | C | E | c | e | f | V | Cw | M | N | S | s | Lu$^a$ | Lu$^b$ | P$_1$ | Le$^a$ | Le$^b$ | K | k | Fy$^a$ | Fy$^b$ | Jk$^a$ | Jk$^b$ | IS | 37C | AHG | check cells |
|---|---|---|---|---|---|---|---|---|---|---|---|---|---|---|---|---|---|---|---|---|---|---|---|---|---|---|---|
| 1. r'r-2 | 0 | + | 0 | + | + | + | 0 | 0 | + | + | 0 | + | 0 | + | 0 | 0 | + | 0 | + | + | 0 | + | + | 0 | 0 | 2+ | |
| 2. R1$^w$R1-1 | + | + | 0 | 0 | + | 0 | 0 | + | + | + | + | 0 | + | + | + | 0 | + | 0 | + | 0 | + | + | 0 | 0 | 0 | 2+ | |
| 3. R1R1-6 | + | + | 0 | 0 | + | 0 | 0 | 0 | 0 | + | 0 | + | 0 | + | + | + | 0 | + | + | 0 | + | + | 0 | 0 | 0 | 2+ | |
| 4. R2R2-8 | + | 0 | + | + | 0 | 0 | 0 | 0 | + | + | + | + | 0 | + | + | 0 | + | + | 0 | 0 | + | 0 | + | 0 | 0 | 0 | ✓ |
| 5. r''r-3 | 0 | 0 | + | + | + | + | 0 | 0 | + | + | + | 0 | 0 | + | + | + | 0 | 0 | + | 0 | + | 0 | + | 0 | 0 | 0 | ✓ |
| 6. rr-32 | 0 | 0 | 0 | + | + | + | + | 0 | + | 0 | + | 0 | 0 | + | + | 0 | 0 | 0 | + | + | + | + | 0 | 0 | 0 | 0 | ✓ |
| 7. rr-10 | 0 | 0 | 0 | + | + | + | 0 | 0 | + | + | + | + | 0 | + | 0 | 0 | + | + | + | 0 | + | + | + | 0 | 0 | 0 | ✓ |
| 8. rr-12 | 0 | 0 | 0 | + | + | + | 0 | 0 | 0 | + | 0 | + | 0 | + | + | 0 | + | 0 | + | + | 0 | 0 | + | 0 | 0 | 0 | ✓ |
| 9. R$_o$-4 | + | 0 | 0 | + | + | + | 0 | 0 | + | 0 | 0 | + | 0 | + | + | + | 0 | 0 | + | + | 0 | 0 | + | 0 | 0 | 0 | ✓ |
| Cord cell | / | / | / | / | / | / | / | / | / | / | / | / | / | / | / | 0 | 0 | / | / | / | / | / | / | | | | |
| Patient | | | | | | | | | | | | | | | | | | | | | | | | 0 | 0 | 0 | ✓ |

*LISS 37C AHG*

**Figure 11–7.** An example of an antibody identification panel depicting an alloanti-C.

DIRECT ANTIHUMAN GLOBULIN TEST

| Poly | *negative* |
|---|---|
| IgG | |
| C3 | |

complicates the process of antibody identification and is discussed briefly in Special Problems in Antibody Identification.

**2. In what phase(s) and at what strength(s) did the positive reactions occur?**

In this case, all positive reactions occurred at the AHG phase and all were 2+, which suggests that a single IgG antibody is present. IgM antibodies are usually detected at the immediate spin reading, whereas reactivity at various strengths and phases may indicate the presence of multiple RBC antibodies.

**3. What antibodies can be ruled out or eliminated as possibilities?**

Antibodies are ruled out when the patient's serum fails to react with an RBC sample known to carry the corresponding antigen. Only cells that gave negative reactions in all phases of testing should be used for ruling out antibodies. In addition, it is best to rule out antibodies using panel cells from homozygous individuals whose RBCs have a double dose of the corresponding antigen because some weakly reactive antibodies may fail to react with cells from heterozygous donors. For example, a weak anti-Jk$^a$ may not react with Jk(a+b+) RBCs because it carries fewer Jk$^a$ antigens than Jk(a+b−) RBCs. Using panel cells from homozygous donors to rule out antibody specificities decreases the chance of missing weakly reactive antibodies. In our example, the patient's serum failed to react with RBC samples 4 through 9. The following antibodies

can be ruled out using cell sample 4 because it is from an individual who is homozygous for the following antigens: Anti-D, anti-E, anti-c, anti-Lu$^b$, anti-Le$^b$, anti-K, anti-Fy$^b$, and anti-Jk$^b$. Continuing with cell 5: anti-f, anti-S, anti-Le$^a$, and anti-k are ruled out; cell 6: anti-e, anti-V, anti-M, and anti-Jk$^a$; and cell 8: anti-N, anti-s, and anti-Fy$^a$. Ruling out specificities makes antibody identification easier because it reduces the possible explanations for the positive results. In this case, ruling out eliminated 20 possible specificities, leaving only anti-C, anti-C$^w$, and anti-Lu$^a$ to be considered.

**4. Does the serum reactivity match any of the remaining specificities?**

The pattern of reactivity usually matches a pattern exactly when a single alloantibody is present. In our example, the serum reactivity perfectly matches the C pattern. The serum gave uniform positive results with all C-positive cells (1, 2, and 3) and negative results with all of the C-negative cells (4 through 9). Cell 2 is also C$^w$-positive, but anti-C$^w$ would not explain the reactions with RBC samples 1 and 3.

The pattern of reactivity does not always match a specific pattern, and there are several reasons for this. The investigator should reexamine the pattern, keeping in mind that weakly reactive antibodies may give positive results only with RBCs from homozygous individuals (e.g., Jk [a+b−]) or cells with strong expression of the antigen (e.g., P$_1$$^{+s}$). Other explanations include the presence of multiple alloantibodies, cold reactive autoantibodies, and antibodies directed at high-frequency and low-frequency antigens. All these possibilities are more fully discussed in Special Problems in Antibody Identification.

### 5. Are all commonly encountered RBC antibodies ruled out?

A patient's serum may contain more than one RBC antibody, and the presence of one specificity may mask or interfere with identification of another. In our example, anti-C is identified and all other specificities are ruled out, with the exception of anti-$C^w$ and anti-$Lu^a$, both of which are antibodies to low-frequency antigens (occurring in less than 5 percent of the population). Antibodies to low-frequency antigens are uncommon because of the small chance of being exposed to the antigen; therefore, it may not be necessary to rule them out. On the other hand, if a commonly encountered antibody is not ruled out, it is important to test selected cells that will rule out the presence of the antibody. For example, if anti-K was not ruled out in this case, an RBC sample that is C-negative and K-positive should be tested. A negative result rules out the anti-K, whereas a positive result suggests the presence of anti-C and anti-K.

### 6. Is there sufficient evidence to prove the suspected antibody?

Conclusive antibody identification requires testing the patient's serum with enough antigen-positive and antigen-negative RBC samples to ensure that the pattern of reactivity is not the result of chance alone. Testing the patient's serum with at least three antigen-positive and three antigen-negative cells will result in a probability ($P$) value of .05. A $P$ value is a statistical measure of the probability that a certain set of events will happen by random chance. A $P$ value of .05 or less is required for identification results to be considered valid, and it means that there is a 5 percent (1 in 20) chance that the observed pattern occurred for reasons other than a specific antibody reacting with its corresponding antigen. Stated another way, it means that the interpretation of the data will be correct 95 percent of the time.

Testing of RBCs selected from other panels is necessary when inadequate numbers of antigen-positive or antigen-negative cells are tested. In our example, the patient's serum reacted with three C-positive cells (1, 2, and 3) but not with six C-negative cells. As a result, selected cells are not required, and the identification of anti-C is conclusive.

### 7. Is the patient lacking the antigen corresponding to the antibody?

Individuals cannot make alloantibodies to antigens that they possess; therefore, the last step in identification studies is to test the patient's RBCs for the corresponding antigen. A negative result is expected and indicates that identification results are correct. If the patient's RBCs are positive for the corresponding antigen, misidentification of the antibody or a false-positive typing are the most likely explanations. Antigen typing

is also useful in the resolution of complex cases because it eliminates many possibilities. For example, an $R_1 R_1$, K-negative, Fy(a−b+), Jk(a+b+), M+N+S+s+ patient could form only anti-c, anti-E, anti-K, or anti-$Fy^a$. It is not practical to do extended typings on all patients with antibodies; however, judicious use of this procedure can be helpful, especially in patients who chronically receive transfusions and are at risk for alloimmunization, such as patients with sickle cell disease or thalassemia. It is important to know whether the patient has received a transfusion in the last 3 months before using this technique because the presence of donor RBCs is likely to result in obtaining mixed-field reactions and in a massively transfused patient may result in false-positive typings.

## PROVIDING COMPATIBLE DONOR UNITS

Once an antibody has been identified, the next task is to provide appropriate units of RBCs for transfusion. When clinically insignificant antibodies are detected, use of crossmatch-compatible RBCs is appropriate. The AABB *Technical Manual*[20] states that no further testing is needed to confirm compatibility when the antibody is anti-M, anti-N, anti-$P_1$, $Le^a$, or $Le^b$. However, when a clinically significant antibody is identified, the blood must be cross-match compatible and confirmed as antigen-negative with reagent antisera. The most economic way of providing such units is to cross-match random units and then confirm that the compatible units are antigen-negative by typing them with reagent antisera. This approach will not work when the antibody is no longer detectable in the patient's serum, and reagent antisera must be used for screening purposes. Knowledge of the incidence of antigens is useful for determining how many units of blood to screen or cross-match for patients with antibodies. For example, if a patient with an anti-$Jk^a$ needed 4 units of blood, how many units would need to be tested to find them? We know that 77 percent of the random population is Jk(a+), or that 23 percent are Jk(a−).[21] As shown here, the number of random units needed for antigen screening is calculated by dividing the number of antigen-negative units desired (4, in this case) by the incidence of antigen-negative individuals in the donor population.

$$Jk (a+) = 0.77$$
$$Jk (a−) = 0.23$$
$$\frac{4 \text{ units Jk(a−) blood needed}}{0.23 \text{ incidence of Jk(a−)}} = 17.4 \text{ units}$$

In this case, testing 17 or 18 random units should yield 4 Jk(a−) units. The same calculations can be used when multiple antibodies are present if the antigen frequencies are first multiplied together. The next example shows that for a patient with an anti-K and anti-$Jk^a$, 10 random units would need to be tested to find 2 that are compatible.

Jk(a+) = 0.77 K positive = 0.09
Jk(a−) = 0.23 K negative = 0.91
Jk(a−) (0.23) × K negative (0.91) = 0.20 Jk(a−) and
K negative
2 units needed = 10 units
0.20 Jk(a−) and Kell negative

Occasionally it is not possible to supply a patient with blood by random screening of banked donor blood. For example, approximately 124 units of blood would need to be screened to find 2 units negative for c, Jk[a], and Fy[a], and 1000 units would need to be tested to find 2 that are k- (Cellano) negative. In these cases, blood suppliers or a rare donor registry would be needed. Blood suppliers have more resources and inventory for finding rare units, and most have a supply of rare units stored in the frozen state. The main purpose of rare donor registries is to locate blood for the most difficult cases by keeping track of rare units and donors across the country. In the United States, a rare donor registry is maintained by a cooperative effort between the American Association of Blood Banks and the American Red Cross. Family members are an important source of potentially compatible RBCs for patients who have an antibody directed against a high-frequency antigen. Siblings from the same parents have a 25 percent chance of also lacking the high-frequency antigen in question and are therefore (if ABO compatible) a good source of compatible RBCs.

## NEWER ROUTINE NON–TEST-TUBE METHODS FOR ANTIBODY DETECTION AND IDENTIFICATION

### The Gel Test

The gel test is a relatively new test, developed and described by Lapierre and coworkers,[22] that has applications for antibody detection and identification as well as other blood bank serologic procedures such as phenotyping, titration, and crossmatching. It utilizes a small plastic card that contains six microtubes, each filled with gel for a specific test. Three kinds of gel are available: specific gel (ABO/Rh, other phenotyping), antiglobulin gel (DAT and IAT tests), and buffered gel (reverse grouping). The gel test is a variation of liquid agglutination technology and uses dextran acrylamide gel and the principle of size exclusion chromatography to separate agglutinated from unagglutinated RBCs. Under centrifugal force, agglutinated RBCs are trapped by the gel, whereas unagglutinated RBCs form a pellet at the bottom of the microtube. The gel has several functions: It serves as a reaction medium that separates agglutinated from unagglutinated RBCs, it entraps RBCs and facilitates a stabilized serologic reaction that can be interpreted many hours after the test is performed, and it entraps unbound IgG so that washing before the AGT is unnecessary. Lapierre and associates wanted the gel test to be a new way to view agglutina-

tion, to decrease false-negative reactions due to resuspension, to improve reproducibility, to improve stability of reactions, and, above all, to have consistent, standardized interpretation of reactions.

The sensitivity of the gel test is greater than that of standard tube tests[22,23] for several reasons. Both the gel and the diluent used have low ionic strength characteristics; there is no washing before the antiglobulin test, so antibody dissociation/or washing away is diminished; and there is no resuspension of RBCs, so weak antigen and antibody bonds are not broken.

Washing with saline before the antiglobulin test is not necessary because the antiglobulin sera is inside (and surrounding) the gel spheres, which contain micropores that permit IgG to diffuse very slowly into the uppermost layer of gel spheres. This results in the trapping of unbound serum IgG. After this happens, nonsensitized RBCs get through the large spaces between the gel spheres and go to the bottom of the microtube with appropriate centrifugation, but sensitized RBCs are trapped in the upper levels of the gel when agglutination occurs.

The procedure for performing a detection or identification by the gel test is to first prepare a 0.8 percent suspension of screening or panel RBCs in the manufacturer's diluent. Label an anti-IgG card with the patient's name and the RBCs to be tested. Add 50 μl of 0.8 percent of RBCs to the appropriate microtubes. Twenty-five microliters of serum or plasma are added to microtubes containing RBCs. Incubate for 15 minutes at 37°C. Centrifuge for 10 minutes. Evaluate reactions and then record results.

Gel test procedures, reactions, and interpretations are more standardized than standard test-tube techniques. In addition, the test is very sensitive, and reactions are more stable and can be evaluated many hours after they are performed. Finally, the hands-on time required to perform the test is reduced, and time saving increases substantially as tests are batched.

### Solid-Phase Techniques

Solid-phase techniques have been recently applied to blood group serology for RBC antibody detection and identification.[24] These assays are performed in microtitration strip wells, and RBC adherence is used as an endpoint instead of hemagglutination. For antibody detection or identification procedures, membranes of RBCs have been bound and dried to the surfaces of the polystyrene microtitration strip wells. The membrane antigens are used to capture RBC-specific IgG antibodies from patient or donor sera or plasma. Following a brief incubation, unbound residual immunoglobulins are rinsed from the wells and replaced with a suspension of anti-IgG-coated indicator RBCs. Centrifugation brings the indicator RBCs in contact with antibodies bound to the reagent RBC membranes. In a positive test, the migration of the indicator RBCs to the bottom of the wells is impeded as anti-IgG–IgG complexes are formed on the surface of the immobilized reagent layer. As a consequence of antibody bridging, the indicator RBCs adhere to the screening cells as a second immobilized layer. In the absence of detectable antigen-antibody interactions (negative test), the indicator RBCs are not impeded during their migration and "pellet" to the bottom of the wells as lightly agglutinated RBC buttons. An antigen profile master list is provided with each product to identify the specificity(ies) of antibody(ies) present. Advantages of solid-phase antibody detection and identification procedures include enhanced sensitivity and the objective endpoint of RBC adherence as compared with agglutination.[24]

## SPECIAL SEROLOGIC TECHNIQUES

### Enzyme Techniques

Treatment of reagent RBCs with enzymes such as trypsin, bromelain, ficin, and papain enhances the reactivity of some antibody specificities but reduces or eliminates the reactivity of others. Anti-Fy$^a$, anti-Fy$^b$, anti-M, anti-N, and anti-S do not react with enzyme-treated cells because their corresponding antigens are removed or denatured by enzyme treatment. Alternatively, the reactivity of Rh, Kidd, Lewis, P$_1$, and I antibodies is enhanced when the reagent RBCs are treated with enzyme; these antibodies are said to be "enhanced by enzymes." Table 11–3 summarizes the effect of proteolytic enzymes on select antigen and/or antibody reaction. Enzyme techniques are performed by adding a solution of enzyme during testing (one-stage technique), or, more commonly, the cells are treated with enzyme before testing (two-stage technique). The two-stage technique is typically used in antibody identification studies because it is more sensitive than the one-stage technique.

Enzyme-pretreated RBC panels are useful in antibody identification studies because they increase detection of some weakly reactive antibodies, help to separate and identify multiple antibodies, and provide clues to the antibody's identity. Despite these advantages, enzyme techniques cannot be used alone because they do not detect anti-M, anti-N, anti-Fy$^a$, or anti-Fy$^b$. In fact, enzyme panels are most informative when the results are compared with the results obtained from the same untreated panel, as illustrated in Figure 11–8. In this example, comparison of the en-

zyme panel results with the LISS panel results shows that more than one antibody is present because the reactivity of the patient's serum with cells 6 and 8 was eliminated, whereas reactivity with cells 1 through 4 and 9 was enhanced. In addition, clues as to the identity of the antibodies are provided by behavior with the enzyme-treated cells. The reactions with cells 6 and 8 are most likely caused by anti-Fy$^a$, anti-Fy$^b$, anti-M, anti-N, or anti-S because these antibodies do not react with enzyme-treated RBCs, whereas the reactions with cells 1 through 4 and 9 must be caused by an Rh, Kidd, Lewis, P$_1$, or I antibody. The example shown in Figure 11–8 is more fully discussed in the section on Multiple Antibodies.

### Elution

A positive DAT result indicates that RBCs were sensitized with antibody or complement in vivo. Positive DAT results may be caused by autoantibodies, alloantibodies (e.g., hemolytic transfusion reactions or hemolytic disease of the newborn), or antibodies to certain medications. Tests with monospecific AHG reagents can determine if IgG or complement, or both, are coating the RBCs, but the antibody specificity cannot be determined while it is bound to the RBC membrane. Elution is a technique used to dissociate IgG antibodies from sensitized RBCs. The recovered antibody is called an eluate and can be tested, like serum, to determine the antibody's specificity. There are numerous elution techniques, but all of them rely on one of the following mechanisms: changing the thermodynamics (temperature), reversing attractive forces between antigen and antibody, or disturbing the structural complementarity of the antigen and antibody.[25] The Landsteiner-Miller heat[26] and Lui freeze-thaw[27] eluates were among the first used to remove antibody from RBCs and to investigate positive DATs. These eluates rely on changes in temperature to disrupt antibody-antigen bonds and to alter the complementarity of the antigen and antibody.[25]

The Landsteiner-Miller heat[26] eluate involves mixing the patient's washed RBCs with an equal volume of fluid (saline or albumin) and heating the mixture to 56°C. The heat causes antibody to dissociate from RBC antigens, and the antibody is released into the fluid. The antibody-containing fluid is the eluate, and it is then separated from the RBCs by centrifugation. Once the eluate is recovered, it is tested against a panel of cells to determine the antibody's specificity. Lui freeze-thaw[27] eluates use the same principle except that the RBC-fluid mixture is frozen and then thawed to disrupt the antibody-antigen bond.

The next generation of eluates involves mixing the patient's washed RBCs with an organic solvent such as ether, xylene, or dichloromethane. The organic solvent is believed to disrupt antibody-antigen bonds by lowering the surface tension of the liquid media, thereby reversing van der Waal forces needed to hold the antibody and antigen together.[28,29] Organic solvent eluates

**Table 11–3.** The Effect of Proteolytic Enzymes on Select Antigen-Antibody Reactions

| Enhanced | Inactivated |
|---|---|
| Rh | Duffy |
| Kidd | MNS |
| Lewis | |
| P$_1$ | |
| I | |

| CELL | D | C | E | c | e | f | V | Cw | M | N | S | s | Lua | Lub | P1 | Lea | Leb | K | k | Fya | Fyb | Jka | Jkb | *LISS* 37C | AHG | *Ficin* 37c | AHG | |
|---|---|---|---|---|---|---|---|---|---|---|---|---|---|---|---|---|---|---|---|---|---|---|---|---|---|---|---|---|
| 1. r'r-2 | O | + | O | + | + | + | O | O | + | + | O | + | O | + | O | O | + | O | + | + | O | + | + | *O* | *3+* | *2+* | *3+* | |
| 2. R1wR1-1 | + | + | O | O | + | O | O | + | + | + | + | O | + | + | + | O | + | O | + | O | + | + | O | *1+* | *3+* | *3+* | *4+* | |
| 3. R1R1-6 | + | + | O | O | + | O | O | O | O | + | O | + | O | + | + | + | O | + | + | O | + | + | O | *1+* | *3+* | *3+* | *4+* | |
| 4. R2R2-8 | + | O | + | + | O | O | O | O | + | + | + | + | O | + | + | O | + | + | O | O | + | O | + | *1+* | *3+* | *3+* | *4+* | |
| 5. r"r-3 | O | O | + | + | + | + | O | O | + | + | + | O | O | + | + | + | O | O | O | + | O | + | O | *O* | *O* | *O* | *O* | ½ ✓ |
| 6. rr-32 | O | O | O | + | + | + | + | O | + | O | + | O | O | + | + | O | O | O | + | + | + | + | O | *O* | *3+* | *O* | *O* | ½ |
| 7. rr-10 | O | O | O | + | + | + | O | O | + | + | + | + | O | + | O | O | + | + | + | O | + | + | + | *O* | *O* | *O* | *O* | ½ ✓ |
| 8. rr-12 | O | O | O | + | + | + | O | O | O | + | O | + | O | + | + | O | + | O | + | + | O | O | + | *O* | *3+* | *O* | *O* | ½ |
| 9. Ro-4 | + | O | O | + | + | + | O | O | + | O | O | + | O | + | O | + | O | O | + | + | O | O | + | *1+* | *3+* | *3+* | *4+* | |
| Cord cell | / | / | / | / | / | / | / | / | / | / | / | / | / | / | / | O | O | / | / | / | / | / | / | | | | | |
| Patient | | | | | | | | | | | | | | | | | | | | | | | | *O* | *O* | *O* | *O* | ½ |

DIRECT ANTIHUMAN GLOBULIN TEST

| Poly | *negative* |
|---|---|
| IgG | |
| C3 | |

**Figure 11–8.** An example of an antibody identification panel depicting anti-D, -C, and anti-Fya.

are more sensitive than the heat or freeze-thaw techniques because they remove more antibody from the RBC. However, they are also time consuming, and the solvents are hazardous.[30]

The third-generation eluates are fast and sensitive and do not use hazardous chemicals.[30] These techniques are called *acid eluates* because they use acidic solutions to decrease pH and disrupt the complementarity of antibody-antigen bonds.[31] The optimal pH for antibody-antigen binding is 6.8 to 7.2.[30] Acid eluates reduce the pH to 3 or less by mixing sensitized RBCs with an acidic solution. The antibody is released from the RBC membrane, and the acidic solution becomes the eluate. The mixture is centrifuged, and the acidic eluate separates from the RBCs. Immediately after separation, the pH is returned to neutral by addition of a buffer, and the eluate is ready for testing. Citric acid, glycine, and digitonin acid are three examples of acid elution techniques, and several commercially available kits are based on this principle.

The above techniques, sometimes appropriately referred to as "total eluates," are performed to prepare an eluate for use in antibody identification studies; RBCs from which the eluates were prepared are usually rendered useless for any other purpose. "Partial eluates" to remove antibody from strongly sensitized RBCs may be performed using ZZAP or chloroquine diphosphate so that the RBCs may be used for other purposes such as autoabsorption or phenotyping, respectively (discussed in more detail later in this chapter).

Testing an eluate against a panel of RBCs helps to determine the exact cause of the positive DAT. Eluates containing warm autoantibodies react with virtually all RBC samples, whereas alloantibodies are recovered from sensitized, transfused RBCs in the patient in hemolytic transfusion reactions or newborn RBCs in hemolytic disease of the newborn. There are many explanations for a nonreactive eluate (all RBC samples negative), such as antibodies to drugs and "nonspecific" binding of proteins to RBC membranes. The evaluation of samples with positive DAT results can be complex and is beyond the scope of this chapter. The reader is referred to appropriate chapters in this book (e.g., Chapters 18, 20, 21) and sources listed in the references.

## Adsorption

In blood banking, adsorption is the process of removing antibody from serum by combining a serum sample with appropriate RBCs under optimal conditions. The serum-cell mixture is incubated, and antibody is removed from the serum as it adsorbs (or binds) to the RBC antigens. Following incubation, the mixture is centrifuged, and the adsorbed serum is separated from the sensitized RBCs.

Adsorptions are most commonly used to remove autoantibodies from serum. Autoantibodies interfere with identification of alloantibodies because they usually react with all reagent and donor RBCs. Autoadsorptions use the patient's own RBCs to remove the autoantibody from the patient's serum without removing any alloantibodies. The temperature at which an autoadsorption is performed depends on the optimal reactivity of the autoantibody. Warm autoadsorptions are performed at 37°C and are used to remove IgG autoantibodies, whereas cold autoadsorptions are carried out at 4°C and will remove IgM autoantibodies. After the autoantibody has been removed from the serum, the autoadsorbed serum can be used for antibody identification and compatibility testing.

Alloadsorptions use RBCs of known phenotypes to selectively remove alloantibodies or autoantibodies from the patient's serum. This technique is especially useful when a serum sample contains multiple antibodies or an antibody to a high-frequency antigen (e.g., anti-$Kp^b$). For example, it may be difficult to find sufficient numbers of $Kp(b-)$ cells to rule out the presence of other alloantibodies when anti-$Kp^b$ is present. Adsorption with $Kp(b+)$ cells removes the anti-$Kp^b$, and the alloadsorbed serum can be tested for other alloantibodies. Cells used in alloadsorptions must be carefully matched to the antibody maker's phenotype in order to avoid removal of other significant alloantibodies. Alloabsorption is also used to adsorb autoantibodies from sera of patients who have been transfused in the past 3 months to determine whether underlying alloantibodies are present. This is a time-consuming but important technique, because as many as 38 percent of patients with warm autoantibodies (and therefore usually positive DATs) have been reported to have underlying alloantibodies.[32] Alloabsorption can theoretically be performed with one cell sample if the patient's RBC phenotype is known and a matching cell sample can be found; however, in most cases, two or three RBC samples of various phenotypes are needed. Just like autoabsorption, these RBC samples are incubated with the patient's serum, and the resulting individual alloabsorbed sera are evaluated against a panel to determine whether the patient's serum has underlying alloantibodies.

## Neutralization

Neutralization uses soluble antigen to inhibit the reactivity of certain antibodies in hemagglutination assays. Soluble antigen is added to serum samples thought to contain the corresponding antibody. The mixture is incubated at room temperature, during which time the soluble antigen neutralizes the antibody by occupying its antigen-binding sites. The neutralized serum is then tested against reagent RBCs, and inhibition of reactivity indicates successful neutralization. A control (dilution control) of serum and saline must be tested in parallel to ensure that the antibody was not simply diluted by the addition of the substance.

Substances containing soluble antigens are available

**Table 11–4.** Sources of Substances for Neutralization for Certain Antibodies

| | |
|---|---|
| Anti-$P_1$ | Hydatid cyst fluid, pigeon droppings, turtledoves' egg whites |
| Anti-Lewis | Plasma or serum |
| Anti-Chido, Anti-Rodgers | Plasma or serum |
| Anti-$Sd^a$ | Urine |

for only a few RBC antibodies. Soluble $P_1$ antigen can be isolated from many sources, such as hydatid cyst fluid, pigeon droppings, turtledove egg whites, and even earthworms![33] Pooled sera or plasma can be used to neutralize anti-Chido and anti-Rodgers as well as Lewis antibodies. In addition, commercial manufacturers sell concentrated $P_1$ and Lewis substances. Finally, urine, which contains high concentrations of soluble $Sd^a$ antigen, is often used to neutralize anti-$Sd^a$. Table 11–4 lists sources of substances for neutralization for certain antibodies.

Neutralization can be used to confirm the identity of these antibodies, but it is most useful when the patient's serum contains multiple antibodies. Figure 11–9 demonstrates the use of Lewis substance in the identification of anti-$Le^b$ and anti-K. In this case, the presence of the anti-$Le^b$ is confirmed because Lewis substance successfully inhibits its reactivity, and the anti-K pattern is easily recognized once the anti-$Le^b$ is inhibited.

## Effect of Chemicals on Antigen Expression

Various chemicals have the ability of inactivating antigen activity. This characteristic can be helpful in antibody identification techniques because RBCs lacking in a specific antigen can be prepared. A partial list of major antigens inactivated by five different chemicals is as follows:[34–36]

1. **Proteolytic enzymes such as ficin and papain.** Inactivates M, N, S, $Fy^a$, $Fy^b$, Fy6, $Yt^a$, Ch, Rg, Pr, $Xg^a$, Pr, JMH, Ge2. Enhances Rh, Kidd, Lewis, and some Kell blood group antigens.
2. **0.2 M dithiothreitol (DTT).** Inactivates Kell blood group antigens (except Kx), $Kn^a$, $Yt^a$, JMH, Hy.
3. **ZZAP.** Inactivates Kell blood group antigens (except Kx) and M, N, S, $Fy^a$, $Fy^b$, Fy6, $Yt^a$, Ch, Rg, Pr, $Xg^a$.
4. **Chloroquine diphosphate (CDP).** Inactivates Bg antigens, some Rh weakened.
5. **Aminoethylisothiouronium bromide (AET).** Inactivates $Yt^a$, Hy, $Kn^a$, $Yk^a$, $Lu^b$, Kell blood group antigens (except Kx).

## Chloroquine Diphosphate

Chloroquine diphosphate (CDP) is a reagent used to remove IgG antibodies from the surface of sensitized RBCs while keeping the RBCs intact and without altering the RBC antigens.[37] This reagent is used to accurately antigen-type RBCs with positive DATs. Red

| CELL | Rh D | C | E | c | e | f | V | Cw | MNS M | N | S | s | Lutheran Lua | Lub | P1 | Lewis Lea | Leb | Kell K | k | Duffy Fya | Fyb | Kidd Jka | Jkb | Albumin 37C | AHG | Control: serum+saline AHG | serum + Lewis substance AHG |
|---|---|---|---|---|---|---|---|---|---|---|---|---|---|---|---|---|---|---|---|---|---|---|---|---|---|---|---|
| 1. r'r-2 | O | + | O | + | + | + | O | O | + | + | O | + | O | + | O | O | + | O | + | + | O | + | + | 0 | 2+ | 2+ | 0 |
| 2. R1wR1-1 | + | + | O | O | + | O | O | + | + | + | + | O | + | + | + | O | + | O | + | O | + | + | O | 0 | 2+ | 2+ | 0 |
| 3. R1R1-6 | + | + | O | O | + | O | O | O | O | + | O | + | O | + | + | + | O | + | O | + | O | + | O | 0 | 2+ | 2+ | 2+ |
| 4. R2R2-8 | + | O | + | + | O | O | O | O | + | + | + | + | O | + | + | O | + | + | O | O | + | O | + | 0 | 2+ | 2+ | 2+ |
| 5. r''r-3 | O | O | + | + | + | + | O | O | + | + | + | O | O | + | + | + | O | O | + | O | + | O | + | 0 | 0 | 0 | 0 |
| 6. rr-32 | O | O | O | + | + | + | + | O | + | O | + | O | O | + | + | O | O | O | + | + | + | + | O | 0 | 0 | 0 | 0 |
| 7. rr-10 | O | O | O | + | + | + | O | O | + | + | + | + | O | + | O | O | + | + | + | O | + | + | + | 0 | 2+ | 2+ | 2+ |
| 8. rr-12 | O | O | O | + | + | + | O | O | O | + | O | + | O | + | + | O | + | O | + | + | O | O | + | 0 | 2+ | 2+ | 0 |
| 9. Ro-4 | + | O | O | + | + | + | O | O | + | O | O | + | O | + | O | + | O | O | + | O | O | O | + | 0 | 0 | 0 | 0 |
| Cord cell | / | / | / | / | / | / | / | / | / | / | / | / | / | / | / | O | O | / | / | / | / | / | / | | | | |
| Patient | | | | | | | | | | | | | | | | | | | | | | | | 0 | 0 | 0 | 0 |

**DIRECT ANTIHUMAN GLOBULIN TEST**

| Poly | *negative* |
|---|---|
| IgG | |
| C3 | |

**Figure 11–9.** Neutralization using Lewis substance of a serum containing anti-Le$^b$ and -K.

blood cells with positive DATs (owing to IgG) cannot be accurately typed for the Kell, Duffy, Kidd, and Ss antigens because the antisera require an AHG reading. Red blood cells with positive DATs are already coated with antibody and always give a positive result when the AHG reagent is added. Antibody can be removed from sensitized RBCs by incubation with CDP for up to 2 hours at room temperature or 30 minutes at 37°C. After incubation, a DAT using monospecific anti-IgG is performed to determine whether or not the antibody was removed. If the DAT result is negative or very weakly positive, the treated RBCs can be phenotyped.

## ZZAP Treatment of RBCs

ZZAP is a mixture of DTT and papain that is used to remove antibody from sensitized RBCs and to enzyme treat them at the same time.[38] ZZAP-treated RBCs are especially suited for autoadsorption (covered later in this chapter) procedures because the treatment results in intact RBCs that have reduced IgG and are enzyme-pretreated. Because of the DTT and enzyme pretreatment, ZZAP-treated RBCs have more antibody sites available, and these sites are more receptive to antibody. ZZAP-treated RBCs should not be used for phenotyping because phenotyping reagents are not li-

censed for use with enzyme-treated RBCs, and false-positive or false-negative reactions may occur.

## Quantification of Antibody

The relative quantity of an RBC antibody can be determined by testing serial twofold dilutions of serum against antigen-positive RBCs. The reciprocal of the highest serum dilution showing macroscopic agglutination is the antibody titer. Table 11–5 illustrates an example of titration studies. In this example, the titer of the first sample is 16 and the second sample 64. Titration studies may also be expressed as antibody scores.[39] The score is calculated by assigning specific numeric value to each reaction, depending on the reaction strength (4+ = 12, 3+ = 10, 2+ = 8, 1+ = 5, and w+ = 3) and adding the numbers.[39] The score reflects variation in the quantity of antibody available to react with each RBC sample (5 versus 8 for a single reaction), whereas the endpoint or titer of the antibody is represented by the total score, the sum of the individual reaction scores.

Titers can be used in antibody identification studies, but most commonly they are used to monitor the quantity of antibody in a woman's serum during pregnancy. Increasing titers of maternal antibody indicate that the fetal RBCs possess the corresponding antigen and that the child is at risk for HDN. Significant in-

**Table 11–5.** Titer and Score of Anti-D*

|  | 1:2 | 1:4 | 1:8 | 1:16 | 1:32 | 1:64 | 1:128 |  |
|---|---|---|---|---|---|---|---|---|
| Previous sample | 2+ | 2+ | 1+ | +w | 0 | 0 | 0 | Titer 16 |
| Score | 8 | 8 | 5 | 3 | 0 | 0 | 0 | Score 24 |
| Current sample | 3+ | 3+ | 2+ | 2+ | 1+ | +w | 0 | Titer 64 |
| Score | 10 | 10 | 8 | 8 | 5 | 3 | 0 | Score 44 |

*Score values: 4+ =12, 3+ = 10, 2+ = 8, 1+ = 5, +w = 3

creases in antibody concentration are indicated when the titer result increases by two tubes (i.e., 4 to 16) or when the score increases by 10 or more.[40]

Titers must be performed in a standardized manner because technical variability greatly influences titer results. The diluent, RBC phenotype, and incubation times must all be the same each time a patient's sample is evaluated. For example, if Kk RBCs are used for the initial titration of anti-K, Kk RBCs must be used for all subsequent evaluations. In addition, parallel testing of previously titered samples (usually stored frozen) helps to control variability in technique from one technologist to the next (e.g., grading reactions, shaking tubes). After testing, the current sample should be frozen so that it can be tested in parallel with the next sample.

## SPECIAL PROBLEMS IN ANTIBODY IDENTIFICATION

### Multiple Antibodies

The presence of multiple alloantibodies should be considered when one or more of the following is true:

1. The observed pattern of reactivity does not fit that of a single antibody.
2. Variations in reaction strengths occur that cannot be explained based on antigen dosage.
3. Different panel cells react at different phases, or the effect of enzyme treatment of the test cell is variable.
4. Unexpected reactions are obtained when attempts are made to confirm the specificity of a single antibody.

As previously discussed, the example shown in Figure 11–8 is an example of a serum with multiple antibody specificities. An enzyme-treated RBC panel was evaluated because the reactions in LISS at 37°C fit the pattern for anti-D, but reactions at the AHG phase are inconclusive. The first step is to use cells with negative results (cells 5 and 7) to rule out or to eliminate possible specificities. Anti-c, anti-e, anti-f, anti-S, anti-Lu[b], anti-P[1], anti-Le[a], anti-Le[b], anti-k, anti-Fy[b], and Jk[b] can be eliminated using homozygous cells. Unfortunately, anti-K can be eliminated on this panel only by using heterozygous cell sample 7 (this is most often the case, inasmuch as KK RBC samples are relatively rare, and even though there is an example of one on this panel,

they are not found on most panels). Next, examine the reactions that are positive in the AHG phase of LISS but negative in the enzyme panel (cells 6 and 8) to see if they are positive for antigens known to be nonreactive with enzyme-treated RBCs. Cells 6 and 8 are Fy(a+). Finally, the reactions in LISS and ficin with cell 1 are still not explained but may be caused by anti-C, which has not been ruled out and is known to be enhanced by enzyme treatment of test RBCs.

After initial evaluation of the panel results, it appears that the patient's serum contains anti-D, anti-C, and anti-Fy[a]; however, additional RBCs selected from other panels are needed for conclusive identification. Cells that are used to confirm the presence of antibodies may be positive for only one of the corresponding antigens. For example, panel cell 6 is D−, C−, and Fy(a+) and can be counted as one of the three Fy(a+) cells needed to prove the anti-Fy[a]; however, cell 1, which is C+ and Fy(a+), cannot be used to confirm the presence of anti-C or anti-Fy[a]. Figure 11–10 represents a panel of selected cells that validate the suspected findings. Cells 1 and 2 are C+, D− and Fy(a−) and confirm the presence of anti-C. Cells 4 and 5 are D+, C−, and Fy(a−) and prove the presence of anti-D. Cells 6 and 7 are Fy(a+), C−, and D−, confirming the presence of anti-Fy[a]. Cell 3 is C−, D−, and Fy(a−) and gives the necessary third negative reaction while also ruling out the presence of anti-s and anti-Jk[a].

The final step in antibody identification studies is to phenotype the patient's RBCs for the corresponding antigens using commercially available antisera. In our example, it would be expected that the patient's RBCs would be D−, C−, and Fy(a−). Although antigen typing is usually the final step in identification studies, the patient's extended phenotype can be of considerable aid in resolution of samples containing multiple antibodies. For example, if this patient's RBCs are rr (cde/cde), the presence of anti-c and anti-e could be eliminated from consideration, whereas anti-D, anti-C, and anti-E would be suspected.

### Antibodies to High-Frequency Antigens

Antigens such as k, Lu[b], and Vel are called high-frequency antigens because they have an incidence of 98 percent or higher (k, 98.8 percent; Lu[b], 99.8 percent; Vel, greater than 99.9 percent[41]). Antibodies directed against high-frequency antigens are uncommon because only the rare individual lacking one of these antigens (1 percent or less of the general population) can

SELECTED CELL PANEL

| CELL | | D | C | E | c | e | f | V | Cw | M | N | S | s | Lua | Lub | P1 | Lea | Leb | K | k | Fya | Fyb | Jka | Jkb | | LISS 37C | AHG | Ficin 37c | AHG |
|---|---|---|---|---|---|---|---|---|---|---|---|---|---|---|---|---|---|---|---|---|---|---|---|---|---|---|---|---|---|
| | | | | | Rh | | | | | | MNS | | | Lutheran | | P1 | Lewis | | Kell | | Duffy | | Kidd | | Others | LISS | | Ficin | |
| R268 | r′r | 0 | (+) | 0 | + | + | + | 0 | 0 | + | 0 | + | + | 0 | + | 0 | 0 | + | 0 | + | 0 | + | + | 0 | | 0 | 3+ | 2+ | 3+ |
| R043 | r′r′ | 0 | (+) | 0 | 0 | + | 0 | 0 | 0 | 0 | + | 0 | + | 0 | + | + | + | 0 | 0 | + | 0 | + | 0 | + | | 0 | 3+ | 2+ | 3+ |
| R192 | rr | 0 | 0 | 0 | + | + | + | 0 | 0 | + | + | 0 | + | 0 | + | + | + | 0 | 0 | + | 0 | + | + | 0 | | 0 | 0 | 0 | 0 |
| R483 | R₂r | (+) | 0 | + | + | + | 0 | 0 | 0 | + | 0 | + | + | 0 | + | 0 | 0 | + | 0 | + | 0 | + | + | + | | 1+ | 3+ | 3+ | 4+ |
| R276 | R₀ | (+) | 0 | 0 | + | + | + | 0 | 0 | + | + | + | + | 0 | + | + | 0 | + | 0 | + | 0 | 0 | + | + | | 1+ | 3+ | 3+ | 4+ |
| R300 | rr | 0 | 0 | 0 | + | + | + | 0 | 0 | + | 0 | + | 0 | 0 | + | 0 | + | 0 | 0 | + | (+) | 0 | 0 | + | | 0 | 3+ | 0 | 0 |
| R305 | rr | 0 | 0 | 0 | + | + | + | 0 | 0 | + | + | + | 0 | 0 | + | + | 0 | + | 0 | + | (+) | 0 | + | + | | 0 | 3+ | 0 | 0 |

**Figure 11–10.** Selected cell panel to confirm anti-D, -C, and Fyᵃ.

produce antibodies to them. Although these antibodies are uncommon, they should be suspected when the patient's autologous control is negative but the serum reacts in a uniform manner (same phase and strength) with all panel and donor RBCs. Resolution of antibodies to high-frequency antigens requires testing of the patient serum against rare reagent RBCs that are missing high-frequency antigens. Most laboratories are unable to maintain an adequate inventory of rare cells, and a reference laboratory may be needed to resolve such problems. Reference laboratories that specialize in resolving difficult antibody problems maintain extensive inventories of rare RBCs.

As with other antibodies, clues to the identity are provided by its serologic characteristics. Room temperature reactivity suggests a high-frequency IgM antibody such as anti-I, anti-H, and anti-HI, whereas in vitro hemolysis may suggest anti-P+P$_1$+P$^k$, anti-Vel, or anti-Jk3. The patient's race and extended phenotype may provide important clues to the identity of antibodies to high-frequency antigens. The lack of certain high-frequency antigens is associated with a particular race (e.g., anti-U and anti-Js$^b$ are usually observed in individuals of African descent, anti-Jk3 in Polynesians, anti-Kp$^b$ in whites, and anti-Di$^b$ in Asian populations). The extended phenotype often provides clues as to which high-frequency antigen the patient is missing (e.g., RBCs from U-negative individuals will type negative for S and s, and those from patients producing anti-Jk3 will type Jk [a−b−]).

Providing compatible units of blood for patients with clinically significant antibodies to high-frequency antigens is often more challenging than identification of the antibody. As previously discussed, blood suppliers, reference laboratories, and rare donor registries are resources used to find rare donor units.

In addition, testing the patient's ABO-compatible siblings is useful because family members are genetically similar and therefore likely to have similar RBC phenotypes.

Some antibodies to high-frequency antigens are not significant because they do not cause shortened survival of antigen-positive units. Antibodies to the Ch$^a$,

Rg$^a$, Kn$^a$, McC$^a$, Cs$^a$, Yk$^a$, and JMH antigens react in vitro with the majority of RBCs tested but do not usually cause RBC destruction in vivo. These antibodies have been referred to as high-titer, low-avidity (HTLA) because they characteristically give very weak reactions (usually microscopic) at the AHG phase but titer to 64 or higher. Although most HTLA antibodies share these serologic characteristics, some investigators find the term misleading because the characteristic weak reactions may be the result of low numbers of antigen sites per RBC, not the result of antibodies with low avidity. Furthermore, the term may be misleading in identification studies because these antibodies do not always yield weak reactions, and they do not always titer to 64. Regardless of what they are called, resolution usually requires testing with reagent RBCs that are missing the corresponding antigens. Panels of enzyme-treated RBCs can provide clues to the specificity because anti-Ch-$^a$, anti-Rg$^a$, and anti-JMH do not react with enzyme-treated cells, and anti-Yk$^a$ may react weaker. Identification of the specificity is not as important as ruling out the presence of other clinically significant alloantibodies that may be masked or hidden. Approximately 25 percent of samples containing these clinically insignificant antibodies also have underlying alloantibodies that are of clinical significance.[42] Once the antibody problem is resolved, units should be selected that are antigen-negative for any clinically significant antibodies and least incompatible by major crossmatch with the clinically insignificant antibody.

### Antibodies to Low-Frequency Antigens

Reactions between a serum and a single-donor or reagent cell sample may be associated with antibodies to low-incidence antigens (e.g., Kp$^a$, Wr$^a$). Other possibilities that should be considered might be that the donor cells are ABO incompatible or have a positive DAT. These more common possibilities should be evaluated first. The serum can then be tested against RBCs with known low-frequency antigens, or the reactive cell can be tested with known examples of antibodies to low-frequency antigens. Reference laboratories are available to assist in the resolution. Transfusion therapy should not be delayed because it will be easy to find compatible donor units.

## Cold Reactive Autoantibodies

Cold reactive autoantibodies are usually of the IgM class and react with antigens found on the patient's own RBCs. Autoanti-I, autoanti-H, and autoanti-HI are the most common specificities, but many others have also been reported. Most adult sera contain cold autoantibodies, but the overwhelming majority are clinically insignificant or benign because they do not react with their corresponding antigens at body temperatures. Cold autoantibodies that are active at or near body temperature are called pathologic and cause an autoimmune hemolytic anemia known as cold hemagglutinin disease (CHD) (see Chapter 21).

Detection of insignificant autoantibodies is common but undesirable because transfusion must be delayed until the presence of significant antibodies is ruled out. Serologic investigation of cold reactive autoantibodies can be difficult and frustrating owing to their tremendous serologic variability. Cold reactive autoantibodies react with reagent RBCs at low temperatures, causing agglutination of saline-suspended RBCs or activation of complement. Cold autoantibodies are easiest to recognize when they cause strong agglutination of all panel cells at the immediate spin reading. Agglutination may also carry over to the 37°C reading, but the reactions usually become weaker with increasing temperature. Cold autoantibodies become difficult to recognize when they bind complement to RBC membranes at low temperatures but do not cause agglutination. In these cases, the immediate spin and 37°C readings are negative, but the anti-complement component of polyspecific AHG reagents results in weak reactions at the AHG phase with a variable number of panel cells. These cases are difficult to resolve because they appear as weakly reactive IgG antibodies, and the reactions are often difficult to reproduce. Evaluation of selected RBC samples at cold temperatures is used to identify or to confirm the presence of cold autoantibodies. A cold antibody screen, as shown in Figure 11–11, involves testing the patient's serum at decreasing temperatures with group O adult RBCs, group O cord RBCs, and ABO-compatible reverse grouping RBCs ($A_1$, $A_2$, and B cells). The patient's serum is combined with appropriate reagent RBCs; then the tubes are centrifuged and read for macroscopic agglutination. The tubes are then placed at room temperature for 15 to 30 minutes, followed by another reading. Readings are also performed after 15- to 30-minute incubations at 18°C and 4°C. Figure 11–11 gives the typical reactions for an autoanti-HI in a group AB individual.

Because they lack clinical significance, the identification of cold reactive autoantibodies is looked on by many workers as being of little value; however, confirmation of their presence will aid in the resolution of the

| CELL | IS | RT | 18°C | 4°C |
|---|---|---|---|---|
| $A_1$ | 0 | 0 | 1+ | 2+ |
| $A_2$ | 1+ | 2+ | 4+ | 4+ |
| B | 0 | 0 | 2+ | 3+ |
| O adult | 2+ | 3+ | 4+ | 4+ |
| O cord | 0 | 0 | 1+ | 2+ |
| Auto | 0 | 0 | 1+ | 2+ |

**Figure 11–11.** A cold antibody screen, illustrating typical reactions for an autoanti-HI in a group AB individual.

antibody problem. Once the presence of a cold autoantibody has been confirmed, a procedure must be selected to detect significant alloantibodies while avoiding interference by the autoantibody. The following section describes four of the more commonly used procedures.

### Avoiding Detection of Cold Autoantibodies

**Use of Monospecific IgG.** The use of monospecific anti-IgG instead of polyspecific AHG is the simplest way to avoid detection of benign cold autoantibodies because membrane-bound complement is not detected at the AHG phase. As previously discussed in the section on AHG reagents, SOP in some laboratories calls for the use monospecific anti-IgG for routine testing to eliminate detection of insignificant cold reactive antibodies. Other workers believe that significant antibodies may be missed by the routine use of monospecific anti-IgG[15,16] and prefer to use polyspecific reagents. The data generated in the 1970s and 1980s supporting the use of polyspecific reagents over monospecific anti-IgG may not be legitimate today, inasmuch as the quality of our anti-IgG reagents has improved and therefore diminished the need for anti-complement to detect clinically significant antibodies.

**Prewarm Procedure.** The prewarm procedure prevents the activation of complement at low temperatures by keeping the test system at 37°C throughout the test procedure. The patient's serum, reagent RBCs, and enhancement media are placed in separate tubes and warmed to 37°C before mixing. Following appropriate incubation at 37°C, the tubes are washed with prewarmed saline (37 to 45°C) three to four times. The tubes should not be allowed to sit with the warmed saline because significant antibodies may dissociate and give false-negative results. Polyspecific or anti-IgG AHG is added following the washing procedure, and the reactions are evaluated as usual. This procedure is simple and easy to use, but significant antibodies may be missed if the procedure is used indiscriminately. There is controversy over the use of prewarming procedures. Clinically significant alloantibodies have been reported to be "prewarmed away." Some workers suggest that prewarming procedures are an inappropriate shortcut and that adsorption techniques are better suited to detect alloantibodies hiding behind cold autoantibodies.[43] Other workers favor the procedure if properly applied and performed.[44]

**Cold Adsorption.** Cold reactive autoantibodies can be selectively removed from patient's serum by adsorption with autologous or rabbit RBCs.[45] Cold autoadsorption involves mixing the patient's serum with an equal volume of packed autologous RBCs and incubating the mixture at 4°C. During the incubation, the autoantibody binds or adsorbs to the RBCs, but alloantibodies remain in the serum. Autologous adsorptions may be performed only when the patient has not had a recent transfusion (in the last 3 months) because alloantibodies may adsorb to donor RBCs present in the patient's blood sample. Rabbit RBCs are rich in I and H antigen and may be used in place of autologous RBCs to remove autoanti-I, autoanti-H, or autoanti-HI. Rabbit erythrocyte stroma is commercially available for this purpose, but there are some reports of weak alloantibodies (anti-D, anti-E, and anti-Le[b]) being adsorbed by these products.[45,46] Following adsorption, the cell-serum mixture is centrifuged and the adsorbed serum separated from the antibody-coated RBCs or stroma. The adsorbed serum can then be used for antibody screening, identification, or crossmatching. Adsorption procedures are time consuming but especially useful for removing strongly reactive cold autoantibodies.

**Dithiothreitol and 2-Mercaptoethanol.** Sulfhydryl compounds such as dithiothreitol (DTT)[47] or 2-mercaptoethanol (2-ME)[48] denature IgM antibodies by breaking the disulfide bonds. A serum that contains cold autoantibodies can be treated with DTT or 2-ME and then evaluated for IgG alloantibodies. IgG agglutinins treated with the sulfhydryl compounds retain their ability to agglutinate RBCs. Equal volumes of DTT or 2-ME and serum are mixed together and incubated for 30 minutes to 3 hours, depending on the strength of the IgM antibody. This mixture is then tested with a panel of RBCs. A control consisting of equal volumes of serum and saline is tested in parallel with the treated serum to ensure that dilution of the antibody is not mistaken for denaturation.

## Warm Autoantibodies

Unlike cold reactive autoantibodies, warm autoantibodies are usually IgG and active at body temperature. These antibodies are uncommon but usually pathologic because they sensitize autologous RBCs in vivo. RBCs that are coated with IgG antibodies become targets of immune destruction and may not survive normally. The rate of RBC destruction depends on the quantity and type of antibody present on the RBCs.[49] For example, autoantibodies composed primarily of IgG subclass 1 or 3 are more pathologic than those composed of IgG subclass 2 or 4. Warm autoimmune hemolytic anemia (WAIHA) results when the rate of RBC destruction exceeds the rate of production by the bone marrow (see Chapter 21).

Warm autoantibodies can interfere with serologic testing because they react with all normal RBCs, including the individual's own RBCs. Patients with warm autoantibodies have RBCs that demonstrate a positive DAT and therefore a positive autocontrol because their cells have been sensitized with IgG antibody in vivo. Mixed-field agglutination is not observed, and use of monospecific AHG reagents gives positive results with anti-IgG and variable results (positive or negative) with anti-C3d. Eluates prepared from the patient's sensitized RBCs usually react uniformly with all normal RBCs.

The serum may or may not contain the autoantibody because the antibody binds to the individual's RBCs once it enters the circulation. As a result, the DAT result may be positive and the eluate may react with all RBCs tested, but results of tests using serum (e.g., the antibody screen) are negative. Alternatively, the autoantibody will be detected in the serum once the amount of antibody produced exceeds the number of antibody-binding sites on the RBCs. These cases are difficult to resolve because, as illustrated in Figure 11–12, the serum reacts with all reagent and donor RBCs tested. To rule out the presence of alloantibodies, the autoantibody must be removed from the serum by adsorption. Warm autoadsorptions are the procedure of choice unless the patient has received a transfusion in the last 3 months. If a patient has had a recent transfusion, it is necessary to perform multiple alloadsorptions, discussed briefly earlier in this chapter.

The efficiency of warm autoadsorptions can be enhanced if the RBCs are pretreated with enzymes or ZZAP before use. ZZAP (mentioned earlier in this chapter) is used to remove antibody from sensitized RBCs and to enzyme-treat them at the same time.[38] Removing bound antibody increases the efficiency by increasing the available antibody-binding sites, whereas enzyme pretreatment of adsorbing RBCs increases the quantity of warm autoantibody that the cells can adsorb.

Once the autoantibody has been removed from the serum, the adsorbed serum can be used for identification of alloantibodies and for compatibility testing. Figure 11–12 demonstrates a case of a warm autoantibody and anti-Jk[a] in a patient's serum. The warm autoantibody masked the presence of the anti-Jk[a] in the initial test, but the anti-Jk[a] pattern is clearly seen in the warm autoadsorbed serum. This patient must receive Jk(a−) units, and crossmatches may be performed with adsorbed serum.

## Antibodies to Reagents and Drugs

Antibodies to a variety of drugs and additives can cause positive results in antibody testing. Several mechanisms may be responsible for this phenomenon. Antibody in the patient's serum can combine with a dye, drug, or chemical in the reagent to form antibody com-

Autoadsorbed Serum

| CELL | D | C | E | c | e | f | V | Cw | M | N | S | s | Lua | Lub | P1 | Lea | Leb | K | k | Fya | Fyb | Jka | Jkb | LISS 37C | AHG | LISS 37C | AHG | check cells |
|---|---|---|---|---|---|---|---|---|---|---|---|---|---|---|---|---|---|---|---|---|---|---|---|---|---|---|---|---|
| 1. r'r-2 | O | + | O | + | + | + | O | O | + | + | O | + | O | + | O | O | + | O | + | + | O | + | + | 0 | 3+ | 0 | 1+ | |
| 2. R1ʷR1-1 | + | + | O | O | + | O | O | + | + | + | + | O | + | + | + | O | + | O | + | O | + | + | O | 0 | 3+ | 0 | 2+ | |
| 3. R1R1-6 | + | + | O | O | + | O | O | O | O | + | O | + | O | + | + | + | O | + | + | O | + | + | O | 0 | 3+ | 0 | 2+ | |
| 4. R2R2-8 | + | O | + | + | O | O | O | O | + | + | + | + | O | + | + | O | + | + | O | O | + | O | + | 0 | 3+ | 0 | 0 | ✓ |
| 5. r″r-3 | O | O | + | + | + | + | O | O | + | + | + | O | O | + | + | + | O | O | + | O | + | O | + | 0 | 3+ | 0 | 0 | ✓ |
| 6. rr-32 | O | O | O | + | + | + | + | O | + | O | + | O | O | + | + | O | O | O | + | + | + | + | O | 0 | 3+ | 0 | 2+ | |
| 7. rr-10 | O | O | O | + | + | + | O | O | + | + | + | + | O | + | O | O | + | + | + | O | + | + | + | 0 | 3+ | 0 | 1+ | |
| 8. rr-12 | O | O | O | + | + | + | O | O | O | + | O | + | O | + | + | O | + | O | + | + | O | O | + | 0 | 3+ | 0 | 0 | ✓ |
| 9. Ro-4 | + | O | O | + | + | + | O | O | + | O | O | + | O | + | O | + | O | O | + | O | O | O | + | 0 | 3+ | 0 | 0 | ✓ |
| Cord cell | / | / | / | / | / | / | / | / | / | / | / | / | / | / | / | O | O | / | / | / | / | / | / | | | | | |
| Patient | | | | | | | | | | | | | | | | | | | | | | | | 0 | 4+ | | | |

DIRECT ANTIHUMAN GLOBULIN TEST

| Poly | 4+ |
|---|---|
| IgG | 4+ |
| C3 | negative |

**Figure 11–12.** Warm autoantibody with underlying alloanti-Jkᵃ.

plexes; the chemicals may bind to the cells; or the cell membrane may be modified so that spontaneous agglutination or aggregation occurs. All tests that employ the offending reagent will yield a positive reaction, including the auto-control. However, the result of the DAT will be negative. Some substances reported to cause this phenomenon are acriflavine, caprylate, thimerosal, LISS, citrate, oxalate, neomycin, and saline.[50] These substances may appear as a portion of the reagent. For example, if a patient has an antibody to caprylate, which is used as a stabilizer in some manufacturers' bovine albumin, all the tubes to which albumin has been added will give a positive reaction. The use of an albumin without caprylate or another enhancement reagent such as LISS will produce negative reactions.

In cases in which patients have a positive DAT because of the immune complex mechanism, reactions with the patient's sera (antibody screens, antibody identification, and crossmatches) may be positive as long as the patient still has circulating drug.[51,52] When the level of drug diminishes (this is different in every case and depends on the half-life of the drug and the patient's ability to metabolize it), reactivity with the patient's serum will become weaker and eventually negative.

## SUMMARY CHART: IMPORTANT POINTS TO REMEMBER (MT/MLT)

- The purpose of the antibody screen is to detect *unexpected* antibodies, which can be classified as allo, auto, or "naturally occurring" and make up approximately 0.3 to 2 percent of the general population and up to 36 percent of certain chronically transfused populations.
- Screening cells are commercially prepared group O cell suspensions obtained from individual donors that are phenotyped for the most commonly encountered and clinically important RBC antigens.
- Red blood cells from a homozygous individual have a double dose of an antigen, which results from the inheritance of two genes that code for the same antigen, whereas heterozygous individuals carry only a single dose of antigen.
- Antibodies in the Kidd, Duffy, and MNSs blood group systems show *dosage* and yield stronger reactions against cells from individuals who have RBCs with a homozygous expression of their corresponding antigen.
- Enhancement reagents, such as LISS and PEG, are solutions added to serum and cell mixtures in the IAT to promote antigen-antibody binding or agglutination.

- Coombs control cells are RBCs coated with human IgG antibody, which is added to all AHG negative tube tests to ensure that the AHG reagent is both present and functional in the test system.
- Conclusive antibody identification is achieved when the serum containing the antibody is reactive with at least three antigen-positive cells (i.e., reagent cells that express the corresponding antigen), negative with at least three antigen-negative cells (i.e., reagent cells that do not express the corresponding antigen), and the patient's RBCs phenotype negative for the corresponding antigen.
- The calculation for determining the number of random-donor units screened for patients with an antibody is described as dividing the number of antigen-negative units desired for transfusion by the incidence of antigen-negative individuals in the donor population.
- The relative quantity of an RBC antibody can be determined by testing serial twofold dilutions of serum against antigen-positive RBCs; the reciprocal of the highest serum dilution showing macroscopic agglutination is the antibody titer.

## REVIEW QUESTIONS

1. Based on the following phenotypes, which pairs of cells would make the best screening cells?
   A. Cell 1: Group A, D+C+c−E−e+, K+, Fy(a+b−), Jk(a+b−), M+N−S+s−
   Cell 2: Group O, D+C−c+E+e−, K−, Fy(a−b+), Jk(a−b+), M−N+S−s+
   B. Cell 1: Group O, D−C−c+E−e+, K−, Fy(a−b+), Jk(a+b+), M+N+S−s+
   Cell 2: Group O, D+C+c−E−e+, K−, Fy(a+b−), Jk(a+b−), M−N+S−s+
   C. Cell 1: Group O, D+C+c+E+e+, K+, Fy(a+b+), Jk(a+b+), M+N−S+s+
   Cell 2: Group O, D−C−c+E−e+, K−, Fy(a−b−), Jk(a+b+), M+N+S−s+
   D. Cell 1: Group O, D+C+c−E−e+, K+, Fy(a−b+), Jk(a−b+), M−N+S−s+
   Cell 2: Group O, D+C−c+E+e−, K−, Fy(a+b−), Jk(a+b−), M+N+S−s−

2. Antibodies are ruled out using cells that are homozygous for the corresponding antigen because:
   A. Antibodies show dosage
   B. Multiple antibodies may be present
   C. It results in a *P* value of .05 for proper identification of the antibody
   D. All of the above

3. A request for 8 units of packed RBCs was received for patient LF. The patient has a negative antibody screen, but one of the 8 units was 3+ incompatible at the AHG phase. Which of the following antibodies may be the cause?
   A. Anti-K
   B. Anti-Le$^a$
   C. Anti-Kp$^a$
   D. Anti-Fy$^b$

4. ES is an Le(a−b−) individual who has produced anti-Le$^a$ and anti-Le$^b$. If ES's serum were to be mixed with pooled plasma before antibody identification tests, the Lewis antibodies would be:
   A. Enhanced
   B. Destroyed
   C. Neutralized
   D. Unchanged

5. Which of the following antibodies is most likely to be detected at low temperatures?
   A. Anti-Fy$^b$
   B. Anti-Jk$^a$
   C. Anti-M
   D. Anti-S

6. A type and screen were ordered for patient DJ. The patient is found to be O Rh-positive with a positive antibody screen. A LISS panel was performed, and all the panel cells reacted 3+ at the AHG phase

| CELL | D | C | E | c | e | f | V | Cw | M | N | S | s | Lua | Lub | P1 | Lea | Leb | K | k | Fya | Fyb | Jka | Jkb | IS | 37 | AHG | Ficin AHG |
|------|---|---|---|---|---|---|---|----|---|---|---|---|-----|-----|----|-----|-----|---|---|-----|-----|-----|-----|----|----|-----|-----------|
| 1. | 0 | + | 0 | + | + | + | 0 | 0 | + | + | 0 | + | 0 | + | 0 | 0 | + | 0 | + | + | 0 | + | + | 0 | 0 | 0 | 0 |
| 2. | + | + | 0 | 0 | + | 0 | 0 | + | + | + | + | 0 | + | + | + | 0 | + | 0 | + | 0 | + | + | 0 | 0 | 0 | 2+ | 0 |
| 3. | + | + | 0 | 0 | + | 0 | 0 | 0 | 0 | + | 0 | + | 0 | + | + | + | 0 | + | + | 0 | + | + | 0 | w+ | w+ | w+ | 1+ |
| 4. | + | 0 | + | + | 0 | 0 | 0 | 0 | + | + | + | + | 0 | + | + | 0 | + | + | 0 | 0 | + | 0 | + | 0 | 0 | 2+ | 0 |
| 5. | 0 | 0 | + | + | + | + | 0 | 0 | + | + | + | 0 | 0 | + | + | + | 0 | 0 | + | 0 | + | 0 | + | w+ | w+ | 3+ | 1+ |
| 6. | 0 | 0 | 0 | + | + | + | + | 0 | + | 0 | + | 0 | 0 | + | + | 0 | 0 | 0 | + | + | + | + | 0 | 0 | 0 | 2+ | 0 |
| 7. | 0 | 0 | 0 | + | + | + | 0 | 0 | + | + | + | + | 0 | + | + | 0 | 0 | + | + | 0 | + | + | + | 0 | 0 | 2+ | 0 |
| 8. | 0 | 0 | 0 | + | + | + | 0 | 0 | 0 | + | 0 | + | 0 | + | + | 0 | + | 0 | + | 0 | + | 0 | + | 0 | 0 | 0 | 0 |
| 9. | + | 0 | 0 | + | + | + | 0 | 0 | + | 0 | 0 | + | 0 | + | 0 | + | 0 | 0 | + | 0 | 0 | 0 | + | w+ | w+ | w+ | 1+ |
| 10. | + | + | 0 | 0 | + | 0 | 0 | 0 | + | 0 | 0 | + | 0 | + | + | 0 | 0 | 0 | + | 0 | + | + | + | 0 | 0 | 0 | 0 |
| AUTO | | | | | | | | | | | | | | | | | | | | | | | | 0 | 0 | 0 | 0 |

**Figure 11–13.** Panel for review questions 7 through 10.

with DJ's serum. The auto-control was negative. Which of the following would be a possible cause for these results? DJ's serum contains:

A. Anti-Kpb
B. A warm autoantibody
C. Anti-K and anti-E
D. Anti-Lua

Refer to Figure 11–13 to answer questions 7 through 10.

7. Which of the following antibodies *cannot* be ruled out using the panel results?
A. Anti-E and anti-K
B. Anti-V, anti-Cw, anti-Lua
C. Anti-S and anti-Lea
D. All of the above

8. Which of the following antibodies best explain the panel results?
A. Anti-E and anti-S
B. Anti-K, anti-E, and anti-Lea
C. Anti-Lea and anti-S
D. Anti-Fyb and anti-Lea

9. What additional selected cells would need to be tested to complete this antibody identification?
A. A Le(a−), S−, E+e− RBC to rule out anti-E
B. A Le(a−), S−, K+ RBC to rule out anti-K
C. A Le(a+), S− cell to prove anti-Lea
D. All of the above

10. What would be the expected results if this patient's RBCs were typed for the Lea and S antigens?
A. The patient's RBCs would be S+ and Le (a−).
B. The patient's RBCs would be S+ and Le (a+).
C. The patient's RBCs would be S− and Le (a−).
D. Information is insufficient to indicate the patient's S or Lea antigen typing.

## ANSWERS TO REVIEW QUESTIONS

1. D (p 255)
2. A (p 262)
3. C (p 270)
4. C (p 267)
5. C (p 260)
6. A (p 267)
7. D (pp 261–263)
8. C (pp 261–263)
9. D (pp 261–263)
10. C (p 263)

## REFERENCES

1. Giblett, ER: Blood group alloantibodies: An assessment of some laboratory practices. Transfusion 17:299, 1977.
2. Boral, L, and Henry, IB: The type and screen: A safe alternative and supplement in selected surgical procedures. Transfusion 17:163, 1977.
3. Orlina, A, Sosler, SD, and Koshy, M: Problems of chronic transfusion in sickle cell disease. J Clin Apheresis 6:243–263, 1991.
4. Ramsey, G, and Smietana,: Long-term follow-up testing of red cell alloantibodies. Transfusion 34:122–124, 1994.
5. Issitt, PD: Applied Blood Group Serology, ed 3. Montgomery Scientific, Miami, 1985, p 309.
6. Ibid, p 324.
7. Walker, RH (ed): Technical Manual, ed 10. American Association of Blood Banks, Arlington, VA, 1990, p 277.
8. Sosler, SD. Mixed-population of RBC antigen. Clin Lab Sci 4:91–92, 1991.
9. Standards for Blood Banks and Transfusion Services, ed 18. American Association of Blood Banks, Bethesda, MD, 1997.
10. Sosler, SD: Enhancement media for transfusion testing. In Ellisor, S, and Wallace, M (eds): Blood Bank Reagents: What to Use and When. American Association of Blood Banks, Arlington, VA, 1997.

11. Hughes-Jones, NC, Gardner, B, and Telford, R: The effect of pH and ionic strength on the reactions between anti-D and erythrocytes. Immunology 7:72, 1964.

12. Atchley, WA, Bhagavan, NV, and Masouredis, SP: Influence of ionic strength on the reactions between anti-D and D positive red cells. Vox Sang 9:396, 1964.

13. Shirey, RS, Boyd, JS, and Ness, PM. Polyethylene glycol versus low-ionic strength solution in pretransfusion testing: A blinded study. Transfusion 34:368–370, 1994.

14. Pollack, W, et al: A study of the forces involved in the second stage of hemagglutination. Transfusion 5:158, 1965.

15. Wright, MS, and Issitt, PD: Anticomplement and the indirect antiglobulin test. Transfusion 19:688, 1979.

16. Howard, JE, et al: Clinical significance of the anti-complement component of antiglobulin antisera. Transfusion 22:269, 1982.

17. Perkins, JT, et al: The relative utility of the autologous control and the antiglobulin phase of the cross-match. Transfusion 30:503–507, 1990.

18. Toy, PTCY, et al: Factors associated with positive direct antiglobulin tests in pretransfusion patient: A case-control study. Vox Sang 49:215, 1985.

19. Judd, WJ, et al: The evaluation of a positive direct antiglobulin test (autocontrol) in pretransfusion testing revisited. Transfusion 26:220, 1986.

20. Vengelen-Tyler, V (ed): Technical Manual, ed 12. American Association of Blood Banks, Bethesda, MD, 1996, p 242.

21. Issitt, PD, op cit, p 279.

22. Lapierre, Y, et al: The gel test: A new way to detect red cell antigen-antibody reactions. Transfusion 30:109–113, 1990.

23. Malyska, H, and Weiland, D: The gel test. Laboratory Medicine 25:81–85, 1994.

24. Plapp, FV, et al: A solid phase antibody screen. Am J Clin Path 82:719–721, 1984.

25. Judd, JW: Elution of antibody from red cells. In Bell, CA (ed): Antigen-Antibody Reactions Revisited. American Association of Blood Banks, Arlington, VA, 1982, p 175.

26. Landsteiner, K, and Miller, CP: Serologic studies on the blood of primates: II. The blood group of anthropoid apes. J Exp Med 42:853, 1925.

27. Eicher, CA, et al: A simple freezing method for antibody elution (abstract). Transfusion 18:647, 1978.

28. van Oss, CJ, Absolom, DR, and Neumann, AW: The "hydrophobic effect": Essentially a van de Waals interaction. Colloid and Polymer Science 1:424, 1980.

29. van Oss, CJ, Absolom, DR, and Neumann, AW: Applications of net repulsive van der Waals forces between different particles, macromolecules or biological cells in liquids. Colloid and Polymer Science 1:45, 1980.

30. South, SF: Use of the direct antiglobulin test in routine testing. In Wallace, ME, and Levitt, JS (eds): Current Application and In-

terpretation of the Direct Antiglobulin Test. American Association of Blood Banks, Arlington, VA, 1988, p 25.

31. Howard, PL: Principles of antibody elution. Transfusion 21:477, 1981.

32. Laine, ML, and Beattie, KM: Frequency of alloantibodies accompanying autoantibodies. Transfusion 25:545–546, 1985.

33. Issitt, PD, op cit, 204.

34. Reid, ME, and Lomas-Frances C: The Blood Group Antigen Facts Book. Academic Press, San Diego, 1997.

35. Daniels, G: Effect of enzymes on and chemical modifications on high frequency red cell antigens. Immunohematology 8:53–57, 1992.

36. Harris, TY: Antibody identification. In Johnson, ST, Rudmann, SV, and Wilson, SM (eds): Serologic Problem Solving Strategies: A Systematic Approach. American Association of Blood Banks, Bethesda, MD, 1996.

37. Edwards, JM, Moulds, JJ, and Judd, WJ: Chloroquine dissociation of antigen-antibody complexes. Transfusion 22:59, 1982.

38. Branch, DR, and Petz, LD: A new reagent having multiple applications in immunohematology (abstract). Transfusion 20:642, 1980.

39. Marsh, WL: Scoring of hemagglutination reactions. Transfusion 12:352, 1972.

40. Walker, RH, op cit, p 568.

41. Issitt, PD, op cit, p 611.

42. Moulds, MK: Special serologic technics useful in resolving high-titer, low-avidity antibodies. In Recognition and Resolution of High-Titer, Low-Avidity Antibodies: A Technical Workshop. American Association of Blood Banks, Washington, DC, 1979.

43. Judd, WJ: Controversies in transfusion medicine prewarmed tests: Con. Transfusion 35:271–275, 1995.

44. Mallory, D: Controversies in transfusion medicine prewarmed tests: Pro—why, when, and how—not if. Transfusion 35:268–270, 1995.

45. Waligora, SK, and Edwards, JM: Use of rabbit red cells for adsorption of cold autoagglutinins. Transfusion 23:328, 1983.

46. Orsini, LA, et al: Removal of serum IgG alloantibodies by rabbit erythrocyte stroma (abstract). Transfusion 25:452, 1985.

47. Pirofsky, B, and Rosner, ER: DTT test: A new method to differentiate IgM and IgG erythrocyte antibodies. VoxSang 27:480, 1974.

48. Deutsch, HF, and Morton, JI: Dissociation of human serum macroglobulins. Science 125:600, 1957.

49. Petz, LD, and Garratty, G: Acquired Immune Hemolytic Anemias. Churchill Livingstone, New York, 1980, p 110.

50. Issitt PD, op cit, p 599.

51. Sosler, SD, et al: Immune hemolytic anemia associated with probenecid. Am J Clin Pathol 84:391–394, 1985.

52. Sosler, SD, et al: Acute hemolytic anemia associated with a chlorpropamide-induced apparent auto-anti-Jk$^a$. Transfusion 24:206–209, 1984.

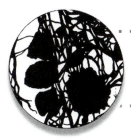

CHAPTER **12**

# COMPATIBILITY TESTING

Mary P. Nix, MS, MT(ASCP)SBB

## OBJECTIVES

*On completion of this chapter, the learner should be able to:*

**1** Recognize the appropriate methods to identify the patient and donor accurately and to collect samples for testing.

**2** Outline the procedure for testing of donor and patient specimens.

**3** Select appropriate donor units based on availability, presence or absence of alloantibody in the patient, unit's age, and unit's appearance.

**4** Compare and contrast crossmatch procedures.

**5** Resolve incompatibilities in the crossmatch.

**6** Explain compatibility testing procedures and protocols in special circumstances.

**7** State the limitations of compatibility testing procedures.

**8** Describe a scheme for effective blood utilization.

**9** List the steps necessary to reidentify the patient before transfusion.

**10** Discuss future issues of compatibility testing.

Blood transfusion has been a part of therapy for less than a century. In the past, transfusions were often performed out of desperation, with no guarantee that patients would benefit or even survive. Donors were chosen solely by availability and willingness.

Today, transfusion therapy is scientific and successful. The concept of antigens and antibodies was unknown until 1900, when Landsteiner described ABO blood groups and recognized their importance in the success or failure of transfusions. By the early 1940s, there were reports of serious transfusion reactions in cases in which the donor and recipient were ABO compatible.[1] It became obvious that not all incompatible reactions could be prevented by ABO group compatibility alone.

As the knowledge of new blood group systems increased, so did the search for more sensitive pretransfusion compatibility testing methods. Pioneer blood bankers mixed the patient's serum and the donor's red cells and observed for direct red cell lysis and/or agglutination. This became known as the major crossmatch test.

The crossmatch became part of a series of pretransfusion tests known as a *compatibility test*. The compatibility test, as we know it today, includes an ABO and $Rh_0(D)$ group on the donor and recipient, screening of the donor's and patient's sera for unexpected antibodies, and a crossmatch. The primary purpose of pretransfusion or compatibility testing is to ensure the best possible results of a blood transfusion. That is, the transfused red cells should have an acceptable survival rate and there should not be significant destruction of the recipient's own red cells. Each of the following is important to ensure safe transfusion therapy and must be considered in any comprehensive review of the process used to select blood for a patient:

1. Identification of the patient and donor and collection of appropriate samples for testing
2. Testing of the donor sample
3. Testing of the patient sample and review of past blood bank records
4. Selection of appropriate donor units
5. Crossmatching
6. Reidentification of the patient before infusion of blood

No testing procedure can prevent sensitization of the recipient to foreign red blood cell antigens or avoid a delayed transfusion reaction caused by antibody present in subdetectable amounts in the pretransfusion serum. Testing cannot guarantee normal survival of transfused cells in the patient's circulation. The potential benefits of transfusion should always be weighed against the potential risks any time this form of therapy is contemplated. Although adverse responses to transfusion cannot always be avoided, results are much more likely to be favorable if pretransfusion testing is carefully performed and results of laboratory testing show no incompatibility between donor and patient.

## COLLECTION AND PREPARATION OF SAMPLES

### Positive Patient Identification

Historically, the major cause of transfusion-associated fatalities was clerical error resulting in incorrect ABO groupings. Today, this fact is virtually unchanged. Forty-eight percent of transfusion deaths are the result of such errors.[2] This disheartening fact shows that clerical errors remain the greatest threat to safe transfusion therapy. The most common cause of clerical errors, and thus transfusion accidents, is misidentification of the patient involved in the transfusion. Errors have resulted from confusion in identification of the patient when the blood sample was drawn, a mix-up of samples during handling in the laboratory, and error in identification of the patient when the transfusion was given.

Exact procedures for proper identification of the patient, patient sample, and donor unit must be established and used by all staff responsible for each aspect of transfusion therapy in order to prevent the occurrence of errors.

To prevent collection of samples from the wrong patient, the blood request form must be used to confirm the patient's identity before phlebotomy is performed. The request form must state the intended recipient's full name and unique hospital identification number.[3] Other information such as age and date of birth, address, sex, and name of requesting physician can be used to further verify patient identity but is not required on the form. Printing must be legible, and indelible nameplate impressions or computer printouts are preferable to handwritten forms.

The patient's wristband identification must always be compared with the requisition form. Any discrepancies must be completely resolved before the sample is taken. Nameplates on the wall or bed labels must never be used to verify identity, inasmuch as the patient specified may no longer occupy that bed.

If the patient does not have a wristband or if the patient's identity is unknown, some form of positive identification must be attached to the patient before collection of samples. This may be a temporary tie tag or a wristband or ankle band, but it should not be removed until proper identification has been attached to the patient and verification of identity is made by the phlebotomist.

In some transfusing facilities, if the patient does not have a wristband and is coherent, it is permissible to ask the patient to state his or her full name and spell it out. If the age or home address is printed on the requisition form, the patient might be asked to state this information. Occasional errors can result from two patients with the same name being mistaken for each other. The phlebotomist should never offer a name and ask the patient to confirm that it is correct (e.g., Are you Mr. Jones?). Some disoriented patients may answer yes to any question. If the patient is very young or is incoherent, some other reliable professional individual who knows the patient must confirm the identity and document this on the requisition form.

Commercially manufactured identification systems using preprinted tags and numbers (Figs. 12–1, 12–2, and 12–3) are especially useful in patient and donor verification procedures. In an effort to improve transfusion safety, an identification system that uses a physical barrier to transfusion, in addition to standard identification procedures, has been described.[4] The physical barrier, a plastic combination lock, is applied to a unit of blood intended for a specific recipient. The lock is opened by nursing or medical personnel at the bedside, where the combination is obtained from the patient's wristband. This system is reported to eliminate the fatal clerical errors that occur outside of the laboratory.

## Collecting Patient Samples

After positive identification has been accomplished, blood samples should be drawn, using careful technique to avoid mechanical hemolysis. Hemolyzed samples cannot be used for testing because hemolysis caused by activation of complement by antigen-antibody complexes will be masked.

Serum or plasma may be used for pretransfusion testing. Most blood bank technologists prefer serum because plasma may cause small fibrin clots to form, and these may be difficult to distinguish from true agglutination. Also, plasma may inactivate complement so that some antibodies may not be detected. About 10 mL of blood is usually sufficient for all testing procedures if there are no known serologic problems.

Tubes must be labeled before leaving the patient's bedside. If imprinted labels are used, they must be compared with the patient's wristband and requisition form before use. Labels should be attached to the tubes in a tamperproof manner that will make removal and reattachment impossible. All writing must be legible and indelible, and each tube must be labeled with the patient's full name, hospital identification number, and the date of sample collection.[5] The phlebotomist must initial or sign the label and add additional pertinent information as required by the standard operating procedure of the facility.

To avoid contamination with materials that may cause confusing serologic results, blood samples should not be taken from intravenous tubing lines. Venous samples should not be drawn from above an infusion

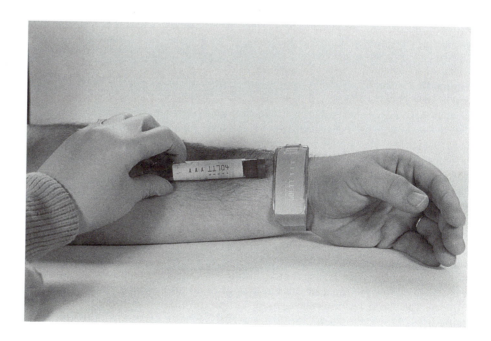

**Figure 12–1.** Commercially manufactured identification systems.

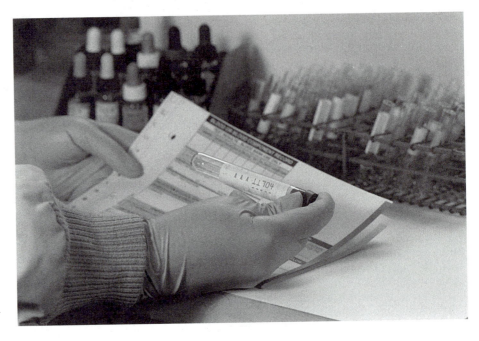

**Figure 12–2.** Commercially manufactured identification systems.

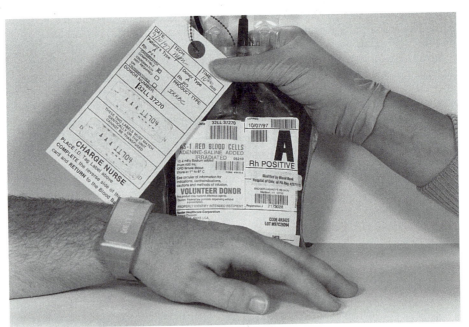

**Figure 12–3.** Commercially manufactured identification systems.

site but may be drawn from below the site. If a sample must be taken from an intravenous line, the line should be disconnected for 5 to 10 minutes, the first 10 mL of blood drawn should be discarded, and then the sample for testing may be obtained. When a specimen is received in the laboratory, a blood bank technologist must confirm that the information on the sample and requisition form agree. All discrepancies must be resolved before the sample is accepted, and if any doubt exists, a new sample must be drawn. Receipt of an unlabeled specimen requires that a new sample be obtained.

Patient samples should be tested as soon as possible after collection, and the serum should be separated from the patient's red cells as soon as possible after the sample has clotted. If testing cannot be performed immediately, samples should be stoppered and kept at 1 to 6°C.

As noted in Chapter 3, recent pregnancy or transfusion indicates an opportunity for a humoral immune response. Antibody production occurs over a predictable range of time, but the exact time will vary from responder (i.e., patient) to responder (i.e., patient). Specimens used in compatibility testing should ideally be collected during the critical phases of the immune response. In an attempt to capture this important time for each patient, serum obtained from samples less than 72 hours after collection must be used for antibody screening and crossmatch testing if the patient was pregnant or received red cell products by transfusion within the last 3 months, or if these histories are unknown.[6]

Patient red blood cells can be obtained from either clotted or anticoagulated samples. They can be washed before use to remove plasma or serum, which may interfere with some testing procedures. A 2 to 5 percent saline suspension of red cells is used for most serologic testing procedures; however, the manufacturer's directions should be consulted for the proper cell concentration to use for typing tests performed with licensed reagents. A method for preparing a button of washed red cells suitable for performing one test is given in Procedural Appendix 1.[7]

## Donor Samples

Samples for donor testing must be collected at the same time as the full donor unit. Depending on the method used for testing, clotted and/or anticoagulated samples are obtained. The donor information and medical history card, the pilot samples for processing, and the collection bag must be labeled with the same unique number code before starting the phlebotomy, and the numbers must be verified again immediately after filling. The donor number is used to identify all records of testing and eventual disposition of all component parts of the unit of blood. More detailed information on donor samples can be found in Chapter 10.

Ideal samples for compatibility testing can be prepared from the segmented tubing through which the donor was bled. The tubing or segments are attached to the collection bag, and each segment is imprinted with the same numbers. These numbers are different from the donor unit number but nonetheless are a positive means of sampling a given unit of blood.

Donor cells can be obtained from the segments in a number of ways that permit several procedures to be performed from the same segment. One technique that works well for sampling is using a lancet to make a tiny hole in the segment through which a single drop of blood can be expressed easily. The hole is essentially self-sealing, so the rest of the blood in the segment remains uncontaminated. Another technique is to cut the red cell end of the segment and use an applicator stick to remove cells, or express a drop by squeezing the tubing. Commercially manufactured segment cutters eliminate the need for scissors and dispense the red cells into a test tube in one motion. The segment may be stored with the cut end down in a properly labeled test tube to minimize contamination. The contents of the segment should preferably not be emptied into a test tube for storage because of the increased risk of contamination.

Regardless of the method used to harvest cells from a segment, it is important that engineering and/or work practice controls be used to eliminate or minimize aerosol production when the segment is cut or opened. Refer to Chapter 14 for additional information on safety procedures.

Both donor and recipient samples must be stored for a minimum of 7 days following transfusion.[8] The samples should be stoppered, carefully labeled, and refrigerated at 1 to 6°C. They should be adequate in volume so that they can be reevaluated if the patient experiences an adverse response to the transfusion.

## COMPATIBILITY TESTING PROTOCOLS

### Testing of the Donor Sample

According to the Code of Federal Regulations (CFR)[9] and the American Association of Blood Banks (AABB) standards,[10] ABO and Rh grouping (including a test for weak D, D$^u$) and tests intended to prevent disease transmission must be performed on a sample of blood taken at the time of collection of the unit of blood from the donor. A screening test for unexpected antibodies to red blood cell antigens is required by AABB Standards on samples from donors revealing a history of prior transfusion or pregnancy.[11] Testing is performed by the facility collecting the donor unit, and results must be clearly indicated on all product labels appearing on the unit.

The transfusing facility is required by AABB Standards[12] to confirm the ABO cell grouping on all units and Rh grouping on units labeled Rh negative. Tests for weak D (D$^u$) are not required to be repeated. The transfusing facility is not required to repeat any other testing procedure. The sample used for this testing must be obtained from an attached segment on the donor unit.

All testing must be performed using in-date, licensed reagents, according to manufacturers' directions and protocol established in the written standard operating procedure of the facility. A detailed explanation of the processing of donor blood can be found in Chapter 10.

### Testing of the Patient Sample

A record of all results obtained in testing patient samples must be maintained. Some large transfusion services keep this information on a computerized retrieval system for ready access. However, when computer records are not available, these transfusion services must have another system that permits retrieval of patient testing results.[13]

Ideally, the same unique identification number should be assigned each time a patient is admitted for treatment. The number can then be used as a method of positive identification for comparing results of previous and current testing. Verification of previous results helps establish that the current samples were collected from the correct individual. Any discrepancies between previous and current results must be resolved before transfusion is initiated. A new sample should be collected from the patient, if necessary, to resolve the problem.

ABO and Rh grouping results should be included in the file. Notations concerning unusual serologic reactions and the identity of unexpected antibodies in the patient's serum should also be included in the file. This is perhaps the most important information. Sometimes subdetectable amounts of antibody may be present in a patient's serum, and previous records are the only source of information regarding its presence and identity and possible clinical significance.

ABO and Rh grouping and antibody screening of the patient's serum can be performed in advance of or at the same time as the crossmatch. If the patient has had a transfusion or has been pregnant within the last 3 months, or if the history is unavailable or uncertain, the sample must be obtained from the patient within 3 days of the scheduled transfusion.[14] An accurate medical history, including information on medications, recent blood transfusions, and previous pregnancies, may help to explain unusual results.

### ABO Grouping

Determination of the patient's correct ABO group is the most critical pretransfusion serologic test. ABO grouping can be performed on slides or in tubes. Tube tests offer greater sensitivity. Testing is performed in a manner similar to that described in Chapter 5, using potent licensed reagents according to the manufacturer's directions. If the cell and serum grouping results do not agree, additional testing must be conducted to resolve the discrepancy. Useful information on resolving ABO grouping discrepancies has been presented in Chapter 5. If the patient's ABO group cannot be satisfactorily determined and immediate transfusion is essential, group O packed red cells should be used.

### Rh Grouping

Rh grouping is performed using anti-D blood grouping serum. Tube or slide tests should be performed according to the manufacturer's directions for the reagent, which may or may not include the use of a suitable diluent control. When indicated, these controls must be run in parallel with Rh grouping tests performed on patient samples, to avoid incorrect designation of Rh-negative patients as Rh-positive. If the diluent control is positive, the result of the Rh grouping test is invalid.[15] In such a case, a direct antihuman globulin test (DAT) should be performed on the patient's red blood cells to determine whether uptake of autoantibodies (or alloantibodies, if the patient has recently received a transfusion) is responsible for the positive control. If a positive DAT is found, accurate Rh grouping can sometimes be performed using saline-active or chemically modified Rh blood grouping serum with an appropriate diluent or 8 percent albumin control. If the Rh group of the recipient cannot be determined and transfusion is essential, Rh-negative blood should be given.

The test for weak D (D^u) is unnecessary when testing transfusion recipients.[16] Individuals typing as Rh-negative in direct testing should receive Rh-negative blood, and those typing as Rh-positive in direct testing should receive Rh-positive blood. Female patients whose red blood cells type as weak D (D^u) are considered Rh-positive (see Chapters 6 and 20) and may receive Rh-positive blood during transfusion.

Some patients who type as Rh-positive, whether by direct or indirect testing, may produce anti-D following transfusion of Rh-positive red blood cell components (see Chapter 6). This occurs rarely and does not justify the routine transfusion of Rh-negative blood to these Rh-positive patients until the antibody is detected.

### Antibody Screening

The patient's serum or plasma must be tested for unexpected antibodies. The object of the antibody screening test is to detect as many clinically significant antibodies as possible. In general, the term *clinically significant antibodies* refers to antibodies that are reactive at 37°C and/or in the antihuman globulin test and are known to have caused a transfusion reaction or unacceptably short survival of the transfused red cells. Table 12–1 lists these antibodies.[17] The incidence of unexpected antibodies in the patient population is low; 1.64 percent in one large study[18] and 0.78 percent in another.[19]

Correct ABO grouping results are much more critical to transfusion safety than antibody screening. Most antibodies, other than anti-A and anti-B, do not cause severe hemolytic transfusion reactions. Therefore, the vast majority of patients would not suffer grave consequences if they received a transfusion of blood from ABO group compatible donors without the benefit of antibody screening tests.

**Table 12–1.** Clinical Significance* of Antibodies[†] Detected at 37°C in Vitro

1. Antibodies regarded as always being potentially clinically significant

| | |
|---|---|
| ABO | Duffy |
| Rh | Kidd |
| Kell | SsU |

2. Antibodies that may sometimes be clinically significant

| | |
|---|---|
| Le^a | Lutheran (Lu^a, Lu^b) |
| MN | Cartwright (Yt^a) |
| P_1 | |

3. Antibodies that rarely, if ever, are clinically significant

| | |
|---|---|
| Le^b | Xg^a |
| Chido/Rodgers (Ch^a/Rg^a) | Bg |
| York (Yk^a) | HTLA |
| Sd^a | |

**Source:** Garratty, G: Mechanisms of immune red cell destruction and red cell compatibility testing. Hum Pathol 14:209, 1983, with permission.
* Clinical significance is defined by proven hemolytic transfusion reactions. This could range from a severe overt reaction to diminished red cell survival as the only sign.
† Very rare antibodies have not been included in this list (e.g., when there is only a single report of an HTR in the literature).

Detection of unexpected antibodies is important, however, for the selection of donor red cells that are likely to survive maximally in the patient's circulation. Weakly reactive antibodies that are capable of reacting with their antigens at 37°C can cause decreased survival of transfused incompatible red cells. Because large numbers of antibody molecules are present in the patient's circulation compared with the number of red cells in a unit of blood, incompatible donor cells are highly vulnerable to destruction by patient antibodies.

Antibody screening offers several advantages over direct crossmatch testing for detection of antibodies:

1. Testing is performed using selected group O red cells that are known to carry optimal representation of important blood group antigens.
2. Testing can be performed well in advance of the anticipated transfusion, allowing ample time for identification of any unexpected antibody and location of suitable donor units lacking the corresponding antigen.

Methods used to detect antibodies in patients' sera must demonstrate all significant coating, hemolyzing, and agglutinating antibodies active at 37°C. Incubation of screening tests at or below room temperature is not advocated, because antibodies that react only at lower temperatures in vitro are usually incapable of complexing with their antigens in vivo.

American Association of Blood Banks Standards stipulate the necessity of performing an antihuman globulin test on patient samples using reagent red cells obtained from single donors.[20] Single-donor screening cells offer increased sensitivity over pooled cell preparations. They are supplied as sets of individual cell samples from two or more donors whose red cell phenotypes have been carefully matched so that they complement each other.

If an antigen is lacking from one cell sample, it is present on the other. Ideally, one sample in each set should carry the products of homozygous genes for antigens such as Jk[a] and c. Antibodies to these antigens sometimes fail to react with cell samples carrying a single dose of the corresponding antigen.

During the late 1970s and early 1980s, polyspecific antihuman globulin (AHG) reagents, containing adequate levels of anti-complement as well as high levels of anti-IgG activity, were the preferred AHG reagents for patient antibody screening and crossmatch testing.[21] It was shown that detection of complement components bound to red cells by antigen-antibody complexing was necessary to demonstrate the presence of some weakly reactive antibodies.[22] In addition, Wright and Issitt[23] found that over 50 percent of antibodies in the Kidd and Duffy blood group systems were detected better when reasonable levels of anticomplement components were present in the AHG serum used. However, polyspecific AHG reagents are known to detect nonspecific and/or insignificant proteins. When used routinely, spurious reactions were investigated, yielding little relevance to patient care, yet increasing costs and consuming valuable technologist time.

The modern blood bank laboratory uses anti-IgG AHG reagents in its compatibility testing procedures. Polyspecific AHG reagents are still used in other tests or procedures. Refer to Chapter 11 for a more complete discussion of the detection and identification of alloantibodies.

To detect false-negative antihuman globulin tests caused by the inactivation of the anti-IgG in the AHG reagent, AABB standards require the addition of IgG-coated red cells (i.e., "check cells") to all tubes with negative AHG test results.[24]

The sensitivity of antibody detection tests can be enhanced by increasing the amount of serum added to the test,[25,26] increasing the length of incubation time at 37°C,[27,28] or adding albumin or another enhancement medium to the test.[29,30] Screening cells can also be treated before use with the proteolytic enzyme solutions such as 0.1 percent papain or ficin to enhance their ability to detect some antibodies.[31,32] However, other antibodies cannot be detected using enzyme-pretreated cell samples, so these cells cannot be used as the only means of screening patients' sera. These serologic factors should be considered when resolving unexpected in vitro results and may be applied to the investigation of incompatible crossmatches, discussed later in this chapter.

Increased sensitivity is especially important when screening the sera of patients who have already formed at least one antibody, inasmuch as they have proved their ability to produce antibodies in response to foreign red blood cell antigens.[33,34] Patients who have had recent transfusions and those who have experienced previously unexplained adverse reactions to blood transfusion are also candidates for more sensitive antibody screening procedures. These patients may have formed antibodies that are too weak to be demonstrable using routine testing procedures. Reexposure to the corresponding antigens on donor red cells may cause a rapid rise in antibody titer and subsequent destruction of circulating incompatible cells. These additional factors, as well as many others, may be kept in mind when dealing with unexpected serologic results.

Antibody screening tests should demonstrate the presence of all potentially significant antibodies in the patient's serum and rapidly indicate the need for further studies. All antibodies encountered must be identified to determine potential clinical significance and to allow a logical decision to be made as to whether there is a need to select antigen-negative units for transfusion.

## SELECTION OF APPROPRIATE DONOR UNITS

In almost all cases, blood and blood components of the patient's own ABO and Rh group should be selected for transfusion. When blood and blood components of the patient's type are unavailable or some other reason precludes its use, units selected must lack any antigen against which the patient has a significant antibody. It is completely acceptable, however, to use blood and blood components that do not contain all of the antigens carried on the patient's own red cells (e.g., group A or B packed red blood cells can be safely given to a group AB recipient). When transfusions of an ABO group different from that of the recipient must be given, packed red cells must be used rather than whole blood, which contains plasma antibodies that are incompatible with the patient's red cells. Group O packed red cells can be safely used for all patients; however, conservation of a limited supply of group O blood should dictate its use for patients of other ABO types only in special circumstances. If ABO-specific blood is not available or is in less than adequate supply, alternate blood groups are chosen as summarized in Table 12–2.

Rh-negative blood can be given to Rh-positive patients; however, good inventory management again should conserve this limited resource for use in Rh-negative recipients. But if the Rh-negative unit is near expiration, the unit should be given rather than wasted. Rh-positive blood should not be given to Rh-negative female patients of childbearing age. Transfusion of Rh-negative male patients and female patients beyond menopause with Rh-positive blood is acceptable as long as no preformed anti-D is demonstrable in their sera. About 80 percent of Rh-negative patients who receive 200 mL or more of Rh-positive blood may respond to such a transfusion by producing anti-D.[35] However, this outcome must sometimes be weighed against the alternatives of not transfusing at all if the supply of Rh-negative blood has been exhausted. If the formation of anti-D is unlikely to be of great significance, for example in an Rh-negative elderly surgical patient, use of Rh-positive blood is judicious in the opinion of many technologists. In these situations, approval by or notification of the blood bank's medical director is necessary, according to the laboratory's standard operating procedure.

When an unexpected antibody is found in the patient's serum during antibody screening, donor units selected at random may be crossmatched with the patient's serum. This may, in fact, assist in the identification of the unexpected antibody. If a clinically significant antibody is identified, the compatible units may be phenotyped with commercial antiserum to verify that they are antigen-negative. There is no need to provide antigen-negative red cells for patients whose sera contain antibodies that are reactive only below 37°C, inasmuch as these antibodies are incapable of causing significant red cell destruction in vivo. Significant or potent examples of anti-$P_1$, anti-Le$^a$, anti-Le$^b$, and other typically cold reactive antibodies in patients' sera can be used to select appropriate donor units that are crossmatch compatible in tests conducted at 37°C.[36]

Potent examples of IgG, warm reactive antibodies in patients' sera can also be used to select suitable donor units by direct testing. Commercially prepared typing reagents must be used to select blood for patients whose sera contain weak examples of antibodies active at 37°C, antibodies that react well only with cell samples carrying homozygous representation of the corresponding antigens, and for patients whose sera no longer exhibit demonstrable in vitro reactivity but which previously were known to contain clinically significant IgG antibodies, such as anti-Jk$^a$, and anti-K, or anti-E.

Donor units should be selected so that the red cells are of appropriate age for the patient's needs and will not expire before use. For efficient inventory management, units that will definitely be transfused should be selected from units close to their expiration date.

Packed red cell units should be selected if the patient does not require volume, only increased oxygen-carrying capacity. Whole blood should be reserved for those occasions when the patient genuinely needs volume expansion, such as in major trauma or surgery. Even in these cases, however, support with appropriate crystalloid solutions and blood components usually produces results equal to or superior to those achieved by transfusion of whole blood. Donor units should be examined visually before compatibility testing for unusual appearance, correct labeling, and hermetic seal integrity. Donor units showing abnormal color change, turbidity, clots, incomplete or improper labeling information, or leakage of any sort should be returned to the collecting facility.

## CROSSMATCHING

The terms *compatibility test* and *crossmatch* are sometimes used interchangeably; they should be clearly differentiated. A crossmatch is only part of a compatibility test. Compatibility testing in the United States consists of (1) review of patient's past blood bank history and records; (2) ABO and Rh grouping of the recipient and donor; (3) antibody screening of the recipient's and donor's serum; and finally (4) the crossmatch. The crossmatch has recently undergone much scrutiny, and there have been thoughts of eliminating it entirely. However, to many blood bankers, the crossmatch still has a definite role.

**Table 12–2.** Choice of Alternative Blood Groups When ABO Identical Donors Are Not Available

| Patient's Blood Group | Alternative Blood Group (Given as Packed Cells) |
|---|---|
| O | None |
| A | O |
| B | O |
| AB | A, B, O* |

Source: Adapted from Widmonn, F (ed): Technical Manual, American Association of Blood Banks, Arlington, VA, 1985.
* Packed cell components of any group are acceptable, but only one of the three should be used for a given antibody, if possible. Group A is more readily available and is thus preferred over group B.

It is important to note that direct crossmatching preceded antibody screening as part of patient pretransfusion testing by several decades. Selected red cells were first used in some laboratories during the late 1950s to screen sera from donors.[37,38] Separate antibody screening of patient sera was not popular as an addition to crossmatching until the early 1960s, when phenotyped red cells for this purpose were marketed commercially. By that time, direct crossmatching was firmly entrenched as a routine procedure that was necessary to ensure the well-being of the recipient. As early as 1964, however, Grove-Rasmussen[39] questioned the need for an antihuman globulin test as part of the crossmatch when antibody screening tests were negative.

Considering that over 99 percent of significant antibodies in patients' sera can be detected by adequate antibody screening procedures, what, then, is the value of performing crossmatching between patient and donor samples? Two main functions of the crossmatch test can be cited:

1. It is a final check of ABO compatibility between donor and patient.
2. It may detect the presence of an antibody in the patient's serum that will react with antigens on the donor red blood cells but that was not detected in antibody screening because the corresponding antigen was lacking from the screening cells.

The current AABB Standards[40] state that tests to detect ABO incompatibility suffice if (1) no clinically significant antibodies were detected in the antibody screening process, and (2) no record exists of the detection of clinically significant unexpected antibodies. Elimination of advance crossmatch testing for patients undergoing surgical procedures in which blood is unlikely to be used has been implemented successfully in many facilities, using the "type and screen" approach or the abbreviated crossmatch discussed in more detail later in this chapter.

## Major and Minor Crossmatch Tests

Historically, crossmatch testing procedures have been divided into two parts: the major crossmatch test, consisting of mixing the patient's serum with donor red cells; and the minor test, consisting of mixing the donor's plasma with patient red cells. As the names imply, the major test is much more critical for ensuring safe transfusion than the minor test.

The minor crossmatch test has been completely eliminated in most blood banks because donor samples are screened beforehand for the more common antibodies. The presence of a low-incidence antibody in the donor's plasma probably would not cause a transfusion reaction because it would be diluted in the recipient's plasma. It is more important to simplify procedures by eliminating the minor crossmatch than to perform it in the belief that it might show some unlikely antibody-antigen reaction.[41]

## Methods for Major Crossmatch Tests

Many different procedures can be used for crossmatch testing. The objective of testing is to select donor units that are able to provide maximal benefit to the patient. This fact should be kept in mind when developing the test protocol. Nothing but delay results from detection of in vitro incompatibilities that are not likely to occur in vivo or use of complicated methods that require several tubes for each unit tested. For this reason, incubation of tests at room temperature has been eliminated in many facilities, and a simple crossmatch test of one tube per unit has become the standard. A sample procedure for a one-tube compatibility test is given in Procedural Appendix 2.[42]

Crossmatch methods can generally be categorized by the test phase in which the procedure ends.

### Immediate Spin Crossmatch

As mentioned previously, when no clinically significant antibodies are detected and there are no previous records of such antibodies, a serologic test to detect ABO incompatibility is sufficient. This is accomplished by simply mixing a patient's serum with donor cells and centrifuging immediately (i.e., immediate spin). Absence of hemolysis or agglutination indicates compatibility.

The type and screen, coupled with an immediate spin crossmatch, are referred to as an abbreviated crossmatch. Studies of the use of an abbreviated crossmatch show that it is a safe and effective method of pretransfusion testing. It has been calculated to be 99.9 percent effective in preventing the occurrence of an incompatible transfusion.[43] Walker[44] was able to show that the frequency with which an incompatible antiglobulin crossmatch follows a negative screen is very low—0.06 percent. Other studies confirm its safety with similar statistics.[45-48]

Recently, however, the ability of this method to detect all ABO incompatibilities has been challenged.[49] False reactions may be seen in the presence of other immediate spin–reactive antibodies (e.g., autoanti-I), in patients with hyperimmune ABO antibodies, when the procedure is not performed correctly (i.e., delay in centrifugation or reading), when rouleaux is observed, or when infants' specimens are tested. Adding ethylenediaminetetraacetic (EDTA) to the test system has been reported to eliminate some of the false-positive reactions, thus improving the sensitivity of the immediate spin crossmatch.[50]

A recent report by Riccardi and coworkers[51] indicated that an electronic (computer) crossmatch to detect ABO incompatibilities was as safe as the serologic immediate spin test. The computer crossmatch compares recent ABO serologic results and interpretations on file for both the donor and the patient being matched and determines compatibility based on this comparison. These investigators noted that, to further decrease the risk of ABO incompatibility, duplicate patient ABO and Rh groupings were needed. Subsequently, anticipating changes in the AABB Standards, Butch and associates[52] produced a model computer crossmatch. Annual savings, reduced sample requirements, reduced handling of biologic materials, and elimination of false reactions associated with the immediate spin crossmatch were additional benefits identified as the result of using the computer crossmatch.

The AABB has indeed changed its standards, which now include statements recognizing the computer crossmatch as an acceptable crossmatch method. The electronic crossmatch may replace the immediate spin crossmatch only when the patient's ABO group has been determined on two occasions. One of the determinations must be done on the current sample. Having a previous ABO result on file may serve as the second occasion. When there are no results on file, testing of the same sample by a second technologist or testing of a second current sample is indicated. Additionally, the computer system must be validated to show that it can detect data entry discrepancies and ABO incompatibilities between patient and donor.[53]

### Antiglobulin Crossmatch

The antiglobulin crossmatch procedure begins in the same manner as the immediate spin crossmatch, continues to a 37°C incubation, and finishes with an antiglobulin test. Several methods are used to enhance antigen-antibody reactions. Albumin may be added before incubation at 37°C to enhance reactivity of some antibodies. Low ionic strength solution (LISS) or polyethylene glycol (PEG) may be added in place of albumin to facilitate complexing of antigens and antibodies.[54] For greatest sensitivity, an AHG reagent containing both anti-IgG and anti-complement may be selected for the final phase of this crossmatch method. However, many laboratories routinely use anti-IgG AHG reagents for reasons previously discussed.

The polybrene (P-AHG) test has been shown to be a rapid and sensitive crossmatch technique.[55-57] It has been used as a method for detecting ABO incompatibility when accompanied by a carefully performed and negative antibody screening on the patient.

An auto-control, consisting of the patient's own cells and serum, may be tested in parallel with the crossmatch test. Although current AABB Standards no longer require an auto-control, some workers still find it useful. Perkins and associates[58] calculated the predictive value of a positive auto-control (3.6 percent) when the antibody screen was negative and decided to continue using the auto-control in pretransfusion testing. Results of the auto-control help clarify possible explanations for positive results in the crossmatches and are discussed later in this chapter.

### Interpretation of Results

Tubes should be carefully labeled so that the contents can be identified at any stage of the procedure. Af-

ter centrifugation of tubes, the supernatant should be examined for hemolysis, which must be interpreted as a positive result. Results should be read against a white or lighted background, and a magnifying mirror or hand lens can be used to facilitate reading, if desired. The button of cells should be gently resuspended. A "wiggle and tilt" method of resuspension is ideal. Violent shaking or tapping of the tubes may yield false-negative results because fragile agglutinates may be disrupted. A jagged button edge is indicative of a positive result, whereas a smooth button edge and swirling free cells indicate the absence of a demonstrable antigen-antibody interaction. After the button has been completely resuspended, the contents of the tube should be interpreted and positive results graded according to a scale used by all technologists in a facility. Uniform grading of reactions allows retrospective analysis of results by supervisory staff, as well as comparison of serial results obtained on samples collected from the same patient. Results can be examined microscopically for verification, if desired. Review **Color Plate 2** for the grading of typical agglutination reactions.

According to the Code of Federal Regulations,[59] all results must be recorded immediately in a permanent ledger using a logical system that allows them to be easily recalled, and actual observations, as well as interpretations, must be recorded. All work should be signed or initialed by the technologist performing the test. If an incompatibility is found, the record should clearly show the location of results of follow-up studies, and additional testing should be performed.

### Resolving Incompatibilities in the Major Crossmatch

The primary objective of the major crossmatch test is to detect the presence of antibodies in the recipient's serum, including anti-A and anti-B, that could destroy transfused red cells. A positive result in the major crossmatch test requires explanation, and the patient should not receive a transfusion until the cause of the incompatibility has been fully determined. When the crossmatch test result is positive, the results of the auto-control and antibody screening test should be reviewed to identify patterns that may help determine the cause of the problem.

### Causes of Positive Results in the Major Crossmatch

A positive result in the major crossmatch test may be caused by any of the following.

1. **Incorrect ABO grouping of the patient or donor.** ABO grouping should be immediately repeated, especially if strong incompatibility is noted in a reading taken after immediate spin. Samples that bear undisputable identity with the original patient sample and the donor bag should be used for retesting.

2. **An alloantibody in the patient's serum reacting with the corresponding antigen on donor red cells.** The auto-control tube will be negative unless the patient has recently received incompatible cells in transfusion. If the antibody screening test is positive, panel studies should allow identification of antibody specificity, which then permits selection of units lacking the offending antigens for compatibility testing. Chapter 11 provides further discussion of antibody detection and identification as well as examples for study.

a. If red cells of all donors tested are incompatible with the patient's serum and the antibody screening test is positive, suspect either an antibody directed against an antigen of high incidence or multiple antibodies in the patient's serum. Consult a reference laboratory if you are unable to identify the specificity. (Note: If the patient has ABO-compatible siblings, they may lack the antigen(s) to which the patient has been sensitized and may be excellent potential donors in an emergency.)

b. If the antibody screening test is negative and only one donor unit is incompatible, an antibody in the patient's serum may be directed against an antigen of relatively low incidence that is present on that donor's red cells. Panel studies of the patient's serum are usually noninformative, and identification of the antibody is academic if other compatible units are easily located.

c. If the antibody screening test is negative, the patient's serum may contain either "naturally occurring" (e.g., anti-$A_1$) or passively acquired ABO agglutinins. Passive acquisition of anti-A, anti-B, or anti-A,B may occur after transfusion of non–ABO-specific blood products (e.g., platelets) or by organ (e.g., liver) or bone marrow transplantation. Checking the serum grouping result to confirm the presence of an unexpected reaction with $A_1$ cells and/or checking the patient's transfusion and transplant histories is helpful in the investigation of these cases.

3. **An autoantibody in the patient's serum reacting with the corresponding antigen on donor red cells.** The auto-control tube will be positive. The antibody screening test and tests of the patient's serum with donor cells will show positive results. Most autoantibodies have specificity for antigens of relatively high incidence. Panel and adsorption studies are important to assess whether underlying alloantibodies are also present. Techniques for management of patients with autoantibodies include autoadsorption of the patient's serum to remove autoantibody activity. Compatibility testing could then be performed using the autoabsorbed serum. Chapter 21 provides further discussion of autoantibodies and their serologic activity.

4. **Prior coating of the donor red cells with protein, resulting in a positive antihuman globulin test.**

If one isolated positive result is obtained, a DAT should be performed on the donor's red cells. Donor cells that demonstrate a positive DAT will be incompatible with all recipients tested in the AHG phase, because the cells are already coated with immunoglobulin and/or complement.

5. **Abnormalities in the patient's serum.**

a. Imbalance of the normal ratio of albumin and gamma globulin (A/G ratio), as in diseases such as myeloma and macroglobulinemia, may cause red cells to stick together on their flat sides, giving the appearance of stacks of coins when viewed microscopically. This is referred to as rouleaux formation (refer to **Color Plate 2**). This property of the serum will affect all tests, including the auto-control. Strong rouleaux may mimic true agglutination; however, clumps are refractile when viewed under the microscope. Rouleaux is usually strongest after 37°C incubation, but does not persist through washing before the AHG test. Problems with rouleaux can often be resolved using the saline replacement technique.[60]

b. The presence of high-molecular-weight dextrans or other plasma expanders may cause false-positive results in compatibility and other tests. However, Bartholomew and colleagues[61] raised doubt that the use of dextran interferes with pretransfusion testing. In scenarios in which plasma expanders interfere, all tests, including the auto-control, are generally affected equally. Saline replacement may be useful to resolve the problem.

c. An antibody against additives in the albumin reagents may cause false-positive results in compatibility tests. Rarely, a patient's serum reacts against the albumin in testing reagents. This occurs when the patient has antibodies to the stabilizing substances, such as caprylate, added to the albumin reagents.[62] Thus, caprylate-free albumin solutions should be used in the testing.

6. **Contaminants in the test system.** Dirty glassware, bacterial contamination of samples, chemical or other contaminants in saline, and fibrin clots may produce positive compatibility test results.

Refer to Table 12–3 for suggestions for investigation of incompatible major crossmatches.

## COMPATIBILITY TESTING IN SPECIAL CIRCUMSTANCES

### Emergencies

Urgent need for transfusion may preclude the performance of usual testing protocol. Several approaches can be utilized in these circumstances. Some laboratories use an "emergency" compatibility testing proce-

**Table 12–3.** Investigation of Incompatible Major Crossmatches

| Observations | Possible Interpretations | Comments |
|---|---|---|
| Major crossmatch:+<br>Auto-control:−<br>Antibody screen:− | ● Incorrect ABO grouping of patient or donor<br><br>● Patient's serum may contain an ABO antibody<br><br>● Alloantibody in patient's serum reacting with antigen donor's red cells but not present on screening cells | ● Repeat ABO grouping: verify identity of sample.<br><br>● Check patient's sample for subgroups; check patient's transfusion and transplantation histories.<br>● Perform antibody identification tests on patient's serum and repeat crossmatch using units negative for the corresponding antigen. If studies are noninformative and patient is incompatible with only 1 unit, locate other compatible units. |
| Major Crossmatch:+<br>Auto-control:−<br>Antibody screen:+ | ● Donor unit may have a positive direct antiglobulin test (DAT)<br>● Alloantibody in patient's serum reacting with antigens on donor's cells and screening cells | ● Perform DAT on donor unit; if positive, do not use the unit.<br>● Perform antibody identification studies on patient's serum and repeat crossmatch using units negative for the corresponding antigen.<br>● If unable to identify antibody specificity, consult a reference laboratory. |
| Major crossmatch:+<br>Auto-control:+<br>Antibody screen:+ | ● Both an autoantibody and alloantibody may be present in the patient's serum<br><br><br>● Abnormalities in patient's serum owing to:<br>1. Imbalance of A/G ratio<br>  ● Plasma expanders<br>  ● Caprylate antibodies<br>  ● Contaminants | ● Perform autoadsorption of patient serum to remove autoantibody (if not recently transfused), perform antibody identification tests, repeat compatibility tests using autoadsorbed serum.<br><br>● If rouleaux is seen, use saline replacement technique.<br>● Obtain new specimen.<br>● Use caprylate-free reagents.<br>● Repeat tests using fresh saline, new bottles of reagent, clean test tubes. |

dure that employs a shortened incubation time, often with addition of LISS to speed antigen-antibody complexing. Others maintain that regular procedures should be used in all circumstances, and blood should be issued before completion of the standard compatibility testing procedure, if necessary. They feel that there is greater danger in using an unfamiliar procedure under pressure than in releasing blood without completed testing. Although both lines of reasoning have merit, the ideal compromise may be to develop regular testing procedures that are concise, so that they can be used in emergency and routine situations alike. Whatever the approach, the protocol for handling emergencies must be decided in advance of the situation and be familiar to all staff in the transfusion service. Adequate pretransfusion samples should be collected before infusion of any donor blood so that compatibility testing, antibody screening, and identification studies, if necessary, can be performed subsequently.

If blood must be issued in an emergency, the patient's ABO and Rh group should be determined, so that group-compatible blood can be given. In extreme emergencies, when there is no time to obtain and to test a sample, group O Rh-negative packed cells can be used. If the patient is Rh-negative and large amounts of blood are likely to be needed, a decision should be made rapidly as to whether inventory allows and the situation demands transfusion of Rh-negative blood. Conversion to Rh-positive is best made immediately if the patient is a man, or a woman beyond childbearing age. Injections of Rh immunoglobulin to prevent formation of anti-D may sometimes be appropriate after the crisis has been resolved. This product is discussed in detail in Chapter 20.

Accurate records of all units issued in the emergency must be maintained. A conspicuous tie tag or label must be placed on each unit indicating that compatibility testing was not completed before release of the unit, and the physician must sign a release authorizing and accepting responsibility for using incompletely tested products, according to the Code of Federal Regulations.[63] Compatibility testing should be completed according to the chosen protocol, and any incompatible result should be reported immediately to the patient's physician and the blood bank medical director.

### Transfusion of Non–Group-Specific Blood

When units of an ABO group other than the patient's own type have been transfused, additional units should be selected after analysis of a freshly drawn patient sample for the presence of unexpected anti-A and anti-B in the recipient's serum. Selection of additional units should always be based on this parameter. When serum from the freshly drawn sample is compatible in the AHG phase with red cells of the patient's own ABO group, group-specific blood may be given for the transfusion. If the AHG phase reveals incompatibility, additional transfusions should be of the alternate blood group. For example, if a group A patient has been given a large number of units of group O packed cells, anti-A may be demonstrable in the serum in the AHG phase. Group O units should therefore be used for any additional transfusions.

## Compatibility Testing for Transfusion of Plasma Products

Compatibility testing procedures are not required for transfusion of plasma products. However, for transfusion of large volumes of plasma and plasma products, a crossmatch test between the donor plasma and patient red cells may be performed, although the current standards do not require a crossmatch test. The primary purpose for testing is to detect ABO incompatibility between donor and patient; therefore, an immediate spin crossmatch is sufficient.

## Intrauterine Transfusions and Transfusions of the Infant

Blood for intrauterine transfusion must be selected to be compatible with maternal antibodies capable of crossing the placenta. If the ABO and Rh groups of the fetus have been determined following amniocentesis, chorionic villus sampling, or percutaneous umbilical blood sampling, group-specific blood could be given provided that there is no fetomaternal ABO or Rh incompatibility. If the ABO and Rh groups of the fetus are not known, then group O Rh-negative red cells should be selected for the intrauterine transfusion. The group O Rh-negative cells must lack any other antigens against which the mother's serum contains antibodies (e.g., anti-Kell, anti-Jk$^a$). Compatibility testing is performed using the mother's serum sample.

Blood for an exchange or regular transfusion of an infant (under 4 months of age) should similarly be compatible with any maternal antibodies that have entered the infant's circulation and are reactive at 37°C. Blood of the infant's ABO and Rh group can be used, provided that the ABO and Rh groups are not involved in fetomaternal incompatibility as judged from studies of maternal and cord samples. An initial pretransfusion specimen from the infant must be typed for ABO and Rh groups (only anti-A and anti-B reagents are required to be used for ABO grouping).[64] Antibody detection testing can be performed using the maternal serum or, alternatively, using the infant's serum (e.g., cord serum) and/or an eluate prepared from the infant's red cells. In addition, when cells selected for transfusion are not group O, the infant's serum or plasma must be tested to demonstrate the absence of anti-A (using A$_1$ cells) and anti-B. This testing must include an antiglobulin phase.[65] It is unnecessary to repeat these pretransfusion tests during any one hospital admission, provided that the infant received only ABO-compatible and Rh-compatible transfusions and had no unexpected antibodies in the serum or plasma.[66] The presence of un-

**Table 12–4. Compatibility Tests for Infants Once per Admission**

*Routine:*
  ABO
  Rh
  Antibody screen
- Using maternal serum *or*
- Using infant's serum, especially when:
  - No maternal specimen available
  - Mother has clinically insignificant antibodies *or*
- Using infant's eluate.

*Additional:*
  IAT using infant serum and A$_1$ and/or B cells
- Cells can be reagent or donor (ie, major crossmatch)
- Must be done if non–group O cells will be transfused
  Antigen typing donor unit
- While infant antibody screen is positive
- Donor units must lack antigen corresponding to antibody

*Every 3 Days*
  Same tests as above when:
- ABO- or Rh-incompatible units are transfused *and/or*
- Unexpected antibodies are demonstrating via antibody screen

expected clinically significant antibodies, including anti-A and anti-B, indicates that cells lacking the corresponding antigen must be selected for transfusion until the antibody is no longer demonstrable in the infant's serum.[67] A crossmatch does not have to be performed in these situations. Table 12–4 summarizes the compatibility tests for infants (less than 4 months old) and how frequently they must be performed.

For both intrauterine and infant (less than 4 months old) transfusions, blood should be as fresh as possible and no older than 7 days to reduce the risk and to increase the benefits of the transfusion. Refer to Chapter 20 for additional information on hemolytic disease of the newborn (HDN).

## Massive Transfusions

When the amount of whole blood or packed cell components infused within 24 hours approaches or exceeds the patient's total blood volume, the compatibility testing procedure may be shortened or eliminated at the discretion of the transfusion service physician following written policy guidelines.[68]

If the patient is known to have an antibody that may be clinically significant, all infused units should be tested and found to lack the offending antigen, if time permits. The antibody in the patient's serum may not be demonstrable because of dilution with large volumes of plasma and other fluids. However, a rapid rise in antibody titer and subsequent destruction of donor red cells may occur if antigen-positive units are infused. The transfusion service physician may decide that it is better to give antigen-untested units than to hold up transfusion waiting for the results of testing. The rationale is that it is important to give the patient a chance to survive and then to treat the immune-mediated anemia induced by massive transfusion of antigen-untested units.

## Specimens with Prolonged Clotting Time

Difficulties may be encountered in testing blood samples from patients who have prolonged clotting times caused by coagulation abnormalities associated with disease or medications. A fibrin clot may form spontaneously when partially clotted serum is added to saline-suspended screening or donor red cells. Complete coagulation of these samples can often be prompted by addition of thrombin. One drop of thrombin, 50 U/mL, to 1 mL of plasma (or the amount of dry thrombin that will adhere to the end of an applicator stick) is usually sufficient to induce clotting.[69] A small amount of protamine sulfate can be added to counteract the effects of heparin in samples of blood collected from patients on this anticoagulant.[70]

## Autologous Transfusion

Autologous transfusion refers to the removal and storage of blood or components from a donor for the donor's own possible use at a later time, usually during or after a surgical procedure. The ABO and Rh groups of the units must be determined by the facility collecting the blood. Tests for unexpected antibodies and tests designed to prevent disease transmission are not required when the blood will be used within the collecting facility.[71] These units must be labeled "For Autologous Use Only."[72]

According to AABB Standards, the pretransfusion testing and identification of the recipient and the blood sample are required and must conform to the protocols mentioned earlier in this chapter. However, tests for unexpected antibodies in the recipient's serum or plasma and a crossmatch test are optional.

## LIMITATIONS OF COMPATIBILITY TESTING PROCEDURES

As mentioned in the introduction to this chapter, no current testing procedure can guarantee the fate of a unit of blood that is to be transfused. Even a compatible crossmatch cannot guarantee that the transfused red cells will survive normally in the recipient. Despite carefully performed in vitro testing, some compatible units will be hemolyzed in the patient. In some cases, even limited survival of donor cells may help to maintain a patient until the patient can begin to produce his or her own cells. Certainly no patient should be denied a transfusion if he or she needs one to survive, and donor cells that appear incompatible by in vitro testing procedures may, in fact, survive quite well in vivo.

In vivo compatibility can be determined using donor red cells labeled with radioactive chromium ($^{51}$Cr) or technetium ($^{99m}$Tc) to measure the likelihood of successful transfusion when standard in vitro testing procedures are inconclusive.[73,74] If a transfusion is needed to save a patient's life and all units are incompatible, and if the $^{51}$Cr studies indicate adequate survival of donor red cells, then transfusion of an in vitro incompatible unit may need to be considered. This decision should be made in consultation with the blood bank medical director and the patient's physician. The blood should be transfused slowly, and the patient should be monitored carefully.[75]

## EFFECTIVE BLOOD UTILIZATION

Many blood bankers are keenly aware of the need to use blood efficiently because of limited blood resources and increasing demands for blood. Technologists observed that there were many surgical procedures—such as dilatation and curettage, and cholecystectomy—for which blood was routinely ordered but rarely used. Blood bankers also pointed out that for many other surgical procedures more units were ordered than used.

The maximum surgical blood order schedule (MSBOS) was developed to promote more efficient utilization of blood. The goal of MSBOS is to establish realistic blood ordering levels for certain procedures. Because variation exists in the surgical requirements of institutions, the standard blood orders should be based on the transfusion pattern of each institution and should be agreed on by the staff surgeons, anesthesiologists, and the blood bank medical director. Refer to Table 12–5 for a sample MSBOS.

Utilization of a type and screen policy is another method to manage blood inventory levels efficiently and to reduce blood banking operating costs.[76–78] With the type and screen methods, the patient's blood sample is completely tested for ABO and Rh groups and unexpected antibodies. The specimen is refrigerated for immediate crossmatching if the need arises. The blood bank must make sure that appropriate donor blood is available in case it is needed. If the patient has blood group alloantibodies, donor blood lacking the corresponding antigens must be available and should be fully crossmatched before surgery or transfusion.

When this type and screen policy is part of the standard operating procedure, and if blood is needed quickly, the blood bank must be prepared to release blood of the same ABO and Rh group as that of the patient and perform the immediate spin (or computer) phase of the crossmatch test before release of the unit, provided that the patient has no unexpected antibodies. Once the blood is issued, both a 37°C incubation and AHG crossmatch are performed using the same tube employed for the immediate spin crossmatch provided the antiglobulin crossmatch is the standard protocol used by the laboratory. If either the 37°C incubation or AHG phase of testing is positive, the patient's physician is notified immediately, and the transfusion of the unit of blood is stopped.

**Table 12–5.** Transfusion Service Guidelines for Elective Surgical Procedures

| Procedure | Units* |
|---|---|
| *General Surgery* | |
| Breast biopsy | T/S |
| Colon resection | 2 |
| Exploratory laparotomy | 2 |
| Gastrectomy | 2 |
| Hernia repair | T/S |
| Laryngectomy | 2 |
| Mastectomy, radical | T/S |
| Pancreatectomy | 4 |
| Splenectomy | 2 |
| Thyroidectomy | T/S |
| *Cardiac-Thoracic* | |
| Aneurysm resection | 6 |
| Coronary artery bypass graft, adults | 4 |
| Coronary artery bypass graft, children | 2 |
| Lobectomy | 2 |
| Lung biopsy | T/S |
| *Vascular* | |
| Aortic bypass with graft | 4 |
| Endarterectomy | T/S |
| Femoral-popliteal bypass with graft | 4 |
| *Orthopedics* | |
| Arthroscopy | T/S |
| Laminectomy | T/S |
| Spinal fusion | 3 |
| Total hip replacement | 3 |
| Total knee replacement | 2 |
| *OB-GYN* | |
| Abdominoperineal repair | T/S |
| Cesarean section | T/S |
| D & C | T/S |
| Hysterectomy, abdominal | T/S |
| Hysterectomy, radical | 2 |
| Labor/delivery, uncomplicated | (Hold) |
| *Urology* | |
| Bladder, transurethral resection | T/S |
| Nephrectomy, radical | 3 |
| Prostatectomy, perineal | 2 |
| Prostatectomy, transurethral | T/S |
| Renal transplant | 2 |

**Source:** From Vengelen-Tyler, V (ed): *Technical Manual.* American Association of Blood Banks, Bethesda, MD, 1996, with permission.
*Numbers may vary with institutional practice.
T/S = Type and antibody screen

## REIDENTIFICATION OF THE PATIENT BEFORE TRANSFUSION

The final link in the chain of events leading to safe transfusion is reestablishment of the identity of the intended recipient and selected donor product. The same careful approach used to identify the patient before collection of samples must be used to verify that the patient is indeed the same person who provided the blood for testing. In addition, the actual product and accompanying record of testing must be verified as relating to the same donor number.

After compatibility testing is completed, two records must be prepared. A statement of compatibility must be retained as part of the patient's permanent medical record if the blood is transfused, and a label or tie tag must be attached to the unit stating the identity of the intended recipient, the results of compatibility testing, and the donor number.[79] This identification must remain on the unit throughout the transfusion.

The original blood request form can be used conveniently to accomplish one or both of these record-keeping requirements. A multipart form is used in some facilities to record the entire history of pretransfusion testing and infusion of the unit. Useful information might include the initials or signature of the phlebotomist taking the sample, the donor numbers, results of compatibility testing, the initials or signature of the technologist performing the testing, and the signatures of the persons who verify the identity of the patient before infusion and who start the infusion. One copy of the form can be placed on the patient's chart after the transfusion is completed and the other returned to the blood bank, if desired, for filing. The last copy of the form might be printed on heavier stock and perforated so that it can be torn off and attached to the unit in the laboratory. The most important feature of this system is that the patient's nameplate impression, rather than a handwritten transcription, identifies all forms used to identify the patient-donor combination.

Other useful systems, mentioned earlier in this chapter, employ numbered strips or other unique coding systems that can be attached to the patient's wristband and to the compatibility form and donor unit. Barcoded identification symbols verified by portable laser scanner devices may be the system of choice in the near future for linking sample, patient, and donor products.

Whatever system is used, the information should be verified at least twice before the infusion of the product actually takes place. A copy of the original blood requisition form, placed on the patient's chart after samples are collected, can be used as the request for release of the units from the blood bank. This allows another check of the nameplate impressions on all forms.

Before blood is taken from the blood bank to the patient treatment area, the following records must be checked: ABO and Rh groupings, clinically significant unexpected antibodies, and adverse reactions to transfusion.[80] In addition, the person releasing and the person accepting the units should verify agreement between the donor numbers and ABO and Rh groups on the compatibility form and on the products themselves. The unit should also be inspected visually for any abnormalities in appearance indicating contamination. If any abnormality is seen, the unit should not be issued unless specifically authorized by the medical director.[81]

Before transfusion is initiated, a reliable professional (and preferably two professionals) must once again verify identity of the patient and donor products. A system of positive patient identification by comparison of wristband identification and compatibility forms must be followed strictly. This is the most critical check and yet the most fallible, because the transfusion may take place in the operating suite or emergency room, where the person responsible for identification may be involved with many other duties as well.

If a unit is returned to the blood bank for any reason, within the specified time frame for that laboratory, it should not be reissued if the container closure was opened or if the unit was allowed to warm above 10°C or to cool below 1°C.[82]

## THE FUTURE OF COMPATIBILITY TESTING

Modern transfusion medicine is a rapidly progressing science. Technological advances will certainly affect the future practice of blood banking.

Developments include the use of red cell substitutes such as modified hemoglobin solutions, currently under investigation.[83,84] These substitutes can provide oxygen-carrying capacity and, because they are biologically inert and nonimmunogenic, can be administered with no requirements for crossmatching. They have been used in coronary angioplasty procedures[85] and could be used instantly at the scene of an accident or in the emergency room.[86] However, further research is needed to develop viable substitutes for blood products, and indications are that a range of products targeted at specific clinical indications, rather than one generic product, will emerge from this research.

Progress in the knowledge of blood group antigen structure may result in the biochemical modification of all non-O blood groups to a phenotypically universal donor blood.[87,88] This could possibly solve the problem of disproportions in certain blood group supplies.

Automation with pretransfusion testing instruments, such as continuous-flow and batch analyzers, has streamlined compatibility testing, especially in large blood centers. Two of the most successful approaches have used microplates to perform either liquid agglutination tests or solid-phase red blood cell adherence tests. These methods provide efficient and economic compatibility tests for processing large numbers of donor specimens.[89] Similar innovations are emerging to streamline blood banking services in hospital transfusion services.

The technology of galvanic testing is in the development stage. With a galvanic biosensor, the energy exploited in an antigen-antibody reaction is measured.[90] This electrochemical procedure could be applied to all immunohematologic tests dependent on antigen-antibody binding, and subsequently to automation.

European, Canadian, and some U.S. and Asian blood banks use a gel test for performing the direct and indirect antiglobulin tests, including the crossmatch. The gel test is sensitive for both antigen testing and antibody detection, is reproducible, and has the potential to be converted to automation.[91-94]

Dipstick tests for determining ABO blood groups are a step in the direction of streamlining services for the hospital transfusion service. These tests are based on the principles of dot immunobinding assays. Studies indicate that their sensitivity and specificity equal those of conventional agglutination tests, and they are fast, stable, inexpensive, and easy to interpret.[95,96]

Researchers from England have identified a dry plate method of ABO and Rh grouping for use in the field or at the patient's bedside. This method, in which monoclonal blood grouping antibodies are dried in a microplate and rehydrated before use, is 99.8 percent accurate and may best be used in developing countries lacking effective refrigeration and in situations where point-of-care testing is needed (e.g., trauma sites).[97]

Preparing for clinical care in space, National Aeronautics and Space Administration (NASA) scientists showed that ABO and Coombs-sensitized standard blood grouping tests can be performed under microgravity. This was done using a closed self-operating system which automatically performed the tests and fixed the results onto filter paper for analysis on earth. Agglutinates were smaller than usual; however, reaction endpoints were clear.[98] While these researchers noted that additional experiments in space were needed to confirm and to quantify their results, these preliminary findings indicate yet another method to perform compatibility testing that is "out of this world."

Perhaps, as information technology continues to grow at the current rate, all aspects of patient care, including compatibility testing, may be computerized. In addition to performing an electronic crossmatch, future computer systems will include electronic identification of the patient, automated testing, and electronic transfer of data. The success of this system lies on interfacing automated testing instruments with bar-code readers and a laboratory computer. The advantages of the system include the issue of blood products that are as safe as, if not safer than, current methods of compatibility testing, and reduction of costs and workload.

Our knowledge of compatibility testing is in a dynamic state, and we look forward to continuing developments in technical procedures to streamline and to safeguard transfusion practice. The challenge of modern blood banking will be to merge new technology with the assurance of beneficial results and positive outcomes for the patient.

## SUMMARY CHART: IMPORTANT POINTS TO REMEMBER (MT/MLT)

**Collection and Preparation of Sample**
- Most fatal transfusion reactions are caused by clerical errors.
- Positive patient identification is very critical.
- Samples and forms must contain patient's full name and unique identity number.
- Writing must be legible and indelible.
- Date of collection must be written on sample.
- Sample must be collected within 3 days of scheduled transfusion.
- Person who drew specimen and confirmed patient identity must sign it.

**Compatibility Testing**
- Confirm blood type of donor.
- Check patient records for results of previous tests.
- Perform ABO grouping, Rh typing, and antibody screening on patient.
- Select donor unit based on ABO group and Rh type of patient; further consider presence of antibodies in patient.
- Perform immediate spin or antiglobulin crossmatch, based on current or historical serologic results.
- Electronic crossmatch can replace immediate spin crossmatch when two blood types on file for the patient.
- Positive results in the crossmatch may be caused by incorrect ABO grouping of patient or donor, alloantibody or autoantibody in patient reacting

with the corresponding antigen on the donor red cells, donor having a positive DAT, abnormalities in patient serum, or contaminants in test system.

**Compatibility Testing in Special Circumstances**
- Emergencies
  —May have to select uncrossmatched, group O, Rh negative
  —May want to give uncrossmatched, group O, Rh positive, if male patient or female patient beyond childbearing years
  —May be able to provide type specific, uncrossmatched blood
- Plasma products units
  —No compatibility testing required
- Transfusion to fetus
  —Compatibility testing performed using mother's sample
  —Donor unit must lack antigen against maternal antibody
  —Group O Rh-negative donor selected when fetal type is unknown or when type is known but is not compatible with mother's type
- Transfusion to infant
  —Maternal sample can be used for compatibility testing.
  —Initial sample from infant typed for ABO (front type) and Rh.
  —Donor unit selected should be compatible with both mother and baby.

## REVIEW QUESTIONS

1. Compatibility testing does which of the following?
   A. Proves that the donor's plasma is free of all irregular antibodies
   B. Detects most irregular antibodies on the donor's red cells that are reactive with patient's serum
   C. Detects most errors in the ABO groupings
   D. Ensures complete safety of the transfusion

2. Which of the following is not true of rouleaux formation?
   A. It is a stacking of red cells to form aggregates.
   B. It can usually be dispersed by adding saline.
   C. It occurs in conditions in which the albumin-globulin serum protein balance is disturbed.
   D. It can occur in normal blood because of the presence of multiple antibodies.

3. What type of blood should be given in an emergency transfusion when there is no time to type the recipient's sample?
   A. O $Rh_0$ (D)-negative, whole blood

B. O $Rh_0$ (D)-positive, whole blood
C. O $Rh_0$ (D)-positive, packed cells
D. O $Rh_0$ (D)-negative, packed cells

4. A patient developed an anti-$Jk^a$ antibody 5 years ago. The antibody screen is negative now. To obtain suitable blood for transfusion, what is the best procedure?
   A. Type the patient for the $Jk^a$ antigen as an added part to the crossmatch procedure.
   B. Crossmatch donors with the patient's serum and release the compatible units for transfusion to the patient.
   C. Type the donor units for the $Jk^a$ antigen and crossmatch the $Jk^a$ negative units for the patient.
   D. Crossmatch the patient with O Rh-negative, "low titer" donor units, because the patient has developed an anti-$Jk^a$ antibody and is a prime candidate to develop many other blood group antibodies.

5. A 26-year-old B $Rh_0$(D)-negative female patient requires a transfusion. No B $Rh_0$(D)-negative donor

units are available. Which of the following should be chosen for transfusion?

A. B $Rh_0(D)$-positive red cells
B. O $Rh_0(D)$-negative red cells
C. AB $Rh_0(D)$-negative red cells
D. A $Rh_0(D)$-negative red cells

6. If all the crossmatches and screening cells are positive, but the auto-control is negative, the cause could be which one or two of the following?
   a. a mixture of antibodies
   b. an antibody to a high-frequency antigen
   c. an antibody to a low-frequency antigen

   A. a and c
   B. a, b, and c
   C. c only
   D. a and b only

7. In crossmatching 5 units of packed cells on a patient, 4 units were compatible, and both the auto-control and antibody screen were negative. One unit, however, was weakly incompatible on the major side of the crossmatch at the antihuman globulin phase. What is the most probable explanation for this problem?
   A. A high-frequency antigen-antibody reaction occurred.
   B. The patient had a positive DAT.
   C. The donor unit had a positive DAT.
   D. A caprylate antibody is suspected.

8. What percentage of Rh-negative individuals would be expected to develop anti-D after transfusion with 1 unit of Rh-positive blood?
   A. 0 to 25 percent
   B. 26 to 50 percent
   C. 51 to 75 percent
   D. 76 to 85 percent

9. Predict compatibility or incompatibility for the following situation. (Assume that the patient has a negative antibody screen and auto-control.)

   |         | Group | $Rh_0(D)$ |
   |---------|-------|-----------|
   | Patient | B     | positive  |
   | Donor   | O     | positive  |

   A. Compatible major side crossmatch
   B. Compatible minor side crossmatch
   C. Incompatible major side crossmatch
   D. Not enough information to predict

10. Blood donor and recipient samples used in crossmatching must be stored for a minimum of how many days following transfusion?
    A. 2
    B. 5
    C. 7
    D. 10

11. Which of the following is *true* regarding compatibility testing for the infant less than 4 months old?
    A. A direct antiglobulin test is required.
    B. A crossmatch is not needed when unexpected antibodies are present.

C. Maternal serum cannot be used for antibody detection.
D. To determine the infant's ABO group, red cells must be tested with reagent anti-A, anti-B, and anti-A,B.

## ANSWERS TO REVIEW QUESTIONS

1. C (p 285)
2. D (p 287)
3. D (p 288)
4. C (p 288, Table 12–3)
5. B (p 284, Table 12–2)
6. D (p 288, Table 12–3)
7. C (p 287)
8. D (p 284)
9. A (p 286)
10. C (p 281)
11. B (p 289, Table 12–4)

## REFERENCES

1. Wiener, AS, and Peters, HR: Hemolytic reactions following transfusions of blood of the homologous group, with three cases in which the same agglutinogen was responsible. Ann Intern Med 13:2304, 1940.
2. Sazama, K: Analysis of causes of blood transfusion fatalities. ASCP Teleconference. December 3, 1992.
3. Standards for Blood Banks and Transfusion Services, ed 17. American Association of Blood Banks, Bethesda, MD, 1993, p 31, I1.000.
4. Wenz, B, and Burns, ER: Improvement in transfusion safety using a new blood unit and patient identification system as part of safe transfusion practice. Transfusion 31:401, 1991.
5. Standards for Blood Banks and Transfusion Services, op cit, p 31, I2.000.
6. Ibid, p 31–32, I4.000.
7. Pittiglio, DH (ed): Modern Blood Banking and Transfusion Practices. FA Davis, Philadelphia, 1983, p 266.
8. Standards for Blood Banks and Transfusion Services, op cit, p 36, J2.OOO.
9. Code of Federal Regulations (CFR), Title 21, Food and Drugs. Office of the Federal Register, National Archives and Records Service, General Services Administration, revised April 1, 1996, Part 610, section 40, and Part 640, section 5.
10. Standards for Blood Banks and Transfusion Services, op cit, p 17, E1.000, E2.000, E5.000.
11. Ibid, p 17.
12. Ibid, p 31, I3000.
13. Ibid, p 48, M1.300.
14. Ibid, p 32, G2.000.
15. White, WB, Issitt, CH, and McGuire, D: Evaluation of the use of albumin controls in Rh typing. Transfusion 14:67, 1974.
16. Standards for Blood Banks and Transfusion Services, op cit, p 32, I4.000.
17. Garratty, G: Mechanisms of immune red cell destruction, and red cell compatibility testing. Hum Pathol 14:204–212, 1983.
18. Giblett, ER: Blood group alloantibodies: An assessment to some laboratory practices. Transfusion 17:299, 1977.
19. Spielmann, W, and Seidl, S: Prevalence of irregular red cell anti-

bodies and their significance in blood transfusion and antenatal care. Vox Sang 26:551, 1974.

20. Standards for Blood Banks and Transfusion Services, op cit, p 32, I4.000.

21. Engelfriet, CP, and Giles, CM: Working party on the standardization of antiglobulin reagents of the expert panel of serology. Vox Sang 38:178, 1980.

22. Petz, LD, and Garratty, G: Antiglobulin sera—past, present and future. Transfusion 18:257, 1978.

23. Wright, MS, and Issitt, PD: Anticomplement and the antiglobulin test. Transfusion 19:688, 1979.

24. Standards for Blood Banks and Transfusion Services, op cit, p 32, I4.000.

25. Beattie, KM: Control of the antigen-antibody ratio in antibody detection and compatibility test. Transfusion 20:277, 1980.

26. Hughes-Jones, NC, et al: Optimal conditions for detecting blood group antibodies by the antiglobulin test. In Pittiglio, DH (ed): Modern Blood Banking and Transfusion Practices. FA Davis, Philadelphia, 1983, p 252.

27. Issitt, PD, and Issitt, CH: Applied Blood Group Serology, ed 2. Spectra Biologicals, Oxnard, CA, 1975, p 41.

28. Steane, EA: The interaction of antibodies with red cell surface antigens: Kinetics, noncovalent bonding and hemagglutination. In Dawson, RD (ed): Blood Bank Immunology. American Association of Blood Banks, Washington, DC, 1977, pp 61–63.

29. Stroup, M, and MacIlroy, M: Evaluation of the albumin antiglobulin technic in antibody detection. Transfusion 5:184, 1965.

30. Reckel, RP, and Harris, J: The unique characteristics of covalently polymerized bovine serum albumin solutions when used as antibody detection media. Transfusion 18:397, 1978.

31. Moulds, JJ: Multiple antibodies and antibodies to high incidence blood group factors. In Dawson, RB (ed): Troubleshooting the Crossmatch. American Association of Blood Banks, Washington, DC, 1977, pp 67–84.

32. McKeever, BG: Antibody screening and identification. In Treacy, M (ed): Pre-Transfusion Testing for the '80s. American Association of Blood Banks, Washington, DC, 1980, pp 409–450.

33. Issitt, PD: On the incidence of second antibody populations in the sera of women who have developed anti-Rh antibodies. Transfusion 5:355, 1965.

34. Issitt, PD, et al: Three examples of Rh-positive good responders to blood group antigens. Transfusion 13:316, 1972.

35. Mollison, PL: Blood Transfusion in Clinical Medicine, ed 7. Blackwell Scientific, Oxford, 1983, p 353.

36. Vengelen-Tyler, V (ed): Technical Manual, ed 12. American Association of Blood Banks, Bethesda, MD, 1996, p 248.

37. Mollison, PF: Factors determining the relative clinical importance of different blood group antibodies. Br Med Bull 15:92, 1959.

38. Giblett, ER: Blood group alloantibodies: An assessment of some laboratory practices. Transfusion 17:299, 1977.

39. Grove-Rasmussen, M: Routine compatibility testing: Standards of the AABB as applied to compatibility tests. Transfusion 4:200, 1964.

40. Standards for Blood Banks and Transfusion Services, op cit, p 33, I5.000.

41. Weisz-Carrington, P: Principles of Clinical Immunohematology. Year Book Medical, Chicago, 1986, p 212.

42. Pittiglio, DH (ed): Modern Blood Banking and Transfusion Practices, op cit, p 266.

43. Henry, JB: Type and screen. In Polesky, HF, and Walker, RH (eds): Safety in Transfusion Practices: CAP Conference, Aspen, 1980. College of American Pathologists, Skokie, IL, 1982, p 191.

44. Walker, RH: On the safety of the abbreviated crossmatch. In Polesky, HF, and Walker, RH (eds): Safety in Transfusion Practices; CAP Conference, Aspen, 1980. College of American Pathologists, Skokie, IL, 1982, p 75.

45. Shulman, IA, et al: Experience with the routine use of an abbreviated crossmatch. Am J Clin Path 82:178–181, 1984.

46. Dodsworth, H, and Dudley, HAF: Increased efficiency of transfusion practice in routine surgery using pre-operative antibody screening and selective ordering with an abbreviated crossmatch. Br J Surg 72:102–104, 1985.

47. Garratty, G: Abbreviated pretransfusion testing (editorial). Transfusion 26:217–219, 1986.

48. Shulman, IA, et al: Experience with a cost-effective crossmatch protocol. JAMA 254:93–95, 1985.

49. Judd, WJ: Are there better ways than the crossmatch to demonstrate ABO incompatibility? (editorial) Transfusion 31:192, 1991.

50. Shulman, IA, and Calderon, C: Effect of delayed centrifugation or reading on the detection of ABO incompatibility by the immediate-spin crossmatch. Transfusion 31:197, 1991.

51. Riccardi, D, et al: Risk of ABO and non-ABO incompatibility by using type and screen and electronic crossmatch (abstract). Transfusion 31:60S, 1991.

52. Butch, SH, et al: The computer crossmatch (abstract). Transfusion 32:5S, 1992.

53. Standards for Blood Banks and Transfusion Services, op cit p 33, I5.000.

54. Slater, JL, et al: Evaluation of the polyethylene glycol-indirect antiglobulin test for routine compatibility testing. Transfusion 29:686, 1989.

55. Mentz, PD, and Anderson, G: Comparison of a manual hexadimethrine bromide-antiglobulin test with saline and albumin-antiglobulin tests for pretransfusion testing. Transfusion 27:134–137, 1987.

56. Steane, EA, et al: A proposal for compatibility testing incorporating the manual hexadimethrine bromide (polybrene) test. Transfusion 25:540–544, 1985.

57. Mentz, PD, and Anderson, G: Comparison of a manual hexadimethrine bromide-antiglobulin test with saline and albumin-antiglobulin tests for pretransfusion testing. Transfusion 27:134–137, 1987.

58. Perkins, JT, et al: The relative utility of the autologous control and the antiglobulin test phase of the crossmatch. Transfusion 30:503, 1990.

59. CFR, op cit, Part 606, section 160.

60. Green, TS: Rouleaux and autoantibodies (or things that go bump in the night). In Treacy, M (ed): Pre-Transfusion Testing for the 80s. American Association of Blood Banks, Washington, DC, 1980, p 93.

61. Bartholomew, JR, et al: A prospective study of the effects of dextran administration on compatibility testing. Transfusion 26:431–433, 1986.

62. Golde, DW, et al: Serum agglutinins to commercially prepared albumin. In Weisz-Carrington, P: Principles of Clinical Immunohematology. Year Book Medical, Chicago, 1986, p 214.

63. CFR, op cit, Part 606, section 160.

64. Standards for Blood Banks and Transfusion Services, op cit, p 35, I8.000.

65. Ibid.

66. Ibid.

67. Ibid.

68. Ibid, p 34, I7.000.

69. Vengelen-Tyler, V (ed): Technical Manual. American Association of Blood Banks, Bethesda, MD, 1996.

70. Ibid.

71. Standards for Blood Banks and Transfusion Services, op cit, p 44, L1.300.

72. Ibid, p 44, L1.400.

73. Mollison, PL: Blood Transfusion in Clinical Medicine, op cit, pp 606–608.

74. Holt, JT, et al: A technetium-99m red cell survival technique for in vivo compatibility testing. Transfusion 23:148–151, 1983.

75. Garratty, G: Mechanisms of immune red cell destruction and red cell compatibility testing. Hum Pathol 3:211, 1983.

76. Shulman, IA, et al: Experience with a cost-effective crossmatch protocol. JAMA 254:93–95, 1985.

77. Davis, SP, et al: Maximizing the benefits of type and screen by continued surveillance of transfusion practice. Am J Med Technol 49:579–582, 1983.

78. Issitt, PD: Applied Blood Group Serology, ed 3. Montgomery Scientific, Miami, 1985, pp 489–492.

79. Standards for Blood Banks and Transfusion Services, op cit, p 36, J1.000.

80. Ibid.

81. Ibid.
82. Ibid.
83. Rudowski, W: Blood Transfusion: Yesterday, Today, and Tomorrow. World J Surg 11:86–93, 1987.
84. Allen, RW, et al: Advances in the production of blood cell substitutes with alternate technologies. In Walls, CH, and McCarthy, LJ (eds): New Frontiers in Blood Banking. American Association of Blood Banks, Arlington, VA, 1986, p 21.
85. Ibid.
86. Rudowski, op cit, pp 88–89.
87. Greenwalt, TJ: Research in transfusion medicine. In Wallis, C, and Simon, TL (eds): Educational Progress in Transfusion Medicine. American Association of Blood Banks, Arlington, VA 1985, pp 55–69.
88. Lenny, LL, et al. Multiple-unit and second transfusions of red cells enzymatically converted from group B to group O: Report on the end of Phase 1 trials. Transfusion 35:899–902, 1995.
89. Plapp, V: New techniques for compatibility testing. Arch Pathol Lab Med 113(3):262–69, March, 1989.
90. Moulds, JJ: Galvanic testing. In Levitt, JS, and Brecher, ME (eds): Emerging Trends in Technology. American Association of Blood Banks, Bethesda, MD, 1992, p 1.
91. LaPierre, Y, et al: The gel test: A new way to detect red cell antigen-antibody reactions. Transfusion 30:109, 1990.
92. Weiland, D: The gel technology: A new approach to blood group serology. In Levitt, JS, and Brecher, ME (eds): Emerging Trends in Technology. American Association of Blood Banks, Bethesda, MD, 1992, pp 3–13.
93. South, SF: Antibody screening and direct antiglobulin testing using BioVue column agglutination technology versus standard tube tests. Immunohematology 9(3):78–80, 1993.
94. Chan, A, et al: The impact of a gel system on routine work in a general hospital blood bank. Immunohematology 12(1): 30–32, 1996.
95. Plapp, FV, et al: Dipsticks for determining ABO blood groups. Lancet i(8496):1465, 1986.
96. Plapp, 1989, op cit.
97. Blakely, D, et al: Dry instant blood typing plate for bedside use. Lancet 336:854, 1990.
98. Morehead, RT, et al: Erythrocyte agglutination in microgravity. Aviat Space Environ Med 60:235, 1989.

## PREPARATION OF WASHED "DRY" BUTTON OF RED CELLS FOR SEROLOGIC TESTS

1. Transfer a small amount of red cells using an applicator stick into a 10- × 75-mm test tube filled with saline. Tube should be prelabeled to identify contents.
2. Centrifuge at high speed until red cells are collected into a tight button at the bottom of the tube.
3. Decant saline by quick inversion of the tube over a receptacle. Flick last drop of saline from cells by giving tube a quick shake while it is still in inverted position. (Reduce aerosol production by using engineering and/or work practice controls.)
4. Add serum directly to "dry" button of cells. Method can be used for antibody screening or identification procedures, compatibility testing, and cell typing using a tube technique.

# PROCEDURAL APPENDIX 2

## MODEL ONE-TUBE-PER-DONOR-UNIT COMPATIBILITY TESTING PROCEDURE

NOTE: No minor side compatibility test is performed.

1. Into an appropriately labeled, 10- $\times$ 75-mm test tube, dispense 1 drop of a washed, 2 to 5 percent suspension of donor red cells. (Alternatively, prepare a washed "dry" button of donor red cells, using the technique in Procedural Appendix 1.)
2. Add 2 or 3 drops of serum to the tube to achieve an approximate 2:1 ratio of serum to red cell. (Droppers used to dispense red cells and serum should be of equivalent size.)
3. Centrifuge at a speed and for a time that have been previously shown to give clear-cut differentiation between positive and negative results (15 seconds in a Serofuge is usually adequate).
4. Observe supernatant for hemolysis that must be considered indicative of an antigen-antibody interaction. Resuspend cell button by *gentle* manipulation of the tube. Grade all positive results. Record observations. STOP HERE FOR IMMEDIATE SPIN CROSS-MATCH.
5. Add 2 drops of 22 percent bovine albumin (or other enhancement medium, such as LISS) to the tube (the enhancement medium may be omitted, if desired). Mix and incubate for 30 minutes at 37°C. Note: If LISS is added to tests at this stage in place of albumin, decrease incubation time to 10 minutes and refer to manufacturer's directions for additional directions.
6. Centrifuge, as above, observe supernatant, resuspend cells, and record results.
7. Wash 3 to 4 times using an automated instrument or manual washing technique. Decant saline completely from last wash.
8. Add 1 to 2 drops of antiglobulin serum to tube. (Follow manufacturer's directions for use of reagent selected.) Centrifuge, resuspend cells, and record results.
9. Add 1 drop IgG-sensitized red cells to each negative test. Centrifuge and examine. Test must be *positive*, or results of procedure are invalid and test must be repeated.

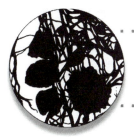

# CHAPTER **13**

# ORIENTATION TO THE ROUTINE BLOOD BANK LABORATORY

Judith Ann Sullivan, MGA, BS, MT(ASCP)SBB

## OBJECTIVES

*On completion of this chapter, the learner should be able to:*

1  Describe the various functional areas of a blood bank.

2  Specify the tests that are performed on a unit of blood during donor processing.

3  Describe the criteria that must be met before a blood product can be labeled.

4  List the components that can be prepared from a unit of whole blood.

5  Compare the methods used for ABO and Rh testing and antibody screening on donor samples versus patient samples.

6  Discuss the tests performed by the reference section of the blood bank laboratory.

## INTRODUCTION

The chapters in this book have, up to this point, been organized into individual units dealing with specific topics in immunohematology. However, it is important to realize that none of these topics exists in a vacuum. To be able to translate the theory of immunohematology into the reality of the laboratory, it is helpful to see how these various pieces interrelate in the actual setting of a blood bank.

To the first-time visitor, a blood bank can be a very confusing and intimidating place. The pressured pace, unfamiliar equipment, and strange and abbreviated terminology can make even those with a theoretic knowledge of immunohematology feel like strangers in a strange land. However, all blood banks do share common characteristics that can serve as points of orientation. Procedures may vary from blood bank to blood bank, reflecting a response to workload, services, and patient population, but all follow requirements and guidelines established by the Food and Drug Administration (FDA) in its *Code of Federal Regulations*,[1] by the American Association of Blood Banks (AABB) in its *Standards for Blood Banks and Transfusion Services*,[2] and by the provisions of the Clinical Laboratories Improvement Act of 1988 (CLIA '88).

The purpose of this chapter is to serve as a tour through the typical blood bank and to describe the various sections within the department and the procedures that are performed there. The intent is to help the reader better understand how the theory learned in this book is applied practically in the laboratory in order to achieve the goals of high-quality patient care and safe transfusion practice.

## ORGANIZATION

For ease of discussion, it is assumed that the blood bank is divided into distinct areas, each with its own

**Table 13–1.** Blood Bank Areas and Functions

| Area | Functions |
|------|-----------|
| Component preparation and storage | ■ Separation of whole blood into packed red blood cells, plasma, platelets, and cryoprecipitate<br>■ Storage of blood products at appropriate temperatures<br>■ Apheresis procedures |
| Donor processing | ■ Donor units tested for:<br> ● ABO and Rh<br> ● Antibody screen<br> ● Serologic test for syphilis<br> ● ALT<br> ● Transfusion-transmitted viruses |
| Main laboratory | ■ Patient samples tested for:<br> ● ABO and Rh<br> ● Antibody screen<br> ● Crossmatch<br> ● DAT<br> ● Prenatal evaluation<br> ● Postpartum evaluation<br> ● Cord blood studies<br>■ Issue of blood products |
| Reference laboratory | ■ Resolution of:<br> ● ABO and Rh discrepancies<br> ● Antibody identification<br> ● Positive DAT<br> ● Warm autoantibodies<br> ● Cold autoantibodies<br> ● Transfusion reaction |

purpose and function (Table 13–1). In reality, with the exception of very large hospitals, these areas are not physically separated but overlap within the overall structure of the laboratory. These areas include the following:

1. **Component Preparation and Storage.** In this area, units of whole blood are separated into their various components and stored under conditions that ensure their optimum viability.
2. **Donor Processing.** Here, the testing that is required to determine the suitability of a blood product for transfusion is performed.
3. **Main Laboratory.** This is the heart of the blood bank, where patient samples are received, testing is performed, and blood and blood components are issued for transfusion.
4. **Reference Laboratory.** Any discrepancies in testing are resolved here.

## COMPONENT PREPARATION AND STORAGE

Depending on their needs, hospitals may choose to collect and process blood components internally, or they may choose to receive blood components collected and processed at outside facilities. Each of these means of obtaining blood products places its own set of demands on blood bank personnel.

## Blood Banks with Collection Facilities

Blood banks that collect their own units of whole blood can use their blood resources more efficiently by separating them into a variety of components, including packed red blood cells, plasma, platelets, and cryoprecipitate (see Chapter 10).

To maximize the number of components derived from 1 unit of blood, processing must occur within 6 to 8 hours of collection, depending on the anticoagulant used. Within this period, the blood can be centrifuged to pack the red blood cells using large floor-model temperature-controlled centrifuges, and the plasma can be expressed and frozen. This is the process by which packed red blood cells and fresh frozen plasma are made. If the unit of blood is maintained at room temperature throughout this process and the appropriate centrifugation times and speeds are observed, a platelet concentrate can also be derived from the expressed plasma before it is frozen (Fig. 13–1). In addition, through a controlled thawing process, the frozen plasma can be further manipulated to yield cryoprecipitate.

Some blood components may also be prepared through a procedure known as apheresis. In apheresis, a donor's blood is removed in a sterile manner through tubing connected to an automated machine that then processes the blood, removes the desired component (platelets, plasma, or white blood cells), and returns the remainder of the components back to the donor via another set of connected tubing (Fig. 13–2). High concentrations of specific components can be removed in this way with minimal removal of red cells (see Chapter 17).

## Blood Banks without Collection Facilities

Blood banks that depend on an outside source for their blood supplies usually receive their products already in component form. However, situations do arise in which products must be modified (Fig. 13–3). For

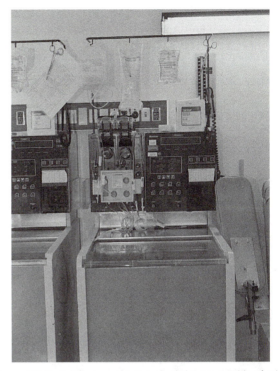

**Figure 13–2.** Apheresis machines such as this are capable of selectively removing a blood component from a donor and returning the remaining components to the donor's circulation. (Courtesy National Institutes of Health, Bethesda, MD.)

```
WHOLE BLOOD -------➤ PACKED RED CELLS

PACKED RED CELLS -------➤ WASHED RED CELLS

RANDOM DONOR PLATELETS -------➤ POOLED PLATELETS

CRYOPRECIPITATE ---➤ THAW -------➤ POOLED CRYOPRECIPITATE

FROZEN RED CELLS ---➤ THAW -------➤ DEGLYCEROLYZED RED CELLS
```

**Figure 13–3.** Additional modifications that blood banks without collection facilities can make to various blood components.

example, a unit received as whole blood may be needed as packed red blood cells. Often, this procedure is as simple as allowing the unit to rest undisturbed until the red cells have settled and then removing the supernatant plasma. However, when time is of the essence, the procedure may be accelerated through centrifugation as previously described.

In some clinical situations, washed red blood cells may be the product of choice for transfusion therapy. Automated cell washers are used to prepare this product. A unit of blood is introduced into a sterile disposable bowl that has tubing connected to a normal saline solution. A portion of this saline is added to the bowl, the cells and saline are mixed, the mixture is centrifuged, and the supernatant is removed through waste tubing. Multiple washes can be performed in this manner.

Blood components such as platelet concentrates and cryoprecipitate may be received as individual units but

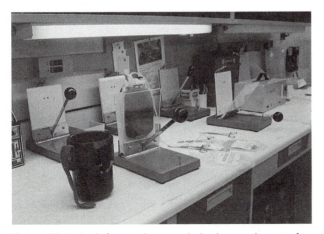

**Figure 13–1.** Fresh frozen plasma and platelets can be manufactured from units of whole blood within 6 to 8 hours of collection.

are more easily administered if pooled before infusion. Such product manipulation is a common occurrence in most blood banks.

If freezers capable of maintaining temperatures at or below −65°C are available, blood banks may choose to freeze rare or autologous units in 40 percent glycerol for long-term storage. The same automated cell washers just mentioned for washing cells can be used to remove the glycerol from these units before transfusion by adding increasingly diluted concentrations of saline to the thawed cells during the procedure (Fig. 13–4).

Regardless of the method used to obtain blood and blood components, all blood banks must follow certain requirements in the storage of their blood products. Therefore, the following equipment is common to most blood banks:

1. Refrigerators maintained at 1 to 6°C for the storage of packed red blood cells and whole blood
2. Freezers maintained at −18°C or lower for the storage of fresh frozen plasma and cryoprecipitate
3. Freezers maintained at −65°C or lower for the storage of red blood cells frozen in 40 percent glycerol
4. Platelet rotators that provide constant gentle agitation at room temperature for the storage of platelet concentrates (Fig. 13–5).

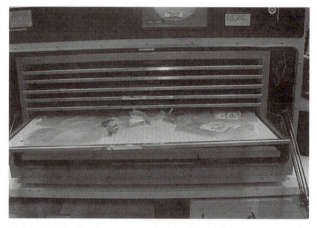

**Figure 13–5.** Platelet rotators provide the conditions necessary for optimum platelet survival. (Courtesy National Institutes of Health, Bethesda, MD.)

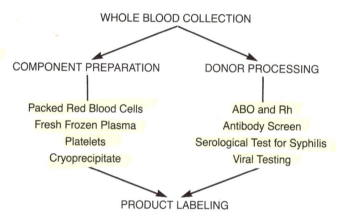

**Figure 13–6.** Processing of whole blood units from collection to labeling. Note that component preparation and donor processing may occur concurrently.

## DONOR PROCESSING

Before a unit of blood can be placed into the general inventory (rendering it available to be used for crossmatching purposes), testing must be performed to determine its suitability for transfusion. This is the responsibility of the donor processing area (Fig. 13–6). Blood banks that collect their own units of blood are required to perform extensive testing to determine the suitability of each of these units. These tests must be performed at each donation regardless of the number of times a donor has previously donated. A separate tube of blood is collected from the donor at the time of donation for this purpose. Required tests include ABO and Rh testing, antibody screen, serologic test for syphilis (STS), and viral testing.

### ABO and Rh testing

This involves forward grouping with anti-A and anti-B, reverse grouping with $A_1$ and B cells, and Rh

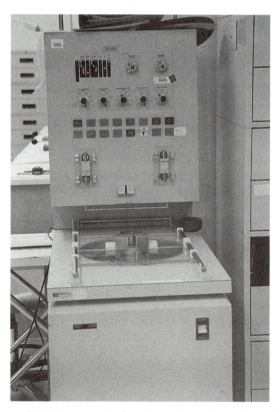

**Figure 13–4.** Automated cell washers such as this may be used to prepare washed red cells or deglycerolize frozen red cells. (Courtesy National Institutes of Health, Bethesda, MD.)

typing with anti-D (including a test to detect weak D when indicated). Monoclonal reagents used for ABO typing that have demonstrated ability to detect weak subgroups of A have streamlined testing, eliminating the need for anti-A,B in the forward group and $A_2$ cells in the reverse group test[3] (see Chapter 5). Anti-D reagents that are blends of monoclonal and polyclonal antibodies have streamlined Rh typing because of their increased sensitivity in detecting D antigens on red cells by immediate spin tests, thereby decreasing the number of tests for weak D that must be performed, and by their lower protein concentrations that make them less prone to false-positive reactions (see Chapter 6).

The ABO and Rh results of the current donation are compared with the results from any previous donations. Any discrepancies must be resolved before the blood components are labeled.

## Antibody Screen

Donor units must be screened in such a way as to detect clinically significant antibodies, because destruction of patient red cells may occur if a large amount of plasma containing a high-titered clinically significant antibody is transfused to a patient whose cells contain the corresponding antigen (see Chapter 10). Some blood banks choose a pooled screening cell for donor antibody detection. This reagent is a pool of two donors chosen so that, between the two, all commonly encountered antigens are expressed. Although not adequately sensitive for patient antibody screens, this pooled screening cell is acceptable for detecting donor antibodies that may cause clinical problems. All units that are identified as containing clinically significant antibodies must be transfused as packed cells, and all plasma-containing components must be discarded or used only for reagent or research purposes.

## Serologic Test for Syphilis (STS)

Blood bankers may choose to perform this test themselves or may send it to another hospital laboratory for completion (see Chapter 10 for further details).

## Viral Testing

Viral testing includes detection of hepatitis B surface antigen (HbsAg) and human immunodeficiency virus, type 1 antigen (HIV-1-Ag), antibodies to hepatitis B core antigen (anti-HBc), human immunodeficiency virus, types 1 and 2 (anti-HIV-1 and anti-HIV-2), human T-cell lymphotropic virus (anti-HTLV), hepatitis C virus (anti-HCV), and measurement of alanine aminotransferase (ALT). All these tests are required by AABB Standards with the exception of ALT and may be performed in a laboratory other than that of the blood bank (see Chapter 19). This list has grown in length over the past 10 years, and as tests are developed to detect additional viral agents that can be transmitted

through blood products, the number of viral tests that must be performed on donor blood will continue to increase.

## Product Labeling

Labeling of blood products may occur only after a careful review of all test results shows the unit to be suitable for transfusion. Suitability requirements include:

1. No discrepancies in the ABO and Rh testing
2. Absence of detectable antibodies in plasma-containing components
3. Nonreactive STS and viral testing
4. ALT values within established limits

When the established criteria are met, the red cells and any other components are labeled with the appropriate ABO, Rh, and expiration date, and the products are stored at their proper temperatures (Fig. 13–7).

It is important to note that the requirements for processing autologous units differ from those just described (see Chapter 10 for additional information).

Units received from an outside source have already undergone the aforementioned required testing and have been deemed suitable for transfusion by the shipping facility. However, because of the serious consequences of transfusing ABO-incompatible blood, the blood bank to which this blood is shipped is required to reconfirm the ABO of each red cell–containing product received. As a cost containment measure, many blood banks confirm group O units using a commercially available mixture of monoclonal anti-A and anti-B in a single reagent and confirm other blood groups using separate anti-A and anti-B reagents. Because of the potential sensitization that may occur if Rh-positive blood is transfused to an Rh-negative patient, the Rh type of all Rh-*negative* units must be reconfirmed. Because no harm will be done if an Rh-negative unit incorrectly labeled as Rh-positive is transfused to an Rh-

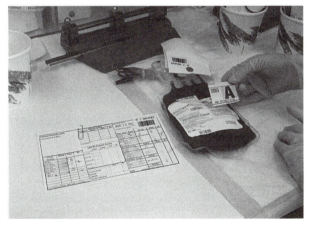

**Figure 13–7.** When all testing requirements are met, a red cell unit can be labeled with ABO group and Rh type and expiration date. (Courtesy National Institutes of Health, Bethesda, MD.)

positive patient, the Rh type of Rh-positive units need not be reconfirmed.

The manner in which donor processing laboratories perform ABO and Rh testing and antibody screening reflects the particular needs of each institution. Thus, hospitals with minimal donor processing may perform all testing using tube methodologies. Blood banks that maintain large blood supplies or collect a large portion of their own blood inventory may choose to conserve time and reagents by performing batch testing using microplates, solid-phase, affinity column, or gel technologies.[4] Expensive automated machinery can generally be justified only by very large donor centers.

Computerization is increasingly an integral part of many donor processing laboratories. Computers may be used for such functions as donor deferral, comparison of ABO and Rh testing with previous donations, input, storage and retrieval of test results, labeling, product inventory, and documentation of process control in a quality program.

## MAIN LABORATORY

Patient care is the primary mission of the main laboratory. Here the testing is performed that determines the compatibility between a patient requiring transfusion and the unit of blood to be transfused. Because of the severe adverse reaction that may occur if the wrong unit of blood is transfused to a patient, great care must be taken not only in the testing performed but also in specimen and unit identification and paperwork. Common approaches are evident in the pretransfusion testing protocols that are established by different blood banks to ensure the orderly, timely, and accurate processing of patient samples (Fig. 13–8).

### Sample Acceptance

Proper patient identification is crucial for any specimen used in blood bank testing. Consequences may be fatal if a blood specimen is labeled with the wrong patient's name. Thus, each specimen and request form the blood bank receives is carefully examined for proper spelling of the patient's name, correct identification number, correct date, and identity of the phlebotomist. Some hospitals employ commercially available systems that provide additional safeguards for proper patient identification.[5]

### Routine Testing

Once a patient sample has been judged acceptable, the testing requested by the patient's physician can be performed. Tests are usually requested as a group, and, for ease in ordering, a shorthand notation designates a group. Some common orders may include those that follow.

### Type and Screen

Many surgical procedures have a very low probability of requiring blood transfusion. To better utilize their blood supplies, blood bankers may choose not to crossmatch units of blood for these procedures but, instead, to use a type-and-screen protocol. ABO and Rh testing and antibody screening are performed using a current patient specimen.

Because only a small percentage of individuals who type as Rh-negative using an immediate spin technique are shown to express a weak D antigen using an antiglobulin technique, many hospitals choose to contain costs and to utilize time more efficiently by eliminating

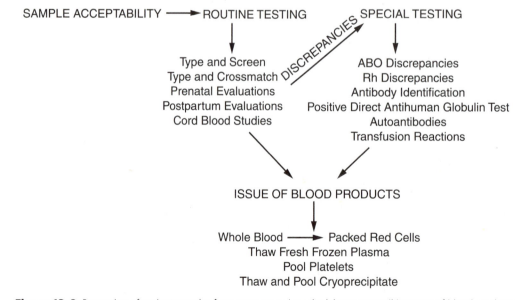

**Figure 13–8.** Processing of patient samples from acceptance into the laboratory until issuance of blood products.

testing of patient samples for weak D and by determining patient Rh types based upon immediate spin results only (see Chapter 6).

To increase the sensitivity of the antibody screen, some blood banks use a three-cell antibody screening set that provides homozygous antigen expression in all major blood group systems. In the absence of a positive antibody screen, if blood is needed on an emergency basis during surgery, it can be released using an abbreviated crossmatch (see further on). If an antibody is detected, identification of that antibody is performed and compatible units are reserved for the patient.

Although not mandated by AABB Standards, some blood banks may choose to include an auto-control or direct antiglobulin test (DAT) in a type-and-screen protocol (see Chapter 11). The decision to include or to eliminate these tests is based on the patient population of the facility, the time and cost involved in the testing, and the amount of useful information the test is expected to provide.[6]

## Type and Crossmatch

When a physician orders units to be crossmatched for a patient, more testing is necessary than the order itself implies. ABO and Rh testing and antibody screening must be performed on a current patient specimen. The same specimen is also used to crossmatch with a segment of the unit intended for transfusion (Fig. 13–9). In the absence of extreme emergency, the unit of blood can be issued for transfusion only if all testing discrepancies are resolved and the crossmatch is compatible. If the result of the antibody screen is positive, the antibody must be identified. If the antibody is clinically significant, antigen-negative units must be chosen for transfusion.

Abbreviated crossmatch protocols have been adopted by some blood banks for routine crossmatching and by others for only emergency situations. In these protocols, ABO and Rh testing and antibody screening are

performed. In the absence of clinically significant antibodies, blood is issued after an immediate spin crossmatch that serves as a confirmation of ABO compatibility. (Compare this with a conventional crossmatch in which an indirect antiglobulin test is performed following incubation at 37°C.)

An electronic or computer crossmatch is yet another method of crossmatching donor and patient that is intended to replace serologic compatibility testing.[7] Two separate ABO and Rh tests are performed on a patient's red cells and entered into a validated computer system; the ABO confirmatory test on a unit of blood is also entered. At the time when the blood is to be issued to the patient for transfusion, the computer electronically verifies the ABO compatibility between the donor unit and the patient and allows the release of the blood. If ABO incompatibilities between the recipient and the donor unit are discovered, the computer alerts the user to the discrepancy so that the blood will not be released.

## Prenatal Evaluation

Accurate serologic testing of obstetric patients is an essential component in the prevention and treatment of hemolytic disease of the newborn (HDN) (Table 13–2). Maternal blood samples are evaluated during pregnancy to determine the ABO group and Rh type of the mother and the presence of serum antibodies that

**Table 13–2.** Blood Bank Testing Protocols for Evaluation of Mothers and Newborns

| Evaluation | Functions |
|---|---|
| Prenatal evaluation | ■ ABO and Rh<br>■ Test for weak D if immediate spin test negative<br>■ Antibody screen<br>■ Antibody identification if screen positive<br>■ Serial titrations if antibody clinically significant |
| Postpartum evaluation | ■ Rh type<br>■ Test for weak D if immediate spin test negative<br>■ Rosette test if mother Rh-negative and baby Rh-positive<br>■ Kleihauer-Betke test if fetomaternal hemorrhage detected |
| Cord blood studies | ■ Routine<br>   ● Rh type<br>   ● Test for weak D if immediate spin test negative<br>■ Mother with clinically significant antibody<br>   ● ABO and Rh<br>   ● DAT<br>■ Baby with symptoms of HDN<br>   ● ABO and Rh<br>   ● Test for weak D if immediate spin test negative<br>   ● DAT<br>   ● Eluate if DAT result positive<br>   ● Antibody identification |

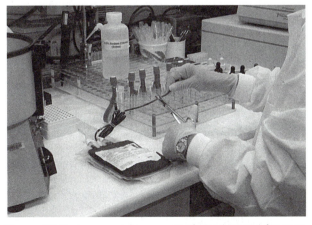

**Figure 13–9.** A segment from a unit of blood is used for crossmatching purposes. (Courtesy National Institutes of Health, Bethesda, MD.)

have the potential to cause HDN.[8] If the woman is classified as Rh-negative after testing for D and weak D, she may be a candidate for antenatal Rh-immune globulin. If the result of the antibody screen is positive, the antibody must be identified. Serial titrations may be performed during the course of the pregnancy if the antibody is considered potentially harmful to the fetus. The obstetrician uses these laboratory results in conjunction with other methods for evaluating the fetal condition to determine the need for clinical interventions such as intrauterine transfusion or early delivery (see Chapter 20).

### Postpartum Evaluation

All women admitted for delivery are required to be tested to determine their Rh status.[1] A test for weak D is performed on any specimen that shows a negative reaction on immediate spin. If the mother is Rh-negative and her baby Rh-positive, the maternal sample is further evaluated to detect a fetomaternal hemorrhage (FMH) in excess of 30 mL of whole blood. (One 300-μg dose of Rh-immune globulin prevents maternal Rh immunization from exposure of up to 30 mL of fetal whole blood.[9]) Commercial kits utilizing rosetting techniques are commonly used for this purpose. Once an FMH in excess of 30 mL of whole blood has been detected, quantification is performed using a Kleihauer-Betke test, flow cytometry, or enzyme-linked antiglobulin test (ELAT) (see Chapter 20). This may be performed in the blood bank or in a separate laboratory. If HDN is suspected, an antibody screen is performed on the mother's serum, and if the result is positive, attempts are made to identify the antibody.

### Cord Blood Studies

Protocols to evaluate cord blood specimens can vary widely from blood bank to blood bank. Cord blood from infants born to Rh-negative mothers is tested for D and for weak D to determine the mother's candidacy for Rh-immune globulin prophylaxis. ABO and Rh typing and DAT are performed on cord samples from infants born to women with clinically significant antibodies. Additional tests may also be performed. Many blood banks follow published guidelines[8] stating that, beyond these circumstances, routine testing of cord samples is not necessary unless the clinical situation warrants it. If an infant develops symptoms that suggest HDN, a full cord blood study is performed that may include ABO and Rh testing (including a test for weak D), DAT, and if the DAT result is positive, an eluate and subsequent antibody identification (see Chapter 11).

### Requests for Other Blood Components

When components that contain large amounts of red blood cells (such as granulocyte concentrates) are requested, pretransfusion testing is identical to that performed for red cell requests (see the previous section).

Orders for platelets and fresh frozen plasma may be filled once the ABO group of the recipient has been determined.

### Issue of Blood Products

After all pretransfusion testing has been completed, blood components may be released for transfusion to the designated recipient. *It is essential that all serologic discrepancies be resolved before issue of blood products, except in extreme emergency.* The individual in the blood bank who will issue the blood product inspects the unit for any abnormal appearance and verifies that all required transfusion forms and labels are complete and adequately identify the transfusion recipient. If another individual is responsible for delivering the blood product to the appropriate location, he or she may also verify that all information is complete. As discussed previously, a computer crossmatch may also be performed at this time. If there are no discrepancies, the component can be released for transfusion. Some form of documentation is used to record the transaction.

Some component preparation may be necessary before the issue of blood products. Fresh frozen plasma may be thawed in a constant-temperature (37°C) water bath, individual platelet concentrates may be pooled into a single bag for ease of transfusion, and individual units of cryoprecipitate may be thawed and then pooled. Because these manipulations shorten the expiration date of the products, it is best that they be performed as close to the time of issue as possible (see Chapter 10).

Blood products may be irradiated before issue to prevent passenger lymphocytes from causing graft-versus-host disease. Blood banks in large medical centers may have an irradiator on the premises (Fig. 13–10); smaller facilities may make arrangements to have the needed products irradiated elsewhere.

As is evident from previous discussions, computers have become an essential part of many transfusion services. Computers may be used not only for crossmatching but also for such functions as input, storage and verification of test results, inventory management, issue of blood products, training of blood bank personnel, statistical analysis, and quality process improvement.

## REFERENCE LABORATORY

Whether it is an entity separate from the main laboratory or, as in most cases, an integrated part, the reference laboratory is the problem-solving section of the blood bank. The goal of the reference laboratory is to ensure that any discrepancies detected in routine testing are resolved in an accurate and time-efficient manner. Other chapters in this book discuss in depth the various problems encountered in serologic testing and strategies for resolving them. Here, then, is a brief summary of some problem situations and common meth-

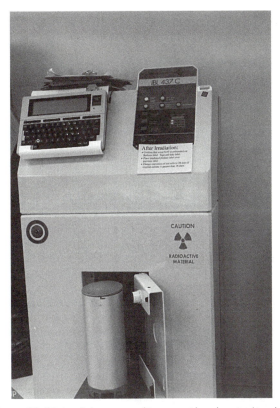

**Figure 13–10.** Irradiators are used to prevent lymphocytes in red cell products from causing graft-versus-host disease in susceptible patient populations. (Courtesy National Institutes of Health, Bethesda, MD.)

ods used in their investigation. It should be noted that before any serologic testing is performed, special testing should always include an investigation of patient diagnosis; age; and pregnancy, drug, and transfusion history.

## ABO Discrepancies

All inconsistencies between forward and reverse group test results must be resolved before an ABO interpretation can be made (see Chapter 5). ABO investigations may include:

1. Variations in incubation times and temperatures
2. Testing with $A_2$ cells or anti-$A_1$ lectin
3. Room temperature antibody identification
4. Adsorption and elution using human sources of anti-A or anti-B
5. Autoadsorption
6. Removal of red cell–bound cold autoantibodies (see Cold Autoantibodies)
7. Secretor studies

## Rh Discrepancies

Problems in Rh typing may occur because of certain clinical conditions or as inherited characteristics (see Chapter 6). Rh investigations may include:

1. Rh phenotyping
2. Adsorption and elution using Rh antisera
3. Isolation of cell populations
4. Use of rare antisera and cells

## Antibody Identification

A positive antibody screen in the absence of a positive auto-control or DAT result indicates possible alloantibody immunization through blood transfusion or pregnancy (see Chapter 11). To establish the identity and clinical significance of an antibody and to provide appropriate blood for transfusion, antibody investigations may include:

1. Antibody identification panels using various enhancement media (such as albumin, low ionic strength solution [LISS], polybrene, or polyethylene glycol [PEG]) and test systems (such as tubes; microplates or capillaries; or solid-phase, affinity column, or gel technologies)
2. Antibody identification panels pretreated with reagents such as enzymes, dithiothreitol (DTT), or 2-aminoethylisothiouronium bromide (AET)
3. Neutralization using substances such as plasma, saliva, urine, or human milk
4. Antigen typing
5. Titration
6. Adsorption and elution
7. Treatment of serum with DTT or 2-mercapto-ethanol (2-ME)
8. IgG subclassing
9. Monocyte monolayer assay (MMA)
10. Use of rare antisera and cells

## Positive Direct Antiglobulin Test (DAT)

A positive DAT may be the result of an immune reaction to a drug, a disease state, or a delayed hemolytic transfusion reaction (see Chapter 4). The investigation of a positive DAT result may include:

1. Use of monospecific reagents (anti-IgG, anti-C3)
2. Elution techniques
3. Antibody identification
4. Removal of red cell–bound antibody using chloroquine diphosphate or other reagents
5. Red cell phenotyping
6. Drug studies
7. Cell separation techniques

## Warm Autoantibodies

In addition to causing a positive DAT result (see previous section), the presence of a warm autoantibody in a patient's serum may mask the presence of clinically significant alloantibodies (see Chapter 21). Tests performed in the investigation of warm autoantibodies may include:

1. Removal of red cell–bound autoantibody followed by serum autoadsorption

2. Heterologous or differential serum adsorptions
3. Elution techniques
4. Autoantibody identification
5. Reticulocyte enrichment or other cell separation techniques

## Cold Autoantibodies

Potent cold autoantibodies may cause discrepancies in ABO testing as well as a positive DAT result (see previous section) and may mask the presence of clinically significant alloantibodies (see Chapter 21). The management of cold autoantibodies may include:

1. Removal of red cell–bound autoantibody using 37°C saline
2. Prewarmed technique
3. Antibody identification
4. Autoadsorption
5. Adsorption using rabbit erythrocyte stroma
6. Treatment of serum or cells with DTT or 2-ME

## Transfusion Reactions

Any adverse reactions to transfusion must be investigated to determine if the reaction is antibody-mediated (see Chapter 18). The extent of transfusion reaction investigations varies widely, depending on policies es-tablished by a particular blood bank and the result of initial testing. If there is strong evidence of an antibody-mediated transfusion reaction, further investigations may include:

1. Elution followed by antibody identification
2. Use of more sensitive techniques for antibody detection in serum and eluates, including enzymes, polybrene, PEG, or ELAT
3. Cell separation techniques

## SUMMARY

On cursory examination, one blood bank may appear to have very little in common with any other blood bank. However, because all blood banks must follow the same requirements and guidelines, and all are committed to providing patients with safe and effective blood products, many common themes become apparent with a more thorough investigation. With varying patient needs, changing technologies, increased regulation, and fluctuating economies, future blood banks may look nothing like the blood banks of today. That same commitment to patient care and excellence in testing, however, will ensure that common underlying themes will still be evident upon closer scrutiny.

---

### SUMMARY CHART: IMPORTANT POINTS TO REMEMBER (MT/MLT)

- In the component preparation and storage department, units of whole blood are separated into their various components and stored under conditions that ensure their optimum viability.
- In the donor processing department, testing is performed to determine the suitability of a blood product for transfusion (e.g., viral marker tests).
- In the main laboratory, patient samples are received and tested, and blood components are issued for transfusion.
- In the reference laboratory, discrepancies in testing are resolved (e.g., ABO subgroups).
- In apheresis, a donor's blood is removed in a sterile manner through tubing connected to an automated machine that then processes the blood, removes the desired component (platelets, plasma, or white blood cells), and returns the remainder of the components back to the donor via another set of tubing.
- Rh-negative units from an outside source must be reconfirmed by the transfusing facility because sensitization may occur if Rh-positive blood is transfused to an Rh-negative patient.

- Cord blood studies may involve ABO and Rh testing (including a test for weak D), DAT, and an eluate and subsequent antibody ID if the DAT result is positive.
- Resolution of ABO discrepancies may include (1) variations in incubation times and temperatures, (2) testing with $A_2$ cells or anti-$A_1$ lectin, (3) room temperature antibody identification, (4) adsorption and elution using human sources of anti-A or anti-B, (5) autoadsorption, and (6) removal of red cell–bound cold autoantibodies.
- Freezers maintained at $-18°C$ or lower are used for the storage of FFP and cryoprecipitate; freezers maintained at $-65°C$ or lower are used for the storage of red blood cells frozen in 40 percent glycerol.
- Refrigerators maintained at 1 to 6°C are used for the storage of packed red blood cells and whole blood.
- Platelet rotators that provide constant gentle agitation at room temperature are used for the storage of platelet concentrates.

## REVIEW QUESTIONS

1. All of the following criteria must be met before a unit of blood can be labeled except which of the following?
   A. ABO and Rh test results must agree with results from previous donations
   B. STS results must be nonreactive
   C. ALT results must be >100 U/L
   D. Viral testing results must be nonreactive

2. Freezers that maintain a temperature of −65°C or below must be used for the storage of which of the following?
   A. Fresh frozen plasma
   B. Red cells frozen in 40 percent glycerol
   C. Cryoprecipitate
   D. Red cells frozen in 20 percent glycerol

3. Which of the following is not required for a type and crossmatch?
   A. ABO testing
   B. Rh testing
   C. Testing for weak D
   D. Antibody screening
   E. Compatibility testing

4. Which of the following products is least likely to cause graft-versus-host disease?
   A. Whole blood
   B. Irradiated packed red cells
   C. Granulocyte concentrates
   D. Apheresis platelets

5. Cryoprecipitate is made by:
   A. Fractionation of plasma
   B. Apheresis
   C. Filtration of fresh frozen plasma
   D. Controlled thawing of fresh frozen plasma

6. Pooled screening cells may be used for antibody screening of:
   A. Donors
   B. Surgical patients
   C. Obstetric patients
   D. Neonates

7. All of the following are included in a routine cord blood evaluation except:
   A. DAT
   B. Fetal screen
   C. ABO
   D. Rh

8. In a prenatal evaluation, what is the significance of an Rh-negative mother?
   A. An indication to transfuse only Rh-positive blood
   B. An indication to transfuse only Rh-negative blood
   C. A potential Rh-immune globulin candidate
   D. A potential immune response to the C antigen

9. A unit of packed cells is issued and transfused to a 29-year-old woman undergoing a hysterectomy. Fifteen minutes into the transfusion, the woman's temperature increases 1.5°C above her baseline and the transfusion is stopped. The floor sends the blood bag and EDTA and serum specimen down to the blood bank. What department of the blood bank would usually test these specimens?
   A. Reference laboratory
   B. Main laboratory
   C. Donor processing
   D. Component preparation and storage

10. To maximize the number of components derived from one unit of blood, processing must occur within:
    A. 1 to 2 hours
    B. 3 to 5 hours
    C. 6 to 8 hours
    D. 10 to 12 hours

## ANSWERS TO REVIEW QUESTIONS

1. C (p 303)
2. B (p 302)
3. C (pp 304–305)
4. B (p 307)
5. D (p 301)
6. A (p 303)
7. B (p 306)
8. C (p 306)
9. A (pp 306–308)
10. C (p 301)

## REFERENCES

1. Code of Federal Regulations. Food and Drugs. Title 21. U.S. Government Printing Office, Washington, DC, 1996 (revised annually).
2. Menitove, JE (ed): Standards for Blood Banks and Transfusion Services, ed 18. American Association of Blood Banks, Bethesda, MD, 1997.
3. Stroup, M: A review: The use of monoclonal antibodies in blood banking. Immunohematology 6:30–36, 1990.
4. Walker, PS: New technologies in transfusion medicine. Lab Med 28:258–262, 1997.
5. Steane, EA, and Steane, SM: Closing the loop: Standardization is the key. Transfusion 36:200–202, 1996.
6. Laird-Fryer, B: Application and interpretation of direct antiglobulin test results as applied to healthy persons and selected patients. In Wallace, E, and Levitt, JS (eds): Current Applications and Interpretations of the Direct Antiglobulin Test. American Association of Blood Banks, Arlington, VA, 1988.
7. Leparc, GF: Electronic crossmatch: Transfusion service's new frontier. Lab Med 25:781–783, 1994.
8. Judd, WJ, et al: Prenatal and perinatal immunohematology: Recommendations for serologic management of the fetus, newborn infant, and obstetric patient. Immunohematology 30:175–183, 1990.
9. Bowman, JM: Historical overview: Hemolytic disease of the fetus and newborn. In Kennedy, MS, and Kelton, JG (eds): Perinatal Transfusion Medicine. American Association of Blood Banks, Arlington, VA, 1990.

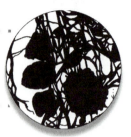

# CHAPTER **14**

# TRANSFUSION SAFETY AND FEDERAL REGULATORY REQUIREMENTS

Mary Ann Tourault, MA, MT(ASCP)SBB

## COMMONLY USED ABBREVIATIONS IN THIS CHAPTER

| | |
|---|---|
| **BLA:** | Biologics License Application |
| **CBER:** | Center for Biologics Evaluation and Research |
| **CDCP:** | Centers for Disease Control and Prevention |
| **CFR:** | Code of Federal Regulations |
| **FDA:** | Food and Drug Administration |
| **FD&C Act:** | Food, Drug and Cosmetic Act |
| **GMP:** | Good Manufacturing Practices |
| **HCFA:** | Health Care Financing Administration |
| **MOU:** | Memorandum of Understanding |
| **NIH:** | National Institutes of Health |
| **PHS:** | Public Health Service |
| **QA:** | Quality Assurance |
| **VMT:** | Viral Marker Test |

## OBJECTIVES

*On completion of the chapter, the learner should be able to:*

1 Describe why laws governing regulation of biologics were enacted.

2 List the requirements for licensing biologic products.

3 List the inspectional authority of FDA.

4 Discuss requirements for FDA registration.

5 List which facilities may ship products interstate.

6 Discuss which facilities will be inspected by FDA and those under the authority of HCFA.

7 Discuss the changes in licensing (BLA).

8 Describe why quality assurance is an FDA guideline.

9 Describe the recall process.

10 Discuss short supply regulations.

## INTRODUCTION

The Public Health Service (PHS) is the principal health agency of the federal government. The mission of PHS is to protect, improve, and advance the health of the American people. The Centers for Disease Control and Prevention and the Food and Drug Administration are organizations of the PHS.

The Food and Drug Administration (FDA) enforces regulations to ensure the safety and efficacy of biologics, drugs, and devices, which include blood and blood components and diagnostic reagents used or manufactured by blood establishments.[1] This chapter describes the history of the regulatory process (Table 14–1), requirements of the FDA, and quality assurance issues. The regulations for blood and blood products promulgated under the Public Health Service Act and the Federal Food, Drug, and Cosmetic (FD&C) Act are found in Parts 211 to 680 of Title 21, Code of Federal Regulations (CFR).

**Table 14–1.** Historical Perspective of the Regulation of Biologics

| | |
|---|---|
| 1902 | Biologics Control Act |
| | Products safe, pure, and potent |
| 1903 | License required for interstate shipment of biologics |
| | Annual inspections |
| 1937 | First blood bank, Cook County |
| 1940 | First US license for Normal Human Plasma |
| 1944 | National Microbiological Institute to National Institutes of Health |
| | Establishment and product license required |
| 1946 | First license for whole blood issued |
| 1955 | Division of Biologic Standards |
| 1962 | First court decision where court ruled blood products are drugs |
| 1970 | Section 351 of PHS Act amended to specifically include blood and blood components and blood derivatives |
| 1972 | Regulation from NIH to FDA |
| 1976 | Medical device amendments |
| 1980 | Transfusion service from FDA to HCFA |
| 1982 | Merger of Bureau of Biologics and Bureau of Drugs |
| 1988 | Center for Drugs and Biologics became two units |
| | Center for Biologics Evaluation and Research |
| | Center for Drug Evaluation and Research |
| 1998 | Single Application for Biologics (BLA) |

These regulations mandate adherence to current Good Manufacturing Practices (cGMP) by following the guidance detailed in standard operating procedures (SOPs). Applicable additional standards for the manufacture of blood and blood products must also be followed. In addition, the regulations address the statutory requirements regarding products licensing and registration as well as product-specific standards for bacterial products, viral vaccines, and human blood and blood products.

## HISTORY AND OVERVIEW OF BIOLOGICS REGULATIONS

Early in the 1900s, biologic drugs were coming into widespread use in the United States after having met with great success in Europe and Russia. Countries such as France, Germany, Italy, and Russia had instituted regulatory controls for such biologics as early as 1895. The regulation of biologic products in the United States began when Congress passed the Biologics Control Act of 1902 (also known as the Virus Toxin Law.)[2]

This act was passed following the deaths of 10 children who had received injections of diphtheria antitoxin contaminated with tetanus.[3] In 1901, there was a serious epidemic of diphtheria resulting in a great demand for the diphtheria antitoxin. Diphtheria was the ninth leading cause of death in the United States. At the time, there was no requirement for safety testing, and, in the rush to provide the needed antitoxin, no safety test had been performed. The horse from which the antitoxin was obtained had contracted tetanus, and the live tetanus organisms were passed on to the children. The 1902 Act required that biologics be manufactured in a manner that ensured safety, purity, and potency.[4] Provisions of the act included:

- Establishment of license requirements
- Product license requirements
- Labeling requirements
- Inspection requirements
- Suspension or revocation of licenses, or both
- Penalties for violations

## Public Health Service

The responsibility for implementing this new law was placed under the Hygienic Laboratory, which was one of the establishments within the Marine Hospital Service (which became the Public Health Service). In 1903, the PHS expanded the regulations to include, among other provisions, that inspections would be unannounced and that licenses were to be issued on the basis of an annual inspection.[5] Today, this act is known as the PHS Act, 42 USC 262 and serves as the legal basis for the Center for Biologics Evaluation and Research (CBER) premarket approval activities for biologic products.

The 1902 Act was amended in 1944. One change included a requirement that a biologic product license could be issued only upon demonstration that both the product and the establishment met standards to ensure the continued safety, purity, and potency of such products. Another change in 1944 was to delegate the responsibility for administering the act to the National Microbiological Institute at the National Institutes of Health (NIH). With the advent of the polio vaccines in the mid-1950s, the focal point for administering the PHS Act was given to the Division of Biologics Standards (DBS) from 1955 to 1972. In 1972, biologics regulation was transferred to the FDA's Bureau of Biologics (BoB). This changed the organization's direction from a research function to one of regulation.

## Drug Regulations

The transfer for the oversight of biologics to the FDA began a merger of the regulatory requirements of the PHS Act and the FD&C Act (21 USC 301 et seq). Biologics were viewed as biologic products under the PHS Act and as drugs under the FD&C Act, subject to inspection according to the good manufacturing practices (GMP) regulations for drugs. During this era, the reagent manufacturers were also inspected under the drug GMP because the device amendments were not enacted until 1976. As a result, administration of the regulatory powers inherent in each of the acts had to be approached with the knowledge that they did not in any way modify the other. Therefore, it was possible for a biologic product to be adulterated or misbranded as a drug or device within the meaning of the FD&C Act. Adulteration has been defined as any deleterious substance that may render a product injurious to health or as any product not manufactured according to GMPs.

Misbranding is defined as any false or misleading labeling.

Another significant change that occurred as a result of the FDA's assuming regulatory responsibility for biologic products was the requirement that biologic establishments, including blood banks, were required to register with the FDA. The GMP regulations for blood and blood products were promulgated under the FD&C Act as well as the PHS Act. Today, one of the major programs of the FDA is to ensure the safety of the nation's blood supply.

## Bureau of Biologics

In 1982, the FDA merged the Bureau of Biologics and the Bureau of Drugs into one agency known as the Center for Drugs and Biologics. In 1988, this organization was divided into two distinct entities, the Center for Biologics Evaluation and Research (CBER) and the Center for Drugs Evaluation and Research (CDER). This division came about as a result of significant events, such as the outbreak of the acquired immunodeficiency syndrome (AIDS), a perceived drugs approval lag in the United States for traditional pharmaceuticals, and the advent of bioengineering-derived and biotechnology-derived products.

CBER has grown in its responsibilities since its beginning as the Hygienic Laboratory for the PHS in 1902, when the technologies for producing biologic products were in their infancy and the primary function was regulation of vaccines. Today the regulation of a wide variety of biologic products and their use as therapeutics requires knowledge of new developments in manufacturing technology, as well as updated approaches to basic research in the relevant biologic disciplines. Even with the infusion of technologic advances into biologics, CBER recognizes that the establishment inspection, which was first used in 1902, will continue to be an integral part of the surveillance effort in regulating new biotherapeutics and new blood products, and monitoring future scientific efforts. Products regulated by CBER are listed in Table 14–2.

## Milestones in the Food and Drug Administration's Regulation of Biologics

Biologic products are defined in Section 351 of the PHS Acts as "any virus, therapeutic serum, toxin, antitoxin, vaccine, blood, blood component or derivative, allergenic product, or analogous product applicable to the prevention, treatment, or cure of diseases or injuries of man."[6] The original statute did not list blood, blood components, or blood derivatives in the definition.

The first blood bank, under the direction of Dr. Bernard Fantus, began in 1937 in Cook County Hospital, located in Chicago, Illinois. The first program addressing blood and blood products was developed during World War II by Drs. Roderick Murray and J. T. Tripp. They established standards and supervised plasma production in commercial establishments

**Table 14–2.** Products Regulated by CBER

Blood and Blood Products
- Whole blood and blood components
- Source plasma
- Plasma derivatives (e.g., antihemophilic factor [AHF], plasma protein fraction [PPF], normal serum albumin [NSA], immune serum globulin [ISG])
- Streptokinase
- Antilymphocyte globulin
- Licensed in vitro reagents (e.g., blood group sera), monoclonal antibodies/recombinant DNA products
- Blood group substances
- Fibrinogen

Bacterial and Viral Products
- Toxoids (e.g., tetanus toxoids)
- Antitoxins (e.g., tetanus antitoxin)
- Bacterial vaccines (e.g., diphtherial and tetanus toxoids and pertussis vaccine [DPT])
- Viral vaccines (e.g., poliovirus vaccine—live, oral, trivalent)
- Allergenic products
- Tuberculin
- Antiviral serum (e.g., antirabies serum)

In Vitro Test Kits
- Anti-HIV, HIV antigen, anti-HTLV-I
- Hepatitis B, HCV expanders

Biotherapeutic Products (Biotechnology-derived)
- Interferons
- Granulocyte colony-stimulating factor (GCSF)
- Granulocyte macrophage colony-stimulating factor (GMCSF)
- Erythropoietin (EPO)
- OKT3-monoclonal antibody

New Drug Application Products (NDA)
- Anticoagulants in blood collection bags
- Plasma volume extenders
- Urokinase
- Perfluorochemicals (e.g., Fluosol)

from blood collected by the American Red Cross. In July 1940, the first federal license for manufacturing Normal Human Plasma was issued. At that time, blood was considered analogous to a therapeutic serum, which was one of the products explicitly covered by Section 351 of the PHS Act. The first license for Whole Blood was issued in May 1946.

Blood and blood components were considered within the ambit of the statutory authority of the FD&C Act as the administrator of the Federal Security Agency (predecessor of Health, Education, and Welfare) ruled on May 31, 1945, that to avoid a duplication of effort, one agency should be responsible for requiring biologic manufacturers to comply with all applicable provisions of the FD&C Act as well as the provisions of the PHS Act. Carrying out this responsibility, the provisions of the FD&C Act were often applied to manufacturers of blood and blood products. For example, pursuant to Section 503(b) of the Act, blood labels were required to carry the legend, "Caution: Federal Law prohibits dispensing without a prescription." In addition, pursuant to Section 502 of the FD&C Act, blood banks were required to supply a package enclosure with the blood that provided instructions for use, indications, contraindications, side effects, and precautions. This is known as the current Circular of Infor-

mation, which should be sent to consignees of blood and blood products at least once each quarter.

In an article for *Transfusion*, Dr. Joel Solomon identifies the first prosecution in 1962 of a biologics manufacturer, which was a commercial blood bank in Westchester County, New York.[7] The Responsible Head, Mr. Calise, was found guilty of record falsification, mislabeling, and adulteration, and, in an unusual precedent, he was prohibited in perpetuity from the practice of blood banking. This was a landmark case because it was the first court decision that ruled that blood products were drugs.

Another milestone in the history of blood bank regulation occurred in 1968 in a legal action brought by the federal government against a commercial blood bank in Dallas, Texas (*United States versus Charles and Maxine Blank*).[8] Maxine Blank and her codefendants were found guilty of false labeling of blood products under Section 351 of the PHS Act and of misbranding a drug (blood) under the FD&C Act. On appeal in 1968, her conviction was reversed on grounds that the products involved were not within the scope of the statute because there was no specific reference to blood or blood products in the biologics statute. The appellate court upheld the conviction for violations of the FD&C Act, which charged misbranding a drug. As a result of this ruling, an amendment was made in 1970 to Section 351 of the PHS Act specifically to include blood, blood components, and blood derivatives, making it clear that Congress intended blood and blood products to be subject to the provisions of the PHS Act.

### Blood Classified as a Drug

Federal courts that have had occasion to consider the issue have held without exception that blood is a drug within the meaning of the FD&C Act. The registration requirement applies not only to establishments that collect or process blood for transfusion but also to those that collect blood and use it or its components in the manufacture of diagnostic laboratory reagents and controls.

In 1976, the FD&C Act was amended to strengthen the FDA's authority to regulate medical devices. The FDA now requires manufacturers of class III medical devices to demonstrate that their products are safe and effective before marketing them. Before 1976, the FDA's authority was limited to removing hazardous or falsely represented products from the market. Under the amendment, blood banks were required to register their establishments with the FDA and to list the products they prepared. In addition, GMPs for blood and blood products were promulgated.

There were also changes in inspectional responsibilities. The FDA has a large network of field offices at the regional, district, and resident post levels across the United States. These field offices are staffed with investigators who perform the inspection and investigation work required of FDA. Because the FDA was charged with the inspection of all blood banks and blood centers in the United States, involvement of the field inspectional force was necessary to share the increased workload. At one time, the inventory of blood-related firms encompassed approximately 7000 locations.

### FDA-HCFA Memorandum of Understanding

Since 1980, the number of blood establishments that the FDA is obligated to inspect has been significantly reduced as a result of an agreement with the Health Care Financing Administration (HCFA). This 1980 Memorandum of Understanding (MOU) between HCFA and the FDA reduced the number of federal agencies inspecting the same facility. If units of blood are collected on a routine basis, including collection of autologous units, blood banks are required to register with, and to be inspected by, the FDA. Those facilities that do not routinely collect blood or that do not prepare blood components are generally inspected under the auspices of HCFA. The preparation of blood components for which a facility would register includes washing, rejuvenating, freezing, or deglycerolyzing red blood cells and irradiating blood products.

Facilities, such as transfusion services, that do not collect blood and do not prepare blood components are generally inspected under the auspices of HCFA. Because HCFA does not have a cadre of inspectors to perform inspections, they have delegated inspections (surveys) to a number of organizations such as the College of American Pathologists, the American Association of Blood Banks, American Osteopathic Association, and state health departments.

### Inspection Authorities and Guidance

Licensed manufacturers of biologic products are inspected under the authorities found in both the PHS Act (42 USC 262[c]) and the FD&C Act (21 USC 374). As discussed earlier, most biologic products also meet the definition of a drug under the FD&C Act. For this reason, the applicable portion of both acts and their implementing regulation are enforced for biologic products. There are also several licensed biologic products, such as blood grouping reagents and viral marker test kits, that meet the definition of a device under the FD&C Act.

Guidance in the form of memoranda issued to all registered blood establishments and inspection guides issued to FDA investigators are available on request from the Congressional and Consumer Affairs Staff, 1401 Rockville Pike, Rockville, MD 20852-1448 (301-594-2000). Compliance programs and compliance policy guides contain instructions to the FDA field investigators, and they are available through the Freedom of Information Office. Compliance programs and compliance policy guides may be obtained by writing to the FOI Officer, HFA-35, 5600 Fishers Lane, Rockville, MD 20856. The compliance programs give guidance to investigators and specify the action points for evaluating regulatory actions such as license suspension or revo-

cation. The FDA Web Resources may be contacted at http://www.fda.gov/.

### Licensing Activities

The application process for biologic products has changed to harmonize with the Center for Drugs Evaluation and Research. In the past, licensing biologics involved issuing licenses for both the biologic product and the establishment that manufactured the product. The review and approval were based on separate application filings for each product, as well as a filing for the establishment. CBER is eliminating the requirement for the establishment filing. The harmonized application form (FDA Form 356h) is a cover sheet for filing an application, and the information, with details of the manufacturing process, is addressed in a listing on the second page of the form.

This change was a result of the FDA's commitment to develop a single, harmonized application for all licensed biologic products and all drug products. The change in CBER began with the publication in the *Federal Register* of May 14, 1996, of the final rule: Elimination of the Establishment License Application for Specified Biotechnology and Specified Synthetic Biological Products. This rule replaced the need for a formal application filing with the demonstration of compliance with regulations which address cGMP. Although this regulation does not specifically name blood and blood products in the final rule, it is used to issue a single license rather than separate establishment and product licenses. The first biologics firm to receive a single license was Genetics Institute for the manufacture of recombinant Factor IX.

The new definition of "manufacturer" is a radical change from the past for CBER. No longer is the definition of manufacturer restricted to the one actually engaged in the manufacturing process. The new definition also includes any legal person or entity who is an applicant for a license where the applicant assumes responsibility for compliance with the applicable product and establishment standards. This expanded definition provides for greater flexibility for all establishments requiring a license from the FDA. The applicant may or may not own the facilities in which the product is manufactured. Another dramatic change is that the new definition eliminates the requirement that each contract facility engaging in significant manufacture obtain a separate license. One result of this change is that it allows a product innovator to be licensed even if the innovator is not engaged in the manufacturing process.

Although changes have been made in the concepts applied to the biotechnology products regulated by CBER, it is important to realize that establishment standards are retained and are an integral part of the licensing process. The need for preapproval of establishment will not be changed.

Guidance documents with directions and descriptions on what is needed to file a single license application are published in the *Federal Register*. The documents follow closely the Center for Drugs Evaluation and Research's established guidance, which includes: (1) a description of the drug substance and drug product, (2) characterization of both the substance and the final product, (3) identification of the manufacturer or manufacturers, and (4) the methods used in manufacturing, validation and process controls employed in the manufacturing, use of any reference standards, release specifications, testing requirements, the container closure system, requirements for shipping, the stability protocol, and environmental assessment.

Applications for blood and blood products licenses may be obtained from CBER, Division of Blood Applications, HFM-370. Before granting a license, CBER staff review applications and, if all necessary data and information are found satisfactory, conduct a prelicense inspection. The application will be reviewed for safety and efficacy, product labeling, and compliance with all applicable regulations. Sample lots must be submitted to CBER for some products, such as HIV tests, and samples may be required from each lot for lot-release testing.

The prelicense inspection is an in-depth review of the physical facilities and the manufacturing methods; SOP manual, records, and equipment; and an evaluation of the training of the staff involved in the manufacturing. This inspection is announced so that it can be a productive time spent with the facility performing the manufacturing of products for which they have requested a license. The inspection is intended to determine the firm's ability to operate in compliance with the applicable regulations. If the results of the prelicense inspection show the firm to be operating in a satisfactory manner and that the product(s) meet applicable standards and regulations for safety and efficacy, a license will be issued. The license must be amended before changing any significant step in manufacturing or making any substantive modification to the facility.

### Changes in Licensing Requirements

In the past, separate federal licenses were issued concurrently for the biologic product license and for the establishment manufacturing the biologic product. The FDA has eliminated the establishment filing, and now a single application filing results in the issuance of a single biologics license. Previously, the definition of "manufacturer" restricted its usage to one actually engaged in the manufacturing process. The new definition includes any legal person or entity who assumes responsibility for compliance with the applicable products and establishment standards. The applicant may or may not own the facility in which the product is manufactured. The new requirement also eliminates the need for each contract facility engaging in significant manufacture to obtain a separate license. This new form has been titled the Biologics License Application (BLA).[9]

The result of the change is that a new blood establishment requesting a license for Whole Blood, Red Blood Cells, Plasma, and Platelets will be required to file one application that describes how the compo-

nents are prepared and controlled. In the past this would have required filing six separate applications.

Within the United States and at foreign establishments holding a U.S. license, ongoing compliance with regulations is secured through inspections of the facilities and products, educational activities, and legal proceedings.

### Sale, Barter, or Exchange

Having a U.S. license allows the establishment to ship products interstate (and internationally) for sale, barter, or exchange. Federal law prohibits unlicensed firms from shipping products from one state to another or out of the United States. Licensed firms may not ship products that have not been included in the licensing process with CBER. The only exception is for documented medical emergencies, and Compliance Policy Guide 7134.11 provides guidance and explains the regulatory aspects of these shipments.

### Authorized Official

Biologic regulations specify that an applicant designate one or more authorized official(s) for each legal manufacturing entity, with authority to represent the manufacturer in all pertinent matters. The official(s) has/have the authority to represent the firm with the FDA. This concept has changed in other parts of the biologics world, such as biotechnology, and the regulations reflect this change and allow greater flexibility.

### Short Supply

A frequently misunderstood area is the concept of short supply. Short supply was introduced in 1948, and the provisions governing short supply are found in 21 CFR 601.22. The short supply provisions of the regulations constitute an exemption from licensure in limited areas and under controlled conditions.

The concept is that certain products, such as Factor VIII, are designated by CBER to be in short supply. It is not that the Recovered Plasma is in short supply, but that the product manufactured using the plasma is in short supply. The short supply provision allows unlicensed source material to be shipped interstate and to be used to manufacture a licensed product. For example, for Factor VIII, the Source Material may be Recovered Plasma, which is not a product that is licensed by the FDA.

The short supply provisions allow manufacturers, such as fractionators, to use an unlicensed product or allow another licensed establishment to perform the initial and partial manufacturing step of collecting the blood or plasma. For Recovered Plasma to be shipped to a fractionator for further manufacture into injectable products, a short supply agreement must exist. This written agreement should be current and state the use of the product, as well as which tests are performed on the units of blood plasma.

**Short Supply Labels.** The use of the product is the

key element in being able to label the product correctly. If the product will be used for further manufacture into an injectable product, the label statement should read: "Caution: For Manufacturing Use Only." If the product will be used for further manufacture into a noninjectable product, the label statement should read: "Caution: For Use in Manufacturing Noninjectable Products Only," and the following statement should also be included: "Not For Use in Products Subject to License Under Section 351 of the Public Health Service Act."

To use the short supply provisions, the manufacturer holding a U.S. license to prepare the finished biologic product must establish with the suppliers the procedures, inspections, tests, or other arrangements necessary to ensure full compliance with the applicable regulation for blood establishments. The short supply agreement must be between the licensed fractionator and the collecting facility. This agreement *may not* be between the licensed fractionator and a broker. The agreement should be updated annually and signed by all parties, including a broker if one is involved. The responsibility for compliance with standards for the source material rests with the licensed manufacturer (i.e., the fractionator) of the finished product, as well as with the supplier. Noncompliance may result in revocation of the short supply exemption as well as other enforcement activities by the FDA. It is advised that the collecting facility have a letter stating the intended use of the product so that it may determine whether the label, often supplied by a broker, is the correct label for the product.

### Recovered Plasma Regulations and Requirements

Recovered Plasma is derived from single units of expired or unexpired Whole Blood or Plasma or is a byproduct of the preparation of blood components from single units of blood as defined in 21 CFR 606.3(c). It is an unlicensed source material intended for use in the manufacture of both licensed and unlicensed products, such as licensed fractionated products for injection (e.g., Factor VIII and clotting factors), licensed diagnostic products, and unlicensed diagnostic products, including clinical chemistry controls. A license is not required to manufacture, distribute, relabel, pool, or repack Recovered Plasma.

Brokers frequently act as an intermediary between the collector and the licensed manufacturer of the final product. Selling plasma to a broker does not relieve the collector of the responsibility of obtaining a short supply agreement if needed or from correctly labeling the product. It is in the best interest of the collector to obtain a letter from the broker stating the intended use of the product. This, of course, is separate from the required short supply agreement between the collector and the licensed fractionator of the product, if the intended use is for an injectable product. Plasma brokers may act as authorized agents and should be identified in the agreement. Brokers that take physical possession of plasma must register with the FDA.

### Testing Laboratories

The FDA regulations require that U.S. licensed blood establishments have testing performed on products at U.S. licensed facilities. Written contracts between the two facilities should designate the number of times a test will be performed and that all viral marker tests will follow the manufacturer's package insert. Strict adherence to an algorithm (manufacturer's instructions and FDA guidance requiring that units be discarded if two of three tests are reactive) is often not fully understood and continues to cause product recalls and other regulatory actions by the FDA.

It is the responsibility of the collecting facility to ensure that tests will follow the manufacturer's instructions. This becomes a problem when tests are sent to laboratories that perform patient testing and have different criteria for determining whether a patient is reactive to a viral marker test. Extreme caution is used by the FDA to protect the blood supply.

## OVERVIEW OF THE INSPECTION PROCESS

A compliance program is written by the CBER headquarters staff to provide guidance to the FDA field investigators, as well as to headquarters staff, concerning surveillance and enforcement activities involving blood establishments.[10] The objective of the compliance program is to ensure that blood and blood products are safe, effective, and adequately labeled. Each inspection should cover the manufacturing operation of the blood bank to ensure that GMPs are being followed. Previously, investigators used a checklist that provided a uniform approach to the inspection. Experienced investigators who were trained in this systematic approach may still use the checklist as a model; however, new staff members do not have this guidance to follow, which results in an uneven inspection process.

In 1991, a CBER review of inspectional findings, error and accident reports, blood product recalls, and enforcement actions indicated a substantial increase in these areas compared with those of the previous five years. This increase prompted the issuance of a memorandum on March 21, 1991, to all registered establishments entitled, "Deficiencies Relating to the Manufacture of Blood and Blood Components." This memorandum listed the most significant deficiencies observed and was provided so that blood establishments could perform audits and correct deficiencies. The significant deficiencies in the donor deferral systems were:

- Deferral records were incomplete, not current, or did not provide for accurate identification of the donor as required by 21 CFR 606.160.
- Donors were not recognized as having multiple reasons for deferral (e.g., HBsAg and serologic test for syphilis).

Blood bank directors and supervisors were urged to review SOPs and manufacturing operations with regard to the potential for errors in testing and deferral lists. One of the reasons for providing the information was so that it could be used for self-audits. The FDA issued a memorandum reminding the blood bank community of the regulation found in 21 CFR 600.14, which requires licensed establishments to report errors to the FDA. A recent regulation also requires unlicensed facilities (transfusion services) to report errors. The number of recalls (Fig. 14–1) and errors (Fig. 14–2) reported to the FDA increased dramatically in 1988 and 1991, respectively, with upward spirals continuing. Figure 14–1 illustrates how the number of recalls stayed at the same low level from 1981 to 1987. With the advent of anti-HIV testing, ALT testing, additional donor suitability criteria associated with signs and symptoms of AIDS, and behaviors that would place donors at increased risk, the number of recalls increased in 1988. The FDA Commissioner, Dr. Frank Young, requested that CBER headquarters staff educate FDA investigators on inspection of viral marker testing. Changes in the focus of the inspections and additional testing requirements resulted in further increases in the number of recalls, beginning in 1989.

In addition to the number of recalls, Figure 14–2 illustrates that an increase in the number of errors reported to the FDA continues to be observed. The increase in error reports is the result of a number of factors. Review and evaluation of the error reports indi-

cates that the sharp increase of reports seen in 1992 results from information received from donors following collection. These reports are listed as postdonation information and account for many of the accident reports received since 1992. Figure 14–3 illustrates the percentages and types of error and accidents reported in fiscal year 1996. Many of the postdonation reports contain information that would have been cause for deferral if the donor had given the information to the collecting facility at the time of donation (Table 14–3). The reports are not considered errors because the information was not given to the collection facility by the donor before the donation. Additional examples of postdonation information are listed in Table 14–4. One area that needs to be addressed is how to get donors to give information before collection that would prevent transfusion of the blood or blood product.

Another area addressed during inspection is fatal transfusion reactions. When a death occurs during or following a transfusion, or in the rare case of blood collection, blood bank staff are often uncertain when they must send a report to CBER.[11] Inasmuch as most transfusions are given to critically ill patients, many patients die while receiving blood or blood products, or shortly after the transfusion. It is not the intent of the fatality regulation that each of these deaths be reported to CBER. The death of the patient or donor may have only a temporal relationship to the transfusion or collection

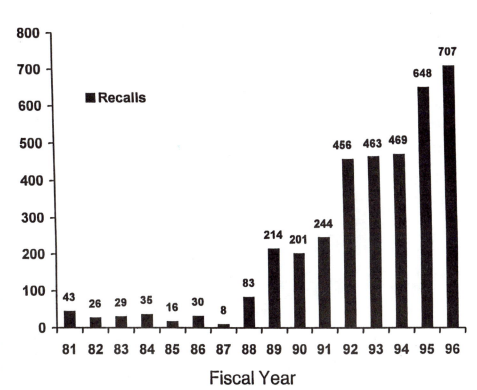

**Recalls
FY81 - FY96**

**Figure 14–1.** Graph demonstrates the increase in biologic products classified by FDA as recalls. The recall figures include a small number of other biologic products such as vaccines, albumin, and bacterial products. The number of products recalled remained at a steady level until 1988.

# Total Number of Error/Accidents

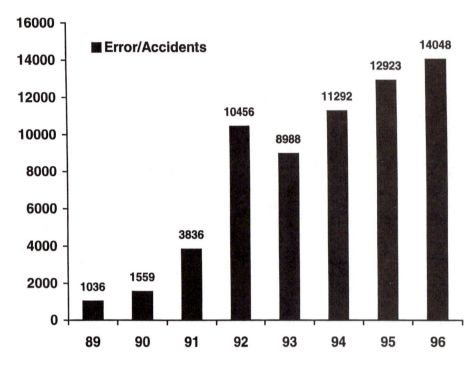

**Figure 14–2.** Graph illustrates an increase in the number of errors/accidents reported to the FDA.

# Error and Accident Reports
# All Blood and Plasma Establishments
# FY96

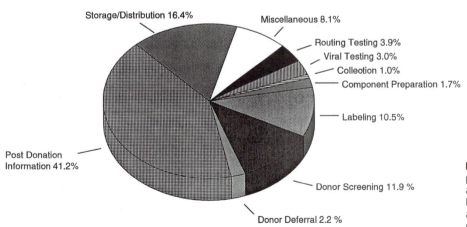

*Reports received (10/1/95 - 9/30/96) = 14,034*

**Figure 14–3.** Graph illustrates the percentages and types of errors and accidents reported to the Center for Biologics Evaluation and Research and Review in fiscal year 1996. Reports submitted from October 1, 1995, to September 30, 1996, are from both blood and plasma establishments.

**Table 14–3.** Postdonation Information Received in Reports Submitted to the Center for Biologics Evaluation and Research in 1996

| Postdonation Information | Blood Establishments | | Total | |
|---|---|---|---|---|
| Tattoo, ear/body piercing, needlestick, or transfusion | 965 | 23.3% | 1030 | 23.5% |
| Travel to malarial endemic area | 572 | 13.8% | 573 | 13.1% |
| IV drug use | 337 | 8.2% | 365 | 8.3% |
| History of cancer | 321 | 7.8% | 322 | 7.4% |
| History of disease/surgery | 317 | 7.7% | 321 | 7.3% |
| Risk factor associated with CJD | 220 | 5.3% | 236 | 5.4% |
| History of hepatitis B/C or jaundice | 187 | 4.5% | 191 | 4.4% |
| Male to male sex | 184 | 4.5% | 203 | 4.6% |
| Received Proscar, Tegison, or Accutane | 161 | 3.9% | 161 | 3.7% |
| Sex with an IV drug user | 138 | 3.3% | 144 | 3.3% |
| Total | 3402 | 82.3% | 3546 | 81.0% |

**Note.** This information was not provided to the collection facility until after the donation. If the information had been provided before donation, the collection facility would have deferred the donor. Only 82.3% of blood establishments reported.

**Table 14–4.** Postdonation Information Report

| Postdonation Information | Blood Establishments | | Total | |
|---|---|---|---|---|
| Illness (not AIDS- or hepatitis-related) | 738 | 63.6% | 741 | 59.6% |
| Diagnosis of cancer, postdonation | 108 | 9.3% | 108 | 8.7% |
| Sex partner tests positive for hepatitis | 43 | 3.7% | 44 | 3.5% |
| Hepatitis-related illness | 34 | 2.9% | 37 | 3.0% |
| Exposure to hepatitis | 32 | 2.8% | 32 | 2.6% |
| Total | 955 | 82.3% | 962 | 77.4% |

**Note:** This information was not provided to the collection facility until after the donation. If the information had been provided before the donation, the collection facility would have disqualified the donor. Not all of the categories would result in permanent deferral of the donor (e.g., illness or exposure to hepatitis A).

of blood. The regulation requires reporting only actions related to a transfusion that may have contributed to the death of a patient or a blood collection error that may have caused a donor fatality.

The purposes of reporting fatalities to CBER are (1) to ensure that the incidents are thoroughly investigated, (2) to determine if appropriate corrective action has been taken to prevent a recurrence, and (3) to evaluate reports for trends that may warrant action by the FDA or HCFA, such as new recommendations or policies or the review of existing approvals or policies.

## Inspection Outcomes

Administrative and legal actions, such as license suspension, injunction, and prosecutions have been an outcome of numerous high-profile inspections. In the majority of inspections, voluntary compliance is the usual course of action.

### Regulatory Sanction and Administrative Actions

When an establishment is found in violation of any of the laws that the FDA enforces, it is usually given an opportunity for voluntary correction before the FDA pursues legal action. When an establishment does not voluntarily correct a public health problem, the FDA may invoke legal sanctions. The regulatory remedies available to the FDA to obtain compliance with the regulations are warning letters and license suspension or revocation of operations under U.S. license. Legal actions include seizure, injunction, and prosecution.

Product recalls are voluntary actions taken by establishments, or in rare instances requested by the FDA, to remove violative products from the market or to correct the labeling of such products. The regulations governing recalls are found in 21 CFR, Part 7.

### Product Recall

Product recall is the most frequent administrative action used by the FDA. The number of recalls classified by the FDA continues to increase as illustrated in Figure 14–1. This increase is the result of increased awareness by the blood bank community as well as by FDA investigators. A recall is a firm's removal or correction of a marketed product when that product violates the laws enforced by the FDA.[12] Recall is far less costly and time consuming than a court procedure, such as seizure of the product, and it removes defective products from the market more quickly.

Recall of blood and blood products is different from that of most drug products because, in the usual course of events, the unit of blood or the blood component has already been transfused, so there can be no physical recall or getting the product back. When a blood product has already been transfused, recall is notification that the product was not labeled correctly. For example, a unit may have had an incorrect and extended expiration date, or a unit may have been labeled as negative for cytomegalovirus (CMV) when, in fact, the test for CMV was positive. Another example with a diagnostic product could involve the information sent with red blood cell antibody screening cells. The information included with the shipment of the product may have listed one of the screening cells as positive or negative for the Kell antigen.

The purpose of the recall is to notify the customer or consignee that the product was not what it was purported to be. The most frequent causes of recalls from blood collection facilities are mistakes in viral marker testing, donor deferral issues, and donor suitability errors. Figure 14–3 depicts the types of recalls that CBER classified in fiscal year recalls for 1996. For example, a donor may admit to having been an intravenous drug user or to having traveled in an area endemic for malaria and the information was not used to defer the donor. This would result in a recall, which would be a notification to the transfusion service of the information.

The recalling firm is always responsible for conducting the actual recall by contacting its consignees by telegram, mailgram, or first-class letters with information that includes:

- The product being recalled
- Identifying information such as lot numbers and serial numbers
- The reason for the recall and any hazards involved
- Instructions to stop distributing the product and what to do with it

The FDA monitors the recall, assessing the firm's efforts in the notification process. Regulations and policy of the FDA require an inspection to review the complaint file, to review the records, to evaluate the corrective action plan, and to evaluate the recall strategy. When the decision is made by the manufacturer or collection facility to recall a product, the FDA district office should be notified, and the district office will send a "24-Hour Alert to Recall Situation," notifying CBER and the FDA's Division of Emergency Operations (DEO) of the recall. Recalls are published by the FDA in the weekly Enforcement Report. A recall is classified as completed or closed when all reasonable efforts have been made to remove or to correct the product. The local FDA district office notifies the firm when FDA considers its recall completed.

There continues to be discussion within the FDA and the blood bank community that the recall procedures are time consuming and should be revised to be tailored to the needs of blood banks and blood centers. It has been suggested that the time spent by the blood bank community and by the FDA on recalls that do not present a hazard to health could be better used by both groups.

### Warning Letter

When deviations from the regulations are documented during an inspection of a blood collection facility or a transfusion service, the violative conditions are documented by the FDA investigator. A report is written and reviewed in the local FDA district office by supervisory investigators and the compliance staff in the district. Any significant deviation from the regulations that indicates a failure to ensure donor protection and product safety, or that represents a continuing pattern of noncompliance, may result in the issuance of a warning letter by the local district office. Because the issuance of warning letters is no longer reviewed by the headquarters staff in CBER before issuance, there is no way to ensure consistent application of the regulations throughout the 21 district offices.

A warning letter is an indication from the FDA that the agency may invoke additional and more severe regulatory sanctions, such as injunction, license suspension, license revocation, seizure, or prosecution, without further notice. After a warning letter has been issued, a follow-up inspection will take place to determine whether corrective action has been taken by the establishment. If appropriate corrective action has not been taken, the agency will consider how best to achieve compliance with the regulations.

### License Suspension or Revocation

The suspension of a license prevents interstate shipment of all biologic products under the establishment's control by requiring immediate cessation of the authority to ship products across state lines. Suspension of a license is considered when conditions jeopardize donor health or product safety, and immediate corrective action is necessary. Suspension may also be an intermediate step to license revocation. Unlike license revocation, which is a lengthy procedure, suspension is a summary action that is very quick and effective in stopping the danger to public safety or health. This administrative action is a very powerful tool and is used with great caution.

The number of establishment license suspensions has remained in the range of 3 to 10 each year since 1977. Most of the license suspensions have involved plasma centers. Fewer than six blood establishments' licenses have been suspended from 1972 to 1997. In one of the blood centers, the FDA found that donors with repeat reactive anti-HIV tests were not placed on a deferral list and that some donors who admitted to intravenous drug use were not deferred as donors. License suspension by the agency is always accompanied by adverse publicity, leading to significant curtailment of overall activities by the firm and immediate correction of the violative conduct leading to the suspension. When suspension does not achieve the necessary corrective action, the next step usually sought by the FDA is a court-ordered consent decree.

### Seizure

Seizure is a civil action to condemn the products, to take custody of the product(s), and to remove them from distribution channels. This is not an effective remedy with blood collection facilities because of the short shelf life of blood and blood components. After seizure, the products may not be tampered with, except by permission of the federal court. The owner or claimant of the seized products is usually given 30 days by the court to decide on a course of action. If nothing is done, the product(s) will be disposed of by the FDA following the instructions of the court. The charges may be contested, and the case will be scheduled for hearings or trial. The owner of the product(s) is required to provide a monetary deposit (i.e., a bond to ensure that the orders of the court will be carried out) and must pay for the FDA supervision of any compliance procedure.

### Injunction

The traditional injunction used by the FDA is the prohibitory injunction. Once ordered by the court, this action prohibits the firm from operating *unless and until* adequate corrections are made and verified by the FDA. The effect of such action is significant and sometimes may result in the complete shutdown of the firm, except in a hospital environment where the firm's transfusion service would continue to process blood from outside sources.

The other type of injunction used by the FDA is a mandatory injunction, in which the court orders the affected firm to address certain specified conditions while the firm continues to operate. This allows a collecting facility to collect and to ship units of blood, thus not adversely affecting the supply of blood for a community.

Injunction is considered when there is a current health hazard or the establishment has a history of uncorrected deviations despite past warnings, and the evidence suggests that serious violations will continue. Injunction may be considered as a legal remedy when the establishment does not hold a U.S. license. If there is no license to suspend, this more formal mechanism is the only remedy left to obtain the needed corrective action. Injunction may also be the course of action with licensed facilities, as recent actions by the FDA indicate. Violations of an injunction are punishable as contempt of court. Any of these types of procedures may be used, depending on the circumstances. Since 1972, there have been approximately six injunctions of volunteer blood establishments, and all but one have been collecting facilities.

The first injunction against a blood bank was in 1972 and concerned a facility that did not hold a U.S. license. The injunction followed a cease-and-desist letter from the FDA commissioner. The FDA filed a complaint for injunction on July 23, 1975, and the firm signed a consent decree of permanent injunction on August 18, 1975. The inspections revealed deviations from GMP in the testing, storage, and use of expired reagents.

The second injunction was in 1979. This was a mandatory injunction, *United States vs John Elliott Blood Bank*. The charges were that the methods, facilities, and controls used for collecting, manufacturing, processing, testing, labeling, and distribution of Whole Blood and blood components failed to comply with current GMP regulations for drugs, found in 21 CFR 211.1 to 211.115 and the biologic products regulations found in 21 CFR 600.3 to 680.16.[13] In 1988, the American Red Cross (ARC) and the FDA entered into a voluntary agreement in which the ARC agreed to correct numerous deficiencies found during inspections in their blood centers. The agreement focused on defects in the ARC computer systems. This voluntary agreement did not correct the problems in the blood centers and resulted in a permanent injunction and consent decree issued by a federal court.

Recent injunctions have included ARC, United Blood Service, and the New York Blood Center. These recent injunctions all have elements in common in that they required a quality assurance unit and adequate training for employees. An important element of the requirement for training is an evaluation of competency. The effectiveness of the training must be measured. This is often an overlooked aspect of training.

## Prosecutions

When fraud, health hazards, or continuing significant violations are encountered, it is the FDA's policy to consider prosecution. Before initiating a prosecution, the FD&C Act in Section 305 provides that individuals be given an opportunity to present their views with regard to the contemplated action. Only under limited and defined conditions will the FDA consider proceeding with prosecution without issuing a notice (e.g., if the violations are fraudulent or if those responsible are likely to flee). Prosecution is a criminal action directed against a firm or responsible individuals or both. It is punitive with the view of punishing past behavior and obtaining future compliance. The courts take a dim view of willful violations of the law and have imposed significant sentences, including incarceration of responsible individuals. The points for evaluation are to determine: (1) whether an individual or the firm has demonstrated a *careless* or *reckless disregard* for the applicable requirements, (2) the seriousness of the violations, (3) the frequency of distribution and amount of violative product distributed, and (4) whether the firm has had a continuous pattern of violative conduct involving repeated significant deviations. Violations should be indicative of more than isolated or sporadic errors and should demonstrate a breakdown in a system that resulted in the release of unsuitable units (e.g., viral marker repeat reactive units).

## Good Manufacturing Practices

Good Manufacturing Practices ensure that products are consistently manufactured according to, and controlled by, the quality standards appropriate for their intended use. Good manufacturing practices encompass both manufacturing and quality control procedures. Quality standards and consistent application of these standards are essential to the quality of blood and blood components. Each unit of blood constitutes one "lot," and it is not feasible to perform quality control on each unit collected from a donor. The concepts are very different for drugs because a very large quantity of an individual drug is manufactured at the same time, in the same laboratory, with the same conditions, using the same raw materials for one lot. For blood products, the donor is the raw material, and, of course, each donor is an individual. Inasmuch as it would be impossible to perform quality control testing on each unit, it is imperative that no variance be allowed in the methods used for collection, storage, testing, and distribution of blood and blood products. Testing is not an end in itself and will not improve the process. Detecting errors after the fact is a costly process. Control of the process is the key to a successful manufacturing process.

The drug regulations found in Title 21 CFR Part 200 were written for manufacturers of pharmaceutical drugs and not for the manufacturer of blood and blood products. There is a notable difference between the language used in Part 200 regulations and that in Part 600. The regulations found in Part 600 specifically address procedures commonly performed in a blood bank, blood center, or transfusion service.

### Quality Assurance Unit

The drug regulations require that each firm must have a quality control unit, which in current terminology would be called a quality assurance (QA) unit. The current thinking of the FDA is that separate QA units are not required for such entities as a small transfusion service or a small blood bank. The expectation for larger facilities is that a separate QA unit is needed and, in fact, this is a major component in the FDA correspondence, such as notice of intent to revoke letters and in consent decrees. Figure 14–4 was used by the FDA to present an overview of the important areas of a QA plan. This could be accomplished in many different ways, such as using QA staff members, peers in other areas of the institution, or persons from other establishments to perform audits of the facility. Regardless of the size and complexity of the firm, establishments must commit time and resources to a quality

assurance program or plan. The structure of a QA unit must be decided by each facility. Allowing individuals within the establishment to perform QA functions may be necessary, but there has to be some separation of the activities.

The responsibilities of the QA unit are identified in the regulations as:

1. To review and to approve procedures, specifications, production records, and final release of the product. In the manufacturing of pharmaceuticals there are fewer lots of each product. One lot may represent a hundred vials or thousands of tablets. In a blood collection facility each unit is a lot. Blood products are traditionally processed in groups or tested as runs, and the concept of batch processing may be adopted in these situations. This concept has been successfully applied by some large collection facilities.

2. To analyze and test raw materials, bulk, in-process product, finished product, and postmarket stability. This language has to be modified when applied to blood collection facilities because the concepts and practices are different. In the drug manufacturing process, production stops and the QA unit tests the product. Necessary adjustments are then made to the batch or lot in process. Blood collection and testing are performed in stages. The donor card review be-

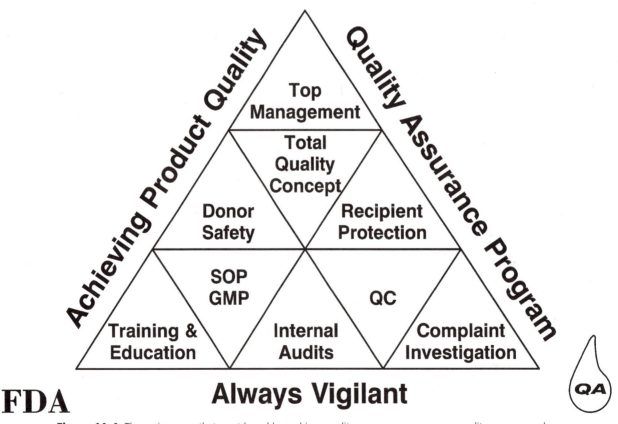

**Figure 14–4.** The major areas that must be addressed in a quality assurance program or quality assurance plan. SOP = Standard Operating Procedure, GMP = Good Manufacturing Practice, QC = Quality Control.

fore collection of the unit of blood, processing, compatibility testing, storage, and distribution are all significant steps in the process, which may be analyzed and tested.

3. To audit by reviewing procedures, records, complaints, and recalls, thereby determining compliance with GMPs and SOPs, and to provide findings to production supervisors. The audit is a very important function and may be met in a number of ways. In a small facility the audit could be performed by the hospital quality team or a supervisor in another section of the laboratory. Error reports should be evaluated to determine the root causes of the error, and SOPs should be changed when appropriate.

4. To review and approve SOPs, record-keeping systems, incoming materials, and equipment validation and maintenance programs. These functions are shared by drug and biologic manufacturers.

5. To monitor SOPs and reagents; verify production at critical control points; and monitor complaints, errors/accidents, and adverse reactions. The GMPs for blood and blood products address errors/accidents and adverse reactions. They require a thorough investigation with documentation.

6. To audit the systems at critical control points, determine compliance with SOPs and GMPs and reinspect for results of corrective actions. Evaluation of corrective action is often an overlooked part of the corrective action plan. The corrective action plan often states that employees will be retrained. The important link in the plan is to determine if the error was a human error or the result of a system that does not work well.

7. To maintain previous SOPs and labels, records or quality control and release testing, investigations of errors, accidents, adverse reactions, complaints, and internal reviews.

8. To review and approve training programs and employee position descriptions and to monitor employee training and performance. These activities are the core of a quality assurance plan. Training programs must be evaluated to determine whether the employees understand the instruction and are following the SOP.

For quality assurance to be an aid in protecting the safety of the nation's blood supply, there must be an understanding that work is a system and in a system no part stands alone.[14] All activities and functions are interrelated; therefore, the way to address a problem is to focus on processes, not individuals. Often solutions to errors are shortsighted and do not identify or remove the underlying causes. Juran and Fryna declare, "Two journeys are required for quality improvement: the diagnostic journey from symptom to cause, and the remedial journey from cause to remedy."[15] Directives for the diagnostic journey are outlined as:

- Use exact language to describe symptoms.
- Observe the defects firsthand and interact with those directly involved.
- Record and quantify data (develop graphic presentations of the data to detect relationship).
- Pick problems with the largest impact.
- Focus on the system because errors are not worker-controlled but system-controlled.
- Develop cause-and-effect diagrams.
- Test theories.

Quality standards should be reviewed annually to determine the need for changes in manufacturing or control procedures. This is required by regulation 21 CFR 211.180(e) of pharmaceutical manufacturers of drug products. The expectation for manufacturers of blood and blood products is that the following will be reviewed: adverse reaction files, fatality reports, complaint files, release of unsuitable products, recalls, error/accident files, product quality records, and returned product files. The review need not be limited to the records listed and should be modified by the individual establishment. The annual review required by 21 CFR 211.180(e) is not viewed as an audit, and records of these reviews may be requested during an inspection by the FDA.

It is not customary for the FDA to examine this review, but the FDA will expect to see evidence that the review has been conducted. The purpose of the review is to determine the need for changes in blood product specifications or manufacturing or control procedures. The re-

**Table 14–5.** Quality Assurance System

| | |
|---|---|
| Critical control point: | QA unit established separate from production |
| Key elements: | Objectives/policies |
| | Product specifications/validation |
| | Standard operating procedures/validation |
| | Training in assigned duties, QA and cGMP for every employee/competency |
| | cGMP/regulatory compliance |
| | Industry standards |
| Critical control point: | Quality control |
| Key elements: | Product testing |
| | Equipment testing |
| | Reagent testing |
| Critical control point: | Audits |
| Key elements: | Responsible personnel |
| | Systems working separately and collectively |
| | Thresholds (limits) |
| | Alert levels/action levels |
| | Written audit reports |
| | Report evaluation/data analysis |
| | Feedback |
| | Corrective action |
| Critical control point: | Equipment maintenance/repair |
| Key elements: | Preventative maintenance |
| | Routine/scheduled maintenance |
| | Maintenance records |
| | Qualification/validation after repair |
| | Repair records |

view would (1) demonstrate trends that could lead to the release of unsuitable product (e.g., decreasing yields in cryoprecipitated AHF, platelets, or deglycerolized red blood cells) and (2) demonstrate that corrective actions taken to prevent recurrence of errors and accidents and the release of unsuitable units are adequate, or to determine whether additional actions need to be taken.

The items listed as critical control points and key elements in the quality assurance guideline are intended to be used as a guide for establishing, enhancing, and assessing systems and process controls for the manufacture of blood and blood components. Table 14–5 lists the critical control points and key elements for a quality assurance system. The goal should be to develop systems that have controls that not only meet those listed in the guideline, as well as the regulations, but also exceed them.

A quality assurance plan is not a quick fix. It is a long-term commitment to improve the entire work process. For a quality plan to be successful, managers and employees must work together and be involved in problem solving.

Chapter 15 defines and describes how a quality plan may be implemented.

---

### SUMMARY CHART: IMPORTANT POINTS TO REMEMBER (MT/SBB)

- The FDA enforces regulations to ensure the safety and efficacy of biologics, drugs, and devices that include blood and blood components and diagnostic reagents used or manufactured by blood establishments.
- The PHS Act requires that any establishment that manufactures or prepares biologic products shipped in interstate commerce for sale, barter, or exchange must be licensed.
- Biologic products are defined as any virus, therapeutic serum, toxin, antitoxin, vaccine, blood, blood component or derivative, allergenic product, or analogous product applicable to the prevention, treatment, or cure of diseases or injuries in humans.
- The Current Circular of Information refers to a package enclosure with blood that provides instructions for use, indications, contraindications, side effects, and cautions as required by the FD&C Act.
- Facilities that do not routinely collect blood or do not prepare blood components are usually inspected under the auspices of HCFA, whereas facilities that collect their own blood on a routine basis are inspected by the FDA.
- The short supply provision allows unlicensed source material to be shipped interstate and to be used to manufacture a licensed product (e.g., Factor VIII).
- A license is not required to manufacture, distribute, relabel, pool, or repack Recovered Plasma derived from single units of expired or unexpired Whole Blood.
- The death of a patient must be reported to the CBER if it is deemed related to a transfusion that may have contributed to the fatality or a blood collection error that led to the demise of the donor.
- Product recalls are voluntary actions taken by the establishments, or as requested by the FDA, to remove violative products from the market or to correct product labeling.
- Seizure is a civil action to condemn the product, to take custody of the product, and to remove it from distribution channels.
- In a mandatory injunction, the court orders the affected firm to address certain specified conditions while the firm continues to operate; a prohibitory injunction halts all operations of the firm until adequate corrections are made and verified by the FDA.
- Current GMPs ensure quality standards of manufactured products for their intended use.

---

### REVIEW QUESTIONS

1. Which of the following is responsible for the safety of the nation's blood supply?
   A. Health Care Financing Administration
   B. Food and Drug Administration
   C. College of American Pathologists
   D. Joint Commission of Accreditation of Health Care Organizations
   E. Occupational Safety and Health Administration

2. Where are the regulations for blood and blood products published?

   A. The AABB *Technical Manual*
   B. CAP checklist for inspection of blood banks
   C. The *Federal Register*
   D. The Code of Federal Regulations
   E. State Inspectional Guidance Documents

3. What was the tragedy that prompted passage of the Public Health Service Act?
   A. Three patients contracted hepatitis C following transfusion.
   B. A child died following transfusion of hemolyzed red blood cells.
   C. A group O patient received group A blood.

D. Ten children died after receiving diphtheria antitoxin contaminated with tetanus.

E. Two patients had adverse reactions after DTP injections.

4. What is required to ship blood and blood products out of the state?
   A. AABB accreditation
   B. CAP certification
   C. State license
   D. HCFA certification
   E. U.S. license

5. A donor calls after collection of a unit of blood to notify the blood bank that he now has a cold. What is the appropriate action?
   A. Place the donor on the permanent deferral list.
   B. Notify the FDA of a recall of product.
   C. Notify the State Health Department.
   D. Send a summary letter to the CDC.
   E. Record the telephone call from the donor and follow the SOP.

6. If a blood center holds a U.S. license to ship blood, can the license number be placed on all of the products manufactured or prepared by the facility?
   A. Only after an inspection by FDA.
   B. Yes, following a successful prelicense inspection by FDA.
   C. No, only those products approved by FDA.
   D. Yes, if the facility is accredited by AABB.
   E. Yes, if the facility has received a state license.

7. When an employee notifies the supervisor of an error, what is the appropriate action?
   A. Follow the SOP that describes how to determine whether the safety of a blood product has been affected and document the error.
   B. Fire the employee.
   C. Retrain the employee.
   D. Counsel the employee.
   E. Call the local FDA office.

8. A patient died following transfusion of ABO-incompatible blood. To whom should this event be reported?
   A. The Center for Biologics Evaluation and Research
   B. The local FDA
   C. The Health Care Financing Administration
   D. The AABB Central Office
   E. The state department of health

9. Which federal group inspects a transfusion service that does not collect blood?
   A. Food and Drug Administration
   B. Centers for Disease Control
   C. Health Care Financing Administration
   D. Occupational Safety and Health Administration
   E. State health department

10. Following registration with the FDA a blood collection facility may ship blood:
    A. To transfusion services in the same city
    B. To facilities within the state
    C. To blood establishments in other states
    D. To transfusion services in other states
    E. As Recovered Plasma

## ANSWERS TO REVIEW QUESTIONS

1. B (p 311)

2. C and D (p 311)

3. D (p 311)

4. E (p 312)

5. E (p 316)

6. C (p 315)

7. A (p 323)

8. A and E (some state laws require reporting of fatalities) (p 317)

9. C (p 314)

10. B and E (p 314)

## REFERENCES

1. Code of Federal Regulations, Title 21 Parts 1-800, FDA. US Government Printing Office, Washington, DC, 1997.
2. Milestones in US Food and Drug History, an FDA Consumer Memo, HHS Publication No(FDA) 85-1063. US Department of Health and Human Services, FDA, Office of Public Affairs, Rockville, MD.
3. The Coroner's Verdict in the St. Louis Tetanus Cases. 1901 New York Medical Journal 74; Special Article: Fatal results from diphtheria antitoxin. Minor comments: Tetanus from antidiphtheria serum. JAMA 37:1255, 1260, 1901.
4. Brady, R, and Kravoc, DA: From diphtheria to cytokine productions: A remarkable scientific journey: An aging regulatory framework. Regulatory Affairs 3:105, 1991.
5. Timm, EA: 75 Years Compliance with Biological Product Regulations. Food Drug Cosmetic Law Journal, May 1978, Washington, DC, p 225.
6. Legislative History of the Regulation of Biological Products, US Department of Health, Education, and Welfare; Public Health Service, FDA Bureau of Biologics, Washington, DC, 1978.
7. Solomon, JM: The evolution of the current blood banking regulatory climate. Transfusion 34:3, 1994.
8. *Blank vs United States* 400 Federal Supplement and 302 (CA 5, 1968).
9. Gustafson, M: Presentation to FDA Blood Products Advisory Committee, March 1997.
10. FDA Compliance Program 7342.001: Inspection of Licensed and Unlicensed Blood Banks. Form FDA 2438f (8/90), insert TN 92-67, Washington, DC, August 3, 1992.
11. Tourault, MA: Fatality reports. AABB Newsbriefs 15:12, 1992.
12. Recall Nordenberg Tamar. FDA Consumer 27, October 1995.
13. *United States vs John Elliott Blood Bank:* Civil No. 79-1807 (SD FDA, 1979).
14. Gambino, R: Most laboratory errors are system dependent—not people dependent. Lab Med 20:123, 1989.
15. Juran, JM, and Fryna, FM: Juran's Quality Control Handbook, ed 4. McGraw-Hill, New York, 1988, p. 17.4.

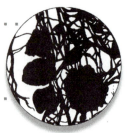

# CHAPTER **15**

# QUALITY IN BLOOD BANKING

Lucia M. Berte, MA, MT(ASCP), SBB, DLM, CQA(ASQ),
and Bonnie Lupo, MS, SBB(ASCP)

**OBJECTIVES**

*On completion of this chapter, the learner
should be able to:*

1 Describe the difference between compliance and
quality management.

2 List three building blocks of quality.

3 Describe the framework of a quality system for
both the blood bank and laboratory.

4 List 10 quality system essentials and the blood
bank operations to which they are applied.

5 Use a flowchart to describe a process or procedure.

6 State the role of validation in introducing a new
procedure.

7 Name at least five blood bank process controls.

8 Explain the causes of variation in a process.

9 Describe the difference between a form and a
record.

10 Explain the importance of document control for
procedures.

11 State the difference between remedial and
corrective action.

12 Describe the role of auditing in a quality system.

13 Identify at least six sources of input for identifying
processes to improve.

14 Define the four steps of a commonly used
problem-solving approach.

15 Explain how to transition a blood bank quality
system into one for the whole laboratory.

Several dictionaries define *quality* as "the degree of excellence." Blood banks must provide quality to their customers in many ways, including:

- Safe, satisfying donation experiences to blood donors
- Accurately labeled and tested blood components to transfusion services
- Timely, accurate transfusion services to physicians and other health care personnel
- Safe and efficacious blood transfusions to patients

To provide a high level of assurance of safe blood donation and transfusion practices to regulatory agencies, accrediting agencies, blood donors, physicians, patients, and patients' families, the following quality philosophy must be embraced by blood centers, hospital blood banks, and transfusion services:

1. Quality, safety, and effectiveness are built into a product.
2. Quality cannot be inspected or tested into a product.
3. Each step in the process must be controlled to meet quality standards.[1]

The method of bringing this quality philosophy into all its operations is for each facility to develop the building blocks of quality: quality control (QC), quality assurance (QA), and quality system (QS). When the building blocks are assembled and the facility's management staff is actively involved in the monitoring and maintenance of the quality system, quality management (QM) has been achieved. Figure 15–1 demonstrates the building blocks of quality and their internationally accepted definitions.[2]

## QUALITY MANAGEMENT VERSUS COMPLIANCE

Blood bank compliance with federal regulations and accreditation standards is required by the Food and Drug Administration (FDA),[3,4] the Joint Commission on Accreditation of Healthcare Organizations (JCAHO),[5,6] the College of American Pathologists (CAP)[7] and the American Association of Blood Banks (AABB).[8] Compliance programs are designed to evaluate how effectively the facility meets the requirements by searching for errors, deficiencies, and deviations. Compliance inspections measure the state of the facility's program with respect to the applicable standards at a single point in time and are usually conducted every 1 to 2 years. Although this process may seem logical, compliance programs alone are inadequate to find and to prioritize a facility's problems. Compliance simply requires the correction of identified deviations and deficiencies and usually leaves the facility with the false sense that it has solved its problems and has been brought into compliance. It should be no surprise, but usually it is, that the same deviations and deficiencies are often found in subsequent inspections. That is because the facility's current QC and QA programs do not identify the structural problems that underlie the devi-

| Quality Management | Activities of the management function that determine the quality policy | |
|---|---|---|
| Quality System | organizational structure, procedures, processes, and resources needed to implement quality management |
| Quality Assurance | planned, systematic activities implemented within the quality system to provide confidence that requirements for quality will be fulfilled |
| Quality Control | operational techniques and activities used to fulfill the requirements for quality |

**Figure 15–1.** The building blocks of quality.

ations and deficiencies. Remember that quality cannot be inspected into a process. Facilities must *prevent* deficiencies and errors.

Quality management, on the other hand, is actively and continuously practiced by the blood bank's leaders, managers, and staff. With QM, the blood bank is always ready for an inspection because it monitors its processes, knows where the problems are, continuously takes action to determine root causes of problems to remove them and to prevent recurrence, and documents its actions. In QM organizations, quality is everyone's job—all the time.

## QUALITY BUILDING BLOCKS

### Quality Control

Most blood bank technologists are familiar with routine blood bank QC procedures, such as daily testing of the reactivity of blood typing reagents; calibration of serologic centrifuges; and temperature monitoring of refrigerators, freezers, and thawing devices. Requirements for the type and frequency of QC are determined in regulations and accreditation standards, operator's manuals and package inserts, and some state and local requirements. Regular performance of QC reveals

when a method, piece of equipment, or procedure is not working as expected.

### Quality Assurance

Quality assurance is a set of planned actions to provide confidence that systems and elements that influence the quality of the product or service are working as expected individually and collectively.[9] Quality assurance looks beyond the performance of a method or piece of equipment at how well a larger process is functioning, particularly those processes that cross functional or departmental lines. For example, a blood center could monitor the number of times and reasons why a set of collected whole blood units transported from the collection site to the component processing site did not arrive in time or was not in an acceptable condition to make blood components. It is important to monitor in the transfusion service the source, number of times, and reason why specimens sent for compatibility testing were not acceptable to the blood bank. Table 15–1 lists common QC and QA activities practiced by most blood banks.[9,10]

### Quality Systems in Blood Banking

Beginning with a quality guideline published for blood banks by the FDA in 1995,[11] there has been a

**Table 15–1.** Common Blood Bank Quality Control Activities and Quality Assurance Indicators

| Quality Control Activities | Quality Assurance Indicators |
|---|---|
| *Whole Blood Collection Equipment*<br>Microhematocrit centrifuge | Number of donor forms with incomplete or incorrect information |
| Hemoglobinometers, cell counters<br>Apheresis equipment | Number and types of unusable units and blood components |
| *Blood Components*<br>Red blood cells hematocrit<br>Cryoprecipitated antihemophilic factor | Number of blood typing discrepancies in donors and patients<br>Number and reasons for invalid test runs |
| Platelet counts in units prepared from whole blood and apheresis | Number of and reasons for component labeling check failures |
| Granulocyte counts in units prepared by apheresis | Number and source of improper and incomplete requests for blood components |
| *Reagents*<br>Copper sulfate<br>Reagent red blood cells<br>Antisera<br>Test kits for donor disease marker testing | Number and location of patients without proper identification at time of specimen collection or transfusion<br>Number, source, and reasons for unacceptable specimens<br>Number of times wrong component or ABO was selected for crossmatch or issue |
| *Laboratory Equipment*<br>Rh view boxes<br>Heating boxes<br>Waterbaths<br>Thawing devices for blood components<br>pH meters<br>Centrifuges and cell washers<br>Blood irradiators<br>Refrigerator, freezers and platelet incubators<br>Blood warmers<br>Shipping containers | Number and type of transfusion complications<br>Number and reasons for testing turnaround time failures |

change in meaning, emphasis, and organization of quality activities. Accrediting agencies such as the JCAHO and AABB are modifying their quality requirements to resemble the quality models used in international manufacturing and service industries. These companies develop and maintain quality systems that are both more comprehensive and more coordinated than either QC or QA. A quality system provides a framework for uniformly applying quality principles and practices across all blood bank operations, starting with donor selection and proceeding through transfusion outcomes.

In its *Standards for Blood Banks and Transfusion Services*,[8] the AABB has defined 10 quality essentials for blood collection and transfusion service facilities and the blood bank operations to which they are applied. Table 15-2 is a list of the quality essentials and blood bank operations on which the AABB assesses blood banks in its accreditation program.

The next sections of this chapter discuss the blood bank's role and responsibilities in fulfilling quality system essentials. It should become apparent that the essentials of a quality system extend far beyond historic QC and QA practices. Figure 15-2 demonstrates the concept in a quality system of applying quality essentials across all blood bank operations.

## QUALITY SYSTEM ESSENTIALS

### Organization

The type and size of the organization determine the configuration of the blood bank's quality system. In hospitals, there is usually already an organization-wide quality function or department that prioritizes and coordinates quality projects, approves resources, and receives reports and information from all hospital

departments. The hospital-based blood bank or transfusion service must participate in blood bank quality-related activities, laboratory-wide quality initiatives, and the hospital's quality improvement program. The blood bank should state in writing its goals, objectives, and policies for each of the quality system essentials and relate them to the bigger laboratory and hospital quality goals. There should be an organization chart showing all relationships within the blood bank, the blood bank's link to the laboratory and hospital, and how it also links to the hospital's quality function.

A free-standing blood center must develop and manage the entirety of its quality system. There may be a quality council represented by top-level management from the various departments. The council develops the blood center's quality goals, objectives, and policies; develops the strategies for quality system implementation; provides resource support; prioritizes identified improvement projects; and provides support for crossfunctional process improvements. There may also be a quality steering committee composed of senior managers and department staff who operationalize the quality strategies and implement process improvements. The blood center must also have written policies for the quality system essentials.

### Personnel

Quality begins and ends with people. All the quality goals, objectives, and policies in the world do not ensure safe and effective blood components and transfusions unless the people involved in blood banking know how their job fits into the organization, are trained to know what to do, and do it right the first time, every time. Blood bank management must work with the human resources departments in blood centers and hospitals to define qualifications for all blood bank jobs and to write job descriptions that include educational qualifications, experience, and federal, state, or local licensing requirements, where applicable, so that qualified persons can be hired. Table 15-3 shows the major types of training that personnel should receive once they are hired. This training extends significantly beyond just the task specifics of a particular job. The competence of personnel to continue to perform their assigned job functions and tasks must also be periodically evaluated and documented. Competence assessment challenges can include direct observation of job task performance, review of records, and written, verbal, or practical tests.

### Equipment Calibration and Maintenance

There should be a process for installing new equipment and ensuring its proper functioning before it is used in daily operations. There must be schedules for calibration, preventive maintenance, and quality control with frequencies determined by laboratory regula-

**Table 15–2.** Quality System Essentials and the Blood Bank Operations to Which They Are Applied

| Quality System Essentials | Blood Bank Operations |
| --- | --- |
| Organization | Donor selection for allogeneic blood |
| Personnel | Collection of blood from the donor |
| Equipment | Preparation of blood components |
| Supplier issues | Testing allogeneic donor blood |
| Process control | Blood and blood component labeling |
| Documents and records | Storage, transportation, and expiration |
| Occurrence management | Apheresis |
| Internal assessment | Compatibility testing/component selection |
| Process improvement | Blood administration/Rh immune globulin |
| Facilities and safety | Investigation of adverse effects |
| | Autologous blood |
| | Information management/records |
| | Histocompatibility and organ transplantation |
| | Tissue storage and dispensing |
| | Hematopoietic progenitor cells |

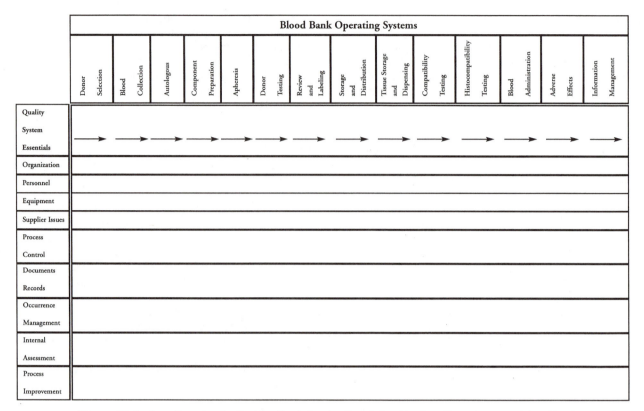

**Figure 15–2.** A quality system for the blood bank showing the relationship of quality system essentials to blood bank operations. (Courtesy Abbott Quality Institute, Abbott Park, IL.)

tions, accreditation standards, operator's manuals, frequency of use, testing volume, and equipment reliability. Instruments such as automated analyzers, readers, pipettors, and washers must also be installed and functioning properly before routine use. Defective equipment and instruments must be identified and repaired when necessary. Records must be kept of all installation, maintenance, and repair activities.

## Supplier Issues

In hospital-based blood banks and transfusion services, contract and purchasing issues are usually handled by the hospital's purchasing department. Blood bank personnel may or may not have control over the specific vendors with which the organization has contracts to purchase blood components and to test reagents, equipment, and other important supplies and materials. At a minimum, hospital-based blood banks and transfusion services must have a process by which incoming blood components and critical supplies (such as blood bags, reagents, test kits, and so forth) are received into the blood bank, inspected before acceptance, and, where required, tested before use.

Blood centers should have specified processes for selecting vendors of equipment, supplies, and services and for entering into and amending contract agreements. In addition, blood centers must also have a process for receipt, inspection, and testing (where required) of in-

**Table 15–3.** Training for New Employees Covers Much Important Information

| Orientation | Safety Training |
|---|---|
| Organization | Emergency preparedness |
| Department | Hazard communications |
| Section | Blood-borne pathogens/tuberculosis |
| | Radiation safety (where applicable) |
| | |
| Quality Training | Job-Specific Procedures Training |
| cGMP* | All SOPs performed in the job |
| Quality system | New SOPs |
| Team skills | Revised SOPs |
| Problem-solving tools | |

*cGMP: current good manufacturing practices.

coming critical materials (such as blood bags and virus testing kits), blood components (such as leukocyte-reduced platelets), and blood products (such as albumin, clotting factor concentrates, and immune globulins).

## Process Control

A *process* can be defined as a set of interrelated resources and activities that transforms inputs into outputs. *Process control* is a set of activities that ensures that a given process will keep operating in a state that is continuously able to meet process goals without compromising the process itself. *Total process control* is the evaluation of the performance of a process, comparison of actual performance with a goal, and action taken on any significant difference. Process control is a means to build quality, safety, and effectiveness into the product from the beginning. It is important to understand the steps of a process, write procedures when needed, test the process to be sure that it works before actual use, measure the process to see that it stays in control, and understand when and why the process has variations.

The FDA has published its requirements for process control as the current Good Manufacturing Practices (cGMP) that are cited in the Code of Federal Regulations (CFR).[3,4] The GMP require that facilities design their processes and procedures to ensure that blood components are consistently manufactured to meet the quality standards appropriate for their intended use.

### Flowcharting

Figure 15–3 is a stepwise flow of the elements of total process control. One of the best tools for understanding a process is to flowchart it. Flowcharting graphically represents the successive steps of a process and shows how inputs are converted into outputs. Flowcharts help to develop a common understanding of a process. Mapping current processes reveals bottlenecks, missing steps, decision points, dead ends, and choices that can lead to errors, delays, and unnecessary work. Mapping a new process facilitates understanding of where resources, human and other, will be needed for its successful accomplishment. Flowcharting can be done on paper or with commercially available software programs for personal computers. Figure 15–4 is a basic flowchart for modifying a unit of whole blood col-

lected in a main bag that has a satellite container. It illustrates different decision points and production choices.

### Standard Operating Procedures

A process usually involves a number of people and activities that take place over a period of time. From a process flowchart, specific procedures can be identified. Procedures are the steps taken, usually by one person who performs just one part of the larger process. For example, the process to provide a physician with a patient's ABO and Rh type involves ordering the test, collecting an appropriate specimen, delivering it to the laboratory, performing the test, and reporting the results. Across a span of time, different people may order the test, collect the specimen, perform the ABO/Rh test, and deliver the results. In this process, there should be specific written procedures for ordering tests manually or on the computer system, collecting and labeling the specimen, delivering the specimen to the laboratory, performing the ABO/Rh testing, and reporting the results.

### Validation

To ensure that new processes will work as needed, they must be validated before being put into use. Validation tests all elements of a new process to provide a high degree of assurance that the process will work as intended. For example, when a new test for a transfusion-transmitted disease (such as HIV antigen) is added to those performed on donated blood units, the new test method—with its associated instruments, test kits, computer functions, and procedures—must be validated in

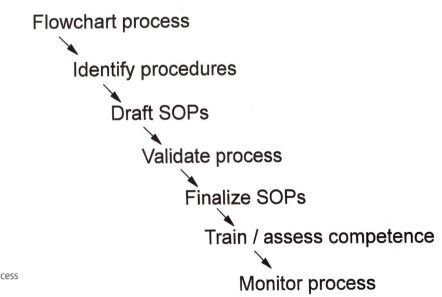

**Figure 15–3.** The steps within total process control.

## Separating Plasma From Whole Blood

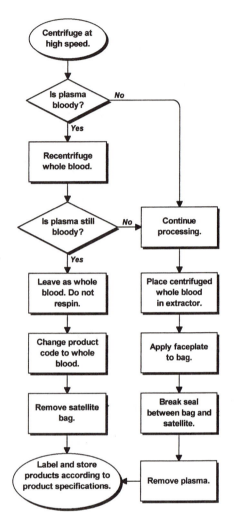

**Figure 15–4.** An example of a flowchart for processing a unit of whole blood collected in a double bag.

each blood bank that will perform the new test. The validation ensures that the new test will perform as expected with that blood bank's instrumentation, written procedures, personnel, and computer systems. The culmination of this validation process is a set of new procedures on which all personnel who will perform the new test must be trained. This training must be documented and personnel determined to be competent in the new test before it is performed on donated blood units, in this example.

### Process Controls

It is essential to monitor a process to ensure that it is performing as required, to correct process problems before they affect output, and to improve processes to meet changing needs and technology. Routine QC procedures, reviews of records, and capture of occurrences when the test did not perform as expected are routine

process control measures that monitor whether a process is functioning as needed.

Proficiency testing is another example of a process control. In proficiency testing, one laboratory's methods and procedures are compared with those of other laboratories for the ability to get the same result on a set of unknown specimens. Regulations require that all laboratories participate in proficiency testing for diagnostic laboratory testing. Blood bank proficiency test challenges include serologic testing for blood types, detection and identification of unexpected antibodies, compatibility of crossmatched blood, and tests for diseases transmitted through blood transfusion.

Other process controls include manual and automated steps to prevent the occurrence of errors. One common process control in serologic testing is the use of green-colored antiglobulin serum to ensure that the antiglobulin serum was indeed added at the antiglobulin phase of testing. Another common process control is the addition of IgG-coated reagent red cells after the antiglobulin phase reading to assure that the antiglobulin serum was indeed working. Computer process controls include automatic comparison of current blood type interpretation with the previous computer records on the same donor or patient to prevent ABO errors and warning signals when ABO-incompatible units are issued for transfusion.

### Process Variations

The performance of a process can vary from day to day, but not every variation is cause for concern. Some minor variation is normal and results from causes that are not easily controlled or changed but are predictable. Such common causes result from many factors, each of which may affect a process to a small degree but collectively have a minimal effect on the process outcome. Certain factors such as changes in the marketplace, sharper competition, and technological improvements may require that a normally functioning process be fine-tuned because the common causes are limiting competitive advancement. Only process redesign removes common causes.

At other times, variations that exceed certain statistically determined operating limits are the results of special causes. The reason for special causes must be quickly determined and corrected because the process is out of control. Special causes can usually be found and eliminated and include variations resulting from malfunctioning equipment, untrained personnel, and defective reagents or supplies.

Control charts and trend analysis tools offer ways to measure and to monitor a process and to determine whether the process is in or out of control. Laboratories have used control charts to monitor test assay performance for several decades. Standards or controls with known values are tested periodically and entered on a chart. Statistical calculations determine the upper and lower limits for the controls' values. Each time the controls are run, it is determined whether or not the process is in control. If the values plotted on the control chart do not exceed the upper and lower limits, then the process is said to be in control. When the values exceed the control limits, the process is considered out of control. An investigation is performed to determine the special cause, and the corrective action is taken and documented. Any tests associated with the out-of-range controls are repeated after the process is brought back into control.

Control charts can be used for any repeatable process that can be measured over time. Figure 15–5 is a sample of a control chart demonstrating upper and lower control limits and common and special causes of variation.

## Documents and Records

Documents are approved information contained in a written or electronic format. Documents define the quality system for external inspectors and internal staff. Examples of documents include written policies, process descriptions, flowcharts, standard operating procedures, forms, computer software, manufacturer package inserts, operator's manuals, and copies of regulations and standards. Records result from capturing the results or outcomes of activities and testing on written forms or electronic media such as manual worksheets, instrument printouts, tags, or labels. Both documents and records must be controlled to provide evidence that regulations and standards are met.

### Document Control

A structured document control system links a facility's policies, processes, and procedures. A typical document control system is structured as a pyramid, as shown in Figure 15–6. The following example best illustrates how a blood bank should link its policies, processes, and procedures.

A blood bank must have a QC program, according to federal regulations and accreditation standards for laboratories and blood banks. The blood bank should have a written policy document stating that it has developed a QC program that meets federal regulations and laboratory/blood bank accreditation standards. A second document should describe the process for the blood bank's QC program. This document describes how the blood bank uses the schedules and requirements of regulations, accreditation standards, operator's manuals, and test/reagent package inserts to determine what QC procedures to perform and when. Several standard operating procedures instruct staff members how to perform the details of QC procedures for equipment, test methods and reagents, and how to record and interpret the results. Manual worksheets and computer screens that are filled in at the time of performing the QC procedures are the records that provide evidence that the facility has a QC program and practices QC as it has described.

There needs to be a mechanism that controls identification, approval, revision, and archiving of a facility's policies, process descriptions, procedures, and related forms. This mechanism includes approved formats for writing SOPs, assigning document identification numbers with version designation, reviewing documents, preparing a master document list, and maintaining document history files. This mechanism is called change control and usually requires the completion and routing of a form that contains information about the reason for a new document or a change to an existing one. Other important change information includes when the change was requested, who wants the change, what other documents, if any, are affected by this change, and approval, training, and in-use dates. A master copy of the new approved version is added to the master file, which contains copies of all previous versions of that same procedure or form. The hard copies in this master file provide a paper backup when

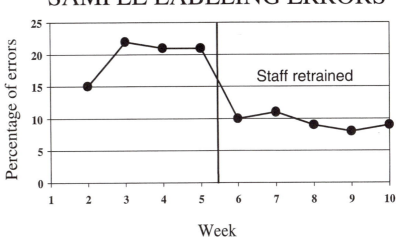

**Figure 15–5.** An example of a control chart used to monitor a process.

## Quality System Documentation

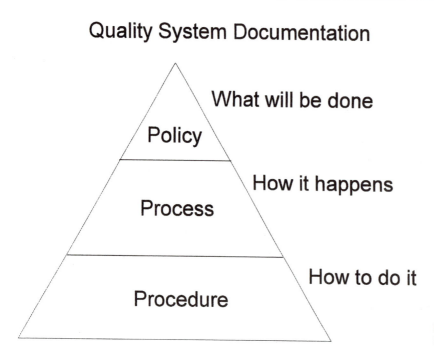

**Figure 15–6.** A simple structure for organizing quality system documents.

electronic files cannot be accessed. The master list is updated with the new version number. When a revised version of a current procedure is ready to be released, there must be control of the distribution process. Copies of the obsolete procedure in working manuals are to be replaced with the new version and then destroyed. Employees should not keep and refer to copies of procedures and forms stashed in lockers, drawers, and personal files. This helps to ensure that only the latest approved version of documents is available for use.

### Records Management

Forms are specially designed documents, either paper or electronic, on which are recorded the results or outcomes of a test or activity. Forms are also controlled documents. The document numbering system should link the form to its respective procedure. Instructions for completion of forms, when needed, can be conveniently placed on the back side of the form. When a form is completed, it becomes a record. Laboratory regulations and accreditation standards require the review of records by supervisory personnel and specify the type of records and length of time they are to be stored for any possible future reference. State, local, and facility requirements for record retention periods may also apply.

### Occurrence Management

Food and Drug Administration regulations require that blood banks report to them any error or accident in the manufacture of blood components that may affect the safety, purity, potency, identity, or effectiveness of the component or that compromises the safety of the blood donor or recipient. Each blood bank must have a process for detecting, reporting, evaluating, and correcting errors and accidents. Occurrence management is one name for such a process.

### Occurrence Reporting

Information about events involving the blood bank that deviate from accepted policy, practice, or procedure should be captured and acted upon. Hospitals usually have in place a risk management program, but this captures mostly information about events involving patients and visitors. An internal blood bank occurrence management system looks at events across the entire path of work flow for blood collection and transfusion service activities.

It is convenient to use the generic terms *occurrence* or *event* to describe an unexpected happening until it is further classified as an error, accident, or other facility-determined definition. Table 15–4 provides some definitions of terms used to further classify blood bank occurrences.

All employees are encouraged to participate in occurrence reporting. It is essential that occurrence reporting not be perceived by the staff as a tool for finger pointing or disciplinary action. Instead, it is important for everyone to understand that occurrences represent parts of the blood bank's process that do not work and thus provide opportunities for improvement. Occurrences may be identified either by staff in the course of routine activities or by supervisors during review of records. Information about all occurrences, including those identified before blood components are distributed or issued, is to be captured. In the reporting process, employees describe the who, where, and when and then briefly describe what happened and what they did at the time to alleviate the problem. A stan-

**Table 15–4.** Common Classifications of Various Types of Occurrences

| Occurrence Type | Definition |
| --- | --- |
| Accident | Occurrence generally not attributable to a person's mistake, such as a power outage or an aged instrument's malfunction |
| Adverse reaction | Complications that occurred to the donor during or after the donation process or to the recipient of transfused blood components |
| Complaint | Expression of dissatisfaction from internal customers (physicians, employees) or external customers (donors, patients) |
| Discrepancy | Difference or inconsistency in the outcomes of a process, procedure, or test results |
| Error | Occurrence attributable to a human or system problem, such as a problem from failure to follow established procedure or a part of a process that did not work as expected |
| Postdonation information | The receipt of information (call or letter) from a donor with additional details regarding his or her donation, such as subsequent illness or neglecting to mention an illness or medication |

dard report form can be used to capture information on all occurrences (Fig. 15–7).

### Investigation and Corrective Action

Supervisors and quality function personnel record the occurrences on a log or spreadsheet so that steps in the resolution process can be tracked. The occurrences are reviewed, investigated, and further classified as errors, accidents, or another definition.

The action initially taken to alleviate the immediacy of the situation is known as remedial action and is meant to be a quick-fix solution. Remedial actions do not address the real cause of the problem, which can be determined only through investigation. Investigation of complaints or errors provides an opportunity to identify factors that contributed to the problem. Process improvement tools (discussed later in this chapter) are used to identify the contributing factors and to determine the best way to remove them through implementing corrective action. Most corrective action involves making changes in the process. All employees performing that process must then be informed of the change and retrained when necessary. Sometimes the corrective action involves only retraining specific individuals who may not have been adequately trained initially or who have been taking unapproved personal deviations from established procedure.

The occurrence-reporting process must be clearly defined so that information is tracked and acted on and feedback is provided. The person responsible for the

quality assurance function in the blood bank (usually called the QA officer) reviews all occurrence reports, assigns an accession number, and forwards the occurrence form to the sections/departments that will be involved in the investigation. The completed report is returned to the QA officer, who reviews it for completeness and appropriateness of corrective action. If an identified error or accident must be reported to the FDA, the appropriate process is initiated.

In a good occurrence management program, occurrences are also linked to the specific processes in the blood bank's path of work flow. This information is trended, manually or with personal computer software, to determine which processes have the most problems. The trending information provides significant support for defending when processes need major changes. Facility staff must make a conscious decision not just to respond with remedial actions but to use occurrence information to take preventive action and to make improvements that truly contribute to the safety and efficacy of transfusion medicine.

### Internal Assessment

The blood bank should have an internal assessment process in place to monitor the effectiveness of its quality system continuously. See Figure 15–2 for a review of the quality system essentials applied to the blood bank path of work flow. Both the quality essentials and the facility's specific operations need to be assessed. Compliance inspection and other checklists[6,7,9] can be used; however, they assess the adequacy of only the listed items. The quality indicators monitored by hospital-based blood banks and transfusion services as part of the laboratory's quality assurance program are also helpful but do not usually cover all important aspects of each operation. Each blood bank should review all its processes and ask the question, What can we monitor on a scheduled basis to ensure that this process is working as needed? Quantitative indicators can then be derived for which the numerator is the number of times the process did or did not work and the denominator is the total number of times the process was performed. Common transfusion service examples include the percentage of specimens received in the compatibility testing laboratory that were not acceptable for testing and the number of times the transfusion service met its established turnaround time for emergency release of uncrossmatched blood to the emergency department. See Table 15–1 for additional examples of quality indicators.

Perhaps the best assessment tool is the performance of an internal audit. Unlike compliance inspections, audits review a specific facility process and determine by examination of documents and records whether the facility is meeting the applicable requirements. In a transfusion service, for example, an auditor could randomly select a unit number for a red blood cell component and track through each step involved in how the component was received, tested, issued, and trans-

# QUALITY ASSURANCE INCIDENT REPORT

ORIGINATOR    ACCESSION # _____    TODAY'S DATE _____

UNIT #(s) _____

DEPARTMENTS(s) _____

NAME OF ORIGINATOR _____

BRIEF DESCRIPTION OF INCIDENT (Attach additional paper, if needed) _____
_____
_____
_____

DATE SENT TO QA_____

INVESTIGATING DEPARTMENT_____

DATE RECIEVED _____ NAME OF INVESTIGATOR(s)_____

ADDITIONAL  DESCRIPTION OF INCIDENT _____
_____
_____
_____

INDICATE CORRECTIVE ACTION TO BE TAKEN  (Attach additional paper if needed) _____
_____
_____
_____
_____
_____

QUALITY ASSURANCE

SIGNATURE OF QA OFFICER _____DATE _____

_____REPORTABLE_____NON-REPORTABLE

DATE SENT TO REGULATORY (If Reportable) _____

REGULATORY AFFAIRS

DATE RECEIVED_____DATE INCIDENT REPORTED_____

**RETURN FORM TO RESPONSIBLE QA OFFICER**

**Figure 15–7.** Incident report form.

fused. The training and competence assessment records of each employee involved in handling the component are reviewed, as are the QC records for the storage refrigerator and the reagents, centrifuges, and heat blocks used in compatibility testing for that unit. The performance on the proficiency test most recent to the unit's testing is reviewed. Copies of procedures and forms used at the workstations for all testing and QC are examined to determine whether they are the most current version, according to the master list. Samples of records are reviewed for inclusion of all required information, interpretations, and required supervisory reviews.

For blood collection operations, a random donor name or number could be selected and the same

process repeated for the donation record, computer files, all related SOPs, training and competence records, component production records, serologic and disease marker testing records, and related QC, labeling, storage, and shipping records.

Audits should be conducted by personnel who have been trained to perform audits and to identify system problems. Auditors should not have responsibility for performing the procedures they are required to audit. In a hospital-based blood bank or transfusion service, there may be insufficient personnel to have a separate quality function, and the supervisor and/or senior personnel may have to perform some auditing activities. A free-standing blood center should have sufficient personnel to designate a QA officer and to separate the quality function from routine operations.

The auditor presents his or her findings to the appropriate management and operations personnel at the closing meeting on a form similar to that in Figure 15–8. The auditor may request corrective action for each finding. A process should be in place for the evaluation and review of the audit by management personnel to ensure that corrective actions will be implemented. The FDA requires that facilities prepare an annual summary of their audit findings and the corrective actions taken.

### Process Improvement

#### Identifying Opportunities for Improvement

Opportunities for improvement for both blood collection facilities and transfusion services can be identified from six main sources:

1. The occurrence trending process pointing to operational areas that are not functioning as well as intended.
2. Customer feedback either as complaints or solicited feedback, from internal (employee) customers and external customers whom the organization serves.
3. Information derived from monitoring quality indicators of operations, particularly when it is compared with peer groups in other institutions (a program known as benchmarking).
4. Internal audit feedback, whereby objective evidence collected by the auditor should support the facility's understanding of why corrective action is needed and should be taken.
5. Feedback from periodic compliance inspections. (However, if the blood bank is already seriously involved in the previous four activities, there should be little new information learned of which the facility is not already aware.)

## QUALITY ASSURANCE INTERNAL AUDIT

| Area/Function Assessed |  |
|---|---|
| **Subject Area** | **Date:** |
| **Key Positive Findings:** |  |
| **Key Opportunity Areas:** |  |
| **Recommendations for Improvement:** |  |
| **Auditors:** | **Date:** |
| **Response:** Planned Actions and Completion Dates |  |
| **Area Mgmt.:** | **Date:** |
| **Approved By:** | **Date:** |

**Figure 15–8.** Internal audit form.

6. Reports from other departments in the hospital's organization-wide quality committee function, such as nursing or emergency department problems in dealing with the blood bank.

### Using Teams

The hospital blood bank or laboratory's quality committee, or the blood center's quality council, should set priorities for the problems that need the most immediate attention. Many organizations have successfully used teams to solve problems or to design process improvements. Names such as process improvement teams, quality action teams, continuous improvement teams, and corrective action teams have all been used to refer to groups of people representing different parts of a given process who have been brought together to identify and to implement ways to remove the problem and to improve the process. Teams need good team skills to perform their assignments successfully. Members of teams should receive team-building and problem resolution training to ensure the most effective outcome for the time and resources expended.[12] Common team "dos and don'ts" are shown in Table 15–5.

### Problem Resolution

Many approaches to the problem-solving process have been published. Several consulting companies provide services for businesses, including hospitals, to learn problem-solving methods in their quality improvement programs. All the problem-solving approaches contain essentially the same steps of problem identification, prioritization, selection, analysis, data

**Table 15–5.** Process Improvement Teams Should Focus on Opportunities to Improve Work Processes

| Teams Should Improve Processes That Affect: | Teams Should Not Work on These Issues: |
| --- | --- |
| Quality of product | Problems governed by or directly related to union contracts |
| Quality and reliability of service to internal and external customers | Grievances and grievance procedures |
| Efficiency and accuracy of job performance | Seniority |
| Waste reduction, scrap, rework, and operating costs | Job assignments |
| Equipment performance, up-time, and reliability | Pay rates or benefits |
| Interdepartmental and intradepartmental communications | Job classifications |
| Improved process controls | |
| Safety, hygiene, and work environment | |
| SOPs and training | |
| Learning new skills, upgrading knowledge of the business, developing personal capabilities, team process | |

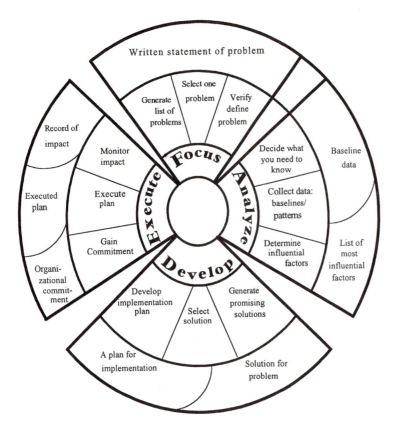

**Figure 15–9.** The FADE cycle. (From Quality Action Teams. Organizational Dynamics Inc., Burlington, MA, 1990, with permission. Copyright 1990, ODI, Burlington, MA.)

collection, identifying possible solutions, implementation, monitoring, and evaluation. Figure 15–9 depicts one such approach—the FADE cycle—to manage the problem-solving process that includes these main steps:

Focus on and define the problems
Analyze those problems
Develop realistic and worthwhile solutions
Execute new procedures and systems

A formalized problem-solving approach is just one piece of process improvement. Figure 15–10 illustrates the whole cycle that encourages continuous improvement.

### Facilities and Safety

In hospitals, the JCAHO mandates an environmental control program that addresses all significant environmental issues for facility management and maintenance such as temperature control, electrical safety, fire protection, and so forth.[5] The JCAHO also requires that hospital laboratories have training programs for all laboratory personnel on emergency preparedness, chemical hygiene, and blood-borne pathogens.[6] Therefore, hospital-based blood banks and transfusion services are already participating in facilities management and safety training. In addition, any blood bank that performs irradiation of blood components must also have a radiation safety program and document appropriate training.

Free-standing blood center facilities must develop their own facilities management programs. All regulations and accreditation standards for emergency preparedness, chemical hygiene, blood-borne pathogens, and radiation safety training and documentation also apply.

## A QUALITY SYSTEM FOR THE MEDICAL LABORATORY

By simply replacing the path of work flow for the blood bank in Figure 15–2 with the path of work flow for the hospital laboratory, a laboratory-wide quality system is derived (Fig. 15–11). All the quality system essentials on the left side of the figure remain the same because these quality elements are universal. A review of the ISO 9000 international quality standards demonstrates that blood bank/laboratory quality system essentials are included in the international standards.[2]

Therefore, all the discussion in the section on quality system essentials in this chapter applies equally to hospital laboratories. It is not only possible but also highly desirable to expand the blood bank's quality system building efforts so that the entire laboratory benefits from improved organization, coordination, and effectiveness of its many processes.[13–18]

## SUMMARY

Today, working in a quality system environment is a requirement, not a luxury, in achieving the standards of excellence necessary to survive the changes facing the

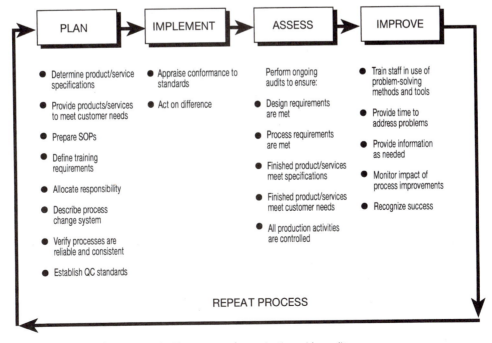

**Figure 15–10.** The process of organization-wide quality assurance.

| Laboratory Operating Systems | | | | | | | | | |
|---|---|---|---|---|---|---|---|---|---|
| Preanalytical | | | | Analytical | | Postanalytical | | Data Systems | |
| Test Requests | Specimen Collection / Labeling | Specimen Transport | Specimen Receipt / Processing | Testing and Review | Interpretation | Results Reporting | Post-Test Specimen Management | Laboratory Information System | Information Management |
| **Quality System Essentials** | | | | | | | | | |
| Organization | | | | | | | | | |
| Personnel | | | | | | | | | |
| Equipment | | | | | | | | | |
| Supplier Issues | | | | | | | | | |
| Process Control | | | | | | | | | |
| Documents | | | | | | | | | |
| Records | | | | | | | | | |
| Occurrence Management | | | | | | | | | |
| Internal Assessment | | | | | | | | | |
| Process Improvement | | | | | | | | | |

**Figure 15–11.** A quality system for the hospital laboratory. (Courtesy Abbott Quality Institute, Abbott Park, IL.)

nation's health care industry. Managed care companies want proof that health care providers such as hospitals and blood centers are involved in organization-wide quality improvement programs. Only those organizations demonstrating measurable quality improvements are approved for contracts for products and ser-

vices. The cultural change from QC/QA to a quality system takes time, and organizations that have not started must begin immediately to keep pace. Consumers of hospital and laboratory services accept no less than total quality. Organizations that provide less will not survive into the next century.

---

### SUMMARY CHART: IMPORTANT POINTS TO REMEMBER (MT/MLT)

- Blood bank compliance with federal regulations and accreditation standards is required by the FDA, JCAHO, CAP, and AABB.
- Compliance inspections measure the state of the facilities program with respect to the applicable standards at a single point in time and are usually conducted every 1 to 2 years.
- Quality control procedures in blood banking may include daily testing of the reactivity of blood typing reagents, calibration of serologic centrifuges, and temperature monitoring of refrigerators, freezers, and thawing devices.
- Quality assurance is a set of planned actions to provide confidence that systems and elements that influence the quality of the product or service are working as expected individually and collectively.
- A quality system provides a framework for uniformly applying quality principles and practices across all blood bank operations starting with donor selection and proceeding through transfusion outcomes.
- Process control is a set of activities that ensures a given process will keep operating in a state that is continuously able to meet process goals without compromising the process itself.

- Current Good Manufacturing Practices require that facilities design their processes and procedures to ensure that blood components are consistently manufactured to meet the quality standards appropriate for their intended use.
- Validation tests all elements of a new process to provide a high degree of assurance that the process will work as intended.
- Routine QC procedures, review of records, and capture of occurrences when the test did not perform as expected are routine process control measures that monitor whether a process is functioning as needed.
- Occurrence management is a name for a process that detects, reports, evaluates, and corrects errors and accidents.
- An internal audit reviews a specific facility process and determines by examination of documents and records whether the facility is meeting the applicable requirements.
- A process improvement team refers to a group of people representing different parts of a given process who have been brought together to identify and to implement ways to solve problems.

---

## REVIEW QUESTIONS

1. A quality system is:
   - A. Synonymous with compliance
   - B. Active and continuous
   - C. Part of quality control
   - D. An evaluation of efficiency

2. Quality system essentials are applied to:
   - A. Just the blood bank's management staff
   - B. Blood bank quality control activities
   - C. Only blood component manufacturing
   - D. The blood bank's path of work flow

3. Current Good Manufacturing Practices (cGMP) refers to:
   - A. Regulations pertaining to laboratory safety
   - B. Validation of testing
   - C. Occurrence reporting
   - D. Manufacturing blood components

4. Common causes of variation are:
   - A. Constant and controllable
   - B. Random and uncontrollable
   - C. Constant and uncontrollable
   - D. Random and controllable

5. The difference between a policy and a procedure is that:
   - A. A policy describes how the process happens
   - B. A procedure simply states what the facility will do
   - C. A procedure informs the reader how to perform a task
   - D. A policy can be flowcharted

6. A blank form is a:
   - A. Record
   - B. Procedure
   - C. Flowchart
   - D. Document

7. An example of a remedial action is:
   - A. Applying the FADE process
   - B. Starting a process improvement team
   - C. Addressing the immediate problem
   - D. Performing an internal audit

8. The FADE cycle is used for:
   - A. Problem resolution
   - B. Process control
   - C. Validation
   - D. Auditing

9. The difference between the blood bank and laboratory quality systems is that:
   A. The laboratory has a different path of work flow
   B. The blood bank does not include computer systems
   C. The quality system essentials are different
   D. The blood bank excludes testing

10. The quality system essentials for the blood bank quality system can be used for the laboratory because:
    A. The paths of work flow are identical
    B. Both the laboratory and blood bank experience accreditation inspections
    C. The quality system essentials are universal
    D. They are required by international standards

## ANSWERS TO REVIEW QUESTIONS

1. B (p 328)
2. D (p 329)
3. D (p 331)
4. B (p 332)
5. C (p 333)
6. D (p 333)
7. C (p 335)
8. A (p 339)
9. A (p 339)
10. C (p 339)

## REFERENCES

1. Food and Drug Administration, Center for Biologics Evaluation and Research: Guideline on General Principles of Process Validation. Food and Drug Administration, Rockville, MD, 1987.
2. International Organization for Standardization: ISO Compendium, ed 6. International Organization for Standardization, Geneva, 1996.
3. Food and Drug Administration, Department of Health and Human Services: Code of Federal Regulations Title 21, Parts 200–299. U.S. Government Printing Office, Washington, revised annually.
4. Food and Drug Administration, Department of Health and Human Services: Code of Federal Regulations Title 21, Parts 600–799. U.S. Government Printing Office, Washington, revised annually.
5. Comprehensive Accreditation Manual for Hospitals. Joint Commission on Accreditation of Healthcare Organizations, Oakbrook Terrace, IL, 1997.
6. Comprehensive Accreditation Manual for Pathology and Laboratory Services. Joint Commission on Accreditation of Healthcare Organizations, Oakbrook Terrace, IL, 1996.
7. Inspection Checklists for Laboratory Accreditation. College of American Pathologists, Northfield, IL, 1996.
8. Menitove, J (ed): Standards for Blood Banks and Transfusion Services, ed 18. American Association of Blood Banks, Bethesda, MD, 1997.
9. The Quality Program. American Association of Blood Banks, Bethesda, MD, 1994.
10. Edelman, B (ed): Accreditation Requirements Manual: Supplement to the 6th Edition. American Association of Blood Banks, Bethesda, MD, 1997.
11. Food and Drug Administration, Center for Biologics Evaluation and Research: Guideline on Quality Assurance in Blood Establishments (Docket no. 91N-0450). Food and Drug Administration, Rockville, MD, 1995.
12. Scholtes, PR, et al: The Team Handbook, ed 2. ASQC Press, Milwaukee, 1996.
13. Berte, LM, and Nevalainen, DE: Quality management for the laboratory. Lab Med 27:232, 1996.
14. Berte, LM, and Nevalainen, DE: Documentation pyramid for a quality system. Lab Med 27:375, 1996.
15. Berte, LM, and Nevalainen, DE: Writing standard operating procedures. Lab Med 27:514, 1996.
16. Berte, LM, and Nevalainen, DE: Self-assessment in a quality system. Lab Med 27:655, 1996.
17. Berte, LM, et al: A quality system for the medical laboratory. J Lab Med 21:44, 1997.
18. Nevalainen, DE, and Berte, LM: Pounding the drum for quality: A new beat. CAP Today 11:10, 1997.

## BIBLIOGRAPHY

Berle, LM (ed): Transfusion Service Manual of SOPs, Training Guides and Competence Assessment Tools, ed 1. American Association of Blood Banks, Bethesda, MD, 1996.
Clinical Laboratory Technical Procedure Manual, ed 3. Approved guideline GP2A-3. NCCLS, Wayne, PA, 1996.
Galloway, D: Mapping Work Processes. ASCQ Press, Milwaukee, 1994.
Nevalainen, DE, and Berte, LM: Training, Verification and Assessment: Keys to Quality Management. Clinical Laboratory Management Association, Malvern, PA, 1993.
Nevalainen, DE and Callery, MF: Quality Systems in the Blood Bank and Laboratory Environment. American Association of Blood Banks, Bethesda, MD, 1994.
Robbins, J (ed): The Quality Program, ed 1. American Association of Blood Banks, Bethesda, MD, 1994.
Tague, NR: The Quality Toolbox. ASQC Press, Milwaukee, 1995.
Training Verification for Laboratory Personnel, ed 1. Approved guideline GP21-A. NCCLS, Wayne, PA, 1995.

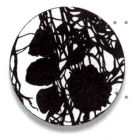

# CHAPTER 16

# TRANSFUSION THERAPY

Melanie S. Kennedy, MD, and Aamir Ehsan, MD

## OBJECTIVES

*On completion of this chapter, the learner should be able to:*

1 Describe the blood components currently available for therapeutic use.

2 Discuss the composition of each blood component and product, including the approximate volume of each product.

3 Select the appropriate blood product for patients with specific disorders.

4 State the expected incremental increase of a patient's:

   a. Hematocrit following transfusion of each unit of packed red cells.

   b. Platelet count following transfusion of each unit of platelets.

5 List the required procedures to prepare each blood component for transfusion.

6 Compare and contrast the two types of filters used for blood transfusion.

7 List the groups of recipients at highest risk of infection from transfusion of cytomegalovirus-positive red blood cells or platelets.

8 Discuss the role of irradiation in the prevention of posttransfusion graft-versus-host disease.

9 State the purpose of the maximum surgical blood order schedule.

10 State the main advantage of autologous transfusion.

11 Review the most important factors to consider when emergency transfusion is indicated.

12 Define *massive transfusion*.

13 Differentiate the various transfusion requirements of oncology and transplantation patients.

14 Compare and contrast hemophilia A and von Willebrand's disease.

15 State the respective blood components of choice for treatment of von Willebrand's disease and hemophilia A.

16 Specify the steps involved in the proper administration of blood.

## BLOOD COMPONENTS

Blood and blood components are considered drugs because of their use in treating diseases. As with drugs, adverse effects may occur, necessitating careful consideration of therapy. The transfusion of blood cells is also transplantation, in that the cells must survive and function after transfusion to have a therapeutic effect. The transfusion of red blood cells (RBCs) is the best-tolerated form of transplantation, but it may cause rejection, as in a hemolytic transfusion reaction. The rejection of platelets, as shown by refractoriness to platelet transfusion, is relatively common in multiply transfused patients.

Transfusion therapy is used primarily to treat two conditions: inadequate oxygen-carrying capacity because of anemia or blood loss, and insufficient coagulation proteins to provide adequate hemostasis. Each patient requires an individualized plan reflecting the patient's changing clinical condition, anticipated blood loss, capacity for compensatory mechanisms, and laboratory results. Some patients do not require transfusion, even in anemia or thrombocytopenia, because their clinical conditions are stable and they have little or no risk of adverse outcomes. An example is a patient with iron-deficiency anemia with minor symptoms.

Component therapy is the transfusion of the specific component needed by the patient. By using blood components, we can treat several patients with the blood from one donor, giving optimal use of every donation of blood. Table 16–1 is a summary of the blood components and products discussed in this chapter.[1,2]

### Whole Blood

The blood collected from a donor is considered whole blood; however, when it is circulating in the donor's blood vessels it is not "whole blood." Instead, whole blood is the donor blood mixed with the anticoagulant and preservative solution, and thus diluted in the proportion of eight parts of blood to one part anticoagulant. The citrate in the anticoagulant chelates ionized calcium, preventing activation of the coagulation system. The glucose, adenine, and phosphate (if present) serve as substrates for RBC metabolism during storage (see Chapter 1).

With the use of component therapy, the use of whole blood is limited to a few clinical conditions. Whole blood should be used to replace the loss of both RBC mass and plasma volume.[1,2] Thus, rapidly bleeding patients can receive whole blood, although most commonly RBCs are used and are equally effective clinically.

A definite contraindication to the use of whole blood is severe chronic anemia. Patients with chronic anemia have a reduced amount of RBCs but have compensated by increasing their plasma volume to restore their total blood volume. Thus, these patients do not need the plasma in the whole blood and, in fact, may adversely respond to the unneeded plasma by developing pulmonary edema and heart failure. This volume overload is more likely to occur in patients with kidney failure or pre-existing heart failure.

For the typical 70-kg (155-lb) human, each unit of whole blood should increase the hematocrit 3 to 5 percent or hemoglobin 1 to 1.5 g/dL. After transfusion, the increase may not be apparent for 48 to 72 hours while the patient's blood volume adjusts to normal. For example, a patient with a 5000-mL blood volume and 25 percent hematocrit has 1250 mL of RBCs. With

**Table 16–1.** Blood Components and Plasma Derivatives

| Component or Product | Composition | Approximate Volume | Indications |
|---|---|---|---|
| Whole blood | RBC (approx. Hct 40%); plasma; WBC; platelets | 500 mL | Increase both red cell mass and plasma volume (WBC and platelets not functional; plasma deficient in labile clotting factors V, VIII) |
| Red blood cells | RBC (approx. Hct 75%); reduced plasma, WBC, and platelets | 250 mL | Increase red cell mass in symptomatic anemia (WBC and platelets not functional) |
| Red blood cells, adenine—saline added | RBC (approx. Hct 60%); reduced plasma, WBC, and platelets; 100 ml of additive solution | 330 mL | Increase red cell mass in symptomatic anemia (WBC and platelets not functional) |
| Leukocyte-reduced RBCs (prepared by filtration) | >85% original volume of RBC; <5 × 10^6 to <5 × 10^8 WBC; few platelets; minimal plasma | 225 mL (Varies) | Increase red cell mass; < 5 × 10^8 WBC to prevent febrile reactions due to leukocyte antibodies; < 5 × 10^6 WBC to decrease the likelihood of alloimmunization to leukocyte or HLA antigens or CMV transmission |
| Washed RBCs | RBC (approx. Hct 75%); <5 × 10^8 WBC; no plasma | 180 mL | Increase red cell mass; reduce risk of allergic reactions to plasma proteins |
| RBCs frozen/deglycerolized | RBC (approx. Hct 75%); <5 × 10^8 WBC; no platelets; no plasma | 180 mL | Increased red cell mass; minimize febrile or allergic transfusion reactions; use for prolonged RBC blood storage |
| Granulocytes, pheresis | Granulocytes (>1.0 × 10^10 PMN/unit); lymphocytes; platelets (>2.0 × 10^11/unit); some RBCs | 220 mL | Provide granulocytes for selected patients with sepsis and severe neutropenia (<500 PMN/μL) |
| Platelet, concentrate (random donor) | Platelets (>5.5 × 10^10/unit); RBC; WBC; plasma | 50 mL | Bleeding due to thrombocytopenia or thrombocytopathy |
| Plateletpheresis | Platelets (>3 × 10^11/unit); RBC; WBC; plasma | 300 mL | Same as platelet concentrate; sometimes HLA-matched or platelet cross-matched |
| Leukocyte-reduced platelets | Platelets (as above); <5 × 10^6 to 5 × 10^8 WBC per final dose of platelets | 300 mL | Same as platelet concentrate; <5 × 10^6 WBC to decrease the likelihood of alloimmunization to leukocyte or HLA antigens or CMV transmission |
| Fresh frozen plasma | Plasma; all coagulation factors; complement (no platelets) | 220 mL | Treatment of some coagulation disorders |
| Plasma | Plasma; stable clotting factors; no platelets | 220 mL | Treatment of stable clotting factor deficiencies (II, VII, IX, X, XI) |
| Cryoprecipitated AHF | Fibrinogen; factors VIII and XIII, von Willebrand's factor | 15 mL | Deficiency of fibrinogen; factor XIII, second choice in treatment of hemophilia A, and von Willebrand's disease |
| Factor VIII (concentrates; recombinant human factor VIII) | Factor VIII; trace amount of other plasma proteins (products vary in purity) | 25 mL | Hemophilia A (factor VIII deficiency); von Willebrand's disease (selected products only) |
| Factor IX complex, factor IX concentrate | Factor IX; trace amount of other plasma proteins (products vary in purity) | 25 mL | Hereditary factor II, IX, or X deficiency, factor VIII inhibitor |
| Anti-inhibitor coagulation complex | Factor VIII inhibitor bypassing activity (FEIBA) | 30 mL | Patients with antibody to factor VIII (note: indications for use not well-established) |
| Albumin/plasma protein fraction | Albumin, some α, β globulins (5% or 25%) | Varies | Volume expansion; fluid mobilization |
| Immune globulin | IgG antibodies; preparations for IV and/or IM use | Varies | Treatment of hypoglobulinemia or agammaglobulinemia; disease prophylaxis; immune thrombocytopenia (IV preparations only) |
| Rh immune globulin | IgG anti-D; preparations for IV and/or IM use | 1 mL | Prevention of hemolytic disease of the newborn due to D antigen; treatment of the auto-immune thrombocytopenia (IV preparations only) |
| Antithrombin III | Antithrombin III; trace amount of other plasma proteins | 10 mL | Treatment of antithrombin III deficiency |
| Alpha₁-proteinase inhibitor (PI) | Alpha₁-PI (alpha₁-antitrypsin); other plasma proteins | Varies | Congenital deficiency of alpha₁-PI with evidence of panacinar emphysema |

*Source:* Lane, T (ed): Blood Transfusion Therapy: A Physician's Handbook. American Association of Blood Banks, Bethesda, MD, 1966, pp 4–5, with permission.

transfusion of 500 mL whole blood, the blood volume will be 5500 mL, or 26.4 percent hematocrit. When the patient's blood volume readjusts to 5000 mL, the hematocrit will be 29 percent (1450 mL divided by 5000 mL). The increase is greater in a smaller person and less in a larger one.

## Red Blood Cells

Red blood cells are indicated for increasing the RBC mass in patients who require increased oxygen-carrying capacity.[1,2] These patients typically have pulse rates greater than 100 beats per minute; respiration rates greater than 30 breaths per minute; and may experience dizziness, weakness, angina (chest pain), and difficulty thinking. The decreased RBC mass may be caused by decreased bone marrow production (leukemia or aplastic anemia), decreased RBC survival (hemolytic anemia), or surgical or traumatic bleeding.

The human body compensates for anemia by increasing plasma volume, increasing heart rate, increasing respiratory rate, and increasing oxygen extraction from the red blood cells. Normally only about 25 percent of the oxygen is extracted, but with increased demand at the organ and tissue level up to 50 percent of the oxygen can be extracted. When the demand exceeds 50 percent of the oxygen content, the compensatory mechanisms fail, and the patient requires transfusion.

There are no set hemoglobin levels that indicate a need for transfusion. Although the level of 8 g/dL has been used for many years for surgical and leukemic patients, the critical level is 6.0 g/dL or lower, except for patients with heart, lung, or cerebral vascular disease.[3,4] Most renal dialysis patients can tolerate 6 g/dL. In fact, healthy individuals could tolerate hemoglobin levels as low as 5.0 g/dL with minimal effects,[4,5] especially if they are placed at bed rest or at decreased levels of activity. Consensus committees suggest trigger values of hemoglobin of less than 6.0 g/dL in the absence of disease and between 8 and 10 g/dL with disease.[6]

Transfusion of RBCs is contraindicated in patients who are well compensated for the anemia, such as those with chronic renal failure. Red blood cells should not be used to treat nutritional anemia, such as iron-deficiency or pernicious anemia, unless the patient shows signs of decompensation (need for increased oxygen-carrying capacity). Red blood cell transfusion is not to be used to enhance general well-being, promote wound healing, prevent infection, expand blood volume when oxygen-carrying capacity is adequate, or prevent future anemia.

Each unit of transfused RBCs is expected to increase the hemoglobin 1 to 1.5 g/dL and the hematocrit 3 to 5 percent in the typical 70-kg (155-lb) human, the same as whole blood. The increase in hemoglobin and hematocrit is evident more quickly than with 1 unit of whole blood, because the adjustment in blood volume is less. In the previous example, the RBC volume would be increased the same, to 1450 mL, but the blood vol-

ume is increased only 300 mL to 5300 mL. The hematocrit is increased immediately to 27.2 percent.

Red blood cells prepared with additive solutions such as additive solution 1 (AS-1) have greater volume than with citrate-phosphate-dextrose (CPD) or citrate-phosphate-dextrose-adenine (CPDA-1), 330 mL versus 250 to 275 mL (see Chapter 1), but the AS-1 unit has less plasma. The RBC mass is the same. Therefore, the hematocrit differs from 70 to 80 percent for CPDA-1 red cells to 55 to 60 percent for AS-1 red cells. The shelf life for CPD RBCs is 21 days; for CPDA-1, 35 days; and for AS-1, 42 days (Table 16–2). AS-1, containing no protein and a minimal amount of oncotic material (mannitol), is quickly eliminated from the body. Neonatal exchange transfusion is generally performed using CPDA-1 anticoagulated blood because of inadequate knowledge about AS-1 and the function of the neonate's cardiovascular and renal systems.

## Leukocyte-Reduced Red Blood Cells

The average unit of RBCs contains approximately $2 \times 10^9$ leukocytes. Donor leukocytes can cause febrile-nonhemolytic transfusion reactions, human leukocyte antigen (HLA) alloimmunization, transfusion-related acute lung injury (TRALI), transfusion-associated graft-versus-host disease (TA-GVHD), and transfusion-related immune suppression. In addition, leukocytes may harbor cytomegalovirus (CMV), Epstein-Barr virus (EBV), human immunodeficiency virus (HIV), or human T lymphotropic virus (HTLV). For these reasons, considerable research has investigated these complications and the reduction of leukocytes in blood components in the attempt to prevent these complications.[7–9]

Reducing the leukocyte content to less than $5 \times 10^8$ prevents most febrile-nonhemolytic transfusion reactions.[10] For the other complications, the leukocyte content must be reduced to less than $5 \times 10^6$, which can be achieved by using one of several third-generation leukocyte reduction filters.[10] With these filters, most blood components are less than $1 \times 10^6$; many are $1 \times 10^4$.

## Washed Red Blood Cells and Frozen/Deglycerolized Red Blood Cells

Patients who have severe allergic (anaphylactic) transfusion reactions to ordinary units of RBCs may benefit from receiving washed RBCs.[1] The washing process removes plasma proteins, the cause of most al-

**Table 16–2.** Red Blood Cell Shelf Life

| Additive Solution | Days |
| --- | --- |
| CPD | 21 |
| CPDA-1 | 35 |
| AS-1 | 42 |

CPD = citrate-phosphate-dextrose; CPDA-1 = citrate-phosphate-dextrose-adenine; AS-1 = Adsol.

lergic reactions. Washed RBCs are used for the rare patient with IgA deficiency and anti-IgA antibodies.

Freezing RBCs allows the long-term storage of rare blood donor units, autologous units, and units for special purposes, such as intrauterine transfusion. Because the process needed to deglycerolize the RBCs removes nearly all leukocytes and plasma, these units, although more expensive, can be used interchangeably with washed RBCs. The 24-hour outdate of washed or deglycerolized RBCs severely limits the use of these components. The expected hematocrit increase for washed or deglycerolized RBCs is the same as that for regular RBC units.

## Platelet Concentrate and Plateletpheresis

Platelets are essential for the formation of the primary hemostatic plug and maintenance of normal hemostasis. Patients with severe thrombocytopenia (low platelet count) or abnormal platelet function may have petechiae, ecchymoses, and mucosal or spontaneous hemorrhage. The thrombocytopenia may be caused by decreased platelet production (e.g., after chemotherapy for malignancy) or increased destruction (e.g., disseminated intravascular coagulation [DIC]). Massive transfusion, which is discussed later in this chapter, may also cause thrombocytopenia because of the rapid use of platelets for hemostasis and the dilution of the platelets by resuscitation fluids and stored blood.

Platelet transfusions are indicated for patients who are bleeding because of thrombocytopenia (Table 16–3) or, in a few cases, owing to abnormally functioning platelets.[11] In addition, platelets are indicated prophylactically for patients who have platelet counts under 20,000/μL.

Each unit of platelet concentrate should increase the platelet count 5000 to 10,000/μL in the typical 70-kg human. Each unit of platelet concentrate must contain at least $5.5 \times 10^{10}$ platelets.[12] Pools of 4 to 6 units, then, will contain roughly $3 \times 10^{11}$ platelets. Massive splenomegaly, high fever, sepsis, disseminated intravascular coagulation, and platelet or HLA antibodies can cause less than expected platelet count increment and survival. The 1-hour posttransfusion platelet count increment is less affected by splenomegaly, high fever, and DIC than by the presence of platelet or HLA antibodies.[13] If the 1-hour increment is less than 50 percent of that expected on two occasions, the patient is considered refractory and should be screened for HLA antibodies or platelet antibodies.[14] If the HLA antibody screen is positive, the patient can be typed for HLA anti-

gens. An HLA-compatible or platelet-crossmatched donor can then be selected for platelet donation by apheresis.

A plateletpheresis component is prepared from one donor and must contain a minimum of $3 \times 10^{11}$ platelets.[12] One plateletpheresis component is equivalent to one dose of random platelet concentrates (e.g., a pool of 4 to 6 units). Components procured by apheresis can be given as random products, platelet crossmatched, or, because of their HLA types, as HLA-matched products.

A corrected count increment using a 1-hour postinfusion platelet count can provide valuable information about patient response to a platelet component.[13] The platelet count increment is corrected for differences in body size so that more reliable estimates of expected platelet increment can be determined.[14] The minimum expected corrected platelet increment is 10,000/μL per $m^2$. One formula for corrected count increment is

$$\frac{\text{Absolute platelet increment/μL} \times \text{body surface area (m}^2)}{\text{Number of platelets transfused (10}^{11})}$$

in which the absolute platelet increment is the posttransfusion platelet count minus the pretransfusion platelet count, the body surface area is expressed as square meters, and the number of platelets transfused is determined by multiplying the number of units (bags) of platelets by 0.55 (the number of platelets in each unit of concentrate expressed in $10^{11}$).

For example, a patient with 10,000/μL platelet count has a body surface area of 1.3 $m^2$. Six units of platelets are given. The 1-hour posttransfusion platelet count is 50,000/μL. Put these into the formula:

$$\frac{(50,000/\text{μL} - 10,000/\text{μL}) \times 1.3}{6 \text{ units} \times 0.55/\text{unit}} = 15,758/\text{μL}$$

The answer shows that the patient has a good increment ($>$10,000/μL) and is not refractory to platelets. An answer of less than 5000/μL indicates refractoriness. The formula can be used for plateletpheresis by using 3 (times $10^{11}$) as the number of platelets in each unit.

In addition to HLA and platelet-specific antigens, ABO antigens are also expressed on the platelet membrane. Often platelets are selected for transfusion without regard to ABO; however, group O recipients may have a lower increment when given group A platelets than when group identical platelets are selected.[15] Group A, B, and AB patients may also develop a positive direct antiglobulin test owing to passive transfer of anti-A, anti-B, or anti-A,B when several ABO-incompatible platelet transfusions are given.

Although platelet membranes do not express Rh antigens, platelet concentrates contain small amounts of RBCs and so can immunize patients to Rh antigens. Rh immune globulin can be given to girls and women of childbearing age to prevent Rh sensitization. Each 300-μg vial is adequate for 30 platelet concentrates or three plateletpheresis.

**Table 16–3.** Indications for Platelet Transfusion

Thrombocytopenia
Chemotherapy for malignancy (decreased production, <20,000/μL)
DIC (increased destruction, <50,000/μL)
Massive transfusion (platelet dilution, <50,000/μL)

DIC = disseminated intravascular coagulation.

For the same reasons as RBCs, platelet components may also be leukocyte-reduced or washed. Special filters are available.[16] Washing platelet components removes some platelets as well as plasma proteins and is an open method, requiring a 4-hour expiration time. Therefore, platelet components should be washed only to prevent severe allergic reactions.

## Granulocytapheresis and Buffy Coat

Patients who have received intensive chemotherapy for leukemia or bone marrow transplant, or both, may develop severe neutropenia and serious bacterial or fungal infection. Without neutrophils (granulocytes), the patient may have difficulty controlling an infection even with appropriate antibiotic treatment. Criteria have been developed to identify patients who are most likely to benefit from granulocyte transfusions: fever, neutrophil counts less than 500/μL, septicemia or bacterial infection unresponsive to antibiotics, reversible bone marrow hypoplasia, and a reasonable chance for patient survival.[1] Prophylactic use of granulocyte transfusions is of doubtful value for those patients who have neutropenia but no demonstrable infection.

Newborn infants may develop overwhelming infection with neutropenia because of their limited bone marrow reserve for neutrophil production. In addition, neonatal neutrophils have impaired function. Recent studies have shown granulocyte transfusions to be beneficial for these patients.[17] Buffy coats prepared from a unit of fresh whole blood are also effective.

For an adult, the usual dose is one granulocytapheresis product daily for 4 or more days. For neonates, a buffy coat or a granulocytapheresis unit is usually given once or twice.

Granulocyte components should be administered as soon as possible and within 24 hours of collection.[18] In most instances, the granulocyte components need to be crossmatched because of a significant content of RBCs.[18] The patient must be followed for resolution of symptoms and clinical evidence of efficacy, inasmuch as the granulocyte count will not noticeably increase in response to infusion of this component.

## Fresh Frozen Plasma

Fresh frozen plasma contains all coagulation factors. Fresh frozen plasma can be used to treat multiple coagulation deficiencies occurring in patients with liver failure, DIC, vitamin K deficiency, warfarin toxicity, or massive transfusion.[19,20]

Vitamin K deficiency or warfarin toxicity should be treated with vitamin K infusion (intravenously or intramuscularly) if liver function is adequate and if enough time exists before a major or minor hemostatic challenge such as surgery. Fresh frozen plasma is given if the patient is actively bleeding or if time is not available for warfarin reversal before surgery.

Congenital coagulation factor deficiencies may also be treated with fresh frozen plasma, although the requirement for surgical procedures and serious bleeding may be so great as to cause pulmonary edema as a result of volume overload, even in a young individual with a healthy cardiovascular system. Factor concentrates (see discussions) currently offer more effective modes of therapy. Factor XI deficiency, however, is still treated by plasma infusion. This disease is milder than hemophilia A or hemophilia B. Factor XI also has a long half-life, so treatment is not needed on a daily basis.

A coagulation factor unit is defined as the activity in 1 mL of pooled normal plasma, so 100 percent activity is 1 unit/mL or 100 units/dL. Less than 50 percent activity of the coagulation factors is required for adequate hemostasis. Thus no more than half of the plasma volume, or about five to six fresh frozen plasma units, is required to correct a hemostatic deficiency. Repeated transfusions, however, would be required for surgical patients until healing has occurred. For example, factor IX has a half-life of 18 to 24 hours, warranting the need for the daily transfusions.

Fresh frozen plasma is sometimes used as a replacement fluid during plasma exchange (plasmapheresis). In cases of thrombotic thrombocytopenic purpura (TTP),[20] hemolytic uremic syndrome (HUS),[20] and the syndrome of hemolysis, elevated liver enzymes, and low platelets (HELLP),[21] fresh frozen plasma provides an unknown substance that the patient's plasma lacks, thus reversing the symptoms. HELLP syndrome occurs in a subgroup of pregnant women who have preeclampsia (pregnancy-induced hypertension and proteinuria) and usually occurs in the postpartum period. Plasmapheresis is used when the disease does not remit on its own.[21]

Fresh frozen plasma should not be used for blood volume expansion or protein replacement because safer products are available for these purposes—serum albumin, synthetic colloids, and balanced salt solutions—none of which transmits disease or causes severe allergic reactions.

Fresh frozen plasma should be ABO-compatible with the recipient's RBCs, but the Rh type can be disregarded.

## Plasma

Plasma was formerly known as a liquid plasma or cryoprecipitate-poor plasma. This component contains variable (usually small) amounts of the labile coagulation factors V and VIII and thus is not recommended for treatment of patients who have deficiency of either or both of these clotting factors. The plasma can be used for treatment of stable coagulation deficiency, especially factor XI deficiency, or as the only source of plasma for patients undergoing plasma exchange for TTP,[22] HUS, or HELLP. Endothelial injury, formation of large von Willebrand's factor molecules, and absence of normal protease inhibitors may play a pathogenic role in TTP and HUS. Some patients apparently respond better to the use of the supernatant plasma from the preparation of cryoprecipitated antihemophilic factor (cryopoor plasma).

For surgical procedures and serious bleeding, the required coagulation factor level may be difficult to achieve owing to volume overload in the patient. Plasma should not be used for blood volume expansion or protein replacement for the same reasons as those for fresh frozen plasma.

## Cryoprecipitated Antihemophilic Factor

Antihemophilic factor (AHF) is also called factor VIII. The cryoprecipitated AHF also contains fibrinogen, von Willebrand's factor (vWF), and factor XIII (Table 16–4); this product can be used to correct the deficiency of some of these coagulation factors.[23] Each unit of cryoprecipitate must contain at least 80 units of factor VIII.[24] However, mild or moderate factor VIII deficiency (hemophilia A) is usually treated with desmopressin acetate (1-deamino-[8-D-arginine]-vasopressin [DDAVP]) or factor VIII concentrates, or both, whereas severe factor VIII deficiency is treated with factor VIII concentrates. Cryoprecipitated AHF is no longer the blood product of choice for von Willebrand's disease, because one manufacturer has available virus-safe factor VIII concentrate with an assayed amount of von Willebrand's factor.

Currently, cryoprecipitated AHF is used primarily for fibrinogen replacement. The American Association of Blood Banks (AABB) has a requirement for at least 150 mg in each unit of cryoprecipitated AHF.[12] Fibrinogen replacement may be required in patients with liver failure or DIC and in rare patients with congenital fibrinogen deficiency. A plasma level of at least 50 mg/dL of fibrinogen is required for adequate hemostasis with surgery or trauma. For example, a patient's fibrinogen must be increased from 30 mg/dL to 100 mg/dL, or 70 mg/dL (100–30 mg/dL). To calculate the amount to be infused, first convert milligrams per deciliter to milligrams per milliliter by dividing by 100 (100 mL/dL). Multiplying this figure, 0.7 mg/mL, by the plasma volume, 3000 mL, we thus require 2100 mg (0.7 mg/mL × 3000 mL). To calculate the bags, divide 2100 mg by 150 mg/bag to get 14 bags. (One can convert the plasma volume to deciliters instead by dividing by 100 mL/dL).

Cryoprecipitated AHF can also be used as a source of fibrin glue,[24,25] which consists of a unit of cryoprecipitate as the source of fibrinogen. Bovine thrombin is mixed with the contents of the bag of cryoprecipitate at the tip of a spray gun (atomizer). The fibrinogen, activated by the thrombin, acts as a fibrin sealant in the area to which it is applied. The glue is applied topically on prosthetic vascular grafts as well as vascular tissue planes in surgery.

## Factor VIII Concentrate

Patients with hemophilia A or factor VIII deficiency have spontaneous hemorrhages that are treated with factor VIII concentrate.[26,27] Factor VIII concentrate is prepared by pharmaceutical firms by fractionation and lyophilization of pooled plasma. The plasma is obtained from paid donors by plasmapheresis or from volunteer whole blood donors. The concentrate is stored at refrigerator temperatures and is reconstituted with saline at the time of infusion. This ease of handling allows home therapy for individuals with hemophilia.

Factor VIII concentrate is prepared in a variety of ways, including anion exchange chromatography, monoclonal antibody purification, and recombinant DNA techniques.[28,29] Factor VIII concentrates are sterilized by different techniques, including pasteurization and solvent-detergent treatment. All of the sterilization methods used ensure sterility for human immunodeficiency virus (HIV) and hepatitis C virus (HCV).[28,29] Cases of hepatitis B still occur, but are rare. The recombinant DNA product is the safest because it is not derived from humans.

The following example illustrates the calculation of the dose of factor VIII: A 70-kg hemophiliac patient with a hematocrit of 30 percent has an initial factor VIII level of 4 percent (4 units/dL, 0.04 units/mL). How many units of factor VIII concentrate should be given to raise his factor VIII level to 50 percent?

$$\frac{(\text{desired factor VIII level in units/mL} - \text{initial factor VIII level in units/mL}) \times \text{plasma volume (mL)}}{= \text{units of factor VIII required}}$$

$$\text{Blood volume} = \text{weight (kg)} \times 70 \text{ mL/kg,}$$
$$\text{so } 70 \text{ kg} \times 70 \text{ mL/kg} = 4900 \text{ mL}$$
$$\text{Plasma volume} = \text{blood volume (mL)} \times (1.0 - \text{Hct}),$$
$$\text{so } 4900 \text{ mL} \times (1.0 - 0.30) = 3430 \text{ mL}$$

Putting into formula:

$$3430 \text{ mL} \times (0.50 - 0.04) = 1578 \text{ units}$$

The assayed value on the label can be divided into the number of units required to obtain the number of vials to be infused.

Only products labeled as containing von Willebrand's factor should be used for patients with von Willebrand's disease.

## Factor IX Concentrate

Factor IX concentrate and factor IX complex (prothrombin complex) concentrate are prepared from pooled plasma using various methods of separation and viral inactivation. The factor IX complex concentrate contains factors II, VII, IX, and X; however, the product is recommended only for factor IX–deficient patients

**Table 16–4.** Cryoprecipitated AHF

| Constituents | Amount |
|---|---|
| Factor VIII | 80–120 U/concentrate |
| Fibrinogen | 150–250 mg/concentrate |
| vWF | 40–70% of original FFP |
| Factor XIII | 20–30% of original FFP |

**Source:** Kennedy, MS (ed): Blood Transfusion Therapy: An Audiovisual Program. American Association of Blood Banks, Arlington, VA, 1985, with permission.

(hemophilia B),[26] patients with factor VII or X deficiency (rare), or selected patients with factor VIII inhibitors.[29] Activated coagulation factors in both the factor IX and the factor IX complex products may cause thrombosis, especially in patients with liver disease. Factor IX concentrates, containing mostly, or only, factor IX, are not useful in cases of factor VIII deficiency with inhibitors but are indicated for only factor IX deficiency.[29]

The dose is calculated in the same manner as that for factor VIII concentrate, using the assayed value of factor IX on the label with the caveat that one-half of any dose of factor IX rapidly diffuses into tissues, whereas the remaining one-half remains within the intravascular space.

### Antithrombin III and Other Concentrates

Antithrombin III is a protease inhibitor with activity toward thrombin.[30] Binding and inactivation of thrombin is enhanced by giving the patient heparin. The hereditary deficiency of antithrombin III is associated with venous thromboses, whereas the acquired deficiency is seen most frequently with DIC. Antithrombin III concentrates are licensed for use in the United States for patients with hereditary deficiency of antithrombin III. The product is pasteurized to eliminate the risk of HIV or HCV infections.[30] Use in acquired deficiency of antithrombin III is currently being evaluated. Liquid plasma and FFP are alternative sources of antithrombin III.

Protein C is a vitamin K–dependent factor and a serine protease inhibitor. Protein C inactivates factors V and VIII, thus preventing thrombus formation. Deficiency (hereditary or acquired) leads to a hypercoagulable state (i.e., prethrombotic state). Protein C concentrates are currently approved for use only in hereditary deficiency states.

Alpha$_1$-proteinase inhibitor concentrates are available for patients with $\alpha_1$-antitrypsin deficiency. This inherited condition is associated with emphysema and liver disease. The product is heat-treated to decrease transmission of viruses.

C1-esterase inhibitor concentrates are not currently approved for use in the United States. Deficiency of C1-esterase inhibitor results in life-threatening angioedema of the mucosa and submucosa of the respiratory and gastrointestinal tracts.

### Albumin and Plasma Protein Fraction

Albumin and plasma protein fraction are prepared by chemical fractionation of pooled plasma. Albumin is available as a 5 percent or a 25 percent solution, of which 96 percent of the protein content is albumin. Plasma protein fraction is available only as a 5 percent solution, containing 83 percent albumin and 17 percent globulins. All products are heat-treated and have proved to be virus-safe over many years of use.

These products may be used to treat patients requiring volume replacement. Controversy surrounds whether these products or crystalloid (i.e., saline or electrolyte) solutions are better for treating hypovolemia. Albumin is used routinely as the replacement fluid in many plasmapheresis procedures, replacing the colloid that is removed during the procedures. Albumin can be used in the treatment of burn patients for replacement of colloid pressure as well.

Albumin and plasma protein fraction can be used with diuretics to induce diuresis in patients with low total protein owing to severe liver or protein-losing disease. The 25 percent solution brings enough extravascular water into the vascular space to dilute the solution to 5 to 6 percent. Thus, patients receiving 25 percent albumin need to have adequate extravascular water and compensatory mechanisms to deal with the expansion of the blood volume.

### Immune Globulin

Immune globulin (Ig) prepared from pooled plasma is primarily IgG. Although small amounts of IgM and IgA may be present in some preparations, others are free of these contaminating proteins.[31] Products are available for intramuscular or intravenous administration. The intramuscular product must not be given intravenously because severe anaphylactic reactions may occur. The intravenous product must be given slowly to lessen the risk of reaction.

Immune globulin is used for patients with congenital hypogammaglobulinemia and for patients exposed to diseases such as hepatitis A or measles.[31] For hypogammaglobulinemia, monthly injections are usually given because of the 22-day half-life of IgG. The recommended dose is 0.7 mL/kg intramuscularly or 100 mg/kg intravenously. For hepatitis A prophylaxis, 0.02 to 0.04 mL/kg intramuscularly is recommended.

The intravenous preparation of immune globulin is used increasingly in the therapy of autoimmune diseases, such as immune thrombocytopenia (ITP),[31] and myasthenia gravis. Various mechanisms of action have been postulated. Basically, the infused immune globulin blocks the reticuloendothelial system or mononuclear phagocytic system.

Various hyperimmune globulins are available for prevention of diseases such as hepatitis B, varicella zoster, rabies, mumps, and others. These are prepared from the plasma of donors who have high antibody titers to the specific virus causing the disease. The dose is recommended in the package insert. It should be remembered that preparations such as hepatitis B hyperimmune globulin provide only passive immunity after an exposure. They do not confer permanent immunity and so must be accompanied by active immunization.

Rh immune globulin (RhIg) was developed to protect the Rh-negative mother who is pregnant with an Rh-positive infant (see Chapter 20). Much of the IgG in this preparation is directed against the D antigen within the Rh system. Administration of this preparation allows attachment of anti-D to any Rh-positive cells of the infant that have entered the maternal circulation. The sensitized cells are subsequently removed by the reticuloendothelial system of the mother, preventing active immunization or sensitization.

An Rh immune globulin product, which can be administered intravenously (or intramuscularly), is approved for use in ITP patients who are Rh-positive.[32] The proposed mechanism of action is blockage of the reticuloendothelial system by anti-D–coated RBCs, thereby reducing the destruction of autoantibody-coated platelets.

Immune globulins may cause anaphylactic reactions (flushing, hypotension, dyspnea, nausea, vomiting, diarrhea, and back pain). Caution should be used in patients with known IgA deficiency and previous anaphylactic reactions to blood components.

## SPECIAL CONSIDERATIONS FOR TRANSFUSION

### Filters for Blood Components

Two types of filters are typically used for blood transfusion: a 170-μm filter or a leukocyte-depletion filter. The 170-μm filter is a "clot-screen" filter that removes gross clots from any blood product and is used in routine blood administration sets. A standard blood administration filter must be used for transfusion of all blood components.

Leukocyte-depletion filters are designed to remove viable white blood cells (WBCs) from RBCs and platelet products.[7] This filter can be used to prevent febrile nonhemolytic transfusion reactions, to prevent or delay the development of HLA antibodies, and to reduce the risk of transfusion of CMV. Filtration in the laboratory, rather than at the bedside, is more reliable for reduction of leukocytes.

### Cytomegalovirus and Blood Components

Cytomegalovirus (CMV) is carried, in a latent or infectious form, in polymorphonuclear neutrophil leukocytes (PMNs) and monocytes. Infusion of these virus-infected cells in a cellular product such as RBCs or platelets can transmit infection. Infection of the patients can be prevented by the removal of leukocytes by filtration[33,34] or by administering a unit from a donor who is CMV antibody–negative. CMV-negative components should be administered to recipients who are CMV-negative and at risk for severe sequelae of CMV infections.[35] Those at established risk include CMV-seronegative pregnant women (mainly for the benefit of the fetus), CMV-seronegative bone marrow transplant recipients, and CMV-seronegative premature infants.[36]

### Irradiated Blood Components

Graft-versus-host disease (GVHD) requires three conditions to occur: (1) transfusion or transplantation of immunocompetent T lymphocytes, (2) histocompatibility differences between graft and recipient (major or minor HLA or other histocompatibility antigens), and (3) usually an immunocompromised recipient.[37] Common after allogeneic bone marrow transplantation, GVHD is a syndrome affecting skin, liver, and gut.

**Table 16–5.** Patients Susceptible to TA-GVHD

SCID
DiGeorge syndrome
Wiskott-Aldrich syndrome
Hodgkin's lymphoma
BMT recipients
Intrauterine transfusions (fetus)
Exchange transfusions (neonate)
Directed donations from blood relatives

SCID = severe combined immunodeficiency disease; BMT = bone marrow transplant; TA-GVHD = transfusion-associated graft-versus-host disease.

Transfusion-associated graft-versus-host disease (TA-GVHD), occurring less frequently, is caused by viable T lymphocytes in cellular blood components (e.g., RBCs and platelets). Mortality is high[37,38]; therefore, prevention is key. Prevention centers on irradiation of cellular components before administration to significantly immunocompromised individuals. Irradiation doses range from 2500 to 5000 cGy, with the higher doses being more effective. Irradiation decreases or eliminates the mitogenic (blastogenic) response of the transfused T cells, rendering these donor T cells immunoincompetent.

Recipients at risk for TA-GVHD are individuals with congenital immunodeficiencies (severe combined immunodeficiency [SCID], DiGeorge syndrome, Wiskott-Aldrich syndrome); individuals with Hodgkin's lymphoma; bone marrow transplant recipients (allogeneic or autologous); fetuses undergoing intrauterine transfusion; neonates undergoing exchange transfusion; and individuals, regardless of immune status, receiving products from blood relatives[37,38] (Table 16–5). In the last case, healthy recipients have experienced TA-GVHD after receiving nonirradiated blood components as directed donations primarily from first-degree relatives. The related donor is homozygous for one of the patient's (host's) HLA haplotypes, so the patient is incapable of rejecting the donor's (graft's) T lymphocytes, which then can act against the HLA antigens encoded by the patient's other haplotype. The donor lymphocytes then reject the host.[39] At this time, neither the level of immunosuppression necessary for a recipient to develop TA-GVHD (although the severe immunosuppression cases listed previously are most at risk) nor the dose of lymphocytes needed for TA-GVHD to occur is known. For the latter reason, prevention is dependent on irradiation and *not* reduction of lymphocytes by filtration.

## TRANSFUSION THERAPY IN SPECIAL CONDITIONS

### Maximum Surgical Blood Order Schedule; Type and Screen

Reviews of blood transfusion practices have found that most surgical procedures do not require blood

**Table 16–6.** Maximum Surgical Blood Order Schedule

| | |
|---|---|
| Purpose | |
| Reduce unnecessary crossmatching | |
| Examples | |
| Type and screen | Two units crossmatched |
| Vagotomy and pyloroplasty | Pulmonary lobectomy |
| Exploratory laparotomy | Hemicolectomy |
| Cholecystectomy | |

**Source:** Kennedy, MS (ed): Blood Transfusion Therapy: An Audiovisual Program. American Association of Blood Banks, Arlington, VA, 1985, with permission.

transfusion. Crossmatching for procedures with a low likelihood of transfusion increases the number of crossmatches performed, increases the amount of blood inventory in reserve and unavailable for transfusion, and contributes to the aging and possible outdating of the blood components. These patients can be better served by performing only a type and antibody screen. If the antibody screen is positive, antibody identification must be completed and compatible units found. However, if the antibody screen is negative, ABO- and Rh-type–specific blood may be released after an immediate spin crossmatch in those rare instances when transfusion is required (Table 16–6).

For a patient who is likely to require blood transfusion, the number of units crossmatched should be no more than twice those usually required for that surgical procedure. Thus, the crossmatch-to-transfusion (C/T) ratio will be between 2:1 and 3:1, which has been shown to be optimal practice. Although individual institutions may vary, general outlines are available concerning the maximum surgical blood-ordering schedule.[40]

### Autologous Transfusion

Autologous (self) transfusion is the donation of blood by the intended recipient; the infusion of blood from another donor is homologous transfusion. The patient's own blood is the safest blood possible, reducing or eliminating the possibility of transfusion reaction or the transmission of infectious disease.[41]

One type of autologous transfusion is the predeposit of blood by the patient (Fig. 16–1). Collected by regular blood donation procedure, the blood can be stored as liquid or, for longer storage, frozen. Patients may donate several units of blood over a period of weeks. They should take iron supplements to replace lost iron and to stimulate erythropoiesis during the time of donation. Predeposit autologous donation is usually reserved for patients anticipating a need for transfusion, such as scheduled surgery. However, patients with multiple RBC antibodies or antibodies to high-incidence antigens may store frozen units for unanticipated future need.

Recombinant erythropoietin (EPO) is available for the treatment of the anemia of chronic renal failure. This preparation is derived from recombinant DNA technology and not from humans. The use of EPO may avoid the transfusion of homologous RBC products.[42] For autologous transfusion, EPO may be used to collect more blood than the usual 2 to 3 units before surgery.[42]

Another type of autologous transfusion, intraoperative hemodilution, is the collection of 1 or 2 units of blood from the patient just before the surgical procedure, replacing the blood volume with crystalloid or colloid solution. Then, at the end of surgery, the blood units are infused into the patient. Care must be taken to label and to store the blood units properly and to identify the blood units with the patient before infusion. This has proved useful with several types of surgical procedures.[43]

Salvage of shed blood may be performed intraoperatively and/or postoperatively for autologous transfusion (see Fig. 16–1). Several types of equipment are available for collecting, washing, and filtering the shed blood before reinfusion. Washing of intraoperative salvage blood is generally recommended to remove the cellular debris, fat, and other contaminants. Heparin or citrate solutions may be used for anticoagulation of the shed blood, although postoperative salvage of thoracotomy blood may not require anticoagulation. For unknown reasons, blood exposed to serosal surfaces,

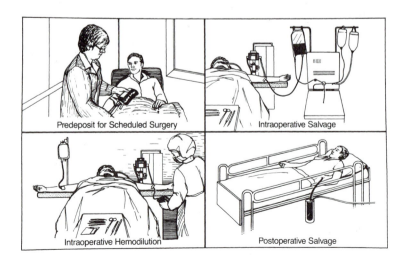

**Figure 16–1.** Types of autologous transfusions. (From Kennedy,[23] with permission.)

such as the pleural lining, is defibrinated. Meticulous salvage of shed blood has allowed surgical procedures that once required many units of blood to be performed without the need for homologous blood.

## Emergency Transfusion

Patients who are rapidly or uncontrollably bleeding may require immediate transfusion. Group O RBCs are selected for patients in whom transfusion cannot wait until the ABO and Rh type of the patient can be determined.[44] Group O–negative RBC units should be used, especially if the patient is a woman of childbearing age. A male patient or an older female patient can be switched from Rh-negative to Rh-positive RBCs if few O-negative units are available and massive transfusion is required.

Patients should be resuscitated with crystalloid or colloid solutions, and transfusions should be reserved for those patients losing more than 20 percent of their blood volume. The condition of most patients allows determination of ABO and Rh type and selection of ABO- and Rh-type–specific blood for transfusion. Delaying blood transfusion in emergency situations may be more dangerous than the small risk of transfusing incompatible blood before the antibody screen and crossmatch are completed.[44] After issuing O blood or type-specific blood, the antibody screen can be completed, and decisions can then be made for the selection of additional units of blood. If the patient has been typed and screened for a surgical procedure and his or her antibody screen is negative, ABO- and Rh-type–specific blood can be selected and given with an immediate spin crossmatch.

## Massive Transfusion

*Massive transfusion* is defined as the replacement of one or more blood volume(s) within 24 hours, or about 10 units of blood in an adult. The strategy for treatment of massive hemorrhage is outlined in Table 16–7. Analysis of the patient's clinical status and laboratory tests is essential for deciding appropriate transfusion therapy. Patients receiving less than one blood volume replacement rarely require platelet or plasma transfusion. Patients receiving two blood volumes usually require platelet and plasma transfusion.[45] If the patient is actively bleeding, platelets are required if the platelet count is less than 50,000/μL, and plasma is needed if the prothrombin time (PT) is greater than 16 seconds (international normalized ratio [INR] 1.5) or the activated partial thromboplastin time (PTT) exceeds 60 seconds. Fibrinogen levels should also be monitored because replacement by cryoprecipitate may be indicated when the fibrinogen level is less than 100 mg/dL.[6] Maintenance of the blood volume is of utmost importance in preventing tissue damage and worsening of thrombocytopenia and coagulopathy because of shock.[44] Extensive monitoring of PT, PTT, platelet count, fibrinogen, hemoglobin, and hematocrit can help direct the choice of the best and most indicated products during the duration of the massive transfusion.

A patient in critical condition and a finite supply of type-specific blood may require a change in ABO or Rh types. An Rh-negative male patient or postmenopausal female patient may be switched from Rh-negative to Rh-positive blood if there is concern about exhausting the inventory of Rh-negative blood. However, an Rh-negative potentially childbearing woman should receive Rh-negative RBC products as long as possible.

## Neonatal Transfusion

Premature infants frequently require transfusion of small amounts of blood to replace blood drawn for laboratory tests. Various methods are available to prepare small aliquots for transfusion. Small aliquots of donor blood can be transferred from the collection bag to a satellite bag or transfer bag, or blood can be withdrawn from the collection bag or transfer bag using an injection site coupler, needle and syringe, or a sterile docking device and syringe.

The aliquot must be labeled clearly with the name and identifying numbers of the patient and donor. The blood must be as fully tested as blood for adult transfusion. Blood units less than 7 days old are preferred to lessen the risk of hyperkalemia and to maximize the 2,3-diphosphoglycerate (2,3-DPG) levels, although, in some instances, CPDA-1 RBCs 14 to 21 days old are used routinely (Table 16–8).

For very–low-birth-weight infants, the blood should be selected to be CMV-seronegative to prevent CMV infection, which can be serious in premature infants. Indeed, pregnant women and new mothers should be given CMV-negative cellular components if they test negative for CMV.

Irradiation of the blood is recommended to prevent possible GVHD when blood is used for intrauterine transfusion, for an exchange transfusion, or for transfusion of a premature (less than 1200 g) neonate. Transfusions in a full-term newborn infant do not require routine irradiation.[37,38]

**Table 16–7.** Treatment Strategy for Massive Hemorrhage

| Condition | Treatment |
| --- | --- |
| Low blood volume* | Crystalloid or colloid |
| Low oxygen-carrying capacity* | RBCs |
| Hemorrhage owing to: | |
| Thrombocytopenia | Platelet concentrates |
| Coagulopathy | Fresh frozen plasma, cryoprecititate (if fibrinogen is low) |

**Source:** Kennedy, MS (ed): Blood Transfusion Therapy: An Audiovisual Program. American Association of Blood Banks, Arlington, VA, 1985, with permission.
*If these occur simultaneously, whole blood may be indicated.

**Table 16–8.** Neonatal RBC Transfusions

Aliquoted units should be:
  Less than 7 days old
  Type O–negative
  CMV-negative
  Irradiated to prevent GVHD
  Hemoglobin S–negative for hypoxic newborns

Infants who are hypoxic or acidotic should receive blood tested and negative for hemoglobin S.

## Oncology and Transplantation

The bone marrow of oncology patients may function poorly because of chemotherapy, radiation therapy, or infiltration and replacement of the bone marrow with malignant cells. Repeated RBC and platelet transfusions may eventuate the need for rare RBC units and/or HLA-matched plateletpheresis components because of incompatibility problems. Platelet use, as well, may necessitate a change from Rh-negative to Rh-positive products. Rh immune globulin may be given to a woman with childbearing potential to protect against immunization by the 5 mL or less of Rh-positive RBCs present in each transfused Rh-positive plateletpheresis component or pool of platelet concentrates. One 300-μg dose of RhIg can neutralize the effects of up to 15 mL of Rh-positive cells. Thus, one dose could be used for three doses or more of platelets.

In addition, some malignancies such as chronic lymphocytic leukemia and lymphoma are frequently complicated by autoimmune hemolytic anemia, increased destruction of RBCs, and pretransfusion testing problems.

Because of immunosuppression therapy, bone marrow transplant patients are at risk for TA-GVHD. Chronic TA-GVHD can cause severe deformity, and both acute and chronic TA-GVHD are usually fatal. Thus irradiation of every blood component containing lymphocytes is essential. Patients receiving transplants other than bone marrow do not require irradiated blood.

Patients having transplants, including bone marrow, kidney, heart, and other organs, may develop severe CMV disease. CMV-seronegative blood units should be selected for transplant patients who are CMV-seronegative.

Liver transplant patients require plasma, RBCs, and sometimes cryoprecipitated AHF during the transplant procedure because of their liver failure (see the next section of this chapter). The plasma must be transfused judiciously, however, because liver function is necessary to metabolize the citrate anticoagulant in the plasma. High citrate levels can result in hypocalcemia, causing disturbed heart contraction and deteriorating heart function.

Transfusion may be contraindicated in patients with certain cancers, apparently because the immune sup-

pression allows the cancer to grow and metastasize more easily.[46,47] Studies are continuing to explore the mechanisms of this effect of blood transfusion.

## Coagulation Factor Deficiencies

Factor VIII is a complex of two proteins: the procoagulant protein (factor VIII) and vWF (Fig. 16–2). Both proteins are necessary for normal hemostasis. Hemophilia A, or classic hemophilia, is a deficiency of the procoagulant portion of the factor VIII complex. The procoagulant portion is measured in functional (clotting) assays of factor VIII. Hemophilia A is seen with factor VIII level less than 30 percent, although clinical disease is generally not apparent unless the factor VIII level is less than 10 percent (normal 80 to 120) (Table 16–9). Individuals with a level less than 1 percent have severe and spontaneous bleeding, typically into muscles and joints. The vWF level is usually normal.

Von Willebrand's disease is characterized by a deficiency of vWF. Type I von Willebrand's disease is manifested by a reduced amount of all sizes of vWF multimers and is milder than type III, in which little or no vWF is produced. Type IIA is characterized by a deficient release of high-molecular-weight multimers,

## VIII—Procoagulant protein, active in clotting

## vWF—von Willebrand Factor

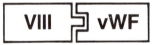

## FACTOR VIII COMPLEX

**Figure 16–2.** Factor VIII complex. (From Kennedy,[23] with permission.)

**Table 16–9.** Differential Diagnosis of Hemophilia A and von Willebrand's Disease

|  | **Hemophilia A** | **von Willebrand's Disease** |
| --- | --- | --- |
| Typical coagulation values | VIII <30%, vWF 50–150% | VIII 2–50%, vWF <40% |
| Bleeding time | Usually normal | Prolonged |
| Clinical course | Bleeding into joints and muscles | Mucosal bleeding |
|  | Bleeding with trauma or surgery | Bleeding with trauma or surgery |

**Source:** Kennedy, MS (ed): Blood Transfusion Therapy: An Audiovisual Program. American Association of Blood Banks, Arlington, VA, 1985, with permission.

whereas type IIB is manifested by abnormal high-molecular-weight multimers that have an increased avidity for binding to platelets. Type I and IIA patients have the ability to make the full spectrum of vWF multimers but do not release them into the circulation in normal amounts. DDAVP, a synthetic vasopressin analog, can stimulate release of the vWF in type I patients as well as in type IIA patients. DDAVP is contraindicated in type IIB. Factor VIII concentrate known to contain vWF is the blood product of first choice. Lyophilized concentrate can be used in type III von Willebrand's disease, or in type I disease when DDAVP treatment has failed.

Hemophilia B is the congenital deficiency of factor IX. Factor IX is activated by factors XIa and VIIa (Fig. 16–3). The activated factor IX (IXa), along with factor VIII, ionized calcium, and phospholipid, promotes the activation of factor X. Factor IX deficiency should be treated with factor IX and factor IX complex concentrates. Factor IX concentrates are made virus-safe by various sterilization techniques.[29,30]

All coagulation factors except vWF are made in the liver. With severe liver failure, multiple coagulation factor deficiencies occur. In addition, some of the coagulation factors produced may be abnormal. The liver also produces many of the thrombolytic proteins, leading to imbalance between the coagulation process and the control mechanism. Fresh frozen plasma, having normal amounts of all these proteins, can be used to treat these patients.

Vitamin K aids in the carboxylation of factors II, VII, IX, and X. With the absence of vitamin K or the use of drugs, such as coumarin, that interfere with vitamin K metabolism, the inactive coagulation factors cannot be carboxylated to active forms (Fig. 16–4). Administration of vitamin K is preferred to fresh frozen plasma administration in order to correct vitamin K deficiency or coumarin overdose. Because several hours are required for vitamin K effectiveness, signs of hemorrhage may require transfusion of fresh frozen plasma.

Disseminated intravascular coagulation is the un-

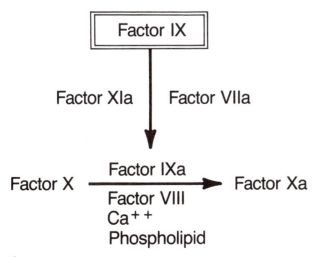

**Figure 16–3.** Factor IX deficiency. From Kennedy,[23] with permission.

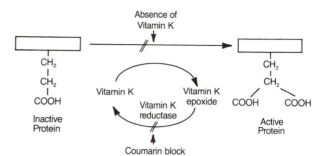

**Figure 16–4.** Mechanism of action of coumarin. From Kennedy,[23] with permission.

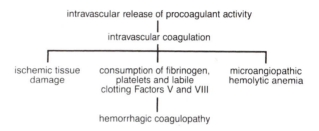

**Figure 16–5.** Pathogenesis of disseminated intravascular coagulation. From Kennedy,[23] with permission.

controlled activation and consumption of coagulation proteins, causing small thrombi within the vascular system throughout the body (Fig. 16–5). Treatment is aimed at correcting the cause of the DIC: sepsis, disseminated malignancy, obstetric complications, or shock. In some cases, transfusion of fresh frozen plasma, platelets, or cryoprecipitate may be required. Monitoring of the PT, PTT, platelet count, fibrinogen, and hemoglobin and hematocrit helps direct therapy and helps with the choice of the next component to be used during the treatment.

Platelet functional disorders may be caused by drugs, uremia, or congenital abnormalities. Platelet transfusions in these patients should be reserved for the treatment of hemorrhage or the impending need for normal hemostasis (such as a surgical procedure) to decrease development of platelet refractoriness. In uremia, DDAVP may be beneficial, as would be dialysis or even platelet transfusions. DDAVP releases fresh, functional vWF from endothelial cells. Dialysis removes by-products of protein metabolism that degrade vWF and coat platelets, thus making both nonfunctional. Platelet transfusions provide a source of fresh and (at least for a while, in the absence of dialysis) functional platelets.

## GENERAL TRANSFUSION PRACTICES

### Blood Administration

Blood must be administered properly for patient safety (Fig. 16–6). The proper identification of the patient, the patient's blood specimen, and the blood unit

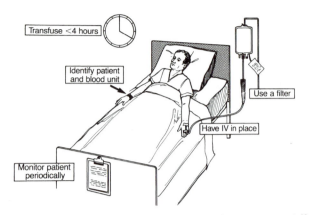

**Figure 16–6.** Blood administration and patient safety. From Kennedy,[23] with permission.

for transfusion are essential. Careful identification procedures prevent a major cause of transfusion-related deaths: ABO incompatibility. Today, clerical errors still represent the main cause of transfusion-related deaths and acute hemolytic transfusion reactions.[48] The identification process begins with proper identification of the patient; that is, asking patients to state or spell their name while you read their armband. A patient identification label is prepared at the bedside after the specimen is drawn. This prevents an empty specimen tube from being labeled with one patient's name and potentially being used for the collection of specimen from another patient. The labels are applied to the specimen tubes before leaving the bedside to avoid labeling the wrong tube.

Proper identification is carried out in the laboratory as work lists (computer or handwritten) are drafted. Another clerical check is performed as blood is issued from the blood bank. At the issue of blood components, two individuals verify the affixing of the proper label to the properly selected and tested blood components. The final clerical check is performed at the patient bedside when the nurse uses the patient armband to compare the patient identification to the patient crossmatch and issuance tags attached to the components to be transfused.

The patient with difficult veins should have the intravenous infusion device in place before the blood is issued from the transfusion service. All blood components must be filtered (170-μm filter) because clots and cellular debris develop during storage. Blood components are infused slowly for the first 10 to 15 minutes while the patient is closely observed for signs of a transfusion reaction. The blood components should then be infused as quickly as tolerated or, at most, within 4 hours. The patient's vital signs (pulse, respiration, blood pressure, and temperature) should be monitored periodically during the transfusion to detect signs of transfusion reaction promptly. These signs are fever with back pain (acute hemolytic transfusion reaction), anaphylaxis, hives or pruritus (urticarial reaction), congestive heart failure (volume overload), and fever alone (febrile nonhemolytic transfusion reaction). A delayed hemolytic transfusion reaction (jaundice, decreasing

hematocrit) may be diagnosed only 7 to 10 days after transfusion and thus is not considered an immediate reaction.

Rapid transfusion, including exchange transfusion, requires blood warming because the cold blood can cause hypothermia in the patient. Patients with paroxysmal cold hemoglobinuria or with cold agglutinins reactive at 37°C during pretransfusion testing may also require blood warming. The blood warmer should have automatic temperature control set with an alarm that will sound if the blood is warmed over 42°C (Fig. 16–7). Blood units must not be warmed by immersion in a waterbath or by a domestic microwave oven because uneven heating, damage to blood cells, and denaturation of blood proteins may occur.

Only isotonic (0.9 percent) saline or 5 percent albumin should be used to dilute blood components, because other intravenous solutions may damage the RBCs and cause hemolysis (dextrose solutions such as 5 percent dextrose in water [$D_5W$]) or initiate coagulation in the infusion set (calcium-containing solutions such as lactated Ringer's solution). In addition, many drugs will cause hemolysis if injected through the blood infusion set.

## Hospital Transfusion Committee

The Joint Commission on Accreditation of Healthcare Organizations (JCAHO) requires all blood transfusions to be reviewed for appropriate use. A hospital transfusion committee, although not required by

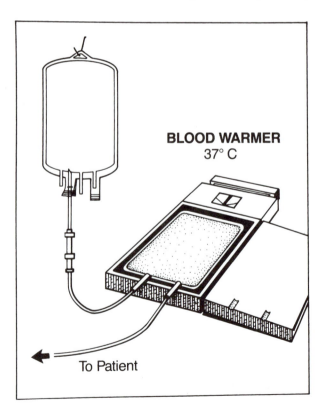

**BLOOD WARMER**
**37° C**

To Patient

**Figure 16–7.** Blood warming. From Kennedy,[23] with permission.

JCAHO, may serve as the peer review group for transfusions. Blood usage review may also be performed prospectively if criteria are approved by the medical staff. The blood bank director may interact and correspond directly with the chair of individual hospital departments concerning medical staff blood component usage patterns. Appropriate criteria for blood transfusion have been published (Table 16–10), serving as a guide for review.[49–52] The results of the review can be used by the transfusion committee to recommend

**Table 16–10.** Criteria for Transfusion Audit

### *All Blood Components*

Review of patients with transfusion reactions of hemolysis, severe allergic signs or anaphylaxis, circulatory overload, or infection
Review of patients with abnormal liver function or diagnosis of hepatitis or abnormal liver function within 6 months of transfusion
Charts of patients with adverse reaction or transfusion-transmitted disease must contain physician evaluation

### *Whole Blood*

| | |
|---|---|
| Indication: | Actively bleeding *and* blood loss >25% total blood volume *or* actively bleeding and received 4 units RBCs |
| Outcome: | H/H <24 hours after transfusion |
| | Surgical procedures: postoperative H/H <preoperative H/H |
| | Review of patients dying within 72 hours of transfusion |

### *Red Blood Cells[52]*

| | |
|---|---|
| Indications: | Hypovolemia and decreased oxygen-carrying capacity secondary to bleeding |
| | *or* acute loss of >15% blood volume |
| | *or* hemoglobin <6 g/dL or hematocrit <18% |
| | *or* symptoms related to anemia *and* a specific chronic anemia, leukemia, lymphoma, Hodgkin's disease, aplastic anemia, thalassemia, or dialysis for renal disease |
| | Review of patients with hemoglobin <6 g/dL, without hypovolemia or hypoxia, and iron-deficiency anemia or pernicious anemia, nutritional deficiency anemia, intestinal malabsorption, or hereditary hemolytic anemia |
| Exceptions: | Patients with chronic disease or specified anemia listed above and hemoglobin >8 g/dL and coronary artery disease, chronic pulmonary disease, or cerebral vascular disease |
| Outcome: | H/H <24 hours after transfusion |
| | Surgical patients: postoperative hemoglobin <preoperative hemoglobin |
| | Review of transfusion reactions and complications |

### *Platelets*

| | |
|---|---|
| Indications: | Platelet count <20,000/μL |
| | *or* operative procedure in <12 hours and platelet count <50,000/μL |
| | Review of patients receiving platelets and with idiopathic (autoimmune) thrombocytopenia purpura, DIC, thrombic thrombocytopenia purpura, or hemolytic uremic syndrome |
| | Review of adults receiving >12 units or <4 units |
| Outcome: | Platelet count immediately before and <18 hours after transfusion |
| | Review of transfusion reactions and complications |

### *Fresh Frozen Plasma*

| | |
|---|---|
| Indications: | Activated PTT >60 seconds |
| | *or* PT >16 seconds |
| | *or* documented coagulation factor deficiency |
| | *and* significant bleeding |
| Outcome: | PT, activated PTT, or coagulation factor assay immediately before and fewer than 4 hours after transfusion |
| | Review of transfusion reactions and complications |

### *Cryoprecipitated AHF*

| | |
|---|---|
| Indications: | Hemophilia A or von Willebrand's disease *or* fibrinogen deficiency *or* factor XIII deficiency |
| Outcome: | Factor VIII, fibrinogen, or factor XIII determination after transfusion |

**Source**: Modified from the National Institutes of Health Consensus Conference. JAMA 257:1777, 1987, and JAMA 253:551, 1985; Silberstein, LE, et al: Strategies for the review of transfusion practices. JAMA 262:1993, 1989; and Simon, TL, et al: Practice parameter for the use of red blood cell transfusions. Arch Pathol Lab Med 122:130, 1998.

H/H = hemoglobin hematocrit.

changes in practice by the hospital staff to improve patient care. The transfusion committee also reviews each transfusion reaction to ensure that adverse reactions are avoidable. In addition, the transfusion committee ensures that appropriate procedures (such as for blood administration) are in place and are followed by hospital personnel.

The transfusion committee is most effective if the various groups who order and administer blood, such as surgeons, anesthesiologists, and oncologists, are represented on the committee. The transfusion committee must have a mechanism for reporting activities and recommendations to the medical staff and hospital administration. Optimally, the transfusion committee ensures that the most appropriate, efficient, and safe use of the blood supply is achieved.

## CASE STUDIES

### CASE 1

A 55-year-old man is contemplating surgery for severe arthritis in the right hip.

1. What should be known to determine how many units of red blood cells should be crossmatched?

2. How could it be determined if the patient can donate blood (autologous predeposit) for use during surgery?

3. The patient has a history of bleeding after a tonsillectomy at age 7. What tests should be done to further study this potential problem?

4. If the patient is found to have von Willebrand's disease, which blood components might be necessary?

*Answers*

1. It is necessary to know the patient's hemoglobin and hematocrit, the surgeon's usual blood usage, whether this is the first surgical procedure on this hip (redo surgery uses more blood), and whether the patient has any pretransfusion compatibility problems.

2. Considerations should be the patient's general health, hemoglobin and hematocrit, amount of time between request for donation and the time of surgery, and whether the patient has infectious diseases that might interfere (e.g., bacterial infections).

3. Tests should include prothrombin time, partial thromboplastin time, platelet count, and von Willebrand's factor workup.

4. If the patient has moderate to severe von Willebrand's disease, he may need either factor VIII concentrate, known to contain von Willebrand's factor, or cryoprecipitate.

### CASE 2

A 45-year-old woman complains of tiredness and weakness. She appears pale. Lab results are as follows: hemoglobin 6.2 g/dL, hematocrit 22 percent, MCV 75 fl, MCHC 38%. On further questioning, she reports excessive menstrual bleeding, sometimes lasting for several weeks.

1. Does this patient need a transfusion? Justify your answer.

2. If the intern decides to give two units of RBCs, what would be the resulting hemoglobin and hematocrit?

*Answers*

1. Yes, her hemoglobin is close to 6.0 g/dL, which is the criteria for RBC transfusion. She will be less tired and weak if she receives a transfusion. No, she is not in any acute distress. She is iron deficient (from blood loss) and should be treated with iron replacement rather than with transfusion, which has higher risks.

2. For adults, each unit of blood should increase the hemoglobin 1 g/dL and the hematocrit 3 percentage points. For accuracy, this is based on a hypothetical 70-kg man. For smaller men and women, the increase is greater; for larger ones, less.

### CASE 3

A 22-year-old woman presents with easy bruising and fatigue. A CBC reveals hemoglobin 9.0 g/dL, hematocrit 27 percent, WBC 15,000/μL, and platelet count 15,000/μL. The hematologist plans to perform a bone marrow biopsy and aspiration.

1. What blood component(s) is (are) indicated? Why?

2. Describe how the dose is calculated. What laboratory result is desired?

3. The patient receives chemotherapy, and 2 weeks later the hemoglobin is 7.0 g/dL and the hematocrit 21 percent. The patient complains of shortness of breath when hurrying to the bus stop. The physician decides to order RBC transfusion. What dose of RBCs is indicated? How is this determined?

*Answers*

1. The platelet count is below 20,000/μL, so a platelet transfusion is indicated. Without the platelet transfusion, she would be at increased risk of bleeding from the site of the bone marrow biopsy. Although the hemoglobin and hematocrit are lower than normal for a woman of this age, an

RBC transfusion is not indicated (hemoglobin >6.0 g/dL in an otherwise healthy young adult).

2. For an adult, each unit (bag) of platelet concentrate should increase the patient's platelet count by 5000 to 10,000/μL. The platelet count should be at about 50,000/μL because a bone marrow biopsy is an invasive procedure. Thus about 4 units of platelet concentrates would be indicated.

3. If it is anticipated that the patient will experience bone marrow recovery soon (after the chemotherapy), just one unit of RBCs is indicated. If, on the other hand, the bone marrow will be suppressed for several weeks, 2 units are indicated, with a recheck in a couple weeks for another possible transfusion. Each unit of RBCs is expected to increase the hemoglobin level about 1 g/dL.

---

## SUMMARY CHART: IMPORTANT POINTS TO REMEMBER (MT/MLT)

- Transfusion therapy is primarily used to treat two conditions: inadequate oxygen-carrying capacity because of anemia or blood loss and insufficient coagulation proteins to provide adequate hemostasis.
- A unit of whole blood or packed RBCs should increase the hematocrit 3 to 5 percent or hemoglobin 1 to 1.5 g/dL.
- Red blood cells are indicated for increasing the RBC mass in patients who require increased oxygen-carrying capacity.
- The shelf life for CPD RBCs is 21 days; for CPDA-1, 35 days; and for AS-1, 42 days.
- Platelet transfusions are indicated for patients who are bleeding because of thrombocytopenia. In addition, platelets are indicated prophylactically for patients who have platelet counts under 20,000/mL.
- Each unit of platelet concentrate should increase the platelet count 5000 to 10,000/mL in the typical 70-kg human; each should contain at least $5.5 \times 10^{10}$ platelets.
- A plateletpheresis product is prepared from one donor and must contain a minimum of $3 \times 10^{11}$ platelets.
- Fresh frozen plasma (FFP) contains all coagulation factors and is indicated for patients with multiple coagulation deficiencies occurring in liver failure, DIC, vitamin K deficiency, warfarin toxicity, or massive transfusion.
- Cryoprecipitated antihemophilic factor (AHF) contains at least 80 units of factor VIII and 150 mg of fibrinogen, von Willebrand's factor, and factor XIII.
- Factor IX complex concentrate contains factors II, VII, IX, and X and is used primarily in the treatment of persons with hemophilia B.
- Immune globulin (Ig) is used in the treatment of congenital hypogammaglobulinemia and patients exposed to hepatitis A or measles.
- Massive transfusion is defined as the replacement of one or more blood volume(s) within 24 hours or about 10 units of blood in an adult.
- Emergency transfusion warrants group O RBCs when patient type is not yet known.

---

## REVIEW QUESTIONS

1. Leukocyte-reduced filters can do all of the following *except*:
   A. Reduce the risk of CMV infection
   B. Prevent or reduce the risk of HLA alloimmunization
   C. Prevent febrile, nonhemolytic transfusion reactions
   D. Prevent TA-GVHD

2. Albumin should *not* be given for:
   A. Burns
   B. Shock
   C. Nutrition
   D. Plasmapheresis

3. Of the following, which blood type is selected when a patient cannot wait for ABO-matched blood?
   A. A
   B. B
   C. O
   D. AB

4. Which patient does not need an irradiated component?
   A. Bone marrow transplant recipient
   B. Neonate less than 1200 g
   C. Healthy adult receiving an RBC transfusion
   D. Healthy adult receiving an RBC transfusion from a blood relative

5. Red blood cell transfusions should be given:
   A. Within 4 hours
   B. With lactated Ringer's solution
   C. With dextrose and water
   D. With cryoprecipitated AHF

6. Which type of transplantation requires all cellular blood components to be irradiated?
   A. Bone marrow
   B. Heart
   C. Liver

D. Pancreas

E. Kidney

7. Characteristics of deglycerolized red blood cells include the following *except*:

A. Inexpensive

B. 24-hour expiration date after thawing

C. Used for rare antigen-type donor blood

D. Used for IgA-deficient recipients

8. Select the appropriate product for the indicated patient or need:

I. Hemophilia A

II. Hemophilia B

III. Fibrinogen deficiency

IV. Bone marrow transplant patient with anemia unresponsive to iron and vitamin $B_{12}$ therapy

V. Increasing oxygen-carrying capacity

VI. Vitamin K deficiency and hemorrhage

VII. Also called AHF

VIII. Directed donation from a blood relative

IX. Repeated febrile transfusion reactions

X. Anaphylaxis

XI. Life-threatening neutropenia

XII. Needlestick accident with infectious blood (hepatitis B)

XIII. Immunodeficiency

XIV. Used for dilution of red blood cells

A. Factor VIII concentrate

B. Cryoprecipitate

C. Fresh frozen plasma

D. Irradiated red blood cells

E. Red blood cells

F. Granulocytapheresis

G. Leukocyte-reduced red cells

H. Washed or deglycerolized red blood cells

I. Immune globulin

J. Hepatitis B immune globulin

K. 0.9 percent saline

L. Lactated Ringer's solution

M. 5 percent dextrose and water solution

N. Factor IX concentrate

## ANSWERS TO REVIEW QUESTIONS

1.  D (p 351)

2.  C (p 350)

3.  C (p 353)

4.  C (p 351)

5.  A (p 356)

6.  A (p 351)

7.  A (p 347)

8.  I A (p 349)

II  N (pp 349–350)

III  B (p 349)

IV  D (p 351)

V  E (p 348)

VI  C (p 348)

VII  B (p 349)

VIII  D (p 351)

IX  G (p 346)

X  H (pp 346–347)

XI  F (p 348)

XII  J (pp 350–351)

XIII  I (pp 350–351)

XIV  K (p 356)

## REFERENCES

1.  Lane, TA (ed): Blood Transfusion Therapy: A Physician's Handbook, ed 5. American Association of Blood Banks, Bethesda, MD, 1996, pp 4–5.

2.  Circular of Information for the Use of Human Blood and Blood Products. American Red Cross, Washington, DC, 1997.

3.  Gould, SA, et al: The physiologic basis of the use of blood and blood products. Surg Annu 16:13, 1984.

4.  Spence, RK, et al: Transfusion guidelines for cardiovascular surgery: Lessons learned from operations in Jehovah's witnesses. J Vascular Surg 16:825, 1992.

5.  Kruskall, MS: Clinical management of transfusions to patients with red cell antibodies. In Nance, SJ (ed): Immune Destruction of Red Blood Cells. American Association Blood Banks, Arlington, VA, 1989, p 263.

6.  Silberstein, LE, et al: Strategies for the review of transfusion practices. JAMA 262:1993, 1989.

7.  Dzik, S: Leukodepletion of blood filters: Filter design and mechanisms of leukocyte removal. Transfus Med Rev 7:65, 1993.

8.  Brand, A: White cell depletion: Why and how? In Nance, SJ (ed): Transfusion Medicine in the 1990s. American Association Blood Banks, Arlington, VA, 1990, p 35.

9.  Kao, K-J, and Bertholf, MF: Leukocyte-depleted blood components for patients with leukemia or aplastic anemia: CON. In Kurtz, SR, Baldwin, ML, and Sirchia, G (eds): Controversies in Transfusion Medicine: Immune Complications and Cytomegalovirus Transmission. American Association Blood Banks, Arlington, VA, 1990, p 13.

10.  Standards for Blood Banks and Transfusion Services, ed 17. American Association Blood Banks, Bethesda, MD, 1996, p 13.

11.  National Institutes of Health Consensus Conference: Platelet transfusion therapy. JAMA 257:1777, 1987.

12.  Standards for Blood Banks and Transfusion Services, ed 17. American Association Blood Banks, Bethesda, MD, 1996, p 15.

13.  Daly, PA, et al: Platelet transfusion therapy: One-hour posttransfusion increments are valuable in predicting the need for HLA-matched preparations. JAMA 243:435, 1980.

14.  McFarland, JG, Anderson, AJ, and Slichter, SJ: Factors influencing the transfusion response to HLA-selected apheresis donor platelets in patients refractory to random platelet concentrates. Br J Haematol 73:380, 1989.

15.  Slichter, SJ: Algorithm for managing the platelet refractory patient. J Clin Apheresis 12:4, 1997.

16.  Kickler, TS, et al: Depletion of white cells from platelet concentrates with a new adsorption filter. Transfusion 29:411, 1989.

17.  Cairo, MS, et al: Role of circulating complement and polymor-

phonuclear leukocyte transfusion in treatment and outcome in critically ill neonates with sepsis. J Pediatr 110:935, 1987.

18. Standards for Blood Banks and Transfusion Services, ed 17. American Association Blood Banks, Bethesda, MD, 1996, p 24.
19. National Institutes of Health Consensus Conference: Fresh-frozen plasma: Indications and risks. JAMA 253:551, 1985.
20. Practice Guidelines Development Task Force: Practice parameter for the use of fresh-frozen plasma, cryoprecipitate, and platelets. JAMA 271:777, 1994.
21. Martin, JN, et al: Postpartum plasma exchange for atypical preeclampsia-eclampsia as HELLP (hemolysis, elevated liver enzymes, and low platelets) syndrome. Am J Obstet Gynecol 172:1107, 1995.
22. Obrador, GT, et al: Effectiveness of cryosupernatant therapy in refractory and chronic relapsing thrombotic thrombocytopenic purpura. Am J Hematol 42:217, 1993.
23. Kennedy, MS (ed): Blood Transfusion Therapy: An Audiovisual Program. American Association of Blood Banks, Arlington, VA, 1985.
24. Casali, B, et al: Fibrin glue from single-donation autologous plasmapheresis. Transfusion 32:641, 1992.
25. Radosevich, M, Goubran, HA, and Burnouf, T: Fibrin sealant: Scientific rationale, production methods, properties, and current clinical use. Vox Sang 72:133, 1997.
26. Julius, C: Coagulation products for hemophilia A, hemophilia B and von Willebrand's disease. In Hackel, E, Westphal, RG, and Wilson, SM (eds): Transfusion Management of Some Common Heritable Blood Disorders. American Association Blood Banks, Bethesda, MD, 1992, p 1.
27. Furie, B, Limentani, SA, and Rosenfield, CG: A practical guide to the evaluation and treatment of hemophilia. Blood 84:3, 1994.
28. Colvin, BT: Guidelines on therapeutic products to treat haemophilia and other hereditary coagulation disorders. Hemophilia 3:63, 1997.
29. Kasper, CK, Lusher, JM, and the Transfusion Practices Committee: Recent evolution of clotting factor concentrates for hemophilia A and B. Transfusion 33:422, 1993.
30. Menache, D, Grossman, BJ, and Jackson, CM: Antithrombin III: Physiology, deficiency, and replacement therapy. Transfusion 32:580, 1992.
31. National Institute of Health Consensus Conference: Intravenous immunoglobulin: Prevention and treatment of disease. JAMA 264:3189, 1990.
32. Bussel, BJ, et al: Intravenous anti-D treatment of immune thrombocytopenic purpura: Analysis of efficacy, toxicity, and mechanism of effect. Blood 77:1884, 1991.
33. Bowden, RA, et al: A comparison of filtered leukocyte-reduced and cytomegalovirus (CMV) seronegative blood products for

the prevention of transfusion-associated CMV infection after marrow transplant. Blood 86:3598, 1995.
34. Van Prooijen, HC, et al: Prevention of primary transfusion-associated cytomegalovirus infection in bone marrow transplant recipients by the removal of white cells from blood components with high-affinity filters. Br J Haematol 87:144, 1994.
35. Reusser, P, et al: Cytomegalovirus infection after autologous bone marrow transplantation: Occurrence of cytomegalovirus disease and effect on engraftment. Blood 75:1888, 1990.
36. Sayers, MH, et al: Reducing the risk for transfusion-transmitted cytomegalovirus infection. Ann Intern Med 116:55, 1992.
37. Anderson, KC, and Weinstein, HJ: Transfusion-associated graft-versus-host disease. N Engl J Med 323:315, 1990.
38. Linden, JV, and Pisciotto, PT: Transfusion-associated graft-versus-host disease and blood irradiation. Transfus Med Rev 6:116, 1992.
39. Otsuka, S, et al: The critical role of blood from HLA-homozygous donors in fatal transfusion-associated graft-versus-host disease in immunocompetent patients. Transfusion 31:260, 1991.
40. Vengelen-Tyler, V (ed): Technical Manual, ed 12. American Association Blood Banks, Bethesda, MD, 1996, p 58.
41. Ibid., p 103.
42. Goodnough, LT, Monk, TG, and Andriole, GL: Erythropoietin therapy. N Engl J Med 336:933, 1997.
43. Stehling, L, and Zauder, HL: Acute normovolemic hemodilution. Transfusion 31:857, 1991.
44. Kruskall, MS, et al: Transfusion therapy in emergency medicine. Ann Emerg Med 17:327, 1988.
45. Leslie, SD, and Toy, TCY: Laboratory hemostatic abnormalities in massively transfused patients given red blood cells and crystalloid. Am J Clin Pathol 96:770, 1991.
46. Blumberg, N, Triulzi, DJ, and Heal, JM: Transfusion-induced immunomodulation and its chemical consequences. Transfus Med Rev 4:24, 1990.
47. Vamvakas, E, and Moore, SB: Preoperative blood transfusion and colorectal cancer recurrence: A qualitative statistical overview and meta-analysis. Transfusion 33:754, 1993.
48. Sazama, K: Reports of 355 transfusion-associated deaths: 1976 through 1985. Transfusion 30:583, 1990.
49. Spence, RK: Surgical red blood cell transfusion practice policies. Am J Surg 170:3S, 1995.
50. American Society of Anesthesiologists Task Force on Blood Component Therapy: Practice guidelines for blood component therapy. Anesthesiology 84:732, 1996.
51. Stehling, L, et al: Guidelines for blood utilization review. Transfusion 34:438, 1994.
52. Simon, TL, et al: Practice parameter for the use of red blood cell transfusions. Arch Pathol Lab Med 122:130, 1998.

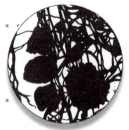

# CHAPTER **17**

# APHERESIS

Francis R. Rodwig, Jr, MD, MPH

**OBJECTIVES**

*On completion of this chapter, the learner should be able to:*

1 Define apheresis, leukapheresis, plateletpheresis, plasmapheresis, erythrocytapheresis, and therapeutic apheresis.

2 Describe the procedures of continuous-flow centrifugation and intermittent-flow centrifugation.

3 Discuss the use of membrane technology in the separation of blood components.

4 State the American Association of Blood Banks requirements for apheresis donations.

5 State the shelf life of platelet concentrates and granulocyte concentrates.

6 List the therapeutic indications for apheresis, differentiating between conditions requiring plasma exchange and those necessitating cytapheresis.

7 Describe the different types of adsorbents and their clinical application.

8 Identify the factors that can be removed by plasmapheresis.

9 Discuss the possible adverse effects of apheresis.

## HISTORY AND DEVELOPMENT

*Apheresis* (or *hemapheresis*) is a term of Greek derivation that means to separate or remove. In an apheresis procedure, blood is withdrawn from a donor or patient and separated into its components. One (or more) of the components is retained, and the remaining constituents are recombined and returned to the individual. Any of the components of blood can be removed, and the procedures are specified by the component selected. Thus the process of removing the plasma from the blood is termed *plasmapheresis*. Similar terms are given to the removal of the other blood components, including platelets (*plateletpheresis* or *thrombocytapheresis*), red blood cells (*erythrocytapheresis*), or leukocytes (*leukapheresis*).

When anticoagulated blood is centrifuged in a test tube, it separates into red blood cells (RBCs), white blood cells (WBCs), platelets, and plasma because of the different weights (specific gravities) of these components (Fig. 17–1). When a pipette is placed at the appropriate level in the test tube, any of these components can be aspirated. The most widely used apheresis equipment applies the same concept, using a machine with a centrifuge bowl or belt. Blood is removed from an individual (usually with a large-bore needle), anticoagulated, and transported directly to the separation mechanism, where it is separated into specific components. Once the components have been separated, any component can be withdrawn. The remaining portions of the blood are then mixed and returned to the donor or patient (Fig. 17–2).

Depending on the goal of the individual procedures (e.g., collecting platelets, removing plasma or RBCs), the instruments must be adjusted appropriately. The variables are (1) centrifuge speed and diameter; (2) length of dwell time of the blood in the centrifuge; (3) the type of solutions added, such as anticoagulants or sedimenting agents; and (4) the cellular content or plasma volume of the patient or donor. By manipulating these variables, the operator can harvest plasma, platelets, white cells, or red cells for commercial or therapeutic purposes. A computerized control panel allows the operator to select the desired procedure and collection parameters. The machines are equipped with optical sensors that detect plasma-cell interfaces and divert components according to the preselected mode.

## METHODOLOGY

Procedures for performing apheresis vary according to the particular component of the blood to be harvested and the equipment that is used. Manufacturers' instructions should always be consulted for specific techniques. The amount of time for a particular procedure can range from 60 to 150 minutes. Currently available machines use disposable equipment, which includes sterile bags, tubing, and collection chambers unique to the machine. Platelets collected using these

**Figure 17–1.** Sedimented blood sample. (Courtesy IBM.)

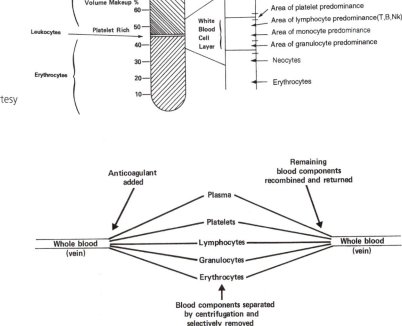

**Figure 17–2.** Principles of apheresis.

systems are considered "closed," with a 5-day dating period. Other sets are composed of sterile tubing and bowls that have to be assembled on the machine prior to use. Such sets are considered an "open" system, and therefore the product has a 24-hour dating period.

The most commonly used instruments employ the centrifugation method of separation. This method can be divided into two basic categories: (1) intermittent-flow centrifugation (IFC) and (2) continuous-flow centrifugation (CFC). Apheresis by membrane filtration techniques is occasionally used.

## Equipment

Intermittent-flow centrifugation (IFC) procedures are performed in cycles (also called passes). Blood is drawn from an individual with the assistance of a pump. To keep the blood from clotting, an anticoagulant is added to the tubing. The blood is pumped into the separation mechanism (in this case, a centrifuge bowl) through the inlet port. The bowl rotates at a fixed speed, separating the components according to their specific gravities. A rotary seal is used, resulting in a closed system. The red cells, which have greater mass, are packed against the outer rim of the bowl, followed by the white cells, platelets, and plasma. The separated component(s) flow from the bowl through the outlet port and are harvested as desired into separate collection bags (Fig. 17–3). The undesired components are diverted into a reinfusion bag and returned to the individual. Reinfusion completes one cycle. The cycles are repeated until the desired quantity of product is obtained. A plateletpheresis procedure usually takes 6 to 8 cycles to collect a therapeutic dose.

One of the advantages of the IFC procedure is that it can be done with only one venipuncture (one-arm procedure; that is, the blood is drawn and reinfused through the same needle). The amount of time for the process can be reduced if both arms are used: one for phlebotomy and one for reinfusion (two-arm procedure). The most widely used machines of this type are manufactured by Haemonetics Corporation. The Mobile Collection Systems (MCS, MCS Plus) are versatile, portable, fully automated, and capable of efficient component collections (Fig. 17–4). The Plasma Collection System (PCS) is designed to collect plasma for transfusions or source plasma.

Continuous-flow centrifugation (CFC) procedures withdraw, process, and return the blood to the individual simultaneously. This is in contrast to IFC procedures, which complete a cycle before beginning the next one. Because blood is drawn and returned continuously during a procedure, two venipuncture sites are necessary. Occasionally, especially with therapeutic procedures, a dual-lumen central venous catheter is used. Blood is drawn from the phlebotomy site with the assistance of a pump, mixed with anticoagulant, and collected in a chamber or belt, depending on the machine. Separation of the components is achieved through centrifugation, and the specific component is diverted and retained in a collection bag. The remainder of the blood is reinfused to the individual via the

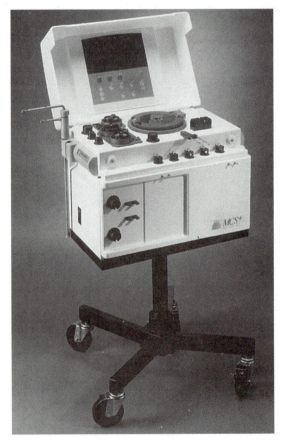

**Figure 17–4.** The Haemonetics MCS Plus LN9000. (Courtesy Haemonetics Corporation, Inc., Braintree, MA.)

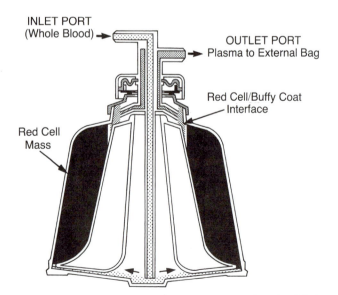

**Figure 17–3.** Cross-section of Haemonetics centrifuge bowl (IFC procedure). (Courtesy Haemonetics Corporation, Braintree, MA.)

second venipuncture site. The process of phlebotomy, separation, and reinfusion is uninterrupted, or continuous. Examples of machines employing this concept are the Fenwal CS-3000 (Fig. 17–5) and the newest model, the Amicus; COBE Spectra (Fig. 17–6); and Fresenius AS-104 (Fig. 17–7).

The IFC and CFC machines have individual advantages and disadvantages.[1] The IFC equipment is usually smaller and more mobile. A single venipuncture may be used with IFC procedures, whereas two venipunctures are usually required with the CFC procedures. New protocols have been developed to allow the CFC equipment to operate with single access. The extracorporeal volume (the amount of blood out of the individual in the centrifuge bowl and tubing) is greater with IFC than with the CFC machines. This may be an important consideration in individuals with small blood volumes (e.g., children and older people). The extra volume removed may lead to difficulties in maintaining proper fluid volume in the individual and may cause adverse effects during the procedure. Because CFC procedures are uninterrupted, the time a person spends on the machine may be less than with IFC machines. The choice of equipment should be based on the functions and needs of the institution and the requirements of the donor or patient.

Membrane filtration technology can also be used to separate blood components. Blood that passes over membranes with specific pore sizes allows passage of plasma through the membrane while the cellular portion passes over it. Filtration has several advantages over centrifugation, including the collection of a cell-free product and the ability to selectively remove plasma components by varying the pore size. However, the newer CFC equipment can perform most varieties of apheresis, whereas the membrane devices are usually limited to plasma collection. Another cell separation technology that combines centrifugation and membrane filtration for plasma collection is found in the Fenwal Autopheresis-C. This intermittent-flow machine collects blood in a small cylinder that is rotating, forcing plasma through a polycarbonate membrane (Fig. 17–8).[2] This system has recently been modified to collect apheresis platelets within a 5-day storage.[3]

Apheresis products may be collected manually, using a refrigerated centrifuge and a specialized multiple plastic bag system. In this procedure, whole blood is collected into a plastic bag, which is then separated from the collection set and centrifuged. The desired component is retained, and the remainder is reinfused. The process is then repeated.[4] Figure 17–9 represents a manual plasmapheresis. This procedure is simple and inexpensive because sophisticated equipment is not required. However, there are disadvantages to this method. The amount of component harvested per procedure is far less than the yield with the automated devices. Because the whole blood must be separated from the collection set to be centrifuged, there is the added risk of returning the red cells to the wrong individual. Consequently, stringent methods to properly identify the red cell unit with the donor must be implemented. This technique is a viable alternative when a person's veins cannot withstand the demands of automated equipment or when such equipment is not available.

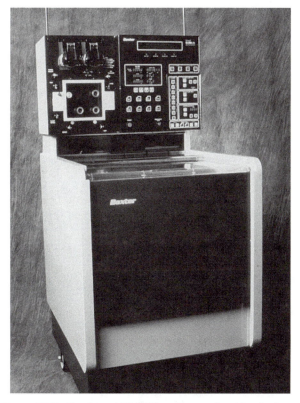

**Figure 17–5.** The Fenwal CS-3000 continuous-flow blood cell separator. (Courtesy Baxter Healthcare Corporation, Deerfield, IL.)

## Fluids

All apheresis procedures use anticoagulants to prevent blood from clotting as it enters the separation mechanism. The most common anticoagulant is acid citrate dextrose (ACD), although heparin is occasionally used. Normal saline is used to prime the system, to keep the line open, and to help maintain fluid volume. For granulocyte collection, a sedimenting agent is added to the blood so that better separation between the white cells and red cells is achieved (because the specific gravities of red cells and white cells are very similar—1.093 to 1.096 for red cells, 1.087 to 1.092 for granulocytes).[5] The most commonly used agent is hydroxyethyl starch (HES). This solution causes red cells to form rouleaux, thus allowing white cells to be harvested more efficiently.

In therapeutic plasmapheresis procedures, large volumes of a patient's plasma are retained. The fluid must be replaced to maintain appropriate intravascular volume and oncotic pressure. Several solutions are available, and the choice is determined by each institution. Crystalloids such as normal saline may be used. Because saline provides less oncotic pressure than

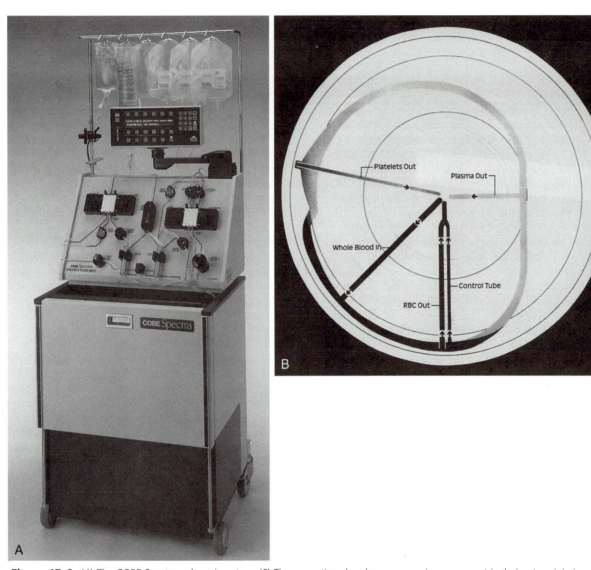

**Figure 17–6.** (*A*) The COBE Spectra apheresis system. (*B*) The separation chamber uses a unique asymmetric design to minimize contamination from red and white blood cells.

plasma, it has the disadvantage that two to three times the volume removed must be used in replacement. Normal serum albumin in a 5 percent solution (NSA) and plasma protein fraction (PPF) are alternatives that may be replaced in a 1:1 ratio. These products provide the proper oncotic properties but increase the cost of the procedure. Plasma protein fraction has been associated with hypotensive reactions[6] and is generally not used in most centers. Neither NSA nor PPF has been implicated in transmission of transfusion-transmitted viruses. Mixtures of normal saline and NSA have also been used. Because NSA can be expensive and is subject to shortages, HES has recently been used successfully as a portion of the replacement fluid.[7] Fresh frozen plasma (FFP) contains all the constituents of the removed plasma and thus would appear to be the optimal replacement fluid. However, frozen plasma has the disadvantages of possible disease transmission, ABO incompatibility, citrate toxicity, and sensitization

to plasma proteins and cellular antigens.[8] It has been implicated in fatal reactions and is now recommended primarily for the treatment of patients with thrombotic thrombocytopenia purpura (TTP) or hemolytic uremic syndrome (HUS). It is postulated that FFP may provide some factor that patients with TTP or HUS are missing, such as a precursor for prostacyclin or other antithrombotic factors.[9] Reports of an unusually large von Willebrand's factor (vWF) as a proposed etiology of TTP or HUS has prompted the use of cryosupernatant fraction of plasma as the replacement fluid, a component deficient in vWF.[10]

## General Requirements

A qualified, licensed physician is responsible for all aspects of the apheresis program. Good equipment and a well-trained, motivated staff are essential to an effective apheresis program. Operators of automated machines

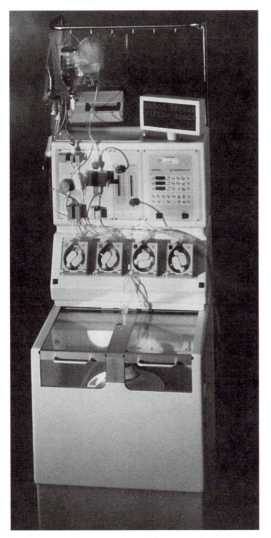

**Figure 17–7.** The Fresenius AS-104. (Courtesy Fresenius USA, Inc., Walnut Creek, CA.)

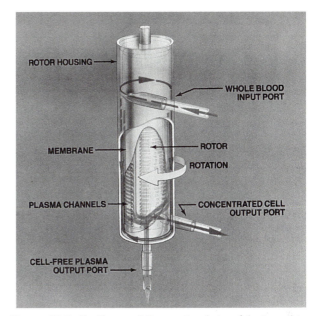

**Figure 17–8.** The Plasmacell-C separation device of the Fenwal Autopheresis-C. (Courtesy Baxter Healthcare Corporation, Deerfield, IL.)

must be knowledgeable in all aspects of operation and troubleshooting. Individuals hired to perform these procedures may be medical technologists or nurses. In some institutions technicians are trained on the job. Regardless of the professional background of the apheresis staff, operators must participate in an intensive orientation program and demonstrate continued competency in all aspects of apheresis.[11,12] This training should include machine operation and quality control, donor selection, familiarity with the standards of the American Association of Blood Banks (AABB)[13] and the Code of Federal Regulations (CFR),[14] documentation, management of complications, and venous access. An apheresis operator should be friendly and outgoing. Because the procedures are often lengthy, complications may be avoided by the operator's ability to relieve the donor's or patient's boredom and anxiety. Although serious complications are unusual, it is essential to have another qualified individual immediately available to assist in case of emergencies. A physician does not have to be in the room but should be within reach if complications should occur.

Written, informed consent must be obtained from donors and patients. The procedure, possible risks and benefits, and alternative modes of therapy must be explained in understandable language. The individual must then be given the opportunity to accept or to reject the procedure.

The apheresis unit must contain an operator's manual with detailed instructions concerning the following:

1. Informed consent process
2. Standardized protocols and policies for component collection (donors) and therapeutic procedures (patients)
3. Quality control of the equipment and apheresis products (component collections)
4. Management of adverse reactions
5. Postapheresis care
6. Proper record keeping; documentation should comply with AABB and CFR regulations

## APPLICATIONS

Blood banks were established for the primary purpose of providing compatible and viable red cells to restore oxygen-carrying capacity to the tissues. Anticoagulant/preservative solutions and plastic bags were developed that allowed maximum storage of red cells with acceptable posttransfusion survival and function. Later, as advances were made in medicine—particularly in the area of chemotherapy—blood banks were faced with the demands for products to overcome the effects of bone marrow depression caused by these drugs. Patients needed platelets and white cells to survive the period of intensive drug therapy. The doses of blood components required to treat such patients effectively could

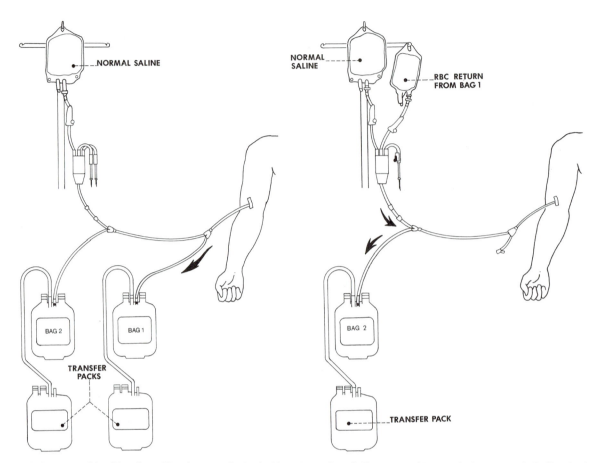

**Figure 17–9.** Venous blood is collected into bag 1 and mixed with anticoagulant (*left*). Bag 1 and its transfer bag are sealed off and taken to a centrifuge for separation into plasma and red blood cells. Meanwhile, the needle and tubing are kept open with normal saline. The red blood cells are attached to the administration set and infused (*right*). The process is then repeated using bag 2. (From Kennedy, MS, and Domen, RE: Therapeutic Apheresis. Vox Sang 45:261, 1983, with permission.)

not be met by products prepared from single whole blood donations. New technology had to be developed to collect larger quantities of a component from a single donor. In addition, increasing concern about transfusion-transmitted diseases and alloimmunization led to the development of programs to reduce the number of donor exposures to the patient. Automated or semiautomated apheresis equipment was the answer to the new demands placed on the blood banks. Component collection thus was the primary application of apheresis equipment.

It was soon realized that the machines also could be used therapeutically to treat patients with certain diseases. The rationale for the procedure was to remove the pathologic component from the blood or patient. Therefore, the use of apheresis technology can be divided into two categories: component collections and therapeutic procedures.

## Component Collections

In component collections, a normal healthy donor undergoes a procedure to obtain a specific blood component that will be transfused to a patient. Apheresis

donors must meet the requirements established by the standards of the AABB.[13] Donors undergoing an occasional procedure (performed no more frequently than once every 4 weeks) must meet the same criteria as a whole blood donor. Exceptions to the requirements are allowed if the product would be of particular value to the patient. In such cases, a physician must verify in writing that the donor's health would not be compromised. More stringent regulations govern the donor who participates in a serial apheresis program (procedure performed more frequently than once every 4 weeks). Careful monitoring of weight, blood cell counts, serum protein levels, and quantitation of immunoglobulins is required. The interval between apheresis procedures should be at least 48 hours, and the amount of red cell loss should not exceed 25 mL per week. The maximum amount of plasma that can be retained during a procedure should not exceed the amount approved by the Food and Drug Administration (FDA). Apheresis procedures should not be performed more than twice in 1 week, or 24 times in 1 year unless approved by the blood bank physician. If the donor's RBCs cannot be reinfused during a procedure, or if the participant donates a unit of whole blood, 4 weeks should elapse before a subsequent cytapheresis procedure, unless the hemoglobin requirement is met and the donor is found acceptable by a blood bank physician.

In component collections, replacement fluids are generally not required. However, careful monitoring of fluid volume in and out is required to prevent complications from shifts in blood volume. The extracorporeal blood volume (volume out of the donor) should not exceed 15 percent of the donor's estimated total blood volume at any time during the procedure. The donor's total blood volume may be obtained from a chart by using the height, weight, and sex of the individual. The extracorporeal volume is calculated from the volume of the apheresis chamber, the donor's hematocrit, and the total blood volume. Several of the modern apheresis machines perform these calculations automatically. If not, the manufacturer must be consulted for the formulas used for each specific machine.

## Plateletpheresis

Platelet transfusions are indicated in patients who are bleeding or at increased risk for bleeding secondary to thrombocytopenia or platelet dysfunction. Platelets for transfusion can be provided by platelet concentrates, which are harvested from routine whole blood donations, or by apheresis. In a plateletpheresis procedure, a portion of the donor's platelets and plasma is removed with the return of the donor's RBCs, WBCs, and remaining plasma. Sedimenting agents are not necessary for this procedure. The platelets are selectively separated from the whole blood and retained in a collection bag manufactured specifically for platelet storage. The platelet yield is related to the donor's initial platelet count and the amount of blood processed. If a plateletpheresis is performed more frequently than every 4 weeks, a platelet count should be obtained and must be more than $150,000/\mu L$ before performing subsequent plateletpheresis. Routinely, the number of platelets in an apheresis product is equivalent to 6 to 10 random platelet concentrates. AABB standards require that 75 percent of plateletpheresis products tested contain a minimum of $3 \times 10^{11}$ platelets, a value approximately six times that of a random platelet concentrate.[13] An apheresis donor for platelets must not have taken aspirin-containing medication within the last 3 days.[15] Aspirin, by inhibiting the enzyme cyclooxygenase in the prostaglandin pathway, prevents adequate platelet aggregation and the release of platelet adenosine diphosphate (ADP). Because an apheresis product would be the sole source of platelets for the patient, careful screening of potential donors is essential for obtaining therapeutically effective products. A routine plateletpheresis procedure usually takes 1 to 2 hours. The product is usually prepared in a closed system, approved for 5 days' storage. If the product is prepared in a open system, it must be transfused within 24 hours. Platelets stored at room temperature (20 to 24°C) should be maintained with continuous, gentle agitation. The pH at the end of the storage period must be 6.2 or greater. If red cell contamination in the product is negligible (less than 5 mL), compatibility testing is not required, but it is recommended that the donor plasma be ABO-compatible with the recipient, especially with a neonate.[13]

Side effects to the donor during plateletpheresis procedures are commonly attributed to citrate toxicity (often termed citrate *effect*). Used to anticoagulate the blood as it enters the separation chamber, citrate is metabolized quickly in the liver. However, if the amount of citrate infused exceeds the body's ability to metabolize it, the donor may feel numbness or tingling around the mouth. The problem can be solved by decreasing the reinfusion rate of the returned components or giving the donor exogenous calcium. Complications may also occur secondary to improper monitoring of fluid volumes, particularly if IFC equipment is used to perform the procedure.

## Leukapheresis

Occasionally granulocytes are needed as a transfusion product for patients who are severely neutropenic and have infections that are unresponsive to traditional therapy. To collect the large numbers of cells needed, apheresis techniques are applied. However, the unique characteristics of the granulocyte present technical problems in their collection. The collection of red cells and platelets is an easier task because of the increased intravascular volume and reduced daily consumption. Neutrophils make up a small portion of the cellular components of the blood, yet 50 percent of the bone marrow is dedicated to their production. The proportion is understandable in view of the daily consumption of neutrophils. Production in a normal adult is about $10^{11}$ cells per day. These cells have a half-life of approximately 6 hours in the blood. A patient with sepsis can increase production to $10^{12}$ cells per day.[16] It is estimated that approximately 230 percent of the neutrophils are replaced daily in a healthy adult, in comparison to only 1 percent of the red cells and 10 percent of the platelets.[17]

Initially, this therapy showed great promise. However, the lack of significant data indicating the clinical benefit of granulocyte transfusions, the difficulties obtaining this product, and its adverse effects have led to a decline in its popularity. The limited success of granulocyte transfusions has been attributed to the inadequate dose of granulocytes obtained. Several techniques have been used to enhance the yield of these cells.

Because the granulocyte layer interfaces with the RBC layer (see Figure 17–1), the use of the sedimenting agent HES allows better separation and improved yield, while minimizing RBC contamination. Although HES is largely removed by the reticuloendothelial system, residual HES has been reported in a donor up to 1 year after granulocytapheresis. However, long-term complications have not been identified. Although a lower-molecular-weight preparation of HES with improved urinary excretion has been used safely,[18] a recent report indicates that this product may be less efficient in collecting granulocytes.[19] Also, HES is a colloidal plasma volume expander and may lead to headaches and peripheral edema as a result of expanded intravascular blood volumes. Each facility should have a policy indicating the maximum cumulative dose of any sedimenting agent within a given time interval.[13] Less than 2 percent of the distribution of granulocytes in the body is present in the circulation, with a small fraction of the marginal pool, and the remainder is in the bone marrow. Corticosteroids, such as prednisone or dexamethasone can increase the number of circulating granulocytes by release of the marginal pool and slow their departure from the intravascular space. The use of steroids in donors before a granulocyte collection may exacerbate certain medical conditions, such as diabetes or hypertension, and should be used under the guidance of the blood bank physician.[20] The use of recombinant hematopoietic growth factors (granulocyte colony-stimulating factor, or G-CSF, and granulocyte-macrophage colony-stimulating factor, or GM-CSF) in granulocyte donors has resulted in marked increases in the collection of granulocytes (up to $1 \times 10^{11}$). This is a significant improvement over the current standard of $1 \times 10^{10}$. Initial studies indicate significant recovery and survival of these granulocytes. Although several side effects have been reported with the use of these growth factors, these are usually well tolerated. The use of this mobilization strategy, as well as a more critical evaluation of the efficacy of this product, has resulted in a recent resurgence of interest in granulocyte transfusions.[21]

The granulocyte concentrate must contain a minimum of $1.0 \times 10^{10}$ granulocytes in at least 75 percent of the units tested. The product has a shelf life of 24 hours but should be transfused as soon as possible after collection for optimal therapeutic effectiveness. The product should be stored at room temperature without agitation. Because of the large numbers of viable lymphocytes present, granulocyte preparations must be irradiated to prevent GVH disease in immunocompromised recipients, or if the donor is related to the recipient. The function of the granulocytes is not affected by the irradiation. Leukocyte depletion filters must not be used. Contamination of granulocyte preparations with RBCs is extremely common. Compatibility testing is required in products containing greater than 5 mL of red cells and should be ABO-compatible with the patient's plasma. Appropriate records of the procedure, yield of granulocytes, and donor information are required.[13]

### Erythrocytapheresis

A significant recent advance in the field of apheresis involves the collection of RBCs by automated apheresis technology.[22] This recently licensed process, developed by the Haemonetics Corporation, allows the col-lection of either two standardized units of RBCs or one unit of RBCs and a large volume unit of fresh frozen plasma during one collection procedure, performed on the Haemonetics MCS Plus. These procedures may be performed on both allogeneic and autologous donors. There are several advantages to automated RBC collection, including (1) a standardized RBC mass collection (180-200 mL); (2) the use of smaller needles for collection; (3) the use of saline compensation, which will reduce the risk of hypovolemia; (4) on-line separation, thus eliminating secondary separation procedures; and (5) reduced costs of testing, data entry, and staffing. Several blood centers are in the process of converting their entire production processes to collection of all components by apheresis.

### Neocytapheresis

Young patients with certain hematologic disorders, especially the thalassemia syndromes, often require continuous red cell transfusion therapy. The benefits of this chronic transfusion support include both prolonged survival and improved quality of life. However, there is a significant complication of this therapy: the accumulation of iron in the body, termed *hemosiderosis.*

Each milliliter (mL) of RBCs contains approximately 1 milligram (mg) of iron. These chronically transfused patients accumulate this iron without an effective physiologic method of excretion. Eventually the iron is deposited in the tissues, leading to organ dysfunction, with significant morbidity and mortality.

The traditional therapy for this complication is an iron-chelating agent, which enhances the urinary excretion of iron. An adjunctive approach in the prevention and treatment of transfusion-associated iron overload is the transfusion of young RBCs, or "neocytes." This method involves the selective removal of the donor's neocytes, or younger cells, found in the upper portion of the red blood cell layer (see Figure 17–1).

A unit of neocytes has a half-life approximately twice that of a regular unit of RBCs, thus reducing the frequency of transfusions in these patients.[23] Various techniques have been developed to collect neocytes, including a form of apheresis termed *neocytapheresis.* Recently a neocyte separation bag system has been described.[24] However, the preparation of these units is time consuming and costly and has not gained wide acceptance.

### Hematopoietic Progenitor Cells

In the field of transfusion medicine there has been significant growth in the use of cytapheresis to collect hematopoietic progenitor cells. Bone marrow transplantation (BMT) is used in the treatment of multiple disorders, including leukemia, solid tumors such as breast cancer, thalassemia, aplastic anemia, and sickle cell anemia, among others. Traditionally, autologous or allogeneic marrow, which includes the progenitor cells, is collected from the patient's or donor's bone marrow. Once harvested, the marrow undergoes extensive processing before storage. The processing can require cell separation, RBC removal, buffy coat concentration, and mononuclear cell purification. In addition, malignant cells in the marrow may be purged by monoclonal antibodies. Techniques have been developed using the currently available apheresis equipment to perform these tasks.[25] Following marrow ablation with myelosuppressive chemotherapy or radiation therapy, or both, the collected progenitor cells are infused to repopulate the marrow, which then begins to redevelop all cell lines.

The primitive progenitor cells that are capable of differentiation are also contained within the peripheral blood and are often termed *peripheral blood stem cells* (PBSCs). These cells can be collected with the use of currently available apheresis techniques. Multiple collections by apheresis are usually needed, and the number and frequency of procedures are determined by the yield of progenitor cells obtained and the patient's condition. Similar to their use in the collection of granulocytes, hematopoietic growth factors are now frequently used to increase the number of circulating stem cells in the peripheral circulation and increase the yield.[26]

There are several advantages to using progenitor cells collected by apheresis over traditional bone marrow collection. Anesthesia is avoided, and the procedures can be performed safely in the outpatient setting. Patients with extensive infiltration of their marrow by a tumor or with myelofibrosis can still undergo progenitor cell collection. Other advantages include a shorter period of cytopenia, decreased transfusion requirements, fewer infectious complications, and decreased length of hospitalization. Disadvantages may include the complications of central venous access, including infection and thrombosis, length of time to collect an adequate dose, the increased volume of the product, and contamination with mature lymphocytes.[27]

Guidelines for the collection of hematopoietic progenitor cells have been published in the AABB standards.[13] Specific information on donor selection, laboratory testing, collection, storage, and infusion are presented in this section. In addition, the procedures for quality management, records, and labeling are provided.

### Plasmapheresis

In a plasmapheresis procedure, the plasma is separated from the cellular components in a collection bag and retained, and then the cells are reinfused to the donor. The procedure may be performed by the manual method described in this chapter or by using automated equipment. For the clinical setting, plasmapheresis may be used to increase the inventory of fresh frozen plasma of a particular ABO group, such as group AB. The procedure may be used to collect immune plasma for patients who are immunosuppressed and have been exposed to varicella or herpes. Reference lab-

oratories perform apheresis to collect rare red and white cell antibodies. Commercially, plasma centers use serial plasmapheresis to draw plasma for manufacturing into such products as plasma derivatives, hepatitis immune globulin, and Rh-immune globulin.

If the procedure is performed no more than once every 4 weeks, the criteria that apply to whole blood donation should be used. However, if the donor is participating in a serial plasmapheresis program (plasma is donated more frequently than once every 4 weeks), AABB standards require additional and continuous assessment of the donor's health.[13] The procedure should not be performed if the total serum protein is less than 6.0 g/dL or if there has been an unexplained weight loss. Every 4 months, all records and laboratory tests must be reviewed and evaluated by a physician, and a serum protein electrophoresis or immunoglobulin level must be determined. If the donor's red cells during a procedure have not been reinfused, 8 weeks must elapse before the donor may be reinstated in the program.

Proper identification of the red cell reinfusion bag is essential, particularly during manual procedures when the bag is separated from the donor. The red cells must be returned within 2 hours of the phlebotomy. Red cell loss must not be greater than 25 mL per week. The amount of whole blood that can be processed must not be greater than 1000 mL (1200 mL if the donor weighs at least 176 lb) in any 48-hour period or 2000 mL (2400 mL if the donor weighs at least 176 lb) in a 7-day period.

### Therapeutic Procedures

When therapeutic apheresis was originally introduced as a treatment modality, it generated enormous enthusiasm and excitement. It was hoped that this new technology would be the answer to many problems, particularly in diseases involving immune-mediated mechanisms. Expectations far exceeded the therapeutic abilities of the procedure. Assessment of effectiveness was difficult because reports in the literature presented data from uncontrolled studies. Most clinical trials were retrospective rather than prospective. However, the last decade has provided the medical field with sufficient data to evaluate apheresis as a form of therapy more realistically and to define its role in the treatment of disease (Table 17–1).[28,29]

Apheresis cannot cure a disease but can be very effective in alleviating the symptoms produced by the underlying disease state. Efficacy of the procedure is enhanced by concomitant drug therapy, particularly immunosuppressive therapy in immune-mediated problems. Duration of the effects of the procedure varies with the individual. The course of therapy may last from several days to several months and is based on the response and tolerance of the patient.

Therapeutic apheresis has placed blood banks in the position of direct medical care for the patient. This situation has necessitated a change in the perspective of

**Table 17-1.** Guidelines for Therapeutic Hemapheresis*

| Category I | Category II | Category III | Category IV |
|---|---|---|---|
| Coagulation factor inhibitors<br>Cryoglobulinemia<br>Goodpasture's syndrome<br>Guillain-Barré syndrome<br>Homozygous familial<br>  hypercholesterolemia<br>Hyperviscosity syndrome<br>Myasthenia gravis<br>Posttransfusion purpura<br>Refsum's disease<br>TTP | Chronic inflammatory<br>  demyelinating<br>  polyneuropathy<br>Cold agglutinin disease<br>Drug overdose and poisoning<br>  (protein-bound toxins)<br>HUS<br>Pemphigus vulgaris<br>Rapidly progressive<br>  glomerulonephritis<br>Systemic vasculitis (primary<br>  or secondary to rheumatoid<br>  arthritis or systemic lupus<br>  erythematosus) | ABO-incompatible organ or<br>  marrow transplantation<br>Maternal treatment of<br>  maternal-fetal<br>  incompatibility (hemolytic<br>  disease of the newborn)<br>Thyroid storm<br>Multiple sclerosis<br>Progressive systemic sclerosis<br>Pure RBC aplasia<br>Transfusion refractoriness<br>  due to alloantibodies<br>  (RBC, platelet, HLA)<br>Warm autoimmune<br>  hemolytic anemia | AIDS (for symptoms of immunodeficiency)<br>Amyotrophic lateral sclerosis<br>Aplastic anemia<br>Fulminant hepatic failure<br>ITP (chronic)<br>Lupus nephritis<br>Polymyositis/dermatomyositis<br>Psoriasis<br>Renal transplant rejection<br>Rheumatoid arthritis<br>Schizophrenia |
| *Cytapheresis* | | | |
| Leukemia with<br>  hyperleukocytosis<br>  syndrome<br>Sickle cell syndrome (also<br>  see category III)<br>Thrombocytosis, symptomatic | Cutaneous T-cell lymphoma<br>  (cytoreduction or<br>  photopheresis)<br>Hairy cell leukemia<br>Hyperparasitemia (e.g.,<br>  malaria)<br>Peripheral blood stem cell<br>  collections for hemopoietic<br>  reconstitution<br>Rheumatoid arthritis | Life-threatening hemolytic<br>  transfusion reactions<br>Multiple sclerosis<br>Organ transplant rejection<br>  (also photopheresis)<br>Sickle cell disease (prophylactic<br>  use in pregnancy) | Leukemia without hyperleukocytosis<br>  syndromes<br>Hypereosinophilia<br>Polymyositis/dermatomyositis |

**Source:** Extracorporeal Therapy Committee: Guidelines for Therapeutic Hemapheresis. American Association of Blood Banks, Bethesda, MD, 1992 (revised 1995), with permission.
*The indications have been divided into four categories as follows: Category I, standard and acceptable under certain circumstances, including primary therapy; category II, sufficient evidence to suggest efficacy, acceptable therapy on an adjunctive basis; category III, inconclusive evidence for efficacy, uncertain benefit/risk ratio; and category IV, lack of efficacy in controlled trials.
HUS = hemolytic uremic syndrome; ITP = idiopathic thrombocytopenic purpura; TTP = thrombotic thrombocytopenic purpura.

the medical director and the technical staff. Clearly defined policies must delineate the responsibility of the blood bank and the attending physician. Issues such as who makes the decision about vascular access, who orders laboratory tests to evaluate and to monitor the patient, and who chooses replacement fluids must be resolved. The medical director should be involved with the attending physician in deciding whether there are clinical indications for the procedure. The technical staff must be properly trained to care for very ill patients. Confidence in handling emergency situations is essential. Attention must be given to the patient's medication schedule. Apheresis may dangerously lower plasma levels of medications given before the procedure. Proper documentation of all facets of the procedure is required. Written informed consent must be properly obtained from the patient.

The rationale of the therapeutic apheresis is based on the following:

1. A pathogenic substance exists in the blood that contributes to a disease process or its symptoms.
2. The substance can be more effectively removed by apheresis than by the body's own homeostatic mechanisms.

The apheresis procedures that reduce the level of the substance involved, and thus improve the symptoms, are classified by the component removed: cytapheresis if the component is cellular, and plasma exchange (or immunoadsorption) if the substance circulates in the plasma. (It should be noted that this text is not intended to provide detailed information on the description or management of specific diseases. If needed, a more thorough review should be consulted).[30]

*Therapeutic Cytapheresis*

Plateletpheresis (thrombocytopheresis) can be used to treat patients who have abnormally elevated platelet counts with related symptoms.[29] This condition has been reported in patients with myeloproliferative disorders such as polycythemia vera. Patients having counts greater than 1,000,000/μL may develop thrombotic or hemorrhagic complications. During a routine apheresis procedure, the platelet count can be decreased by as much as one-third to one-half the initial value.[31] The procedure can be repeated as frequently as necessary until drug therapy becomes effective and the symptoms disappear.

Leukapheresis has been used to treat patients with

leukemia. This therapy is particularly indicated in patients with impending leukostasis, in which leukocyte aggregates and thrombi may interfere with pulmonary and cerebral blood flow. Leukocyte counts in excess of 100,000/$\mu$L are considered appropriate indications for instituting apheresis therapy. The greatest therapeutic benefits are seen in acute cases under the following conditions: (1) drug therapy was just started and has not yet taken effect, (2) drug therapy is contraindicated, or (3) patients have become refractory to drug treatment. Lymphocytapheresis (the removal of lymphocytes) has been investigated as a means of producing immunosuppression in conditions with a cellular immune mechanism such as rheumatoid arthritis, systemic lupus erythematosus, kidney transplant rejection, and autoimmune and alloimmune diseases. These procedures are not used routinely, and further studies are required to determine efficacy and to assess possible long-term complications from the procedure.

The therapeutic uses of cytapheresis mentioned earlier involve depletion of cellular constituents without replacement. Erythrocytapheresis, however, is considered an exchange procedure. A predetermined quantity of red cells is removed from the patient and replaced with homologous blood. The procedure has been used successfully to treat various complications of sickle cell disease, such as priapism and impending stroke.[32] Other indications are rare. Successful therapy has been reported in patients with severe parasitic infections from malaria and babesiosis.[33,34]

### Therapeutic Plasmapheresis (Plasma Exchange)

*Plasmapheresis* is the removal and retention of the plasma, with return of all cellular components to the patient. This therapeutic procedure has become synonymous with the term *plasma exchange*, which describes the protocol more accurately. The purpose is to remove the offending agent in the plasma causing the clinical symptoms. The larger volume of plasma that is removed must be replaced or exchanged, thus the term *plasma exchange*. It has been postulated that beneficial effects of the procedure, particularly in diseases that involve malfunction of the immune system, may be attributed to the removal of the factors listed in Table 17-2.[35]

**Table 17-2.** Factors Removed by Plasmapheresis

1. Immune complexes (e.g., systemic lupus erythematosus)
2. Autoantibodies or alloantibodies (e.g., factor VIII inhibitors)
3. Antibodies causing hyperviscosity (e.g., Waldenström's macroglobulinemia)
4. Inflammatory mediators (e.g., fibrinogen and complement)
5. Antibody blocking the normal function of the immune system
6. Protein-bound toxins (e.g., barbiturate poisoning)
7. Lipoproteins
8. Platelet-aggregating factors (e.g., possible role in TTP)

TTP = thrombotic thrombocytopenic purpura.

The efficiency of a plasma exchange is related to the amount of plasma removed. This effect is diluted by the necessity to replace the plasma to maintain the patient's fluid volume. A procedure that removes an amount of plasma equal to the patient's plasma volume is called a *one-volume exchange*. The actual amount of plasma removed may vary from 2 to 4 L, depending on the patient's size. A one-volume exchange should reduce the unwanted plasma component to 30 percent of its initial value. If a second plasma volume is removed as part of the same procedure, the procedure becomes less efficient, reducing the component from 30 percent to only 10 percent.[8] Because of the diminishing effect of increased plasma removal, it is recommended that approximately 1 to 1.5 plasma volumes be exchanged per procedure.[36]

Synthesis and catabolism of the pathologic component, as well as its distribution between the extravascular and intravascular space, are factors affecting the outcome of a plasma exchange. If the antibody that causes the patient's symptoms is IgM, apheresis can be an effective therapeutic tool. IgM is primarily intravascular and is synthesized slowly, whereas IgG is equally distributed in the intravascular and extravascular spaces. Reappearance of IgG in the plasma occurs more quickly because of reequilibration. Removal of IgG with apheresis can lead to increased antibody synthesis (rebound phenomenon). Because of this effect, therapeutic procedures performed to remove IgG antibodies are most effective when combined with immunosuppressive drugs.

### Immunoadsorption

Immunoadsorption refers to a method in which a specific ligand is bound to an insoluble matrix in a column or filter. Plasma is then perfused over the column, with selective removal of the pathogenic substance and return of the patient's own plasma. The removal is usually mediated by an antigen-antibody or chemical reaction. Both off-line and on-line procedures have been developed using the current apheresis equipment. A diagram of the process is shown in Figure 17-10.

A number of adsorptive matrices have been used with varying specificity. Table 17-3 lists some of the adsorbents, the substance removed, and the clinical applications of each.

Staphylococcal protein A as an immunoadsorbent has gained greater acceptance in clinical use. This ligand has an affinity for IgG classes 1, 2, and 4 as well as IgG immune complexes. The immunoaffinity column currently has federal licensure to treat patients with idiopathic thrombocytopenic purpura (ITP).[37] The column has also shown promise in the treatment of a variety of other disease processes, including human immunodeficiency virus (HIV)-associated thrombocytopenia,[38] chemotherapy-induced TTP/HUS,[39] and alloimmunization resulting in platelet refractoriness.[40] A number of adverse reactions, including fever, chills, and rash, have been reported, as have several fatalities.[41]

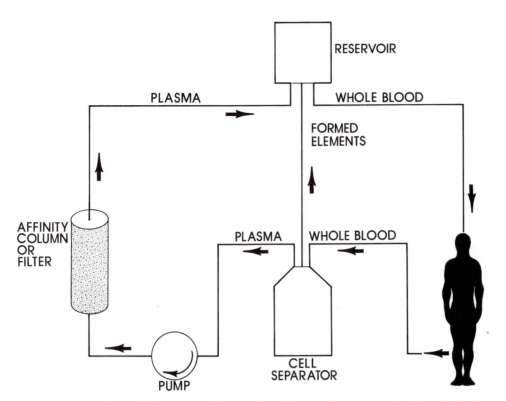

**Figure 17–10.** Perfusion of plasma over columns or filters. (From Berkman, EM, and Umlas, J (eds): Therapeutic Hemapheresis: A Technical Workshop. American Association of Blood Banks, Washington, DC, 1980, p 142, with permission.)

The mechanism of action of these columns is not well established. Removal of IgG and immune complexes alone cannot explain the clinical benefit of the treatment. There appears to be a significant immunomodulatory effect of this treatment, with enhanced anti-idiotypic antibody regulation and activated cellular immune function.[42]

Familial hypercholesterolemia, associated with abnormal metabolism of the low-density lipoprotein (LDL) and increased plasma cholesterol levels, is a significant cause of morbidity and mortality from premature atherosclerotic cardiovascular disease. Plasma exchange therapy is only partially effective in this disorder. LDL-apheresis, using either dextran sulfate cellulose adsorption[42] or heparin-induced extracorporeal LDL precipitation (HELP),[43] has been associated with regression of cardiovasular disease.

### Photopheresis

Photopheresis is a recently developed leukocytapheresis technique, requiring a special intermittent-flow machine utilizing the bowl technology. This treatment has been shown to be efficacious against cutaneous T-cell lymphoma, a malignant skin disorder characterized by an abnormal proliferation of CD4 lymphocytes. Before the procedure, the patient ingests the drug psoralen, which binds to the deoxyribonucleic acid (DNA) of all nucleated cells. Following the leukocytapheresis, the collected white blood cells are exposed

**Table 17–3.** Types of Adsorbents and Their Clinical Application

| Adsorbent | Substance Removed | Application |
|---|---|---|
| Charcoal | Bile acids | Cholestatic pruritus |
| A and B antigens | Anti-A, anti-B | Transplantation |
| Anti-LDL, heparin | LDL | Hypercholesterolemia |
| DNA | ANA, immune complexes | Systemic lupus erythematosus |
| Protein A | IgG, immune complexes | ITP, cancer, HUS |

ANA = antinuclear antibodies; HUS = hemolytic uremic syndrome; ITP = idiopathic thrombocytopenic purpura; LDL = low-density lipoproteins.

to ultraviolet light, which activates the psoralen and prevents replication. These treated cells are then returned to the patient, inducing an immune response against the abnormal lymphocyte clone.[44] Photopheresis has been used in several other immunologically mediated conditions, including scleroderma,[45] rheumatoid arthritis,[46] and chronic heart transplant rejection.[47]

## ADVERSE EFFECTS

Apheresis is accepted as a relatively safe procedure, but complications do occur. Adverse effects may be observed in component collections as well as in therapeutic procedures. In the latter case, it is sometimes difficult to evaluate whether the deleterious effects were caused by the procedure or by the underlying disease entity. Some of the problems encountered are listed in Table 17–4.

Citrate toxicity is usually observed during cytapheresis component collections when anticoagulated plasma is returned at a rapid rate. If fresh frozen plasma is used as replacement fluid during a therapeutic plasma exchange, this phenomenon is more likely to occur. Decreasing the reinfusion rate usually alleviates the symptoms. Some centers have switched to using a lower percent citrate solution. The most common initial complaint of citrate toxicity is tingling around the mouth. Citrate binds to calcium, and the lowering of the body's ionized calcium leads to the symptoms. Intravenous calcium is not recommended on a routine basis. If unattended, the symptoms can lead to tetany and cardiac arrythmia.

Complications of the vascular access needed for apheresis procedures are relatively common and include hematoma formation, localized or systemic infections, phlebitis, and neuropathies. Vasovagal reactions often can be avoided by attentive, receptive apheresis operators. Individuals undergoing these procedures require assurance from the operators. Hypovolemia is observed more frequently with IFC equipment. These machines require a greater extracorporeal volume (fluid volume out of the individual and into the separation chamber and tubing must not exceed 15 percent of the patient's total blood volume) than do the CFC machines. Careful monitoring of the volume in and out is necessary to prevent not only hypovolemia but also hypervolemia. Allergic reactions are related to the replacement fluids. This is generally observed in cases in which fresh frozen plasma is administered, but it has also been reported with albumin. Hemolysis is usually caused by a mechanical problem with the equipment, such as a kink in the plastic tubing. Observing the return line is critical to avoid this problem. Air embolism and clotting factor deficiencies are not commonly observed.

Deaths resulting from therapeutic apheresis procedures have been reported.[48] The majority of these have been caused by circulatory (cardiac arrest) or respiratory distress. Of the 50 cases reported, 25 had received plasma as part or all of the replacement fluid. Because plasma has been associated with fatalities, its use is recommended only in cases of TTP or HUS in which there is a specific indication for its use. Plasma is also capable of transmitting diseases such as hepatitis and the human immunodeficiency viruses.

Donors undergoing multiple plateletpheresis procedures in a short period of time may experience significant decreases in lymphocyte counts.[9] The long-term effects of lymphocyte reduction following plateletpheresis are minimal.[49]

## SUMMARY

The field of apheresis continues to evolve, as do all areas of transfusion medicine. Emerging technology has resulted in dramatic advances in the understanding of the immune response and the diseases associated with immune abnormalities. Also, innovative apheresis techniques, such as the collection of red blood cells and leukocyte-reduced platelet collections, further our ability to produce the optimal component for patients. Transfusion and transplantation practices have benefited from this knowledge and will continue to rely on the collection of cellular or plasma components by apheresis for transfusion or therapeutic purposes.

**Table 17–4.** Adverse Effects of Apheresis

1. Citrate toxicity
2. Vascular access complications (hematoma, sepsis, phlebitis, neuropathy)
3. Vasovagal reactions
4. Hypovolemia
5. Allergic reactions
6. Hemolysis
7. Air embolus
8. Depletion of clotting factors
9. Circulatory and respiratory distress
10. Transfusion-transmitted diseases
11. Lymphocyte loss
12. Depletion of proteins and immunoglobulins

---

## SUMMARY CHART: IMPORTANT POINTS TO REMEMBER (MT/SBB)

- In an apheresis procedure, blood is withdrawn from a donor or patient and separated into its components. One or more of the components is retained, and the remaining constituents are recombined and returned to the individual.
- The process of removing plasma from the blood is termed *plasmapheresis*; removal of platelets is termed *plateletpheresis* or *thrombocytopheresis*; removal of red blood cells is termed *erythrocytapheresis*; removal of leukocytes is known as *leukapheresis*.
- The variables of automated apheresis instruments include (1) centrifuge speed and diameter, (2) length of dwell time of the blood in the centrifuge, (3) the type of solutions added (anticoagulants), and (4) the cellular content or plasma volume of the donor.
- Apheresis equipment that uses intermittent-flow centrifugation (IFC) requires only one venipuncture, in which the blood is drawn and reinfused through the same needle. Once the desired component is separated, the remaining components are reinfused to the donor, and one cycle is complete. Therapeutic procedures usually require many cycles to reach an acceptable dose.

- Continuous-flow centrifugation (CFC) procedures withdraw, process, and return the blood to the individual simultaneously. Two venipuncture sites are necessary. The process of phlebotomy, separation, and reinfusion is uninterrupted.
- Membrane filtration technology uses membranes with specific pore sizes, allowing the passage of plasma through the membrane while the cellular portion passes over it.
- The most common anticoagulant used in apheresis is acid citrate dextrose (ACD).
- In therapeutic plasmapheresis procedures the replacement fluids used to maintain appropriate intravascular volume and oncotic pressure include normal saline, FFP, and 5 percent NSA.
- Granulocyte concentrates must contain a minimum of $1.0 \times 10^{10}$ granulocytes in at least 75 percent of units tested.
- Plateletpheresis products should contain a minimum of $3 \times 10^{11}$ platelets, which is equivalent to 6 to 10 random platelet concentrates in 75 percent of units tested.

---

## REVIEW QUESTIONS

1. American Association of Blood Bank standards requires that plateletpheresis products:
   A. Prepared in a closed system be transfused within 24 hours
   B. Contain $3 \times 10^{11}$ platelets in 75 percent of the units tested
   C. Have a compatibility test performed before transfusion
   D. Have a pH of 6.0 or greater on the day of collection

2. Therapeutic cytapheresis is used in patients with:
   A. Sickle cell disease to reduce the number of crises
   B. Systemic lupus erythematosus to remove immune complexes
   C. Leukemia to help increase granulocyte production
   D. Polycythemia vera to decrease the red blood cell count

3. The minimum interval allowed between plateletpheresis component collection procedures is:
   A. 24 hours
   B. 48 hours
   C. 7 days
   D. 8 weeks

4. A donor weighing 75 kg is undergoing a plasmapheresis procedure. What is the maximum amount of whole blood that can be processed over a 7-day period?
   A. 1000 mL
   B. 1200 mL
   C. 2000 mL
   D. 2400 mL

5. In a plasma exchange, the therapeutic effectiveness is:
   A. Greatest with the first plasma volume removed
   B. Affected by the type of replacement fluid used
   C. Enhanced if the unwanted antibody is IgG rather than IgM
   D. Independent of the use of concomitant immunosuppressive therapy

6. The replacement fluid indicated during plasma exchange for TTP or HUS is:
   A. Normal (0.9%) saline
   B. HES
   C. FFP
   D. PPF
   E. NSA (5%)

7. The most common adverse effect of plateletpheresis collection is:
   A. Allergic reactions
   B. Hepatitis

C. Hemolysis

D. Citrate effect

E. Air embolism

8. Apheresis can be used to collect all of the following except:
   A. Leukocytes
   B. Macrophages
   C. Neocytes
   D. Platelets
   E. Lymphocytes

9. Platelets collected in a closed apheresis system have a shelf life of:
   A. 35 days
   B. 24 hours
   C. 5 days
   D. 21 days
   E. 7 days

10. Peripheral blood stem cells are:
    A. Responsible for phagocytosis of bacteria
    B. Removed during erythrocytapheresis
    C. Pluripotential hematopoietic precursors that circulate in the peripheral blood
    D. Immature RBCs used for transfusion in patients with thalessemia
    E. Lymphocytes involved with the immune response

11. Advantages of CFC over IFC include:
    A. Portability
    B. Greater extracorporeal volume
    C. Two venipunctures needed
    D. Single venipuncture needed
    E. Lower extracorporeal volume

## ANSWERS TO REVIEW QUESTIONS

1. B (p 369)

2. A (p 373)

3. B (p 368)

4. C (p 371)

5. A (p 373)

6. C (p 366)

7. D (p 369)

8. B (p 371)

9. C (p 369)

10. C (p 371)

11. E (p 365)

## REFERENCES

1. Price, TH: Centrifugal equipment for the performance of therapeutic hemapheresis procedures. In MacPherson, JL, and Kaspirisin, DO (eds): Therapeutic Hemapheresis, Vol 1. CRC Press, Boca Raton, FL, 1985, p 123.

2. Rock, G, Tittley, P, and McCombie, N: Plasma collection using an automated membrane device. Transfusion 26:269–271, 1986.

3. Simon, T, et al: Storage and transfusion of platelets collected by an automated two-stage apheresis procedure. Transfusion 32:624, 1992.

4. Blood collection, storage and component preparation. In Walker, RH (ed): Technical Manual, ed 10. American Association of Blood Banks, Arlington, VA, 1990, pp 642–644.

5. Heustis, DW, et al: Use of hydroxyethyl starch to improve granulocyte collection in the Latham blood processor. Transfusion 15:1559, 1975.

6. Alving, BM, et al: Hypotension associated with prekallikrein activator (Hageman-factor fragments) in plasma protein fraction. N Engl J Med 299:66, 1978.

7. Brecher, ME, and Owen, HG: Washout kinetics of colloidal starch as a partial or full replacement for plasma exchange. J Clin Apheresis 11:123–126, 1996.

8. McCullough, J, and Chopek, M: Therapeutic plasma exchange. Lab Med 12:745, 1981.

9. Westphal, RG: Complications of hemapheresis. In Westphal, RG, and Kaspirisin, DO (eds): Current Status of Hemapheresis: Indications, Technology and Complications. American Association of Blood Banks, Arlington, VA, 1989.

10. Byrnes, JJ, et al: Effectiveness of the cryosupernatant fraction of plasma in the treatment of refractory thrombocytopenic purpura. Am J Hematol 34:169–174, 1990.

11. Quality Program, vols 1 and 2. American Association of Blood Banks, Bethesda, MD, 1994.

12. Food and Drug Administration: Guideline for Quality Assurance in Blood Establishments, July 1995.

13. Menitove, JE, ed: Standards for blood banks and transfusion services, 18th ed. American Association of Blood Banks, Bethesda, MD, 1997.

14. Code of Federal Regulations, 21 CFR 606.100 (b). US Government Printing Office, Washington, DC, 1996 (revised annually).

15. Hemapheresis. In Vengelen-Tyler, V (ed): Technical Manual, ed 12. American Association of Blood Banks, Bethesda, MD, 1996, pp 115–133.

16. Klock, JC: Granulocyte transfusion physiology. In Mielke, CH (ed): Apheresis: Development, Applications, and Collection Procedures. Alan R Liss, New York, 1981, p 14.

17. Wright, DG: Leucocyte transfusions: Thinking twice. Am J Med 76:637, 1984.

18. Strauss, RG, et al: Selecting the optimal dose of low-molecular weight hydroxyethyl starch (Pentastarch) for granulocyte collection. Transfusion 27:350, 1987.

19. Lee, JH, et al: A controlled study of the efficacy of hetastarch and pentastarch in granulocyte collections by centrifugal leukapheresis. Blood 86:4662–4666, 1995.

20. Hinckley, ME, and Heustis, DW: Premedication for optimal granulocyte collection. Plasma Therapy 2:149–152, 1981.

21. Strauss, RG: Clinical perspectives of granulocyte transfusions: Efficacy to date. J Clin Apheresis 10:114–118, 1995.

22. Meyer, D, et al: Red cell collection by apheresis technology. Transfusion 33:819–824, 1993.

23. Propper, RD: Neocytes and neocyte-gerocyte exchange. In Volger, WR (ed): Cytapheresis and Plasma Exchange Clinical Indications. Alan R Liss, New York, 1982, p 227.

24. Collins, AF, et al: Comparison of a transfusion preparation of newly formed red cells and standard washed red cell transfusions in patients with homozygous B-thalassemia. Transfusion 34:517, 1994.

25. Areman, EM, and Sacher, RA: Bone marrow processing for transplantation. Transfus Med Rev 5:214–227, 1991.

26. Bishop, MR, et al: High-dose therapy and peripheral blood progenitor cell transplantation: Effects of recombinant human granulocyte-macrophage colony-stimulating factor on the autograft. Blood 83:610, 1994.

27. Badarenko, N, et al: Apheresis: New opportunities. Clin Lab Med 16(4):907–929, 1996.

28. Report of the AMA panel on therapeutic plasmapheresis: Current status of therapeutic plasmapheresis and related techniques. JAMA 253:819, 1985.
29. Taft, EG: Therapeutic apheresis. Hum Pathol 14:235, 1983.
30. Strauss, RG, et al: Clinical applications of therapeutic apheresis: Report of the Clinical Applications Committee. J Clin Apheresis 8:4, 1993.
31. Goldfinger, D: Clinical applications of therapeutic cytapheresis. In Berkman, EM, and Umlas, J (eds): Therapeutic Hemapheresis. American Association of Blood Banks, Washington, DC, 1980, p 67.
32. Kleinman, SH, and Goldfinger, D: Erythrocytapheresis (ERCP) in sickle cell disease. In MacPherson, JL, and Kaspirisin, DO (eds): Therapeutic Hemapheresis, Vol 2. CRC Press, Boca Raton, FL, 1985, p 129.
33. Yarrish, RL, et al: Transfusion malaria. Treatment with exchange transfusion after delayed diagnosis. Arch Intern Med 142:187, 1982.
34. Cahill, KM, et al: Red cell exchange: Treatment of babesiosis in a splenectomized patient. Transfusion 21:193, 1981.
35. Patten, E: Pathophysiology of the immune system. In Kilins, J, and Jones, JM (eds): Therapeutic Apheresis. American Association of Blood Banks, Arlington VA, 1983, p 19.
36. Klein, HG: Effect of plasma exchange on plasma constituents: Choice of replacement solutions and kinetics of exchange. In MacPherson, JL, and Kaspirisin, DO (eds): Therapeutic Hemapheresis, Vol 2. CRC Press, Boca Raton, FL, 1985, p 5.
37. Snyder, HW, Jr, et al: Experience with protein A–immunoadsorption in treatment-resistant adult immune thrombocytopenia purpura. Blood 79:2237, 1992.
38. Mittelman, A, et al: Treatment of patients with HIV thrombocytopenia and hemolytic uremic syndrome with protein A (Prosorba® Column) immunoadsorption. Semin Hematol 26 (Suppl 1):15–18.
39. Snyder, HW, Jr, et al: Successful treatment of cancer-chemotherapy associated thrombotic thrombocytopenic purpura/hemolytic uremic syndrome (TTP/HUS) with protein A immunoadsorption. Blood 76(Suppl1):4679, 1990.
40. Christie, DJ, et al: Protein A column therapy in the treatment of immunologic refractoriness to platelet transfusion. Blood 76 (Suppl 1):4679, 1990.
41. Pineda, AA: Immunoaffinity apheresis columns: Clinical applications and therapeutic mechanisms of action. In Sacher, RA, et al: Cellular and Humoral Immunotherapy and Apheresis. American Association of Blood Banks, Arlington, VA, 1991, p 31.
42. Gordon, BR, and Saal, SD: Low-density lipoprotein apheresis using the Liposorber dextran sulfate cellulose system for patients with hypercholesterolemia refractory to medical therapy. J Clin Apheresis 11:128–131, 1996.
43. Lees, RS, et al: Treatment of hypercholesterolemia with heparin-induced extracorporeal low-density lipoprotein precipitation (HELP). J Clin Apheresis 11:132–131, 1996.
44. Edelson, R, et al: Treatment of cutaneous T-cell lymphoma by extracorporeal photochemotherapy—Preliminary results. N Engl J Med 316:297–303, 1987.
45. Rook, AH, et al: Treatment of systemic sclerosis with extracorporeal photochemotherapy. Arch Dermatol 128:337–346, 1992.
46. Malawista, SE, Trock, DH, and Edelson, RL: Treatment of rheumatoid arthritis by extracorporeal photochemotherapy: A pilot study. Arthritis Rheum 34:646–654, 1991.
47. Constanza-Nordin, MR, et al: Successful treatment of heart transplant rejection with photopheresis. Transplantation 53:808–815, 1992.
48. Heustis, DW: Risks and safety practices in hemapheresis procedures. Arch Pathol Lab Med 113:273–278, 1989.
49. Boograerts, MA: Side effects of hemapheresis. Trans Med Rev 1:186, 1987.

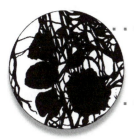

# CHAPTER 18

# ADVERSE EFFECTS OF BLOOD TRANSFUSION

Patricia Joyce Larison, MA, MT (ASCP)SBB, and Lloyd O. Cook, MD

## OBJECTIVES

*On completion of this chapter, the learner should be able to:*

1 Define *transfusion reaction.*

2 Discuss risks of transfusions.

3 Compare and contrast immediate hemolytic transfusion reactions (IHTR) with delayed hemolytic transfusion reactions (DHTR).

4 List the types of immediate and delayed transfusion reactions.

5 Differentiate clinical signs and symptoms of each described transfusion reaction.

6 List laboratory findings associated with IHTR and DHTR.

7 For each type of transfusion reaction, discuss definition, pathophysiology, signs, symptoms, therapy, prevention, and clinical work-up.

8 List antibodies most associated with immediate and delayed hemolytic transfusion reactions.

9 Identify procedures to follow at a patient's bedside in the event of a suspected transfusion reaction.

10 Discuss the importance of the patient's history in relationship to medications, transfusion history, and pregnancies.

11 List logical steps and procedures to follow in a laboratory investigation of transfusion reactions.

12 Discuss reporting of transfusion reaction work-ups.

13 List accreditation agencies involved in determining policies regarding transfusion reactions.

14 State regulatory record requirements and procedure to follow in reporting a fatal transfusion reaction.

## INTRODUCTION

*Transfusion* is an irreversible event that carries potential benefits and risks to the recipient. A *transfusion reaction* is any unfavorable transfusion-related event occurring in a patient during or after transfusion of blood components.[1] In addition to proper recognition, appropriate therapy and prevention of transfusion reactions require that the clinical and laboratory staff understand various types of reactions. Transfusion reactions are divided into immune-mediated and non–immune-mediated and are categorized according to their relationship to the time of transfusion as immediate or delayed. By knowing the rapidity of onset and mechanism of action, transfusionists can better assess current and future risks along with proper treatment and preventive measures.

## RISKS OF TRANSFUSION

As with any medical or technical procedure, the act of blood component transfusion has the potential for both benefit and risk to the patient. Table 18–1 lists specific adverse consequences of transfusions. The risk of fatality from noninfectious causes was analyzed using transfusion-associated death reports from registered blood establishments submitted to the Food and Drug Administration (FDA) from 1976 through 1985.[2] Table 18–2 lists typical causes of transfusion-associated deaths. Of

**Table 18–1.** Immediate and Delayed Noninfectious Transfusion Reaction Effects

| Immediate | Delayed |
|---|---|
| *Immune Effects* | |
| IHTR | DHTR |
| FNHTR | Alloimmunization |
| Allergic reaction | PTP |
| Anaphylaxis and anaphylactoid reactions | TA-GVHD |
| NCPE  *TRALI* | Immunosuppression |
| *Nonimmune Effects* | |
| Bacterial contamination | Iron overload |
| TACO | |
| Physical RBC damage | |
| Depletion and dilution of coagulation factors and platelets | |

IHTR = immediate hemolytic transfusion reaction; DHTR = delayed hemolytic transfusion reaction; FNHTR = febrile nonhemolytic transfusion reaction; PTP = Posttransfusion purpura; TA-GVHD = transfusion-associated graft-versus-host disease; NCPE = noncardiogenic pulmonary edema; TACO = transfusion-associated circulatory overload.

**Table 18–2.** Some Typical Causes of Transfusion-associated Deaths

Acute hemolysis (ABO-incompatible blood components)
Acute pulmonary edema
Bacterial contamination of product
Delayed hemolytic reactions
Anaphylaxis
External hemolysis (e.g., temperature exceeded 40°C)
Acute hemolysis; damaged blood component (e.g., nondeglycerolized, improper solution)
Transfusion-associated graft-versus-host disease

**Table 18–3.** Diseases Simulating Transfusion Reactions

1. Paroxysmal nocturnal hemoglobinuria
2. Autoimmune hemolytic anemia
3. Glucose-6-phosphate dehydrogenase (G-6-PD) deficiency
4. Malignant hyperthermia
5. Hemoglobinopathies
6. RBC membrane defects

the 256 immediate hemolysis deaths reported to be caused by noninfectious complications, clerical error was the prime factor determined as the fundamental flaw. Diseases that can cause red blood cell (RBC) hemolysis and might be misinterpreted for a hemolytic transfusion reaction are listed in Table 18–3.

## Rates of Risks

Occurrence rates of the various transfusion reaction types, along with their signs and symptoms, are useful in determining the most probable type of reaction a patient may be experiencing.

A National Institute of Health (NIH) Consensus Conference panel[3] reviewed occurrence data for common immune transfusion reactions and assigned the following rates of occurrence per unit transfused: (1) nonhemolytic febrile transfusion reaction (NHFTR), 1 to 2 percent; (2) allergic, 1 to 2 percent; (3) immediate hemolytic transfusion reaction (IHTR) and delayed hemolytic transfusion reaction (DHTR), 1:6000; (4) fatal immediate, 1:100,000. A review of rates of risk, including occurrence of reactions and fatality episodes, summarized the following frequencies: (1) acute hemolytic reaction, 1:25,000; (2) delayed hemolytic reaction, 1:2500; (3) noncardiogenic pulmonary edema, 1:1000; (4) transfusion-associated graft-versus-host disease (TA-GVHD) and related donor, 1:7000, and (5) TA-GVHD and unrelated donor, 1:39,000.[4] Linden and coworkers[5] reviewed transfusion data collected by the New York State Department of Health (NYS/DOH) for the period 1990 to 1995, along with comparison data collected by the Food and Drug Administration (FDA) for the calendar year 1994. These data were analyzed for the frequency of death resulting from various types of transfusion reactions. Some of the data compiled by Isbister[4] and Linden and associates[5] are collated in Table 18–4. General, everyday types of fatality risks, collected by Isbister, are included for perspective on degree of risk.

## Error Analysis

An internal study of the 355 reports received by the FDA of transfusion-associated fatality cases for the period 1976 through 1982 sought to identify where errors occurred in preventable transfusion-associated deaths.[6] Table 18–5 identifies transfusion locations where errors associated with transfusion reactions have occurred. Four leading causes of preventable laboratory

errors were (1) improper specimen identification, (2) improper patient identification, (3) antibody identification error, and (4) crossmatch procedure error. For nursing, anesthesia, and medical staff errors, improper patient identification was by far the major cause of transfusion death. Thus, adherence to proper transfusion standards, policies, and procedures is essential to reduce transfusion-associated fatalities. Table 18–6 summarizes frequent error causes associated with transfusion reactions.

Some studies have demonstrated wide variability in the rate of occurrence of DHTR,[7] which can be attributed to reduced clinical recognition of DHTR and the nonspecific clinical evidence of DHTR in complicated patient cases with fever, jaundice, anemia, and so forth which may be linked to other disease processes. Although rare, there have been single-case reports of death attributable to DHTR, with the incidence of DHTR fatalities about one-sixth (1:600,000) that of IHTR fatalities.[8]

**Table 18–4.** Frequency of Death for Selected Transfusion Reactions[4, 5]

| Type of Reaction | NYS/DOH | FDA |
|---|---|---|
| Acute hemolytic | 1:1,700,000 | 1:1,300,000 |
| Delayed hemolytic | 0 | 1:560,000 |
| Noncardiogenic pulmonary edema | 1:3,000,000 | 1:6,600,000 |
| TA-GVHD | 0 | 1:10,000,000 |

**Risk of Death for Selected General Situations**

| | |
|---|---|
| Lifetime risk | 1:1 |
| Cancer | 1:4 |
| Coronary artery bypass surgery | 1:33 |
| Admission to a hospital | 1:200 |
| Driving a car | 1:5000 |
| Flying on a commercial airline | 1:500,000 |

**Table 18–5.** Locations of Preventable Transfusion-associated Deaths, in Order of Occurrence

Laboratory
Nursing service
Anesthesia service
Clinical staff

**Table 18–6.** Summary of Frequent Error Causes Associated with Transfusion Reactions

1. Patient misidentification
2. Sample error
3. Wrong blood issued
4. Transcription error
5. Administration error
6. Technical error
7. Storage error

Anaphylactic and anaphylactoid reactions are immediate immune reactions.[9] About 1 in 700 of healthy
individuals in the general population is immunoglobin A (IgA) deficient. Despite this relatively large risk
group, anaphylactic and anaphylactoid reactions occur
at very low rates, about 1 in 20,000 transfusions.[10] Errors in clinical diagnosis and case reporting do not allow calculation of an accurate risk rate.[11]

Acute pulmonary injury accounted for 15 percent of
the fatal transfusion-associated reports and was the
third most reported cause of transfusion-associated
deaths.[12] Bacterial contamination of blood components and nonimmune hemolysis accounted for the
next largest number of cases reported to the FDA during the 1976 to 1985 period.

## HEMOLYTIC TRANSFUSION REACTIONS

Hemolytic transfusion reactions (HTRs) can occur
either at the time of transfusion (immediate) or a few
days after transfusion (delayed).

### Immediate Hemolytic Transfusion Reaction

#### Definition

Most commonly, an IHTR occurs very soon after the
transfusion of incompatible RBCs. The cells are rapidly
destroyed, releasing hemoglobin and RBC stromata
into the circulation. In an anesthetized patient, hemoglobinuria, abnormal bleeding at the surgical wound
site, and hypotension may be the only warning signs of
IHTR. The reaction period varies from 1 to 2 hours.[13]
However, signs and symptoms can occur within minutes after starting the transfusion. ABO-incompatible
transfusions may be life threatening, causing shock,
acute renal failure, and disseminated intravascular coagulation (DIC). Prompt diagnosis and treatment are
essential.

#### Pathophysiology

The underlying cause of immune IHTR is transfusion
of an immunologically incompatible whole blood or
RBC product to a recipient. The four most commonly
identified RBC antibody specificities causing IHTR are
anti-A, anti-Kell, anti-Jk[a], and anti-Fy[a].[14] These four antibodies are traditionally considered binders of complement to RBC surfaces and have efficient in vitro lytic
properties. Immune-mediated IHTR can destroy RBCs
by one of two mechanisms: (1) intravascular hemolysis or (2) extravascular hemolysis.[15] In both, the initial
event is the binding of patient antibody to the transfused incompatible RBCs, which forms an antigen-
antibody (Ag-Ab) complex on the RBC surface. Intravascular RBC lysis releases hemoglobin, RBC stromata, and intracellular enzymes, manifesting in hemoglobinemia and hemoglobinuria. Figure 18–1 is an
overall view of the gross pathology of kidneys, demon-

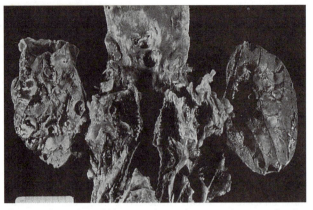

**Figure 18–1.** Gross kidney specimens from a patient experiencing
hemolysis. Note the sclerotic glomeruli, fibrosis of the cortex.

strating sclerotic glomeruli, fibrosis of the cortex, and
tubular necrosis. Figure 18–2 is an overall view of gross
pathology of the liver, demonstrating portal fibrosis
and necrotic hepatocytes. Both organs are from a patient who experienced acute intravascular hemolysis.
Figure 18–3 depicts the intravascular hemolysis pathway.

Extravascular immune-mediated IHTR is characterized by Ag-Ab complex formation on RBCs with incomplete activation of complement. Because RBC lysis
does not occur intravascularly, there is no release into
the circulation of free hemoglobin, RBC enzymes, or
RBC stromata.

#### Signs, Symptoms, and Clinical Work-up

For immune-mediated IHTR with intravascular hemolysis, signs and symptoms can be profound. Table
18–7 lists clinical signs and symptoms that can occur
in IHTR and can usually be observed in a conscious patient. Several important clinical findings include:[16]

1. 35 percent of patients with IHTR experience fever,
   with or without chills.

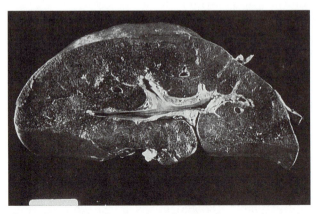

**Figure 18–2.** Gross liver specimen from a patient experiencing hemolysis. Note the portal fibrosis and necrotic hepatocytes.

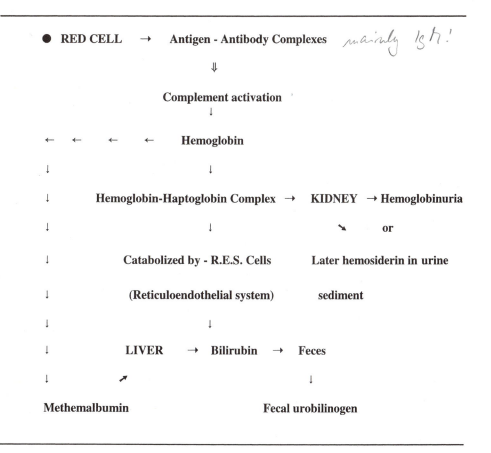

● RED CELL → Antigen - Antibody Complexes *mainly IgM!*

⟱

Complement activation

↓

← ← ← ← Hemoglobin

Hemoglobin-Haptoglobin Complex → KIDNEY → Hemoglobinuria

or

Catabolized by - R.E.S. Cells     Later hemosiderin in urine

(Reticuloendothelial system)     sediment

LIVER → Bilirubin → Feces

Methemalbumin     Fecal urobilinogen

**Figure 18–3.** Intravascular hemolysis pathway.

2. 34 percent experience oliguria with complete recovery.
3. 13 percent develop anuria.
4. 10 percent die, with sustained hypotension being the primary clinical finding.
5. 8 percent experience coagulopathy.

Signs and symptoms associated with extravascular IHTR are usually mild and not life-threatening. Fever, chills, jaundice, unexpected anemia, and decreased haptoglobin are usual findings. Once an immune-mediated IHTR is suspected, immediate action is mandatory. Table 18–8 abbreviates guideline bedside procedures for handling suspected IHTR.

## Therapy and Prevention

Patient care in IHTR is focused on prevention and supportive measures. The physician should closely monitor the patient for risk factors to DIC, hypotension, and acute renal failure.[17] Traditionally, mannitol has been the agent of choice to induce renal diuresis and to prevent renal failure.[18] More recent investigations using ethacrynic acid and furosemide indicate that these agents both improve renal blood flow and induce diuresis.[19] Hypotension is treated with intravenous fluids and vasoactive drugs (e.g., dopamine), as

**Table 18–7.** Clinical Signs and Symptoms That May Be Caused by Immediate Hemolytic Transfusion Reactions

| | |
|---|---|
| Fever | Hemoglobinemia |
| Chills | Hemoglobinuria |
| Facial flushing | Shock |
| Chest pain | Anemia |
| Back or flank pain | Oliguria or anuria (renal failure) |
| Hypotension | Pain at transfusion site |
| Abdominal pain | Generalized bleeding |
| Nausea | Urticaria |
| Dyspnea | Diarrhea |
| Vomiting | Disseminated intravascular coagulation |

**Table 18–8.** Immediate Transfusion Reaction Bedside Procedures

1. *Stop the transfusion.*
2. Keep intravenous line open with physiologic saline.
3. Notify patient's physician and transfusion service.
4. Take care of patient per physician's orders.
5. Perform bedside clerical checks.
6. Return unit, set, and attached solution to blood bank.
7. Collect appropriate blood specimens for evaluation.
8. Document reaction.

**Table 18–9.** Preventive Transfusion Reaction Measures

Store RBCs only in blood bank–monitored refrigerators.
Never warm RBCs above 37°C for transfusion.
Do not transfuse blood if patient or donor identification is not
  accurate.
Never sign out blood by name only.
Do not add medications to blood.
Follow procedures for issuing blood components.
Follow protocol for specimen collection, labeling, and testing.
Follow transfusion policies and procedures.

necessary. Blood component therapy, such as fresh frozen plasma, cryoprecipitate, and platelet concentrates, should be used in patients having a bleeding diathesis or significant coagulation abnormalities. Extravascular IHTR usually does not require therapeutic intervention. To ensure the patient's welfare, the vital signs, coagulation status, and renal output should be monitored.

Because most IHTRs are caused by clerical (i.e., human) error, they are potentially preventable. All policies and procedures should be followed to ensure proper patient identification, sample collection and labeling, unit identification, patient testing, handling, and correct transfusion at the bedside. Table 18–9 lists preventive measures to minimize transfusion reactions.

## Delayed Hemolytic Transfusion Reaction

### Definition

Delayed hemolytic transfusion reaction (DHTR) is most often the result of an anamnestic response in a patient who has previously been sensitized by transfusion, pregnancy, or transplant and in whom antibody is not detectable by standard pretransfusion methods.[20] Clinical signs and symptoms are usually mild, and severe DHTR cases and fatalities are uncommon. Unexpected or unexplained decreases in hemoglobin or hematocrit values following transfusion should be investigated as possible DHTR.

### Pathophysiology

Two different types of DHTR have been identified: (1) secondary (anamnestic) response to transfused RBCs and (2) primary alloimmunization. In DHTR caused by a secondary response, a period of about 3 to 7 days from the time of transfusion is necessary for enough antibody to be produced by the patient to cause clinical signs and symptoms of extravascular red cell hemolysis.[21] In DHTR caused by primary alloimmunization, the patient has no past history of pregnancy, transfusion, or transplant. It should be noted that the time from transfusion to the onset of clinical signs and symptoms of hemolysis and detection of the causative antibody is longer for DHTR than for IHTR.[22]

Extravascular hemolysis is the mechanism of RBC destruction for both types of DHTR. Figure 18–4 depicts the extravascular hemolysis pathway. Patient antibody attaches to the specific foreign donor RBC antigen, causing sensitization of RBCs, which are removed by the reticuloendothelial system (RES), commonly called the monocyte-macrophage system. Table 18–10 groups common and uncommon antibodies implicated in DHTR.[23] Delayed hemolytic transfusion reaction is also reportedly associated with bone marrow transplantation and may be caused by HLA antibodies in some cases.[24]

### Signs, Symptoms, and Clinical Work-up

Clinical signs and symptoms of DHTR are mild compared with those of IHTR because of the extravascular hemolysis and may be undetected clinically. In DHTR, complement is not activated; therefore, no intravascular hemolysis occurs, as is observed in IHTR.[25] If clinically detected, DHTR is most commonly manifested by mild fever or fever with chills, and moderate jaundice may be observed. Oliguria and DIC are rare.[26] Table 18–11 lists signs and symptoms that have been observed in DHTR.

When DHTR is suspected, blood specimens (both clotted and anticoagulated) should be sent to the blood

● RED CELL → Antigen - Antibody → Hemoglobin catabolized by

　　　　　　　　Complexes　　　　　　　Reticuloendothelial cells

　　　　　　　　　　　　　　　　　　　　　　↓

　　　　　　　　　　　　　　　　　　LIVER - conjugated bilirubin

　　　　　　　　　　　　　　　　　　　　　　↓

　　　　　　　　　　　　　　　　　　Fecal urobilinogen

**Figure 18–4.** Extravascular hemolysis pathway.

**Table 18–10.** Antibodies Implicated in DHTR

| Common Antibodies | Uncommon Antibodies |
|---|---|
| Anti-Jkᵃ | Anti-A₁ |
| Anti-E | Anti-P₁ |
| Anti-D | |
| Anti-C | IgG |
| Anti-K | |
| Anti-Fyᵃ | |
| Anti-M IgM | |

**Table 18–11.** Clinical Signs and Symptoms of DHTR

| Common Signs and Symptoms | Unusual Signs and Symptoms |
|---|---|
| Fever | Hemoglobinemia |
| Anemia | Hemoglobinuria |
| Mild jaundice | Shock |
| | Renal failure |

bank for posttransfusion reaction investigation. Other laboratory testing for DHTR may include hemoglobin, hematocrit, and coagulation studies, and renal function tests. The patient should be closely observed for signs and symptoms indicating severe complications.

### Therapy and Prevention

The goal of therapy is to prevent and, if necessary, treat severe complications of DHTR. Renal function can be supported with intravenous fluid therapy to maintain a normovolemic status.[27] Only symptomatic anemia should be treated with RBC transfusions. Clinical signs and symptoms of hemolysis or DIC should be monitored to reduce the risk of renal failure.

Because DHTR is usually caused by an anamnestic response, a thorough medical history including previous transfusions, pregnancies, transplants, and transfusion reactions should be taken. The blood bank should be alerted to any previously reported complicating factors. Ideally, a type and screen should be performed at the time of admission on patients who may need transfusion, who have previously received blood, or who have known risk factors, such as pregnancy or previous red cell exposure.

## IMMEDIATE NONHEMOLYTIC TRANSFUSION REACTIONS

The common types of immediate nonhemolytic transfusion reactions are febrile and allergic. Anaphylaxis, anaphylactoid reaction, and noncardiogenic pulmonary edema occur less frequently. Although the immune system is a common pathway for each of these reactions, intravascular or extravascular RBC hemolysis does *not* occur.

## Febrile Nonhemolytic Transfusion Reaction

### Definition

Febrile nonhemolytic transfusion reaction (FNHTR) occurs in about 1 percent of transfusions. Along with allergic reactions, FNHTR is the most commonly encountered type of transfusion reaction. Several common definitions are used regarding FNHTR, based on increases in temperature after transfusion. The American Association of Blood Banks (AABB) *Technical Manual* defines FNHTR as a 1°C temperature rise associated with transfusion and having no medical explanation other than blood component transfusion.[28] Others[29] define FNHTR as (1) any 1°C or greater temperature increase above the patient's baseline temperature, during or within 24 hours after transfusion with a minimum recorded temperature of 38°C; or (2) a 1°C temperature increase above the patient's baseline pretransfusion temperature during or within 8 hours after the end of the transfusion.

### Pathophysiology

Febrile nonhemolytic transfusion reactions are caused by antileukocyte antibodies present in the patient's plasma. The antileukocyte antibodies are commonly directed against antigens present on monocytes, granulocytes, and lymphocytes.[30] Alloimmunization by prior blood transfusion, tissue transplantation, or pregnancy is the causative stimulus for antibody formation. These antibodies are predominantly HLA or lymphocytotoxic antibodies.[31]

The febrile mechanism still is not fully elucidated. The febrile reaction may follow activation of the complement system, producing C5a, which causes production and release of the pyrogen interleukin-1 (IL-1) from the patient's macrophages and monocytes.[32] Interleukin-1 may initiate synthesis of prostaglandins (PGE₂) in the hypothalamic cells, resulting in an additional pyrogenic effect.[33] Release of pyrogens from the transfused white blood cells (WBCs) also plays a role in fever development and other clinical signs and symptoms.

### Signs, Symptoms, and Clinical Work-up

The most frequent expressions of FNHTRs are fever with or without chills and, rarely, hypotension. Most symptoms are mild and benign. Occasionally a patient may briefly exhibit pronounced pallor. Severe reactions may include hypotension, cyanosis, tachycardia, tachypnea, dyspnea, cough, limited fibrinolysis, and transient leukopenia.[34]

Febrile nonhemolytic transfusion reaction is a diagnosis of exclusion, inasmuch as the nonspecific signs and symptoms can have many other causes. For example, fever can be caused by IHTR, bacteremia, drugs taken by the patient, or another underlying illness. Past medical history for transfusion, transplantation, pregnancy, and drug therapy is important for accurate diagnosis. Tests to evaluate FNHTRs may vary from one laboratory to another. When an FNHTR is suspected, the transfusion should be stopped, but the intravenous line should be kept open with normal saline to support treatment in the event of a severe complication.

### Therapy and Prevention

Because leukocyte antibodies are the primary cause of FNHTR, leukocyte-poor ("leukopoor") blood components are indicated. A variety of methods have been developed that effectively remove enough leukocytes from blood components to prevent FNHTR, including laboratory or bedside filtration using leukopoor blood filters, washed RBCs, deglycerolized RBCs, or centrifugation.[35] Because approximately one in eight patients reacts to the next unit transfused following an FNHTR, many recommend documenting two or more FNHTRs before ordering leukocyte-poor blood components. Antipyretics such as aspirin or acetaminophen can be used to premedicate a patient before transfusion. It should be noted that aspirin is contraindicated in patients with thrombocytopenia and thrombocytopathy.

Even with WBC reduction in blood components, not all FNHTRs can be prevented. Premedication may be beneficial to patients with documented histories of FNHTR. As leukopoor filter cost declines, more aggressive use of these bedside filters will eventually reduce the incidence of FNHTR.

## Allergic (Urticarial) Transfusion Reactions

### Definition

Allergic, or urticarial, transfusion reactions are as commonly reported as FNHTRs. If clinical signs and symptoms appear within minutes of exposure, the allergic reaction is of the immediate hypersensitivity type. Anaphylactic and anaphylactoid reactions are also of the immediate hypersensitivity type but are clinically more severe and will be discussed later.

### Pathophysiology

Despite the fact that allergic reactions are one of the two most commonly reported transfusion reactions, the definitive causes are still not known. Two possible etiologies have been proposed,[36] based on the passive transfer of donor plasma to a patient after transfusion of a blood component:

1. The donor plasma has a foreign protein (allergen) with which immunoglobulin E reagin (IgE) or immunoglobin G (IgG), or both, antibodies in patient plasma react.
2. The donor plasma has reagins (IgE or IgG or both) that combine with allergens in the patient plasma.

Histamine appears to be the primary mediator of the allergic response.[37] Histamine is released when the allergen-reagin complex attaches to the surface of tissue mast cells. On release from mast cells, histamine in-

creases vascular dilation and permeability, allowing vascular fluids to escape into tissues. This causes swelling and raised red welts that may itch (pruritus). Another group of mediators that may participate in allergic reactions is leukotrienes, which have been estimated to be about 1000 times more potent than histamine.[38]

### Signs, Symptoms, and Clinical Work-up

The majority of allergic reactions are mild and not life-threatening. Most common signs and symptoms include local erythema (redness), pruritus (itching), and hives (raised, firm, red welts). Fever may or may not be present. Rarely, allergic reactions can be severe, with angioneurotic edema, laryngeal edema, and bronchial asthma.

No reliable laboratory tests are available to identify the offending allergens or reagins causing an allergic reaction. Bedside observation focuses on identifying the manifestations of an allergic reaction, monitoring for severe effects, and instituting supportive care.

### Therapy and Prevention

Treatment with an antihistamine such as diphenhydramine (Benadryl) is often sufficient for mild forms of allergic reactions. In patients with histories of repeated allergic reactions, removal of plasma from blood components is often used (washed RBCs; washed platelets). Premedication with antihistamines before transfusion is also common. For severe allergic reactions, the use of aminophylline, epinephrine, or corticosteroids may be necessary. Some clinicians permit temporary cessation of blood component transfusion when a mild allergic reaction is observed, while antihistamine treatment is given. After antihistamine administration, the same component transfusion is resumed. Because some allergic reactions can be severe, some blood banks recommend following the same transfusion reaction protocol as in other transfusion reactions and observing the patient for any severe reaction effects.

Allergic reactions cannot be completely prevented. For patients with suspected or documented histories of allergic reactions, premedication, plasma-deficient blood components, or all three, are the usual prevention strategies.

## Anaphylactic and Anaphylactoid Reactions

### Definition

Anaphylactic and anaphylactoid reactions are of the immediate hypersensitivity type of immune system response. Anaphylaxis can range from mild urticaria (hives) and pruritus to severe shock and death. Any organ of the body can be involved, such as the lungs, blood vessels, nerves, skin, and gastrointestinal tract.[39] Two significant features distinguish anaphylactic and anaphylactoid reactions from other types of transfusion reactions: (1) fever is absent, and (2) clinical signs and symptoms occur after transfusion of just a few milliliters of plasma or plasma-containing blood components.

## Pathophysiology

Anaphylactic and anaphylactoid reactions are attributed to IgA deficiency in patients who have developed anti-IgA antibodies by sensitization from transfusion or pregnancy.[40] Despite the fact that about 1 in 700 people have some level of IgA deficiency, anaphylactic and anaphylactoid reactions are quite rare.[41]

As discussed previously in allergic transfusion reactions, immune hypersensitivity reactions are mediated by histamines and leukotrienes.

## Signs, Symptoms, and Clinical Work-up

These hypersensitivity reactions have been divided into two categories: (1) anaphylactic, in patients deficient in IgA who have class-specific IgA antibodies; and (2) anaphylactoid, in patients having normal levels of IgA but a limited type-specific anti-IgA that reacts with light chain (kappa or lambda) of the donor's IgA. Anaphylactic reactions are sudden in onset with pronounced symptoms that may include coughing, dyspnea, nausea, emesis, bronchospasm, flushing of skin, chest pain, hypotension, abdominal cramps, diarrhea, possibly shock, loss of consciousness, and death. Anaphylactoid reactions are usually less severe and are characterized by urticaria, periorbital swelling, dyspnea, or perilaryngeal edema.

There is no predictive test to determine who is at risk for either anaphylactic or anaphylactoid reactions. If either type of reaction is suspected, a patient serum sample can be immunoelectrophoresed to determine IgA levels, or immunodiffusion techniques may identify subclass antibodies.

## Therapy and Prevention

Treatment measures must be prompt:

1. Stop the transfusion, and do not restart transfusion of the blood component.
2. Keep the intravenous line open with normal saline.
3. Immediately give epinephrine (usually about 0.5 mL of 1:1000 solution).
4. For severe reactions, corticosteroids or aminophylline, or both, may be indicated. Airway patency must be maintained, and vital signs must be stabilized by appropriate means.

Because the diagnosis of anaphylactic and anaphylactoid reactions is retrospective, in patients with documented or suspected histories of these reactions special measures must be taken. If a plasma-containing blood component has been implicated in the anaphylactic or anaphylactoid reactions and the patient requires transfusions, two transfusion approaches may be considered: (1) remove all plasma from the blood component before transfusion, or (2) transfuse blood components from donors lacking IgA. Even a small amount of plasma found in fibrin glue preparation may cause anaphylactic reactions.[42] In a prospective study, colloid transfusion products also caused a risk of anaphylactoid reactions (plasma-protein solutions, 0.003 percent; hydroxyethyl starch (HES), 0.006 percent; dextran, 0.008 percent; and gelatin solution, 0.038 percent).[43] Therefore, any transfusible source of IgA antigenic material can precipitate anaphylactic or anaphylactoid reactions.

## Noncardiogenic Pulmonary Edema Reactions

### Definition

Several terms have been used to identify pulmonary complications associated with blood component transfusion: noncardiogenic pulmonary edema (NCPE), transfusion-related acute lung injury (TRALI), pulmonary hypersensitivity reaction, and allergic pulmonary edema. The clinical picture of NCPE is similar to that of adult respiratory distress syndrome (ARDS).

### Pathophysiology

Although the cause of NCPE is not well understood, the most consistent finding is antileukocyte antibodies in donor or patient plasma. Several mechanisms for lung injury have been postulated and include the following: (1) antileukocyte antibodies in donor or patient plasma could initiate complement-mediated pulmonary capillary endothelial injury, and (2) antileukocyte antibodies could react with leukocytes to trigger the complement system to produce C3a and C5a. This, in turn, would cause tissue basophils and platelets to release histamine and serotonin, resulting in leukocyte emboli aggregating in the lung capillary bed.[44] Whatever the mechanism, capillary damage induces interstitial edema and fluid in alveolar air spaces, causing decreased gas exchange and hypoxia.

### Signs, Symptoms, and Clinical Work-up

Noncardiogenic pulmonary edema is usually characterized by chills, cough, fever, cyanosis, hypotension, and increasing respiratory distress shortly after transfusion of blood component volumes that usually do not produce hypervolemia. Clinical signs and symptoms may be mild, resolving after a few days, or severe, resulting in rapidly progressive pulmonary failure. Sera from both the donor and patient should be tested for antileukocyte antibodies. The diagnosis of NCPE is a diagnosis of exclusion. Conditions that should be excluded are heart failure, volume overload, bacterial sepsis, and myocardial infarction.

### Therapy and Prevention

If clinical signs and symptoms occur during the transfusion, the transfusion should be discontinued and not restarted. Explicit instructional procedures should be followed for handling the transfusion reaction. With adequate respiratory and hemodynamic supportive treatment, NCPE pulmonary infiltrates usually clear after several days.[45]

If NCPE is caused by patient antileukocyte antibodies, then leukopoor blood component preparations should be used. If NCPE is caused by donor antileukocyte antibodies, no special blood component preparations appear to be indicated for the patient in the future. Deferral of donors associated with NCPE cases is a complicated and controversial issue. At present, no standard has been set for acceptance or deferral of donors associated with NCPE cases.

## Transfusion-associated Circulatory Overload

### Definition

Transfusion-associated circulatory overload (TACO) is a good example of an iatrogenic (physician-caused) transfusion reaction. Patients at significant risk include children, elderly patients, and patients with chronic normovolemic anemia, cardiac disease, thalessemia major, or sickle cell disease.[46]

### Pathophysiology

The most frequent cause of circulatory overload is transfusion of a unit at too fast a rate. Hypervolemia associated with transfusion leads to congestive heart failure and pulmonary edema (which may or may not be reversible).[47]

### Signs, Symptoms, and Clinical Work-up

Clinical circulatory overload effects include dyspnea, coughing, cyanosis, orthopnea, chest discomfort, headache, restlessness, tachycardia, systolic hypertension (greater than 50 mm Hg increase), and abnormal electrocardiograms.

The transfusion should be stopped immediately. If transfusion is critical to patient therapy, the slowest possible infusion rate must be used. The intravenous line should be maintained, and the patient may be placed in a sitting position. Electrocardiogram and chest x-ray examinations to assess cardiac and pulmonary status should be considered. If possible, central venous pressure and peripheral vital signs should be closely monitored.

### Therapy and Prevention

Rapid reduction of hypervolemia and patient respiratory and cardiac support are primary goals. Oxygen therapy and intravenous diuretics should be used appropriately. If more rapid fluid volume reduction is necessary, therapeutic phlebotomy can be used. Cardiac arrhythmias or decreased myocardial function should be corrected.

The usual rate of transfusion is about 200 mL per hour. In patients at risk or with histories of circulatory overload, rates of 100 mL per hour or less are appropriate. Donor units should be split into aliquots to permit transfusion for longer time periods. Red blood cells should be used instead of whole blood. Washed or frozen washed RBCs have been advocated to reduce plasma oncotic load to the patient.[48] In some patients with chronic normovolemic anemia having hematocrits in the range of 10 to 20 percent, a therapeutic phlebotomy to reduce plasma volume equal to the intended transfusion volume should be considered.

## Bacterial Contamination Reactions

### Definition

Although the frequency of bacterial contamination of blood components is low, this type of septic reaction can have a rapid onset and lead to death. Of the deaths caused by bacterial contamination of blood components reported to the Centers for Disease Control (CDC), most are caused by blood components contaminated by *Yersinia enterocolitica*. Since 1987, 20 cases have been reported to the CDC, with 12 deaths caused by this organism. Cases have been reported with transfused RBCs,[49] platelets,[50] and other blood components as well as with manufactured products such as intravenous solutions and HES.[51]

### Pathophysiology

Transfusion reactions attributed to bacterial contamination reactions are commonly caused by endotoxin produced by bacteria capable of growing in cold temperatures (psychrophilic) such as *Pseudomonas* species, *Escherichia coli*, and *Y. enterocolitica*.[52]

### Signs, Symptoms, and Clinical Work-up

Clinical signs and symptoms of septic reactions usually appear rapidly during transfusion or within about 30 minutes after transfusion. Clinically, this type of reaction is termed warm and is characterized by dryness and flushing of the patient's skin. Additional manifestations include fever, hypotension, shaking, chills, muscle pain, vomiting, abdominal cramps, bloody diarrhea, hemoglobinuria, shock, renal failure, and DIC.

Rapid recognition of sepsis caused by bacterial contamination is essential. At the first sign of the reaction, the transfusion must immediately be stopped, the intravenous line kept open, and instructions for handling transfusion reactions followed. The blood component unit and any associated fluids and transfusion equipment should be sent immediately to the blood bank for visual inspection, Gram stain, and cultures. In addition, blood cultures should be drawn from the patient as soon as possible for detection of aerobic or anaerobic organisms.

## Therapy and Prevention

Broad-spectrum antibiotics should be immediately administered intravenously. Therapy for shock, steroids, and vasopressors such as dopamine, fluid support, respiratory ventilation, and maintenance of renal function may be indicated.

Bacterial contamination of blood components usually occurs at the time of phlebotomy, during the component preparation or processing, or during thawing of blood components in waterbaths. Strict adherence to policies and procedures regarding blood component collection, storage, handling, and preparation is essential to reducing risk. Visual observation of RBC units for color change at the time of issue for transfusion is required, but this step alone cannot guarantee that there is no bacterial contamination.[53] Visual inspection of components before release from the transfusion service includes looking for the presence of brown or purple discoloration, visible clots, or hemolysis. However, gross observation is often inadequate in detecting the presence of bacterial contamination. One preventive measure is to make sure the blood components are infused within standard allowable maximum time limits (usually 4 hours). Adherence to good component production methods and prudent transfusion practices is currently the best strategy to reduce the risk of bacterial contamination and sepsis.[54]

## Physically or Chemically Induced Transfusion Reactions

### Definition

Patients are at risk of experiencing a transfusion reaction caused by a broad range of physical or chemical factors that either affect a blood component or are a consequence of the transfusion event. Physically or chemically induced transfusion reactions (PCITRs) are a heterogeneous group and can include physical RBC damage, depletion and dilution of coagulation factors and platelets, hypothermia, citrate toxicity, and hypokalemia or hyperkalemia (decreased or increased ionized serum potassium level in the patient). Because the clinical signs and symptoms of PCITR can be subtle, the transfusionist must be alert to identify and to correct these reaction effects. Table 18–12 lists physical, mechanical, and inherited induced nonhemolytic transfusion reaction examples.

### Pathophysiology

Red cells are susceptible to membrane damage and intravascular lysis by hypertonic or hypotonic solutions, heat damage from blood warmers, freezing damage in the absence of a cryoprotective agent, or mechanical damage such as that caused by roller pumps in a blood pump.[55] During massive transfusion (replacement of patient's total blood volume within a 24-hour period), rapid depletion and dilution of platelets

**Table 18–12.** Nonhemolytic Transfusion Reactions: Physically, Chemically, and Inherited Induced Examples

*Physical Damage to Red Blood Cells*
Intravascular lysis by hypertonic or hypotonic solutions
Heat damage from blood warmers, during shipping, in hot rooms
Freeze damage in absence of cryoprotective agent, during shipping

*Mechanical Damage*
Blood pumps, roller pumps
Infusion under pressure through small-bore needles

*Patients with Intrinsic Abnormal Cells*
Congenital hemolytic anemias such as G-6-PD deficiency
Patients in sickle cell crisis
Patients with paroxysmal nocturnal hemoglobinuria (PNH) or
  autoimmune hemolytic anemia (AIHA)

and plasma coagulation factors can occur.[56] Hypothermia, a core body temperature of less than 35°C, is usually associated with large volumes of cold fluid transfusions.[57] Excess citrate from transfusions can act on the patient's plasma-free ionized calcium and may result in hypocalcemia.[58] Transfusion-associated hyperkalemia can be caused by the intracellular loss of potassium from RBCs during storage in the blood unit plasma.[59] Transfusion-induced hypokalemia is most likely to be caused by infusion of intracellular potassium-depleted RBC blood components, such as washed RBCs or frozen washed RBCs.[60]

Mechanical or chemical damage of transfused RBCs can result in intravascular hemolysis. The resulting free hemoglobin is rapidly cleared by the kidneys. Usually the resulting RBC stroma does not induce DIC, but DIC is a possibility.[61] Coagulation factors, especially factor VIII, decline in activity level during blood component storage, and factor levels can be reduced by use of fluid replacement solutions such as colloids and crystalloids during massive transfusions.[62] Hypothermia inhibits the immune system function, intensifies lactic acidosis and cardiac arrhythmias, and can cause coagulopathies.[63] Citrate toxicity is caused by the rapid lowering of plasma-free calcium ions caused by chelation with citrate. Massive transfusion is seldom a cause of citrate toxicity, but automated apheresis procedures using large amounts of citrate anticoagulant are a more likely cause.[64] Hyperkalemia and hypokalemia can cause cardiac arrhythmias and seizures.

### Signs, Symptoms, and Clinical Work-up

Many of the clinical signs and symptoms of PCITR are nonspecific. The more common signs and symptoms include facial numbness, chills, generalized numbness, muscle twitching, cardiac arrhythmias, nausea, vomiting, perioral tingling, altered respirations, and anxiety. Laboratory tests for PCITR investigation may include electrolyte levels, serum ionized calcium, blood pH, blood glucose, urinalysis, hemoglobin, hematocrit, platelet count, prothrombin time, and activated partial thromboplastin time.

## Therapy and Prevention

Treatment is directed at correcting the underlying cause of the signs and symptoms. For example, hypothermia could be treated by placing the patient on a warming blanket and giving supportive care to any cardiac arrhythmias or electrolyte imbalance. Heparin might be indicated for DIC caused by physical RBC lysis. Citrate toxicity is often rapidly self-correcting, but administration of a calcium-rich product such as milk or an antacid with calcium gluconate (e.g., Tums) is usually adequate.

Precautionary measures are the best strategies to avoid PCITR. Blood warmers can be used to avoid hypothermia. Prudent use of platelet concentrates and fresh frozen plasma may avoid rapid depletion and dilution of coagulation factors during massive transfusion. Monitoring the patient's mental status and vital signs may prove valuable in detecting rapid changes in levels of calcium and potassium. The close monitoring of RBCs transfused through blood pumps can avoid mechanical destruction. In general, attention to proper transfusion practices can greatly reduce the risk of PCITRs.

## DELAYED NONHEMOLYTIC TRANSFUSION REACTIONS

### Alloimmunization

#### Definition

Alloimmunization may result from prior exposure to donor blood components. As an adverse effect of blood component transfusion, alloimmunization is a significant complication. Even very small amounts of donor antigenic RBCs can elicit an alloimmune response.[65] Adverse effects may include difficulty in finding compatible RBC units because of the presence of clinically significant RBC antibodies, transfusion reactions, or platelet refractoriness.[66]

#### Pathophysiology

Because no two humans (except identical twins) have the same genetic inheritance, exposure to foreign antigens by blood component transfusions, tissue transplantation, or pregnancy may cause a patient's immune system to produce alloantibodies.

With the first exposure to foreign antigen, lymphocyte memory is invoked. This results in a moderate production of IgM and IgG antibodies. Secondary exposure elicits rapid production of large amounts of IgG class antibody rising rapidly in the first two days after reexposure to the antigen. The antibody produced attaches to the antigenic surface and may interact with the complement system or RES.[67]

#### Signs, Symptoms, and Clinical Workup

Clinical signs and symptoms may be mild, including slight fever and falling hemoglobin and hematocrit levels; or severe, including platelet refractoriness with bleeding. To detect an alloimmunization state in a patient, several tests can be of benefit. The antibody screen test is used to detect clinically significant RBC antibodies. If HLA antibodies are suspected, lymphocyte panels and lymphocytotoxic antibody procedures can be performed on the patient's serum. However, a thorough patient history of past transfusions, transplantations, and pregnancies is important.

### Therapy and Prevention

Treatment depends on the type and severity of the transfusion reaction. Most reactions are mild and often missed clinically. Severe reactions should be treated promptly, as appropriate. Alloimmunization cannot be completely prevented. With the advent of third-generation bedside leukocyte filters, delay—if not prevention—of antileukocyte antibody production is now possible.[68] The matching of donor and patient RBC phenotypes to avoid sensitization in chronically transfusion-dependent patient populations has also been recommended to prevent the formation of RBC antibodies by the patient.[69] Table 18–13 lists occurrence of alloimmunization and other transfusion reactions.

### Posttransfusion Purpura

#### Definition

A rare complication of blood transfusion, usually involving platelet concentrates (PC), posttransfusion purpura (PTP) is characterized by a rapid onset of thrombocytopenia as a result of anamnestic production of platelet alloantibody. Posttransfusion purpura usually occurs in multiparous females. The lag time between transfusion and onset of thrombocytopenia is approximately 7 to 14 days.

**Table 18–13.** Relative Occurrence of Transfusion Reaction Effects

| Type of Reaction | Common | Less Common | Unusual |
|---|---|---|---|
| Allergic reaction | × | | |
| Alloimmunization | × | | |
| Febrile reaction | × | | |
| Depletion and dilution of coagulation factors and platelets | | × | |
| DHTR | | × | |
| TACO | | × | |
| Anaphylaxis and anaphylactoid reactions | | | × |
| Bacterial contamination | | | × |
| Immediate hemolytic transfusion reactions | | | × |
| Iron overload | | | × |
| Noncardiogenic pulmonary edema | | | × |
| Physical RBC damage | | | × |
| Posttransfusion purpura | | | × |
| TA-GVHD | | | × |

## Pathophysiology

The platelet antibody specificity most frequently identified is HPA-1a (anti-PL$^{A1}$). About 2 percent of people are negative for the PL$^{A1}$ platelet-specific antigen. Other implicated antibody specificities are HLA-A2 and lymphocytotoxic antibodies.

Platelet alloantibody attaches to the platelet surface, which permits extravascular destruction by the RES in the liver and spleen. The patient's autologous platelets are destroyed, enhancing the thrombocytopenia. The exact mechanism of platelet destruction is still not fully explained.[70]

## Signs, Symptoms, and Clinical Work-up

Purpura and thrombocytopenia occur about 1 to 2 weeks after transfusion. Thrombocytopenia can be severe, with platelet counts of less than 10,000/mm$^3$. Hematuria, melena, and vaginal bleeding have also been reported. Diagnosis is retrospective because the purpura and thrombocytopenia start a week or 2 weeks after transfusion. Platelet counts and coagulation support should be considered. The thrombocytopenia is usually self-limited. Platelet transfusions should be reserved for severe cases, inasmuch as they usually are not beneficial. Patient sera should be tested for platelet-specific antibodies, HLA antibodies, and lymphocytotoxic antibodies.

## Therapy and Prevention

Three types of therapy have been advocated: corticosteroids, exchange transfusions, and plasmapheresis.[71] Intravenous immunoglobulin therapy has also been advocated.[72] Review of the PTP literature does not yield a strong consensus of opinion on treatment of PTP. In an acute, bleeding patient with concomitant lesions, the most likely therapeutic regimen would be moderate-dose corticosteroids (prednisone), intravenous immunoglobulin G (IV IgG), and plasmapheresis (personal communication, L. Lutcher, MD). Exchange transfusions would be reserved for cases in which initial therapy was considered a failure. Platelet transfusion should be avoided as much as possible during the PTP treatment period. Furthermore, there are no good ways to prevent posttransfusion purpura. A thorough patient history of prior transfusion and any adverse reactions should be taken before all blood component therapy. In suspicious cases with possible risk, appropriate antibody studies should be considered.

## Transfusion-associated Graft-versus-Host Disease

### Definition

Transfusion-associated graft-versus-host-disease (TA-GVHD) is a complication of blood component therapy or bone marrow transplantation. Although TA-GVHD is a rare complication of transfusion, significant populations of patients are at risk, and mortality is significant. Some of the at-risk groups include patients experiencing lymphopenia or bone marrow suppression, fetuses receiving intrauterine transfusions, newborn infants receiving exchange transfusions, individuals with congenital immunodeficiency syndromes, patients with certain hematologic and oncologic disorders, and patients receiving blood components from blood relatives.[73] The fatality rate for transfusion-associated TA-GVHD has been documented at 84 percent, with a median survival period of 21 days posttransfusion.[74] Death is usually caused by infection or hemorrhage secondary to bone marrow aplasia.

### Pathophysiology

Transfusion-associated graft-versus-host disease is caused by a proliferation of T-cell lymphocytes derived from the donor blood immunologically responding to major and minor histocompatibility antigens in the patient. Patients with cell-mediated immunodeficiency are at risk of not being able to reject transfused lymphocytes. Another risk group includes patients who have an HLA type that is haploidentical with that of the donor; these are usually first-degree relatives.[75] The mechanism of TA-GVHD has not been fully explained.

### Signs, Symptoms, and Clinical Work-up

Most clinical signs and symptoms of TA-GVHD appear in about 3 to 30 days after transfusion.[76] Pancytopenia is a clinically significant indication of TA-GVHD. Other effects include fever, elevated liver enzymes, copious watery diarrhea, erythematous skin rash progressing to erythroderma, and desquamation.

Tissue biopsies and laboratory tests assessing liver function status should be considered if histologic changes indicative of TA-GVHD are found in the liver, gastrointestinal tract, skin, and bone marrow. Close observation for infection or coagulation abnormalities should be monitored because these complications are responsible for most TA-GVHD fatalities. Human leukocyte antigen cell typing to confirm the presence of donor cells in the patient's circulation is used to confirm diagnosis.[77]

### Therapy and Prevention

Various therapeutic treatments have been used in patients with TA-GVHD, including corticosteroids, cyclosporine, methotrexate, azathioprine, and antithymocyte globulin. To date, the clinical efficacy of these and other experimental agents have not proved adequate in TA-GVHD. Because there is no adequate therapy for TA-GVHD, prevention is the only way to avoid potential fatalities. Blood component gamma irradiation has been demonstrated as the best current technology to reduce the risk of TA-GVHD.[78] The usual dosage range is 25 Gray (Gy) to 35 Gy (1 Gray = 100 rads).[79] Irradiation of the blood component before transfusion results in inactivation of the lymphocytes in the blood components, inhibiting lymphocyte blast transformation and mitotic activity. Table 18–14 details recipients who would be candidates for irradiated blood components before transfusion to reduce the risk of TA-GVHD.

### Iron Overload

#### Definition

A long-term complication of RBC transfusion is iron overload, also known as transfusion hemosiderosis. Each unit of RBCs has about 225 mg of iron as part of the hemoglobin molecules. Patients with certain diseases are chronically dependent on RBC transfusion support as part of therapy. Some of these diseases include congenital hemolytic anemias, aplastic anemia, and chronic renal failure.

#### Pathophysiology

Accumulated iron begins to affect the function of heart, liver, and endocrine glands. The full mechanism of iron overload leading to hemosiderosis is not yet fully elucidated. A likely pathologic effect is interference of mitochondrial function by excess iron accumulation.

#### Signs, Symptoms, and Clinical Work-up

Clinical signs and symptoms of hemosiderosis may include muscle weakness, fatigue, weight loss, mild jaundice, anemia, mild diabetes, and cardiac arrhythmias. A long history of chronic RBC transfusion should be a strong clinical indicator for diagnosis of iron overload. Assessment of storage iron levels such as ferritin levels and other iron studies should be performed. Tissue stains specific for iron in tissue biopsies should be considered.

#### Therapy and Prevention

Removal of accumulated tissue iron stores without lowering patient hemoglobin levels is the treatment of choice. Subcutaneous infusion of deferoxamine, an iron-chelating agent, has been tried with some success.

**Table 18–14.** Blood Component Irradiation: Clinical Indications for Transfusion Recipients to Reduce the Risk of Graft-versus-Host Disease

Bone marrow or peripheral blood stem cell recipients
Fetuses receiving intrauterine transfusions
Selected immunocompromised or immunodeficient recipients
Recipients of donor units known to be from a blood relative
Recipients of HLA-selected platelets or platelets known to be HLA-homozygous
Other—per physician order and transfusion service physician approval

Chronically transfusion-dependent patients should be exposed to as few units of RBCs as possible. One promising strategy is hypertransfusion using units rich in neocytes (young RBCs) to reduce the frequency of transfusion.[80]

### Immunosuppression

#### Definition

Immunosuppression is a generalized, nonspecific effect diminishing the activity of the recipient's immune system soon after blood component(s) transfusion. Since the early 1970s, immunosuppression of the transfusion recipient's immune system has been observed.[81] Individuals receiving RBC transfusions before renal transplantation were noted to have better graft survival than individuals who did not receive RBC transfusions. Some studies have linked postsurgical bacterial infections with blood component transfusions.[82,83] Also, transfusions have been associated with tumor recurrence in colorectal cancer patients.[84] Thus, immunosuppression has a potentially wide range of effects on the transfusion recipient. However, a review of over 60 articles reporting results on immunosuppression, some using a statistical tool called meta-analysis, did not define a posttransfusion immunosuppressive effect.[85] Obviously, this is an area of controversy that only further research will resolve as to the substance and degree of blood component immunosuppression.

#### Pathophysiology

To date, no specific mechanism or mechanisms have been definitely proven as the pathway for posttransfusion immunosuppression. Several theories have been put forward, such as rapid uptake of blood component cellular matter into the reticuloendothelial system (RES), but no supportive proof has been developed to identify a cause-and-effect relationship.

#### Signs, Symptoms, and Clinical Work-up

No specific signs or symptoms have been attributed to immunosuppression. Given the generalized nature of the immunosuppressive response, no specific work-up has been defined. The importance is realizing that blood component transfusion may impart an increased risk of a suppressive effect on the transfusion recipient's immune system. The transfusionist must always keep in mind any potential, as well as likely, adverse effects of transfusion, with the goal to minimize such adverse effects, if possible.

#### Therapy and Prevention

Currently, because of the limited knowledge base on immunosuppression, no specific therapy regimen is available. Prevention centers around the basic principle of transfusing a patient only when necessary with the appropriate blood component(s) in the dosage amounts most likely to have a beneficial effect. Thus, benefit must exceed risk for the transfusion to be justifiable, and the patient is properly required to assume this potential risk. Table 18–15 identifies commonly transfused blood components, functions, and associated transfusion reaction complications.

## TRANSFUSION REACTION INVESTIGATION

Adverse clinical manifestations after transfusion of blood components must be evaluated promptly and to the extent considered appropriate by the medical director. The exceptions to this rule are circulatory overload and allergic reactions, which do not have to be evaluated to the same extent as hemolytic transfusion reactions.[86] The transfusionist must first recognize that a transfusion reaction is occurring and then must take action immediately by initiating appropriate established procedures for transfusion reaction responses. Investigations of transfusion reactions are necessary for (1) diagnosis, (2) selection of appropriate therapy, (3) transfusion management, and (4) prevention of future transfusion reactions. Investigation should include correlations of clinical data with laboratory results.[87] Transfusion reaction protocols may vary according to the patient's clinical signs and symptoms, federal regulations, and assessment by the medical director and the patient's physician. In the investigation, one should remember that absence of evidence is not evidence of the absence of a transfusion reaction!

Any investigation of a suspected transfusion reaction must include investigation of clinical data to include (1) diagnosis; (2) medical history of pregnancies, transplants, and previous transfusions; (3) current medications; and (4) clinical signs and symptoms of the reaction. The transfusion history may give clues as to the possible cause of the transfusion reaction.[88] During the investigation, the following questions related to the transfusion and medical information may be included:

1. How many milliliters of RBCs or blood component were transfused?
2. How fast and for how long was the unit transfused?
3. Were RBCs given cold or warmed?
4. Was the transfusion given under pressure, and what size needle was used?
5. How was it given? Was a filter used, and if so, what type? What other solutions were given?
6. Were any drugs given at the time of transfusion?

A transfusion reaction form should be completed for each reaction and include the patient's pretransfusion and posttransfusion vital signs, type of reaction, time of occurrence, amount transfused, and other pertinent information.

The transfusion service must have a procedure manual detailing instructions to follow when a transfusion reaction occurs.[89] Table 18–16 details standard operating transfusion reaction procedures to include in manuals. To investigate a suspected HTR, the transfusion service should receive promptly after the transfusion a clotted blood sample, properly collected (avoiding hemolysis) and labeled, along with a nonclotted ethylenediaminetetraacetic acid (EDTA) specimen. Tests considered appropriate for an investigation are determined by the transfusion service medical director, indicated by the patient's clinical signs and symptoms, or ordered by the patient's physician.

Depending on the preliminary investigation results, more specimens may be required:

1. A clotted blood specimen drawn 5 to 7 hours after transfusion for unconjugated indirect bilirubin determination.

**Table 18–15.** Commonly Transfused Blood Components, Functions, and Associated Transfusion Reaction Complications

| Component | Function | Potential Reactions |
|---|---|---|
| Red blood cells | Carry oxygen to tissues and restore red cell mass following hemorrhage. | Allergic, febrile, hemolytic, bacterial contamination, alloimmunization, GVHD, circulatory overload, iron overload, anaphylactic, metabolic complications, and immunosuppression. |
| Platelets | Treat bleeding thrombocytopenic patients with severely decreased or functionally abnormal platelets, or patients with dilutional thrombocytopenia, or some patients with platelet consumption (DIC). | Same as red blood cells. After repeat transfusions, refractoriness to platelets may develop. |
| Fresh frozen plasma | Patients requiring labile coagulation plasma factors, used in dilutional coagulopathy, and in plasma exchanges for TTP. | Allergic, anaphylactic, fever, bacterial contamination, circulatory overload, and metabolic complications. |
| Cryoprecipitate | Control of bleeding associated with factor VIII deficiency, for von Willebrand's disease, and replacement of fibrinogen or factor XIII. | Same as for red blood cells. A positive DAT may develop if ABO-incompatible cryoprecipitate is given, rarely hemolysis. |

GVHD = graft-versus-host disease; DIC = disseminated intravascular coagulation; TTP = thrombotic thrombocytopenic purpura; DAT = direct antiglobulin test.

**Table 18–16.** Standard Operating Procedures for Transfusion Reactions

*Transfusion Service Manual*
Detection, reporting, and evaluation SOPs
Specimen requirements
Clerical and technical check procedures
Return of bag, solutions, filter-set, and intact tubing
Immediate and extended investigation procedures
Test procedures and record policies
Interpretations, reporting, and notification procedures

*Nursing Manual*
Recognition and response SOPs
Signs and symptom descriptions
Stop the transfusion instructions
Patient care responsibilities
Notification to physician and transfusion service

SOP = standard operating procedures.

2. The first voided posttransfusion urine collection.
3. Other specimens collected at various times that are considered appropriate to the transfusion reaction investigation.

### Immediate Laboratory Investigation

Laboratory transfusion reaction investigative procedures vary, but all begin with immediate preliminary procedures. Based on the preliminary investigative results and the patient's clinical condition, further testing may be necessary. Table 18–17 outlines immediate as-required and extended procedures that may be performed in investigating HTR.[90] Immediate transfusion reaction procedures include clerical checks, visual inspection, and direct antiglobulin test (DAT).

### Clerical Checks

Because many of the transfusion reactions reported have resulted from clerical errors (mislabeling and misidentification), immediate investigation should always begin with clerical checks.[91] Clerical checks should identify any possible errors or discrepancies in patient or donor identification.[92] Clerical checks may include patient and specimen identification data, blood unit inspection, tubing, filter, and solution examination, and label and record checks. Table 18–18 itemizes posttransfusion verification procedures.

### Visual Inspection

Visually observe the serum of the patient's pretransfusion and posttransfusion reaction blood specimens. The color of pretransfusion reaction serum and immediate posttransfusion recipient serum or plasma should be compared for evidence of RBC hemolysis. This is critical to investigation of an HTR. Normal serum or plasma appears pale yellow in color. If plasma or serum contains 0.2 g/L (20 mg/dL) of free hemoglobin, it will appear pink. If free hemoglobin exceeds

**Table 18–17.** Laboratory Investigation Outline for HTR

*Immediate Procedures*
Clerical checks
Visual inspection of serum and plasma for free hemoglobin (pretransfusion and posttransfusion)
Direct antiglobulin test—posttransfusion EDTA sample

*"As Required" Procedures*
ABO grouping and RH typing, pretransfusion and posttransfusion
Major compatibility test, pretransfusion and posttransfusion specimens
Antibody screen test, pretransfusion and posttransfusion specimens
Alloantibody identification
Antigen typings
Free hemoglobin in first voided-urine posttransfusion
Unconjugated (indirect) bilirubin 5–7 hours posttransfusion

*Extended Procedures (as Indicated)*
Gram stain and bacterial culture of unit(s)
Quantitative serum hemoglobin
Serum haptoglobin on pretransfusion and posttransfusion specimens
Serial hemoglobin, hematocrit, and platelet counts
Peripheral blood smear
Coagulation and renal output studies
Hemoglobin electrophoresis
Urine hemosiderin

EDTA = ethylenediaminetetraacetic acid.

**Table 18–18.** Posttransfusion Reaction Verifications

Rule out the possibility that the patient received the wrong blood component.
Verify the fact that the appropriate blood component was selected, accurately tested, and properly issued within expiration period.
Verify accuracy of patient and donor ABO and Rh type.
Verify accuracy of labels and records.
Rule out the possibility that any other patient or blood component was involved.

1 g/L (100 mg/dL), the plasma or serum will appear red.[93] During visual color observation, if only the posttransfusion specimen shows pink or red discoloration, a hemolytic process can be presumed. The posttransfusion plasma sample should be spectrophotometrically measured to quantitate the amount of free plasma hemoglobin. If the sample was not collected immediately after the transfusion, hemoglobin can be converted to bilirubin, which changes the plasma color to a bright yellow. The maximum bilirubin concentration occurs usually 3 to 6 hours after a hemolytic transfusion episode.[94] Myoglobin can cause serum to appear pink. If crush injuries exist, differentiation of myoglobin from hemoglobin should be determined. In the absence of extensive muscle trauma, myoglobin is unlikely.[95] Figure 18–5 depicts pretransfusion and posttransfusion reaction specimens from a patient with sickle cell disease experiencing a DHTR that demonstrates visually discernible free hemoglobin in the posttransfusion specimen.

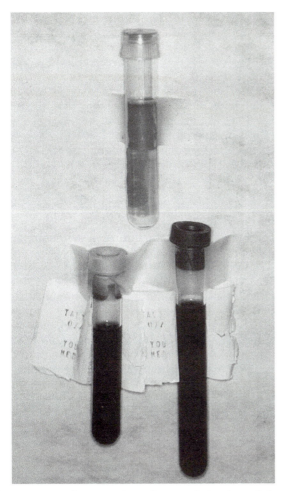

**Figure 18–5.** Color comparison of pretransfusion (top tube) and posttransfusion (bottom tubes) blood specimens from a sickle cell patient experiencing a DHTR.

A visual inspection of the return blood bag(s), solution(s), and attached tubing and filter set(s) may rule out hemolysis from nonimmunologic causes. Red blood cell hemolysis has been reported from open-heart bypass surgery machines, blood pumps, infusion through small-bore needles, infusion of blood under high pressure, drugs or solutions added to blood lines, heating or freezing blood improperly, and bacterial contamination.

### Direct Antiglobulin Test

In suspected immediate or delayed hemolytic reactions, a DAT should be performed on the posttransfusion specimen. The DAT result may be negative if the incompatible transfused cells have been immediately destroyed. In both immediate and delayed reactions, the DAT result may be positive, show mixed-field reactions, or be negative. When the DAT result appears as mixed-field agglutination, there are mixtures of agglutinated transfused donor cells along with unagglutinated patient cells. Table 18–19 summarizes some approaches to DAT testing.

## Additional Testing, as Indicated

If the immediate procedures suggest hemolysis, or if the results are misleading or negative but the patient's signs and symptoms suggest immune hemolysis, then additional testing is necessary. Testing may include the following procedures.

### ABO Grouping and Rh Typing

The recipient pretransfusion and posttransfusion reaction blood specimens and donor segments should be tested, and misidentification of any other patient sample or donor unit should be ruled out.

### Compatibility Test

When indicated, testing should include the pretransfusion and posttransfusion reaction samples tested with RBCs from donor units involved. An incompatible crossmatch with the pretransfusion sample indicates an original error (clerical or technical) with recipient or donor specimens. Incompatibility with only the posttransfusion specimen indicates a possible anamnestic response (as seen in DHTR), or a patient sample identification problem.

### Antibody Screen and Alloantibody Identification

To determine whether the transfusion reaction was the result of an antibody, the antibody screening tests should be repeated on the pretransfusion and posttransfusion reaction specimen and donor unit. Table 18–20 identifies causes of false-negative antibody screen results that should be considered in transfusion reaction investigations. Unexpected alloantibodies found in the patient's serum should be identified and any posttransfusion reaction-positive DAT result investigated. If the pretransfusion or posttransfusion antibody screening tests are reactive, identification is essential to determine antibody specificity to avoid another reaction when the patient requires further transfusion. Once antibody specificity is determined, all donor units must be tested for the corresponding antigen before additional transfusions are performed.

**Table 18–19.** Approaches to DAT

*DAT Result Positive*
Perform an elution and determine specificity.
Repeat DAT on several specimens to detect rising antibody titers.

*DAT Result Negative*
Perform an elution, if clinical hemolysis present.
If there exist too few antibody molecules to detect, perform an elution and concentrate antibody.
If all incompatible RBCs are destroyed, screen serum, perform clerical and technical checks, and repeat DAT later with new specimen.

DAT = direct antiglobulin test; RBC = red blood cell.

**Table 18–20.** Causes of False-Negative Antibody Screen Results

---

Failure to detect antibody in original test procedure
Test not sensitive enough to detect antibody
Clerical or technical error
Antibody screening cells represented a single dose of antigen (donor screen cells from a heterozygote)
Antibody identified in posttransfusion specimen only (may represent anamnestic response or patient sample identification problem)

---

## Urine Test

The first voided posttransfusion reaction specimen should be examined for the presence of free hemoglobin. Intact RBCs (hematuria) represent bleeding, not hemolysis. When unexplained hemoglobinemia occurs, the urine can be examined for hemoglobinuria. Table 18–21 indicates responses when using reagent strips to test urine for free hemoglobin and urobilinogen in suspected HTRs.

A week or more after suspected HTR investigation, the patient's urine can be examined for hemosiderinuria. Hemosiderin can appear in urine when the level exceeds 0.25 g/L (25 mg/dL) as free hemosiderin.[96]

## Bilirubin Test

A change from a pretransfusion normal pale yellow serum to a posttransfusion reaction bright or deep yellow serum should prompt an investigation for RBC hemolysis. The maximum concentration of bilirubin following hemolysis is not evident until approximately 3 to 6 hours after transfusion.[97] The posttransfusion result for indirect bilirubin should be compared with the pretransfusion result. Bilirubin excretion may return to normal within 24 hours.

## Hemoglobin and Hematocrit

Hemoglobinemia occurs when large excesses of free hemoglobin are released into the blood. The hemoglobin and hematocrit can be monitored to detect a drop in hemoglobin or failure of the transfusion to raise the hematocrit. Table 18–22 summarizes laboratory evidence supporting a diagnosis of DHTR. Hemoglobinemia immediately after a transfusion reaction confirms hemolysis, provided that an acceptable blood specimen was collected. Serial hematocrits and hemoglobin testing may be necessary to demonstrate therapeutic or nontherapeutic responses.[98] Table 18–23 lists suggested times when some tests may be performed when investigating a possible HTR.

Extended testing depends on analysis and interpretations of tests performed and the patient's clinical condition.

## Reporting Transfusion Reaction Workups

If the laboratory evaluation or test interpretations suggest an HTR or a bacterial contamination, the patient's physician and transfusion service medical director must be notified immediately. After the medical director of the transfusion service has evaluated the laboratory results, interpretations must be recorded in the patient's chart. The transfusion service must maintain the testing results, interpretations, and reaction classification for referral if the patient requires further transfusion therapy. The AABB standards require that transfusion records of patients with difficult blood typing, clinically significant antibodies, and adverse reactions to transfusions be retained indefinitely. The standards also require that before blood is issued for transfusion, a comparison of the patient's current records with the past 12 months' records must be made for ABO and Rh typings, clinically significant antibodies, and any severe adverse transfusion reactions; and the comparison must be documented.[99]

Both federal regulatory and voluntary accreditation agencies require investigation and reporting of recipient adverse transfusion reactions. The FDA states in the Code of Federal Regulations (CFR) the requirements for transfusion reaction reporting. If a reaction results in a fatality, the Director of the Office of Compliance for the Center of Biologic Evaluation and Research must be notified by telephone or telegraph as soon as possible. A required written report to the director must follow within 7 days of the investigation.[100] Other voluntary agencies requiring investiga-

**Table 18–21.** Urine Reagent Strip (Multistix) Chart for Suspected HTR

| | Reaction | Identify Reason | Microscopic (Rule Out Intact RBCs) | Monitor Patient's Renal Function | Test Sensitivity |
|---|---|---|---|---|---|
| Free hemoglobin | Positive | ✔ | ✔ | ✔ Evaluate further | 0.0015–0.0062 mg/dL Equivalent to 5–10 intact RBCs |
| Urobilinogen unit[†] (<1 Ehrlich or unit[†] is normal) | Positive (pink-red)* | ✔ | | ✔ Evaluate further | 0.02–1.0 Ehrlich test immediately Store in dark container* |

*Reagent strips utilizing p-dimethylaminobenzaldehyde are subject to interference by Ehrlich unit.
[†]1 mg/dL = 1 Ehrlich unit.

**Table 18–22.** Laboratory Evidence Suggesting DHTRs

Positive DAT result after transfusion; pretransfusion DAT result
  negative
Posttransfusion indirect bilirubin elevation
Posttransfusion hemoglobin decrease 2 g/dL or more
Hemoglobinuria or hemosiderinuria
Antibody present 3 to 5 days (or more) after transfusion, antibody
  absent before transfusion

DAT = direct antiglobulin test.

**Table 18–23.** Times to Perform Laboratory Test to Investigate IHTRs and DHTRs

| | Immediate | 1–3 Hours | 3–6 Hours | 24 Hours | Days |
|---|---|---|---|---|---|
| *Blood* | | | | | |
| Antibody IHTR | ✔ | ✔ | ✔ | ✔ | ✔ |
| Antibody DHTR | | | | | ✔ |
| Direct Coombs IHTR | ✔ | | | | May need to repeat |
| Direct Coombs DHTR | | | | | ✔ ✔ |
| Hemoglobinemia | ✔ | ✔ | ✔ | | ✔ |
| Haptoglobin | | | ✔ | ✔ | ✔ |
| Bilirubin | | | ✔ 3–12 hours | | ✔ |
| Methemalbumin | | ✔ | ✔ | ✔ | ✔ 1–2 days |
| *Urine* | | | | | |
| Hemoglobin | ✔ | ✔ | ✔ | | |
| Urobilinogen | | | | ✔ | ✔ |
| Hemosiderin | | | | | ✔ |

IHTR = immediate hemolytic transfusion reaction; DHTR = delayed hemolytic transfusion reaction.

tion and internal reporting of transfusion reactions include the College of American Pathologists (CAP) and the AABB. These agencies require that written transfusion reaction policies and procedures include steps for detection, evaluation, and reporting of adverse transfusion reactions.

## SUMMARY

This chapter has outlined posttransfusion difficulties associated with blood components. The transfusion service should establish policies and procedures that optimize transfusion practices and provide safety to transfusion recipients with reduced risk of morbidity and mortality. Continuous quality improvement of transfusion practices for the patient's safety requires constant review and surveillance of procedures, practices, and standards. The summary chart lists key points to remember.

## TRANSFUSION REACTION CASE STUDIES

### CASE 1

#### Clinical History

A 45-year-old man was admitted to the hospital with gastrointestinal bleeding from recurrent peptic ulcers. The patient had received a transfusion 4 months earlier for the same symptoms.

#### Hospital Course

The patient's hemoglobin on admission was 70 g/L (7 g/dL). Four units of blood were ordered and crossmatched, found to be compatible, and transfused. Five days after the transfusion, the patient appeared pale and mildly jaundiced and had a fever of 39°C. A complete blood count (CBC) and a blood culture were ordered by the physician.

#### Laboratory Findings

*Hematology Test Rests*

The patient's 5-day posttransfusion hemoglobin was 50.0 g/L (5 g/dL); hematocrit 0.15 L/L (15 percent). Spherocytes were present on the peripheral blood smear. Because of the low hemoglobin, 2 units of blood were ordered by the patient's physician.

*Blood Bank Test Results*

Five days after transfusion 2 units of blood were crossmatched and found to be incompatible. The antibody screen was positive at this time. Five days previously, the antibody screen test result had been negative. A transfusion reaction work-up was initiated.

*Clerical Checks*

No clerical errors were revealed.

*Technical Results*

Repeat ABO and Rh typings on pretransfusion and posttransfusion reaction specimens confirmed original results. Repeat crossmatch test on pretransfusion and posttransfusion patient specimens with donor units revealed no incompatibility. The pretransfusion DAT result was negative, but the posttransfusion DAT result was positive because of IgG sensitization. Panels completed on the patient's serum and eluate revealed the following antibody identification:

Serum: Anti-Jk^a by enzyme technique
Eluate: Anti-Jk^a by enzyme technique
Phenotyping of patient's RBCs for Jk^a antigen (pretransfusion specimen)
Patient's test results: Jk^a negative

*Microbiology Results*

Results of the patient's blood culture, Gram stain, and culture of the donor unit were negative.

*Interpretation*

This case illustrates the laboratory results of a DHTR. Anti-Jk$^a$ is known for its transient properties of appearing and disappearing and for its enhancement by enzymes. The reaction occurred at a time when transfusion was least suspected as the cause. The transfusion caused a secondary immune stimulus, resulting in rise in antibody titer. In DHTR from transfused donor RBCs, destruction is usually gradual. The patient experienced anemia, fever, and mild jaundice 3 to 7 days after the transfusion. If the patient should require future transfusion, blood lacking Jk$^a$ antigen would be required.

## Conclusion

The patient had DHTR caused by Jk$^a$ antibody.

## CASE 2

### Clinical History

A 55-year-old man was hospitalized to have abdominal surgery for carcinoma. The patient had no previous history of transfusion.

*Hospital Course*

The patient's admission hemoglobin was 100 g/L (10 g/dL). Two units of RBCs were ordered for the surgery. The patient was blood group O-positive. The antibody screen result was negative. Two units of RBCs were crossmatched and found compatible. During surgery, after receipt of the first unit of RBCs, the patient experienced oozing at the surgical site. His blood pressure fell from a pretransfusion level of 120/70 mm Hg to 80/40 mm Hg after the transfusion. The transfusion was immediately stopped and the hypotension treated. A new blood sample was sent to the blood bank, and four more units of RBCs were requested immediately.

*Laboratory Findings*

The blood bank technologist, on typing the new posttransfusion sample, obtained the following results:

| Reactions of Cells | | Reaction of Serum with RBCs | | |
|---|---|---|---|---|
| Anti-A | Anti-B | A$_1$ | B | O |
| +mf | neg | ++ | +++ | neg |
| mf = mixed field, + = positive, neg = negative | | | | |

Repeat typing of the patient's pretransfusion blood specimen confirmed the blood group as originally designated O-positive. The posttransfusion reaction specimen revealed mixed-field agglutination when tested with anti-A antisera. The surgeon was notified by the medical director that a potential immune-hemolytic reaction may be in progress.

*Clerical Checks*

Clerical checks were performed in both the blood bank and the operating room. On completion of the clerical checks, it was determined that the wrong unit of blood had been selected for this patient. Two patients with similar names were undergoing surgery at the same time. The unit had been selected from the operating room refrigerator by name only and had not been checked to include hospital identification number before transfusion. It was additionally determined that two persons had not checked the unit before transfusion as required by the hospital transfusion policy. Investigation eliminated the possibility that any other patient was at risk for a similar incident at that time. The inadvertently transfused unit was determined to be group A–positive.

*Laboratory Investigation*

The postreaction DAT test was negative, indicating rapid destruction of the incompatible transfused RBCs. The pretransfusion and posttransfusion antibody screen test results were negative. The crossmatch on the pretransfusion specimens with the original group O donor units revealed no incompatibility. Hemoglobinemia and hemoglobinuria were present, with free hemoglobin demonstrated in the first posttransfusion urine specimen.

The patient developed a hemorrhagic coagulopathy with afibrinogenemia. His platelets decreased, with a concomitant increase in fibrinogen and fibrin degradation products. He soon became anuric, producing only 50 mL of urine in 12 hours. The patient's condition deteriorated despite attempts to control the hemorrhagic process, and he died. Autopsy findings 4 days posttransfusion revealed hemoglobin casts in the renal tubules of the patient's kidneys.

*Interpretation*

In an anesthetized patient the only symptoms of an HTR may be oozing, bleeding, or hypotension, as experienced by this patient. The erroneously transfused group A donor unit RBCs reacted with the patient's anti-A antibody, resulting in destruction of the transfused donor cells. The coagulation system was activated, resulting in a hemorrhagic diathesis with resultant acute renal failure and death.

To prevent HTR, identity of the patient and donor blood component by two persons is essential to ensure that the appropriate blood component is transfused. Blood must never be released if it is identified by a patient's name. There must be not only verification policies but also monitoring to ensure that established policies are adhered to. At the first sign of a transfusion reaction, the transfusion must be stopped, a line left open for normal saline administration, the patient immediately attended to, and an immediate investigation initiated. Most errors in ABO mismatch of blood transfusion are misidentification of either the patient or blood sample. Human errors resulting in serious or fatal transfusion reactions are often litigated, not excused.

## Conclusion

This patient had an immune acute hemolytic transfusion reaction caused by ABO incompatibility.

## CASE 3

### Clinical History

A 45-year-old woman was admitted to the hospital for a hysterectomy. The patient had been pregnant four times and had no history of transfusions. She was taking no medications.

The patient's admission complete blood count (CBC) revealed a low hemoglobin of 70 g/L (7.0g/dL). The physician ordered a unit of RBCs to be given before surgery to correct her anemia before an elective hysterectomy.

### Laboratory Test

A unit of group O Rh-positive RBCs was crossmatched and found compatible. The patient's antibody screen test result was negative.

### Hospital Course

A transfusion of group O Rh-positive compatible RBCs was begun at 1:45 PM and given through a standard 170-μm blood infusion set. After receiving approximately half of the RBCs, the patient experienced chills, and her temperature rose from a pretransfusion temperature of 37.2°C to 39.4°C. She had a severe headache and felt anxious and uncomfortable. The blood transfusion was stopped and the patient's physician notified. A transfusion reaction investigation was initiated.

### Laboratory Findings

#### Clerical Checks

No clerical errors were detected. Donor and patient identifications were verified.

#### Serologic Findings

Examination of the patient's pretransfusion and posttransfusion blood and urine specimens revealed no visible hemolysis. The DAT result on the posttransfusion blood specimen was negative. No RBC alloantibodies were detected in the serum of the patient or the donor. Repeat blood typings and crossmatch tests on the pretransfusion and posttransfusion specimens and donor unit confirmed the original test results. No incompatibility was demon-

strated. Results of the serum bilirubin test 5 hours after the transfusion were normal. Bacterial contamination was ruled out by a negative culture and Gram stain.

### Interpretation

Because serologic test results did not indicate a hemolytic reaction, blood group incompatibility, or bacterial contamination, other causes were considered. The patient's four pregnancies and transfusion reaction signs and symptoms suggested that a reaction to donor leukocytes had occurred. Leukocytes in RBC and platelet transfusions have been associated frequently with adverse effects (1 to 3 percent) when transfused to recipients who are alloimmunized from previous pregnancies, transfusions, or organ transplantation. The reactions are frequently associated with alloimmunization to HLA class I or leukocyte-specific antigens. Red blood cell transfusions contain approximately 2 to $5 \times 10^9$ leukocytes. Using adsorption RBC filters to transfuse the RBCs through, leukocyte removal can achieve up to a 3-log (99.9 percent) leukocyte reduction. This reduction can prevent recurrent NHFTRs and delay of alloimmunization to leukocyte antigens in selected patients requiring long-term transfusion therapy.

## Conclusion

This patient had an NHFTR. If she should experience two or more similar reactions, leukocyte-poor prepared blood or an in-line leukocyte reduction filter should be used. Although there are a number of ways to prepare leukocyte-poor blood, third-generation adsorption filters that remove leukocytes by adherence can achieve profound leukocyte reduction.

## CASE 4

### Clinical History

A 38-year-old man arrived at the hospital emergency department (ED) complaining of abdominal pain. A CBC was ordered. His hemoglobin level was found to be 70 g/L (7 g/dL). The physician determined evidence of bleeding and ordered 2 units of RBCs immediately. The patient had no history of prior transfusion and was taking no medications.

### Laboratory Findings

Two units of RBCs were crossmatched and found compatible. The patient's antibody screen test was negative. One compatible donor unit was released to the ED.

### Hospital Course

After proper identification of the unit of RBCs with the patient by two persons, vital signs were checked and recorded, and the transfusion was initiated. Thirty minutes after the transfusion had begun, the patient experienced a slight rash and itching. No other associated adverse effects were noted. The patient was given diphenhydramine (Benadryl). While the medication took effect, the transfusion was discontinued and normal saline transfused. Once the symptoms subsided (15 to 20 minutes), the transfusion was continued with no ill effects noted.

### Interpretation

Urticarial reaction is the only immediate immunologic adverse effect of transfusion in which the transfusion can continue, provided that no other adverse effects occur. This type of reaction is likely to be caused by the passive transfer of IgE or IgG antiatopen (e.g., hay fever reaction to pollen), or both, from the donor plasma to the recipient. Histamine is presumed the mediator because it is released from antigen attached to the mast cell along with the IgE antibody. If the signs and symptoms are more severe (pulmonary edema, asthma, facial edema, hives over entire body) or become more severe after medicative treatment, the transfusion must be stopped immediately and investigated.

### Conclusion

This patient had an urticarial reaction, which was treated effectively with Benadryl.

## CASE 5

### Clinical History

A teenage girl undergoing chemotherapy for an adenosarcoma developed pancytopenia. The patient had a history of multiple transfusions of blood components.

### Hospital Course

On admission the patient was found to have small petechiae on her arms, face, mouth, chest, and conjunctiva. The admitting physician ordered an emergency platelet count, and on receiving the results ordered eight irradiated pooled platelet concentrates immediately. Within several minutes of the platelet transfusion, the patient developed tightness in the chest, flushing of the skin, respiratory distress, coughing, and hypotension. The transfusion was stopped, and the patient was given epinephrine according to physician's orders. The patient's physician consulted with the transfusion service medical director concerning a therapeutic approach for additional platelet transfusions.

### Laboratory Data

The patient's platelet count at admission was 11.2 $\times 10^9$/L, and the WBC count was 33.4 $\times 10^9$/L.

### Clerical Checks

No clerical errors were found.

### Technical Results

Platelet studies after transfusion revealed no patient or donor antibodies to specific platelet or WBC antigens, and the patient's serum contained normal levels of IgA.

### Interpretation

This patient experienced severe, immediate, and generalized reaction symptoms to transfused pooled platelet concentrates resolved by treatment with epinephrine. She also experienced a severe anaphylactoid reaction to plasma proteins in the platelet concentrates. After consultation with the transfusion service medical director, the patient was given irradiated washed platelet concentrates prepared using the COBE 2991 blood cell processor.

### Conclusion

After the washed irradiated platelets were transfused through a leukocyte-reduction filter, the patient experienced no further adverse reactions to transfused platelets.

## CASE 6

### Clinical History

A pregnant woman (primigravida) with a history of sickle cell disease had been followed in the hospital clinic for over 11 years. She had had many past sickle cell crises requiring medical attention. The patient had previously received multiple transfusion of RBCs.

### Transfusion Service Laboratory

Two units of group O Rh-negative RBCs were ordered, crossmatched, and found compatible. The patient's antibody screen test result was negative.

### Clinic Course

At 22 weeks' gestation, the patient was given a prophylactic transfusion of 2 units of compatible RBCs in the clinic. Seven days later she received another transfusion of 2 additional compatible units of RBCs.

### Hospital Course

Sixteen days after transfusion of the initial 2-unit transfusion, the patient returned to the clinic complaining of pain. She was afebrile but icteric, and was admitted to the hospital. During days 16 to 23, the patient had a marked decrease in hemoglobin concentration.

### Laboratory Findings

#### Serologic Findings

Blood samples submitted to the transfusion service revealed that the patient had a positive direct antiglobulin test (DAT) result. An elution test was performed. Antibody panel results of the elution study revealed that the patient had developed anti-Co$^b$ antibody. Twenty-seven days after the initial transfusion of 2 units of RBCs, the antibody screen test remained positive.

### Hematology and Urinalysis Findings

The patient's total hemoglobin concentration decreased from 11.0 g/dL to 6.0 g/dL during days 16 to 23. Her hemoglobin A concentration at 23 days was 2.0 g/dL. Urinalysis results 16 days after transfusion of the two initial RBC units showed an elevation of bilirubin.

### Interpretation

After transfusion of 2 RBC units, this patient developed anti-Co$^b$ antibody. This antibody is usually IgG in nature and can cause hemolytic transfusion reactions. Approximately 11 percent of random donor units would be incompatible if a patient had detectable anti-Co$^b$. Co$^b$ is a low-incidence antigen in the Colton blood group system.

### Conclusion

This patient suffered a DHTR caused by anti-Co$^b$. She experienced a fall in hemoglobin concentration accompanied by a positive antibody screen and positive DAT test. Anti-Co$^b$ was identified in the patient's serum and eluate, prepared from her RBCs.

---

## SUMMARY CHART: IMPORTANT POINTS TO REMEMBER (MT/MLT)

- Transfusion reactions range from benign to fatal.
- Any suspected transfusion reaction must be evaluated promptly.
- If a death occurs as a consequence of transfusion, notify the FDA within 24 hours.
- At the first sign of a transfusion reaction, stop the transfusion.
- Rule out wrongly transfused blood in anesthetized patients with bleeding at the surgical site, hypotension, and hemoglobinuria.
- Recipients of any transfused blood component may produce alloantibodies.
- Alloimmunization and infection are major adverse transfusion complications.
- FNHTRs have undefined temperature increase greater than 1°C during or hours after transfusion.
- Fatal HTRs caused by errors in patient identification are associated with ABO incompatibility.
- TA-GVHD can be prevented by irradiating blood components before transfusion.
- Transfusion-associated circulatory overload (TACO) can be lessened by defined transfusion criteria and conservative fluid management.
- An anamnestic antibody response may be elicited about 7 to 10 days posttransfusion in DHTR patients who were previously immunized.
- Do not add drugs or incompatible solutions to RBCs to avoid hemolysis.
- Transfusions can save lives; however, one must be aware of transfusion risks; recognize reactions, causes, and means of management; and ensure proper identification and administration.

---

## REVIEW QUESTIONS

1. Plasma that contains free hemoglobin in quantities of 100 mg/dL has a color that appears as:
   - A. Straw yellow
   - B. Faint pink
   - C. Deep, bright yellow
   - D. Red
   - E. Blue

2. Transfused plasma constituents resulting in immediate erythema, itching, and hives best typify which of the following transfusion reactions?
   - A. HTR
   - B. DHTR
   - C. Allergic
   - D. Iron overload
   - E. Alloimmunization

3. Which listed transfusion reaction may result from an anamnestic response following a secondary exposure to donor RBCs?
   - A. IHTR
   - B. Alloimmunization
   - C. Anaphylactoid reaction

   - D. TACO
   - E. TA-GVHD

4. Patients at greatest risk of developing TACO may include:
   - A. Children
   - B. Elderly people
   - C. Patients with chronic normovolemic anemia
   - D. Patients with sickle cell disease
   - E. All of the above

5. Which listed transfusion reaction is most associated with transfused patients lacking IgA immunoglobulin?
   - A. Anaphylactic
   - B. Hemolytic
   - C. Febrile
   - D. TACO
   - E. Allergic

6. The result of the DAT after a delayed transfusion reaction may be:
   - A. Positive
   - B. Mixed-field
   - C. Positive because of complement coating only

D. Negative
E. All of the above

7. A transfusion reaction that usually appears rapidly during transfusion termed "warm" and may result in fever, shock, or death is which one of the following listed reactions?
   A. Hemolytic
   B. Bacterial contamination
   C. TACO
   D. Allergic
   E. FNHTR

8. After an IHTR, the recipient's serum bilirubin may return to normal in:
   A. 5 hours
   B. 12 hours
   C. 48 hours
   D. 3 hours
   E. 24 hours

9. Which of the following antibodies is most responsible for IHTR?
   A. Anti-Le$^a$
   B. Anti-N
   C. Anti-A
   D. Anti-M
   E. Anti-D

10. Fatal transfusion reactions are most frequently caused by:
    A. Clerical errors
    B. Improper refrigeration
    C. Overheating blood
    D. Mechanical trauma
    E. Filters

11. When a suspected hemolytic reaction occurs, the first thing to do is:
    A. Slow the transfusion rate and call the physician
    B. Administer medication to stop reaction
    C. Stop the transfusion, but keep the intravenous line open with saline
    D. First inform the laboratory to begin an investigation
    E. Begin technical checks

12. Which of the following are symptoms of FNHTR?
    A. Shock, hemoglobinuria, hypotension
    B. Respiratory distress, vascular instability, shock
    C. DIC, renal failure, hemoglobinuria
    D. Temperature rise of 1°C with transfusion
    E. Temperature rise of 2°C or more with transfusion

13. If a patient experiences two or more FNHTRs, with each reaction becoming more severe, the easiest preventive approach for transfusion of RBCs is to:
    A. Administer the RBCs slowly
    B. Use specialized filters that remove most of the WBCs
    C. Use washed RBCs
    D. Administer smaller amounts of RBCs
    E. Use phenotypically matched RBCs

14. FNHTR is characterized by which of the following descriptions?
    A. Occurring in 50 percent of transfusions
    B. Rarely occurring after transfusions
    C. Occurring in about 1 percent of transfusions
    D. Occurring in 99 percent of transfusions
    E. Resulting from clerical errors

15. DHTRs from anamnestic responses usually occur within which time period?
    A. 5 hours
    B. 24 hours
    C. Several weeks after transfusion
    D. 3 to 7 days after transfusion
    E. 48 hours posttransfusion

16. Pretransfusion irradiation of all blood products in certain patients is done to prevent which of the following?
    A. CMV
    B. TA-GVHD
    C. FNHTR
    D. PNH
    E. HTR

17. If a fatality results directly from a transfusion complication, what organization must be notified within 24 hours of the fatality?
    A. FDA
    B. CAP
    C. AABB
    D. CDC
    E. JCAHO

18. The most common reason for transfusion of leukocyte-poor blood is that the recipient:
    A. Has RBC alloantibodies
    B. Has a positive DAT result
    C. Has been pregnant
    D. Has experienced an urticarial reaction
    E. Has had two or more FNHTRs

19. When a patient receiving platelet transfusion experiences purpura, the most likely cause is:
    A. RBC alloantibodies
    B. Platelet antigens
    C. Contaminating leukocytes in the platelet component
    D. Platelet antibodies
    E. Plasma proteins in blood component

20. Symptoms of an IHTR in an anesthetized patient may present only as:
    A. Unexplained hypotension and abnormal bleeding
    B. Unexplained hypertension and thrombocytopenia
    C. Pale skin color
    D. Abdominal distention
    E. Respiratory distress

21. Of the transfusion reaction types listed, which results in thrombocytopenia owing to platelet alloantibody?
    A. IHTR
    B. TA-GVHD

C. FNHTR
D. PTP
E. DHTR

22. Bacterial contamination of blood components can occur:
    A. At the time of phlebotomy
    B. During the component preparation
    C. In components stored at room temperature
    D. During thawing in waterbaths
    E. All of the above

23. A patient was suspected of having an adverse reaction to a transfusion. The patient experienced urticaria. Which is the most likely associated etiology for urticaria?
    A. Plasma proteins
    B. Leukoagglutinins
    C. Platelet antibodies
    D. Antibody-induced intravascular hemolysis
    E. Antibody-induced extravascular hemolysis

24. A patient was suspected of having TA-GVHD as a result of transfusion therapy. What may cause TA-GVHD?
    A. Transfused contaminated blood components
    B. Functional T lymphocytes in cellular blood components
    C. Hypersensitivity reaction
    D. Results from platelet-specific antibody following transfusion
    E. Results from transfused serum proteins (IgE) reacting with recipient antibodies

25. IHTR reactions resulting from ABO-incompatible transfused RBCs are usually associated with which of the following findings?
    A. Intact RBCs in the urine
    B. Presence of leukoagglutinins
    C. Hemoglobinuria
    D. Extravascular hemolysis
    E. An increase in the serum haptoglobin concentration

26. Red blood cell alloimmunization can result from:
    A. Pregnancy
    B. Platelet transfusions
    C. Leukocyte transfusions
    D. RBC transfusions
    E. All of the above

27. Transfusion reactions can be caused by:
    A. Citrate toxicity
    B. Hyperkalemia
    C. Overheating donor blood
    D. Adding drugs to donor unit
    E. All of the above

28. What electrolyte may fall in level as a result of citrate toxicity from massive transfusions?
    A. Calcium
    B. Phosphorus
    C. Sodium
    D. Potassium
    E. Magnesium

29. In looking at the first voided postreaction urine specimen, hematuria (representing bleeding, not hemolysis) would be represented by the finding of:
    A. Free hemoglobin
    B. Hemosiderin
    C. Urobilinogen
    D. Intact RBCs
    E. All of the above

30. A patient was suspected of having an adverse reaction to a transfusion of RBCs. The patient experienced an FNHTR. Which is the most likely associated etiology?
    A. Plasma proteins
    B. Leukoagglutinins
    C. Platelet antibodies
    D. Antibody-induced intravascular hemolysis
    E. Antibody-induced extravascular hemolysis

## ANSWERS TO REVIEW QUESTIONS

1. D (p 394)
2. C (p 386)
3. B (p 390)
4. E (p 388)
5. A (p 387)
6. E (p 395)
7. B (p 388)
8. E (p 396)
9. C (p 382)
10. A (p 394)
11. C (p 383, Table 18–8)
12. D (p 385)
13. B (p 386)
14. C (p 385)
15. D (p 384)
16. B (p 391)
17. A (p 396)
18. E (p 386)
19. D (p 390)
20. A (p 382)
21. D (p 390)
22. E (p 388)
23. A (p 387)
24. B (p 391)

25. C (p 382)

26. E (p 390)

27. E (p 390)

28. A (p 389)

29. D (p 396)

30. B (pp 385–396)

## REFERENCES

1. Standards for Blood Banks and Transfusion Services, ed 18. American Association of Blood Banks, Bethesda, MD, 1997, p 41, K2.000.
2. Sazama, K: Reports of 355 transfusion associated deaths: 1976 through 1985. Transfusion 30:583, 1990.
3. NIH Consensus Conference: Perioperative red cell transfusion. JAMA 260:2700, 1988.
4. Isbister, JP: Risk management in transfusion medicine. Transfus Med Rev 10:183, 1996.
5. Linden, JV, Tourault, MA, and Scribner, CL: Decrease in frequency of transfusion fatalities. Transfusion 37:243, 1997.
6. Pritchard, E: Transfusion-associated Fatalities: Review of Bureau of Biologic Reports 1976–1982. Health Care Finance Administration Regional Office, Philadelphia, 1982.
7. Moore, SB, et al: Delayed hemolytic transfusion reactions: Evidence of the need for an improved pretransfusion compatibility test. Am J Clin Pathol 74:94, 1980.
8. Sazama, K, op cit, p 585.
9. Vengelen-Tyler, V (ed): Technical Manual, ed 12. American Association of Blood Banks, Bethesda, MD, 1996, p 549.
10. Pineda, AA, and Taswell, HF: Transfusion reactions associated with anti-IgA antibodies: Report of four cases and review of the literature. Transfusion 15:10, 1975.
11. Taswell, HF: Hemolytic transfusion reactions: Frequency and clinical and laboratory aspects. In Bell, CA (ed): A Seminar on Immune Mediated Cell Destruction. American Association of Blood Banks, Washington, DC, 1981, p 71.
12. Sazama, K, op cit, p 583.
13. Holland, PV: The diagnosis and management of transfusion reactions and other adverse effects of transfusion. In Petz, LD, and Swisher, SN (eds): Clinical Practice of Transfusion Medicine, ed 2. Churchill Livingstone, New York, 1989, p 714.
14. Taswell, HF, op cit, p 76.
15. Pisciotto, PT (ed): Blood Transfusion Therapy: A Physician's Handbook, ed 4. American Association of Blood Banks, Bethesda, MD, 1993, p 77.
16. Pineda, AA, Brzica, SM, and Taswell, HF: Hemolytic transfusion reaction: Recent experience in a large blood bank. Mayo Clin Proc 53:378, 1978.
17. Popovsky, MA, Abel, MD, and Moore, SB: Transfusion-related acute lung injury associated with passive transfer of antileukocyte antibodies. American Review of Respiratory Disease 128:185, 1983.
18. Barry, KG, and Malloy, JP: Oliguric renal failure: Evaluation and therapy by the intravenous infusion of mannitol. JAMA 179:510, 1962.
19. Hammerschmidt, DE, and Jacob, HS: Adverse pulmonary reactions to transfusion. Adv Intern Med 27:511, 1983.
20. Mollison, PL, Engelfriet, CP, and Contreas, M: Blood Transfusion in Clinical Medicine, ed 9. Blackwell Scientific, Oxford, 1993, p 527.
21. Davenport, RD: Hemolytic transfusion reactions. In Popovsky, MA (ed): Transfusion Reactions. American Association of Blood Banks, Bethesda, MD, 1996, p 24.
22. Patten, E, et al: Delayed hemolytic transfusion reaction caused by a primary immune response. Transfusion 22:248, 1982.
23. Furling, MB, and Monaghan, WP: Delayed hemolytic episodes due to anti-M. Transfusion 21:45, 1981.
24. Panzer, S, et al: Haemolytic transfusion reactions due to HLA antibodies. Lancet 1:474, 1987.
25. Chaplin, H, Jr: The implication of red-cell bound complement in delayed hemolytic transfusion reactions. Transfusion 24:185, 1984.
26. Holland, PV, and Wallerstein, RO: Delayed hemolytic transfusion reaction with acute renal failure. JAMA 204:1007, 1968.
27. Levin, MW: Furosemide and ethacrynic acid in renal insufficiency. Med Clin North Am 55:107, 1971.
28. Vengelen-Tyler, V, op cit, p 548.
29. Wenz, B: Microaggregate blood filtration and febrile transfusion reaction: A comparative study. Transfusion 23:95, 1983.
30. Gleichmann, H, and Greininger, J: Over 95% sensitization against allogenic leukocytes following single massive blood transfusion. Vox Sang 28:66, 1975.
31. Moore, SB, et al: Transfusion-induced alloimmunization in patients awaiting renal allografts. Vox Sang 47:354, 1984.
32. Okusawa, S, et al: C5a induction of human interleukin-1: Synergistic effect with endotoxin or interferon-α. J Immunol 139:2635, 1987.
33. Dinnarello, CA, and Wolff, SM: Molecular basis of fever in humans. Am J Med 72:799, 1982.
34. Brubaker, DB: Immunologically mediated immediate adverse effects of blood transfusions (allergic, febrile nonhemolytic, and noncardiogenic pulmonary edema). Plasma Therapeutics and Transfusion Technology 6:19, 1985.
35. Wenz, B: Clinical and laboratory precautions that reduce the adverse reactions, alloimmunization, infectivity, and possibly immunomodulation associated with homologous transfusions. Tranfus Med Rev 4:3, 1990.
36. Seldon, TH: Untoward reactions and complications during transfusions and infusions. Anesthesiology 22:810, 1961.
37. Thompson, JS: Urticaria and angioedema. Ann Intern Med 69:361, 1968.
38. Dahler, SE, et al: Leukotrienes promote plasma leakage and leukocyte adhesion in postcapillary venules: In vivo effects with relevance to the acute inflammatory response. Proc Natl Acad Sci USA 78:3887, 1981.
39. Bochner, BS, and Lichtenstein, LM: Anaphylaxis. N Engl J Med 324:1785, 1991.
40. Vyas, GN, et al: Serologic specificity of human anti-IgA and its significance in transfusion. Blood 34:573, 1969.
41. Mollison, PL, op cit, p 690.
42. Milde, LN: An anaphylactic reaction to fibrin glue. Anesth Analg 69:684, 1989.
43. Ring, J, and Messmer, K: Incidence and severity of anaphylactoid reactions to colloid volume substitutes. Lancet 1:466, 1977.
44. Hammerschmidt, DE, et al: Association of complement activation and elevated plasma-C5a with adult respiratory distress syndrome. Lancet 1:947, 1980.
45. Holland, PV: Other adverse effects of transfusion. In Petz, LD, and Swisher, SN (eds): Clinical Practice of Blood Transfusion. Churchill Livingstone, New York, 1981, p 783.
46. Barton, JC: Noninfectious transfusion reactions. In Dutcher, JP (ed): Modern Transfusion Therapy. CRC Press, Boca Raton, FL, 1990, p 71.
47. Goldfinger, D: Adverse reactions to blood transfusion. In Mayer, K (ed): Guidelines to Transfusion Practices. American Association of Blood Banks, Washington, DC, 1980, p 144.
48. Goldfinger, D, and Lowe, C: Prevention of adverse reactions to blood transfusion by the administration of saline washed red blood cells. Transfusion 21:277, 1981.
49. Wagner, SJ, et al: Transfusion-associated bacterial sepsis. Clin Microbiol Rev 7:290–302, 1994.
50. Wagner, SJ, et al: Comparison of bacteria growth in single and pooled platelet concentrates after deliberate inoculation and storage. Transfusion 35:298–302, 1995.
51. Klein, HG, et al: Current status of microbial contamination of blood components: Summary of a conference. Transfusion 37:95–101, 1997.
52. Buckholz, DH, et al: Detection and quantitations of bacteria in platelet products stored at ambient temperature. Transfusion 13:268, 1985.

53. Kim, DM, et al: Visual identification of bacterially contaminated red cells. Transfusion 32:221, 1992.
54. Hoppe, PA: Interim measures for detection of bacterially contaminated red cell components. Transfusion 32:199, 1992.
55. Linden, JV, et al: In vitro and in vivo evaluation of an electromechanical blood infusion pump. Lab Med 19:574, 1988.
56. Miller, RD, et al: Coagulation defects associated with massive blood transfusion. Ann Surg 174:794, 1971.
57. Reuler, JB: Hypothermia: Pathophysiology, clinical settings, and management. Ann Intern Med 89:519, 1978.
58. Gibson, JG, Gregory, CB, and Button, LN: Citrate-phosphate-dextrose solutions for preservation of human blood: A further report. Transfusion 1:280, 1961.
59. Valeri, C: Viability and function of preserved red cells. N Engl J Med 284:81, 1971.
60. Mammen, E, and Walt, A: Eight years of experience with massive blood transfusion. J Trauma 11:275, 1971.
61. Quick, AJ: Influence of erythrocytes on the coagulation of blood. Am J Med Sci 239:101, 1960.
62. Barton, JC: Massive transfusion: Complications and their management. J Tenn Med Assoc 68:895, 1975.
63. Best, R, Syverud, S, and Novak, RM: Trauma and hypothermia. Am J Emerg Med 3:48, 1985.
64. Silberstein, LE, et al: Calcium homeostasis during therapeutic plasma exchange. Transfusion 26:151, 1986.
65. Wolfowitz, E, and Schechter, Y: More about alloimmunization by transfusion of fresh-frozen plasma. Transfusion 24:544, 1984.
66. Cox, JV, et al: Risk of alloimmunization and delayed hemolytic transfusion reactions in patients with sickle cell disease. Arch Intern Med 148:2488, 1988.
67. Salama, A, and Mueller-Eckhardt, C: Delayed hemolytic transfusion reactions: Evidence for complement activation involving allogeneic and autologous red cells. Transfusion 24:188, 1984.
68. Kooy, MVM, et al: Use of leukocyte-depleted platelet concentrates for the prevention of refractoriness and primary HLA alloimmunization: A prospective, randomized trial. Blood 77:201, 1991.
69. Vichinsky, EP, et al: Alloimmunization in sickle cell anemia and transfusion of racially unmatched blood. N Engl J Med 322:1617, 1990.
70. Kickler, TS, et al: Studies on the pathophysiology of posttransfusion purpura. Blood 68:347, 1986.
71. Cimo, PL, and Aster, RH: Posttransfusion purpura: Successful treatment by exchange transfusion. N Engl J Med 287:290, 1980.
72. Mueller-Eckhardt, C, et al: High-dose intravenous immunoglobulin for posttransfusion purpura (abstract P12–21). Eighteenth Congress of the International Society of Blood Transfusion, 1984, p 194.
73. Brubaker, DB: Human posttransfusion graft-versus-host disease. Vox Sang 45:401, 1983.
74. Anderson, KC, and Weinstein, HJ: Transfusion-associated graft-versus-host disease. N Engl J Med 323:315, 1990.
75. Linden, JV, and Pisciotto, PT: Transfusion-associated graft-versus-host disease and blood irradiation. Transf Med Rev 6:116, 1992.
76. Rosen, RC, Huestis, DW, and Corrigan, JJ: Acute leukemia and granulocyte transfusion: Fatal graft-versus-host disease following transfusion of cells obtained from normal donors. J Pediatr 93:268, 1981.
77. Siimes, MA, and Hoskimies, S: Chronic graft-versus-host disease after blood transfusions confirmed by incompatible HLA antigens in bone marrow. Lancet 1:42, 1982.
78. Button, LN, et al: The effects of irradiation on blood components. Transfusion 21:419, 1981.
79. Anderson, KC, et al: Variation in blood component irradiation practice: Implications for prevention of transfusion-associated graft-versus-host disease. Blood 77:2096, 1991.
80. Propper, RD, Button, LN, and Nathan, DG: New approach to transfusion management of thalassemia. Blood 55:55, 1980.
81. Opelz, G, et al: Effect of blood transfusions on subsequent kidney transplants. Transplant Proc 5:253, 1973.
82. Graves, A, et al: Relationship of transfusion and infection in a burn population. J Trauma 29:948, 1989.
83. Heal, JM, and Cohen, HJ: Do white cells in stored blood components reduce the likelihood of posttransfusion bacterial sepsis? Transfusion 31:581, 1991.
84. Blumberg, N, and Heal, JM: Effects of transfusion on immune function: Cancer recurrence and infection. Arch Pathol Lab Med 118:371, 1994.
85. Vamkas, EC: Perioperative blood transfusion and cancer recurrence: Meta-analysis for explanation. Transfusion 35:760, 1995.
86. Standards for Blood Banks and Transfusion Services, op cit, p 42, K2.200.
87. Judd, WJ: Investigation and management of immune hemolysis: Autoantibodies and drugs. In Wallace, ME, and Levitt, JS (eds): Current Applications and Interpretations of the Direct Antiglobulin Test. American Association of Blood Banks, 1988, Arlington, VA, p 47.
88. Laird-Fryer, B: Application and interpretation of direct antiglobulin test results as applied to healthy persons and selected patients. In Wallace, ME, and Levitt, JS (eds): Current Applications and Interpretations of the Direct Antiglobulin Test. American Association of Blood Banks, Arlington, VA, 1988, p 123.
89. Accreditation Requirement Manual of the American Association of Blood Banks, ed 6. Bethesda, MD, 1995, p 134.
90. Davenport, RD, op cit, p 18.
91. Sacher, RA, McPherson, RA, and Campos, JM: Transfusion medicine. In Sacher, RA (ed): Widmann's Clinical Interpretation of Laboratory Tests. FA Davis, Philadelphia, 1991, p 299.
92. Bacon, JM, and Young, IF: ABO incompatible blood transfusion. Pathology 21:181, 1989.
93. Mollison, PL, op cit, p. 540.
94. Ibid, p 541.
95. Vengelen-Tyler, V, op cit, p 554.
96. Mollison, PL, op cit, p 518.
97. Ibid, p 541.
98. Vengelen-Tyler, op cit, p 415.
99. Standards for Blood Banks and Transfusion Services, op cit, pp 32, 33, 50.
100. Code of Federal Regulations, Title 21, Part 606.170. Food and Drugs. US Government Printing Office, Washington, DC, 1995.

## BIBLIOGRAPHY

Ciavarella, D (ed): Symposium on leukocyte-depleted blood products. Transfus Med Rev (suppl 1)4, 1990.
Dutcher, JP (ed): Modern Transfusion Therapy. CRC Press, Boca Raton, FL 1990, Vols 1 and 2.
Miale, JB (ed): Laboratory Medicine: Hematology, ed 6. CV Mosby, St Louis, MO, 1982.
Mollison, PL, Engelfriet, CP, and Contreras, M: Blood Transfusion in Clinical Medicine, ed 9. Blackwell Scientific, Boston, 1993.
Petz, LD, and Swisher, SN (eds): Clinical Practice of Transfusion Medicine, ed 6. Churchill Livingstone, New York, 1989.
Popovsky, MA: Transfusion Reactions. American Association of Blood Banks, Bethesda, MD, 1996.
Rutnam, RC, and Miller, WV (eds): Transfusion Therapy: Principles and Procedures. Aspen Systems Corporation, Rockville, MD, 1981.
Turgeon, ML: Fundamentals of Immunohematology: Theory and Technique. Lea & Febiger, Philadelphia, 1989.

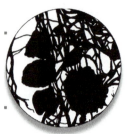

# CHAPTER **19**

# TRANSFUSION-TRANSMITTED VIRUSES

Herbert F. Polesky, MD

## OBJECTIVES

*On completion of this chapter, the learner should be able to:*

**1** List the criteria for donor selection.

**2** List the tests performed on donor blood.

**3** Describe procedures for look-back and recipient follow-up.

**4** Describe the nature of various hepatitis viruses and the diseases they cause.

**5** Discuss the current theories regarding transfusion-associated hepatitis.

**6** Characterize the human immunodeficiency virus.

**7** Discuss the nature of the acquired immunodeficiency syndrome and its relation to blood products.

**8** Name and describe the laboratory tests performed on donor blood to detect human immunodeficiency virus infection.

**9** Describe the dangers of cytomegalovirus and Epstein-Barr virus contamination of blood components.

**10** Discuss the various laboratory tests for the detection of viruses with reference to their sensitivity and accuracy.

## INTRODUCTION

The decision to transfuse must be based on weighing the therapeutic benefits against any potential risks to the recipient. Although small, the possibility of transmitting one or more viruses to a recipient continues to be one of the major complications of transfusion (Table 19–1). In spite of this possible risk, if the source of blood and blood components is limited to individuals who meet carefully chosen clinical criteria, the safety of giving blood greatly exceeds the harm of not transfusing.

## DONOR SELECTION

Ensuring that blood and its components are as safe as possible requires having systems in place to minimize the chance of an infectious unit getting into the inventory of components available for transfusion. The first and most important step in ensuring that transfused blood will not transmit a pathogenic virus is careful selection of the donor. Part of this selection process is the inducement used to motivate the donation. Before the availability of tests to detect hepatitis B surface antigen (HBsAg), it was clearly shown that eliminating donors motivated by cash payment significantly decreased the risk of hepatitis B virus (HBV) infection in recipients.[1] With the recognition that acquired immune deficiency syndrome (AIDS) could be transmitted by blood and in the absence of any serologic screening test, requesting potential donors to self-defer based on predonation information about activities that could increase their chance of being infected with human immunodeficiency virus (HIV) had a major impact on the safety of blood.[2]

Selection of blood and organ donors to prevent disease transmission includes evaluation of the individual's medical history. Potential donors who may need to be deferred include those who have:

1. Had an exposure in the past 12 months to individuals with a viral illness that could be transfusion-transmitted (TTV)
2. Been implicated as a donor in a case of TTV

**Table 19–1.** Risk of Transfusion-transmitted Viral Disease from Test Negative Units (1996 Estimates)

| Viral Agent | Risk per Million Units (+/− 95% CI) |
|---|---|
| HIV-1 | 2.03 (0.34–4.95) |
| HIV-2* | <0.0001 |
| HTLV-I | 1.56 (0.50–3.91) |
| HTLV-II | <0.001 |
| HBV | 15.9 (6.80–32.3) |
| HCV | 9.7 (3.47–35.7) |

**Source:** Schreiber, GB, et al: The risk of transfusion-transmitted viral infections. N Engl J Med 334:1685, 1996.
*CDC: MMWR CDC Surveill Summ 44:603, 1995.

3. A past history of hepatitis after age 10
4. Engaged in risk behaviors that are associated with infection by HIV
5. Signs and symptoms suggestive of hepatitis or AIDS
6. Received a blood transfusion, a coagulation concentrate, or human tissue graft in the past 12 months
7. Traveled to or been born in certain countries where HIV subtypes not detected by current tests are present
8. Been treated for or had syphilis in the past 12 months
9. Been incarcerated or institutionalized in the last year
10. Received pituitary growth hormone of human origin, had a dura mater transplant, or have a family history of Creutzfeldt-Jakob disease (CJD).

Direct questions about possible risk behaviors and review of past deferrals are essential parts of the donor evaluation process. The current edition of the American Association of Blood Banks (AABB) standards and memorandum from the Food and Drug Administration (FDA) should be consulted to determine specific criteria for disqualifying donors.[3,4]

The brief donor physical examination must include inspection of both arms for possible signs of intravenous drug use and evaluation of the donor's health status. During the donor interview, it is important to be sure the donor understands the importance of self-deferral if he or she might be putting a recipient at risk. A mechanism for privately indicating that the donated blood is not suitable for transfusion, confidential unit exclusion (CUE), or a call-back system is used by many collection facilities to allow self-deferral for those who feel compelled by peer pressure to donate.

## DONOR TESTING

Testing donor blood for specific and surrogate markers of TTV is another important step in ensuring the safety of a unit of blood and its component parts. Specific tests discussed in this chapter include HBsAg, antibody to hepatitis B core antigen (anti-HBc), antibody to hepatitis C virus (anti-HCV), antibodies to HIV (anti-HIV 1/2), HIV p24 antigen, antibody to human T-cell lymphotropic virus types I and II (anti-HTLV-I/II), and antibody to cytomegalovirus (anti-CMV). Alanine aminotransferase (ALT) levels on donors are used in some countries as a surrogate test for liver damage that might be associated with some forms of transmissible hepatitis. Testing by the polymerase chain reaction (PCR) to detect viral genome markers associated with HIV and HCV has been proposed for routine screening of donor blood.[5] In performing these tests, appropriate quality-control methods and documentation must be used. These tests are screening procedures that determine whether a unit can be released for transfusion.

Most blood banks require additional confirmation tests to establish the specificity of the result and to aid in counseling the donor. A system must be in place to ensure that only units from acceptable donors whose tests are negative for all mandated markers be released for transfusion.[4]

Although most of the tests are very sensitive (true-positive/true-positive + false-negative [TP/TP + FN]) and have good specificity (true-negative/true-negative + false-positive [TN/TN + FP]), none can detect all carriers of a virus. The efficacy of each test can be determined by calculating the predictive value of a positive or negative test. For example, in the case of HCV screening, if 95 of 100 reactive screening tests are confirmed as true-positives by supplementary testing, the predictive value of a positive test (chance that the donor is an HCV carrier) is 95/100 or 0.95 (95 percent). In the case of anti-HIV testing by enzyme-linked immunosorbent assay (ELISA), which is very sensitive (99.8 percent) and has good specificity (99.5 percent), most positive tests will be false-positives because the prevalence of the disease in the donor population is very low (0.01 percent). The ratio of true-positives to false-positives will be 1:50, and the predictive value of a positive test equal to 1.6 percent.[6]

## RECIPIENT FOLLOW-UP

Another way to increase the safety of the blood supply is to eliminate from the donor pool individuals who have negative tests but are implicated in TTV. The AABB Standards[3] require that the donor of blood or component given to a recipient who develops clinical or laboratory evidence of transfusion-associated hepatitis (TAH), infection with HIV, or HTLV-I/II infection must be permanently deferred if his or her unit was the only unit administered. Identifying recipients who have developed viral complications after transfusion is not easy. Many of the patients transfused at tertiary care facilities may not be followed up at the same hospital or by the physician who ordered the transfusions. Patients may die of complications of their primary illness during the incubation period of the TTV illness. In addition, the long incubation time between infection and disease recognition may result in failure to consider transfusion as the source of infection. This is a particular problem in the case of hepatitis C virus (HCV) infection, with which liver disease may not be recognized for 20 or more years after a transfusion event. Treating physicians should be reminded periodically of the need to suspect and report cases of TTV.

## LOOK-BACK (INVENTORY, DONOR, RECIPIENT)

When a donor is found to have a reactive test for a TTV or reports development of a transfusion-transmissible disease, it is important to determine the status of any units previously donated by the individual. If components are still in inventory, these must be quarantined and/or discarded.

As discussed previously, when a recipient develops a transfusion-associated viral infection, it is important to identify implicated donors. Because most patients get units from multiple donors and donors who give frequently are at a greater risk of being implicated, the decision to defer all or some of the donors is often difficult. A mathematical approach taking into account the total number of donors and other factors in the case allows assignment of a risk factor to each donor.[7,8] This is particularly useful when the same donor is implicated in more than one case.

If an individual who develops HIV infection (detected because of seroconversion on a subsequent donation or by clinical history) has been a blood donor, it is necessary to determine prior recipients of components from this donor and notify them of the risk of infection. The FDA has mandated that collection facilities have a process in place to notify consignees (hospitals or other facilities) to quarantine any previous units from the donor in inventory.[9] If the donor is confirmed as positive, the Health Care Financing Administration has issued regulations that require a transfusion service to take specific steps to identify and to notify prior recipients of the need for HIV testing and counseling.[10] Similar programs of directed look-back have been mandated for donors who seroconvert when tested for HCV, as well as recipients of blood since 1987 who may have been exposed to components at risk of transmitting HCV.[11] Look-back and recipient notification are also necessary when there is a possibility of HTLV-I/II infection in the donor.[3] It is also important to initiate tracing of other potential recipients when a patient with a transplant develops a viral disease that may have been transmitted by the tissue. In many cases organs and tissues from the donor have been used for multiple patients.

## TRANSFUSION-ASSOCIATED HEPATITIS

At least four viruses have been associated with hepatitis occurring after transfusion:

1. Hepatitis A virus (HAV)
2. Hepatitis B virus (HBV)
3. Hepatitis C virus (HCV)
4. Hepatitis D virus (HDV)

Several other viruses causing hepatitis have been identified. Hepatitis E virus has been identified as the cause of epidemic hepatitis associated with contaminated water. This agent, found in many underdeveloped areas of the world, has not been associated with transfusion-associated hepatitis (TAH).[12] The majority of TAH cases have been caused by either HBV or HCV; however, in a few cases, testing for hepatitis A to E viruses is negative, suggesting that non–A to E virus or viruses exist. Recently a hepatitis virus (HGV) and its strain variant, the GB agent (GBV-C), have been identified.[13] These agents are found in donors and are transmitted by transfusion, although it is unclear as to whether they result in non–A to E hepatitis.[14]

The frequency with which hepatitis occurs after transfusion (see Table 19–1) is difficult to establish. Many patients who develop TAH are asymptomatic and are likely to be recognized only if they are prospectively followed or if they are incidentally found to have an abnormal test such as an elevated ALT. It is estimated that less than one-third of patients with TAH develop clinical signs and symptoms of the disease, which can include jaundice, abdominal tenderness, nausea, vomiting, weakness and fatigue, dark urine, and acholic (light) stools. Before routine testing for HBsAg, the frequency of hepatitis following transfusion had been variously reported to be as high as 18 percent of recipients to as low as 0.1 percent.[15] Several factors influence the rates reported. These include geographic differences in the frequency of hepatitis carriers in the population, the tests used to screen the donor blood, and the adequacy of reporting of cases. Recent data suggest that less than 1 in 15,000 (0.008 percent) recipients of blood screened for HBsAg, anti-HBc, and anti-HCV will develop TAH.[16]

The severity of TAH is also quite variable. Most patients are asymptomatic. Of those who develop acute illness, most recover; however, about 1 to 2 percent of this group may die from the disease. Table 19–2 indicates that both mortality and morbidity are increased when hepatitis occurs in individuals over age 40. A very rare occurrence is the development of acute fulminant hepatitis. About 70 percent of these patients die during their acute illness. Another severe form of TAH is superinfection by HDV. This fulminant form of hepatitis is a special problem in chronic receivers of transfusion who are also carriers of HBV. Although about 10 percent of patients infected with HCV after transfusion are also carriers of HGV, there does not appear to be any worsening of the course of their HCV.[17]

Sequelae of TAH include the development of chronic active hepatitis (CAH) or chronic persistent hepatitis (CPH). These occur more commonly when there is infection with HCV and can, over many years, progress to cirrhosis and/or hepatocellular carcinoma.[1] The chronic liver problems can occur in asymptomatic patients as well as in those with acute disease that appears to resolve. In a large group of patients followed for 18 years after a diagnosis of non-A, non-B (NANB) TAH, there was no difference in mortality as compared with controls who were selected from transfused patients who did not develop TAH.[18] There were twice as many deaths from liver disease in the TAH group (3.2 percent) as compared with controls (1.5 percent), but in both groups 70 percent of the liver-related deaths occurred in patients with chronic alcoholism.[19]

Interferon therapy should be considered for selected patients with chronic hepatitis C. The decision to treat will depend on the age of the patient, whether he or she has a persistently abnormal ALT, a positive HCV RNA, and the histologic findings on a liver biopsy. In some cases with decompensated cirrhosis, liver transplantation should be considered.[19]

## CHARACTERISTICS OF HEPATITIS VIRUSES

### Hepatitis A Virus

The virus causing hepatitis A (HAV), or infectious hepatitis, is a 27-nm RNA virus in the family Picornaviridae. This virus does not have a lipid capsule. The virus replicates in infected liver cells and may be shed in the stools of acutely ill patients.[20] There is no chronic carrier state in humans. Infection is usually spread by the oral-fecal route. Outbreaks can usually be traced to contamination of food or water or person-to-person spread where hygiene is compromised (e.g., day-care centers).

Transfusion-transmitted HAV infection has occurred, but it is very rare.[21] An outbreak of HAV infection has been reported in recipients of solvent detergent-treated coagulation factor.[22] Infection by transfusion requires that the donor have viremia and the recipient be susceptible to the virus. Viremia, if it occurs, is usually brief and at the time of onset of acute illness. Antibodies to HAV regularly appear after infection (Fig. 19–1), and thus a large percentage of the population has immunity. The frequency with which anti-HAV is found increases with age and is inversely related to the level of sanitation.

Hepatitis A infection can be actively prevented by administration of an inactivated vaccine. Passive prophylaxis can be achieved by giving intramuscular immune serum globulin (ISG) after exposure (ideally within 2 weeks) or before travel to endemic areas. The rarity of infection after transfusion does not warrant routine testing of donors or the use of IG in recipients.

### Hepatitis B Virus

Hepatitis B virus (HBV) is in the family Hepadnaviridae. These deoxyribonucleic acid (DNA) viruses

**Table 19–2.** Epidemiologic and Clinical Characteristics of Patients with Hepatitis*

| Patient Characteristics | Hepatitis B (%) | | Hepatitis C/NANB (%) | |
| --- | --- | --- | --- | --- |
| | All Ages (3714 Patients) | Age > 40 yr (994 Patients) | All Ages (856 Patients) | Age > 40 yr (260 Patients) |
| Blood transfusion | 0.8 | 2.0 | 2.3 | 4.3 |
| Jaundice | 81.5 | 76.9 | 66.9 | 60.1 |
| Hospitalized | 28.2 | 36.0 | 32.9 | 41.7 |
| Died | 1.4 | 2.1 | 1.9 | 4.5 |

Data from Hepatitis Surveillance Report No. 56, Centers for Disease Control and Prevention, Atlanta, GA, 1996, pp 27–32.
*Centers for Disease Control and Prevention Viral Hepatitis Surveillance Program, 1993.
NANBH = non-A, non-B hepatitis.

Markers in HAV Infection

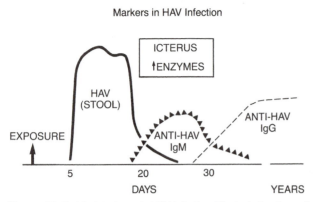

**Figure 19–1.** Markers in acute HAV infection. The typical pattern of HAV infection includes early shedding of virus in the stool, appearance of IgM anti-HAV, and immunity on recovery.

have been found in the Peking duck, woodchuck, and some ground squirrels.[23] In humans the virus is a 42-nm particle consisting of a 28-nm core with double-stranded circular DNA and DNA polymerase. The core is surrounded by a coat protein—HBsAg—which also occurs free in the serum as 22-nm spheres and 22- to 200-nm filaments (Fig. 19–2). Several polypeptides are associated with this virus, including the hepatitis B e antigen (HBeAg). The polypeptide making up the coat protein was described by Blumberg and coworkers[24] in 1965, when they discovered a precipitin line between serum from a multitransfused hemophiliac patient and a sample from an Australian aborigine. Initially this antigen was called Australia antigen (Au) and was thought to be associated with leukemia. Its subsequent association with hepatitis led to the terms hepatitis-associated antigen (HAA) and HBsAg.

When an individual is infected by HBV, several of the antigens and antibodies can be detected by serologic tests (Table 19–3). Usually the first marker of HBV to

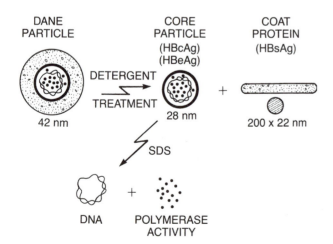

**Figure 19–2.** Diagram of the intact Dane particle (HB virion) as seen by electron microscopy. Detergent treatment disrupts the particle, releasing DNA (double- and single-stranded) and DNA polymerase activity.

appear is HBsAg (Fig. 19–3). This marker is also found in the 5 to 10 percent of infected patients who become chronic carriers of HBV. This polypeptide is very complex, and several antigenic subtypes have been defined. The subtypes occur with different frequencies in various parts of the world and can be helpful in epidemiologic studies. The subtypes are related to the viral strain, not the host. In addition, all strains have a common determinant.

Shortly after infection and before clinical signs and symptoms or biochemical changes in liver function occur, two other markers—HBeAg and anti-HBc—are usually detectable in serum from infected individuals. Initially the anti-HBc is an immunoglobulin M (IgM) antibody; however, as the infection progresses, IgG antibody appears. This latter antibody persists in persons who recover from HBV infection (Table 19–3). HBeAg usually disappears when the patient enters the convalescent phase. In individuals who do not develop immunity to HBV (usually persons infected vertically [transplacentally] or with immunosuppression), HBeAg, HBsAg, and anti-HBc can be present. In others with chronic infection (persistence of HBsAg for longer than 6 months), HBeAg is cleared, and anti-HBe is found. This group of patients, unlike those with HBsAg, are more likely to have normal liver function tests and have minimal histologic evidence of disease.

Immunity to HBV develops in most individuals who have acute or asymptomatic infection. As with HAV infection, immunity to HBV is specific; individuals do not usually have a second infection with HBV, although they are not immune to infection from another hepatitis virus, such as HAV, HCV, or rare variants of HBV.[25] Individuals who have recovered from HBV infection will have anti-HBs and/or anti-HBc in their sera. The frequency of these markers depends on the population studied.

Two approaches have been used to prevent HBV infection. An immune globulin prepared from persons with a high titer of anti-HBs called hepatitis B immune globulin (HBIG) has been used to provide passive immunity to healthcare workers and others who are exposed to patients with HBV infection. Extensive studies of HBIG after accidental needlestick exposure showed that its effect was to prolong the incubation and to reduce the severity of the disease. In 1982 a vaccine made from HBsAg isolated from human plasma was licensed.[26] This material has been shown to be very effective in preventing HBV infection in cases of accidental needlestick, in infants whose mothers are HBsAg, HBeAg-positive, and in homosexual men. About 90 to 95 percent of those given vaccine in the deltoid muscle (it is less effective if given in the gluteal muscle) develop anti-HBs, which can subsequently be detected for several years (note: anti-HBc does not develop as a response to vaccination). In 1987 a recombinant vaccine prepared from common baker's yeast (*Saccharomyces cerevisiae*) infected with a plasmid containing the gene for HBsAg was licensed.[27] This vaccine has minimal side effects and is recommended for all newborns

**Table 19–3.** Serologic Tests in the Diagnosis of Viral Hepatitis

| Hepatitis Agent | Diagnostic Test | | | | | | Interpretation |
|---|---|---|---|---|---|---|---|
| HAV | Total (IgM × IgG) and/or IgM anti-HAV | | | | | | Acute hepatitis A |
| | Total (IgM + IgG) only | | | | | | Previous hepatitis A |

| | | | *Anti-HBc* | | | | |
|---|---|---|---|---|---|---|---|
| | *HBsAg* | *Anti-HBs* | *Total* | *IgM* | *HBeAg* | *Anti-HBe* | |
| HBV | + | − | (+/−) | (+/−) | (+/−) | − | Early acute hepatitis B, before symptoms |
| | + | − | (+/−) | (+/−) | + | − | Acute hepatitis B with high infectivity |
| | − | − | ++ | + | (+/−) | + | Early convalescence from hepatitis B |
| | + | (−/+)* | + | − | + | − | Carrier state (infectious?) |
| | + | (−/+) | + | − | − | + | Chronic HBsAg carrier (years) |
| | − | + | + | − | − | (−/+) | Previous hepatitis B (recovered) |
| | − | + | − | − | − | − | Previous hepatitis B (recovered) or vaccination with HBsAg |
| | − | − | + | − | − | − | Previous hepatitis B or false-positive |

| | *Total (IgG)* | | *IgM†* | | | | |
|---|---|---|---|---|---|---|---|
| HDV | +/− low titer | | + low titer (rising) acute delta hepatitis | | | | Acute delta hepatitis |
| | + high titer (persistent) | | + high titer (persistent) | | | | Chronic delta hepatitis |
| | + | | − | | | | Previous delta hepatitis |

| | *ELISA* | | *RIBA* recombinat immuno blot assay | | | | |
|---|---|---|---|---|---|---|---|
| HCV | + | | + | | | | Acute or chronic |
| | + | | − or Ind‡ | | | | Possible false-positive or early infection |
| Non–A to E | None available | | Exclude HAV, HBV, HCV, HDV, HEV, CMV, EBV | | | | Acute and chronic |
| HGV | Anti-HGV and HGV RNA available for research use only! | | | | | | Questionable hepatitis |

(−/+) usually negative, but in some cases positive
†Not available commercially
‡Indeterminate

(note: it can be given in combination with other newborn vaccines), all healthcare workers and public safety personnel who are likely to be exposed to blood or body fluid, sexually active teenagers, and individuals who will be chronic transfusion recipients or treated with coagulation concentrates. Usually the vaccine is given in three doses. In individuals lacking immunity who are exposed to HBV (through needlestick or in the case of a newborn of an HBsAg positive mother), it is recommended that both HBIG and the vaccine be administered in different sites. Follow-up vaccine is given 1 month and 6 months later. No recommendations have been made regarding when and if persons should be given a booster of HBV vaccine. If a previously vaccinated individual accidentally exposed to HBV-positive blood or body fluid has no evidence of anti-HBs, he or she is probably protected; however, it is common to give a booster in this circumstance.

Prevention of HBV infection through universal vac-

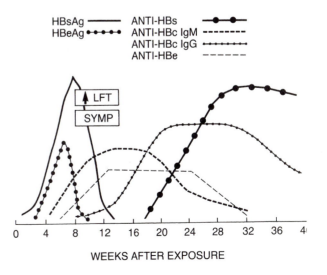

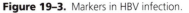

**Figure 19–3.** Markers in HBV infection.

cination is a goal of several current public health initiatives.[28] Because this virus is often sexually transmitted, early vaccination can eliminate the morbidity associated with acute disease, prevent long-term sequelae (in endemic areas, long-term HBV infection is associated with a high incidence of hepatoma [primary liver cell cancer]) and eliminate the risk of vertical transmission.

## Hepatitis D Virus

The delta agent, first described by Rizzetto[29] in 1977, is a particle about 35-nm in diameter. This ribonucleic acid (RNA) virus can infect and replicate, but it appears to require HBV virus to cause hepatocellular damage.[30] Infection with HDV can occur simultaneously with HBV infection (coinfection) or in a carrier of HBV (superinfection). This latter infection is of particular concern in chronically transfused patients who may have been previously exposed to HBV.

Most delta infections occur in drug addicts. At least one report documents the occurrence of HDV infection in a small percentage of patients with TAH.[31] The illness associated with delta infection is usually severe, and antibody to HDV occurs more frequently than expected in patients with fulminant hepatitis.

The diagnosis of delta hepatitis depends on finding antidelta in the serum or demonstrating the antigen (HDAg) by use of immunofluorescence on liver biopsy material. Individuals who recover after HDV infection usually become seronegative. Methods that prevent HBV infection should be effective in reducing the risk of HDV infection as well.

## Hepatitis C Virus

In 1989 after an extensive testing of a gene library with serum taken from a chimpanzee infected with non-A, non-B hepatitis (NANBH), a fusion peptide that represents a portion of the HCV genome was identified.[32] Further studies have revealed that HCV is an enveloped positive-strand RNA virus. The 9.6-kd genome codes for a polyprotein of about 3000 amino acids. A diagram of the proposed genome is shown in Figure 19–4. This virus, which has not been cultured, is classified in the family Flaviviridae. Direct intrahepatic inoculation of transcribed RNA from clones isolated from a patient have been found to be infectious and to cause disease in chimpanzees.[33] Using recombinant technology and peptide synthesis, several test systems were developed that made it possible to identify an antibody, anti-HCV, that is present in more than 80 percent of patients having transfusion-associated or community-acquired NANB hepatitis.[34-36] Studies with first-generation tests (anti-HCV 1.0) showed that some patients with TAH did not have detectable antibody for up to 30 weeks after onset of acute illness or a significant rise in ALT.[37] Modifications of the test systems (anti-HCV 2.0, anti-HCV 3.0) have increased the number of viral determinants detected, making it possible to detect seroconversion at about 70 to 80 days.[38] Routine screening

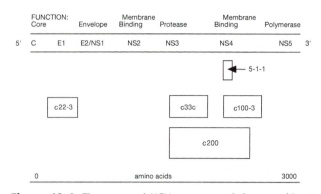

**Figure 19–4.** The proposed HCV genome and the recombinant proteins used to test for HCV. The HCV 1.0 test detects antibody to C100-3. The HCV 2.0 test detects antibody to C200 (including C33c and C100-c) and C22-3. Supplementary tests, such as the recombinant immunoblot assay (RIBA), detect antibody to specific gene products including C22-3, C33c, C100-3, and 5-1-1. (Adapted from package insert for the HCV 2.0 test. Ortho Diagnostic Systems, Raritan, NJ.)

of blood donors in the United States with anti-HCV 1.0 started in May of 1990. Second-generation reagents (anti-HCV 2.0) became routinely available in March of 1992. A modified second-generation test (anti-HCV 3.0) was introduced in June of 1996. A major problem associated with donor screening for anti-HCV 3.0 is the lack of a licensed confirmatory assay for further evaluation of reactive donors. Three supplemental tests are available. One is based on neutralization of antibody. Another, known as recombinant immunoblot assay (RIBA), is based on reaction of specific antibodies with antigen fixed to a membrane. Although these tests are helpful in providing counseling to donors, reentry of donors who may have a false-positive screening result can be done only if the confirmation and screening test are licensed to be used together. The most sensitive method for detecting HCV is PCR. Hepatitis C virus RNA may be detected 10 days after onset of infection.[38] Subtyping and quantitation of HCV RNA by PCR are used to predict and evaluate the response of infected individuals treated with antiviral drugs.[39]

Probably one or more other viral agents cause some of the clinical disease formerly called NANB hepatitis. About 10 to 15 percent of NANB hepatitis is negative for hepatitis A to E.[40] There is also evidence that these cases are not caused by HGV.

Prior to the routine screening of donated blood for anti-HCV in the United States, between 5 and 10 percent of NANB hepatitis was found in individuals with a history of blood transfusion, about 40 percent occurred in drug addicts, and less than 5 percent occurred because of a household or occupational exposure.[41] Thus, a large percentage of HCV cases seems to have no identified risk factor. Studies have shown that, unlike the situation with HBV and HIV, heterosexual and homosexual transmission of HCV is rare. One epidemiologic study has shown a correlation between HCV-positive NANB hepatitis and low socioeconomic status.[35]

The time from infection by HCV to onset of symptoms is quite variable. In transfusion recipients, HCV hepatitis has an incubation period of 40 to 60 days, which is considerably shorter than the 90 to 180 days associated with HBV infection. Many patients are asymptomatic and may be identified as having HCV infection only by the presence of mild liver function abnormalities, such as an elevated ALT, or because of a positive anti-HCV test. A major problem with HCV is that more than 80 percent of infected individuals may develop chronic liver disease. In some individuals this results in cirrhosis and/or hepatocellular carcinoma. The lag time between the acute infection and recognition of the chronic liver disease may be as long as 20 years. In selected patients with chronic liver disease caused by HCV infection, treatment with recombinant alpha interferon may induce both biochemical and histologic improvement.[19] Preliminary studies with combinations of interferon and other viricidal drugs such as ribavirin suggest that prolonged response (normal ALT and absence of HCV RNA) can be achieved in more than the 30 percent of patients who respond to a 1-year course of interferon alpha 2b alone. The effect of treatment following acute HCV hepatitis is also being evaluated.[19]

Before the development of a specific test for anti-HCV, surrogate test systems were introduced in an attempt to reduce this transfusion complication. Alanine aminotransferase/serum glutamate pyruvate transaminase (ALT/SGPT) and anti-HBc were mandated as screening tests for donors in 1986. In 1996 a National Institutes of Health (NIH) consensus panel recommended that ALT testing be discontinued.[42] Evaluation of recipients given anti-HCV-negative blood and components showed that eliminating donors with elevated ALT did not contribute to preventing non–A to E hepatitis. Alanine aminotransferase screening using higher cutoff values continues to meet European regulatory requirements for blood derivatives made from plasma used in further manufacturing.

Prospective studies also showed that NANB-TAH was also more likely to occur if the recipient was given anti-HBc-positive donor blood.[43] Epidemiologic studies show that up to one-third of patients with acute HCV infection have evidence of a prior HBV infection. Several studies of donors with anti-HCV have failed to show a correlation with this marker and the presence of anti-HBc. It has been suggested that anti-HBc may be present in some donors capable of transmitting HBV who have a negative test for HBsAg.[44] One effect of using surrogate tests is that many donors with a long history of safe donation become ineligible because of these tests. Anti-HBc is positive in a large number of healthy donors who have recovered from an asymptomatic infection with HBV. These donors are also anti-HBs-positive. Another group of donors are anti-HBc-positive with the screening test used, but when tested with another manufacturer's reagent they are usually nonreactive.[45]

## Hepatitis G Virus

Two groups of investigators have recently described hepatitis G viruses, HGBV-C and HGV.[46,47] Both are positive single-stranded RNA viruses. They are distantly related to the hepatitis C virus and are organized like Flaviviridae. Inasmuch as both isolates have a large percentage of their nucleotides and deduced amino acid sequences in common, they probably are the same virus.[40]

Based on a test for HGV RNA, it has been shown that HGV is present in 1.4 percent of randomly selected blood donors, can be transmitted by transfusion, and is not causally related to hepatitis.[17] In community-acquired non–A to E hepatitis (about 3 percent of hepatitis cases), less than 10 percent were HGV-positive.[48] It also appears that 10 to 20 percent of patients with HCV infection are also reactive for HGV. In these cases the HGV did not seem to affect the course of the HCV disease. Studies of intravenous (IV) drug users with an antibody to an envelope protein (E2) of HGV showed that more than 40 percent were reactive, though few had HGV RNA.[49] Based on the studies done through mid-1997, there is some question as to whether the designation of this agent as a hepatitis virus is premature.[14]

## THE HUMAN IMMUNODEFICIENCY VIRUS TYPES 1 AND 2

The HIV of the family Retroviridae is a lentivirus that causes chronic infection and grows slowly. The HIV virus is a 100-nm sphere with an envelope consisting of a lipid membrane through which glycoproteins protrude. The core of the virus contains the genomic RNA and reverse transcriptase (Fig. 19–5).[50] Various types of HIV virus, such as HIV-1 and HIV-2, have different envelope and core proteins (Table 19–4) and can produce different clinical and serologic responses in the host.

### Serologic Response to HIV Infection

Figure 19–6 is a schematic representation of the usual serologic findings in an individual who develops HIV-1 infection.[38,51] Shortly after exposure, the core protein, p24, has been found in some individuals. Within a few weeks antibodies to both envelope (gp41) and core (p24) proteins appear in almost all infected individuals. During the early phase of infection a nonspecific acute "viral illness" may occur. Once antibody appears, it seems to increase in titer even though the host is asymptomatic. During this phase of infection viral cultures of isolated lymphocytes demonstrate the presence of virus. As infection progresses, changes in

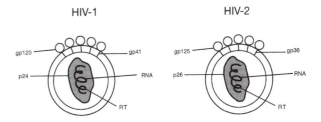

**Figure 19–5.** Schematic representation of the human immunodeficiency virus genomes, HIV-1 and HIV-2. RT = reverse transcriptase.

**Table 19–4.** Components of the HIV Virus

| Gene | Bands Observed | | Protein |
| | HIV-1 | HIV-2 | |
| --- | --- | --- | --- |
| Gag | p18, p24, p15 | p16, p26, p55 | Core |
| Pol | p31 | | Endonuclease |
| | p51, p65 | p68 | Reverse transcriptase |
| Env | gp41 | gp36 | Transmembrane protein |
| | gp120, gp160 | gp140, gp125 | Envelope unit |

p = protein; gp = glycoprotein (number indicates molecular weight).

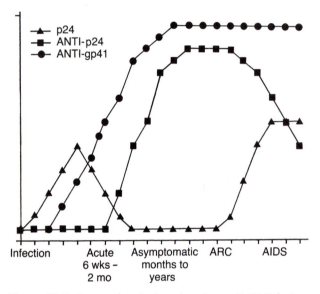

**Figure 19–6.** Pattern of serologic markers detected in HIV infection. ARC = AIDS-related complex.

the ratio of T-lymphocytes with specific surface markers, CD4 (helper) to CD8 (suppressor) cells, are observed. The number or percent of CD4+ T cells in an HIV- seropositive individual is useful as a guide to clinical and therapeutic management. Under classification guidelines issued by the Centers for Disease Control and Prevention (CDC), HIV-positive persons with fewer than 200 CD4+ T cells per microliter are considered as having AIDS in the absence of symptoms and/or opportunistic infection.[52] Depending on the host and other factors not yet identified, the type of symptoms and length of time before severe illness occurs vary. In patients with terminal illness, antibody to the core proteins may fall in titer and even disappear.

**Transfusion-associated AIDS (TAA)**

There is no question as to the infectivity of blood and components from individuals infected with HIV.[53] Recipients have developed AIDS after receiving a single contaminated unit of whole blood or any of its components. Derivatives from human blood such as albu-

min and immune globulins have not been reported to transmit HIV infection. Coagulation concentrates if heat-treated and/or purified by chemical or antibody methods have little risk of transmitting HIV infection when these products are made from donor plasma that has been screened for anti-HIV.

As of January 1, 1997, transfusion and tissue transplantation have been reported as the only identifiable risks in 8261 AIDS cases (1.4 percent of all cases) reported to the CDC.[54] In addition, 4674 cases have occurred in patients with hemophilia. Except for a very few cases (36 transfusion and 12 transplant recipients reported as of December 31, 1996), the transfusions were given before routine testing for anti-HIV was available. All cases reported from blood collected in the United States have been caused by HIV-1.

The mean incubation period between the time of transfusion and diagnosis of AIDS was estimated to be 4.5 years, with a range of 2 to 14 years.[55] This long incubation period and a high mortality among transfusion recipients (approximately 50 percent within 6 months) makes it difficult to determine the actual risk of TAA from blood and components collected prior to the availability of serologic tests for anti-HIV. The risk of infection from HIV-1 or HIV-2 and HIV p24 Ag–tested blood in the United States is less than 2 to 3 in a million units transfused.[16,38]

## HUMAN T-LYMPHOTROPIC VIRUS TYPES I AND II

Human T-cell lymphotropic virus type I is an oncogenic retrovirus that causes adult T-cell leukemia (ATL) and a neuromuscular wasting syndrome called HTLV-I-associated myelopathy (HAM), or tropical spastic parapersis (TSP). This RNA virus is endemic in southern Japan, the Caribbean basin, Brazil, and sub-Saharan Africa.[56] It has rarely been associated with transfusion-transmitted disease; however, seroconversion (development of anti-HTLV-I) has been observed in recipients of red blood cells less than 14 days old and platelets prepared from seropositive donors.[57]

HTLV-II is a retrovirus with a genome that has a high homology to HTLV-I. It was initially isolated from a patient with hairy cell leukemia. High rates of seropositivity have been observed in IV drug users. It is endemic in various populations, including some Native American groups. In some individuals HTLV-II has been associated with a HAM/TSP myelopathy.[56]

Routine testing of all donors was instituted because infection with HTLV-I or HTLV-II causes a lifelong carrier state and because of concerns related to the long incubation period of ATL and other HTLV-associated syndromes. There is a high percentage of crossreactivity between HTLV-I and HTLV-II in most screening tests. The FDA mandated that by February 1998 donor screening tests had to be specific for both viruses. In many countries HTLV screening tests are done only on first-time donors.[58]

## CYTOMEGALOVIRUS AND EPSTEIN-BARR VIRUS

Two viruses in the family Herpesviridae—cytomegalovirus (CMV) and Epstein-Barr virus (EBV)—can cause disease following transfusion.[59] These are DNA viruses that can persist in the host and cause latent infection. Antibodies to these agents are found with high frequency, indicating that they are prevalent in many populations (CMV, 40 to 90 percent; EBV, 90 percent). Inasmuch as a large percentage of recipients are carriers of these viruses, transmission by donor blood should not be a significant route of infection. This is true for EBV, which rarely causes infectious mononucleosis-like illness following cardiopulmonary bypass.

Transfusion-associated CMV infection is a problem, particularly in neonates and immunosuppressed patients. Convincing evidence exists that low-birth-weight infants (less than 1250 g) born to anti-CMV-negative women have less morbidity and mortality when they receive transfusions of blood and components lacking anti-CMV or those from which white cells have been removed (e.g., filtered, freeze thawing, washing).[60] The effects of CMV on transplant recipients is less clear. In some patients immunosuppression can reactivate latent infection; in others the organ is the source of infection; and in others transfusion plays a role. Cytomegalovirus infection is a serious complication in patients given an allogeneic bone marrow transplant.

Prevention of CMV complications requires testing of donors or filtration of cellular components. Testing of potentially at-risk patients is also useful. If the mother of a low-birth-weight infant has anti-CMV, it is not worthwhile to give blood tested for anti-CMV. The use of tested blood or leuko-reduced blood in transplant patients depends on the protocol and the CMV status of the recipient.[61]

## TESTING FOR VIRAL MARKERS

Several test systems are available to detect the presence of markers of viral infection. Each test varies in sensitivity and specificity and requires careful quality control. A reactive screening test on a sample from a blood donor requires quarantine of the blood and components pending further investigation. Confirmation tests are important to determine how to counsel a healthy blood donor and whether or not it might be necessary to initiate notification of prior recipients. The general scheme shown in Figure 19–7 for anti-HIV testing can be applied to other markers as well. The general principles of the tests are shown in Table 19–5 and Table 19–6. In almost all systems detection is based on a labeled antibody or antigen. In the case of HBV, HCV, and HIV, although the tests are very sensitive, not all infectious units are detectable. It is also possible that an infectious individual early in the incubation phase (window period) of the disease may not have de-

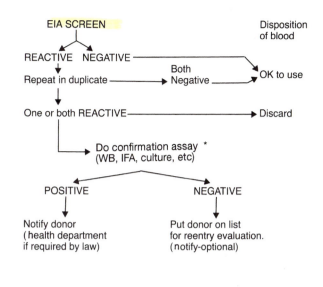

* If the screening test is a combination (anti-HIV-1/HIV-2) additional testing with anti-HIV-1 and anti-HIV-2 reagents is indicated.

**Figure 19–7.** 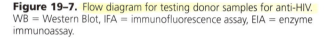 Flow diagram for testing donor samples for anti-HIV. WB = Western Blot, IFA = immunofluorescence assay, EIA = enzyme immunoassay.

tectable antibody or antigen when tested (see Figures 19–3 and 19–6).

### Testing for HIV

The enzyme immunoassay (EIA) systems developed to screen blood donors (see Table 19–6) for anti-HIV have been based on indirect detection of antibody similar to the antihuman globulin method for detecting red cell antibodies. Material containing the appropriate viral epitopes is coated onto a solid phase, such as a bead or microtiter well. First-generation tests used antigen derived from viral cultures by disruption of the infected host cell. This material was then purified and treated to eliminate the risk of infectivity. Subsequent tests (second and third generation) with increased sensitivity and specificity use blends of recombinant material and/or synthetic polypeptides containing the desired epitopes. Reagents that detect donor antibody bound to the antigen on the solid phase are polyspecific or monospecific antihuman immunoglobulin (goat, murine monoclonal) labeled with enzyme (horseradish peroxidase, alkaline phosphatase). A chromogenic substrate is used to obtain a colorimetric reaction that can be read in a spectrophotometer. Most tests also require a blocking agent to be used as part of the sample diluent. These include combinations of various animal proteins, powdered milk, and proprietary substances, which are intended to prevent nonspecific attachment of immunoglobulin in the unknown to the coated solid phase. A stop solution (1 $N$ sulfuric acid, sodium hydroxide) is usually used to terminate the color development after a specified time interval. Also available are direct testing systems, which

**Table 19–5.** Tests for Viral Hepatitis Markers: Principles and Calculations

| Principle | Method | | | | Calculation RIA/EIA | Test For |
|---|---|---|---|---|---|---|
| *Direct* | Antibody-coated solid phase | + Unknown | + labeled antibody | − ↑cpm ↑OD | A/A | HBsAg HBeAg |
| (Sandwich) | Antigen-coated solid phase | + Unknown | + labeled antigen | − ↑cpm ↑ OD | A/A | Anti-HBs |
| (Sandwich) | Antigen-coated solid phase | + Unknown | + labeled anti-IgG | − ↑OD | NA/A | Anti-HCV |
| Antigen capture | Anti-IgM–coated solid phase | + Unknown (specific Aby-IgM class) | + Antigen + labeled antibody | − ↑cpm ↑OD | B/B | IgM: Anti-HAV Anti-HBc |
| *Indirect* | Antigen-coated solid phase | + Unknown + labeled antibody | | − ↓cpm ↓OD | C/C | Anti-HBc Anti-HAV |
| Competitive | Antibody-coated solid phase | + Unknown + antigen | + labeled antibody | − ↓cpm ↓OD | C/C | Anti-HBe |

Method of calculating negative cutoff: RIA tests
A. Factor (e.g., 2.1) × mean control cpm
B. Mean negative control cpm + 0.1 (mean positive control cpm)
C. $\dfrac{\text{Mean negative control cpm} + \text{mean positive control cpm}}{2}$

EIA Tests
A. Factor (e.g., .05) + mean negative control optical density (OD)
B. (Factor × mean positive control OD) + mean negative control OD
C. Factor (mean negative control OD) + factor (mean positive control OD)

NA = Not available.
cpm = Counts per minute.

**Table 19–6.** Principles of Test Methods—Detection of HIV Antibodies and Antigens

| Enzyme-labeled Antiglobulin | Western Blot | Antigen Capture |
|---|---|---|
| Antigen on solid phase* | Separate viral lysate in SDS—PAGE Transblot to a membrane | Anti-HIV on solid phase |
| Diluted unknown serum | Incubate with unknown serum | Unknown sample Antibody to specific HIV protein (probe) |
| Labeled antihuman Ig or antigen Substrate-chromogen Measure color (proportional to amount of anti-HIV) | Labeled antihuman Ig Substrate-chromogen Evaluate bands present | Labeled antiprobe Ig Substrate-chromogen Measure color (proportional to amount of captured antigen) |

*Viral lysate, recombinant, or synthetic peptide.

depend on antibody in the unknown attaching to antigen on the solid phase. Detection of bound antibody depends on binding of labeled purified antigen. These methods are often referred to as *sandwich systems.*

Because the number of false-positive test results compared with true-positives is high when screening normal donors with a low prevalence of disease and because there can be lot-to-lot variation in the specificity of the test reagents, protocols have been developed by the FDA to allow reentry of donors whose subsequent anti-HIV or HBsAg tests are nonreactive.[62] These reentry schemes require a defined interval between the reactive test and the subsequent test. This is based on the observation that seroconverters whose initial test was weakly positive will show increased reactivity over time. Other requirements for reentry include use of multiple reagents and negative results with specified confirmation assays.

## CONFIRMATION ASSAYS: WESTERN BLOTTING, RECOMBINANT IMMUNOBLOT ASSAY, IMMUNOFLUORESCENCE, NEUTRALIZATION, AND POLYMERASE CHAIN REACTION

Transblotting was first described by E. M. Southern (hence the term *Southern blots*) as a method to study DNA. It is referred to as Western blotting (WB) when applied to proteins. This technique is useful in detecting the presence of anti-HIV and in determining with which viral components the antibodies react. This test is both sensitive and specific, but its technical complexity precludes using it as a screening test.

The various components of a purified, heat-treated, viral lysate dissolved in sodium dodecyl sulfate (SDS) are separated electrophoretically on polyacrylamide gel

(PAGE). The viral components are distributed according to their molecular weight. The proteins are then transferred (transblotted) from the gel to a membrane. The membrane is divided into multiple strips. These are incubated with blocking agents before the sample is added. Incubation and rotation of the unknown with the strip is followed by washing. If antibodies in the unknown have reacted with the viral proteins, the bands will be detected by the indicator system (i.e., biotinylated antihuman IgG). After incubation and washing, avidin-labeled alkaline phosphatase is added. This is followed by a nitro blue tetrazolium, 5-bromo-4-chloro-3-iodophosphate substrate/stain. Known anti-HIV-positive and anti-HIV/negative samples must be run with each membrane. It is also useful to run molecular weight standards when doing electrophoresis and transblotting. Interpretation of WB results depends on the bands detected (Table 19–4).[63] Most patients with AIDS and donors with anti-HIV show multiple bands, including p17/18, p24, p31, gp41, p65, gp120, and gp160. In some cases very few bands are seen. Usually these blots are called indeterminate, and repeat samples are requested. In healthy donors without other risk factors, indeterminate blots that do not change over 6 months are considered false-positive, although the individual is not eligible as a donor.

Recombinant immunoblot assay (RIBA) is a confirmation system that uses recombinant proteins placed on a membrane in strips. The sample containing antibody is incubated with the membrane. If antibody to the specific protein is present, it will bind to the membrane. The presence of antibody is detected using a labeled antiglobulin that gives a colorimetric reaction. A weak or strong positive control on the membrane makes it possible to grade the intensity of the bound antibody. The pattern of reactivity indicates the specificity of the antibodies in the sample.

Immunofluorescence assays (IFAs), based on the reaction of unknown sera with cells infected with HIV, have been shown to have good sensitivity and specificity. Reactive samples are detected by using a fluorescent-labeled antibody, which gives a distinct pattern when anti-HIV reacts with the cells on a coated slide.

Neutralization assays are used to confirm the presence of antigen (HBsAg or HIV-1 p24) when the screening test is repeatedly reactive. The procedure requires incubation of the donor or patient sample with specific antibody before testing for antigen. If antigen is present, antibody-antigen complexes will form and the reaction in the antigen test will become nonreactive or significantly weaker. Controls to correct for dilution of the sample with the neutralizing antibody must be included in the test run.

The most sensitive assay for the detection of HIV infection is the polymerase chain reaction (PCR).[64] This test depends on the amplification of HIV integrated in the DNA of infected cells. Polymerase chain reaction systems require several cycles with a thermostable polymerase at carefully controlled temperatures and need specific primers present as templates for the amplified DNA. The detection of the amplification product is by a labeled probe in an immunoblot assay. This method, though extremely sensitive, requires very careful control to ensure that positive reactions are specific. Because PCR detects HIV infection before tests for antigen or antibody and thus further shortens the window period (time between infection and detection), PCR screening tests for blood donors are being developed. Although routine PCR tests may have only a small impact on blood safety with regard to HIV, the potential for closing the window period for HCV infection is significant.

Implementation of routine PCR testing of individual donors will require development of automated systems that will eliminate the time-consuming steps necessary to extract DNA and to prepare samples. Several protocols based on testing pooled donor samples have been evaluated. Various matrices are used so that, if a pool is positive, only a small number of samples will need further testing. Because several outbreaks of HCV infection have been reported after the administration of intravenous immunoglobulin (IVIG), the FDA has recommended that pools of donors used and/or the final product be tested for HCV RNA by PCR.

## VIRAL INACTIVATION

Numerous strategies to modify blood and components have the potential to provide increased safety of blood and components. An unexpected benefit of the heating of albumin to 60°C for stabilizing it during storage was the elimination of the risk of hepatitis.[65] Wet heating combined with monoclonal antibody purification significantly reduces the risk of coagulation concentrates that are made from large pools of donor plasma.[66] Solvent detergent treatment of plasma destroys enveloped viruses.[67] This technique can be applied to fresh frozen plasma with minimal loss of coagulation factors. Several methods are under investigation to apply combinations of chemicals, physical treatments such as ultraviolet (UV) irradiation and/or filtration to inactivate or to remove viral and other infectious agents from cellular components.[68] These methods combined with hemoglobin substitutes, components produced by recombinant technologies, more sensitive and specific donor tests, and the judicious use of blood and components can eliminate many of the risks of transfusion-transmitted viruses.

## SUMMARY CHART: IMPORTANT POINTS TO REMEMBER (MT/MLT)

- The first and most important step in ensuring that transfused blood will not transmit a pathogenic virus is careful selection of the donor.
- *Look-back* is a process mandated by the FDA that directs collection facilities to notify donors who test positive for viral markers and to notify prior recipients of components of the possibility of infection, as well as quarantining or discarding current components in inventory.
- Hepatitis A virus is usually spread by the oral-fecal route and in communities where hygiene is compromised.
- On infection with hepatitis B virus, the first serologic marker to appear is HBsAg, followed by HBeAg and IgM anti-HBc within the first few weeks of exposure.
- HBIG is an immune globulin prepared from persons with a high titer of anti-HBs and is used to provide passive immunity to healthcare workers and others who are exposed to patients with HBV infection.
- Hepatitis D virus infection is common among drug addicts and can occur simultaneously with HBV infection; diagnosis depends on finding anti-delta in the serum or demonstrating the antigen (HDAg) by use of immunofluorescence on liver biopsy material.
- In transfusion recipients, hepatitis C virus has an incubation period of 40 to 60 days; the most sensitive test for detecting HCV is the polymerase chain reaction (PCR), in which HCV RNA can be detected 10 days after onset of infection.
- Diagnosis of HIV-1 and HIV-2 infection is dependent on the presence of antibodies to both envelope and core proteins; HIV-positive persons with less than 200 CD4+ T cells per $\mu$L are considered as having AIDS in the absence of symptoms.
- Transfusion-associated CMV infection is a concern for low-birth-weight neonates born to anti-CMV-negative women and immunocompromised patients.
- The Western blot confirmation test detects the presence of anti-HIV and determines with which viral proteins the antibodies react.
- The polymerase chain reaction can detect HIV infection before tests for antigen or antibody and therefore shortens the window period.

## REVIEW QUESTIONS

1. Which of the following has the greatest impact in ensuring that transfused blood is safe?
   A. Using the most sensitive testing techniques available
   B. Using the most specific testing techniques available
   C. Careful selection of blood donors
   D. Careful selection of the recipient

2. The oral-fecal route is common in transmission of which of these hepatitis viruses?
   A. HAV
   B. HBV
   C. HDV
   D. HCV

3. Which of the following is the component of choice for a low-birth-weight infant with a hemoglobin of 8 g/dL if the mother is anti-CMV negative?
   A. Whole blood from a donor with anti-CMV
   B. Red cells from a donor who is anti-CMV negative
   C. Leuko-reduced platelets
   D. Solvent detergent-treated plasma

4. Testing donors for anti-HBc is thought to prevent transmission of which of the following infections?
   A. Hepatitis A
   B. Hepatitis B
   C. Hepatitis C
   D. Non–A to E hepatitis

5. Which of the following tests is useful to confirm that a patient or donor is infected with HCV?
   A. ALT + anti-HBc
   B. Anti-HIV 1/2
   C. Lymph node biopsy
   D. RIBA (recombinant immunoblot assay)

6. The test for HIV p24 antigen is used for which of the following reasons?
   A. It identifies donors with late-stage HIV who lack antibody.
   B. It confirms the presence of anti-HIV in asymptomatic HIV-infected donors.
   C. It is positive in recently HIV-infected individuals before current tests detect the presence of antibody.
   D. It closes the HIV window phase better than tests based on PCR.

7. When a donor sample is found to be positive for anti-HCV, which of the following steps should be taken first?
   A. Notify all recipients of previous components from this donor.
   B. Check current inventory for previous components from this donor.

C. Advise the donor to have a liver biopsy.
D. Notify public health officials of the test result.

8. Patients developing non–A to E hepatitis after transfusion usually have which of the following?
   A. Fulminant hepatitis
   B. A positive test for one of the HGV agents
   C. Normal liver function tests
   D. No clear evidence for an etiologic agent

## ANSWERS TO REVIEW QUESTIONS

1. C (p 407)

2. A (p 409)

3. B (p 415)

4. B (p 413)

5. D (p 412)

6. C (p 417)

7. B (p 408)

8. D (p 409)

## REFERENCES

1. Alter, HJ: You'll wonder where the yellow went: A 15-year retrospective of post transfusion hepatitis. In Moore, SB (ed): Transfusion Transmitted Viral Disease. American Association of Blood Banks, Arlington, VA, 1987, pp 53–86.
2. Pindyk, J, et al: Measures to decrease the risk of acquired immunodeficiency syndrome transmission by blood transfusion: Evidence of volunteer blood donor cooperation. Transfusion 25:3, 1985.
3. Klein, HG (ed): Standards for Blood Bank and Transfusion Services, ed 18. American Association of Blood Banks, Bethesda, MD, 1997.
4. Code of Federal Regulations: Current edition. 21 Food and Drugs, parts 600–700. Washington, DC: U.S. Government Printing Office.
5. Hewlett, IK, and Epstein, JS: Food and Drug Administration conference on the feasibility of genetic technology to close the HIV window in donor screening. Transfusion 37:346, 1997.
6. Galen, RS, and Gambino, SR: Beyond Normality: The Predictive Value of and Efficiency of Medical Diagnosis. John Wiley & Sons, New York, 1975.
7. Hanson, M, and Polesky, HF: A method for calculating the risk of donors implicated in transfusion-associated hepatitis. Proceedings International Hepatitis Workshop, 1982, pp 99–100.
8. Ladd, DJ, and Hillis, A: A new method for evaluating the hepatitis risk of the multiply-implicated donor. Transfusion 24:80, 1984.
9. 21 CFR Parts 606 and 610; Current good manufacturing practices for blood and blood components. Notification of consignees receiving blood and blood components at increased risk for transmitting HIV infection. Final Rule. Federal Register 61, 175: 47413, 1996 (Sep 9).
10. 42 CFR Parts 482 Medicare and Medicaid programs; hospital standards for potentially infectious blood and blood products. Final Rule. Federal Register 61, 175:47423, 1996 (Sep 9).
11. Guidance for industry: Current good manufacturing practice for blood and blood components: 1. Quarantine and disposition of units from prior collections from donors with repeatedly reactive screening tests for antibody to hepatitis C virus (anti-HCV); 2. Supplemental testing and the notification of consignees and blood recipients of donor test results for anti-HCV. FDA, CBER, Rockville, MD, Sept 23, 1998.
12. Chauhan, A, et al: Hepatitis E virus transmission to a volunteer. Lancet 341:149, 1993.
13. Mikakawa, Y, and Mayumi, M: Hepatitis G virus—a true hepatitis virus or an accidental tourist? N Engl J Med 336:795, 1997.
14. Alter, HJ: G-pers creepers, where'd you get those papers? A reassessment of the literature on the hepatitis G virus. Transfusion 37:569, 1997.
15. Polesky, HF, and Hanson, M: Transfusion-associated hepatitis: A dilemma. Lab Med 14:717, 1983.
16. Schreiber, GB, et al: The risk of transfusion-transmitted viral infections. N Engl J Med 334:1685, 1996.
17. Alter, HJ, et al: The incidence of transfusion-associated hepatitis G virus infection and its relation to liver disease. N Engl J Med 336:747, 1997.
18. Seeef, LB, et al: Long-term mortality after transfusion-associated non-A, non-B hepatitis. N Engl J Med 327:1906, 1992.
19. NIH Consensus Statement: Management of Hepatitis C. March 27, 1997.
20. Aach, RD: Primary hepatic viruses: Hepatitis A, hepatitis B, delta hepatitis and non-A, non-B hepatitis. In Insalaco, SJ, and Menitove, JE (eds): Transfusion-transmitted Viruses: Epidemiology and Pathology. American Association of Blood Banks, Arlington, VA, 1987, pp 17–40.
21. Hollinger, FB, et al: Posttransfusion hepatitis type A. JAMA 250:2313, 1983.
22. Centers for Disease Control: Hepatitis A among persons with hemophilia who received clotting factor concentrates: United States, September–December 1995. MMWR 45:29, 1996.
23. Mason, WS, Seal, G, Summers, J: Virus of Peking ducks with structural and biological relatedness to human hepatitis B virus. J Virol 36:829, 1980.
24. Blumberg, BS, Alter, HJ, and Visnich, S: A "new" antigen in leukemia sera. JAMA 191:541, 1965.
25. Carmen, WF, Korula, J, and Wallace, L: Fulminant reactivation of hepatitis B due to envelop protein mutant that escaped detection by monoclonal HBsAg ELISA. Lancet 345:1406, 1995.
26. Szmuness, W, et al: Hepatitis B vaccine: Demonstration of efficacy in a controlled clinical trial in a high risk population in the United States. N Engl J Med 303:833, 1980.
27. Stevens, CE, et al: Yeast-recombinant hepatitis B vaccine: Efficacy with hepatitis B immune globulin in prevention of perinatal hepatitis B virus transmission. JAMA 257:2612, 1987.
28. Centers for Disease Control: Immunization Practices Advisory Committee recommendations for hepatitis B virus: A comprehensive strategy for eliminating transmission in the United States through universal childhood vaccination. MMWR 40:11, 1991.
29. Rizzetto, M: Biology and characterization of the delta agent. In Szmuness, W, Alter, H, and Maynard, J (eds): Viral Hepatitis 1981 International Symposium. Franklin Institute, Philadelphia, 1982, pp 355–362.
30. Craig, JR: Hepatitis delta virus: No longer a defective virus. Am J Clin Pathol 98:552, 1992.
31. Rosina, F, Saracco, G, and Rizzetto, M: Risk of post transfusion infection with the hepatitis delta virus: A multi-center study. N Engl J Med 312:1488, 1985.
32. Choo, Q-L, et al: Isolation of a clone derived from blood-borne non-A, non-B viral hepatitis genome. Science 244:359, 1989.
33. Kolykhalov, AA, et al: Transmission of hepatitis C by intrahepatic inoculation with transcribed RNA. Science 277:570, 1997.
34. Kuo, G, et al: An assay for circulating antibodies to a major etiologic virus of human non-A, non-B hepatitis. Science 244:363, 1989.
35. Alter, MJ, et al: The natural history of community-acquired hepatitis C in the United States. N Engl J Med 327:1899, 1992.
36. Aach, RD, et al: Hepatitis C virus infection in post-transfusion hepatitis: An analysis with first- and second-generation assays. N Engl J Med 325:1325, 1991.
37. Esteban, JI, et al: Evaluation of antibodies to hepatitis C virus in a study of transfusion-associated hepatitis. N Engl J Med 323:1107, 1990.

38. Kleinman, S, et al: The incidence/window period model and its use to assess the risk of transfusion-transmitted human immunodeficiency virus and hepatitis C virus infection. Transfus Med Rev 11:155, 1997.

39. Isopet, J, et al: Baseline level and early suppression of serum HCV RNA for predicting sustained complete response to alpha-interferon therapy. J Med Virol 54:86–91, 1998.

40. Alter, MJ, et al: Acute non-A-E hepatitis in the United States and the role of hepatitis G virus infection. N Engl J Med 336:741, 1997.

41. Alter, MJ, et al: Risk factors for acute non-A, non-B hepatitis in the United States and association with hepatitis C virus infection. JAMA 264:2231, 1990.

42. NIH Consensus Development Panel on Infectious Disease Testing for Blood Transfusions: Infectious disease testing for blood transfusions. JAMA 274:1374, 1995.

43. Stevens, CE, et al: Hepatitis B antibody in blood donors and occurrence of non-A, non-B hepatitis in transfusion reagents: An analysis of the transfusion-transmitted viruses study. Ann Intern Med 104:488, 1984.

44. Hoofnagle, JH: Posttransfusion hepatitis B. Transfusion 30:384, 1990.

45. Hanson, MR, and Polesky, HF: Evaluation of routine anti-HBc screening of volunteer blood donors: A questionable surrogate test for non-A, non-B hepatitis. Transfusion 27:107, 1987.

46. Linnen, J, et al: Molecular cloning and disease association of hepatitis G virus: A transfusion-transmissible agent. Science 271:505, 1996.

47. Leary, TP, et al: Sequence and genomic organization of GBV-C: A novel member of the Flaviviridae associated with human non-A-E hepatitis. J Med Virol 48:60, 1996.

48. Alter, HJ: The cloning and clinical implications of HGV and HGBV-C. N Engl J Med 334:1536, 1996.

49. Tacke, M, et al: Detection of antibodies to a putative hepatitis G virus envelope protein. Lancet 349:318, 1997.

50. Smith, TF: Structure, classification and replication of viruses. In Insalaco, SJ, and Menitove, JE (eds): Transfusion-transmitted Viruses: Epidemiology and Pathology. American Association of Blood Banks, Arlington, VA, 1987, pp 1–16.

51. Allain, JP, et al: Serologic markers in early stages of human immunodeficiency virus infection in haemophiliacs. Lancet 2:1233, 1986.

52. Centers for Disease Control and Prevention: 1993 revised classification system for HIV infection and expanded surveillance case definition for AIDS among adolescents and adults. MMWR 41/RR-17: 1–19, Dec 18, 1992.

53. Busch, MP: Retroviruses and blood transfusions: The lessons learned and the challenge yet ahead. In Nance, SJ (ed): Blood Safety: Current Challenges. American Association of Blood Banks, Bethesda, MD, 1992, pp 1–44.

54. Centers for Disease Control and Prevention: HIV/AIDS surveillance report, March 1997:1–23.

55. Lui, KJ, et al: A model-based approach for estimating the mean incubation period of transfusion-associated acquired immunodeficiency syndrome. Proc Natl Acad Sci 83:3051, 1987.

56. Vrielink, H, Zaaijer, HL, and Reesink, HW: The clinical relevance of HTLV type I and II in transfusion medicine. Transfus Med Rev 11:173, 1997.

57. Okachi, K, Sato, H, and Himuma, Y: A retrospective study in transmission of adult T cell leukemia virus by blood transfusion: Sero-conversion in recipients. Vox Sang 46:245, 1984.

58. Whyte, GS: Is screening of Australian blood donors for HTLV-I necessary? Med J Aust 166:478, 1997.

59. Tegtmeier, GE: The role of blood transfusion in the transmission of herpes viruses. In Insalaco, SJ, and Menitove, JE (eds): Transfusion-transmitted Viruses: Epidemiology and Pathology. American Association of Blood Banks, Arlington, VA, 1987, pp 41–68.

60. Eisenfeld, L, Silver, H, and McLaughlin, J: Prevention of transfusion-associated cytomegalovirus infection in neonatal patients by removal of white cells from blood. Transfusion 32:205, 1992.

61. Lehman, CM, Becker, JL, and Wilkinson, DS: Red cells and platelets. Clin Lab Med 16:781, 1996.

62. Zoon, KC: Revised Recommendations for Prevention of Human Immunodeficiency Virus (HIV) Transmission by Blood and Blood Products. Food and Drug Administration, Center for Biologics Evaluation and Research, Bethesda, MD, 1–21, April 23, 1992.

63. Centers for Disease Control: Interpretive criteria used to report Western blot results for HIV-1-antibody testing—United States. MMWR 40:692–695, 1991.

64. Jackson, JB: The polymerase chain reaction in transfusion medicine. Transfusion 30:51–57, 1990.

65. Kendrick, DB: Blood Program in World War II. Washington, DC, Office of Surgeon General, Department of the Army, 1964.

66. Kasper, CK, and Lusher, JM: Recent evolution of clotting factor concentrates for hemophilia A and B. Transfusion 33:422, 1993.

67. Horowitz, B, et al. Solvent/detergent-treated plasma: A virus-inactivated substitute for fresh frozen plasma. Blood 79:826, 1990.

68. Corash, L: Virus inactivation in cellular components. Vox Sang (suppl 3) 70:9, 1996.

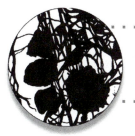

CHAPTER **20**

# HEMOLYTIC DISEASE OF THE NEWBORN AND FETUS

Melanie S. Kennedy, MD, and
Abdul Waheed, MS, MT(ASCP)SBB

## OBJECTIVES

*On completion of this chapter, the learner should be able to:*

1 State the definition and characteristics of hemolytic disease of the newborn.

2 Describe the role of the technologist in the diagnosis and clinical management of hemolytic disease of the newborn.

3 Compare and contrast ABO versus Rh hemolytic disease of the newborn in terms of:

  a Pathogenesis

  b Incidence

  c Blood types of mother and baby

  d Severity of disease

  e Laboratory data: anemia, direct antiglobulin test, bilirubin

  f Prevention and treatment

4 Define Rh immune globulin and describe its function.

5 Identify the requirements that must be met before a woman can receive Rh immune globulin.

6 List the tests used for detection of fetomaternal hemorrhage.

7 Outline the protocol for testing of maternal and cord blood in cases of suspected hemolytic disease of the newborn.

8 Given maternal and infant ABO blood group phenotypes, state the possible ABO donor blood group(s) you would select for an exchange transfusion. Be specific as to donor blood groups for both the plasma and red blood cells.

9 State the blood components and the maximum age of the donor unit preferred for intrauterine or exchange transfusions.

10 State with whom (mother and child) the cross-match for a neonate must always be compatible.

Hemolytic disease of the newborn and fetus (HDN) is the destruction of the red blood cells (RBCs) of the fetus and neonate by antibodies produced by the mother. The mother can be stimulated to form the antibodies by previous pregnancy or transfusion; a small number occur during the pregnancy itself. Previously, about 95 percent of the cases were caused by antibodies in the mother directed against the Rh antigen D or $Rh_0$. The incidence of the disease caused by anti-D has steadily decreased since 1968 with the introduction of Rh immune globulin (RhIg). Currently, $Rh_0(D)$ incompatibility is still the most common, although other RBC incompatibilities are increasing in incidence at referral centers.[1] Because $Rh_0(D)$ incompatibility was the major concern for many years, the diagnosis and treatment of HDN caused by anti-D has been the emphasis of much investigation. These findings can be applied to other clinically significant RBC antibodies causing HDN, except for ABO antibodies, which will be discussed separately.

In addition to the use of RhIg, many other advances have been made in the diagnosis and treatment of HDN. Ultrasound and percutaneous umbilical blood sampling have greatly increased the success of accurately diagnosing and adequately treating this disease.

## ETIOLOGY

### Historical Overview

Although the changes in the fetus and newborn were noted as early as the seventeenth century, it was not until 1939 that Levine and Stetson reported a transfusion reaction from transfusing the husband's blood to a postpartum woman. They postulated that the mother had been immunized to the father's antigen through the fetus.

Then, in 1940, Landsteiner and Wiener conducted the experiments immunizing rabbits and guinea pigs to rhesus monkey RBCs. Using the serum from these experiments, Levine demonstrated that the mother who had the transfusion reaction was rhesus-negative, and the father, rhesus-positive. In addition, the mother's serum agglutinated the father's RBCs.

### Disease Mechanism

Hemolytic disease of the newborn and fetus is caused by the destruction of the RBCs of the fetus by antibodies produced by the mother. Only antibodies of the immunoglobulin G (IgG) class are actively transported across the placenta; other classes, such as IgA and IgM, are not. Most IgG antibodies are directed against bacterial, fungal, and viral antigens, so the transfer of IgG from the mother to the fetus is beneficial. However, in HDN, the antibodies are directed against those antigens on the fetal RBCs that were inherited from the father.

## Rh HEMOLYTIC DISEASE OF THE NEWBORN AND FETUS

Usually in the case of Rh disease, the Rh-positive firstborn infant of an Rh-negative mother is unaffected because the mother has not yet been immunized. During gestation, and particularly at delivery when the placenta separates from the uterus, variable numbers of fetal RBCs enter the maternal circulation (**Color Plate 15**). These fetal cells, carrying Rh antigen inherited from the father, immunize the mother and stimulate the production of anti-D. Once the mother is immunized to Rh antigen, all subsequent offspring inheriting the D antigen will be affected. The maternal anti-D crosses the placenta and binds to the fetal Rh-positive cells (Fig. 20–1). The sensitized RBCs are destroyed by the fetal reticuloendothelial system, resulting in anemia.

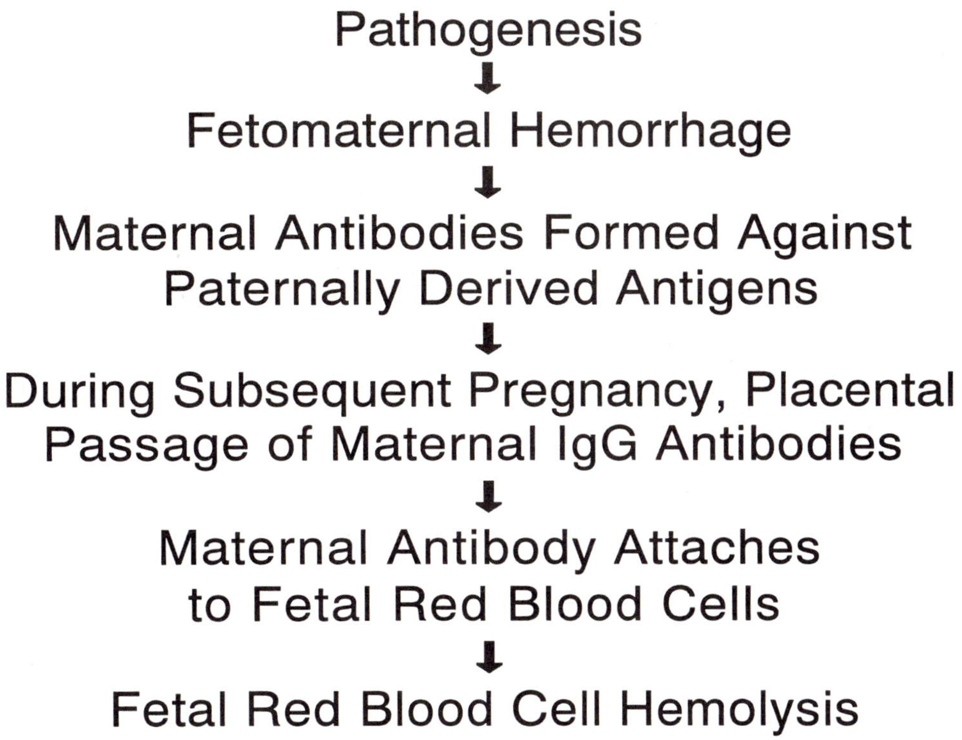

# Pathogenesis
↓
# Fetomaternal Hemorrhage
↓
# Maternal Antibodies Formed Against Paternally Derived Antigens
↓
# During Subsequent Pregnancy, Placental Passage of Maternal IgG Antibodies
↓
# Maternal Antibody Attaches to Fetal Red Blood Cells
↓
# Fetal Red Blood Cell Hemolysis

**Figure 20–1.** Pathogenesis of hemolytic disease of the newborn and fetus.

## Factors Affecting Immunization and Severity

### Antigenic Exposure

Transplacental hemorrhage of fetal RBCs into the maternal circulation occurs in up to 7.0 percent of women during gestation.[2] Using molecular biology techniques, 50[3] to 65 percent[4] of pregnant women have nucleated fetal cells in their peripheral blood. In addition, interventions such as amniocentesis and chorionic villus sampling, as well as trauma to the abdomen, increase the risk of fetomaternal hemorrhage. At delivery, the incidence is more than 50 percent. In the majority of cases, the volume of fetomaternal hemorrhage is small; however, as little as 1 mL of fetal RBCs can immunize the mother.

Fetomaternal hemorrhage during pregnancy can cause significant increases in maternal antibody titers, leading to increasing severity of HDN. In addition, the number of antigenic sites on the fetal RBCs corresponds to heterozygous RBCs, inasmuch as all fetal antigens incompatible with the mother must have been inherited from the father, who can give only one gene to the fetus. Generally, heterozygous RBCs have fewer antigenic sites than homozygous RBCs.

### Host Factors

The ability of individuals to produce antibody in response to antigenic exposure varies, depending on complex genetic factors. In Rh-negative individuals who are transfused with 1 unit (500 mL) of Rh-positive RBCs, about 80 percent form anti-D.[5] Nearly all of the nonresponders will fail to produce anti-D even with repeated exposures to Rh-positive blood. On the other hand, the risk of immunization is only about 10 percent for an Rh-negative mother after an Rh-positive pregnancy if RhIg is not administered.

### Immunoglobulin Class

Immunoglobulin class and subclass of the maternal antibody affect the severity of the HDN. Of the immunoglobulin classes (IgG, IgM, IgA, IgE, and IgD), only IgG is transported across the placenta. The active transport of IgG begins in the second trimester and continues until birth. The IgG molecules are transported via the Fc portion of the antibodies.

Of the four subclasses of IgG antibody, $IgG_1$ and $IgG_3$ are more efficient in RBC hemolysis than are $IgG_2$ and $IgG_4$. Therefore, the subclass(es) in the mother can affect the severity of the hemolytic disease.

### Antibody Specificity

Of all the RBC antigens, Rh(D) is the most antigenic. For this reason, only Rh-negative blood is transfused to Rh-negative women of childbearing age. Other antigens in the Rh system, such as C(rh'), E(rh"), and c(hr'), are also potent immunogens (although less potent than D) (Table 20–1). These other Rh antibodies have been associated with moderate to severe cases of HDN. Anti-E in particular has caused HDN severe enough to require intervention and treatment.

Of the non–Rh-system antibodies, anti-Kell is con-

**Table 20–1.** Antibodies Identified in Prenatal Specimens

| | Cause of HDN | |
|---|---|---|
| **Common** | **Rare** | **Never** |
| anti-D | anti-Fy[a] | anti-Le[a] |
| anti-D + C | anti-s | anti-Le[b] |
| anti-D + E | anti-M | anti-I |
| anti-C | anti-N | anti-IH |
| anti-E | anti-S | anti-P[1] |
| anti-c | | |
| anti-e | | |
| anti-K | | |

sidered the most clinically significant in its ability to cause HDN. Almost any IgG RBC antibody is capable of causing HDN, although the disease caused by these antibodies is usually moderate in severity. Nevertheless, all pregnant women with IgG RBC antibodies should be followed closely for HDN. Vengelen-Tyler[6] lists and discusses 64 different RBC antibody specificities reported to cause HDN.

### Influence of ABO Group

When the mother is ABO-incompatible with the fetus (major incompatibility), the incidence of detectable fetomaternal hemorrhage decreases. Investigators noted many years ago that the incidence of Rh immunization is less in mothers with major ABO incompatibility with the fetus. The ABO incompatibility protects somewhat against Rh immunization apparently by the hemolysis in the mother's circulation of ABO-incompatible Rh-positive fetal RBCs before the Rh antigen can be recognized by the mother's immune system.

## PATHOGENESIS

### Hemolysis, Anemia, and Erythropoiesis

Hemolysis occurs when maternal IgG attaches to specific antigens of the fetal RBCs (see Figure 20–1, **Color Plate 16:** untreated). The antibody-coated cells are then removed from the circulation by the macrophages of the spleen. The rate of destruction depends on antibody titer and specificity, as well as the number of antigenic sites on the fetal RBCs. Destruction of fetal RBCs and the resulting anemia stimulate the fetal bone marrow to produce RBCs at an accelerated rate, even to the point that immature RBCs (erythroblasts) are released into the circulation. The term *erythroblastosis fetalis* was used to describe this finding. When the bone marrow fails to produce enough RBCs to keep up with the rate of RBC destruction, erythropoiesis outside the bone marrow is increased in the hemopoietic tissues of the spleen and liver. The spleen and liver become enlarged (he-

patosplenomegaly), resulting in portal hypertension and hepatocellular damage.

Severe anemia along with hypoproteinemia caused by decreased hepatic production of plasma proteins leads to the development of high-output cardiac failure with generalized edema, effusions, and ascites, a condition known as *hydrops fetalis*. In severely affected cases, hydrops can develop at 18 to 20 weeks' gestation. In the past, hydrops fetalis was almost uniformly fatal; currently, most fetuses with this condition can be successfully treated.[1,7]

The process of RBC destruction goes on even after such an infant is delivered alive—in fact, as long as maternal antibody persists in the newborn infant's circulation. The rate of RBC destruction after birth decreases because no more maternal antibody is entering the infant's circulation through the placenta. However, IgG is distributed both extravascularly and intravascularly and has a half-life of 25 days, so sensitization and hemolysis of RBCs continue for several days to weeks after delivery.

### Bilirubin

The RBC destruction releases hemoglobin, which is metabolized to bilirubin (Fig. 20–2). This bilirubin is called "indirect" because indirect methods are required to measure the bilirubin in the laboratory. The indirect bilirubin is transported across the placenta and conjugated in the maternal liver to "direct" bilirubin. The conjugated bilirubin is then excreted by the mother. Although levels of total bilirubin in the fetal circulation and in the amniotic fluid may be elevated, these do not cause clinical disease in the fetus. However, after birth, accumulation of metabolic by-products of RBC destruction can become a severe problem for the newborn infant. The newborn liver is unable to conjugate bilirubin efficiently, especially in premature infants. With moderate to severe hemolysis, the unconjugated or indirect bilirubin can reach levels toxic to the infant's brain (generally, more than 18 mg/dL) and, if left untreated, can cause kernicterus or permanent damage to parts of the brain.

## DIAGNOSIS AND MANAGEMENT

The diagnosis and management of HDN require close cooperation among the pregnant patient, her obstetrician, her spouse or partner, and the personnel of the clinical laboratory performing the serologic testing. Serologic and clinical tests performed at appropriate times during the pregnancy can accurately determine the level of antibody in the maternal circulation, the potential of the antibody to cause hemolytic disease, and the severity of RBC destruction during gestation (Fig. 20–3). If clinical and serologic data indicate that the fetus is becoming severely anemic, interventions such as intrauterine transfusion can be used to treat the anemia and prevent the development of severe disease.

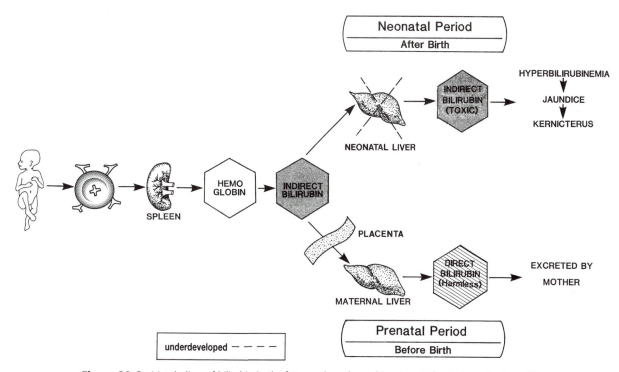

**Figure 20–2.** Metabolism of bilirubin in the fetus and newborn. (Courtesy Ortho Systems, Raritan, NJ.)

## Serologic Testing

The recommended obstetric practice is to perform a type-and-antibody screen at the first prenatal visit, preferably during the first trimester. At that time, the pregnant woman can be asked about previous pregnancies and their outcomes. Previous severe disease and poor outcome predict similar findings in the current pregnancy.

### ABO and Rh Testing

The testing of the specimen should include ABO and Rh testing for D antigen. The Rh test should include weak D if no immediate reaction with anti-D occurs. The patient's RBCs should also be tested simultaneously with Rh control reagent while testing for weak D. If weak D–positive, the patient can be considered Rh-positive. In rare cases, weak D phenotype is caused by missing a part of the Rh antigen (see Chapter 6). Such patients may produce anti-D as an alloantibody, which has been reported to cause HDN.

### Antibody Detection Test (Antibody Screen)

The test conditions must be able to detect clinically significant IgG alloantibodies that are reactive at 37°C and in the antiglobulin phase. At least two separate reagent screening cells, covering all common blood group antigens, should be used. An antibody-enhancing medium such as albumin or low ionic strength saline solution (LISS) can increase sensitivity of the assay. Many prenatal patients produce clinically in-

significant antibodies, such as anti-Le$^a$ and/or anti-Le$^b$. Therefore, many workers in this field encourage omitting immediate spin and room temperature incubation phases and using anti-IgG, rather than broad-spectrum, antiglobulin reagent. These steps reduce detection of IgM antibodies, which cannot cross the placenta.

If the antibody screen in nonreactive, repeat testing is recommended at 20 to 24 weeks' gestation and again at delivery.

### Antibody Specificity

If the antibody screen is reactive, the antibody specificity must be determined. Follow-up testing will depend on the antibody specificity. Cold reactive IgM antibodies such as anti-I, anti-IH, anti-Le$^a$, anti-Le$^b$, and anti-P$_1$ can be ignored. As mentioned earlier, Lewis system antibodies are rather common in pregnant women but have not been reported to cause HDN.

Antibodies such as anti-M and anti-N can be IgM or IgG, or a combination of both. Both anti-M and anti-N rarely can cause mild to moderate HDN. To establish the immunoglobulin class, the serum can be treated with sulfhydryl reagents such as dithiothreitol (DTT) or 2-mercaptoethanol and then retested with appropriate controls. Immunoglobulin M antibodies will be destroyed by this treatment; IgG antibodies will remain.

Many Rh-negative pregnant women have weakly reactive anti-D, particularly during the third trimester. Most of these women have received RhIg (see subsequent text), either after an event with increased risk of fetomaternal hemorrhage or at 28 weeks' gestation. The passively administered anti-D will be weakly reac-

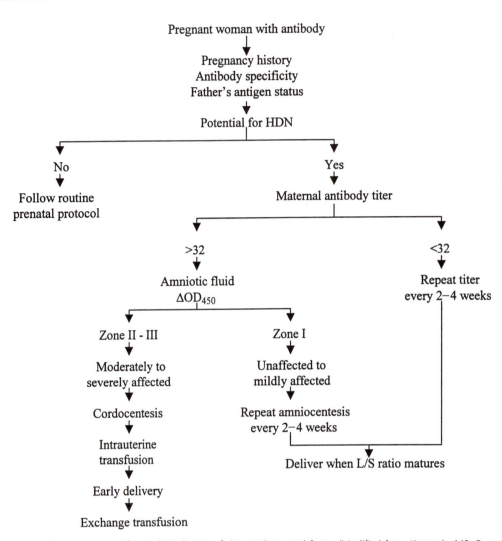

**Figure 20–3.** Diagnosis and management of hemolytic disease of the newborn and fetus. (Modified from Kennedy, MS: Essentials of immunohematology and blood therapy. In Zuspan, FP, and Quilligan, EJ (eds): Practical Manual of Obstetrical Care. CV Mosby, St Louis, 1982, p 119, with permission.)

tive in testing and will remain demonstrable for 2 to 3 months or longer. This must be distinguished from active immunization. A titer higher than 4 almost always indicates active immunization. With a titer under 4, active immunization cannot be ruled out but is less likely.

If the antibody specificity is determined to be clinically significant and the antibody is IgG, further testing is required. Other than anti-D, the most common and most significant antibodies are anti-K, anti-E, anti-c, anti-C, and anti-Fy^a (see Table 20–1).

### Paternal Phenotype

A specimen of the father's blood should be obtained and tested for the presence and zygosity of the corresponding antigen. If the mother has anti-D and the father is D-positive, a complete Rh phenotype can help determine his chance of being homozygous or heterozygous for the D antigen. The information is helpful in planning further testing of the mother and in counseling her.

In cases of antibody specificity other than D, testing the father can save a great deal of time, expense, and worry if he is shown to lack the corresponding antigen. The mother must be counseled in private as to the paternity of the fetus.

### Amniocyte Testing

If the mother has anti-D and the father is most likely to be heterozygous for the D antigen, amniocentesis can be done as early as 10 to 12 weeks' gestation to determine whether the amniocytes carry the gene for the D antigen. Amniocytes can be similarly tested for the genes coding c, e, C, E, and K.

### Antibody Titers

The relative concentration of all antibodies capable of crossing the placenta and causing HDN must be determined by antibody titration. The patient serum is serially diluted and tested against appropriate RBCs to determine the highest dilution at which a reaction occurs. The method must include the indirect antiglobulin phase using anti-IgG reagent. The result is expressed as either the reciprocal of the titration endpoint or as a titer score.

The titration must be performed exactly the same way each time the patient's serum is tested. The RBCs used for each titration should be of the same genotype (preferably from the same donor), approximately the same storage time, and the same concentration. The first serum specimen should be frozen and run in parallel with later specimens. Only a difference of greater than 2 dilutions or a score change of more than 10 should be considered as a significant change in titer.

Each laboratory should develop its own critical titer levels by reviewing the outcome of a number of pregnancies complicated by HDN. In general, a titer of 32 is considered significant. If the initial titer is 32 or higher, a second titer should be done at about 18 to 20 weeks' gestation. A titer reproducibly and repeatedly at 32 or above represents an indication for amniocentesis or percutaneous umbilical blood sampling between 20 and 24 weeks' gestation.

When the titer is 16 or less, the titer should be repeated monthly during the second trimester, beginning at 18 to 20 weeks' gestation, and biweekly during the third trimester. The last determination should be made within a week of the expected date of delivery.

Antibody titer in itself cannot predict severity of HDN. In some sensitized women, the antibody titer may remain moderately high throughout pregnancy while the fetus is becoming more and more severely affected. Similarly, a previously sensitized woman may have consistently high antibody titer whether pregnant or not and, if pregnant, whether the fetus is Rh-positive or Rh-negative. In others, the titer may rise rapidly, which portends increasing severity of HDN. However, antibody titers consistently below the laboratory's critical level throughout the pregnancy reliably predict an unaffected or only moderately affected fetus.

## Amniocentesis and Cordocentesis

At about 18 to 20 weeks' gestation, further diagnosis and treatment are begun. Patients with a history of a severely affected fetus or early fetal death may require earlier intervention. Under ultrasound guidance, amniocentesis is done to assess the status of the fetus. The concentration of bilirubin pigment in the amniotic fluid correlates with the degree of fetal anemia. The amniotic fluid is subjected to a spectrophotometric scan at steadily increasing wavelengths, so that the change in

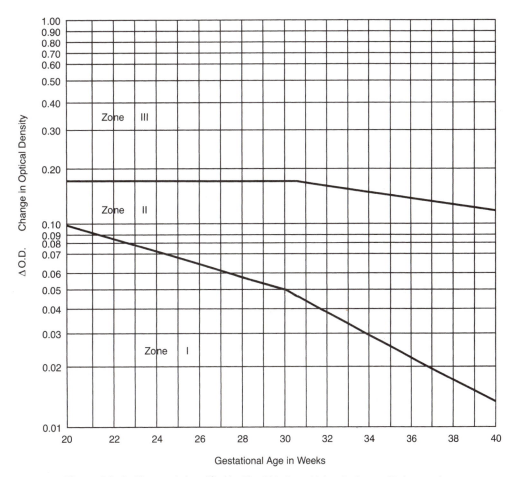

**Figure 20–4.** Liley graph (modified by The Ohio State University Prenatal Laboratory).

the optical density (ΔOD) at 450 nm (the absorbance of bilirubin) can be calculated. The measurement is plotted on the Liley graph (Fig. 20–4) according to gestational age. The optical density of the amniotic fluid is high in the second trimester and steadily decreases until delivery. An increasing or unchanging ΔOD 450 nm as pregnancy proceeds predicts worsening of the fetal hemolytic disease and the need for frequent monitoring and intervention if indicated. Values in zone III indicate severe and often life-threatening hemolysis and require urgent intervention. In zone II, most fetuses have moderate disease that may require intervention. Values in zone I predict mild or no disease, which do not require intervention.

Amniotic fluid analysis, although a useful tool, still represents an indirect prediction of the severity of fetal anemia. Recent advances in sonography have allowed clinicians to obtain a sample of the fetal blood through a procedure called *percutaneous umbilical blood sampling,* or *cordocentesis.* Using high-resolution ultrasound with color Doppler enhancement of blood flow, the umbilical vein is visualized at the level of the cord insertion into the placenta (Fig. 20–5). A needle is inserted into the umbilical vessel and a sample of the fetal blood is obtained. The fetal blood sample can then be tested for hemoglobin, hematocrit, blood type, and direct antiglobulin test.

### Intrauterine Transfusion

Intervention in the form of intrauterine transfusion becomes necessary when one or more of the following conditions exists:

1. Amniotic fluid ΔOD 450 nm results are in high zone II or in zone III.
2. Cordocentesis blood sample has hemoglobin level less than 10 g/dL.
3. Fetal hydrops is noted on ultrasound examination.

Intrauterine transfusion can be performed intraperitoneally by injecting the RBCs into the fetal peritoneal cavity, where the RBCs can be absorbed into the circulation. More recently, cordocentesis has been used to inject donor RBCs directly into the fetal umbilical vein.[7] Once intrauterine transfusion is initiated, the procedure is repeated every 2 to 4 weeks until 34 to 36 weeks' gestation, or until the fetal lungs are mature, when early delivery can be performed.

Amniocentesis and cordocentesis have several risks, among them trauma to the placenta, which may cause increased antibody titers because of antigenic challenge to the mother through fetomaternal hemorrhage.

### Early Delivery

Early delivery was used for many years for moderate to severe disease to interrupt the transport of maternal antibody to the fetus and to allow exchange transfusion. With the use of repeated and frequent intravenous transfusions in the fetus, delivery before the lungs are mature usually can be avoided.

### Phototherapy

After delivery, phototherapy with ultraviolet light can be used. In infants with mild to moderate hemolysis, the use of phototherapy may avoid the need for exchange transfusion to treat hyperbilirubinemia.

### Serologic Testing of the Newborn Infant

#### ABO Grouping

ABO antigens are not fully developed in newborn infants and thus may give weak reactions. In addition, the infant does not have his or her own isoagglutinins but may have those of the mother, so reverse grouping cannot be used to confirm the ABO group.

#### Rh Typing

If the direct antiglobulin test result is strongly positive, Rh reagents with high-protein media can give false-positive results. Therefore, saline reagents are recommended for all RBCs with a positive direct antiglobulin test. In addition, red cells heavily sensitized with anti-D can give a false-negative Rh type, or what has been called "blocked Rh." An eluate from these red cells will reveal anti-D, and typing of the eluted red cells will show reaction with anti-D.

#### Direct Antiglobulin Testing

The most important serologic test for diagnosis of HDN is the direct antiglobulin test with anti-IgG

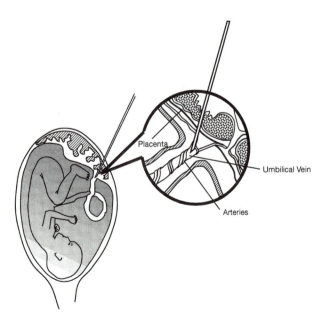

**Figure 20–5.** Technique of percutaneous umbilical blood sampling (cordocentesis). (From Ludomirski,[7] p 91, with permission.)

reagent. The positive test result indicates antibody is coating the infant's RBCs; however, the strength of the reaction does not correlate well with the severity of the HDN. A positive test result may be found in infants without clinical or other laboratory evidence of hemolysis.

### Elution

The routine preparation of an eluate of all infants with a positive direct antiglobulin test result is unnecessary. Elution in cases of known HDN and postnatal ABO incompatibility (see discussion later) is not needed, inasmuch as eluate results do not change therapy. The preparation of an eluate may be helpful when the cause of HDN is in question. As noted earlier, the resolution of a case of "blocked Rh" will require an eluate.

### Newborn Transfusions

The newborn infant may receive small aliquot transfusions or exchange transfusions, or both. Small aliquots can be used to correct anemia when the bilirubin level is not high enough to warrant an exchange transfusion. Exchange transfusions are used primarily to remove high levels of unconjugated bilirubin and thus to prevent kernicterus. Premature newborn infants are more likely than full-term infants to require exchange transfusions for elevated bilirubin because their livers are less able to conjugate bilirubin. Other advantages of exchange transfusion include the removal of part of the circulating maternal antibody, removal of sensitized RBCs, replacement of incompatible RBCs with compatible RBCs, and suppression of erythropoiesis (Table 20–2). All of these help interrupt the bilirubin production caused by hemolysis; however, the suppression of erythropoiesis by small aliquot or exchange transfusions may cause anemia to occur after the immediate neonatal period.

Although full-term newborn infants normally have rather high hemoglobin levels (14 to 20 g/dL), below 12 g/dL is considered anemia that may require transfusion. Below 8 g/dL is considered severe anemia and corresponds to zone III of the Liley graph, whereas 8 to 12 g/dL corresponds to zone II. A cord blood sample closely correlates with the levels during gestation. If the obstetrician infuses placenta blood after delivery, the infant's hemoglobin level will be higher than the cord sample.

**Table 20–2.** Beneficial Effects of Exchange Transfusion

Removal of bilirubin
Removal of sensitized RBCs
Removal of incompatible antibody
Replacement of incompatible RBCs with compatible RBCs
Suppression of erythropoiesis (reduced production of incompatible RBCs)

### Selection of Blood

Most centers handling HDN use group O RBCs for intrauterine as well as neonatal transfusions. Donors are usually cytomegalovirus (CMV) seronegative as well. Physicians in these centers are usually transfusing neonates for other indications, such as RBC replacement for blood samples taken for laboratory tests. This allows a small inventory of group O CMV-seronegative donor units to be set aside for intrauterine and neonatal transfusions. Rh-negative units are selected for fetuses and neonates whose blood type is unknown or is Rh-negative.

For exchange transfusions, one practice is to prepare RBCs from whole blood units and then to replace the plasma with group AB plasma to reduce the amount of blood group antibodies transfused. This procedure may be avoided if both the fetus or neonate and the mother are the same ABO group.

Blood transfused to the fetus and premature infant should also be gamma-irradiated to prevent graft-versus-host disease (see Chapter 16). It is also recommended that blood for exchange transfusion not contain hemoglobin S, because the decreased oxygen tension that may occur early in the neonatal period may cause hemoglobin S–containing blood to sickle. Traditionally, blood units less than 7 days from collection from the donor are selected. Special circumstances, such as the need for units of mother's blood when high-incidence antibodies are involved, have shown that older blood units can be safe and effective for the newborn.

## Rh IMMUNE GLOBULIN

Active immunization induced by RBC antigen can be prevented by the concurrent administration of the corresponding RBC antibody. This principle has been used to prevent immunization to Rh(D) antigen by the use of high-titered RhIg.

During pregnancy and delivery, mixing of fetal and maternal blood occurs. If the mother is Rh-negative and the fetus is Rh-positive, the mother has up to a 9 percent chance of being stimulated to form anti-D[2]. As little as 1 mL of fetal RBCs can elicit a response. Before delivery, the risk of sensitization is 1.5 to 1.9 percent of susceptible women, indicating that a significant amount of fetal RBCs can enter the maternal circulation during pregnancy.[1] However, the greatest risk of immunization to Rh is at delivery.

### Mechanism of Action

The administered RhIg attaches to the fetal Rh-positive RBCs in the maternal circulation (**Color Plate 16**). The antibody-coated RBCs are trapped in the maternal spleen, where they take up more antibody from the circulating plasma. This activates suppressor cells or causes the production of blocking antibody, or both. The amount of antibody necessary for the suppressor effect has been determined experimentally and is known to be less than that required to saturate all D antigen sites.

## Indications

### Postpartum

The Rh-negative unsensitized mother should receive RhIg soon after delivery of an Rh-positive infant. The recommended time interval is within 72 hours after delivery, based on experiments conducted many years ago. Even if more than 72 hours have elapsed, RhIg should still be given, inasmuch as it may be effective and is not contraindicated.

The mother should be D-negative as well as weak D-negative (Fig. 20–6). The infant should be D-positive or weak D-positive. If the type of the infant is unknown (e.g., if the infant is stillborn), RhIg should also be administered. Antibody titers are not recommended because the amount of circulating RhIg does not correlate with effectiveness of the immune suppression or with the amount of fetomaternal hemorrhage.[8]

### Antenatal

Because of the known risk of Rh immunization during pregnancy, RhIg should be given early in the third trimester, or at about 28 weeks' gestation. The dose does not pose a risk to the fetus, inasmuch as this amount will cause a titer of only 1 or 2 in the mother.[1] However, a positive direct antiglobulin test (DAT) result may be observed in the newborn.

If the infant is Rh-positive, a second dose is indicated after delivery. The half-life of IgG is about 25 days, so only about 10 percent of the original dose will be present at 40 weeks' gestation. It is essential that the anti-D from antenatal RhIg present at delivery not be interpreted erroneously as active rather than passive immunization. Omission of the indicated dose after delivery may lead to active immunization.

Other conditions may pose a risk of Rh immunization and therefore require RhIg administration (Table 20–3). The microdose can be used for abortions and ectopic pregnancies before the twelfth week of gestation.[9]

## Dose and Administration

The regular-dose vial in the United States contains sufficient anti-D to protect against 15 mL of packed RBCs or 30 mL of whole blood. This is equal to 300 μg of the World Health Organization (WHO) reference material. The regular-dose vial in the United Kingdom contains about 100 μg, which appears to be adequate for postpartum prophylaxis. The microdose (equivalent to 50 μg) is sufficient for abortion, amniocentesis, and ectopic rupture at up to 12 weeks' gestation. The total fetal blood volume is estimated to be less than 5 ml at 12 weeks.

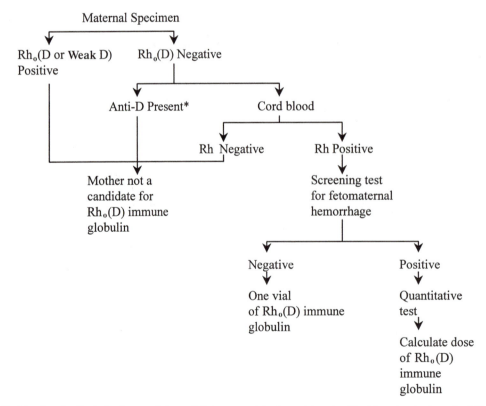

**Figure 20–6.** Decision tree for the indications and dose of Rh immune globulin as determined by laboratory test results. If the cord or neonatal blood specimen is unavailable, assume the fetus is D positive. (Modified from Kennedy,[9] p 235, with permission.)

**Table 20–3.** Additional Indications for RhIg

Amniocentesis
Chorionic villus sampling
Abortion (spontaneous and induced)
Ectopic pregnancy
Abdominal trauma
Accidental or inadvertent transfusion

Recently, an intravenous (IV) preparation of Rh immune globulin has been approved for use in the United States. This product also contains 300 µg in each vial and can be administered either intramuscularly or intravenously. Additional manufacturing steps are required to allow intravenous use, so the product is more expensive.

Massive fetomaternal hemorrhages of more than 30 mL of whole blood occur in fewer than 1 percent of deliveries. These massive hemorrhages can lead to immunization if adequate RhIg is not administered. Massive fetomaternal hemorrhages can be detected by the routine use of a screening test, such as the rosette technique. Quantitation of the actual amount of hemorrhage must be done by a test such as the Kleihauer-Betke. In this test, a maternal blood smear is treated with acid (or alkali) and then stained with a counterstain. Fetal cells contain hemoglobin that is resistant to acid or alkali and will remain red. The maternal cells will appear as ghosts. After 2000 cells are counted, the percentage of fetal cells is determined, and the volume of fetal hemorrhage is calculated using the formula:

$$\frac{\text{Number of fetal cells} \times \text{Maternal blood volume}}{\text{Number of maternal cells}} =$$

Volume of fetomaternal hemorrhage

The calculated volume of fetomaternal hemorrhage is then divided by 30 to determine the number of required vials of RhIg. A simpler way of calculating the dose is to multiply the percentage of fetal cells by 50, which gives the volume of fetomaternal hemorrhage in milliliters.

The number of vials for transfusion accidents is calculated by dividing the volume of Rh-positive packed RBCs transfused by 15 mL, the amount of RBCs covered by one vial. The number of vials can be large, so the entire dose is often divided and administered in several injections at separate sites. Another approach is to perform an exchange transfusion with Rh-negative blood and then calculate the dose based on the number of Rh-positive RBCs remaining in the circulation. For platelet concentrates, one vial is sufficient for 30 or more units (bags), because each unit contains less than 0.5 mL RBCs. The dose for leukocyte concentrates can be calculated by obtaining the hematocrit and volume of the product from the supplier.

The RhIg must be injected according to the product label. The IV product can also be given intramuscularly (IM). The IM form must be given IM only. Intravenous injections of IM preparations can cause severe anaphylactic reactions because of the anti-complementary activity of these products.

## Other Considerations

Rh immune globulin is of no benefit once a person has been actively immunized and has formed anti-D. Care must be taken, however, to distinguish women who have been passively immunized by antenatal administration of RhIg from those who have been actively immunized by exposure to Rh-positive RBCs.

Care must also be taken so that fetal Rh-positive RBCs in the maternal circulation is not interpreted as maternal, because then the mother would be assumed erroneously to be weak D positive. The difference is distinguished by a quantitative test such as the Kleihauer-Betke.

RhIg is not indicated for the mother if the infant is found to be D negative and weak D negative. The blood type of fetuses in abortions, stillbirths, and ectopic pregnancies usually cannot be determined; therefore, RhIg should be administered in these circumstances. RhIg must not be given to the newborn infant.

There is no risk of transmission of the viral diseases hepatitis A and B and human immunodeficiency virus (HIV).[10] Several investigators have reported transmission of non-A, non-B hepatitis and hepatitis C, however. RhIg has been reported to contain antibody to hepatitis A, B, and C, and thus may cause false-positive hepatitis serology.[11]

## ABO HEMOLYTIC DISEASE OF THE NEWBORN

ABO incompatibility between the mother and newborn infant can cause HDN. Maternal ABO antibodies that are IgG can cross the placenta and attach to the ABO-incompatible antigens of the fetal RBCs. However, destruction of fetal RBCs leading to severe anemia is extremely rare. More commonly, the disease is manifested by the onset of hyperbilirubinemia and jaundice within 12 to 48 hours of birth. The increasing levels of bilirubin can be treated with phototherapy. Severe cases requiring exchange transfusion are extremely rare. A comparison of ABO versus Rh HDN is shown in Table 20–4.

As the incidence of HDN caused by $Rh_0(D)$ has declined, ABO incompatibility has become the most common cause of hemolytic disease. Statistically, mother and infant are ABO-incompatible in one of every five pregnancies.

### Factors Affecting Incidence and Severity

ABO antibodies are present in the sera of all individuals whose RBCs lack the corresponding antigen. These antibodies, the result of environmental stimulus, occur more frequently as high-titered IgG antibodies in

**Table 20–4.** Comparison of ABO versus Rh HDN

| Characteristic | ABO | Rh |
|---|---|---|
| First pregnancy | Yes | Rare |
| Disease predicted by titers | No | Yes |
| Antibody IgG | Yes (anti-A,B) | Yes (anti-D, etc.) |
| Bilirubin at birth | Normal range | Elevated |
| Anemia at birth | No | Yes |
| Phototherapy | Yes | Yes |
| Exchange transfusion | Rare | Common |
| Intrauterine transfusion | None | Sometimes |
| Spherocytosis | Yes | Rare |

group O individuals than in group A or B individuals. Hence, ABO HDN is nearly always limited to A or B infants of group O mothers with potent anti-A,B. Most occur in group A infants in white populations. In the black population, however, group B infants are more often affected, and the overall incidence of ABO HDN is several times greater than in other groups.

The mother's history of prior transfusions or pregnancies seems unrelated to the occurrence and severity of the disease. Thus, ABO HDN may occur in the first pregnancy and in any, but not necessarily all, subsequent pregnancies. However, tetanus toxoid administration and helminth parasite infection during pregnancy have been linked to the production of high-titered IgG ABO antibodies and severe HDN.

Even high-titered IgG antibodies that are transported across the placenta seem incapable of causing significant RBC destruction in an ABO-incompatible fetus. These infants are delivered with mild anemia or normal hemoglobin levels. The mild course of ABO HDN is related more to the slow development of ABO antigens on fetal RBCs than the characteristics of the maternal antibody. That ABO antigens are not fully developed until after the first year of life is well demonstrated by the A antigen. Group A infant RBCs are serologically more similar to $A_2$ adult cells, with group $A_2$ infant RBCs much weaker. The weakened A antigen on fetal and neonatal RBCs is more readily demonstrable with human than with monoclonal anti-A reagents. As expected, group $A_2$ infants are less likely to have ABO HDN.

The laboratory findings in ABO HDN differ from those in Figure 20–3 for Rh disease. Microspherocytes and increased RBC fragility in the infant are characteristic of ABO HDN but not of Rh HDN. The severity of the disease is independent of the presence of a positive direct antiglobulin test result or demonstrable anti-A, anti-B, or anti-A,B in the eluate of the infant's RBCs.

The bilirubin peak is later, at 1 to 3 days, as well. Phototherapy is usually sufficient for slowly rising bilirubin levels. With rapidly increasing bilirubin levels, exchange transfusion with group O RBCs may be required. The serious consequences of Rh and other blood groups causing HDN, such as stillbirth, hydrops fetalis, and kernicterus, are extremely rare in ABO HDN.

## Prenatal Screening

Many workers have tried to use the immunoglobulin class and titer of maternal ABO antibodies to predict ABO HDN. These tests are laborious and at best demonstrate the presence of IgG maternal antibody but do not correlate well with the degree of fetal RBC destruction. Consequently, detection of ABO HDN is best done after birth.

## Postnatal Diagnosis

No single serologic test is diagnostic for ABO HDN. When a newborn infant develops jaundice within 12 to 48 hours after birth, various causes of jaundice need to be investigated, and ABO HDN is only one. The DAT on the cord or neonatal RBCs is the most important diagnostic test. In all cases of ABO HDN requiring transfusion therapy, the DAT result has been positive.[12] On the other hand, the DAT result can be positive even in the absence of signs and symptoms of clinical anemia in the newborn infant. However, these infants may have compensated anemia, or the RBCs may not be destroyed by the reticuloendothelial system.

Collecting cord blood samples on all delivered infants is highly recommended. The sample should be collected by venipuncture to avoid contamination with Wharton's jelly and maternal blood and should be anticoagulated for storage. If the neonatal infant develops jaundice, ABO, Rh, and DAT results can be assessed. The DAT result is neither strongly nor consistently positive, although 90 percent of the cases complicated by jaundice are positive.[13] When the DAT result is negative but the infant is jaundiced, other causes of jaundice should be investigated. In the rare cases in which ABO incompatibility can be the only cause of neonatal jaundice but the DAT result is negative, the eluate of the cord RBCs always reveals ABO antibodies. The eluate can also be helpful when the mother's blood specimen is not available.

### CASE STUDY

At a rural hospital near a migrant farm camp, a 32-year-old Hispanic woman has just delivered a severely anemic infant. At 6 weeks' gestation, the mother had been typed as A-negative, with positive antibody screen. The antibody was identified as anti-D, titer 256. A report stated that she had an intrauterine transfusion 3 weeks earlier at a university hospital in another state. The cord blood collected at delivery was typed as A-negative. On a heelstick specimen, the infant's hemoglobin was reported as 4.3 g/dL, and bilirubin, as 3.9 mg/dL. Typing results of this specimen are as follows:

| Anti-A | Anti-B | Anti-A,B | Anti-D | Anti-D | DAT |
|---|---|---|---|---|---|
| 0 | 0 | 0 | (IS)0 | (AHG)+ | +/− |

IS-immediate spin
AHG-antihuman globulin

What is the infant's blood type? Why is the infant so anemic? What further testing is indicated?

*Answer*

First of all, the blood types of the cord blood and heelstick specimens are different—A negative versus O weak D positive. The severely anemic infant could have HDN, although the cord blood results do not indicate severe disease (DAT $+/-$). On the other hand, a large fetomaternal hemorrhage could have occurred. Further testing showed the following:

|  | Cord Blood | Heelstick |
|---|---|---|
| Anti-I | 4 + | 3 + |
| Kleihauer-Betke | 0/1000 | 23/1000 |

The results indicate that the cord blood specimen is all adult blood and the heelstick specimen is nearly all adult blood. How could that happen?

*Answer*

Cord blood should be collected by needle and syringe from the umbilical cord vein. Collecting the specimen by allowing blood from the placenta or cord to drip into the tube can contaminate the specimen with maternal blood. In this case, the tube marked "cord blood" could have been a mislabeled maternal sample.

The heelstick is nearly all adult blood because of the recent intrauterine transfusion. Group O blood is usually used. As discussed in this chapter, transfusion causes suppression of erythropoiesis and therefore the production of few fetal RBCs. The cells produced are being hemolyzed by the high-titered maternal antibody. This leads to anemia, in this case quite severe, with elevated bilirubin levels indicating that hemolysis is occurring.

Further testing was done on the heelstick specimen.

|  | Anti-A | Anti-B |
|---|---|---|
| 4°C | 0 | + |

| RBC Eluate |
|---|
| Anti-D |

These results indicate that the infant is probably B-positive and has HDN caused by anti-D.

---

## SUMMARY CHART: IMPORTANT POINTS TO REMEMBER (MT/MLT)

- Hemolytic disease of the newborn (HDN) is the destruction of the red blood cells of the fetus and neonate by IgG antibodies produced by the mother.
- Only antibodies of the IgG class are actively transported across the placenta.
- In Rh HDN the Rh-positive firstborn infant of an Rh-negative mother is unaffected because the mother has not yet been immunized; in subsequent pregnancies fetal cells carrying the Rh antigen immunize the Rh-negative mother and stimulate production of anti-D.
- In ABO HDN the firstborn infant may be affected as well as subsequent pregnancies in which the mother is group O and the newborn is group A or B; the IgG antibody, anti-A,B in the mother's circulation crosses the placenta and attaches to the ABO-incompatible antigens of the fetal RBCs.
- Erythroblastosis fetalis describes the presence of immature RBCs or erythroblasts in the fetal circulation because the splenic removal of the IgG-coated RBCs causes anemia; the term commonly used now is *hemolytic disease of the newborn* (HDN).
- Although anti-D is the most antigenic of the Rh antibodies, anti-Kell is considered the most clinically significant of the non–Rh-system antibodies in the ability to cause HDN.
- Prenatal serologic tests for obstetric patients include an ABO, Rh, and antibody screen during the first trimester of pregnancy.
- A cord blood work-up includes an ABO, Rh, and DAT; the most important serologic test for diagnosis of HDN is the DAT with anti-IgG reagent.
- Rh immune globulin (RhIg) administered to the mother within 72 hours following delivery is used to prevent active immunization by the Rh(D) antigen on fetal cells; RhIg attaches to fetal Rh-positive RBCs in maternal circulation, blocking immunization and subsequent production of anti-D.
- A Kleihauer-Betke test is used to quantitate the number of fetal Rh-positive cells in the mother's circulation as a result of a fetomaternal hemorrhage.

## REVIEW QUESTIONS

1. Hemolytic disease of the newborn is characterized by:
   - A. IgM antibody
   - B. Nearly always anti-D
   - C. Different RBC antigens between mother and father
   - D. Antibody titer less than 32

2. The main difference between the fetus and the newborn is:
   - A. Bilirubin metabolism
   - B. Maternal antibody level
   - C. Presence of anemia
   - D. Size of RBCs

3. Kernicterus is caused by the effects of:
   - A. Anemia
   - B. Unconjugated bilirubin
   - C. Antibody specificity
   - D. Antibody titer

4. The advantages of cordocentesis include all of the following except:
   - A. Allows measurement of fetal hemoglobin and hematocrit levels
   - B. Allows antigen typing of fetal blood
   - C. Allows direct transfusion of fetal circulation
   - D. Decreases risk of trauma to the placenta

5. Amniocentesis is used to:
   - A. Measure bilirubin in milligrams per deciliter
   - B. Determine fetal blood type
   - C. Determine change in optical density
   - D. Measure hemoglobin in grams per deciliter

6. Blood for intrauterine transfusion should be all of the following except:
   - A. More than 7 days old
   - B. Screened for CMV
   - C. Gamma-irradiated
   - D. Compatible with maternal serum

7. Rh immune globulin is indicated for:
   - A. Mothers who have anti-D
   - B. Infants who are Rh-negative
   - C. Infants who have anti-D
   - D. Mothers who are Rh-negative

8. Rh immune globulin is given without regard for fetal Rh type in all of the following conditions except:
   - A. Ectopic pregnancy rupture
   - B. Amniocentesis
   - C. Induced abortion
   - D. Full-term delivery

9. A Kleihauer-Betke test indicates 10 fetal cells per 1000 adult cells. For a woman with 5000 mL blood volume, the proper dose of RhIg is:
   - A. One regular-dose vial
   - B. Two regular-dose vials
   - C. One microdose vial
   - D. Two microdose vials

10. Rh immune globulin is indicated in the following circumstances:
   - A. Mother weak D positive, infant D positive
   - B. Mother D negative, infant D positive and weak D positive
   - C. Mother D positive and weak D positive, infant D negative
   - D. Mother D negative, infant D negative and weak D negative

11. ABO HDN is usually mild because:
   - A. ABO antigens are poorly developed in the fetus
   - B. ABO antibodies prevent the disease
   - C. ABO antibodies readily cross the placenta
   - D. ABO incompatibility is rare

## ANSWERS TO REVIEW QUESTIONS

1. C (p 422)
2. A (p 424)
3. B (p 424)
4. D (p 428)
5. C (pp 427–428)
6. A (p 429)
7. D (p 429)
8. D (p 429)
9. B (p 431)
10. B (p 430)
11. A (p 432)

## REFERENCES

1. Bowman, JM: Historical overview: Hemolytic disease of fetus and newborn. In Kennedy, MS, Wilson, S, and Kelton, JG (eds): Perinatal Transfusion Medicine. American Association of Blood Banks, Arlington, VA, 1990, p 1.
2. Mollison, PL, Engelfriet, CP, and Contreras, M: Blood Transfusion in Clinical Medicine, ed 9. Blackwell Scientific, London, 1993, p 543.
3. Dennis, YM, et al: Two-way cell traffic between mother and fetus: Biologic and clinical implications. Blood 88:4390, 1996.
4. Little, M-T, et al: Frequency of fetal cells in sorted subpopulations of nucleated erythroid and CD34+ hematopoietic progenitor cells from maternal peripheral blood. Blood 89:2347, 1997.
5. Mollison, PL, Engelfriet, CP, and Contreras, M: Blood Transfusion in Clinical Medicine, ed 9. Blackwell Scientific, London, 1993, p 218.
6. Vengelen-Tyler, V: The serological investigation of hemolytic disease of the newborn caused by antibodies other than anti-D. In Garratty, G (ed): Hemolytic Disease of the Newborn. American Association of Blood Banks, Arlington, VA, 1984, p 145.
7. Ludomirski, A: The anemic fetus: Direct access to the fetal circulation for diagnosis and treatment. In Kennedy, MS, Wilson, S, and Kelton, JG (eds): Perinatal Transfusion Medicine. American Association of Blood Banks, Arlington, VA, 1990, p 89.

8. Ness, PM, and Salamon, JL: The failure of postinjection Rh immune globulin titers to detect large fetal-maternal hemorrhages. Am J Clin Pathol 85:604, 1986.

9. Kennedy, MS: Rho(D) immune globulin. In Rayburn, W, and Zuspan, FP (eds): Drug Therapy in Gynecology and Obstetrics, ed 3. CV Mosby, St. Louis, 1991, p 297.

10. Lack of transmission of human immunodeficiency virus through Rho(D) immune globulin (human). MMWR CDC Surveill Summ 36:728, 1987.

11. Tabor, E, Smallwood, LA, and Gerety, RJ: Antibodies to hepatitis A and B virus antigen in Rho(D) immune globulin. Lancet 1:322, 1986.

12. Issitt, PD, and Anstee, DJ: Applied Blood Group Serology, ed 4. Montgomery Scientific, Durham, NC, 1998, p 1045–1083.

13. Walker, RH: Relevancy in the selection of serologic tests for the obstetric patient. In Garratty, G (ed): Hemolytic Disease of the Newborn. American Association of Blood Banks, Arlington, VA, 1984, p 173.

# CHAPTER 21

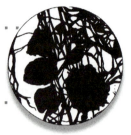

# AUTOIMMUNE HEMOLYTIC ANEMIAS

Denise M. Harmening, PhD, MT(ASCP), CLS(NCA),
Lee Ann Prihoda, MEd, MT (ASCP)SBB, and
Ralph E. B. Green, BAppSci, FAIMS, MACE

## OBJECTIVES:

*On completion of this chapter, the learner
should be able to:*

1 Define *autoantibody* and compare the types of
immune hemolytic anemias with respect to
thermal amplitude, red cell destruction, and the
type of protein (antibody or complement) coating
the red cells.

2 Characterize autoantibodies that react at
temperatures below 37°C and identify the
common specificities of benign cold
autoagglutinins.

3 Discuss problems encountered in laboratory
testing of specimens containing cold
autoagglutinins, and outline testing procedures
that can differentiate between specificities.

4 Discuss pathologic cold autoagglutinins,
including laboratory testing and treatment.

5 Differentiate between idiopathic warm
autoimmune hemolytic anemia (WAIHA) and
drug-induced immune hemolytic anemia.

6 Illustrate the clinical and laboratory findings in
WAIHA, including red cell hemolysis, difficulties
in serologic testing, and selection of blood for
transfusion.

7 Compare the four classic mechanisms for drug-
induced hemolysis, and give examples of
medications causing each type.

*Immune hemolytic anemia* is defined as shortened red
cell survival mediated through the immune response,
specifically by humoral antibody. Immune hemolysis
represents the result of an acquired abnormality of the
red blood cell membrane associated with demonstrable antibodies, as opposed to intracorpuscular defects
such as enzyme deficiencies and hemoglobinopathies,
which represent intrinsic abnormalities of the patient's
red blood cells.

Numerous classifications of immune hemolytic anemias have been proposed; however, three broad categories are generally used:

1. Alloimmune
2. Autoimmune
3. Drug-induced

In an alloimmune response, patients produce alloantibodies to foreign red cell antigens introduced
into their circulation, most often through transfusion
or pregnancy. For a discussion of alloantibody production, refer to Chapters 18 and 20.

This chapter focuses on the latter two categories:
autoimmune hemolytic anemia and drug-induced
hemolytic anemia. An autoimmune response occurs
when a patient produces antibodies against his own
red cell antigens. A drug-induced hemolytic anemia is
the result of a patient's production of antibody to a particular drug or drug complex, with ensuing damage to
the patient's red cells.

## AUTOANTIBODIES

### Definition

Antibodies that are directed against the individual's
own red cells are autoantibodies or autoagglutinins.
Most autoantibodies react with high-incidence antigens; they agglutinate, sensitize, or lyse red blood cells
(RBCs) of most random donors as well as those of the
antibody producer. Red cell survival may be shortened
by this circulating humoral antibody.

Studies in animal models indicate that production of
antibodies against "self" occurs because of a failure of
the mechanisms regulating the immune response.[1,2]
Briefly, under normal circumstances, immunoglobulins are made by B lymphocytes. Another type of lymphocyte, the T lymphocyte, modulates the activity of
the antibody-producing cells. Helper T cells assist immunocompetent B cells in making antibody against
foreign antigens. Another population of T lymphocytes, suppressor T cells, has the opposite effect on
B-cell activity; they prevent excessive proliferation of B
cells and overproduction of antibodies. Suppressor
T cells are thought to act through a feedback mechanism.
An increasing concentration of antibody activates these
T cells and suppresses further antibody production.[3]

Autoantibody production may be prevented through
a similar mechanism. Suppressor T cells induce tolerance to "self" antigens by inhibiting B-cell activity.
Conversely, loss of suppressor T-cell function could result in autoantibody production. Support for this concept comes from animal studies[2] and patients taking
the drug alpha-methyldopa.[4] The cause of dysfunction
of the regulatory system is not understood, but microbial agents and drugs have been suggested.[5] For further
discussion of the immune response, the reader is referred to Chapter 3.

Autoantibodies are important for two reasons. First,
they can cause destruction of red cells in vivo. In addition, when an individual's cells are coated with autoantibody and the serum contains autoantibody that
is reactive with the cells of most random donors, it may
be difficult to correctly interpret routine cell typing, antibody detection and identification, and compatibility
tests. The effect of autoantibodies on routine testing
and techniques to resolve the difficulties are discussed
below. It is important to note that the serologic and
clinical problems can be found separately or together.

### Characterization

The presence of autoantibodies in a patient's serum
or coating a patient's cells may be indicative of autoimmune hemolytic anemia (AIHA), but additional
information is needed before one draws this conclusion. One must establish that RBCs are being destroyed
by an immune-mediated process. Individuals who experience immune red cell destruction may or may not
be anemic (decreased hemoglobin/hematocrit levels),
depending on whether red cell production has in-

creased to compensate for the loss. The reticulocyte count, unconjugated bilirubin levels, and lactate dehydrogenase (LDH) levels are increased, whereas the haptoglobin levels are decreased. With intravascular red cell destruction, hemoglobinemia and hemoglobinuria may occur. There are other causes of hemolysis (e.g., heriditary spherocytosis, hemoglobinopathies, and RBC enzyme defects); therefore, AIHA must be confirmed by additional serologic testing. Diagnostic tests include (1) the direct antiglobulin test (DAT), using polyspecific and monospecific antiglobulin reagents; and (2) characterization of the autoantibody in the serum and/or eluate. Based on these results and the clinical evaluation of the patient, AIHA can be diagnosed and classified as cold-reactive, warm-reactive, or drug-induced. The expected laboratory findings for each type are discussed in the following section. Petz and Garratty[6] devote a chapter in their book, *Acquired Immune Hemolytic Anemias*, to the diagnosis of the hemolytic anemias and another to drug-induced immune hemolytic anemia. The reader is referred to this text for a complete discussion.

Individuals may have autoantibodies in their sera and on their red cells but display no evidence of decreased RBC survival. For example, the incidence of positive DATs in normal blood donor populations has been reported to be as high as 1 in 1000 in the U.S. population,[7] whereas the incidence in hospitalized patients ranges from 0.3 to 1.0 percent (using anti-IgG antiglobulin reagent)[8,9] to 15 percent (using polyspecific antiglobulin reagent).[10] Many of the latter group have only anti-complement bound to the red cells. The differences between individuals who are affected (i.e., have AIHA) and those who are unaffected by autoantibodies are not clearly understood. Among the possibly significant factors are:

1. Thermal amplitude of antibody reactivity[11]
2. IgG subclass of the antibody[12]
3. Amount of antibody bound to the red cells[12]
4. Ability of the antibody to fix complement in vivo[13]
5. Activity of the individual's macrophages[6]
6. Quantitative or qualitative change in Band 3 and proteins 4.1 and 4.2 in the RBC membrane structure.[14]

The opposite situation also occurs; in some patients with hemolytic anemia, autoantibodies cannot be demonstrated by routine techniques. Some patients have more IgG on their RBCs than normal but less than the amount detectable by the routine antiglobulin test.[15] In other cases, the patient's red cells are sensitized with anti-IgA or anti-IgM.[16-18] Because polyspecific antihuman globulin reagents must contain only anti-IgG and anti-C3d,[19] antibodies to other immunoglobulins are not consistently present, and cells sensitized with IgA or IgM may not give a positive test. Finally, prior to current requirements for polyspecific antiglobulin reagents, many commercial reagents did not routinely agglutinate cells coated with complement components.[20] Therefore, a negative DAT was not an unusual finding in patients with cold agglutinin hemolytic anemia. The reader is cautioned, however, to note the date of a publication in which AIHA associated with a negative DAT is reported.

As earlier stated, autoantibodies can be divided into two main groups, depending on the optimal temperature of reactivity. About 70 percent of the reported cases of AIHA are those that react best at warm temperatures (37°C), and cold-reactive (4 to 30°C) autoagglutinins account for about 18 percent. Drug-induced autoagglutinins are present in about 12 percent of the reported cases of AIHA. Characterization of autoantibodies is important because treatment of the patient and resolution of the serologic problems differ according to the optimal temperature of reactivity. The remainder of this chapter details clinical and laboratory aspects of cold-reactive, warm-reactive, and drug-induced autoantibodies.

## COLD-REACTIVE AUTOANTIBODIES

### Benign Cold Autoantibodies

The most commonly encountered autoantibody is a benign cold agglutinin that is demonstrable in the serum of most normal, healthy individuals when testing is done at 4°C. Normally it presents no serologic problem, inasmuch as routine tests are not done at this temperature. The typical cold agglutinin has a relatively low titer: at 4°C it is less than 64. Occasionally, the antibody has increased thermal amplitude and will agglutinate cells at room temperature (20 to 24°C). However, even in this situation one obtains the strongest reactions at 4°C. Table 21–1 compares the characteristics of benign (normal) cold autoantibodies with those of pathologic cold autoagglutinins. Most cold agglutinins react best with enzyme-treated cells; therefore, cold agglutinins are quite likely to be detected when using ficin-treated cells. Cold autoantibodies are of the IgM class and can activate complement in vitro. Reactions may be seen in the antiglobulin phase when using polyspecific antiglobulin reagents. Table 21–2 shows reactions typical of cold autoagglutinins.

### *Laboratory Tests Affected by Cold Autoagglutinins*

Cold agglutinins sometimes interfere with routine serum and cell testing performed at room temperature. The degree to which they cause problems depends on how strongly the antibody reacts at this temperature (i.e., the concentration and thermal amplitude of the antibody). Although the normal cold autoantibody found in the serum of most people usually does not interfere with testing, it is one of the more common causes of serologic problems. Therefore, one should be familiar with the recognition and methods of resolution of problems associated with these antibodies.

**Table 21–1.** Comparison of Characteristics of Normal Cold and Pathologic Cold Autoantibodies

| Characteristic | Normal | Pathologic |
|---|---|---|
| Thermal amplitude | <22°C | Broad; up to 32°C |
| Spontaneous autoagglutination (in anticoagulated tube of blood) | None | Significant degree which disperses upon warming to 37°C |
| Titer | <64 (seldom >16 at 4°C) | >1000 at 4°C |
| Enhancement by albumin | None | Enhances reactivity |
| Clonality of antibody | Polyclonal | Idiopathic = monoclonal |
| | | Secondary to infection = polyclonal |
| Clinical significance | None | Causes cold AIHA |
| Common antibody specificity | Anti-I | Anti-I |
| Direct antiglobulin test | Negative or weakly positive with polyspecific antiglobulin reagent | 2+ to 3+ with polyspecific antiglobulin reagent |

*Source:* Adapted from Harmening, DM: Clinical Hematology and Fundamentals of Hemostasis, ed 3. FA Davis, Philadelphia, 1997, p 227, with permission.
AIHA = autoimmune hemolytic anemia.

**ABO Typing.** If an individual's RBCs are heavily coated with cold agglutinins, they may agglutinate spontaneously. Consequently, one can obtain false-positive reactions with the routine ABO reagents. In most cases, valid results can be obtained using the patient's cells washed once or twice with normal saline warmed to 37°C. The cold autoantibody elutes from the cells during washing. For example, group O cells coated with cold autoantibody might give the following reactions before and after washing:

| | Anti-A | Anti-B |
|---|---|---|
| Serum suspended RBCs | + | + |
| Saline-washed, suspended RBCs | 0 | 0 |

If more potent autoagglutinins are present, the specimen can be kept at 37°C after collection and the cells washed with 37 to 45°C saline to remove the autoantibody.[21] In the rare situation in which washing with warm saline is not effective, thiol reagents (e.g., dithiothreitol) can be used to disperse the autoagglutination.[22] (See Procedure A of the Procedural Appendix of this chapter.)

Because ABO serum grouping is done at room temperature, cold autoagglutinins can cause discrepancies in the reverse typing also. In the following example, the forward typing results indicate the cells to be group AB. Therefore, one does not expect the serum to agglutinate either the $A_1$ or B cells. Although a number of explanations for this discrepancy exist, a cold agglutinin is a likely cause. Autologous cells should also be tested and will most likely be positive if a cold autoagglutinin is present.

| | Anti-A | Anti-B | |
|---|---|---|---|
| RBCs | 4+ | 4+ | |
| | $A_1$ cells | B cells | Autologous cells |
| Serum | + | + | + |

Such a discrepancy is easily resolved if the serum is prewarmed before testing or if the cold-reactive autoantibody is removed by an autoadsorption technique, and

the tests with the $A_1$ and B cells are repeated with autoadsorbed serum. (See Procedure B in the Procedural Appendix of this chapter.)

| | $A_1$ cells | B cells | Autologous cells |
|---|---|---|---|
| Autoadsorbed serum | 0 | 0 | 0 |

**Rh (D) Typing.** As in ABO cell grouping, one can find false-positive reactions with Rh reagents when testing RBCs coated with cold autoagglutinins. In typing with anti-D (high-protein reagent), the Rh control may be positive, rendering the test invalid. Today, the commonly used monoclonal blend anti-D reagents (low-protein) normally yield valid results. When this type of reagent is used, a negative reaction with any of the ABO reagents serves as the control for the D typing. As stated previously, if a discrepancy exists in the ABO typing, washing the cells in warm saline usually gives acceptable results. This also holds true when testing with low-protein anti-D. Thiol reagents may be used when washing with warm saline is ineffective.

Cold autoagglutinins can activate the complement cascade in vitro, causing complement components to be bound to the RBC and leading to false-positive reactions in the weak D test if a polyspecific antiglobulin reagent is used. The Rh control will also be positive. The use of monospecific anti-IgG for weak D testing or use of RBCs collected into ethylenediaminetetra-acetic

**Table 21–2.** Serologic Reactions of a Typical Cold Autoagglutinin

| Serologic Reactions | O Cells (Screening Cells) | Autologous Cells |
|---|---|---|
| 4°C | 4+ | 4+ |
| RT | + | + |
| 37°C | 0 | 0 |
| AHG (polyspecific) | w+ | w+ |
| AHG (anti-IgG) | 0 | 0 |

RT = room temperature reactions, 20–24°C; AHG = antihuman globulin phase.

acid (EDTA), so that complement cannot bind in vitro, can eliminate the problems of cold agglutinins in D typing. The following examples illustrate these results.

| Testing | Anti-D | Rh Control | Comments |
|---|---|---|---|
| Immediate spin | 0 | 0 | |
| Antihuman globulin (polyspecific) | + | + | Detects complement components |
| Antihuman globulin (anti-IgG) | 0 | 0 | Does not detect complement |
| Red cells collected in EDTA | 0 | 0 | Complement not bound |

Similar problems can be encountered in other phenotyping tests (e.g., K, Fy$^a$) that require the use of an antiglobulin test. Use of an anti-IgG antiglobulin reagent and/or a sample collected in EDTA is recommended when cold autoagglutinins are present.

**Direct Antiglobulin Test.** When a properly collected specimen is used (EDTA), the DAT on a patient with benign cold autoagglutinins is negative. However, one frequently obtains a positive result using polyspecific antiglobulin if a clotted specimen is used, because complement can be activated in vitro. If monospecific reagents are used, these cells are agglutinated by anti-C3 but not by anti-IgG. As discussed in the previous section, one can obtain false-positive antigen typings when clotted specimens and polyspecific antiglobulin reagents are used.

**Antibody Detection and Identification.** The frequency with which cold autoagglutinins interfere with detection and identification of red cell alloantibodies depends to a large extent on the routine procedures used in patient testing. As shown in Table 21–2, cold agglutinins react best at 4°C but are not detected because routine testing is not done at this temperature. Room temperature–reactive autoantibodies will not usually be detected if the laboratory no longer performs routine antibody detection at this phase. Antibodies reactive only at room temperature are usually not clinically significant. Benign cold autoagglutinins do not react at 37°C, but they may interfere with testing at the antiglobulin phase if polyspecific antiglobulin reagent is used. They bind to cells at lower temperatures when the serum and cells are mixed together initially or during centrifugation following the 37°C incubation, and complement is activated. The antibody elutes during the incubation or washing phases, but complement remains attached. Polyspecific antiglobulin reagent will agglutinate the cells coated with C3. When enzyme-treated cells are used, reactions in all phases may be stronger.

Many antibodies capable of causing accelerated red cell destruction are detected by the antiglobulin test; therefore, reactions in this phase may be significant and must be investigated. The reactions caused by a cold autoagglutinin can mask those of an alloantibody. The use of anti-IgG antiglobulin reagent will eliminate most problems with cold autoagglutinin reactivity in the antihuman globulin (AHG) phase.

Other techniques useful in differentiating between cold autoantibodies and alloantibodies are prewarming tests or performing tests with autoadsorbed serum.[21] By prewarming the cells and serum before mixing, avoiding room temperature centrifugation after 37°C incubation, and washing with 37 to 45°C saline, one can prevent the reaction between the cold autoagglutinin and the antigen, thus preventing complement activation. Alloantibodies that are reactive at 37°C, however, can bind to the cells and cause agglutination at the AHG phase. (See Procedure C in the Procedural Appendix of this chapter.) An example of the results of testing a serum that contains a cold autoagglutinin and an anti-Fy$^a$ by routine antiglobulin technique using polyspecific antiglobulin and by the prewarmed technique is shown in Table 21–3. Reactions are present at AHG with both Fy$^a$(+) and Fy$^a$(−) cells. In a prewarmed test, only the reactions expected of the anti-Fy$^a$ are evident. The weak reactions of the cold autoagglutinin are eliminated by prewarming the test. The prewarming technique is simple and successful in most cases. If the autoantibody is very potent, it may be difficult to maintain the cells and serum at 37°C through each phase of testing to avoid the antigen-antibody interaction and complement activation.

Although it is very helpful in resolving problems caused by cold autoagglutinins, the prewarmed technique should not be used indiscriminately. Cases have been reported in which clinically significant alloantibodies have been missed after prewarming.[23] Prewarming should be used only when the reactions obtained indicate the likely presence of a cold autoagglutinin (i.e., autocontrol positive and reactions noted below 37°C). A cold autoagglutinin is not apt to be the answer if only weak reactions are present in the antiglobulin phase with the anti-IgG.

When strong cold autoantibodies are present or if one wishes to identify a room temperature–reactive alloantibody, an absorption must be done to remove the autoantibody. An autologous absorption, described in Procedure B in the Procedural Appendix of this chapter, may be done if the patient has *not* been recently transfused (within 2 to 3 months). An aliquot of patient cells is incubated with an equal aliquot of the patient's serum at 4°C. Autoantibody is removed, and alloantibody remains in the serum. It may be necessary

**Table 21–3.** Reactions Observed with a Serum Containing anti-Fy$^a$ and a Cold Autoagglutinin

| Reagent RBCs | Standard AHG Technique* | Prewarmed AHG Technique |
|---|---|---|
| Fy(a+) | + | + |
| Fy(a−) | +w | 0 |
| Fy(a+) | + | + |
| Fy(a−) | + | 0 |
| Fy(a−) | +w | 0 |
| Fy(a+) | + | + |

*Using polyspecific AHG reagent.

to repeat the absorption several times if the autoantibody is particularly strong. The patient's red cells may be treated with enzymes before absorption to increase the amount of autoantibody removed by the absorption. Autologous absorption is not recommended if a patient has been recently transfused, inasmuch as donor RBCs will be present in the patient's circulation. Alloantibodies, as well as autoantibodies, will be adsorbed if an autoadsorption is performed. In this situation, it is best to use the prewarmed technique or adsorption using rabbit erythrocyte stroma (see Procedure D in the Procedural Appendix of this chapter).

If anti-IgG antiglobulin reagent is used, one can avoid the problem caused by most cold agglutinins. However, one can miss very rare clinically significant alloantibodies that are detected only with polyspecific antiglobulin because they bind complement. Use of anti-IgG reagents is an attractive alternative when prewarming is not effective and there is not enough time to adsorb the serum.

**Compatibility Testing.** The difficulties encountered in antibody detection and identification tests are also found in compatibility tests because the most commonly encountered autoantibody (autoanti-I) is directed against an antigen that is found on the RBCs of most random donors as well as on most reagent red cells. Compatibility tests, like antibody identification tests, can be done with prewarmed or autoadsorbed serum or using anti-IgG antiglobulin reagent.

Two of the other common cold autoagglutinins, anti-IH and anti-H, distinguish between reagent RBCs and random donor cells. As discussed in the following section on specificity, anti-IH and anti-H react best with group O cells; they react less well with group $A_1$ and $A_1$B cells. Anti-IH and anti-H are found most often in the serum of group $A_1$ and $A_1$B persons; therefore, the units selected for compatibility testing (group A or AB) are those which give the weakest, if any, reactivity. On the other hand, group O cells (antibody screening cells) give the strongest reactions.

### Specificity of Cold Autoagglutinins

**Anti-I, Anti-i.** Most cold-reactive autoantibodies have anti-I specificity. The I antigen is fully expressed on the RBCs of virtually all adults, whereas it is only weakly expressed on cord RBCs. At birth, the infant has the i antigen on the cells. As an infant matures, the i antigen is converted to I antigen; the amount of I antigen increases until the adult levels are reached at about 2 years of age.[21] Very rarely do adults lack the I antigen; and if they do lack it, they are termed "i adults" and may produce alloanti-I.

The reactivities of several examples of anti-I are given in Table 21–4. As shown, anti-I specificity may be apparent when a serum is tested with adult and cord cells. Serum 1, for example, reacts with adult cells but not with cord cells. Serum 2 reacts with both adult and cord cells, but the preference for the adult cells is still obvious. Alloanti-I is frequently present in the serum of i adults.[24]

**Table 21–4.** Reactions of Sera Containing Anti-I with Adult and Cord Cells

| Sera | Serum Dilution | RBCs | |
|---|---|---|---|
| | | Adult | Cord |
| Serum 1 | Neat | 3+ | 0 |
| Serum 2 | Neat | 4+ | 2+ |
| | 1:2 | 4+ | + |
| | 1:4 | 3+ | 0 |
| | 1:8 | 2+ | 0 |

Anti-i is a relatively uncommon autoantibody. As shown in Table 21–5, this antibody reacts in an antithetical manner to anti-I. Cord cells and i adult cells have the most i antigen; adult I cells have the least.

**Anti-H, Anti-IH.** Cold agglutinins found in the serum of group $A_1$ and $A_1$B individuals (and rarely group B) may have the specificity of an anti-H. This antibody distinguishes between cells of various ABO groups. Group O and $A_2$ cells react best because they have the most H substance. Group $A_1$ and $A_1$B cells have the least H antigen, so they react weakly. The pattern of reactivity seen with anti-H is shown in Table 21–5. See Chapter 5 for a discussion of the ABO system and H substance.

It is very important not to confuse cold-reactive anti-H with the anti-H found in the serum of $O_h$ (Bombay) individuals who lack the H antigen. Cold-reactive anti-H is an autoantibody even though the cells of the antibody maker ($A_1$ or $A_1$B) may give considerably weaker reactions. The anti-H in the $O_h$ person is a potent alloantibody, reacts at 4 to 37°C, and is capable of causing rapid intravascular RBC destruction.

Anti-IH, another of the usually harmless cold autoagglutinins, is also found more commonly in the serum of $A_1$ and $A_1$B individuals. This antibody agglutinates only RBCs that have both the I and the H antigens. As with anti-H, group O and group $A_2$ cells react best. The difference between these two antibodies is that group O $i_{cord}$ cells and group O $i_{adult}$ cells react as strongly as group O $I_{adult}$ cells with anti-H, but not with anti-IH (see Table 21–5).

**Table 21–5.** Relative Strengths of Serologic Reactions of Cold Autoagglutinins at 4°C

| RBC Phenotype | Anti-I | Anti-i | Anti-H | Anti-IH |
|---|---|---|---|---|
| O I (adult) | 4+ | + | 4+ | 4+ |
| $A_1$ I (adult) | 4+ | + | + | + |
| $A_2$ I (adult) | 4+ | + | 2+ | 2+ |
| $O_h$ I (adult) | 4+ | + | 0 | 2+ |
| O i (cord) | + | 3+ | 4+ | + |
| O i (adult) | + | 4+ | 4+ | + |
| $A_1$ i (adult) | + | 4+ | + | 0 |
| $A_2$ i (adult) | + | 4+ | 2+ | + |
| $O_h$ i (adult) | + | 4+ | 0 | 0 |

*Sera are ABO compatible with RBCs.

## Other Cold-Reactive Autoagglutinins

A number of other less commonly encountered cold autoagglutinins have been described, such as anti-Pr, anti-Gd, and anti-Sd$^x$ (anti-R$_x$). The reader is referred to the review by Marsh[25] for additional information. Cold autoantibodies with the specificity of anti-M have also been described.[26] Most workers agree that specificity of cold-reactive autoantibodies is primarily of academic interest and usually not clinically important. However, development of autoantibodies with specificities for integral components of the RBC membrane, such as the glycophorins or Band 3, may be precursors for development of other autoimmune disorders, such as systemic lupus erythematosus or rheumatoid arthritis.[27]

## Pathologic Cold Autoagglutinins

### Cold Hemagglutinin Disease (Idiopathic Cold AIHA)

Most cold autoagglutinins do not cause RBC destruction, but in some patients they can cause hemolytic anemia that varies in severity from mild to life-threatening intravascular lysis. Cold-reactive immune hemolytic anemia may be a chronic, idiopathic (no identifiable cause) condition or an acute, transient disorder often associated with an infectious disease, such as *Mycoplasma pneumoniae* pneumonia or infectious mononucleosis. Cold agglutinin syndrome (CAS), also called cold hemagglutinin disease (CHD) or idiopathic cold AIHA, represents approximately 16 percent of the cases of AIHA. A moderate chronic hemolytic anemia is produced by a cold autoantibody that optimally reacts at 4°C but also reacts between 25 and 31°C. The antibody is usually an IgM immunoglobulin, which quite efficiently activates complement.

**Clinical Picture.** Cold hemagglutinin disease occurs predominantly in older individuals, with a peak incidence in those over 50 years of age. Antibody specificity in this disorder is almost always anti-I, less commonly anti-i, and rarely anti-Pr. It is rarely severe and is usually seasonal, inasmuch as the winter months often precipitate the signs and symptoms of a chronic hemolytic anemia. Acrocyanosis of the hands, feet, ears, and nose is frequently the patient's main complaint, along with a sense of numbness in the extremities. Changes take place when the person is exposed to the cold, because the cold autoantibody agglutinates the patient's RBCs as they pass through the skin capillaries, resulting in localized blood stasis. During cold winter weather, the temperature of an individual's blood falls to as low as 28°C in the extremities, activating the cold autoantibody in these patients. The antibody then agglutinates the RBCs and fixes complement as the cells flow through the capillaries of the skin, causing autoagglutination and signs of acrocyanosis. These patients may also experience hemoglobinuria, because the complement fixation may result in intravascular hemolysis. Figure 21–1 illustrates the relation between LDH concentration, a reflection of the severity of hemolysis, and ambient temperature in such a patient over a period of 18 months.[28] However, this intravascular hemolytic episode is not associated with fever, chills, or acute renal insufficiency, any one of which is characteristic of patients with paroxysmal cold hemoglobinuria (PCH) or severe warm AIHA.

Patients usually display weakness, pallor, and weight loss, which are characteristic symptoms of a chronic anemia. Cold hemagglutinin disease usually remains quite stable, and if it does progress in severity, it is insidious in intensity. Physical findings such as hepatosplenomegaly are infrequent because of the mechanism of hemolysis.

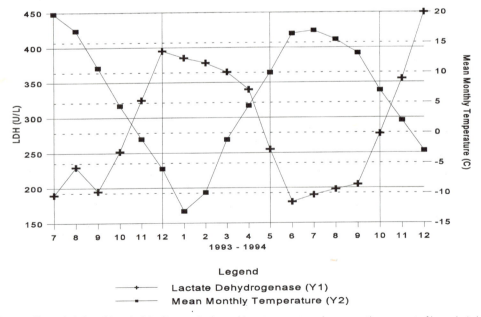

**Figure 21–1.** Seasonal hemolysis in cold agglutinin disease. As the ambient temperature decreases, the amount of hemolysis (reflected in serum lactate dehydrogenase levels) increases. During warmer months, LDH levels return to normal.

Other clinical features of CHD include jaundice and Raynaud's phenomenon (symptoms of cold intolerance, such as pain and bluish tinge in the fingertips and toes as a result of vasospasm). Patients with severe CHD usually live more comfortably in warmer climates.

**Laboratory Findings.** Laboratory findings in CHD include reticulocytosis and a positive DAT resulting from complement coating only. It is suggested that a simple serum-screening procedure be performed initially to test the ability of the patient's serum to agglutinate autologous saline-suspended red cells at 18 to 20°C. If this test result is positive, further steps may be taken to determine the titer and thermal amplitude of the patient's cold autoantibody. If it is negative, the diagnosis of CHD is unlikely. The peripheral smear of a patient with CHD may show agglutination, polychromasia, mild to moderate anisocytosis, and poikilocytosis (**Color Plate 19**). Autoagglutination of anticoagulated whole blood samples is characteristic of CHD and occurs quickly as the blood cools to room temperature, causing the binding of cold autoantibodies to the patient's red cells. As a result of this autoagglutination, performance of automated blood counts and preparation of blood smears are extremely difficult with these patient samples. Leukocyte and platelet counts are usually normal.

Table 21–6 summarizes the clinical criteria for diagnosis of CHD.

**Selection of Blood for Transfusion.** Most patients with CHD do not require transfusion; however, when they do, it is sometimes difficult to select blood. As previously described, potent cold autoantibodies interfere with most routine tests. Perhaps the most difficult problem is to detect and identify alloantibodies. Procedures to manage these problems were described earlier in this chapter. It is important to give red cells compatible with any clinically significant alloantibodies. Most patients receive transfusion of blood that is positive for the autoantibody. Units of $i_{adult}$ RBCs are extremely rare and should be reserved for patients with alloanti-I.

The issue of transfusion in CHD patients is most relevant in patients undergoing surgical procedures that use hypothermia (lowering of the body temperature to 22 to 30°C), such as cardiac procedures. For patients with CHD, blood for transfusion can be warmed through an approved blood warmer, or the operative procedures can be performed without subjecting the patient to hypothermia.[29]

### Cold Autoantibodies Related to Infection (Secondary Cold AIHA)

Cold hemagglutinin disease can also occur as a transient disorder secondary to infection. Episodes of cold autoimmune hemolytic anemia often occur after upper respiratory infections. Approximately 50 percent of patients suffering from pneumonia caused by *Mycoplasma pneumoniae* have cold agglutinin titers of greater than 64. In the second or third week of the patient's illness, CHD may occur in association with the infection, and a rapid onset of hemolysis is observed. Pallor and jaundice are characteristically present. Acrocyanosis and hemoglobinuria are uncommon and not consistently present. Usually, resolution of the episode occurs within 2 to 3 weeks because the hemolysis is self-limiting. The offending cold autoantibody is an IgM immunoglobulin with a characteristic anti-I specificity. Very high titers of cold autoagglutinins are seen almost exclusively in patients with *M. pneumoniae*. It has been reported that the cold agglutinin produced in this infection is an immunologic response to the mycoplasma antigens, and this antibody crossreacts with the red cell I antigen.

The antibodies produced in primary CHD and in this disorder secondary to *M. pneumoniae* both have anti-I specificity, and the RBCs are sensitized with complement components. If the complement cascade does not proceed to C9 (cell death by lysis), the macrophages of the reticuloendothelial system can still clear the sensitized RBCs through their receptors for C3b fragments, thereby causing hemolysis.

Infectious mononucleosis also may be associated with a hemolytic anemia resulting from a cold autoantibody. Although it occurs infrequently, it has been well documented that a high-titered IgM anti-i with a wide thermal range plays a major role in hemolytic anemia associated with this viral infection. Acute illness with a sore throat and a high fever, followed by weakness, anemia, and jaundice is a characteristic feature of infectious mononucleosis. Lymphadenopathy and hepatosplenomegaly are common findings. A larger percentage of patients with infectious mononucleosis have been reported to develop anti-i, but only a small number of these patients develop the antibody of sufficient titer and thermal amplitude to induce in vivo hemolysis. Table 21–7 reviews the cold autoantibody

---

**Table 21–6.** Clinical Criteria for the Diagnosis of Cold Agglutinin Disease

1. Clinical signs of an acquired hemolytic anemia, with a history (which may or may not be present) of acrocyanosis and hemoglobinuria on exposure to cold
2. A positive DAT result using polyspecific antisera
3. A positive DAT result using monospecific anti-C3 antisera
4. A negative DAT result using monospecific anti-IgG antisera
5. The presence of reactivity in the patient's serum due to a cold autoantibody
6. A cold agglutinin titer of 1000 or greater in saline at 4°C with visible agglutination of anticoagulated blood at room temperature

*Source:* Adapted from Harmening, DM: Clinical Hematology and Fundamentals of Hemostasis, ed 3. FA Davis, Philadelphia, 1997, p 229, with permission.
DAT = direct antiglobulin test.

---

**Table 21–7.** Secondary Cold AIHA

| Type of Infection | Cold Autoantibody Specificity |
|---|---|
| *Mycoplasma pneumoniae* | Anti-I |
| Infectious mononucleosis | Anti-i |

specificity most commonly found in the infections that cause secondary CHD.

**Treatment.** Therapy for CHD is generally unnecessary. Most patients require no treatment and are instructed to avoid the cold, keep warm, or move to a milder climate. Patients with moderate anemia are given the same instructions, urging them to tolerate the symptoms rather than to use drugs on a therapeutic trial basis. There is some advantage to the use of plasma exchange in more severe cases, inasmuch as IgM antibodies have a predominantly intravascular distribution. However, response to plasma exchange is still variable in this patient population. Corticosteroids also have been used but generally have a poor effect. In some patients whose red cells are strongly coated with C3, successful results have been reported with corticosteroids. Some favorable responses also have been reported with the alkylating drug chlorambucil. Splenectomy is generally considered ineffective.

### Paroxysmal Cold Hemoglobinuria

Paroxysmal cold hemoglobinuria (PCH) is the least common type of AIHA, with an incidence of between 1 and 2 percent. It is, however, more common in children in association with viral illnesses such as measles, mumps, chickenpox, infectious mononucleosis, and the ill-defined "flu syndrome." Originally, PCH was described in association with syphilis, with an autoantibody formed in response to the *Treponema pallidum* infection. However, with the effective treatment of syphilis with antibiotics, PCH is no longer commonly reported in relation to syphilis.

Red cell destruction is caused by a cold autoantibody referred to as a *biphasic autohemolysin,* which binds to the patient's red cells at low temperatures and fixes complement. Hemolysis occurs when the body temperature rises to 37°C and the sensitized cells undergo complement-mediated intravascular lysis. In contrast to the other cold-reactive autoagglutinins, the antibody in PCH is an IgG immunoglobulin with biphasic activity. The classic antibody produced in PCH is called the Donath-Landsteiner antibody and has the specificity of an autoanti-P. Other specificities have been reported, including anti-i[30] and anti-Pr-like.[31]

To confirm the diagnosis of PCH, the Donath-Landsteiner test is performed in the laboratory. This test involves the collection of two blood specimens from the patient. One specimen, the control, is maintained at 37°C for 60 minutes after collection. The second sample is cooled at 4°C for 30 minutes and then incubated at 37°C for an additional 30 minutes. Both samples are then centrifuged and observed for hemolysis. In a positive Donath-Landsteiner test, hemolysis is demonstrable in the sample placed at 4°C and then at 37°C, whereas no hemolysis is observed in the control sample. Table 21–8 summarizes the reactions of the Donath-Landsteiner test.

As the name of PCH implies, paroxysmal or intermittent episodes of hemoglobinuria occur on exposure

**Table 21–8.** Donath-Landsteiner Test

|  | Whole Blood Sample 1 (Control) | Whole Blood Sample 2 (Test) |
|---|---|---|
| *Procedure:* |  |  |
| 1. 30 min | 37°C | 4°C |
| 2. 30 min | 37°C | 37°C |
| 3. Centrifuge and observe |  |  |
| *Results:* |  |  |
| Positive | No hemolysis | Hemolysis |
| Negative | No hemolysis | No hemolysis |
| Inconclusive | Hemolysis | Hemolysis |

*Source:* Harmening, DM: Clinical Hematology and Fundamentals of Hemostasis, ed 3. FA Davis, Philadelphia, 1997, p 230, with permission.

to cold. These acute attacks are characterized by sudden onset of fever, shaking chills, malaise, abdominal cramps, and back pain. All the signs of intravascular hemolysis are evident, along with hemoglobinemia, hemoglobinuria, and bilirubinemia, depending on the severity and frequency of the attack (Fig. 21–2). This results in a severe and rapidly progressive anemia with hemoglobin levels frequently around 4 to 5 g/dL. Polychromasia, nucleated red blood cells, and poikilocytosis are demonstrated in the peripheral smear, findings that are consistent with hemolytic anemia. These signs and symptoms, as well as hemoglobinuria, may resolve in a few hours or persist for days. Splenomegaly, hyperbilirubinemia, and renal insufficiency may also develop.

Paroxysmal cold hemoglobinuria is an acute hemolytic anemia occurring almost exclusively in chil-

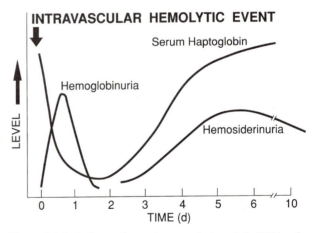

**Figure 21–2.** Indicator of acute intravascular hemolysis. Within a few hours of an acute hemolytic event, free hemoglobin is cleared from plasma and the serum haptoglobin falls to undetectable levels. Hemoglobinuria ceases soon after this. If no further hemolysis occurs, the serum haptoglobin level recovers and methemalbumin disappears within several days. The urinary hemosiderin can provide more lasting evidence of the hemolytic event. (From Hillman, RS, and Finch, CA: Red Cell Manual, ed 7. FA Davis, Philadelphia, 1996, p 112, with permission.)

**Table 21–9.** Comparison of PCH and Cold Agglutinin Syndrome

|  | PCH | Cold Agglutinin Syndrome |
|---|---|---|
| Patient population | Children and young adults | Elderly or middle-aged adults |
| Pathogenesis | Following viral infection | Idiopathic; lymphoproliferative disorder; following *Mycoplasma pneumoniae* infection |
| Clinical features | Hemoglobinuria: acute attacks upon exposure to cold (symptoms resolve in hours to days) | Acrocyanosis; autoagglutination of blood at room temperature |
| Severity of hemolysis | Acute and rapid | Chronic and rarely severe |
| Site of hemolysis | Intravascular | Extravascular/intravascular |
| Autoantibody class | IgG (anti-P specificity)—biphasic hemolysin | IgM (anti-I/i) monophasic |
| DAT | 2–3+ polyspecific AHG; neg IgG; 3–4+ C3 monospecific AHG | 2–3+ polyspecific AHG; neg IgG; 3–4+ C3 monospecific AHG |
| Thermal range | Moderate (<20°C) | High (up to 30–31°C) |
| Titer | Moderate (<64) | High (>1000) |
| Donath-Landsteiner Test | Positive | Negative |
| Treatment | Supportive (disorder terminates when underlying illness resolves) | Avoid cold |

*Source:* Harmening, DM: Clinical Hematology and Fundamentals of Hemostasis, ed 3. FA Davis, Philadelphia, 1997, p 230, with permission.

dren and young adults, and almost always represents a transient disorder. Table 21–9 compares and contrasts PCH with CHD.

**Treatment.** For chronic forms of PCH, protection from cold exposure is the only useful therapy. Acute postinfection forms of PCH usually terminate spontaneously after resolution of the infectious process. Steroids and transfusion may be required, depending on the severity of the attacks.

Paroxysmal nocturnal hemoglobinuria (PNH) is often confused with PCH because of the similarity of the names and acronyms. An autoantibody has not been implicated in PNH; a membrane defect is thought to be involved. Red cell destruction in PNH is complement-mediated because of the absence or reduced amounts of some complement regulatory proteins.[32] The only reason for this comment is to alert the reader to a common error in relating PCH and PNH.

## WARM-REACTIVE AUTOANTIBODIES

Autoantibodies that react best at 37°C are not found as often as the almost universal cold autoanti-I. However, many more of the true autoimmune hemolytic anemias are of the warm type (70 percent) than of the cold-reactive type (16 percent).[6] As with the cold-reactive autoantibodies, some individuals have apparently harmless warm autoantibodies. However, the harmless autoantibodies are serologically indistinguishable from the harmful ones. There are no diagnostic tests to determine which autoantibodies will cause red cell destruction. When a warm-reactive autoantibody is encountered, it should be characterized as such and reported to the patient's physician. The presence of the antibody may alert the physician to an underlying autoimmune disease.

## Clinical Findings

Patients with warm AIHA present a different problem to the blood bank than those with cold AIHA. A significant percentage of cases suffer from an anemia of sufficient severity to require transfusion. The degree of anemia is variable; however, hemoglobins less than 7 g/dL are not uncommon. The onset of warm AIHA is usually insidious and may be precipitated by a variety of factors such as infection,[33] trauma, surgery, pregnancy,[34] or psychological stress. In other patients the onset is sudden and unexplained. Warm AIHA may be idiopathic, with no underlying disease process, or secondary to a pathologic disorder. Table 21–10 lists the disorders commonly associated with AIHA.

Signs and symptoms appear when a significant anemia has developed. Pallor, weakness, dizziness, dyspnea, jaundice, and unexplained fever are occasionally presenting complaints. Hemolysis is usually acute at

**Table 21–10.** Disorders Reported to Be Frequently Associated with Warm AIHA

1. Reticuloendothelial neoplasms, such as chronic lymphocytic leukemia, Hodgkin's disease, non-Hodgkin's lymphomas, thymomas
2. Collagen disease, such as systemic lupus erythematosus, scleroderma, and rheumatoid arthritis
3. Infectious diseases, such as viral syndromes in childhood and adults
4. Immunologic diseases, such as hypogammaglobulinemia, dysglobulinemia, and other immune-deficiency syndromes
5. Gastrointestinal diseases, such as ulcerative colitis
6. Benign tumors, such as ovarian dermoid cysts
7. Pregnancy

*Source:* Adapted from Petz, LD, and Garratty, G: Acquired Immune Hemolytic Anemias. Churchill Livingstone, New York, 1980, p 32, with permission.
AIHA = autoimmune hemolytic anemia.

onset and may stabilize or continue to accelerate at a variable rate.

The peripheral blood smear usually displays polychromasia, reflecting reticulocytosis, which is characteristic of a hemolytic anemia (Color Plate 20). Spherocytosis and occasionally red cell fragmentation, indicating extravascular hemolysis, can be demonstrated along with nucleated red blood cells. An uncommon manifestation of warm AIHA is reticulocytopenia. This may be associated with a hypoplastic marrow that is secondary to an underlying disease state. Because antigenic determinants on erythrocyte precursors also can react with the patient's red cell autoantibodies, reticulocytes can be destroyed as they are released from the bone marrow. Reticulocytopenia at the time of intense hemolysis, therefore, is associated with a high mortality. Products of hemolysis such as bilirubin (particularly the unconjugated or indirect fraction) and urinary urobilinogen are increased. In severe cases, depleted serum haptoglobin, hemoglobinemia, hemoglobinuria, and increases in LDH may be demonstrated.

## Red Cell Hemolysis

In 80 percent of cases of warm AIHA, the antibody causing the hemolysis is an IgG immunoglobulin, with IgG subclasses 1 and 3 found in patients demonstrating clinical signs of hemolytic anemia. The subclasses or isotypes of IgG are distinguished by the number of disulfide bonds present in the hinge region of the molecule, accounting for their different electrophoretic mobility and biologic properties. Refer to Chapter 3 for a complete discussion of the properties of the IgG subclasses. All IgG subclasses possess the ability to bind complement via the classical pathway of activation, with IgG3 being more efficient than IgG1, which in turn is more efficient than IgG2. Macrophages possess receptors for the Fc region of IgG1 and IgG3.

Immune red cell destruction resulting from sensitization with IgG antibody is primarily extravascular, taking place in the fixed reticuloendothelial system (RES) cells of the liver and spleen. However, the spleen is 100 times more efficient in removal of IgG-sensitized red cells. Macrophages are equipped with two important biologic receptors on their membranes: (1) receptors for the Fc fragments of IgG1 and IgG3 immunoglobulins, and (2) receptors for the C3b fragment of complement. Sensitized red cells are phagocytized by interaction with RES mononuclear phagocytes, depending on which protein coats the erythrocytes. If only IgG coats the red cells, gradual phagocytosis of the erythrocytes occurs. If both IgG and C3b are coating the red cells, there is a rapid phagocytosis, because the C3b fragment augments the action of IgG, enhancing sequestration and phagocytosis of the coated erythrocytes. If only C3b is coating the red cells, transient immune adherence occurs. It has been estimated that more than 100,000 molecules of the complement fragment would be required to induce phagocytosis. Therefore, the activity of the macrophages

**Table 21–11.** Factors Affecting Activity of Macrophages

1. Subclass of IgG, especially IgG1 and IgG3
2. Presence of complement (C3b) fragments
3. Quantity of immunoglobulin or complement
4. Number and activity of helper T cells (CD4)
5. Number and activity of suppressor T cells (CD8)

*Source:* Adapted from Pittiglio, D, and Sacher, RA: Clinical Hematology and Fundamentals of Hemostasis. FA Davis, Philadelphia, 1987, p 153, with permission.

and the severity of hemolysis via phagocytosis of sensitized RBCs are dependent on various factors, summarized in Table 21–11.

## Serologic Characteristics

Because warm-reactive autoantibodies are typically IgG immunoglobulins, they react best by the antiglobulin technique. As a rule, they do not agglutinate saline-suspended RBCs after 37°C incubation. However, if one adds albumin or another agglutination potentiator to the reaction mixture, one may observe agglutination in this phase. They may activate complement and are usually enhanced by enzyme techniques. Most of these autoantibodies react with a high-incidence antigen and often have a general specificity within the Rh blood group system, but there are reports of autoantibodies associated with most of the other blood group systems. Identification of autoantibodies is discussed in the following section. The typical reactions of warm autoantibodies are shown in Table 21–12.

### Laboratory Tests Affected by Warm-Reactive Autoantibodies

Warm-reactive autoantibodies can interfere with most routine blood bank tests, and they may present more of a dilemma than cold autoagglutinins. Most cold autoantibodies can be avoided if testing is performed at 37°C or if anti-IgG antiglobulin is used. In the case of warm AIHA, however, both significant alloantibodies and the autoantibodies react best at 37°C. Therefore, one may have to use more complicated and time-consuming procedures to resolve the problems.

**Table 21–12.** Serologic Reactions of Typical Warm Autoantibodies

| Reaction Phase | Screening Cells | Autologous Cells |
|---|---|---|
| RT | 0 | 0 |
| 37°C* | 0 | 0 |
| AHG | 2–3+ | 4+ |

*Agglutination may be observed if the RBCs are suspended in albumin or low ionic strength solution or if they are enzyme-treated.
RT = room temperature; AHG = antihuman globulin.

**ABO Typing.** Because warm-reactive autoantibodies are not direct agglutinins, ABO grouping is usually not affected. Even though the patient's cells may be heavily coated with antibody, they normally do not agglutinate spontaneously when reagent anti-A and anti-B are added. Similarly, warm autoantibodies in the serum usually do not agglutinate saline-suspended $A_1$ and B cells.

**Rh (D) Typing.** False-positive D typing tests can be a problem when the patient's cells are coated with warm-reactive autoantibodies. Agglutination potentiators are added to many Rh typing reagents (the slide/modified tube reagents) so that D-positive cells, once coated with anti-D, will directly agglutinate. Potentiators are beneficial because they allow one to perform an immediate spin test for the D antigen. The disadvantage of adding potentiators is that cells coated with any antibody may be agglutinated, including D-negative cells coated with autoantibody. For this reason a control test, consisting of patient cells and the matched Rh diluent, must be performed in parallel with the D typing test when using the high-protein (slide/modified tube) reagents. The results of the D antigen typing are valid only when the control is negative.

Similar problems that occur with cold autoagglutinins can be easily resolved by washing the cells with warm saline. Warm-reactive autoantibodies cannot be easily removed from the cells, so other approaches must be used. Most of the time, valid results can be obtained using a low-protein anti-D reagent (the monoclonal/polyclonal blend-IgG or saline-reactive IgM). As stated previously in this chapter, a negative reaction among the ABO forward typing results serves as a control for the low-protein anti-D reagents. If the patient types as AB, D-positive (all tubes in the ABO forward and D typings are positive), a separate Rh control (matched diluent or 6 percent albumin) must be tested along with the anti-D to ensure that the D antigen typing is valid. (Refer to Chapter 6.) In an extreme situation, the cells may be treated with chloroquine diphosphate according to the procedure by Edwards and others[35] to remove the IgG antibody from the cells before typing. (See Procedure E in the Procedural Appendix of this chapter.)

If one wishes to test for the weak expression of the D antigen, one may use special techniques for removal of the autoantibody before performance of the weak D test. Monospecific anti-IgG antiglobulin is of no help in this situation because the autoantibody is IgG in nature. Chloroquine-treated cells, as described previously, may be used. Another technique, the rosette test commonly used in detection of fetal-maternal hemorrhage, may also be used to detect D-positive cells. (Refer to Chapter 20, "Hemolytic Disease of the Newborn," for discussion of the rosette test.) This screening test, used to detect fetal D-positive cells in the circulation of the D-negative mother, will also detect D-positive cells in any cell population. If the patient's cells are D-positive, the rosette test will be strongly positive. Inasmuch as the rosette test does not incorporate an antiglobulin phase, a patient with a positive DAT can be accurately typed for the D antigen by this method.

It is important to note that it is not absolutely necessary to determine the correct weak D typing of a patient with warm AIHA, inasmuch as D-negative RBCs can be transfused if necessary.

**Direct Antiglobulin Test (DAT).** A positive DAT is expected in association with warm-reactive autoantibodies. As autoantibody is produced, it adsorbs onto the associated antigens present on the patient's own RBCs. The RBCs may then be coated with IgG alone (20 percent), IgG and complement (67 percent), or complement alone (13 percent).[6] In rare cases, the DAT may be negative or cells coated only with IgA or IgM.[16-18]

**Antibody Detection and Identification.** The serum of a patient with warm autoagglutinins may contain only autoantibody or a mixture of autoantibody and alloantibody, if the patient has previously received a transfusion or has been pregnant. When smaller amounts of autoantibody have been produced, all of the autoantibody may be adsorbed onto the patient's cells in vivo, and no free autoantibody will be detectable in the serum.

When warm-reactive autoantibodies are present in the serum or on the patient's cells, the extent of the testing should be based upon the patient's history. It must be determined that the antibody coating the patient's cells is an autoantibody, and limited testing should be performed to determine the specificity. If the patient has had a previous transfusion or has been pregnant, efforts must be made to detect clinically significant alloantibodies that might be masked by the autoantibody.

*Evaluation of Autoantibody.* A positive DAT can result from RBC alloantibodies or drug-induced antibodies as well as from RBC autoantibodies. IgG may be present on the cells in each case, and antibody may not be present in the serum. It is important to differentiate the origins of a positive DAT because selection of RBCs for transfusion and treatment protocols differ. To make the distinction between these causes, one must have the patient's medical history, including previous transfusions and pregnancies, diagnoses, and medications. When a patient has had a recent transfusion, one must consider the possibility that alloantibodies are coating the remaining transfused donor cells. In most cases, by examining the DAT microscopically for mixed-field agglutination and by determining the specificity of the antibody in the eluate, one can establish alloantibodies as the cause (see Chapter 18, "Adverse Effects of Blood Transfusion," in this text). Inasmuch as warm autoantibodies are frequently associated with certain diseases, such as systemic lupus erythematosus (SLE), and with medications, such as Aldomet, the patient's diagnosis and drug history are informative. As discussed below, the specificity of the antibody may be helpful in differentiating between autoantibody and alloantibody.

To identify the specificity of a warm-reactive autoantibody, one must test an eluate prepared from the patient's RBCs, in addition to the patient's serum, against a panel of reagent red cells. (See Procedure F in the Procedural Appendix of this chapter for instructions in preparing a digitonin-acid eluate.) If the patient has not been recently transfused (within the past 2 to 3 months), one can assume that any antibody activity in the eluate is autoantibody. The serum may contain alloantibody in addition to autoantibody.

The reactions of an autoantibody may be different in the serum and in the eluate. Warm autoantibodies may have an apparent autoanti-e specificity in the serum but may show panagglutination of RBCs tested with the eluate because the concentration of antibody removed from the cells in the elution process may be greater than that in the serum. Table 21–13 illustrates an example of such reactivity. Differing elution techniques may also yield varying results in testing eluate (i.e., a heat eluate generally reacts more weakly than an acid eluate or one of the "chemical" eluates, such as dichloromethane or ether).

Many warm-reactive autoantibodies have a complex Rh-like specificity similar to those shown in Table 21–14. They may react with all RBCs of normal Rh phenotype (e.g., cde/cde, CDe/cDE). To categorize them as anti-nl (normal), anti-pdl (partially deleted), or anti-dl (deleted), one must use very rare RBCs; for example, partially deleted ($-D-/-D-$) and fully deleted ($Rh_{null}$) cells.[36] Classification in this manner is purely academic.

There are numerous reports of autoantibodies with specificities other than Rh, many of which appear to be directed against antigens of high incidence. Among the other specificities are autoanti-U, $-Wr^a$, $-En^a$, $-Kp^b$,[37] $-Vel$,[38] and $-Ge$.[39] The reader is referred to Chapter 7 of Petz and Garratty[6] for a detailed discussion of autoantibody specificity. Apparent specificities

such as these can cause confusion, especially when the patient has had a recent transfusion. Determination of the patient's phenotype is crucial to classifying the antibody as auto or allo.

Most workers agree that it is not necessary to do extensive studies to identify autoantibodies, but they do recommend limited testing. By testing a commercial red cell panel, one can identify an antibody of simple specificity. This information may be useful in evaluating whether the antibody is autoantibody or alloantibody. On the other hand, an antibody that is reactive with all cells is probably an autoantibody. There are, however, many exceptions to these interpretations. The need to consider the medical history cannot be overemphasized. Specificity may also be helpful in selecting blood for transfusion. Some workers prefer to transfuse RBCs that are compatible with the autoantibody when, for example, the specificity is anti-e-like. However, because the transfused cells are most likely to be destroyed as rapidly as the patient's own cells, regardless of phenotype, it is best to reserve e-negative RBCs for those patients with alloanti-e.

*Detection and Identification of Alloantibodies.* All workers agree that detection and identification of all alloantibodies are of primary concern when one must give a transfusion to a patient with warm AIHA, especially when the patient has had a previous transfusion or pregnancy. When autoantibody is found in the serum, it will typically mask any alloantibodies present. In this situation one can use several techniques:

1. If the autoantibody demonstrates a specificity, such as anti-e, test a panel of cells negative for the corresponding antigen (e-negative, in this case) and positive for other important antigens—Kell, Duffy, Kidd, S, and s.
2. If the patient has *not* had a recent transfusion (within the past 2 to 3 months), remove the autoantibody by adsorption with autologous RBCs.
3. If the patient has had a recent transfusion or if the patient is severely anemic, determine the patient's phenotype for the common RBC antigens (Rh, Kell, Kidd, Duffy, MNSs) and adsorb the autoantibody with RBCs of selected phenotypically similar donors (allogeneic absorption).

When autoantibodies have a broader specificity, an absorption technique must be employed. See discussion below of considerations in using an autoadsorption procedure. In a warm autoadsorption, the patient's serum and autologous cells are incubated at 37°C, allowing the autoantibody to be bound to the autologous cells and leaving any alloantibody in the serum. To improve the uptake of autoantibody, some of the antibody that has coated the cells in vivo can be removed by a gentle elution at 45°C, or the cells can be treated with the ZZAP reagent, a mixture of proteolytic enzyme and thiol reagent. If there is a large amount of autoantibody in the serum, more than one absorption may be necessary (see Procedure G in the Procedural Appendix of this chapter). Table 21–15 gives an exam-

**Table 21–13.** Serologic Reactions of Serum and Eluates Containing Warm Autoantibodies

| RBC Phenotype | Antiglobulin Reactions | | |
|---|---|---|---|
| | Serum | Acid Eluate | Heat Eluate |
| Dce/DCe | + | 4+ | 2+ |
| DcE/DcE | 0 | 3+ | + |
| dce/dce | + | 4+ | 2+ |
| Dce/dce | + | 4+ | 2+ |
| dcE/dcE | 0 | 3+ | + |

**Table 21–14.** Serologic Reactions of Warm Autoantibodies with RBCs of Selected Rh Phenotypes

| | RBC Phenotype | | |
|---|---|---|---|
| | Normal (cde/cde, etc.) | Partially Deleted $-D-/-D-$, etc. | Fully Deleted ($Rh_{null}$) |
| Anti-nl | + | 0 | 0 |
| Anti-pdl | + | + | 0 |
| Anti-dl | + | + | + |

**Table 21–15.** Antibody Detection Using Unabsorbed and Autoabsorbed Serum

| Reagent | *Unabsorbed* | | *Absorbed × 1* | | *Absorbed × 2* | |
| --- | --- | --- | --- | --- | --- | --- |
| Red Cells | 37°C | AHG | 37°C | AHG | 37°C | AHG |
| I | + | 3+ | 0 | + | 0 | 0 |
| II | + | 3+ | 0 | + | 0 | 0 |

AHG = antihuman globulin.

**Table 21–16.** Differential Absorption Technique for Detecting Alloantibodies in the Serum of a Patient with Warm-Reactive Autoantibodies

| Donor | RBC Phenotype of Adsorbing Cells | Antibody Remaining in Absorbed Serum |
| --- | --- | --- |
| A | R1R1, Ss, Fy(a−b+), Jk(a+b−), kk | c, E, Fy$^a$, Jk$^b$, K |
| B | R2R2, ss, Fy(a+b+), Jk(a−b+), kk | C, e, S, Jk$^a$, K |
| C | rr, SS, Fy(a+b−), Jk(a+b+), kk | C, D, E, s, Fy$^b$, K |

ple of antibody-detection tests using unadsorbed, once-adsorbed, and twice-adsorbed serum. In this example, one adsorption failed to remove all the autoantibody, but two adsorptions were effective. No underlying alloantibodies are evident in this example.

There are several difficulties to consider with autoadsorptions. First, if the patient has been recently transfused, donor RBCs in the patient specimen may remove alloantibody during the absorption procedure. Autoadsorption would not be recommended in this instance. Second, if the patient is severely anemic, one may not be able to obtain autologous cells for multiple adsorptions. Third, whenever an absorption is done, whether with autologous or allogeneic cells, the serum is diluted to some degree. Some saline remains in "packed" RBCs. A weakly reactive alloantibody could be diluted and missed if multiple adsorptions are performed.

When the patient has had a recent transfusion or is severely anemic, one can use cells of selected phenotypes for absorption. If the patient's phenotype is unknown and cannot be determined, adsorptions can be performed using a trio of selected cells (R1R1, R2R2, rr). They should also lack the antigens for the more commonly encountered clinically significant alloantibodies (e.g., Kell, Duffy, Kidd, Ss). As shown in Table 21–16, if one adsorbs the patient's serum with cells from donors A, B, and C and then tests the adsorbed sera, one can detect many important alloantibodies.

Alternatively, if a pretransfusion phenotype is available for the patient, phenotypically matched RBCs can be used to adsorb. (See discussion of antigen typing the patient with a positive DAT.) For example, examine the patient's RBC phenotype in Table 21–17. The patient should not form alloantibodies to RBC antigens that he or she possesses; therefore, we are concerned about the antigens the patient lacks. The patient is negative for the following antigen: c, E, Fy$^b$, Jk$^a$, N, and s. If donor cells are selected that are also negative for c, E, and Jk$^a$, and if we enzyme-treat the cells to destroy the Duffy and MNSs antigens, we can adsorb the autoantibody and leave the common alloantibodies that the patient might form. In this example, the patient has an underlying alloanti-E.

It is impossible to detect all clinically significant alloantibodies, like those directed against high-incidence antigens. For example, an anti-K2 (Cellano) would be adsorbed onto virtually all random donor cells, inasmuch as the K2 antigen is present on the cells of more than 99 percent of the population (such as cells A, B, and C in Table 21–16 and the phenotypically matched donor in Table 21–17). An antibody such as this would be differentiated from the autoantibody only if a cell negative for the high-incidence antigen happened to be present among the cells used for adsorption.

When alloantibodies are found or suspected in the serum of a patient with warm AIHA, it is necessary to test the patient's red cells for the absence of the corresponding antigen. Inasmuch as the patient has a posi-

**Table 21–17.** Adsorption Using Phenotype-matched Cells

| Patient's phenotype: | R1R1, K−, Fy(a+b−), Jk(a−b+), MMSs |
| --- | --- |
| Adsorbing cell: | R1R1, K−, Jk(a−b+) - enzyme-treated |

Initial panel results: 2+ reactions with all cells tested.
Selected cell panel tested with adsorbed serum:

| Cell | D | C | E | c | e | M | N | S | s | K | k | Fy$^a$ | Fy$^b$ | Jk$^a$ | Jk$^b$ | 37° | AHG |
| --- | --- | --- | --- | --- | --- | --- | --- | --- | --- | --- | --- | --- | --- | --- | --- | --- | --- |
| 1 | + | + | 0 | 0 | + | + | 0 | 0 | + | 0 | + | 0 | + | + | + | 0 | 0 |
| 2 | + | 0 | + | + | 0 | 0 | + | + | 0 | 0 | + | + | 0 | 0 | + | 0 | 1+ |
| 3 | + | + | 0 | 0 | + | 0 | + | + | 0 | + | + | 0 | 0 | + | 0 | 0 | 0 |
| 4 | 0 | 0 | 0 | + | + | + | 0 | 0 | + | 0 | + | + | 0 | + | + | 0 | 0 |
| 5 | 0 | 0 | 0 | + | + | + | + | + | + | 0 | + | + | + | 0 | + | 0 | 0 |
| 6 | + | 0 | + | + | + | 0 | + | 0 | + | + | + | + | + | + | 0 | 0 | 1+ |

Interpretation: Alloanti-E present in adsorbed serum.
AHG = Antihuman globulin.

tive DAT, usually with IgG coating the cells, antigen typing using an antiglobulin test (such as typing for Kell, Duffy, and Kidd antigens) will be invalid. Chloroquine-treated cells may be used in these situations to obtain valid antigen typings. Chloroquine diphosphate will remove much of the coating IgG while leaving the antigens intact. Careful attention should be paid to the procedure, following instructions on the package insert of commercially available chloroquine reagents, to ensure that certain antigens will not be destroyed or weakened.

## Selection of Blood for Transfusion

Many patients with warm AIHA never require transfusion; they can be managed with medical treatment. Occasionally, however, the anemia is so severe that transfusion cannot be avoided.[6] Patients who have a nonhemolytic warm AIHA pose problems when blood is needed for a surgical procedure. In these cases, compatibility with any alloantibodies in the patient's serum is the primary concern.

Compatibility with the autoantibody is controversial. If the autoantibody shows a simple specificity, such as anti-e, local practice may be to select donor units that are negative for the corresponding antigen. However, one must ensure that the cells selected do not possess an antigen that is likely to result in stimulation of the patient to form alloantibodies. For example, because virtually all D-negative cells are e-positive, a D-negative patient with autoanti-e specificity should not receive a transfusion of D-positive RBCs to have cells lacking the e antigen.[40] Singh and colleagues[41] report hemoglobin increments in patients with AIHA comparable to the expected increment even when e-positive units are transfused to patients with an apparent autoanti-e. Finding compatible units for patients with a broad-specificity warm autoagglutinin is virtually impossible. "Least incompatible" red cells may be selected for transfusion. In all cases, the transfused donor cells are likely to be destroyed as rapidly as the patient's own red cells. Units that are compatible with any present alloantibodies should be selected using the techniques described in the previous section.

## Treatment

Therapy is generally aimed at treating the underlying disease first, if one is present. General measures to support cardiovascular function are important in patients who are severely anemic. Transfusion is generally avoided, if possible, inasmuch as this may only accelerate hemolysis instead of ameliorating the anemia. However, transfusion should not be avoided in situations of life-threatening anemia. In many cases, small amounts of transfused RBCs (one-half to one unit) are sufficient to relieve the symptoms of the anemia.[42]

The forms of treatment described in the discussions following are generally used, depending on the severity of the disorder.

## Corticosteroid Administration and Use of Intravenous Immunoglobulin

One form of therapy involves the use of corticosteroids, such as prednisone. Initially, high doses of 100 to 200 mg of prednisone are maintained until the patient's hematocrit stabilizes. Patients who have not had transfusions respond to steroid therapy more rapidly than those who are transfused. Several mechanisms have been proposed for the action of prednisone, including (1) reduction of antibody synthesis, (2) altered antibody activity, and (3) alteration of macrophage receptors for IgG and C3, which reduces the clearance of antibody-coated RBCs.[43]

The dosage of prednisone should be reduced when the hematocrit begins to rise and the reticulocyte count drops. Finally, the steroids are withdrawn slowly over a period of 2 to 4 months. A beneficial response to the administration of prednisone is demonstrated in 50 to 65 percent of all cases of warm AIHA. An androgenic steroid, danazol, has also been beneficial in prednisone-resistant cases.[43] The use of intravenous immune globulin in patients unresponsive to corticosteroid treatment is controversial and appears to have limited efficacy.[44]

## Splenectomy

If steroid therapy fails, or if a patient requires large doses of steroids to control hemolysis, splenectomy is usually recommended. The decision to perform splenectomy requires clinical evaluation and judgment. There are three reasons for performing splenectomy: (1) failure of steroid therapy, (2) need for continuous high-dose steroid maintenance, and (3) complications of steroid therapy. Splenectomy results in decreased production of antibody and removes a potent site of red cell damage and destruction. Patients who had a good initial response to steroids respond better with splenectomy than do those who failed initial steroid therapy.

It has been reported that as many as 60 percent of patients with warm AIHA benefit from splenectomy if steroid dosages greater than 15 mg per day are also used to maintain remission.

## Immunosuppressive Drugs

This is usually the last approach used in management of warm AIHA. Azathioprine (Imuran) and cyclophosphamide are examples of immunosuppressive drugs that interfere with antibody synthesis by destroying dividing cells.

Experience in using this therapy is limited. The most detrimental side effect that threatens the common use of these drugs is a potential for neoplastic growth as a result of the defective immune surveillance of immunosuppressed patients.

Table 21–18 reviews and compares the characteristics of cold and warm autoimmune hemolytic anemias.

**Table 21–18.** Comparison of Warm and Cold Autoimmune Hemolytic Anemias

| | Warm AIHA | Cold AIHA |
|---|---|---|
| Optimal reaction temperature | >32°C | <30°C |
| Immunoglobulin class | IgG | IgM |
| Complement activation | May bind complement | Binds complement |
| Site of hemolysis | Usually extravascular (no cell lysis) | Usually intravascular (cell lysis) |
| Frequency | 70–75% of cases | 16% of cases (PCH: 1–2%) |
| Specificity | Frequently broad Rh-like | Ii system (PCH: autoanti-P) |

*Source:* Adapted from Harmening, DM: Clinical Hematology and Fundamentals of Hemostasis, ed 3. FA Davis, Philadelphia, 1997, p 231, with permission.

## DRUG-INDUCED IMMUNE HEMOLYTIC ANEMIA

Drugs can cause a variety of side effects, including immune destruction of RBCs and other blood cells, although the incidence is rare. Hemolytic anemia, leukopenia, and thrombocytopenia can occur separately, but in some patients more than one cell line can be affected. The cells may be coated with antibody, antibody and complement, or complement alone. The discussion in this section is limited to RBC problems, but many of the same principles also apply to platelets and leukocytes.

Drug-mediated problems may come to the attention of the blood bank technologist in one of two ways:

1. A request for diagnostic testing on a patient with a possible hemolytic anemia.
2. Unexpected results in routine testing; for example, a positive autologous control in the antiglobulin phase of antibody screening or compatibility testing or a positive DAT.

Drugs should be suspected as a possible explanation for immune hemolysis or a positive DAT when there is no other reason for the serologic and hematologic findings and if the patient has a history of taking drugs. Other causes should be considered first, because, with the exception of Aldomet-induced problems, drug-induced positive DATs and hemolytic anemia are relatively rare. Petz and Garratty[6] review the four classic mechanisms proposed to account for drug-induced problems: immune complexes, drug adsorption, membrane modification, and autoantibody formation. Specific drugs have been commonly associated with one particular mechanism but may work by another.[45,46] Currently, other theories postulate combining aspects of these earlier proposed mechanisms.[47] Drug-related positive DATs may be additionally classified as "drug-dependent" or "drug-independent." A discussion of the classical categories of drug-induced hemolytic anemias

follows, including elements of these new hypotheses. Representative drugs associated with each mechanism, as well as those known to act by multiple mechanisms, are listed in Table 21–19.

## Immune Complex ("Innocent Bystander") Mechanism

Although the occurrence is rare, many drugs have been implicated in causing immune-mediated problems by the immune complex mechanism. This mechanism was first described in the early 1960s, and it was thought that drugs operating through this mechanism combine with plasma proteins to form immunogens.[48] The antibody (IgG or IgM) subsequently produced recognizes determinants on the drug. If the patient ingests the same drug (or a drug bearing the same haptenic group) after immunization, the formation of a drug-antidrug complex may occur. The complement cascade may be activated because of this antigen-antibody interaction. Red blood cells are thought to be involved in this process only as "innocent bystanders."[49] The soluble drug-antidrug complex nonspecifically adsorbs loosely to the red cell surface. Complement, when activated, sensitizes the cell and may cause lysis (Fig. 21–3).

More recently, however, the concept of "neoantigen"

**Table 21–19.** Representative Drugs Implicated in Positive Direct Antiglobulin Tests and/or Hemolytic Anemia

| Drug-Dependent | | |
|---|---|---|
| **Drug Adsorption** | **Immune Complexes** | |
| Penicillin | Carboplatin | Minocycline |
| Cephalosporins | Cefotaxime | Nomifensine |
| Carbimazole | Cefotetan | Quinidine |
| Carboplatin | Ceftazidime | Phenacetin |
| Carbromal | Ceftriaxone | Sulindac |
| Cianidanol | Chlorinated hydrocarbons | Teniposide |
| Cisplatin | Diclofenac | Tolmetin |
| Erythromycin | Fludarabine | Sulfonamides |
| Streptomycin | Galfenine | Zomepirac |
| Tolbutamide | Latamoxef | |

| Membrane Modification | | |
|---|---|---|
| Cephalosporins | | |

| Drug-Independent | Drug-Independent/Dependent | |
|---|---|---|
| Alpha methyldopa | Azapropazone | Galfenine |
| Levodopa | Carbimazole | Latamoxef |
| Ibuprofen | Carboplatin | Nomifensine |
| Procainamide | Cefotetan | Phenacetin |
| Mefenamic acid | Cefoxitin | Streptomycin |
| Chlorpromazine | Chlorinated hydrocarbons | Teniposide |
| Fenfluramine | Cianidanol | Tolmetin |
| | Diclofenac | |

Some drugs act by more than one mechanism.
List not meant to be all-inclusive. For more detailed lists, see references 6, 21, 47, 51.

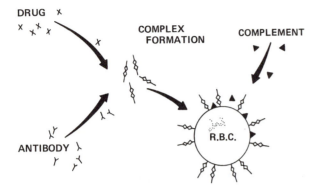

DRUG

COMPLEX
FORMATION

COMPLEMENT

R.B.C.

ANTIBODY

**Figure 21–3.** Immune complex mechanism. (From Petz and Garratty,[6] p 272, with permission.)

formation has been proposed. In this model, the drug interacts in a noncovalent manner with a specific membrane component and forms a new determinant consisting of both drug and membrane components.

Because complement activation is involved in the immune complex, clinically affected patients frequently present with acute intravascular hemolysis.[21] When other causes for hemoglobinemia and hemoglobinuria have been excluded (e.g., ABO hemolytic transfusion reactions or cold autoimmune hemolytic anemia), one should consider a drug-antidrug reaction. When obtaining the drug history, it is important to realize that this group of patients needs to take only small doses of the drug to be affected. The patient recovers rapidly once the drug is withdrawn.

The patient's DAT when polyspecific antiglobulin reagent is used will usually be positive. If monospecific reagents are used, agglutination usually occurs with anti-complement, but not with anti-IgG. Tests with anti-IgG are negative, even when the antibody is of the IgG class, because the drug-antidrug complex is thought to elute from the cell during the washing procedure before the antiglobulin test.[50,51] Other routine blood bank tests are negative in all phases; the antibody is directed against a drug or the drug-RBC membrane "neoantigen," not a true red cell antigen. Therefore, the antibody screen and compatibility tests are negative, unless an alloantibody is also present. An eluate tested against reagent red blood cells will also be negative. A summary of typical serologic results is given in Table 21–20.

To confirm that a drug-antidrug reaction through this mechanism is responsible for a positive DAT, one must demonstrate the antibody in the patient's serum. The patient's serum can be incubated with a solution of the drug in question and ABO-compatible red cells. Complement activation is the usual indicator of an antigen-antibody reaction; therefore, one should observe for hemolysis after incubation and use reagents containing anti-C3 activity for the antiglobulin test. A general procedure for demonstrating antibodies reacting by the immune complex mechanism, suggested by Garratty,[52] is given in Procedure H of the Procedural Appendix of this chapter.

For the test results to be interpreted correctly, adequate controls must be performed. The patient's serum must not react with the cells when saline or the diluent used to dissolve the drug is substituted for the drug solution, and the drug solution must not hemolyze the suspension of cells nonspecifically. Examples of typical reactions with the patient's serum and control are given in Table 21–21.

An eluate from the patient's cells is usually nonreactive even if the drug and a source of complement are added. Very little antibody, if any, remains on the cells after washing.

In most blood banks, confirmatory testing is done only when the patient has hematologic complications and not when the patient simply has a history of taking the drug and a positive DAT. Some of the drugs known to cause immune complex–mediated problems are in frequent use, and there are a large number of patients with a positive DAT and no evidence of hemolysis. Therefore, a full work-up is of only academic interest and is not required before release of RBCs for transfusion.

**Table 21–20.** Serologic Reactions Observed with Drug-induced Positive DATs

| Mechanism | Direct Antiglobulin Test | | | Serum | Eluate |
|---|---|---|---|---|---|
| | Polyspecific | Anti-IgG | Anti-C3 | | |
| Immune complex | + | 0* | + | Routine antibody screens negative; antibody demonstrable if serum, drug, complement incubated with RBCs | Antibody not demonstrable even in presence of drug |
| Drug adsorption | + | + | 0* | Routine antibody screens negative; high-titered antibody demonstrable if serum tested with drug-coated RBCs | Antibody demonstrable using drug-coated RBCs |
| Membrane modification | + | + | + | Routine antibody screens negative; nonimmunologic mechanism | Eluate nonreactive |
| Autoantibody formation | + | + | 0* | Autoantibody reactive with normal RBCs may or may not be present | Eluate reactive with normal RBCs |

*May occasionally be positive.

**Table 21–21.** Interpretation of Tests to Confirm Presence of Antidrug Antibody Acting by Immune Complex Mechanism

| Test | Patient's Serum | Fresh Serum* | Drug | RBCs | Results[†] | Interpretation |
|------|-----------------|--------------|------|------|-----------|----------------|
| 1 | X | X | X | X | Positive | Antidrug antibody present if controls working |
| 2 | X | X | X | X | Negative | Antidrug antibody not present; drug not present in proper concentration, etc. |
| *Controls (to be run)* | | | | | | |
| 1 | X | O | O | X | Negative | No alloantibody against these RBC antigens present |
| 2 | O | X | X | X | Negative | No alloantibody against RBC or drug present in serum of random donor |
| 3 | O | O | X | X | Negative | Drug solution does not cause RBCs to agglutinate or lyse |

*Source of complement.
[†]Based on presence of hemolysis, agglutination.
X = present in the test tube.
O = not present in the test tube.

Treatment involves discontinuing the use of the drug. Although hemolysis by this mechanism is rare, the onset is usually sudden and may be characterized by intravascular hemolysis and renal failure. Therefore, immediate cessation of the drug is essential. Steroid treatment may also be given.

## Drug-Adsorption (Hapten) Mechanism

Unlike drugs acting through the immune complex mechanism, drugs operating through the drug-adsorption mechanism bind firmly to proteins, including the proteins of the red cell membrane (Fig. 21–4). Presumably because of their ability to bind to proteins, these drugs are better immunogens. For example, antibodies to penicillin, the drug most commonly associated with this mechanism, are found in about 3 percent of hospitalized patients receiving large doses of penicillin; of these, fewer than 5 percent develop a hemolytic anemia.[21] Even with the relatively high incidence of antipenicillin antibodies and the ability of the drug to bind to the red cell membrane, penicillin-induced positive DATs are rare.[10] The low incidence may reflect the fact that the patient must receive massive doses (10 million units per day) of penicillin for the cells to be coated adequately. Also, most penicillin antibodies are IgM and therefore not detected by the antiglobulin test. The penicillin antibody responsible for a positive DAT is IgG. Complement activation does not occur.

The laboratory results are consistent with this description of the mechanism (see Table 21–20). Cells from patients with a positive DAT are usually coated with IgG alone. However, sometimes both IgG and complement are present on the cells. The patient's serum and eluate are nonreactive with reagent red cells and random donor cells. Therefore, the antibody screen is negative, and crossmatches are compatible in all phases. However, if the serum and eluate are tested against penicillin-coated cells, agglutination does occur in the antiglobulin phase. The procedure for preparing the penicillin-coated cells is given in Procedure I of the Procedural Appendix of this chapter.[52] Because many patients have penicillin antibodies, Garratty emphasizes that the serum antibody must be high titered and the eluate must be positive before the findings are definitive. Interpretation of the confirmatory tests to demonstrate antipenicillin antibodies is outlined in Table 21–22.

Only a small percentage of those patients with penicillin-induced positive DATs exhibit hematologic complications. The clinical features of such a hemolytic episode differ from those of immune complex–mediated problems in several ways. Because the complement cascade is usually not activated, cell destruction is predominantly extravascular rather than intravascular. Therefore, the anemia develops more slowly and is not life-threatening unless the cause for the hemolysis is not recognized and the penicillin therapy is continued. Penicillin-induced hemolysis occurs only when the patient receives massive doses of the antibiotic, in contrast to the small amounts of drug that are necessary for hemolysis due to immune complexes. The patient

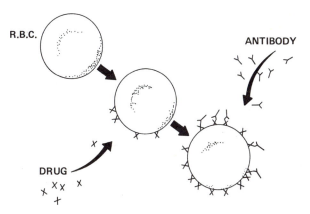

**Figure 21–4.** Drug adsorption mechanism. (From Petz and Garratty,[6] p 280, with permission.)

**Table 21–22.** Interpretation of Screening Tests for Presence of Antidrug Antibody Acting by Drug Adsorption Mechanism

| Test | Patient's Serum/Eluate | Drug-Coated RBC | Uncoated RBC* | Results[†] | Interpretation |
|------|------------------------|-----------------|---------------|---------|----------------|
| 1 | X | X | O | Positive | Antidrug antibody present if controls working; antibody in serum usually high-titered |
| 2 | X | X | O | Negative | Antidrug antibody not present |
| *Controls (to be run)* | | | | | |
| 1 | X | O | X | Negative | No alloantibody against these RBC antigens present in serum or eluate |
| 2 | O | X | O | Negative | Drug-coated RBCs do not spontaneously agglutinate or lyse |

*Same RBCs as those coated with drug.
[†]Based on presence of agglutination or hemolysis.
X = present in the test tube
O = not present inthe test tube

improves once the drug is withdrawn, but hemolysis continues at a decreasing rate until cells heavily coated with penicillin are removed. The DAT may remain positive for several weeks. Mixed-field agglutination will be seen in the DAT because some cells are penicillin-coated but others are not. The antibody may crossreact with ampicillin and methicillin.

Other drugs cause a positive DAT and hemolytic anemia by this mechanism, most notably the cephalosporins (see Table 21–19). Distinguishing between cephalosporin-induced problems and penicillin-induced problems is technically difficult because the drugs have antigenic determinants in common, and antipenicillin is frequently in the serum. Antipenicillin reacts with Keflin-treated cells; anti-Keflin with penicillin-coated cells. Garratty[52] suggests that comparing the strength of the reactivity of the serum or eluate (titer or score) with penicillin-coated and Keflin-coated cells may be of value.

Reports of severe hemolytic episodes associated with the newer second- and third-generation cephalosporins appear to be increasing.[47,53–55] Several of these cases appear to involve aspects of both the immune complex and the drug-adsorption mechanisms. The immune-mediated hemolysis has occurred rapidly after administration of only a small amount of the drug. Because these antibiotics are routinely used in both adult and pediatric populations, any evidence of intravascular hemolysis should be noted and evaluated.

### Membrane Modification (Nonimmunologic Protein Adsorption)

It is hypothesized that the cephalosporins, especially cephalothin (Keflin), in addition to operating through the drug-adsorption mechanism, are able to modify red cells so that plasma proteins (e.g., IgG, IgM, IgA, and complement) can bind to the membrane (Fig. 21–5).[56] Consequently, RBCs from approximately 3 percent of patients receiving Keflin may exhibit a positive DAT with polyspecific and monospecific reagents. The uptake of immunoglobulins or complement components is not the result of an antigen-antibody reac-

tion, so this mechanism is nonimmunologic. Inasmuch as antibody is not involved, tests with the patient's serum and eluate are negative (see Table 21–20). Numerous cases of cephalosporin-associated hemolytic anemia have been reported, but, as stated earlier, RBC destruction seems to have been mediated through the drug adsorption or immune complex mechanism rather than the membrane modification mechanism. There is no treatment approach because hemolytic anemia associated with the ingestion of these drugs has not been described in relation to membrane modification.

### Autoantibody Formation

Unlike the drugs acting through the previously described mechanisms which induce production of an *allo*antibody against a determinant on a drug or on a combination of the drug and RBC membrane, alpha-methyldopa (Aldomet) induces the production of an *auto*antibody that recognizes RBC antigens.[57,58] The antibodies produced are serologically indistinguishable from those seen in patients with warm AIHA (see previous section). Presence of the drug is not required to obtain positive reactions. Positive DATs are encoun-

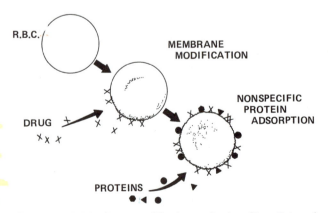

**Figure 21–5.** Membrane modification mechanism. (From Petz and Garratty,[6] p 284, with permission.)

**Table 21–23.** Proposed Theories for Methyldopa-induced or Procainamide-induced Mechanism of Immune Hemolytic Anemia

1. The drug interferes with the function of T suppressor cells, allowing proliferation of B cells, which produce IgG antibody against self.
2. The drug causes subtle alteration of intrinsic RBC antigens, creating new epitopes that are no longer recognized as self.
3. The drug acts as a hapten, resulting in the production of antibodies that cross-react with normal red cell antigens.
4. The drug interferes with normal immunoregulation.
5. The drug elicits production of an antibody that recognizes a binding site sufficiently similar to normal RBC membrane structures.

tered in approximately 10 to 20 percent of patients receiving this Aldomet as an antihypertensive. However, very few (0.5 to 1.0 percent) of this group of patients subsequently develop significant immune hemolytic anemia.[6,59] Other drugs that also cause autoantibody production are L-dopa, mefenamic acid, procainamide, and diclofenac[59,60] (see Table 21–19).

Several mechanisms by which Aldomet causes the production of autoantibodies have been proposed (Table 21–23).[3,51,58] Kirtland, Horwitz, and Mohler[4] propose that methyldopa alters the function of T-suppressor cells and suggest that this upset in the immune system would allow production of antibody against self. Worlledge and associates[58] suggest that the drug alters RBC membrane components, similar to the theory of the "neoantigen" formation. However, at this time there is little evidence to support either of the theories. Much more work is needed to determine the true mechanisms involved in the production of drug-induced autoantibodies.

The serologic features of this type of drug-induced problem are very different from those of the other drug-related immune hemolytic anemias. As shown in Table 21–20, the antibody in the eluate *does* react with normal red cells in the absence of the drug. Antibody of similar specificity and reactivity may be found in the serum. The patient's RBCs are usually coated with IgG, rarely with complement components.

Because the serology of Aldomet-induced positive DAT/immune hemolytic anemia is identical to that of the idiopathic warm AIHA, one cannot establish in the laboratory that Aldomet is the cause of the problem. However, if the patient is receiving the drug, one should be highly suspicious. If Aldomet is withdrawn, autoantibody production will eventually stop, but it may be several months before the DAT is negative.

## Treatment

Discontinuation of the drug is the treatment of choice for patients with a drug-induced hemolytic anemia. The presence of a positive DAT result does not nec-

**Table 21–24.** Mechanisms Leading to Development of Drug-Related Antibodies

| Mechanism | Prototype Drugs | Ig Class | DAT Result | Eluate | Frequency of Hemolysis |
|---|---|---|---|---|---|
| Immune complex formation ("innocent bystander") | Quinidine Phenacetin | IgM or IgG | Positive (often complement only; however, IgG may be present) | Often negative | Small doses of drugs may cause acute intravascular hemolysis with hemoglobinemia and hemoglobinuria; renal failure is common |
| Drug adsorption (hapten) | Penicillins Cephalosporins Streptomycin | IgG | Strongly positive | Often negative | 3–4% of patients on large doses (10,000,000 U) of penicillin, which is one of the most common causes of immune hemolysis, usually extravascular in nature |
| Membrane modification (nonimmunologic protein adsorption) | Cephalosporins | Numerous plasma proteins (nonimmunologic sensitization) | Positive because of a variety of serum proteins | Negative | No hemolysis; however, 3% of patients receiving the drug develop a positive DAT |
| Methyldopa-induced (unknown) | Methyldopa (Aldomet) | IgG | Strongly positive (because of IgG sensitization) | Positive (warm autoantibody identical to that found in WAIHA) | 0.8% develop a hemolytic anemia that mimics a warm AIHA (depends on the drug dose); 15% of patients receiving methyldopa develop a positive DAT |

*Source:* Adapted from Harmening, DM: Clinical Hematology and Fundamentals of Hemostasis, ed 3. FA Davis, Philadelphia, 1997, p 232, with permission.
AIHA = autoimmune hemolytic anemia.

**Table 21–25.** Summary of Antibody Characteristics in AIHA

|  | Warm-Reactive Autoantibody | Cold-Reactive Autoantibody | Paroxysmal Cold Hemoglobinuria | Drug-related Autoantibody |
|---|---|---|---|---|
| Immunoglobulin characteristics | Polyclonal IgG; occasionally IgM and IgA may be present | Polyclonal IgM in infection; monoclonal kappa chain IgM in cold agglutinin disease | Polyclonal IgG | Polyclonal IgG |
| Complement activity | Variable | Always | Always | Depends on mechanism of drug, antibody, and red cell interaction |
| Thermal reactivity | 20–37°C (optimum 37°C) | 4–32°C; rarely to 37°C (optimum 4°C) | 4–20°C; biphasic hemolysin | 20–37°C (optimum 37°C) |
| Titer of free antibody | Low (<32); may be detectable only with enzyme-treated cells | High (>1000 at 4°C) | Moderate to low (<64) | Depends on mechanism of drug, antibody, and red cell interaction |
| Reactivity of eluate with antibody screening cells | Usually panreactive | Nonreactive | Nonreactive | Panreactive with methyldopa type; nonreactive in all other cases |
| Most common specificity | Anti-Rh precursor; anti-common Rh; anti-LW; anti-En$^a$/Wr$^b$; anti-U | Anti-I Anti-i Anti-Pr | Anti-P | Anti-"e"-like; methyldopa antidrug |
| Site of red cell destruction | Predominantly spleen with some liver involvement | Predominantly liver, rarely intravascular | Intravascular | Intravascular and spleen |

*Source:* Adapted from Harmening, DM: Clinical Hematology and Fundamentals of Hemostasis, ed 3. FA Davis, Philadelphia, p 233, with permission.

essarily imply that the drug must be discontinued, if the effects of the drug are of therapeutic benefit and significant hemolysis is not present. In general, however, other drugs should be substituted and the patient observed for resolution of the anemia to confirm a drug-induced hemolytic process. If the patient has a positive DAT without hemolysis, continued administration of the drug is optional.

Generally, the prognosis for patients with drug-induced hemolytic anemia is excellent. In Table 21–24, the four recognized mechanisms leading to the development of drug-related antibodies are compared. Table 21–25 contrasts the antibody characteristics of the various types of autoimmune hemolytic anemias.

## SUMMARY

By understanding the mechanisms by which drugs can cause a positive DAT or immune hemolytic anemia, one can quickly decide which laboratory tests are most likely to be informative. Many other drugs have been cited as a cause for hemolytic anemia; however, the majority of these have only one reported case and the association between the hemolytic anemia and the drug may be unclear. Before any special testing is done, one should proceed in the following manner:

1. Obtain the patient's medical history, including transfusions, pregnancies, medications, and diagnosis.
2. Perform a DAT using RBCs collected in EDTA. Test the cells with a polyspecific antiglobulin reagent and monospecific reagents.
3. Screen the patient's serum for RBC alloantibodies.
4. Prepare and test an eluate for RBC alloantibodies if the patient has been recently transfused.

After evaluating this information, one can decide whether drugs are a possible cause of the problem and which of the mechanisms is involved. It is wise to also note that many drugs cause an immunologic reaction by both drug-dependent and drug-independent mechanisms. When other causes (e.g., transfusion reaction) have been excluded and the clinical situation warrants additional testing, drug-coated cells or solutions of the drug can be prepared for confirmatory tests.

Distinguishing autoimmune hemolytic anemias, drug-induced as well as cold-reactive and warm-reactive, from a transfusion reaction caused by an alloantibody is of the utmost importance. However, extensive workup of autoimmune antibodies is usually unnecessary. The most important concern in evaluation of autoantibodies is detection and identification of underlying clinically significant alloantibodies.

## CASE STUDIES

### CASE 1

#### Part A

A 77-year-old woman was admitted for treatment of a severe upper respiratory infection. Her past medical history is unremarkable, and she has been in excellent health for many years. Twelve days before admission, she developed "a bad cold." Her symptoms have grown progressively worse until today, when she felt "too weak to get out of bed," and she is noted to be slightly jaundiced. She had three uneventful pregnancies and normal deliveries, and she has never had a transfusion. Her admission laboratory results follow:

| | | WBC differential: | |
|---|---|---|---|
| Hemoglobin: | 7.5 g/dL | | |
| Hematocrit: | 23.2% | Segmented | |
| | | neutrophils: | 56% |
| White blood cells: | 15.3 $\times$ | Immature | |
| | $10^3/mm^3$ | neutrophils: | 8% |
| Platelets: | 125,000 | Lymphocytes: | 33% |
| | $/mm^3$ | | |
| RBC morphology: | | Eosinophils: | 2% |
| Normocytic, | | Basophils: | 1% |
| normochromic, few | | | |
| spherocytes, rare | | | |
| schistocytes | | | |

The physician orders a crossmatch for two units of packed RBCs. The initial transfusion service results are given below:

| Antisera | | | Cells | |
|---|---|---|---|---|
| $-A$ | $-B$ | $-D$ | $A_1$ | B |
| 4+ | 0 | 3+ | 1+ | 4+ |

| | IS | 37° | Anti-IgG |
|---|---|---|---|
| Screening cell I | 1+ | 0 | 0 |
| Screening cell II | 1+ | 0 | 0 |
| Screening cell III | 1+ | 0 | 0 |
| Crossmatch 1 | w+ | 0 | 0 |
| Crossmatch 2 | 2+ | 0 | 0 |
| IS = Immediate spin. | | | |

1. What problem do you note in the initial testing results?

2. What are possible explanations for these results?

3. What further testing must be performed before release of blood for transfusion?

4. Does the patient history give any clues as to the cause of the testing results?

#### Part B

An auto-control is tested at immediate spin, along with repeating the reverse grouping, with the following results:

| | |
|---|---|
| $A_1$ cells: | 1+ |
| B cells: | 4+ |
| Autologous cells: | 1+ |

A DAT is also tested to obtain more information about this apparent autoantibody:

| | |
|---|---|
| Polyspecific AHG: | 3+ |
| Anti-IgG: | 0 |
| Anti-C3d: | 3+ |

The reverse grouping, antibody screen, and compatibility testing are repeated using a prewarmed technique. The immediate spin results are shown below:

| Cells | IS |
|---|---|
| $A_1$ | 0 |
| B | 4+ |
| Auto | 0 |
| SC I | 0 |
| SC II | 0 |
| SC III | 0 |
| XM #1 | 0 |
| XM #2 | 0 |

1. What is the patient's true ABO type and the result of the antibody screen?

2. What conclusions can you draw regarding the clinical significance of this antibody?

3. Is this antibody likely to cause hemolysis of the transfused RBCs?

#### Case 1 Answers

*Part A*

1. The forward and reverse typing do not match. The forward result is that typical of a group A, but the reverse is that of a group O (with a weak reaction between the patient's serum and the $A_1$ cells). There is also an unexpected reaction in the immediate spin phase of the antibody screening test and the compatibility testing.

2. a. The patient may be a subgroup of A with anti-$A_1$ in the serum. Anti-$A_1$ would not, however, explain the reactions with the antibody screening cells.

   b. The patient may have an alloantibody reactive at room temperature, such as anti-Le$^a$ or $-$Le$^b$, $-M$, $-N$, or $-P_1$. The reverse grouping cells are quite likely to be positive for any of these antigens, inasmuch as those cells are produced from pools of donors. An RBC panel must be tested to determine whether one of the antibodies might be responsible for the reactions.

c. The patient may have a cold autoantibody that reacts with the reverse grouping cells as well as with the antibody screening cells and the donor units. An auto-control would be helpful in determining if this might be the case. If the auto-control is positive, a DAT is indicated to determine the nature of the protein coating the patient's RBCs.

3. As described in Question 2, an auto-control, tested at immediate spin, and possibly an antibody identification panel must be performed in order to resolve the discrepancy. If the auto-control is positive, a prewarmed technique may be used to obtain valid reactions without interference from the cold autoantibody.

4. The patient has an upper respiratory infection. It is known that infections with *Mycoplasma pneumoniae* are associated with cold hemagglutinin disease (CHD) due to anti-I. The patient's clinical symptoms and laboratory evidence of anemia would also be consistent with CHD.

*Part B*

1. The patient is A, D positive, and the antibody screen is negative for clinically significant antibodies.

2. This antibody is most likely an autoanti-I, possibly produced in response to infection by *M. pneumoniae*. The antibody will cause hemolysis of the autologous cells, on some occasions resulting in clinical anemia. Because the antibody is IgM, causing sensitization of the cells with complement, there is no reaction in the antibody screen or compatibility testing with anti-IgG reagent. In this case, the use of a prewarmed technique eliminates all aberrant reactions and allows the provision of crossmatch-compatible RBCs for transfusion if needed.

3. If it is determined that this patient truly needs a transfusion, the RBCs may be administered through a blood warmer. If the RBCs are kept at 37°C, there should be minimal hemolysis. In this case, the hemolytic process is transient and will resolve within 2 to 3 weeks with treatment of the primary disease. Supportive care and avoiding cold are the best therapy.

## CASE 2

### Part A

A 45-year-old man was admitted with complaints of extreme fatigue and back pain. Admission test results are as follows:

| | |
|---|---|
| Hemoglobin | 4.5 g/dL |
| Reticulocyte count | 15% |
| Total bilirubin | 6.8 mg/dL |

The attending physician orders 4 units of packed RBCs for transfusion as soon as possible. Records indicate that 3 years ago the patient received a transfusion of 4 units of RBCs following an automobile accident. No serologic problems were noted at that time. Initial pretransfusion testing follows:

| Anti-A | Anti-B | Anti-D | A₁ cells | B cells | |
|---|---|---|---|---|---|
| 0 | 0 | 3+ | 4+ | 4+ | |
| | | | IS | 37° | AHG |
| Antibody screen I | | | 0 | 0 | 3+ |
| II | | | 0 | 0 | 3+ |
| III | | | 0 | 0 | 3+ |
| Crossmatches 1 | | | 0 | 0 | 3+ |
| 2 | | | 0 | 0 | 3+ |
| 3 | | | 0 | 0 | 3+ |
| 4 | | | 0 | 0 | 3+ |

IS = immediate spin; AHG = antihuman globulin.

1. In light of the patient history and results, what kind of problems might be present in this patient?

2. What further information or testing would be helpful?

### Part B

Direct antiglobulin testing was performed on the patient's cells:

Anti-IgG    4+
Anti-C3b    Negative

A panel was performed on the patient's serum and all cells reacted (3+). An auto-control was also 4+, as expected. The patient's history was investigated and the following points were noted:

The only known transfusion was that contained in the previous record (3 years ago).
Patient has had problems with hypertension and is currently taking methyldopa.

1. What explanation for the serologic problems can you now propose?

2. What additional testing must be done to provide blood for this patient if the physician decides to transfuse?

3. What advice would you give the patient's physician regarding transfusion?

### Part C

Inasmuch as the patient has not been recently transfused, his cells were treated with ZZAP reagent, and an autoadsorption was performed. The antibody screen and crossmatches were repeated with the following results:

| Adsorbed serum | | IS | 37° | AHG |
|---|---|---|---|---|
| Screening cell | I | 0 | 0 | 0 |
| | II | 0 | 0 | 2+ |
| | III | 0 | 0 | 0 |
| Crossmatch | 1 | 0 | 0 | 0 |
| | 2 | 0 | 0 | 0 |
| | 3 | 0 | 0 | 2+ |
| | 4 | 0 | 0 | 0 |

IS = Immediate spin; AHG = antihuman globulin.

A panel was performed and the results are shown at the right.

1. What antibody specificities are evident?

2. What further testing must be done before release of blood for transfusion?

3. What additional tests might be helpful in providing blood for this patient in the future?

## Case 2 Answers

### Part A

1. The significantly decreased hemoglobin and increased reticulocyte count are indicative of a hemolytic episode. The serologic results reveal a panagglutinin, reactive with all cells tested at the antiglobulin phase. This patient may have a warm autoimmune hemolytic anemia.

2. A DAT should be performed to determine whether the antibody in the serum is autoantibody or alloantibody. If positive, anti-IgG and anti-C3 should be tested to identify the protein coating the cells. We know that the patient has not had a recent transfusion. We also need information about his diagnosis and any medications he has been taking. A panel should be performed to determine if the antibody shows a specificity.

### Part B

1. From the serologic results and the history of methyldopa therapy, it is evident that the patient must have methyldopa-associated warm AIHA.

2. Because the patient has had a transfusion in the past, it is essential to ensure that he has no underlying alloantibodies before providing blood for transfusion. We can perform a warm autoadsorption, inasmuch as he has not been recently transfused. This will remove the autoantibody, leaving any alloantibodies to be identified.

3. If at all possible, transfusion should be delayed until any alloantibodies that may be present are detected. Transfusion will complicate the sero-

Panel performed using adsorbed serum:

| Cells | D | C | E | c | e | M | N | S | s | K | k | Fya | Fyb | Jka | Jkb | 37° | AHG |
|---|---|---|---|---|---|---|---|---|---|---|---|---|---|---|---|---|---|
| 1 | 0 | + | 0 | + | + | 0 | + | + | 0 | 0 | + | + | 0 | 0 | + | 0 | 0 |
| 2 | + | + | 0 | 0 | + | + | + | 0 | + | 0 | + | + | + | + | 0 | 0 | 0 |
| 3 | + | + | 0 | 0 | + | + | 0 | 0 | + | 0 | + | 0 | 0 | + | + | 0 | 0 |
| 4 | + | 0 | + | + | 0 | + | + | + | 0 | + | + | + | 0 | + | + | 0 | 2+ |
| 5 | 0 | 0 | + | + | + | 0 | + | + | + | 0 | + | 0 | + | 0 | + | 0 | 0 |
| 6 | 0 | 0 | 0 | + | + | 0 | + | + | 0 | 0 | + | 0 | + | + | 0 | 0 | 0 |
| 7 | 0 | 0 | 0 | + | + | + | 0 | 0 | + | + | 0 | + | 0 | + | 0 | 0 | 2+ |
| 8 | 0 | 0 | 0 | + | + | 0 | + | + | + | 0 | + | + | 0 | + | + | 0 | 0 |
| 9 | + | 0 | 0 | + | + | + | + | + | + | 0 | + | 0 | 0 | + | + | 0 | 0 |
| 10 | + | + | 0 | + | + | + | 0 | + | 0 | 0 | + | 0 | + | 0 | + | 0 | 0 |

AHG = antihuman globulin.

logic picture and make it difficult to provide additional compatible RBCs. The transfused cells will be destroyed as rapidly as the patient's own cells. An alternative therapy for his hypertension should be started. After the patient stops taking the methyldopa, his clinical status will improve, although not rapidly. The autoantibody may be present in the patient's serum for up to 2 years. Panel performed using adsorbed serum:

*Part C*

1  An alloanti-K1 is present in this patient.

2. Any units released for transfusions should be verified as K1-negative. The patient should also be typed for K1 to prove that the antibody is truly an alloantibody. Because the patient has a positive DAT and the test of K1 requires the antiglobulin phase, his cells must be chloroquine-treated, as discussed below, before testing. The units can be crossmatched with the adsorbed serum.

3. To prepare for future transfusions, it may be helpful to determine the patient's complete RBC phenotype using chloroquine-treated cells. The patient could make alloantibodies to only those antigens he lacks, so this information would be valuable in future antibody identification. When using the chloroquine method of removing IgG from RBCs, one must keep in mind the evidence that some antigens may be weakened by chloroquine treatment. Cells should be treated in accordance with manufacturer's directions if using a commercially prepared reagent or by an approved procedure.

## CASE 3

A 36-year-old woman was seen by her obstetrician 3 weeks after delivery of her third child and was given a diagnosis of a severe urinary tract infection. The physician prescribed a 10-day course of ceftriaxone. On day 4, the woman returned, complaining of weakness on exertion and dark urine. Her hemoglobin and hematocrit values were 7.4 g/dL and 22%, respectively. The physician ordered direct and indirect antiglobulin tests. The DAT was 2+ with anti-IgG and 1+ with anti-C3. The antibody screen was negative at all phases.

1. What is the most likely explanation for the patient's symptoms and for the serologic results?

2. What further testing is necessary?

3. What therapy is needed at this time?

**Case 3 Answers**

1. This patient is most likely to be experiencing a drug-induced hemolytic episode. The third-generation cephalosporins (of which ceftriaxone is an example) are known to cause rapid hemolysis in some patients. Cephalosporins have been shown to cause a positive DAT by formation of immune complexes, by drug adsorption, and by membrane modification. Most likely this hemolytic event is caused by a combination of immune complex formation and drug adsorption. The presence of both complement and IgG on the cells supports this assumption.

2. No additional testing is required. Testing with drug-coated cells or determination of the presence of immune complexes would be purely academic and not essential to treatment.

3. Ceftriaxone should be stopped immediately and another antibiotic substituted. The patient should recover after the drug is ceased. If the physician feels that transfusion is necessary, there should be no problems with compatibility testing.

---

## SUMMARY CHART: IMPORTANT POINTS TO REMEMBER (MT/MLT)

- Immune hemolytic anemia is defined as shortened red cell survival mediated through the immune response, specifically by humoral antibody.
- In alloimmune hemolytic anemia, patients produce alloantibodies to foreign red cell antigens introduced into their circulation, most often through transfusion or pregnancy.
- In autoimmune hemolytic anemia, patients produce antibodies against their own red cell antigens.
- In drug-induced hemolytic anemia, patients produce antibody to a particular drug or drug complex, with subsequent damage to red cells.
- AIHA (autoimmune hemolytic anemia) may be classified as cold-reactive (18%), warm-reactive (70%), or drug-induced (12%); diagnostic tests include the DAT and characterization of the autoantibody in the serum and/or eluate.
- The common antibody specificity in both benign and pathologic cold autoagglutinins is anti-I.
- In CHD (cold hemagglutinin disease), the DAT will be positive because of complement coating of the red cells; an antibody titer greater than 1000 may cause visible agglutination of anticoagulated blood.
- The classic antibody produced in PCH (paroxysmal cold hemoglobinuria) is called the Donath-Landsteiner antibody and has the specificity of autoanti-P. This biphasic antibody binds to patient red cells at low temperatures and fixes complement. Hemolysis occurs when coated cells are warmed to 37°C, and complement-mediated intravascular lysis occurs.
- In 80% of warm AIHA, the antibody causing the hemolysis is an IgG immunoglobulin with IgG subclasses 1 and 3 found in association with most cases of hemolytic anemia.
- Warm-reactive autoantibodies may activate complement, are enhanced by enzyme techniques, and often react with a general specificity within the Rh blood group system.
- When transfusing a patient with warm AIHA, the primary concern is detection and identification of all alloantibodies that are masked by the warm autoantibody.
- In the immune complex drug mechanism, the soluble drug-antidrug complex nonspecifically adsorbs loosely to the red cell surface, yielding a positive DAT with polyspecific AHG and anti-C3.
- In the drug-adsorption (hapten) mechanism, drugs such as penicillin bind firmly to proteins of the red cell membrane. The DAT will show reactivity with polyspecific AHG and anti-IgG.
- In the membrane modification drug mechanism, drugs such as the cephalosporins modify the red cells so that plasma proteins can bind to the membrane nonimmunologically. The DAT will demonstrate reactivity with both anti-IgG and anti-C3.
- In the autoantibody drug mechanism, the drug alpha-methyldopa (Aldomet) induces production of an autoantibody that recognizes RBC antigens. Both the autoantibody and eluate are reactive with normal RBCs. The DAT is reactive with polyspecific AHG and anti-IgG.

---

## REVIEW QUESTIONS

1. Immune hemolytic anemias may be classified in which of the following categories?
   A. Alloimmune
   B. Autoimmune
   C. Drug-induced
   D. All of the above

2. When preparing cells for a cold autoadsorption procedure, it is helpful to pretreat the cells with which of the following?
   A. Dithiothreitol
   B. Ficin
   C. Phosphate-buffered saline at pH 9.0
   D. Bovine albumin

3. The blood group involved in the autoantibody specificity in paroxysmal cold hemoglobinuria is:
   A. P
   B. ABO
   C. Rh
   D. Lewis

4. Which of the following blood groups reacts best with an anti-H or anti-IH?
   A. $A_1B$
   B. B
   C. $A_2$
   D. $A_1$

5. With cold-reactive autoantibodies, the protein coating the patient's cells and detected in the direct antiglobulin test is:
   A. C3
   B. IgG
   C. C4
   D. IgM

6. Problems in routine testing caused by cold-reactive autoantibodies can usually be resolved by all of the following *except*:
   A. Prewarming
   B. Washing with warm saline
   C. Using anti-IgG antiglobulin serum
   D. Collecting clotted blood specimens

7. Pathologic cold autoagglutinins differ from common cold autoagglutinins in:
   A. Immunoglobulin class
   B. Thermal amplitude
   C. Antibody specificity
   D. DAT results on EDTA specimen

8. Cold autoimmune hemolytic anemia is sometimes associated with infection by:
   A. *Staphylococcus aureus*
   B. *Mycoplasma pneumoniae*
   C. *Escherichia coli*
   D. Group A *Streptococcus*

9. Many warm-reactive autoantibodies have a broad specificity within which of the following blood groups?
   A Kell
   B. Duffy
   C. Rh
   D. Kidd

10. Valid Rh typing can usually be obtained on a patient with warm autoimmune hemolytic anemia using all of the following reagents or techniques *except*:
    A. Slide and modified tube anti-D
    B. Chloroquine-treated RBCs
    C. Rosette test
    D. Monoclonal blend anti-D

11. In pretransfusion testing for a patient with warm autoimmune hemolytic anemia, the primary concern is:
    A. Treating the patient's cells with chloroquine for reliable antigen typing
    B. Adsorbing out all antibodies in the patient's serum to be able to provide compatible red cells
    C. Determining the exact specificity of the autoantibody so that compatible red cells can be found
    D. Discovering any existing significant alloantibodies in the patient's circulation

12. Penicillin given in massive doses has been associated with red cell hemolysis. Which of the classic mechanisms is involved in the hemolytic process?
    A. Immune complex
    B. Drug adsorption
    C. Membrane modification
    D. Autoantibody formation

13. Which of the following drugs has been associated with complement activation and rapid intravascular hemolysis?
    A. Penicillins
    B. Quinidine
    C. Alpha-methyldopa
    D. Cephalosporins

14. A patient is admitted with a 5.6 g/dL hemoglobin. Initial pretransfusion work-up appears to indicate

the presence of a warm autoantibody in the serum and coating his red cells. He received 6 U of RBCs in transfusion 2 years ago after an automobile accident. Which of the following would be most helpful in performing antibody detection and compatibility testing procedures?
   A. Adsorb the autoantibody using the patient's enzyme-treated cells.
   B. Perform an elution and use the eluate for compatibility testing.
   C. Crossmatch random units until compatible units are found.
   D. Collect blood from relatives who are more likely to be compatible.

15. A patient who is taking Aldomet has a positive direct antiglobulin test. An eluate prepared from his red cells would be expected to:
    A. React only with Aldomet-coated cells
    B. Be neutralized by a suspension of Aldomet
    C. React with all normal cells
    D. React only with $Rh_{null}$ cells

## ANSWERS TO REVIEW QUESTIONS

1. D (p 437)
2. B (p 440)
3. A (p 444)
4. C (p 441)
5. A (p 440)
6. D (pp 440–441)
7. B (p 439, Table 21–1)
8. B (p 443)
9. C (p 447)
10. A (p 448)
11. D (pp 448–449)
12. B (p 453)
13. D (p 454)
14. A (pp 448–449)
15. C (pp 454–455)

## REFERENCES

1. Izui, S: Autoimmune hemolytic anemia. Curr Opin Immunol 6:926, 1994.
2. Barthold, DR, Kysela, S, and Steinberg, AD: Decline in suppressor T cell function with age in female NZB mice. J Immunol 112:9, 1974.
3. Banacerraf, B, and Unanue, ER: Textbook of Immunology. Williams & Wilkins, Baltimore, 1979.
4. Kirtland, HH, Horwitz, DA, and Mohler, DN: Inhibition of suppressor T cell function by methyldopa: A proposed cause of autoimmune hemolytic anemia. N Engl J Med 302:825, 1980.

5. van Loghem, JJ: Concepts on the origin of autoimmune diseases: The possible role of viral infection in the etiology of idiopathic autoimmune diseases. Semin Hematol 9:17, 1965.

6. Petz, LD, and Garratty, G: Acquired Immune Hemolytic Anemias. Churchill Livingstone, New York, 1980.

7. Allan, J, and Garratty, G: Positive direct antiglobulin tests in normal blood donors (abstract). Proceedings of the 16th Congress of the International Society of Blood Transfusion, Montreal, 1980.

8. Okuno, T, Germino, F, and Newman, B: Clinical significance of autologous control (abstract). American Society Clinical Pathologists 16, 1984.

9. Lau, P, Haesler, WE, and Wurzel, HA: Positive direct antiglobulin reaction in a patient population. Am J Clin Pathol 65:368, 1976.

10. Judd, WJ, et al: The evaluation of a positive direct antiglobulin test in pretransfusion testing. Transfusion 20:17, 1980.

11. Garratty, G, Petz, LD, and Hoops, JK: The correlation of cold agglutinin titrations in saline and albumin with haemolytic anaemia. Br J Haematol 35:587, 1977.

12. Engelfriet, CP, et al: Autoimmune hemolytic anemias. I. Serological studies with pure anti-immunoglobulin reagents. Clin Exp Immunol 3:605, 1968.

13. Rosse, WF: Quantitative immunology of immune hemolytic anemia. II. The relationship of cell-bound antibody to hemolysis and the effect of treatment. J Clin Invest 50:734, 1971.

14. De Angelis, V, et al: Abnormalities of membrane protein composition in patients with autoimmune haemolytic anaemia. Br J Hematol 95:273, 1996.

15. Gilliland, BC, Baxter, E, and Evans, RS: Red cell antibodies in acquired hemolytic anemia with negative antiglobulin serum tests. N Engl J Med 285:252, 1971.

16. Garratty, G: Autoimmune hemolytic anemia. In Garratty, G (ed): Immunobiology of Transfusion Medicine. Marcel Dekker, New York, 1994, p 493.

17. Stratton, F, et al: Acquired hemolytic anemia associated with IgA anti-e. Transfusion 12:197, 1972.

18. Sturgeon, P, et al: Autoimmune hemolytic anemia associated exclusively with IgA of Rh specificity. Transfusion 19:324, 1979.

19. Hoppe, PA: The role of the Bureau of Biologics in assuring reagent reliability. In Considerations in the Selection of Reagents. American Association of Blood Banks, Washington, DC, 1979, p 1.

20. Garratty, G, and Petz, LD: An evaluation of commercial antiglobulin sera with particular reference to their anticomplement properties. Transfusion 11:79, 1971.

21. Vengelen-Tyler, V (ed): Technical Manual, ed 12. American Association of Blood Banks, Bethesda, MD, 1996, p 379.

22. Reid, ME: Autoagglutination dispersal utilizing sulfhydryl compounds. Transfusion 18:353, 1978.

23. Judd, WJ: Controversies in transfusion medicine: Prewarmed tests: Con. Transfusion 35:271, 1995.

24. Chaplin, H, et al: Clinically significant allo-anti-I in an I negative patient with massive hemorrhage. Transfusion 26:57, 1986.

25. Marsh, WL: Aspects of cold-reactive autoantibodies. In Bell, CA (ed): A Seminar on Laboratory Management of Hemolysis. American Association of Blood Banks, Washington, DC, 1979, p 79.

26. Combs, MR, et al: An auto-anti M causing hemolysis in vitro. Transfusion 31:756, 1991.

27. Garratty, G: Target antigens for red-cell-bound autoantibodies. In Nance, ST (ed): Clinical and Basic Science Aspects of Immunohematology. American Association of Blood Banks, Arlington, VA, 1991, p 33.

28. Lyckholm, LJ, and Edmond, MB: Seasonal hemolysis due to cold-agglutinin syndrome. N Engl J Med 334:437, 1996.

29. Aoki, A, et al: Cardiac operation without hypothermia for the patient with cold agglutinin. Chest 104:1627, 1993.

30. Shirey, RS, et al: An anti-i biphasic hemolysin in chronic paroxysmal cold hemoglobinuria. Transfusion 26:62, 1986.

31. Judd, WJ, et al: Donath-Landsteiner hemolytic anemia due to an anti-Pr-like biphasic hemolysin. Transfusion 26:423, 1986.

32. Reid, M: Association of red blood cell membrane abnormalities with blood group phenotype. In Garratty, G (ed): Immunobiol-

ogy of Transfusion Medicine. Marcel Dekker, New York, 1994, p 257.

33. Salloum, E, and Lundberg, WB: Hemolytic anemia with positive direct antiglobulin test secondary to spontaneous cytomegalovirus infection in healthy adults. Acta Hematol 92:39, 1994.

34. Benraad, CEM, Scheerder, HAJM, and Overbeeke, MAM: Autoimmune haemolytic anaemia during pregnancy. Eur J Obstet Gynecol Reprod Biol 55:209, 1994.

35. Edwards, JM, Moulds, JJ, and Judd, WJ: Chloroquine dissociation of antigen-antibody complexes: A new technique for typing red blood cells with a positive direct antiglobulin test. Transfusion 22:59, 1982.

36. Weiner, W, and Vos, GH: Serology of acquired hemolytic anemias. Blood 22:606, 1963.

37. Win, N, et al: Autoimmune haemolytic anaemia in infancy with anti-Kp$^b$ specificity. Vox Sang 71:187, 1994.

38. Becton, DL, and Kinney, TR: An infant girl with severe autoimmune hemolytic anemia: Apparent anti-Vel specificity. Vox Sang 51:108, 1986.

39. Reynolds, MV, Vengelen-Tyler, V, and Morel, PA: Autoimmune hemolytic anemia associated with auto anti-Ge. Vox Sang 41:61, 1981.

40. Wilkinson, SL: Serological approaches to transfusion of patients with allo- or autoantibodies. In Nance, ST (ed): Immune Destruction of Red Blood Cells. American Association of Blood Banks, Arlington, VA, 1989, pp 227.

41. Singh, M, Thompson, H, and Pallas, C: Response to transfusions in autoimmune hemolytic anemia. Abstracts of South Central Association of Blood Banks Annual Meeting, Tucson, AZ, 1997.

42. Jeffries, LC: Transfusion therapy in autoimmune hemolytic anemia. Hematol Oncol Clin North Am 8:1087, 1994.

43. Anderson, DR, and Kelton, JG: Mechanisms in intravascular and extravascular cell destruction. In Nance, ST (ed): Immune Destruction of Red Blood Cells. American Association of Blood Banks, Arlington, VA, 1989, p 39.

44. Flores, G, et al: Efficacy of intravenous immunoglobulin in the treatment of autoimmune hemolytic anemia: Results in 73 patients. Am J Hematol 44:237, 1993.

45. Kerr, RO, et al: Two mechanisms of erythrocyte destruction in penicillin-induced hemolytic anemia. N Engl J Med 298:1322, 1972.

46. Ries, CA, et al: Penicillin-induced immune hemolytic anemia. JAMA 233:432, 1975.

47. Garratty, G: Review: Immune hemolytic anemia and/or positive direct antiglobulin tests caused by drugs. Immunohematology 10:41, 1994.

48. Shulman, NR: Mechanism of blood cell destruction in individuals sensitized to foreign antigens. Transactions of the Association of American Physicians 76:72, 1963.

49. Dameshek, W: Autoimmunity: Theoretical aspects. I. Ann N Y Acad Sci 124:6, 1965.

50. Petz, LD, and Mueller-Eckhardt, C: Drug-induced immune hemolytic anemia. Transfusion 32:02, 1992.

51. Garratty, G: Drug-induced immune hemolytic anemia. In Garratty, G (ed): Immunobiology of Transfusion Medicine. Marcel Dekker, New York, 1994, p. 523.

52. Garratty, G: Laboratory Investigation of Drug-induced Immune Hemolytic Anemia and/or Positive Direct Antiglobulin Tests. American Association of Blood Banks, Washington, DC, 1979.

53. Eckrich, RJ, Fox, S, and Mallory, D: Cefotetan-induced immune hemolytic anemia due to the drug-adsorption mechanism. Immunohematology 10:51, 1994.

54. Bernini, JC, et al: Fatal hemolysis induced by ceftriaxone in a child with sickle cell anemia. J Pediatr 126:813, 1995.

55. Lascari, AD, and Amyot, K: Fatal hemolysis caused by ceftriaxone. J Pediatr 126:816, 1995.

56. Spath, P, Garratty, G, and Petz, LD: Studies on the immune response to penicillin and cephalothin in humans. II. Immunohematologic reactions to cephalothin administration. J Immunol 107:860, 1971.

57. Carstairs, KC, et al: Incidence of a positive direct Coombs' test in patients on alpha-methyldopa. Lancet 2:33, 1966.

58. Worlledge, SM, Carstairs, KC, and Dacie, JV: Autoimmune he-

molytic anemia associated with methyldopa therapy. Lancet 2:135, 1966.

59. Petz, LD: Drug-induced hemolytic anemia. Transfus Med Rev 7:242, 1993.
60. Lopez, A, et al: Autoimmune hemolytic anemia induced by diclofenac. Ann Pharmacother 29:787, 1995.
61. Harmening, DM: Clinical Hematology and Fundamentals of Hemostasis, ed 3. FA Davis, Philadelphia, 1997, pp 221–243.

## BIBLIOGRAPHY

Calvo, R, et al: Acute hemolytic anemia due to anti-i; frequent cold agglutinins in infectious mononucleosis. J Clin Invest 44:1033, 1965.

Carter, P, Koval, JJ, and Hobbs, JR: The relation of clinical and laboratory findings to the survival of patients with macroglobinaemia. Clin Exp Immunol 28:241, 1977.

Chaplin, H, and Avioli, LV: Autoimmune hemolytic anemia. Arch Intern Med 137:346, 1977.

Dacie, JV: Autoimmune hemolytic anemia. Arch Intern Med 135:1293, 1975.

Dameshek, W: Alpha-methyldopa red cell antibody: Cross reaction or forbidden clone. N Engl J Med 276:1382, 1967.

Evans, RS, Baxter, E, and Gilliland, BC: Chronic hemolytic anemia due to cold agglutinins: A 20-year history of benign gammopathy with response to chlorambucil. Blood 42:463, 1973.

Forbes, CD, Craig, JA, and Mitchell, R: Acute intravascular hemolysis associated with cephalexin therapy. Postgrad Med J 48:186, 1972.

Frank, MM, Atkinson, JP, and Gadek, J: Cold agglutinins and cold agglutinin disease. Ann Rev Med 28:291, 1977.

Freedman, J, and Lim, FC: An immunohematologic complication of isoniazid. Vox Sang 35:126, 1978.

Garratty, G: Drug-induced immune hemolytic anemia and/or positive direct antiglobulin tests. Immunohematology 2:6, 1985.

Garratty, G: Target antigens for red-cell-bound autoantibodies. In Nance, ST (ed): Clinical and Basic Science Aspects of Immunohematology. American Association of Blood Banks, Arlington, VA, 1991, pp 33–72.

Gottlieb, AJ, and Wurzel, HA: Protein-quinone interaction: In vivo induction of indirect antiglobulin reactions with methyldopa. Blood 43:85, 1974.

Gralnick, HR, McGinniss MH, and Elton, W: Hemolytic anemia associated with cephalothin. JAMA 217:1193, 1971.

Habibi, B: Drug induced red blood cell autoantibodies co-developed with drug specific antibodies causing haemolytic anaemias. Br J Haematol 61:139, 1985.

Harmening-Pittiglio, DM: Warm auto immune hemolytic anemia: A review of clinical and laboratory considerations. Immunohematology 1, 1984.

Hendry, EG: Osmolarity of human serum and of chemical solutions of importance. Clin Chem 7:156, 1961.

Jeannet, M, et al: Cephalothin-induced immune hemolytic anemia. Acta Haematol 55:109, 1976.

Kaplan, K, Reisburg, B, and Weinsteins, L: Cephaloridine studies of therapeutic activity and untoward effects. Arch Intern Med 121:17, 1968.

Kickler, TS, et al: Probenecid induced immune hemolytic anemia. J Rheumatol 13:208, 1986.

Kramer, MR, Levine, C, and Hershko, C: Severe reversible autoimmune haemolytic anaemia and thrombocytopenia associated with diclofenac therapy. Scandinavian Journal Haematology 36:118, 1986.

Leddy, JP, and Swisher, SN: Acquired immune hemolytic disorders (including drug-induced immune hemolytic anemia). In Samter, M (ed): Immunological Diseases, ed 3, Vol 2, 1978, p 1187.

Marchand, A: Charting a course for hemolytic anemia. Diagn Med 1981.

Marchand, A: Immune hemolytic anemia. Part I: Classification, manifestations and mechanism of destruction. Diagnostic Medicine 1982.

Marchand, A: Immune hemolytic anemia. Part II: Test procedures and strategy. Diagnostic Medicine 1983.

Petz, LD, and Branch, DR: Immune Hemolytic Anemias. Churchill Livingstone, Edinburgh, 1985.

Seldon, MR, et al: Ticarcillin-induced immune haemolytic anaemia. Scand J Haematol 28:459, 1982.

Silberstein, LE (ed): Autoimmune Disorders of Blood. American Association of Blood Banks, Bethesda, MD, 1996.

Tafani, O, et al: Fatal acute immune haemolytic anaemia caused by nalidixic acid. Br Med J 285:936, 1982.

Tanowitz, HB, Robbins, N, and Leidich, N: Hemolytic anemia: Associated with severe *Mycoplasma pneumoniae* pneumonia. N Y State J Med 78:2231, 1978.

Tuffs, L, and Mancharan, A: Flucloxacillin-induced haemolytic anaemia (letter). Med J Aust 144:559, 1986.

Wallace, ME, and Green, TS (eds): Selection of Procedures for Problem Solving. American Association of Blood Banks, Arlington, VA, 1983.

Wallace, ME, and Levitt, JS: Current Applications and Interpretations of the Direct Antiglobulin Test. American Association of Blood Banks, Arlington, VA, 1988.

Worlledge, SM: Immune drug-induced haemolytic anemias. Semin Hematol 6:181, 1969.

## A—USE OF THIOL REAGENTS TO DISPERSE AUTOAGGLUTINATION*

### Application

Thiol reagents, which cleave the intersubunit disulfide bonds of pentameric IgM molecules, can be used to disperse agglutination caused by cold-reactive autoantibodies. Treating spontaneously agglutinated red cells with 2-mercaptoethanol (2-ME) or dithiothreitol (DTT) provides a nonagglutinated specimen for use in blood grouping tests.

### Materials

1. 0.01 M DTT or 0.1 M 2-ME
2. Phosphate-buffered saline (PBS) at pH 7.3
3. Packed red cells to be treated, washed three to four times

### Method

1. Dilute washed red cells to a 50 percent concentration in PBS.
2. Add an equal quantity of 0.01 M DTT in PBS, or 0.1 M 2-ME in PBS, to the red cells.
3. Mix and incubate at 37°C for 15 minutes for DTT or 10 minutes for 2-ME.
4. Wash red cells three times.
5. Dilute the treated red cells to a 3 to 5 percent concentration in saline and use in blood grouping tests.

## B—COLD AUTOADSORPTION†

### Application

Autoadsorption can be used to remove cold-reactive autoantibodies, allowing detection of clinically significant alloantibodies.

### Materials

1. 1 percent ficin or 1 percent papain
2. 2 mL of serum to be adsorbed
3. 3 mL of packed autologous red cells

### Method

1. Wash the red cells four times in warm saline and divide into three equal aliquots in 13 × 100 mm test tubes. Completely remove supernatant after last wash.
2. Add an equal volume of 1 percent ficin or 1 percent papain to each aliquot of washed cells.
3. Mix, and incubate at 37°C for 15 minutes.
4. Wash the red cells three times in saline. Centrifuge the last wash for 5 minutes at 1000 × g, and remove as much of the supernatant saline as possible (see note).
5. To one tube of enzyme-treated red cells add 2 mL of the autologous serum.
6. Mix, and incubate at 4°C for 30 to 60 minutes.

---

*Adapted from Reid, ME. Autoagglutination dispersal utilizing sulfhydryl compounds. Transfusion 18:353, 1978.

†Adapted from Beattie, K, et al: Immunohematology Methods. American Red Cross, Rockville, MD, 1993.

7. Centrifuge at 1000 × g for 5 minutes, and transfer the serum into a second tube of enzyme-treated autologous red cells.
8. Mix and incubate at 4°C for 30 to 40 minutes.
9. In most cases, two adsorptions are sufficient to remove the autoantibody. If the autoantibody is particularly strong, repeat steps 7 and 8 using the third tube of enzyme-treated red cells.
10. After the final adsorption, test the serum for alloantibody activity.

NOTES:

1. To avoid dilution of the serum and possible loss of weak alloantibody activity during the adsorption process, it is important to remove as much of the residual saline as possible in step 4. Placing a narrow strip of filter paper into the packed red cells helps remove saline that surrounds the packed cells.
2. Autoadsorption should not be used when the patient has recently received a transfusion. Adsorption with rabbit erythrocyte stroma may be used in this situation.

## C—PREWARMED TECHNIQUE FOR TESTING SERUM CONTAINING COLD AGGLUTININS*

### Application

The reactivity of IgM cold autoantibodies can be reduced or eliminated by performing prewarmed tests. Most problems encountered in compatibility testing, antibody detection, and identification tests that are caused by cold agglutinins can be resolved with the use of this technique. By preventing the reaction between the cold agglutinin and the red cell at room temperature (during centrifugation, and so on), one prevents complement activation. The anti-C3 in polyspecific antihuman globulin reagent reacts with the remaining C3, making detection of significant AHG-reactive antibodies difficult. Prewarming of the serum, cells, and additive will hinder the binding of the cold autoantibody and the resulting complement activation.

### Materials

1. Normal saline, warmed to 37°C
2. Patient's serum
3. Additive solution (bovine albumin, low ionic strength solution, polyethylene glycol, etc.), if any
4. Cells to be tested (screening or panel cells, donor cells)

### Method

1. Label 1 tube for each reagent or donor cell sample to be tested.
2. Add 1 drop of the appropriate 2 to 4 percent cell suspension to each tube.
3. Place the tubes containing the red cells, a tube containing a small amount of patient's serum, and a tube containing the additive solution, if any, at 37°C for 5 to 10 minutes.
4. Transfer 2 drops of prewarmed serum into each tube containing prewarmed red cells. Mix without removing the tubes from the incubator.
5. Incubate at 37°C for at least 30 minutes with no additive, or the appropriate time for the additive used.

---

*Adapted from Vengelen-Tyler, V (ed): Technical Manual, ed 12. American Association of Blood Banks, Bethesda, MD, 1996, p 379.

6. Without removing the tubes from the incubator, fill all tubes with prewarmed saline (37°C). Centrifuge and wash two to three more times with warm saline.
7. Add anti-IgG antiglobulin reagent, centrifuge, and record reactions.

NOTES:

1. Use of the anti-IgG antiglobulin reagent ensures that positive reactions caused by cold autoagglutinins with complement binding only will not be detected. Most significant antibodies react in the antiglobulin phase with anti-IgG reagent.
2. A prewarmed technique should be used only in situations in which a true cold autoagglutinin appears to be present. See reference 23.

## D—ADSORPTION OF COLD AUTOANTIBODIES WITH RABBIT ERYTHROCYTE STROMA*

### Application

Autoadsorption procedures are not recommended when a patient has recently received a transfusion. Rabbit erythrocytes are known to possess the I antigen, and stroma made from rabbit erythrocytes is commercially available for use in adsorption techniques.

### Materials

1. Rabbit erythrocyte stroma (REST$^R$, BCA, a division of Biopool International, West Chester, Pa)
2. Patient's serum containing cold autoantibodies

### Method

1. Centrifuge for at least 2 minutes to pack the rabbit stroma and completely remove the supernatant.
2. Add 1 mL of the serum to be adsorbed.
3. Stopper and mix well using a vortex mixer.
4. Incubate at 4°C for 15 to 60 minutes, mixing occasionally.
5. Centrifuge for at least 2 minutes, and transfer the adsorbed serum to a clean tube.
6. Perform antibody screening, antibody identification, or compatibility testing according to routine procedures.

NOTES:

1. In addition to the I antigen, rabbit erythrocyte stroma carries the B antigen, P system antigens, and H antigens. Therefore, serum adsorbed with rabbit RBC stroma should not be used for ABO reverse typing.
2. Some alloantibodies, including anti-D, anti-E, and anti-Le$^b$, have been reported to be adsorbed onto rabbit RBC stroma.

---

*Adapted from Waligora, SK, and Edwards, JM: The use of rabbit red blood cells for the adsorption of cold autoagglutinins. Transfusion 23:328, 1983.

# E—DISSOCIATION OF IgG BY CHLOROQUINE

## Application*

Red cells with a positive DAT cannot be used directly for blood grouping with antisera, such as anti-K1, anti-Fy$^a$, and $-$Fy$^b$ and others, that require the use of an indirect antiglobulin technique. Under controlled conditions, chloroquine diphosphate dissociates IgG from red cells with little or no damage to the red cell membrane. Use of this procedure permits complete phenotyping of DAT-positive red cells, including tests with antisera solely reactive by the indirect antiglobulin test.

## Materials

1. Chloroquine diphosphate solution prepared by dissolving 20 g of chloroquine diphosphate in 100 mL of saline (pH 5.1)
2. Red cells with a positive DAT due to IgG coating
3. Control red cells heterozygous for the antigen for which the test sample is to be phenotyped
4. Anti-IgG antiglobulin reagent

## Method

1. To 1 volume of washed packed IgG-coated test red cells add 4 volumes of chloroquine diphosphate solution. Treat the control sample similarly.
2. Mix and incubate at room temperature for 30 minutes.
3. Remove a small aliquot (e.g., 1 drop) of the treated red cells, and wash four times with saline.
4. Test the washed cells with anti-IgG.
5. If nonreactive with anti-IgG, wash the entire sample of treated test red cells and the control sample three times in saline, and use for phenotyping with antiglobulin-reactive antisera. Use an anti-IgG reagent when testing these cells.
6. If the treated red cells react with the anti-IgG after the 30-minute incubation, repeat steps 3 and 4 at 30-minute intervals (for a maximum incubation of 2 hours), until the red cells are nonreactive with anti-IgG. Proceed as described in step 5.

NOTES:

1. Chloroquine diphosphate does not dissociate complement components from red cells. If cells are coated with both IgG and C3 in vivo, test performed after chloroquine treatment should be done using anti-IgG.
2. Incubation of red cells in chloroquine diphosphate should not be extended beyond 2 hours. Prolonged incubation at room temperature, or incubation at 37°C, may result in hemolysis and damage to or loss of red cell antigens. An alternate procedure described by Beaumont and associates recommends incubation at 30°C for 90 minutes or 37°C for 30 minutes. The reader is referred to this article for details.
3. Some denaturation of Rh antigens may occur. This is most often noted when red cells have hemolyzed following incubation with chloroquine diphosphate. Use high-protein antisera and control reagent when Rh-typing chloroquine-treated cells.
4. Include an inert control reagent when phenotyping chloroquine-treated red cells.

---

*Adapted from Beaumont, AE, et al: An improved method for removal of red-cell bound immunoglobulin using chloroquine solution. Immunohematology 10:22, 1994.

## F—DIGITONIN-ACID ELUTION*

### Application

Removal of antibodies bound to red cell antigens is used in investigation of a positive DAT associated with warm-reactive (IgG) autoantibodies or alloantibodies, and for the separation of mixtures of IgG antibodies.

### Materials

1. Digitonin (0.5 percent w/v), prepared by dissolving 0.5 g of digitonin in 100 mL of distilled water. Store at 4°C.
2. Glycine (0.1 M, pH 3.0), prepared by dissolving 3.754 g of glycine in 500 mL of distilled water. Adjust pH to 3.0 with 12 N HCl. Store at 4°C.
3. Phosphate buffer (0.8 M, pH 8.2), prepared by dissolving 109.6 g of $Na_2HPO_4$ and 3.8 g of $KH_2PO_4$ in approximately 600 mL of distilled water. Adjust pH, if necessary, with either 1 N NaOH or 1 N HCl. Dilute to a final volume of 1 liter with distilled water. Store at 4°C.
4. Bovine serum albumin, 30 percent.
5. Packed red cells (1 mL), washed six times in saline.
6. Supernatant saline from last wash.

### Method

1. Warm reagents to 37°C before use, and mix well.
2. Mix 1 mL of washed packed red cells and 9 mL of saline in a 16 × 100 mm test tube.
3. Add 0.5 mL of digitonin, and mix by inversion until all red cells are hemolyzed (at least 1 minute).
4. Centrifuge at 1000 × g for 5 minutes, and discard the supernatant.
5. Wash the red cell stroma at least five times, or until it appears white. Centrifuge for at least 2 minutes during the washing process.
6. Discard the final supernatant wash solution, and add 2 mL of glycine to the stroma.
7. Mix by inversion for at least 1 minute.
8. Centrifuge the tube at 1000 × g for 5 minutes.
9. Transfer the supernatant eluate to a clean test tube, and add 0.2 mL of phosphate buffer.
10. Mix and centrifuge at 1000 × g for 2 minutes.
11. Transfer the supernatant into a clean test tube, and add one-third volume of 30 percent bovine serum albumin. Test in parallel with the last wash saline.

NOTES:

1. The low pH of the acid buffer enhances elution of antibody from the red cell stroma. Phosphate buffer is added to restore neutrality to the acidic eluate. Persisting acidity may cause lysis of red cells added to the eluate. Adding bovine albumin to the eluate protects against hemolysis.
2. Ensure that digitonin is well mixed and warmed to 37°C before use.
3. Use centrifugation times of at least 2 minutes when washing stroma.
4. Phosphate buffer will crystallize on storage at 4°C. Redissolve at 37°C before use.

---

*Adapted from Jenkins, DE, and Moore, WH: A rapid method for the preparation of high-potency auto- and alloantibody eluates. Transfusion 17:110, 1977.

# G—AUTOLOGOUS ADSORPTION OF WARM-REACTIVE AUTOANTIBODIES

## Application

Warm-reactive autoantibodies may mask the presence of coexisting alloantibodies in a serum. Adsorbing the serum with autologous red cells can remove autoantibody from the serum, permitting detection of underlying alloantibodies. Circulating autologous cells, however, are already coated with autoantibody. Some of the autoantibody must be removed from the surface of the autologous red cells in order to achieve maximum removal of autoantibody by the adsorption process. Autoadsorption should not be performed if a patient has recently received a transfusion because the circulating transfused cells may absorb out alloantibodies.

### a. Heat and Enzyme Method*

*Materials*

1. Six percent bovine albumin, prepared by diluting 22 percent or 30 percent bovine albumin with saline
2. One percent ficin or 1 percent cysteine-activated papain
3. Blood sample containing warm-reactive autoantibodies

*Method*

1. Wash 2 mL of red cells four times in saline, and discard the final supernatant.
2. Add an equal volume of 6 percent albumin to the packed red cells. Mix and incubate at 56° C for 3 to 5 minutes. Gently agitate the mixture during this time.
3. Centrifuge at 1000 × g for 2 minutes and harvest the supernatant. This may be used for eluate if the patient's cells are in short supply.
4. Wash the cells three times in saline, and discard the final supernatant.
5. Add 1 mL of 1 percent ficin or papain to the red cells. Mix and incubate at 37° for 15 minutes.
6. Wash the red cells three times in saline. Centrifuge the last wash for at least 5 minutes at 1000 × g. Use suction to remove as much of the supernatant as practical.
7. Divide the red cells into two equal aliquots.
8. To 1 aliquot add 2 mL of patient's serum. Mix and incubate at 37° C for 30 minutes.
9. Centrifuge at 1000 × g for 2 minutes and transfer the serum to the second aliquot of enzyme-treated red cells. Mix and incubate at 37° C for 30 minutes.
10. Centrifuge at 1000 × g for 2 minutes, and harvest the adsorbed serum.
11. Test the adsorbed serum for antibody activity using an indirect antiglobulin technique.

### b. ZZAP Method†

*Materials*

1. One percent cysteine-activated papain
2. Phosphate-buffered saline (PBS) at pH 7.3

---

*Morel, PA, Bergren, ML, and Frank, BA: A simple method for detection of alloantibody in the presence of autoantibody (abstract). Transfusion 18:388, 1978.
†Branch, DR, and Petz, LD: A new reagent (ZZAP) having multiple applications in immunohematology. Am J Clin Pathol 78:161–167, 1982.

3. 0.2 M dithiothreitol (DTT) prepared by dissolving 1 g of DTT in 32.4 mL of pH 6.5 PBS. Dispense into 2.5-mL aliquots and store at or below $-20°C$
4. Blood samples containing warm-reactive autoantibodies.

*Method*

1. Prepare ZZAP reagent by mixing 0.5 mL cysteine-activated papain with 2.5 mL DTT and 2 mL pH 7.3 PBS. Alternatively, use 1 mL ficin, 2.5 mL DTT, and 1.5 mL pH 6.5 PBS.
2. To two tubes, each containing 1 mL of packed red cells, add 2 mL of ZZAP reagent. Mix and incubate at 37°C for 30 minutes.
3. Wash the red cells three times in saline. Centrifuge the last wash at least 5 minutes at $1000 \times g$. Use suction to remove as much of the supernatant as practical.
4. Proceed as from step 8 in Procedure a above.

*Interpretation*

A twofold autologous adsorption usually removes sufficient autoantibody from the serum so that alloantibody, if present, is readily apparent. Occasionally, two adsorptions are insufficient. If the patient's red cells can be shown to have a negative DAT following heat treatment (Procedure a), ZZAP treatment (Procedure b), or after treatment with chloroquine diphosphate, such red cells may be used to check the efficacy of the adsorption process. For example, if Procedure a was used and the heat-treated cells obtained after step 4 have a negative DAT, the autoadsorbed serum should be tested against them and two group O red cell samples (screening cells).

Results can be interpreted as follows:

1. When there is no reactivity against the group O reagent red cells, it is unlikely that alloantibody is present.
2. If there is reactivity against both the patient's heat-treated red cells and the group O cells, further adsorptions are necessary to remove the autoantibody.
3. When the adsorbed serum reacts with one or both of the group O reagent red cells and not with the autologous red cells, the serum contains alloantibody, and antibody identification studies should be undertaken on the adsorbed serum.

NOTES:

1. ZZAP reagent should be prepared immediately before use.
2. ZZAP treatment destroys all Kell system antigens except Kx, in addition to M, N, S, s, Fy$^a$, Fy$^b$, and other receptors that are destroyed by protease.
3. There is no need to wash red cells before treatment with ZZAP.

## H—DEMONSTRATION OF DRUG-INDUCED IMMUNE COMPLEX FORMATION*

### Application

Certain drugs and their respective antibodies form immune complexes and attach weakly to red cells. These nonspecifically bound immune complexes activate complement, which may lead to hemolysis in vivo. This procedure provides a means to demonstrate in vitro the immune complex formation associated with drug-antidrug interactions.

---

*Adapted from Garratty, G: Laboratory Investigation of Drug-induced Immune Hemolytic Anemia and/or Positive Direct Antiglobulin Tests. American Association of Blood Banks, Washington, DC, 1979.

## Materials

1. Drug under investigation, in the same form (tablet, solution, capsules) that the patient is receiving
2. Phosphate-buffered saline (PBS) at pH 7.0–7.4
3. Patient's serum
4. Fresh normal serum known to lack unexpected antibodies, as a source of complement
5. Group O red cells, both untreated and treated with a proteolytic enzyme

## Method

1. Prepare a 1 mg/mL suspension of the drug in PBS. Centrifuge and adjust the pH of the supernatant fluid to 7.0 with either 1 $N$ NaOH or 1 $N$ HCl, as required.
2. Using 0.2 mL of each reactant, prepare the following test mixtures:
   a. Patient's serum + drug
   b. Patient's serum + complement (normal serum) + drug
   c. Patient's serum + complement (normal serum) + PBS
   d. Normal serum + drug
   e. Normal serum + PBS
3. To 3 drops of each test mixture, add 1 drop of a 5 percent saline suspension of group O red cells. To another 3 drops of each test mixture, add 1 drop of a 5 percent saline suspension of enzyme-treated group O reagent red cells.
4. Mix and incubate at 37°C for 1 to 2 hours with periodic gentle mixing.
5. Centrifuge and examine for hemolysis/agglutination.
6. Wash the red cells four times in saline and test with a polyspecific antiglobulin reagent.

## Interpretation

Hemolysis, agglutination, or coating can occur. Such reactivity in any of the tests containing patient's serum to which the drug was added, and absence of reactivity in the corresponding control tests containing PBS instead of the drug, indicates a drug-antidrug interaction.

NOTES:

1. The use of a mortar and pestle (if the drug is in tablet form), incubation at 37°C, and vigorous shaking of the solution may help dissolve the drug.
2. Many drugs will not dissolve completely, but enough may be dissolved to react in serologic tests. Other methods, obtained from the manufacturer or other publications, may be needed to dissolve adequate quantities of some drugs.

## I—DETECTION OF ANTIBODIES TO PENICILLIN OR CEPHALOTHIN*

### Application

Red blood cells can be coated with penicillin or cephalosporins and tested to investigate a positive DAT associated with these antibiotics.

---

*Adapted from Garratty, G: Laboratory Investigation of Drug-induced Hemolytic Anemia and/or Positive Direct Antiglobulin Tests. American Association of Blood Banks, Washington, DC, 1979.

## Materials

1. Barbital-buffered saline (BBS) at pH 9.6, prepared by dissolving 20.6 g of sodium barbital in 1 liter of saline. Adjust to pH 9.6 with 0.1 $N$ HCl. Store at 4°C.
2. Penicillin ($1 \times 10^6$ U per 600 mg)
3. Cephalothin sodium (Keflin)—400 mg
4. Washed, packed group O red cells (2 mL)
5. Serum or eluate to be tested

## Method

1. Prepare penicillin-coated red cells by incubating 1 mL of red cells with 600 mg of penicillin in 15 mL BBS for 1 hour at room temperature. Wash three times in saline and store in Alsever's solution at 4°C.
2. Prepare cephalothin-coated red cells by incubating 1 mL of red cells with 400 mg of cephalothin sodium in 10 mL of BBS for 2 hours at 37°C. Wash three times in saline and store in Alsever's solution at 4°C.
3. Mix 2 or 3 drops of serum or eluate with 1 drop of a 5 percent suspension of drug-coated cells. Dilute serum 1:20 with saline for tests with cephalothin-coated cells.
4. Test in parallel uncoated red cells from the same donor.
5. Incubate the tests at 37°C for 30 to 60 minutes. Centrifuge and examine macroscopically for agglutination. Grade, and record results.
6. Wash the red cells four times in saline and test by the indirect antiglobulin technique using polyspecific or anti-IgG reagent.

## Interpretation

Antibodies to penicillin or cephalothin will react with drug-coated cells but not with uncoated cells. Antibodies to either drug may cross-react with red cells coated with the other drug (e.g., antipenicillin antibodies cross-react with cephalothin-coated red cells and vice versa).

NOTES:

1. Phosphate-buffered saline at pH 7.3 may be substituted for BBS in the preparation of cephalothin-coated red cells.
2. All normal sera react with cephalothin-coated red cells, since such red cells absorb all proteins nonimmunologically. This reactivity does not occur with incubation times as short as 15 minutes, or if the serum is diluted 1:20 with saline before testing.
3. Eluates do not contain enough protein to be absorbed nonimmunologically by cephalothin-coated red cells. Reactivity of an eluate with cephalothin-coated red cells indicates antibody to cephalosporins, which may cross-react with penicillin-coated red cells.

CHAPTER **22**

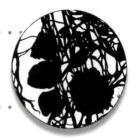

# POLYAGGLUTINATION

Phyllis S. Walker, MS, MT(ASCP)SBB

## OBJECTIVES

*On completion of this chapter, the learner should be able to:*

### MICROBIALLY ASSOCIATED FORMS OF POLYAGGLUTINATION: T, TK, AND ACQUIRED B

1 List the bacterial organism(s) associated with T, Tk, and acquired-B forms of polyagglutination.

2 Describe the mechanism, including the specific microbial product that produces each polyagglutinable state.

3 List the clinical conditions that are associated with each form of polyagglutination.

4 Discuss the clinical significance of the polyagglutinable state.

5 List the laboratory results that are expected in each form of polyagglutination (e.g., ABO grouping, reactions following enzyme treatment, reactions with various lectins).

### NONMICROBIALLY ASSOCIATED POLYAGGLUTINATION: TN

1 Describe the alteration that characterizes the polyagglutinable state.

2 Discuss the clinical significance of the polyagglutinable state.

3 List the laboratory results that are expected in this form of polyagglutination (e.g., ABO grouping, reactions following enzyme treatment, reactions with various lectins).

### INHERITED POLYAGGLUTINATION: CAD AND HEMPAS (HEREDITARY ERYTHROBLASTOSIS MULTINUCLEARITY WITH A POSITIVE ACIDIFIED SERUM) TEST (HAM'S TEST)

1 State the form of inheritance.

2 Describe the alteration that is seen in the condition.

3 Discuss the clinical significance of the polyagglutinable state.

4 List the laboratory results that are expected (e.g., I/i antigenic expression, reactions following enzyme treatment, reactions with various lectins).

## INTRODUCTION

Polyagglutination refers to the agglutination of altered red cells by a large proportion of ABO-compatible adult human sera. Alterations in the red cell membrane may be acquired after microbial (bacterial or viral) activity, associated with certain forms of aberrant erythropoiesis, or inherited. In the microbially induced forms of polyagglutination, microbial enzymes alter the structure of the normal red cell membrane by removing carbohydrate residues and thus exposing cryptic (hidden) antigens, or *cryptantigens*. Naturally occurring IgM antibodies (polyagglutinins) found in normal adult human sera react with these cryptantigens, caus-

ing the altered cells to be polyagglutinable. Polyagglutinins are considered "naturally occurring," but their production is probably stimulated by intestinal flora, particularly gram-negative organisms, which have antigenic similarities to the red blood cell (RBC) cryptantigens. Cryptantigen exposure can be detected before polyagglutination by testing the red blood cells in vitro with specific lectins.[1] Polyagglutination, which requires significant cryptantigen exposure, is a rare condition; however, detectable cryptantigen exposure is not. Microbially induced polyagglutination may occur in vitro or in vivo. When polyagglutination occurs in vivo, the condition is usually transient. The microbial organisms may be present in the bloodstream, or the enzymes may enter the bloodstream from an extravascular site of infection. For polyagglutination to occur, the enzymes must be present in excess of the amount required to neutralize normal plasma enzyme inhibitors.[1] Microbially induced forms of polyagglutination include T, Th, Tk, Tx, acquired B, acquired microbial polyagglutination caused by passive adsorption, and probably Vienna. A nonmicrobial form of acquired polyagglutination, Tn, is caused by the somatic mutation of a faulty hematopoietic stem cell clone. This form of polyagglutination is usually a persistent condition. Finally, some forms of polyagglutination are inherited, including Cad, hemoglobin M-Hyde Park, hereditary erythroblastic multinuclearity with a positive acidified serum (HEMPAS), and NOR. The inherited forms of polyagglutination are permanent conditions.

Historically, polyagglutination was first described as an in vitro phenomenon caused by bacterial contamination of red cell suspensions. The first report, by Hübener, appeared in 1926.[2] Later, polyagglutination was described by Thomsen and Friedenreich,[3] and it became known as the Hübener-Thomsen-Friedenreich phenomenon. The cryptantigen exposed by the action of the bacterial enzyme became known as the T receptor (in honor of Thomsen). Over the past 70 years, other forms of polyagglutination have been described. Recognition and classification of polyagglutinable cells may be complicated by variations in the strength of the antigens and antibodies. Also, it is not uncommon to find several forms of polyagglutination existing simultaneously in vivo. This chapter discusses the most common types, including the serologic recognition of polyagglutination and the classification of polyagglutinable red cells by using lectins.

## CATEGORIES OF POLYAGGLUTINABLE CELLS

### Microbially Associated

#### T Polyagglutination

T transformation is a transient, acquired form of polyagglutination, usually found in patients with septicemia, gastrointestinal lesions, or wound infections. Occasionally T transformation has been observed in apparently healthy blood donors[4]; however, it is usually considered a pathologic finding—possibly an early symptom of a latent disease condition. It has been more frequently observed in infants and children than in adults. T activation of red blood cells is caused by the action of neuraminidase, which is produced by bacteria such as pneumococci, *Clostridium perfringens*, and *Vibrio cholerae* and viruses such as the influenza virus.[5] Neuraminidase cleaves terminal *N*-acetylneuraminic acid (NeuNAc) residues from red cell membrane glycoproteins and glycolipids, exposing the subterminal T receptor.[6] One structure on the red cell membrane that can be altered to express the T receptor is the alkali-labile tetrasaccharide of Thomas and Winzler.[7] These tetrasaccharides are found on the MN-sialoglycoprotein (SGP), the Ss-SGP, other minor red blood cell SGPs, and on gangliosides.[8] Figure 22–1 illustrates the biochemical structures of the tetrasaccharide of Thomas and Winzler and the neuraminidase-modified structure that expresses the T receptor. T activation may occur in vitro or in vivo. In vitro, T activation may be produced by bacterial contamination of blood samples or by the deliberate addition of neuraminidase to red cell suspensions. When T receptors on red blood cells are exposed, the cells are agglutinated by almost all normal adult sera which contain naturally occurring anti-T. Patients who have T polyagglutination generally lack anti-T in their sera and therefore are expected to have negative autologous controls. The degree of T activation or cryptantigen exposure depends on the amount of neuraminidase that gains access to the

bloodstream, the amount of inhibitor present in the patient's plasma, and the number of NeuNAc residues that are removed by the enzymes.[9] In addition to red blood cells, T receptors may be found as cryptantigens on leukocytes,[10] platelets,[10] tissue cells,[11] and in body fluids.[12] T activation is a transient condition in vivo. When the microbial organism is eliminated, the polyagglutinable property of the red cells usually disappears.

### Th Polyagglutination

Th polyagglutination is probably another microbially induced form of polyagglutination. This form of polyagglutination was first observed in septic patients by Bird and coworkers in 1978.[13] Several microbial organisms were isolated from these patients, including clostridia, bacteroides, *Escherichia coli*, and proteus. Because the polyagglutinins anti-T and anti-Tk were found in normal amounts in the sera of these patients, it was apparent that Th polyagglutination is different from T polyagglutination and Tk polyagglutination. In an in vitro experiment, Sondag-Thull and associates[14] produced Th-transformed red blood cells using the neuraminidase produced by *Corynebacterium aquaticum*. They showed that the neuraminidase associated with Th transformation is weaker than the neuraminidase that produces T transformation, and they concluded that Th-transformed red blood cells express a weakened expression or an early stage of the T transformation.

Alkali-labile tetrasaccharide of Thomas and Winzler:

Gal-β (1–3) - GalNAc - - - - α - - - - Serine or Threonine

α (2–3)     α (2–6)

NeuNAc     NeuNAc

T receptor:

Gal-β (1–3) - GalNAc - - - - α - - - - Serine or Threonine

Gal = Galactose

GalNAc = *N*-acetylgalactosamine

NeuNAc = *N*-acetylneuraminic acid

**Figure 22–1.** Structure of the alkali-labile tetrasaccharide of Thomas and Winzler and the neuraminidase-modified structure that expresses the T receptor in the terminal position.

## Tk Polyagglutination

Like other forms of microbially associated polyagglutination, Tk transformation is a transient, acquired form of polyagglutination, usually found in patients with septicemia, gastrointestinal lesions, and wound infections. Initially, enzymes produced by a certain strain of *Bacteroides fragilis* were associated with Tk polyagglutination.[15] Later, cultures of *Serratia marcescens*, *Aspergillus niger*, and *Candida albicans* were also shown to produce endo-β-galactosidases and exo-β-galactosidases that are capable of producing Tk transformation. The enzymes cleave a galactose residue from the paragloboside structure, exposing *N*-acetylgluosamine (GluNAc), the Tk receptor.[16,17] Paragloboside is a precursor in the biosynthetic pathways of the ABH, Lewis, Ii, and P1 antigens. Thus, Tk-polyagglutinable red cells may have altered expressions of these antigens, resulting in decreased antigen expression.[18] Figure 22–2 illustrates the biochemical structures of paragloboside and the Tk receptor. Tk transformation can be produced in vitro or in vivo.[16] When Tk receptors on red blood cells are exposed, the cells are agglutinated by almost all normal adult sera, which contain naturally occurring anti-Tk. When the microbial organism is eliminated, the polyagglutinable property of the red cells usually disappears.

## Tx Polyagglutination

Tx transformation was first described in children with pneumococcal infections.[19] The mechanism of Tx transformation has not been explained. A second report of Tx transformation described a child with acute hemolytic anemia.[20] Tx transformation of the child's red blood cells was observed, but no direct association with the anemia could be proved. Examination of family members showed Tx polyagglutination of the red blood cells of two siblings. The polyagglutination was transient, lasting 4 to 5 months. The Tx transformation

could have been caused by an unidentified bacterial or viral infection; however, blood, nasopharyngeal, urine, and rectal cultures were all negative.

## Acquired-B Polyagglutination

Like T activation, acquired B is considered a transient, acquired form of polyagglutination, usually found in patients with septicemia, gastrointestinal lesions, and wound infections. Also like T activation, acquired B has been found in apparently healthy blood donors,[21] but the condition is considered a pathologic finding. The acquired-B antigen is caused by enzymes produced by certain strains of *Escherichia coli*,[22] *Clostridium tertium*,[22] and probably by certain strains of *Proteus vulgaris*.[23] The microbial enzyme causes deacetylation of α-*N*-acetyl-D-galactosamine (group A determinant) with the production of α-D-galactosamine. α-D-Galactosamine is similar to α-D-galactose (group B determinant) and can cross-react with human anti-B typing sera and some monoclonal anti-B typing reagents.[24,25] Figure 22–3 illustrates the biochemical structures of α-*N*-acetylgalactosamine and α-D-galactosamine, the acquired B determinant. Acquired B may be produced in vitro or in vivo. In vitro, acquired B can be produced by coating group A or O red cells with lipopolysaccharides from *E. coli* $O_{86}$ or *P. vulgaris* $0 \times 19$. In vivo, acquired B is a transient condition, occurring only on red blood cells that have the A antigen. When the microbial organism is eliminated, the cross-reactivity with anti-B typing reagent usually disappears.

## Passive Adsorption of Bacterial Products

Very rarely, polyagglutination may be caused by the passive adsorption of bacterial products onto red blood cells. Such coated cells can be polyagglutinable because human sera sometimes contain antibodies to the bacteria. Chorpenning and Dodd reported a severe transfusion reaction that was probably caused by this mechanism.[26]

Paragloboside:

Gal-β (1–4) - GluNAc-β (1–3) - Gal-β (1–3) - Glu - Ceramide

Tk receptor:

GluNAc-β (1–3) - Gal-β (1–3) - Glu - Ceramide

Gal = Galactose

GluNAc = *N*-acetylglucosamine

Glu = Glucose

**Figure 22–2.** Structure of paragloboside and the enzymatically modified structure that expresses the Tk receptor in the terminal position.

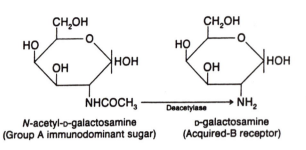

**Figure 22–3.** Structure of the group A determinant (*N*-acetyl-D-galactosamine) and the enzymatically modified structure (D-galactosamine) that expresses the acquired-B receptor.

N-acetyl-D-galactosamine
(Group A immunodominant sugar)

D-galactosamine
(Acquired-B receptor)

Deacetylase

## VA Polyagglutination

VA polyagglutination is rare, and it has not been well characterized. It was first described in a 20-year-old man from Vienna, (VA) who had had hemolytic anemia most of his life.[27] The H antigens of VA polyagglutinable red cells are significantly depressed. The action of a microbial α-fucosidase could account for the depressed H antigens; however, the presence of a microbial enzyme has not been proved.[9] VA polyagglutinability appears to be a persistent condition.

## Nonmicrobially Associated

### Tn Polyagglutination

Tn polyagglutinability is believed to be caused by a mutation in the hematopoietic tissue. The mutation gives rise to a clone of cells that lack β-3-D-galactosyl-transferase,[28] the transferase that is needed to complete the biosynthesis of the normal structure of the alkali-labile tetrasaccharide of Thomas and Winzler.[7] This tetrasaccharide structure is found on the MN-SGP and the Ss-SGP.[29] Inasmuch as this form of polyagglutination is caused by a mutation, it is considered permanent and irreversible. The mutant clone coexists with normal hematopoietic tissue, and, therefore, this form of polyagglutination is characterized by a mixed-field appearance.[30] Only the cells produced by the mutant clone are agglutinated by the naturally occurring anti-Tn, which is found in normal adult sera. Tn polyagglutination occurs only in vivo, and it may occur in apparently healthy people. When the transferase is absent, the crypt Tn antigen (α-GalNAc) is exposed. In addition to red blood cells, the Tn receptor may be found as a cryptantigen on leukocytes,[31] platelets,[31] and tissue cells.[11] Figure 22–4 illustrates the biochemical structures of the

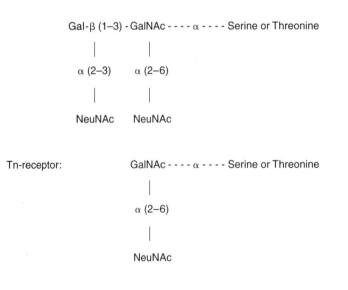

Alkali-labile tetrasaccharide of Thomas and Winzler:

Gal-β (1–3) - GalNAc - - - - α - - - - Serine or Threonine

α (2–3)        α (2–6)

NeuNAc      NeuNAc

Tn-receptor:                    GalNAc - - - - α - - - - Serine or Threonine

α (2–6)

NeuNAc

Gal = Galactose

GalNAc = *N*-acetylgalactosamine

NeuNAc = *N*-acetylneuraminic acid

**Figure 22–4.** Structure of the alkali-labile tetrasaccharide of Thomas and Winzler and the incomplete structure that expresses the Tn receptor in the terminal position.

tetrasaccharide of Thomas and Winzler and the incomplete structure that expresses the Tn receptor.[32]

## Inherited Forms of Polyagglutination

### Cad

Cad polyagglutination was first described in 1968 by Cazal and coworkers.[33] Cad is an inherited autosomal dominant condition that gives rise to a permanent polyagglutinable state. The amount of Cad antigen varies on red blood cells, and based on the amount of Cad antigen present, red cells can be divided into four Cad phenotypes.[34] In 1971, Sanger and associates[35] reported that Cad-positive red blood cells are agglutinated by anti-Sd$^a$. It is known that the structure that includes the Cad determinant is a potent inhibitor of anti-Sd$^a$; however, it is not clear whether this means that Cad and Sd$^a$ are identical or that a concentrated isolate of a structure similar to Sd$^a$, with GalNAc as the terminal residue, has the ability to cross-react with anti-Sd$^a$.[36] Inasmuch as anti-Sd$^a$ is present as an autoantibody in most normal adult sera, Cad cells can be classified as polyagglutinable. Cad polyagglutination is quite uncommon. This form of polyagglutination appears to have little clinical significance; however, Cad-positive cells show considerable resistance to invasion by merozoites of *Plasmodium falciparum*.[37] Cad polyag-

glutinable red cells have normal sialic acid levels. The Cad determinant on the red cell membrane and the Sd$^a$ antigen isolated from Sd(a+) urine share a nonreducing trisaccharide.[38-40] The Cad receptor, a pentasaccharide, is produced when an additional sugar is added to the alkali-labile tetrasaccharide of Thomas and Winzler.[38] Figure 22–5 illustrates the biochemical structures of the tetrasaccharide of Thomas and Winzler and the modified structure that expresses the Cad receptor.

### Hemoglobin M-Hyde Park

Polyagglutination associated with hemoglobin M-Hyde Park was initially reported in a South African family of mixed race.[41] The red cells of 12 members of the family were weakly agglutinated, often mixed-field pattern, by many ABO-compatible human sera. All 12 family members who had hemoglobin M-Hyde Park had polyagglutinable red blood cells; however, polyagglutination was absent in 23 other family members who had normal hemoglobin. Because all of the family members were apparently healthy, it is unlikely that the polyagglutinability was caused by in vivo bacterial or viral activity. King and others[42] reported that the polyagglutinability associated with M-Hyde Park red blood cells is caused by two unrelated abnormalities. They found heterogeneity in the molecular size of SGPs

Alkali-labile tetrasaccharide of Thomas and Winzler:

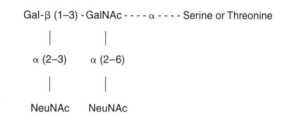

Gal-β (1–3) - GalNAc - - - - α - - - - Serine or Threonine

α (2–3)      α (2–6)

NeuNAc     NeuNAc

Cad receptor:

GalNAc-β (1–4) - Gal-β (1–3) - GalNAc - - - - α - - - - Serine or Threonine

α (2–3)      α (2–6)

NeuNAc     NeuNAc

Gal = Galactose

GalNAc = *N*-acetylgalactosamine

NeuNAc = *N*-acetylneuraminic acid

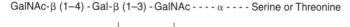

**Figure 22–5.** Structure of the alkali-labile tetrasaccharide of Thomas and Winzler and the modified structure that expresses the Cad receptor.

and a mild reduction in the sialylation of O-linked oligosaccharide chains on the M-Hyde Park membrane components. Also, these red blood cells showed incomplete biosynthesis with exposure of terminal *N*-acetylglucosamine (GluNAc) on polylactosamine-type, *N*-linked carbohydrate chains of Band 3.

## HEMPAS

HEMPAS, which stands for *Hereditary Erythroblastic Multinuclearity with a Positive Acidified Serum test* (Ham's test), is also known as congenital dyserythropoietic anemia type II (CDA II). HEMPAS is an autosomal-recessive condition that is characterized by abnormal red cell membranes, multinucleated erythroblasts in the bone marrow, and red blood cells that have a second membrane internal and parallel to the external membrane.[43,44] HEMPAS red blood cells have increased amounts of i-antigen and decreased amounts of H antigen and sialic acid, and they show increased susceptibility to lysis by anti-i and anti-I in the presence of complement. Many normal human sera contain a naturally occurring, IgM, complement-binding alloantibody that reacts with HEMPAS cells. For this reason, HEMPAS cells are considered polyagglutinable.[9] A specific HEMPAS determinant has not been described.

## NOR

NOR, an inherited dominant form of polyagglutination, was discovered when the red blood cells of a 19-year-old blood donor from Norfolk, Virginia, were unexpectedly incompatible with the majority of adult sera tested. NOR cells were compatible with cord sera. Tests with lectins and other reagents ruled out other known forms of polyagglutination, and this donor's serum contained the expected naturally occurring antibodies to other forms of polyagglutination. No lectin has been found that agglutinates NOR cells. Possibly NOR-polyagglutination is related to the P blood group system, inasmuch as it has been observed that anti-NOR is inhibited by hydatid cyst fluid and avian P1 substance. Anti-NOR is a naturally occurring IgM antibody that is found in approximately 75 percent of normal adult sera.[45] The NOR determinant has not been described.

## LABORATORY TESTING: DETECTION, CONFIRMATION, AND CLASSIFICATION

### Detection

In the past, cryptantigen expression and polyagglutination were sometimes detected by ABO discrepancies in which polyagglutinins in the typing sera reacted with polyagglutinable cells. Similarly, false-positive direct antiglobulin tests were sometimes observed when polyagglutinins in the antiglobulin reagent reacted with polyagglutinable cells. When minor crossmatches were commonly performed, incompatible minor crossmatches could lead to the detection of polyagglutination, resulting from polyagglutinable recipient's cells reacting with polyagglutinins in the donor's serum.

Today, monoclonal antisera have replaced human ABO reagents, and these antisera fail to recognize polyagglutination because they lack the naturally occurring polyagglutinins that are found in adult human serum. Similarly, monoclonal antiglobulin reagents lack the polyagglutinins, and the minor crossmatch is rarely performed. Cryptantigen exposure would not be detected during routine compatibility testing unless the donor's cells demonstrated cryptantigens. If donor samples became bacterially contaminated in vitro, the samples could become polyagglutinable, and sometimes apparently healthy donors have Tn or one of the inherited forms of polyagglutination. In these cases, if the number of receptors on the donor cells and the amount of antibody in the patient's serum were adequate, polyagglutination could be detected—especially if the immediate-spin, room temperature crossmatch is used.

The Tn receptor in Tn polyagglutination, which is produced by a mutant clone of hemopoietic cells, is *N*-acetylgalactosamine. This is the same sugar that defines the A antigens on group A cells. In the past, human anti-A reagent was used, and Tn polyagglutination was sometimes detected, when the anti-A antiserum cross-reacted with the Tn receptors. These reactions appeared like an "acquired A"—a mixed-field population of A cells in a group O individual or a weak subgroup of AB in a group B individual. Although some monoclonal antibodies have been produced that react with both A cells and Tn polyagglutinable cells, commercial manufacturers of monoclonal anti-A reagents have formulated their typing sera to avoid this cross-reactivity (personal communications).

Acquired B is a relatively rare form of polyagglutination that is produced when bacterial deacetylase enzymatically converts the A antigen, *N*-acetylgalactosamine, into galactosamine, which cross-reacts with anti-B reagents. When monoclonal reagents replaced the human antisera, there was a sharp increase in the detection of acquired B by one particular clone, ES4.[46] ES4 detected many examples of acquired B that were previously nonreactive when tested with human anti-B reagents. Because the transfusion of group AB blood to a group A recipient who had acquired-B polyagglutination could result in a serious transfusion reaction, the three manufacturers who currently produce ES4-containing anti-B reagents quickly reformulated their antisera to avoid detecting acquired B. The detection of acquired B by ES4 is avoided by lowering the pH of the reagent; however, it is important to note that it is possible to inadvertently reverse the pH if unwashed red blood cells are typed with ES4 reagents.

Because many monoclonal reagents are used in the transfusion laboratory today and the minor crossmatch is rarely performed, it is unlikely that polyagglutination would be detected during testing. It is more likely that unexplained hemolysis following a blood transfusion would be the first clue that the patient has polyagglutination.

## Confirmation

When polyagglutination is suspected, the red blood cells should be tested with several cord blood sera and with several normal group AB adult sera. If the red cells are agglutinated by most of the adult sera and are not agglutinated by the cord sera, polyagglutination has been established. The cord sera used for polyagglutination studies must be pretested to determine that they lack maternal alloantibodies, which might produce misleading results. The adult sera must be pretested to determine that they are free of unexpected antibodies.

Polyagglutinins are naturally occurring antibodies in adult serum; however, the amount of antibody varies from one individual to another. For this reason, several adult sera should be used. Polyagglutinins usually react best at lower temperatures by direct agglutination. Because polyagglutinins are unstable, it is important to use fresh adult sera. The auto-control in individuals who have polyagglutinable red blood cells is usually nonreactive. Polyagglutinins in most normal adult sera are low-titered. As polyagglutinable red cell transformation begins, the polyagglutinin antibodies are adsorbed onto the transformed cells until the antibodies have been completely removed from circulation. At that time, the auto-control is expected to be negative.

*N*-acetylneuraminic acid (sialic acid) is a normal component of the red cell membrane. Certain forms of polyagglutination (T and Tn) show decreased amounts of sialic acid. It is possible to quantitate sialic acid levels, but such testing is not practical in routine serology laboratories. Instead, sialic acid levels are usually determined qualitatively with Polybrene and *Glycine soja* lectin. Polybrene, a positively charged polymer, acts by neutralizing the negative charge on normal red cells and causing them to aggregate nonspecifically. Because the negative charge is almost entirely caused by sialic acid groups, cells that lack sialic acid (T and Tn) are not aggregated by Polybrene. Conversely, *G. soja* lectin does not react with normal cells, but it strongly agglutinates sialic acid–deficient red cells (T and Tn) as well as Cad cells.

## Classification

### Enzymes

Enzymes may be useful in the classification of polyagglutinable red cells. Generally, agglutination of Tk-, Cad-, and NOR-polyagglutinable cells is enhanced following enzyme treatment. HEMPAS, VA-, and T-polyagglutinable cells show no change in their agglutination by normal adult sera following enzyme treatment. Tn- and Th-polyagglutinable cells show decreased agglutinability following enzyme treatment. Table 22–1 summarizes the findings with normal cells versus polyagglutinable cells.

### Lectins

Lectins are routinely included in the classification of polyagglutinable red cells. Lectins are proteins present in plants (usually seeds), invertebrate animals, and lower vertebrates. Lectins bind specifically to carbohydrate determinants; agglutinating erythrocytes by binding their cell surface oligosaccharide. Highly concentrated lectins may react nonspecifically with all red cells; however, with careful standardization a battery of lectin reagents will permit the accurate classification of most forms of polyagglutination. Table 22–2 summarizes the differentiation of polyagglutinable cells using lectins.

## Typing Polyagglutinable Red Cells

Typing polyagglutinable red cells is usually uncomplicated when monoclonal reagents are used. These antisera contain antibodies that are specific for the desired antigen, and they lack contaminating polyagglu-

**Table 22–1.** Normal versus Polyagglutinable Cells

| | Screening Methods | | | | |
| | Fresh Adult Sera | Cord Sera | Polybrene | Agglutination after Papain Treatment | Duration |
| --- | --- | --- | --- | --- | --- |
| Normal group O | 0 | 0 | + | Usually enhanced | — |
| T | + | 0 | 0 | No effect | Transient |
| Tn | + | 0 | 0/+ mf | Decreased | Persistent |
| Tk | + | 0 | + | Enhanced | Transient |
| Cad | Sometimes + | 0 | + | Enhanced | Permanent |
| Acquired-B | + | 0 | | | Transient |
| VA | +w | 0 | + | No effect | Persistent |
| Th | + | 0 | + | Decreased | Transient |
| NOR | + | 0 | + | Enhanced | Permanent |

0 = no reactivity; + = reactivity/aggregation; +w = weak reactivity/aggregation; +mf = mixed-field reactivity; Transient = cells revert to normal state after primary condition is resolved; Persistent = essentially permanent, but rare cases have been reported in which the cells returned to normal; Permanent = cells remain permanently altered and polyagglutinable.

**Table 22–2.** Differentiation of Polyagglutinable Cells Using Lectins

| | Glycine soja | Arachis hypogaea | Dolichos biflorus | Salvia sclarea | Salvia horminum | Griffonia simplicifolia (GS II)* | Vicia graminea (N_VG Receptor) |
|---|---|---|---|---|---|---|---|
| Normal group O | 0 | 0 | 0 | 0 | 0 | 0 | — |
| T | + | + | 0 | 0 | 0 | 0 | Enhanced |
| Tn | + | 0 | + | + | + | 0 | Depressed |
| Tk | 0 | + | 0 | 0 | 0 | + | No effect |
| Cad | 0/+w | 0 | + | 0 | + | 0 | |
| Acquired-B | | 0 | | 0 | 0 | 0 | |
| VA | 0 | 0 | 0 | 0 | 0 | 0 | |
| Th | 0 | + | 0 | 0 | 0 | 0 | |
| NOR | 0 | 0 | 0 | 0 | 0 | 0 | |

*Previously known as *Bandeiraea simplicifolia* (BS II).

tinins that are found in normal human-derived antisera. Typing polyagglutinable red cells may be difficult if the cells are strongly polyagglutinable and only human, polyclonal antisera are available. Several approaches to typing cells under these conditions are available and are described in the following discussions.[47]

## Adsorption

Some polyagglutinable cells can be prepared in vitro (T, Th, Tk, Tx, and acquired B), and these cells may be used to adsorb the polyagglutinins from human typing reagents.

## Enzymes

Some polyagglutination receptors are destroyed by enzymes (Tn and Th). In these forms of polyagglutination, the polyagglutinable cells may be enzyme-treated before typing. This approach would be limited to typing the cells for antigens that are not destroyed by enzymes, and controls must be used carefully to avoid false interpretations caused by unexpected, enzyme-reactive antibodies in the human typing sera.

## Cord Sera

ABO-compatible cord sera that contain the desired antibody specificity may be used as typing reagents. Polyagglutinins are expected to be absent from cord sera.

## Aged Sera

Polyagglutinins are unstable, and time-expired or aged human sera often lack the polyagglutinins. Such sera may be used as typing reagents if the desired antibodies are still demonstrable.

## Dilution

It may be possible to dilute human antisera beyond the endpoint of the polyagglutinins and still retain the desired specificity.

## Sulfhydryl Compounds

If the desired antibody in the human antiserum is IgG, it may be possible to treat the typing serum with 2-mercaptoethanol (2-ME) or dithiothreitol (DTT) to destroy IgM antibodies, such as the polyagglutinins, without affecting the desired IgG antibody.

## Adsorption and Elution

Adsorption and elution techniques may be used to determine the correct blood type of polyagglutinable red cells. After incubating the polyagglutinable red cells with typing serum, an elution is performed. If the specificity of the typing serum is demonstrable in the eluate, the cells may be considered positive for the antigen.

## CLINICAL SIGNIFICANCE

Polyagglutination is a condition with both serologic and clinical significance. When cells are altered to expose cryptantigens, they are susceptible to agglutination by most adult sera. The reaction between the cryptantigens and the naturally occurring polyagglutinins produces antibody-coated cells that may have clinical significance. In addition to sepsis, polyagglutination has been associated with leukemia, breast cancer, and other malignancies.

### Sepsis

Polyagglutination has been reported in patients with sepsis, upper respiratory infections, wound infections, intestinal infections, and malignancies. Some of the bacterial and viral organisms that have been associated with polyagglutination are *Aspergillus niger, Bacteroides fragilis, Candida albicans, Clostridium perfringens, Clostridium tertium, Corynebacterium aquaticum, E. coli,* pneumococci, *Proteus vulgaris, Serratia marcescens, Vibrio cholerae,* and viruses such as the influenza virus. Bird[9] pointed out that microbes do not have to be in the bloodstream to cause polyagglutination and that an extravascular site of infection can produce enzymes that enter the bloodstream in amounts greater than can be neutralized by normal serum inhibitors.

In infants with suspected necrotizing enterocolitis (NEC), cryptantigen exposure provides diagnostic information and may serve as an early guide to the causative organism and to antibiotic therapy. A simple test for cryptantigen exposure using a two-lectin panel (*A. hypogaea* and *G. soja*) should be performed using cells from any infant that is suspected of NEC. Positive tests for cryptantigen exposure should be quantified because the amount of exposure correlates with the severity of the NEC and the likelihood of intestinal perforation.[48]

### Case Report

A 7-month-old girl was admitted to the hospital with acute intestinal obstruction. The child's hematocrit was 22 percent (reference range 33 to 43 percent), and a 90-mL transfusion of packed red blood cells was ordered. Immediately after the transfusion, hemoglobinemia and hemoglobinuria were noted; however, immediate surgery was performed to remove a segment of necrotic small intestine. During surgery, 250 mL of whole blood was administered. Following the transfusion, the patient's temperature rose from 37° to 39°C, and evidence of hemolysis persisted. A transfusion reaction work-up was ordered. The results of the laboratory tests indicated that the child's pretransfusion and posttransfusion antibody screen and crossmatches were nonreactive. The direct antiglobulin test was negative pretransfusion, but posttransfusion the patient's red blood cells were weakly coated with complement. An antibody identification panel using the pretransfusion serum was nonreactive, and an eluate from the patient's posttransfusion red blood cells was also nonreactive. Because the source of the hemolysis was unexplained, a lectin panel was performed to test for possible polyagglutination. The patient's red blood cells were strongly agglutinated by *A. hypogaea* and *G. soja* lectins. T transformation was confirmed.

### Hemolytic Anemia and Hemolytic Uremic Syndrome

When cryptantigen exposure occurs in vivo, the patient's own IgM, complement-binding polyagglutinins can initiate intravascular hemolysis by binding to the transformed cells. In addition, the transfusion of plasma products containing normal levels of polyagglutinins may intensify the hemolysis. In rare cases, disseminated intravascular coagulation (DIC) and hemolytic uremic syndrome have been reported.[49,50] Hemolytic anemia has been more commonly reported in T polyagglutination[51-54]; however, Th polyagglutination[55] has also been implicated in severe intravascular hemolysis and DIC. The presence of cryptantigens on red blood cells, white blood cells, platelets, and tissue cells accounts for the anemia, thrombocytopenia, and renal dysfunction. Naturally occurring polyagglutinins

are absent in newborns, and because these antibodies are IgM, they do not cross the placenta.[56] Consequently, hemolysis is not seen in newborns with neonatal necrotizing enterocolitis (NEC) or other cryptantigen-exposing conditions unless they are transfused with plasma products.

### Leukemia, Breast Cancer, and Other Malignancies

Tn polyagglutination has been found in apparently healthy people; however, it has also been reported in patients with acute myelocytic leukemia.[57-59] One apparently healthy person who was found to have Tn polyagglutination later developed acute leukemia. In two of the leukemia patients, chemotherapy resulted in a clinical remission of the leukemia and the disappearance of the Tn-polyagglutinable red cells.[58] Thus, it could be concluded that Tn may be a preleukemic state. Although several healthy individuals are known who have had Tn polyagglutination for a number of years, Ness and coworkers[58,59] recommend that these individuals be hematologically monitored. Monoclonal antibody FBT3 is a mouse IgM monoclonal antibody that reacts specifically with Tn-transformed red blood cells by hemagglutination and by direct immunofluorescence. Roxby and colleagues[60] recommended using immunohistochemical staining with FBT3, which is far more sensitive than hemagglutination, to detect Tn antigen expression in bone marrow aspirates and peripheral blood. By monitoring bone marrow aspirates and peripheral blood from patients who have leukemia using FBT3, it may be possible to detect small numbers of leukemic cells and to predict relapse.

The cryptantigens T and Tn have been found on malignant tissue cells from breast, colon, and urinary bladder and in metastatic lesions.[11] The presence of these cryptantigens on malignant tissue has been attributed to the incomplete synthesis of MN glycoproteins.[61] The amount of the expressed antigen usually parallels the cancer malignancy and invasiveness.[60,62] The finding of T and Tn cryptantigens and/or a decrease in their respective serum antibodies may serve as an immunologic marker, with diagnostic and therapeutic implications.

### Cryptantigens in the Absence of Apparent Infection

Two cases of transient Tn polyagglutination were described in apparently healthy neonates.[63] Delayed maturation of the sialyltransferase system was postulated as the cause of the cryptantigen exposure. Similarly, both Tn and Th cryptantigens were detected in a patient with myelodysplasia.[64] These cryptantigens were detectable over a 5-year period, and the patient showed no apparent bacterial or viral infection. In a study of maternal and cord bloods, Wahl and others[65] reported that a significant number of normal mothers and their newborn infants had Th-activated red blood cells without polyagglutination. This study suggested that Th activation could be a normal change in pregnancy and that the Th antigen could be a marker for fetal hematopoiesis that is enhanced by some conditions during pregnancy and in utero development. Similarly, Rodwell and Tudehope[48] reported that T, Th, and Tn are all expressed on fetal red blood cells during the first trimester and that Th and Tn are thought to be developmental markers. Herman and colleagues[66] reported that Th activation may be a red cell developmental marker present in congenital hypoplastic anemias. This study suggested that Th is a more specific marker for congenital hypoplastic anemia than i antigen expression or other fetal red cell characteristics.

### Case Report

A 19-year-old woman donated blood for the first time at a company-sponsored blood drive. She was apparently healthy, her medical history was unremarkable, and all of the tests performed on her blood by the laboratory were normal. These tests included ABO typing, Rh typing, screening for unexpected antibodies, a serologic test for syphilis, and viral marker tests for HBsAg, anti-HBc, anti-HCV, anti-HIV-1/2, HIV p24 antigen, and anti-HTLV-I/II. However, the hospital transfusion service discovered that her unit of blood was incompatible with three patients who had no unexpected antibodies using an immediate-spin, room temperature compatibility test. A direct antiglobulin test, which is not included in the routine testing, was performed on the unit, and the results were negative. Finally, testing for polyagglutination was performed using the two-lectin panel (*A. hypogaea* and *G. soja*). The red blood cells of the unit were agglutinated by *G. soja* but not by *A. hypogaea*. Tn polyagglutination was confirmed.

### Blood Transfusion

In conclusion, polyagglutination is a rare condition; however, cryptantigen exposure is not. Cryptantigen exposure can be detected before polyagglutination develops by testing the patient's red blood cells in vitro with specific lectins. A screening test using a two-lectin panel of *A. hypogaea* and *G. soja* is simple to perform and detects most of the causes of polyagglutination: T, Th, Tk, Tn, and Tx.[53] Patients with a potential risk of developing cryptantigen exposure and polyagglutination (i.e., patients with various infections, malignancies,[67] unexplained anemias, and infants with necrotizing enterocolitis[48,68]) should be screened for cryptantigen exposure using the two-lectin panel. When cryptantigen exposure is detected, Rodwell and Tudehope[48] recommend quantitating the amount of exposure to serve as a guide for transfusion options. If there is marked (3 to 4+) activation, washed red blood cells should be supplied to avoid potentially fatal intravascular hemolysis. If the activation is only moderate (1 to 2+), it may be possible to select plasma-containing products for transfusion using the minor crossmatch technique.[48,67–70] The minor crossmatch using the patient's red blood cells and potential donors' plasma would detect plasmas containing the specific polyagglutinin and identify compatible units that could be selected for transfusion.

## SUMMARY CHART: IMPORTANT POINTS TO REMEMBER (MT/MLT)

- Polyagglutination refers to the agglutination of altered red cells by a large proportion of ABO-compatible adult human sera caused by microbial (bacterial or viral) activity, certain forms of aberrant erythropoiesis, or inherited alterations in the red cell membrane.
- Microbially associated forms of polyagglutination include T, Th, Tk, Tx, acquired-B, and VA. Nonmicrobial forms of polyagglutination include Tn, Cad, hemoglobin M-Hyde Park, HEMPAS, and NOR.
- In acquired-B polyagglutination, enzymes produced by *E. coli*, *C. tertium*, and *P. vulgaris* cause deacetylation of the group A determinant on red cells ($\alpha$-*N*-acetyl-D-galactosamine) to a produce a structure similar to the group B determinant (D-galactose), which cross-reacts with human anti-B typing reagents.
- In T polyagglutination, the enzyme neuraminidase produced by bacteria such as pneumococci cleaves terminal *N*-acetylneuraminic acid residues from the red cell membrane, exposing the (hidden) T antigen.
- Tk polyagglutination may lead to decreased expression of the ABH, Ii, Lewis, and P1 antigens because of microbial enzymatic action on galactose present on the paragloboside structure.
- HEMPAS (hereditary erythroblastic multinuclearity with a positive acidified serum test) red blood cells have increased amounts of i-antigen decreased amounts of H antigen and sialic acid and are susceptible to lysis by anti-i and anti-I in the presence of complement.
- Polyagglutination is investigated through the use of cord blood sera, fresh group AB adult sera, an auto-control, enzymes, and lectin studies. Polyagglutinins are naturally occurring and react best at lower temperature via direct agglutination.
- The clinical significance of polyagglutination is most related to sepsis, leukemia, and breast cancer.
- Blood transfusion options for persons exhibiting polyagglutinable red cells include washed red blood cells and minor crossmatch techniques to detect plasma-compatible units that do not contain the polyagglutinin.

## REVIEW QUESTIONS

1. Polyagglutinable cells are agglutinated by the majority of adult human sera, irrespective of:
   A. Temperature
   B. pH
   C. Incubation time
   D. Blood group
   E. Serum/cell ratio

2. T activation is:
   A. A preleukemic state
   B. Bacterially induced
   C. Persistent and irreversible
   D. Characterized by increased i antigen
   E. An inherited condition

3. The T receptor is:
   A. Nonreactive with cord blood sera
   B. *N*-acetylgalactosamine
   C. Cross-reactive with anti-B typing serum
   D. Cross-reactive with anti-A typing serum
   E. Exposed by deacetylase

4. The T receptor is:
   A. Reactive with *Dolichos biflorus*
   B. Reactive with *Salvia sclarea*
   C. Destroyed by enzymes
   D. Reactive with *Salvia horminum*
   E. Reactive with *Arachis hypogaea*

5. T activation is a form of polyagglutination that is caused by microorganisms that produce_____ as a metabolic by-product.
   A. Fucosidase
   B. Deacetylase
   C. Galactosidase
   D. Glucosidase
   E. Neuraminidase

6. Th polyagglutination is:
   A. Reactive with *Glycine soja*
   B. Persistent and irreversible
   C. Considered clinically benign
   D. Produced by neuraminidase
   E. Enhanced by enzymes

7. Tk polyagglutination is:
   A. An autosomal dominant inheritance
   B. A mutation in the hematopoietic tissue
   C. Associated with altered ABH, Lewis, Ii, and P1 antigens
   D. An autosomal recessive inheritance
   E. Permanent and irreversible

8. Tx polyagglutination is associated with:
   A. *Vibrio cholerae*
   B. *Clostridium perfringens*
   C. *Candida albicans*
   D. Pneumococcus
   E. *Serratia marcescens*

9. Which of the following is associated with acquired-B polyagglutination?
   A. Mutation in the hematopoietic tissue
   B. Bacterially induced
   C. Permanent and irreversible
   D. Increased hemolysis with anti-I in the presence of complement
   E. Cross-reacts with anti-A typing serum

10. VA polyagglutination was found in a patient with:
    A. Pneumococcal infection
    B. Leukemia
    C. Breast cancer
    D. Thrombocytopenia
    E. Hemolytic anemia

11. Tn polyagglutination is:
    A. A preleukemic state
    B. Bacterially induced
    C. An inherited condition
    D. Found in vitro and in vivo
    E. Enhanced by enzymes

12. The Tn receptor is:
    A. Cross-reactive with anti-A typing serum
    B. Cross-reactive with anti-B typing serum
    C. Exposed by the action of bacterial metabolites
    D. Galactose
    E. Reactive with *Arachis hypogaea*

13. From the following list, select a form of polyagglutination that is genetically inherited:
    A. Cad
    B. T activation
    C. Acquired B
    D. Tn polyagglutination
    E. Tk polyagglutination

14. Which of the following describes Cad polyagglutination?
    A. Autosomal-recessive inheritance
    B. Reacts with anti-Sd$^a$
    C. Associated with hemolytic anemia
    D. Associated with HUS
    E. Associated with breast cancer

15. HEMPAS is:
    A. An autosomal-dominant inherited condition
    B. An autosomal-recessive inherited condition
    C. Bacterially induced
    D. Caused by a mutation in the hematopoietic tissue
    E. A condition that occurs in vitro and in vivo

16. HEMPAS red blood cells are characterized by:
    A. Increased amounts of i antigen
    B. Increased amounts of H antigen
    C. Resistance to lysis
    D. Resistance to *Plasmodium falciparum*
    E. Increased amounts of sialic acid

17. NOR polyagglutination is caused by:
    A. Bacterial infection
    B. Viral infection
    C. Mutation in the hematopoietic tissue
    D. Autosomal-dominant inheritance
    E. Autosomal-recessive inheritance

18. Lectins are:
    A. Antibodies
    B. Plant extracts
    C. Enzymes
    D. Bacterial metabolites
    E. Antigens

19. Sialic acid is decreased in which polyagglutinable states?
    A. T and Tn
    B. Acquired-B and T
    C. Tk and Tn
    D. Cad and Tk
    E. Acquired-B and Tk

20. Patients with in vivo polyagglutination should be given transfusions of:
    A. Whole blood
    B. Packed cells
    C. Washed red blood cells
    D. Fresh frozen plasma
    E. Platelets

## ANSWERS TO REVIEW QUESTIONS

1. D (p 475)
2. B (pp 475–476)
3. A (p 481)
4. E (p 482, Table 22–2)
5. E (p 476)
6. D (p 476)
7. C (p 477)
8. D (p 477)
9. B (p 477)
10. E (p 478)
11. A (p 478)
12. A (p 480)
13. A (p 479)
14. B (p 479)
15. B (p 480)
16. A (p 480)
17. D (p 480)
18. B (p 481)
19. A (p 481)
20. C (p 484)

# REFERENCES

1. Bird, GWG: Clinical aspects of red blood cell polyagglutinability of microbial origin. In Salmon, CH (ed): Blood Groups and Other Red Cell Surface Markers in Health and Disease. Masson, New York, 1982.
2. Hübener, G: Untersuchungen über Isoagglutination mit besonderer Berücksichtigung scheinbarer Abweichungen vom Gruppenschema. Zeitschrift für Immunitäts Forschung 45:223, 1926.
3. Friedenreich, V: Production of a Specific Receptor Quality in Red Cell Corpuscles by Bacterial Activity: The Thomsen Hemagglutination Phenomenon. Levin and Munskgaard, Copenhagen, 1930.
4. Stratton, F: Polyagglutinability of red cells. Vox Sang 4:58, 1954.
5. Levene, C, et al: Red cell polyagglutination. Transfus Med Rev 2:176, 1988.
6. Uhlenbruck, G, et al: On the specificity of lectins with broad agglutination spectrum. II. Studies on the nature of the T antigen and the specific receptors for the lectin Arachis hypogaea (ground nut). Zeitschrift für Immunitäts Forschung, Allergie Klinische Immunologie 138:423, 1969.
7. Thomas, DB, and Winzler, RJ: Structural studies on human erythrocyte glycoproteins: Alkali-labile tetrasaccharides. J Biol Chem 244:5943, 1969.
8. Anstee, DJ: Blood group MNSs: Active sialoglycoproteins of the human erythrocyte membrane. In Sandler, SG, et al (eds): Immunobiology of the Erythrocyte: Progress in Clinical Biological Research. Liss, New York, 1980.
9. Bird, GWG: Lectins and red cell polyagglutinability: History, comments, and recent developments. In Beck, ML, and Judd, WJ (eds): Polyagglutination. American Association of Blood Banks, Washington, DC, 1980.
10. Hicklin, BL, and Beck, ML: Latent polyagglutinable receptors on leukocytes and platelets (abstract). Transfusion 14:508, 1974.
11. Anglin, Jr, JH, et al: Blood group-like activity released by human mammary carcinoma cells in culture. Nature 269:254, 1977.
12. Kline, WE, and Issitt, CH: T substance in body fluids (abstract). Transfusion 16:527, 1976.
13. Bird, GWG, et al: Th, a "new" form of erythrocyte polyagglutination. Lancet 1:1215, 1978.
14. Sondag-Thull, D, et al: Characterization of a neuraminidase from Corynebacterium aquaticum responsible for Th polyagglutination. Vox Sang 57:193, 1989.
15. Inglis, G, et al: Effect of Bacteroides fragilis on the human erythrocyte membrane: Pathogenesis of Tk polyagglutination. J Clin Pathol 28:964, 1975.
16. Dôinel, C, et al: Tk polyagglutination produced in vitro by an endo-beta-galactosidase. Vox Sang 38:94, 1980.
17. Judd, WJ: The role of exo-β-galactosidases in Tk-activation (abstract). Transfusion 20:622, 1980.
18. Andreu, G, et al: Induction of Tk polyagglutination by Bacteroides fragilis culture supernatants: Associated modifications of ABH and Ii antigens. Revue Française de Transfusion et Immuno-hématologie Blood Transfusion and Immunohematology 22:551, 1979.
19. Bird, GWG, et al: Tx, a "new" red cell cryptantigen exposed by pneumococcal enzymes. Proceedings of the 16th Kongress Deutsche Gesamte Hämatologie 25:215, 1982.
20. Wolach, B, et al: Tx polyagglutination in three members of one family. Acta Haematol 78:45, 1987.
21. Kline, WE, et al: Acquired-B antigen and polyagglutination in a healthy blood donor. Transfusion 19:648, 1979.
22. Gerbal, A, et al: Immunologic aspects of the acquired-B antigen. Vox Sang 28:398, 1975.
23. Garratty, G, et al: Acquired-B antigen associated with Proteus vulgaris infection. Vox Sang 21:45, 1971.
24. Salmon, C, and Gerbal, A: The acquired-B antigen. In Handbook of Clinical Laboratory Science. CRC Press, Cleveland, 1977, Vol 1, sect D, p 193.
25. Judd, WJ: Review: Polyagglutination. Immunohematology 8:58, 1992.
26. Chorpenning, FW, and Dodd, MC: Polyagglutinable erythrocytes associated with bacteriogenic transfusion reactions. Vox Sang 10:460, 1965.
27. Graninger, W, et al: "VA": A new type of erythrocyte polyagglutination characterized by depressed H receptors and associated with hemolytic anemia. I. Serological and hematological observations. Vox Sang 32:195, 1977.
28. Dahr, W, et al: Cryptic A-like receptor sites in human erythrocyte glycoproteins: Proposed nature of Tn-antigen. Vox Sang 27:29, 1974.
29. Lee, LT, et al: Immunochemical studies on Tn erythrocyte glycoprotein. Blood 58:1228, 1981.
30. Myllylä, G. et al: Persistent mixed-field polyagglutinability: Electrokinetic and serological aspects. Vox Sang 20:7, 1971.
31. Beck, ML, et al: Observations on leukocytes and platelets in six cases of Tn-polyagglutination. Medical Laboratory Sciences 34:325, 1977.
32. Dahr, W, et al: Molecular basis of Tn-polyagglutinability. Vox Sang 29:36, 1975.
33. Cazal, P, et al: Polyagglutinabilitié héréditaire dominante: antigène privé (Cad) correspondent à un anticorps public et à une lectine de Dolichos biflorus. Revue Française de Transfusion et Immuno-hématologie Blood Transfusion and Immunohematology 11:209, 1968.
34. Cazal, P, et al: Les antigènes Cad en 1976. Revue Française de Transfusion et Immuno-hématologie Blood Transfusion and Immunohematology 20:165, 1977.
35. Sanger, R, et al: Plant agglutinin for another human blood group. Lancet i:1130, 1971.
36. Herkt, F, et al: Structure determination of oligosaccharides isolated from Cad erythrocyte membranes by permethylation analysis and 500-MHz $^1$H-NMR spectroscopy. Eur J Biochem 146:125, 1985.
37. Issitt, PD: The antigens Sd$^a$ and Cad. In Moulds, JM, and Woods, LL (eds): Blood Groups: P, I, Sd$^a$ and Pr. American Association of Blood Banks, Arlington, VA, 1991.
38. Blanchard, D, et al: Comparative study of glycophorin A derived O-glycans from human Cad, Sd(a+), and Sd(a−) erythrocytes. Biochem J 232:813, 1985.
39. Donald, ASR, et al: The human blood group Sd$^a$ determinant: A terminal non-reducing carbohydrate structure in N-linked and mucin type glycoproteins. Biochem Soc Trans 12:596, 1984.
40. Williams, J, et al: Structural analysis of the carbohydrate moieties of human Tamm-Horsfall glycoprotein. Carbohydr Res 134:141, 1984.
41. Bird, AR, et al: Haemoglobin M-Hyde Park associated with polyagglutinable red blood cells in a South African family. Br J Haematol 68:459, 1988.
42. King, MJ, et al: Enhanced reaction with Vicia graminea lectin and exposed terminal N-acetyl-D-glucosaminyl residues on a sample of human red cells with Hb M-Hyde Park. Transfusion 28:549, 1988.
43. Crookston, JH, et al: Red cell abnormalities in HEMPAS (hereditary erythroblastic multinuclearity with a positive acidified serum test). Br J Haematol 23:83, 1972.
44. Gockerman, JP, et al: The abnormal surface characteristics of the red blood cell membrane in congenital dyserythropoietic anemia type II (HEMPAS). Br J Haematol 30:383, 1975.
45. Harris, PA, et al: An inherited RBC characteristic, NOR, resulting in erythrocyte polyagglutination. Vox Sang 42:134, 1982.
46. Beck, ML, et al: High incidence of acquired-B detectable by monoclonal anti-B reagents (abstract). Transfusion 32:17S, 1992.
47. Issitt, PD: Applied Blood Group Serology, ed 3. Montgomery Scientific Miami, 1985, pp 456–476.
48. Rodwell, R, and Tudehope, DI: Screening for cryptantigen exposure and polyagglutination in neonates with suspected necrotizing enterocolitis (Editorial comment). Journal of Paediatrics and Child Health 29:16–18, 1993.
49. Fischer, K, et al: Neuramindase-induzierte Alteration der Erythrozyten und Gefässendothelium—eine Ursache des hämolytische urämischen Syndroms. Proceedings of the 16th Kongress Deutsche Gesamte Hämatologie, Bad Neuheim, 1972.
50. Rumpf, KW, et al: Hemolytic-uremic syndrome in an adult with T-cryptantigen liberation. Deutsche Medizinische Wochenschrift 115:1270, 1990.

51. van Loghem, Jr, JJ, et al: Polyagglutinability of red cells as a cause of a severe haemolytic transfusion reaction. Vox Sang 5:125, 1955.

52. Moores, P, et al: Severe hemolytic anemia in an adult associated with anti-T. Transfusion 15:329, 1975.

53. Levene, C, et al: Intravascular hemolysis and renal failure in a patient with T polyagglutination. Transfusion 26:243, 1986.

54. Judd, WJ, et al: Fatal intravascular hemolysis associated with T-polyagglutination. Transfusion 22:345, 1982.

55. Levene, NA, et al: Th polyagglutination with fatal outcome in a patient with massive intravascular hemolysis and perforated tumor of colon. Am J Hematol 35:127, 1990.

56. Novak, RW: The pathobiology of red cell cryptantigen exposure. Pediatric Pathology 10:867, 1990.

57. Bird, GWG, et al: Erythrocyte membrane modification in malignant disease of myeloid and lymphoreticular tissues. I. Tn-Polyagglutination in acute myelocytic leukemia. Br J Haematol 33:289, 1976.

58. Ness, PM, et al: Tn Polyagglutination preceding acute leukemia. Blood 54:30, 1979.

59. Ness, PM: The association of Tn and leukemia. Haematologia (Budap) 16:93, 1983.

60. Roxby, DJ, et al: Expression of the Tn antigen in myelodysplasia, lymphoma and leukemia. Transfusion 32:834–838, 1992.

61. Buskila, D, et al: Exposure of cryptantigens on erythrocytes in patients with breast cancer. Cancer 61:2455, 1988.

62. Springer, GF: T and Tn, General carcinoma autoantigens. Science 224:1198, 1984.

63. Rose, RR, et al: Transient neonatal Tn-activation: Another example (abstract). Transfusion 23:422, 1983.

64. Janvier, D, et al: Concomitant exposure of Tn and Th cryptantigens on the red cells of a patient with myelodysplasia. Vox Sang 61:142, 1991.

65. Wahl, CM, et al: Th activation of maternal and cord blood. Transfusion 29:635, 1989.

66. Herman, JH, et al: Th activation in congenital hypoplastic anemia. Transfusion 27:253, 1987.

67. Sigler, E, et al: Polyagglutination: A rare mechanism for intravascular hemolysis (letter). Am J Med 92:113, 1992.

68. Marshall, LR, et al: A fatal case of necrotizing enterocolitis in a neonate with polyagglutination of red blood cells. Journal of Paediatrics and Child Health 29:63–65, 1993.

69. Buskila, D, et al: Polyagglutination in hospitalized patients: A prospective study. Vox Sang 52:99, 1987.

70. Adams, M, et al: Exposure of cryptantigens on red blood cell membranes in patients with acquired immune deficiency syndrome or AIDS-related complex. J Acquir Immune Defic Syndr Hum Retrovirol 2:224, 1989.

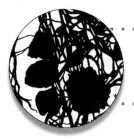

CHAPTER **23**

# THE HLA SYSTEM

Donna L. Phelan, BA, CHS(ABHI), MT(HEW)

**OBJECTIVES**

*On completion of this chapter, the learner should be able to:*

1 Define the abbreviations HLA, MLR, MLC, and MHC.

2 Define the standard method used for HLA typing.

3 Describe the three regions of the HLA complex located on the short arm of chromosome 6.

4 List the important characteristics of the HLA genes.

5 List the three exceptions to the practice of naming all serologic specificities on the basis of correlation with an identified sequence that eliminates the need for a provisional "w" designation.

6 Describe the current nomenclature for HLA genes.

7 List two clinical situations in which HLA typing is important.

8 Define the term *haplotype*.

9 Describe the difference between HLA phenotype and HLA genotype.

10 List the characteristics of HLA class I and class II gene products.

11 Describe the characteristics of HLA antibodies.

12 Define linkage disequilibrium, a characteristic of HLA antigens.

13 Describe the techniques used for HLA antigen detection.

14 Describe the techniques for HLA antibody detection.

15 Describe the role of HLA typing in paternity testing, disease association, platelet transfusion, and transplantation.

## INTRODUCTION

Human leukocyte antigen (HLA) is a specialized branch or division of immunology for human histocompatibility testing. The laboratory discipline supports a number of clinical specialties in transplantation, transfusion, and immunogenetics. Because of its specialized nature, HLA is given relatively little attention in most training programs such as nursing or medical technology.

This chapter is intended to serve as an introduction to basic concepts of HLA and clinical applications of HLA testing. It is written for the reader with some training in the biomedical sciences and familiarity with general immunology concepts.

The emphasis of the chapter is on principles and concepts of HLA structure and function, HLA procedures, and the clinical application of HLA testing to immunogenetics (paternity and disease association), transfusion practices, and transplantation. Inasmuch as it is an overview of a technologically complex area, it lacks a great deal of detail. References are provided that will introduce a path to further information.

Evidence for human leukocyte blood groups was first advanced in 1954 by Dausset,[1] who observed that patients whose sera contained leukoagglutinins had received a larger number of blood transfusions than other patients. He observed that these agglutinins were not autoantibodies as had been thought previously but, rather, alloantibodies produced by the infusion of cells bearing alloantigens not present in the recipient.

Dausset[2] also observed that the sera from seven patients with multiple transfusions agglutinated leukocytes from about 60 percent of the French population but not the leukocytes of the seven patients. He termed the leukocyte antigen defined by leukoagglutination techniques MAC, and family studies showed that leukocyte antigens were genetically determined. At about the same time, Payne[3] showed that the sera of patients with febrile nonhemolytic transfusion reactions often contained leukoagglutinins.

The microdroplet lymphocytotoxicity test was introduced by Terasaki and McClelland[4,5] at the First International Histocompatibility Workshop as a means to define MAC specificity clearly. The microdroplet technique was adopted as the standard method of typing because of the unreliability of the leukoagglutination test. In various modifications this test is still the major HLA-typing serologic technique. The development of HLA typing was further aided by the introduction of computer analysis programs by van Rood and van Leeuwen[6] to study the serologic complexities. Despite numerous false-positive and false-negative serologic reactions, certain specificities could be discerned by computer analysis.

Van Rood applied computer analysis techniques to define specific HLA alleles. He tested approximately 66 sera containing leukoagglutinating antibodies against a random panel of 100 cells. Using two-by-two chi-square analysis, he compared reactivity of each serum with that of every other serum. In this way he was able to identify several groups of sera that were detecting common specificities. In addition, one group of sera having high chi-square values with each other but low values with other serum groups suggested products of allelic genes. Van Rood called this diallelic system 4, with $4^a$ and $4^b$ as alleles.

After the discovery of the first leukocyte antigens and a suitable test system, the number of defined serologic specificities increased rapidly. By 1967 they were all clearly shown to belong to the same genetic system, and the term HL-A (human leukocyte antigen, or HLA— the hyphen has since been deleted) was approved by the World Health Organization (WHO) Committee on Nomenclature.[7] The WHO Committee was formed to establish worldwide uniform nomenclature for the HLA antigens. The committee meets after each international workshop and uses the data from the workshop to update and to assign new names for antigens. These workshops, which are collaborative efforts to advance the field of histocompatibility, are held approximately every 2 to 3 years (Table 23–1). Standardized name assignments aid the rapid but orderly development in this field.

By 1967, it was generally accepted that the HLA antigens were coded for by two closely linked loci, each coding for a multiple number of alleles.[8,9] Antigens were assigned to one of the loci, based upon large population studies and segregation analysis within families. In 1970, the existence of a third locus was defined, which codes for only 10 different serologic alleles to date.[10] Additional research disclosed that the lymphocytes from two different individuals would undergo blast transformation and divide when mixed and cultured in vitro. This cellular response is known as the mixed-lymphocyte reaction (MLR).[11,12] In 1967, Bach and Amos[13] discovered that the MLR was negative when leukocytes from a pair of HLA identical siblings were mixed together, indicating that HLA gene products were responsible for the MLR activity. The tech-

**Table 23–1.** International Workshops

| Year | Location | Advances |
|------|----------|----------|
| 1964 | Durham, North Carolina | Test techniques |
| 1965 | Leiden, The Netherlands | Antigens and transplantation |
| 1967 | Turin, Italy | Family typing studies |
| 1970 | Los Angeles, California | Common serum sets |
| 1972 | Evian, France | Population studies |
| 1975 | Arhus, Denmark | MLC, class II antigens |
| 1977 | Oxford, United Kingdom | Class II genetics |
| 1980 | Los Angeles, California | DR serology, haplotype analyses |
| 1984 | Munich, Germany, and Vienna, Austria | HTC, DNA technology |
| 1987 | Princeton, New Jersey, and New York, New York | RFLP, cellular typing |
| 1991 | Yokohama, Japan | DNA technology |
| 1996 | Paris, France | Molecular nomenclature typing techniques |

nique used to test for MLR activity is the mixed-lymphocyte culture (MLC). Mixed-lymphocyte culture data revealed that there might be a fourth locus (D) very closely linked with the HLA complex. The Seventh International Histocompatibility Workshop in 1977 clearly established the D locus and also a new DR locus defined by serologic methods.[14] Most significantly, the typing of B lymphocytes for their DR specificities was accomplished. The letter *R* in DR indicates *related*, for this locus was found to be either identical with or similar to the D locus identified by the MLC technique.

Evidence suggests that a separate HLA-D locus, defined only by MLR, does not exist. HLA-D assignments are the result of the combined effect of the HLA-DR, HLA-DQ, and HLA-DP determinants, subregions on the class II molecule.

## NOMENCLATURE

The HLA genetic region is a series of closely linked genes that determine major histocompatibility factors; that is, surface antigens or receptors that are responsible for the recognition and elimination of foreign tissues. The region is also referred to as the major histocompatibility complex (MHC). The HLA complex contains an estimated 35 to 40 genes physically grouped into three regions located on the short arm of chromosome 6 (Fig. 23–1). The class I region encodes genes for the classic transplantation molecules, HLA-A, HLA-B, and HLA-C. It also encodes for additional non-classic genes, including HLA-E, HLA-F, and HLA-G. The class II region encodes genes for the molecules HLA-DR, HLA-DP, and HLA-DQ composed of both α and β chains. DP molecules are the product of DPA1 and DPB1 alleles (Fig. 23–2); DPB2 and DPA2 are pseudo-genes, genes with mutations that prevent gene activation or transcription. DQ molecules are the product of DQA1 and DQB1 alleles. Lastly, DR molecules use DRA but can use alleles coded by either DRB1 (the classic DR specificities), DRB3 (DR52 molecules), DRB4 (DR53), and DRB5 (DR51).

The class III region encodes structurally and functionally diverse molecules, including C2, C4, Bf (the com-

## CLASS II

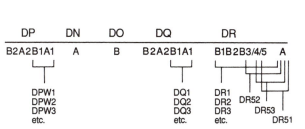

**Figure 23–2.** The loci that code for the major categories of HLA class II gene products. (From Rodey, GE: HLA beyond Tears. De Novo, Atlanta, 1991, p 12, with permission.)

plement factors), 21-hydroxylase, and tumor necrosis factor. In addition, two other genes, glyoxalase-1 (GLO) and phosphoglucomutase-3 (PGM-3), are linked with the HLA complex.

One very important characteristic of the HLA genes is that they are highly polymorphic, and several alleles exist at each locus. The allelic specificities are designated by numbers following the locus symbol (e.g., HLA-A1, HLA-A2, HLA-B5, HLA-B7, and so on). Provisionally identified or tentative specificities, before the 1991 International Workshop, carried the initial letter w (for workshop) inserted between the locus letter designation and the temporary allele specificity number. The w specificities required further definition and confirmation. For example, HLA-Bw53 indicated that the definition of the Bw53 specificity was not fully agreed upon by the WHO Committee on HLA nomenclature. After the 1991 workshop, however, the WHO Committee agreed that all serologic specificities with the letter w indicating provisional status would, with three exceptions, drop the letter w.[15] In the future, all serologic specificities will be named on the basis of correlation with an identified sequence, eliminating the need for a provisional w designation. The three exceptions are (1) Bw4 and Bw6 to distinguish them as epitopes different from other B locus alleles, (2) the C locus specificities where the w is retained to maintain distinction between HLA-C locus alleles and the complement components, and (3) the D and DP specificities defined by mixed-lymphocyte reaction (MLR) and primed lymphocyte typing (PLT).

Table 23–2 lists the current specificities of the HLA system recognized by the WHO committee. Note that specificities within the A and B loci are not numbered consecutively, as are those within the C, DR, DQ, and DP loci. This is because many of the A and B specificities were established before the discovery of the latter loci, and, to avoid renumbering, the existing numbers for the A and B loci were retained.

Also note in Table 23–2 that many of the broad specificities are subdivided into two or more different specificities because of the detection of discrete gene products by monospecific antisera. Monospecific antisera by definition react only with antigenic determi-

## HUMAN CHROMOSOME 6

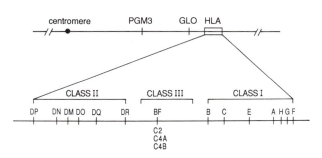

**Figure 23–1.** The HLA complex on the short arm of chromosome 6.

**Table 23–2.** HLA Serologic and Cellular Specificities Officially Recognized Following the Twelfth International Histocompatibility Workshop

| A | B | C | D | DR | DQ | DP |
|---|---|---|---|----|----|-----|
| A1 | B5 | Cw1 | Dw1 | DR1 | DQ1 | DPw1 |
| A2 | B7 | Cw2 | Dw2 | DR103 | DQ2 | DPw2 |
| A203 | B703 | Cw3 | Dw3 | DR2 | DQ3 | DPw3 |
| A210 | B8 | Cw4 | Dw4 | DR3 | DQ4 | DPw4 |
| A3 | B12 | Cw5 | Dw5 | DR4 | DQ5 (1) | DPw5 |
| A9 | B13 | Cw6 | Dw6 | DR5 | DQ6 (1) | DPw6 |
| A10 | B14 | Cw7 | Dw7 | DR6 | DQ7 (3) | |
| A11 | B15 | Cw8 | Dw8 | DR7 | DQ8 (3) | |
| A19 | B16 | Cw9 (w3) | Dw9 | DR8 | DQ9 (3) | |
| A23 (9) | B17 | Cw10 (w3) | Dw10 | DR9 | | |
| A24 (9) | B18 | | Dw11 (w7) | DR10 | | |
| A2403 | B21 | | Dw12 | DR11 (5) | | |
| A25 (10) | B22 | | Dw13 | DR12 (5) | | |
| A26 (10) | B27 | | Dw14 | DR13 (6) | | |
| A28 | B2708 | | Dw15 | DR14 (6) | | |
| A29 (19) | B35 | | Dw16 | DR1403 | | |
| A30 (19) | B37 | | Dw17 (w7) | DR1404 | | |
| A31 (19) | B38 (16) | | Dw18 (w6) | DR15 (2) | | |
| A32 (19) | B39 (16) | | Dw19 (w6) | DR16 (2) | | |
| A33 (19) | B3901 | | Dw20 | DR17 (3) | | |
| A34 (10) | B3902 | | Dw21 | DR18 (3) | | |
| A36 | B40 | | Dw22 | | | |
| A43 | B4005 | | Dw23 | DR51 | | |
| A66 (10) | B41 | | | | | |
| A68 (28) | B42 | | Dw24 | DR52 | | |
| A69 (28) | B44 (12) | | Dw25 | | | |
| A74 (19) | B45 (12) | | Dw26 | DR53 | | |
| A80 | B46 | | | | | |
| | B47 | | | | | |
| | B48 | | | | | |
| | B49 (21) | | | | | |
| | B50 (21) | | | | | |
| | B51 (5) | | | | | |
| | B5102 | | | | | |
| | B5103 | | | | | |
| | B52 (5) | | | | | |
| | B53 | | | | | |
| | B54 (22) | | | | | |
| | B55 (22) | | | | | |
| | B56 (22) | | | | | |
| | B57 (17) | | | | | |
| | B58 (17) | | | | | |
| | B59 | | | | | |
| | B60 (40) | | | | | |
| | B61 (40) | | | | | |
| | B62 (15) | | | | | |
| | B63 (15) | | | | | |
| | B64 (14) | | | | | |
| | B65 (14) | | | | | |
| | B67 | | | | | |
| | B70 | | | | | |
| | B71 (70) | | | | | |
| | B72 (70) | | | | | |
| | B73 | | | | | |
| | B75 (15) | | | | | |
| | B76 (15) | | | | | |
| | B77 (15) | | | | | |
| | B78 | | | | | |
| | B81 | | | | | |
| | Bw4 | | | | | |
| | Bw6 | | | | | |

nants unique to the specific antigen. This process of "splitting" previously recognized antigens is still going on. Table 23-3 lists the broad specificities and their designated split specificities. Also listed are associated antigens (#), which are variants of the original broad specificity and not splits as previously defined.

There are no 4 or 6 allelic assignments within the A and B loci, because these numbers were reserved for the

**Table 23–3.** Broad Specificities, Their Splits, and Associated Antigens

| Original Broad Specificities | Splits and Associated Antigens (#) |
|---|---|
| A2 | A203#, A210# |
| A9 | A23, A24, A2403# |
| A10 | A25, A26, A34, A66 |
| A19 | A29, A30, A31, A32, A33, A74 |
| A28 | A68, A69 |
| B5 | B51, B52, B5102#, B5103# |
| B7 | B703# |
| B12 | B44, B45 |
| B14 | B64, B65 |
| B15 | B62, B63, B75, B76, B77 |
| B16 | B38, B39, B3901#, B3902# |
| B17 | B57, B58 |
| B21 | B49, B50, B4005# |
| B22 | B54, B55, B56 |
| B27 | B2708# |
| B40 | B60, B61 |
| B70 | B71, B72 |
| Cw3 | Cw9, Cw10 |
| DR1 | DR103# |
| DR2 | DR15, DR16 |
| DR3 | DR17, DR18 |
| DR5 | DR11, DR12 |
| DR6 | DR13, DR14, DR1403#, DR1404# |
| DQ1 | DQ5, DQ6 |
| DQ3 | DQ7, DQ8, DQ9 |
| Dw6 | Dw18, Dw19 |
| Dw7 | Dw11, Dw17 |

**Table 23–4.** Bw4 and Bw6 Associated Specificities

| | |
|---|---|
| Bw4: | B5, B5102, B5103, B13, B17, B27, B37, B38 (16), B44 (12), B47, B49 (21), B51 (5), B52 (5), B53, B57 (17), B58 (17), B59, B63 (15), B77 (15) and A9, A23, A24 (9), A2403, A25 (10), A32 (19) |
| Bw6: | B7, B703, B8, B14, B18, B22, B2708, B35, B39 (16), B3901, B3902, B40, B4005, B41, B42, B45 (12), B46, B48, B50 (21), B54 (22), B55 (22), B56 (22), B60 (40), B61 (40), B62 (15), B64 (14), B65 (14), B67, B70, B71 (70), B72 (70), B73, B75 (15), B76 (15), B78, B81 |

example, the serologically defined HLA-B27 specificity is actually made up of seven distinct allelic variations. These alleles are now defined as HLA-B *2701 through *2707. The nomenclature of certain alleles contains a fifth digit, such as HLA-Cw *02021 and *02022. The fifth digit indicates that the two variants differ by a silent nucleotide substitution, but not in amino acid sequence.

Some examples of current HLA genetic nomenclature are provided in Table 23–5.

## ANTIGENS AND ANTIBODIES

It is necessary to evaluate the HLA antigen composition in prospective donor-recipient pairs before organ transplantation and in candidates for platelet therapy refractory to random donor platelets. Even more important is the evaluation and identification of HLA antibodies in the serum of recipients before transplantation and transfusion. Evidence clearly indicates that presensitization to HLA antigens may cause rapid rejection of transplanted tissue or poor platelet survival following transfusion.[16] HLA-antigen testing is also used in disease correlation, paternity testing, and anthropologic studies.

Each person has two alleles for each locus. Both alleles or gene products of a locus are expressed codominantly; that is, there is equal expression of both alleles. The presence of one allele does not suppress the expression of the other. If there are two different alleles on one locus, the person is heterozygous. If both alleles on that locus are the same, the person is homozygous.

leukocyte antigen systems under active investigation at the time the nomenclature was established. The antigens originally called 4 and 6 are now termed Bw4 and Bw6. Every HLA-B locus molecule and some HLA-A locus molecules carry either the Bw4 or the Bw6 antigenic determinant. The distribution of Bw4 and Bw6 determinants on HLA-A and HLA-B locus gene products is found in Table 23–4.

Current nomenclature was recommended during the Tenth International Histocompatibility Workshop in 1987; minor modifications were made in 1990, and total implementation was achieved after the Eleventh International Workshop in 1991. Many HLA allelic variants were discovered by nucleotide and amino acid sequence data that are not detectable by traditional serologic techniques. This complexity necessitated the development of the following nomenclature for HLA genes:

1. HLA- designates the MHC.
2. A capital letter indicates a specific locus (A, B, C, D, etc.) or region. All genes in the D region are prefixed by the letter D and followed by a second capital letter indicating the subregion (DR, DQ, DP, DO, DN, etc.).
3. Loci coding for the specific class I peptide chains are next identified (A1, A2, B1, B2).
4. Specific alleles are designated by * followed by a two-digit numeral defining the unique allele. For

**Table 23–5.** Examples of Current HLA Nomenclature

| Serologic Specificity | Gene Locus | Allelic Variation | Number of Gene Products |
|---|---|---|---|
| HLA-A3 | HLA-A | A*0301, A*0302, A*0303 | 3 |
| HLA-B14 | HLA-B | B*1401, B*1402 | 2 |
| HLA-DR15 | HLA-DRB1 | DRB1*15011   DRB*1503<br>DRB1*15012   DRB1*1504<br>DRB1*15021   DRB1*1505<br>DRB1*15022   DRB1*1506 | 8 |
| HLA-DQ2 | HLA-DQB1 | DQB1*0201<br>DQB1*0202<br>DQB1*0203 | 3 |

The entire set of A, B, C, DR, DQ, and DP antigens located on one chromosome is called a *haplotype*. Genetic crossovers and recombination in the HLA region are uncommon (less than 1 percent), and thus a complete set of antigens located on a chromosome is usually inherited by children as a unit (haplotype).

Figure 23–3 illustrates the segregation of HLA haplotypes in a family. The two haplotypes of the father are labeled a and b, and the mother's c and d. Each offspring inherits two haplotypes, one from each parent. Thus only four possible haplotypes—ac, ad, bc, and bd—can be found in the offspring. It can be calculated that 25 percent of the offspring will have identical HLA haplotypes, 50 percent will share one HLA haplotype, and 25 percent will share no HLA haplotypes. An important corollary is that a parent and child can share only one haplotype, making an identical match between the two unlikely. It should also be apparent that uncles, grandparents, and cousins are very unlikely to have identical haplotypes with any given child. These are important factors when looking for a well-matched organ or blood donor.

The HLA phenotype, then, represents the surface markers or antigens detected in histocompatibility testing of a single individual. The HLA genotype represents the association of the antigens on the two C6 chromosomes as determined by family studies, and the term *haplotype* refers to the antigenic makeup of a single C6 chromosome, illustrated in Figure 23–4.

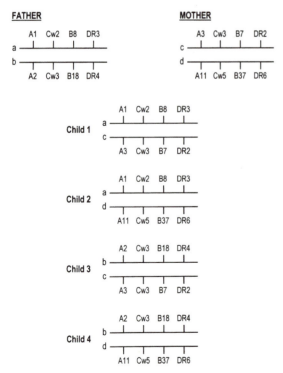

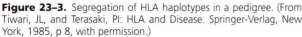

**Figure 23–3.** Segregation of HLA haplotypes in a pedigree. (From Tiwari, JL, and Terasaki, PI: HLA and Disease. Springer-Verlag, New York, 1985, p 8, with permission.)

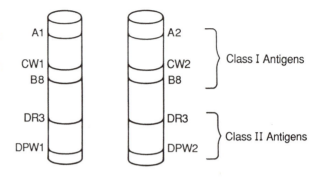

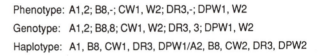

Phenotype: A1,2; B8,-; CW1, W2; DR3,-; DPW1, W2

Genotype: A1,2; B8,8; CW1, W2; DR3, 3; DPW1, W2

Haplotype: A1, B8, CW1, DR3, DPW1/A2, B8, CW2, DR3, DPW2

**Figure 23–4.** Schematic representation of the HLA loci on the short arm of chromosome 6. (From Miller, WV, and Rodey, G: HLA without Tears. American Society of Clinical Pathologists, Chicago, 1981, p 10, with permission.)

## HLA Gene Products

### Structure

Human leukocyte antigen gene products are globular glycoproteins, each composed of two noncovalently linked chains. Class I (HLA-A, HLA-B, and HLA-C) molecules consist of a heavy chain of 45,000 dalton molecular weight associated noncovalently with $\beta_2$-microglobulin, a nonpolymorphic protein of 12,000 dalton molecular weight found in serum and urine. The heavy chain folds into three domains and is inserted through the cell membrane via a hydrophobic sequence.[17]

Class II (HLA-DR, HLA-DQ, and HLA-DP) molecules consist of two similar-sized chains of 33,000 (alpha) and 28,000 (beta) dalton molecular weight associated noncovalently throughout their extracellular portions. In these molecules, both chains are inserted through the membrane via hydrophobic regions. The extracellular portions of these chains fold into two domains.[18,19]

Class I molecules are present on all nucleated cells and platelets, whereas class II molecules have a much more restricted distribution. They are found only on B lymphocytes, macrophages, monocytes, and endothelial cells. Although class I and class II molecules have some obvious structural differences, they are thought to be very similar in overall three-dimensional configuration (Fig. 23–5). Class I and class II molecules are also alike in that most of the polymorphism is expressed in the portion of the molecule farthest from the cell membrane.[20]

Early structural models of class I molecules indicated that the α-1 and α-2 domains consisted of stretches of amino acids that were arranged into helical structures rather than sheets typical of globular proteins. The crystallography studies of Bjorkman and colleagues[21] elu-

CLASS I         CLASS II

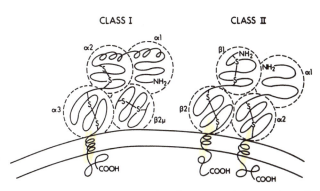

**Figure 23–5.** Three-dimensional configurations of class I and II molecules. $\beta2\mu$ = B$_2$-microglobulin. (From Rodey, GE: HLA beyond Tears. DeNovo, Atlanta, 1991, p 17, with permission.)

cidated the three-dimensional structure of the class I, HLA-A2 molecule. The $\alpha_1$ and $\alpha_2$ domains form a platform overlaid by two helical structures to form the peptide binding site (Fig. 23–6). This groove holds processed peptides for presentation to T cells.

The surface topography, created by the folding of globular proteins into three-dimensional configurations, is large and irregular, containing multiple, nonrepeating sites (antigenic determinants or epitopes) that are potentially immunogenic. It is possible that the entire surface of the HLA molecule consists of these multiple, overlapping epitopes. An epitope is estimated to involve a minimum of five to six amino acid residues, but larger sequences are often necessary to construct the appropriate conformation.

Epitopes that differ among individual members of the same species are alloepitopes. Human leukocyte antigen alloepitopes are defined with well-characterized alloantibodies and cloned T lymphocytes. Serologically defined epitopes are located primarily in and around the peptide groove and are finite in number. The epi-

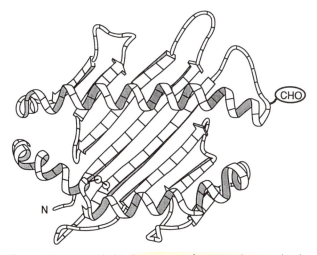

**Figure 23–6.** Peptide binding groove of an HLA class I molecule. CHO = attached carbohydrate unit. N = amino terminus. (The author thanks Dr. Peter Parham for providing this illustration.)

topes recognized by T lymphocytes are less precisely mapped, very numerous, and distinct from the serologically defined ones.[22]

## Function

The primary role of the adaptive arm of the immune system is to recognize and to eliminate foreign antigens. An essential feature of this specific function is the immune system's ability to discriminate between self and nonself or foreign antigens. Major histocompatibility complex class I and II molecules play a crucial role in the process of discrimination at the molecular, cellular, and species levels between self and nonself elements.

## Antibodies

The majority of HLA alloantibodies are IgG. Antibodies to HLA molecules can be divided into two groupings: (1) those that detect a single HLA gene product ("private" antibodies binding to an epitope unique to one HLA gene product) and (2) those that detect more than one HLA gene product. These may be "public" (binding to epitopes shared by more than one HLA gene product) or "cross-reactive" (binding to structurally similar HLA epitopes).[23]

Monoclonal HLA antibodies (moabs) are produced by fusing HLA antibody-producing B cells with plasmacytoma lines.[24] Plasmacytoma cells arise from the malignant transformation of plasma cells or differentiated B cells. These cells continue to secrete antibody after transformation. Moabs detect a broader range of epitopes because they are derived through xenoimmunization—immunization across different species.

## Crossing Over

An event that infrequently complicates HLA-typing interpretation and haplotype determination is crossing over, or recombination. During meiosis, exchange of material between the paired chromosomes can occur. During chromosomal replication, replicated chromosomes often overlay each other, forming X-shaped chiasmata (Fig. 23–7). When the chromosomes are pulled apart during meiotic division, breaks can occur at the crossover site, resulting in complementary exchange of genetic material. The farther apart two loci are on a given chromosome, the more likely it is that genetic exchanges will take place. For example, recombination between HLA-A and HLA-DP occurs commonly, whereas recombination between HLA-DQ and HLA-DR is a

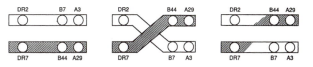

**Figure 23–7.** Schematic of a recombination event between HLA-B and -DR.

rare event. Crossing over has the effect of rearranging the genes on the chromosome to produce new haplotypes in the general population.

## Linkage Disequilibrium

An important characteristic of HLA antigens is the existence of linkage disequilibrium between the alleles of the loci. Linkage disequilibrium is the occurrence of HLA genes more frequently in the same haplotype than would be expected by chance alone. In the Rh system, the blood groups C, D, and e are found together more often than one would expect based on their individual gene frequencies. This is commonly found within the HLA system. In a randomly mating population at Hardy-Weinberg equilibrium,[25] the occurrence of two alleles from closely linked genes will be the product of their individual gene frequencies. If the observed value of the joint frequency is significantly different from the expected frequency (the product of the individual allele frequencies), the alleles are said to be in linkage disequilibrium. For example, if HLA-A1 and HLA-B8 gene frequencies are 0.16 and 0.1, respectively, in a population, the expected occurrence of an HLA haplotype bearing both A1 and B8 should be 0.16 × 0.1 × 100, or 1.6 percent. In certain white populations, however, the actual occurrence of this haplotype is as high as 8 percent, far in excess of the expected frequency. The HLA alleles frequently associated through disequilibrium are listed in Table 23–6. Disequilibrium between the B and DR loci alleles may account for problems in correlating B-locus serotyping with allograft survival

**Table 23–6.** HLA Alleles Frequently Associated through Disequilibrium in Different Populations

| HLA-A, HLA-C, HLA-B | HLA-A, HLA-B, HLA-DR |
|---|---|
| *White* | |
| A1, Cw7, B8 | A1, B8, DR3 |
| A3, Cw7, B7 | A3, B7, DR2 |
| A2, Cw5, B44 | A29, B44, DR7 |
| A1, Cw6, B57 | A3, B35, DR1 |
| A11, Cw4, B35 | A1, B17, DR7 |
| A30, Cw6, B13 | A30, B13, DR7 |
| *Black* | |
| A36, Cw4, B53 | A1, B8, DR3 |
| A1, Cw7, B8 | A30, B42, DR3 |
| A11, Cw2, B35 | A28, B64, DR7 |
| A24, Cw4, B35 | A2, B58, DR11 |
| A2, Cw2, B72 | A28, B58, DR14 |
| A2, Cw7, B58 | A3, B7, DR3 |
| *Asian* | |
| A30, Cw6, B13 | A24, B52, DR2 |
| A2, Cw1, B46 | A33, B44, DR14 |
| A24, Cw1, B54 | A24, B7, DR1 |
| A33, Cw3, B58 | A33, B44, DR13 |
| A24, Cw7, B7 | A30, B13, DR7 |
| A11, Cw4, B62 | A24, B54, DR4 |

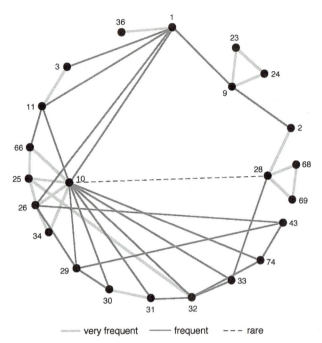

**HLA-A LOCUS CREGS**

— very frequent — frequent - - - rare

**Figure 23–8.** Cross-reactions within the HLA-A locus. (From Bender, K: The HLA System. Biotest Diagnostics, 1991, p 21, with permission.)

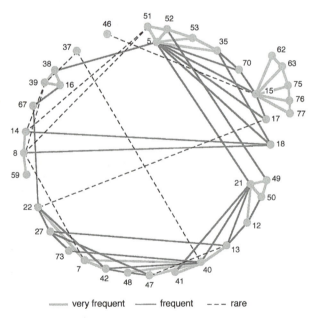

**HLA-B LOCUS CREGS**

— very frequent — frequent - - - rare

**Figure 23–9.** Cross-reactions within the HLA-B locus. (From Bender, K: The HLA System. Biotest Diagnostics, 1991, p 22, with permission.)

and disease associations, inasmuch as matching or typing for B-locus alleles would, by disequilibrium, often result in matching or typing for D-locus alleles as well. D-locus and DR-locus matching has been found to be clinically significant to allograft survival.

## Cross-Reactivity

Cross-reactivity is a phenomenon in which an antiserum directed against one HLA antigenic determinant reacts with other HLA antigenic determinants as well. Cross-reactive antigens share important structural elements with one another but retain unique, specific elements. Human leukocyte antigen serologists recognized very quickly that many of the HLA alloantibodies were serologically cross-reactive with HLA specificities.[26–28] Dausset and his colleagues[29] suggested in 1967 that these antibodies might detect public specificities shared by multiple HLA gene products. The broadly reactive antibodies used in van Rood and von Leeuwen's original computer-derived HLA clusters also defined many of the currently defined major cross-reactive groups, or CREGs.

The majority of cross-reactive alloantibodies detect HLA specificities of allelic molecules coded by the same locus. On the basis of these reactions, most specificities can be grouped into major CREGs (Figs. 23–8 and 23–9).[30,31] For example, the HLA-A locus antigens A2, A23, A24, and A28 share a common determinant and therefore make up the A2 CREG, or A2c. HLA-A28 also shares a common determinant with A26, A33, and A34, defining the A28 CREG. There are also at least three interlocus cross-reactions detected by alloantisera and moabs that occur between the HLA-A and HLA-B loci: HLA-A23, HLA-A24, HLA-A25, and HLA-A32 with HLA-Bw4[32–35]; HLA-A11 with HLA-Bw6[36]; and HLA-A2 with HLA-B17.[37–39] Recently, cross-reactive groups have been defined molecularly using amino acid residues. Table 23–7 lists the residues identified and their correlative HLA-A,B antigens and representative CREGs.

## TECHNIQUES OF HISTOCOMPATIBILITY TESTING

The principles used in histocompatibility testing are basically similar to those used for red cell testing; that is, known sera are used to type HLA antigens on test cells, recipient serum is screened for the presence of HLA antibodies, and cross-matching of donor cells and recipient sera is performed to determine compatibility.

Preformed antibodies to tissue of both donor and recipient may cause significant complications in transplantation or transfusion. Recipient lymphocytotoxic HLA antibodies to donor antigens have been associated with accelerated graft rejection and with poor response to platelet transfusion. Antibody in donor plasma to recipient leukocytes has been associated with severe pulmonary infiltrates and respiratory distress following transfusion.

Cross-matching involves both serologic and cellular procedures. Serologic cross-matching is performed by cytotoxicity and flow cytometric techniques.[39] Lymphocyte-defined compatibility is determined by the mixed-lymphocyte reaction or one of its modifications.

Over the past 10 years, practical techniques have been developed to characterize gene structure and specific alleles. The techniques of molecular genetics have revolutionized the field of molecular biology.

## HLA Antigen Detection

The agglutination methods initially used to define the HLA complex have given way to a precise microlymphocytotoxicity test.[40] Cytotoxicity techniques require only 1 to 2 μL of serum and are sensitive and reproducible.

Acid-citrated dextrose (ACD) or phenol-free heparinized blood is used for testing. A purified lymphocyte suspension is prepared by layering whole blood on a Ficoll-Hypaque gradient and centrifuging. Residual red cells and granulocytes are forced to the bottom of the gradient, and platelets remain in the supernatant. Lymphocytes collect at the gradient's interface and can be harvested, washed, and adjusted to appropriate test concentrations (Fig. 23–10). HLA-A, HLA-B, and HLA-C typing is performed on this lymphocyte suspension. HLA-DR typing requires a purified B-lymphocyte suspension.

B-lymphocyte suspensions were generally prepared in two ways: (1) nylon wool separation[41,42] and (2)

**Table 23–7.** HLA-A, B Residues and Corresponding CREGs

| Residue | A, B Antigens | CREG |
|---------|---------------|------|
| R114 | A1, A3, A11, A29, A36 | A1C |
| K127 | A2, A9, A23, A24, A28, A68, A69 | A2C |
| A71–D74 | B7, B22, B27, B42, B46, B54, B55, B56, B67 | B7C |
| T69–S77 | B8, B14, B16, B39, B64, B65, B78 | B8C |
| T41 | B12, B13, B21, B40, B41, B44, B45, B47, B49, B50, B60, B61 | B12C |
| R83 | A9, B5, A23, A24, A25, A32, B12, B13, B17, B21, B27, B37, B38, B44, B47, B49, B51, B52, B53, B57, B58, B59 | Bw4 |
| N80 | B7, B8, A11, B14, B15, B16, B18, B22, B35, B39, B40, B41, B42, B45, B46, B48, B50, B54, B55, B56, B60, B61, B62, B64, B65, B67, B70, B71, B72, B75, B76, B78, B79 | Bw6 |

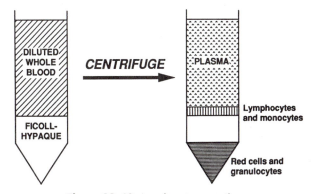

**Figure 23–10.** Lymphocyte separation.

fluorescent labeling.[43] The nylon wool separation of B lymphocytes was based on the observation that B cells adhere preferentially to nylon wool, from which they can be eluted, whereas T lymphocytes do not adhere to the wool. Fluorescent labeling involved the incubation of lymphocytes with fluorescein isothiocyanate-labeled anti-immunoglobulin. B lymphocytes developed distinct fluorescent caps owing to the binding of the labeled anti-immunoglobulin to the cell surface immunoglobulin found on B cells and not on T cells. A major advantage of the fluorescent labeling technique was that it did not involve the physical separation of T and B cells, in contrast to nylon wool separation.

Techniques currently used are immunomagnetic beads to positively select (target cells rosetted on beads) lymphocyte subpopulations for use in HLA typing, both for class I and II antigens.[44] These techniques provide rapid isolation of cells with a high degree of purity and use immunofluorescence lymphocytotoxicity. The technique for isolation of either T or B cells depends on the moab for bead coating.

HLA testing is performed in 60-well or 72-well microtiter trays. Antiserum test trays are prepared by dispensing 1 μL of serum into the bottom of each well, which contains mineral oil. Mineral oil is used to prevent evaporation of antisera during test incubations. Antiserum trays are frozen at −70°C until just before use. On use, they are removed from the freezer and thawed for 3 to 5 minutes.

Every laboratory performing HLA typing uses some form of complement-dependent microlymphocytotoxicity (CDC) (Fig. 23–11). In this procedure 1 μL of antisera is mixed with 1 μL of cells and incubated at room temperature for 30 minutes. Rabbit serum (5 μL) is added as a source of complement, and the cells are further incubated at room temperature for 60 minutes. Complement-mediated cell membrane injury that is induced in cells binding HLA antibody is visualized by the uptake or release of eosin-Y or trypan blue dye. The test is a tertiary binding assay that depends heavily upon many factors—that is, time, temperature, antibody

strength—that influence the efficiency with which the antibodies will activate the complement cascade.

Trays are usually read on inverted phase-contrast microscopes. Under properly adjusted phase, cells that have not been injured appear small, bright, and refractile. Injured cells that have taken up eosin-Y or trypan owing to antibody and complement flatten and appear large, dark, and nonrefractile. The percent of cell death is coded numerically: the number 8 is used for a strong positive with essentially all cells killed; the number 1 is used for a negative reaction in which cell viability is the same as in the negative control. By scoring the reaction of each known serum with test cells, a phenotype can be assigned. Antigen assignment is made by looking at the specificity of the defined HLA antibody in the positive wells. For example, if all wells containing HLA-A3 antibody are positive (eight reactions), the A3 antigen is assigned to the phenotype.

## HLA-D Typing

Because allografted tissue is rejected by a lymphocyte-mediated immune response, as well as by antibody response, tests have been developed that use a biologic response of lymphocytes to foreign antigens as a measure of histocompatibility. The mixed-lymphocyte reaction (MLR) test is especially important because it provides an in vitro model in which lymphocytes can be used both as responders (recipient cells) to foreign HLA-alloantigens and as stimulators (donor cells) carrying those antigens.[11] For example, lymphocytes of the recipient are mixed with lymphocytes of the donor, after donor lymphocytes have been treated with mitomycin C or x-irradiation to inhibit DNA synthesis. The response of the recipient cells to these treated donor cells in the MLR is measured by the incorporation of radioactive thymidine into the responding cells during cell division. If the responding cells have been stimulated, large amounts of labeled thymidine are incorporated into the newly synthesized DNA. This incorporation can be quantitated in a liquid scintillation counting device. Appropriate controls and replicate samples must be tested. The MLR reaction recognizes the antigenic differences on stimulator cells; therefore, it follows that cells bearing the same antigens as the responding cell will cause no stimulation. This indicates that the stimulator and the responder cells have the same HLA-D type.

To type for HLA-D antigens, stimulator cells from individuals known to be homozygous for HLA-D series antigens are used. Initially, these homozygous D-typing cells were obtained from HLA-identical children of first-cousin marriages. More recently, similar cells have been found, although infrequently, in the general population. Cells of both types are referred to as homozygous-typing cells (HTC). To perform D typing, HTCs of each known phenotype are set up in MLR as stimulators against the test cells. Lack of response in MLR to specific cell types indicates that the test cell bears the same antigen as those HTC.

**COMPLEMENT-DEPENDENT LYMPHOCYTOTOXICITY (CDC) ASSAYS**

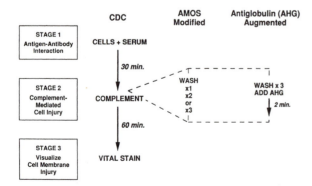

**Figure 23–11.** Complement-dependent microlymphocytotoxicity assay with two variations: three-wash AMOS and antiglobulin.

## HLA Antibody Detection Techniques

Detection and identification techniques of HLA antibodies are similar to those of red cell antibodies. The unknown serum is tested against a panel of cells of known HLA phenotype. Cells from a large panel of donors must be selected if antibodies to all HLA specificities are to be detected. A panel of at least 30 carefully selected cells is required for initial screening in the determination of panel reactive antibody (PRA), and a panel of at least 60 cells is required for accurate antibody identification. Serum can be screened using freshly prepared lymphocytes or lymphocytes frozen in bulk or in trays. Lymphocytes frozen in trays have the advantage of rapid preparation, enabling serum to be screened in just a few hours.

The test serum is evaluated by a microlymphocytotoxicity technique. The method depends on the purpose of the screen. When looking for alloantisera to be used as typing reagents, it is essential to screen using the method to be used in the typing procedure, the standard CDC being the most common. When screening recipient serum samples, a more sensitive technique—Amos-modified, extended incubation, or antihuman globulin—should be employed. The Amos-modified technique introduces a wash step after the initial serum-cell incubation. The wash step removes anti-complementary activity, aggregated immunoglobulin in the serum which can activate complement, making it unavailable for binding on the cell membranes. Standard CDC tests rarely detect 100 percent of the antigen-binding specificities of cross-reactive antibodies.[45,46] Sensitivity of the CDC test can be greatly enhanced by the addition of an antihuman globulin reagent following serum and cell incubation.[45] The addition of goat antihuman kappa chain increases the likelihood of complement binding and subsequent cell injury, especially in circumstances in which the amount of HLA-antibody binding is below the threshold of detection in the standard technique. The antihuman globulin test functions like a complement-independent technique with respect to HLA alloantibodies. If antibodies to class II molecules (DR and DQ) are to be identified, then separated or labeled B-lymphocyte suspensions of known phenotype must be used.

## HLA Crossmatch Techniques

Numerous techniques have been described and applied as crossmatch procedures for transplantation and transfusion. Lymphocytotoxicity is the most widely used technique because the assays are rapid and reproducible, and they use small volumes of recipient antisera and small numbers of donor cells. The primary purpose of crossmatching before transplantation or transfusion is to identify antibodies in the serum of the potential recipient to antigens present on donor tissues.

To facilitate detection of low levels of antibodies in potential recipients, sensitive techniques must be used, as in recipient serum screens. The correlation between hyperacute rejection and the presence of serum[16] antibody against donor tissue is well established. Cases of irreversible rejection during the first days after transplantation may be a result of low levels of antibody undetected by less sensitive techniques.[47-48] Thistlewaite and colleagues[49] have observed that T-cell crossmatches performed with an immunofluorescence flow cytometric technique are highly sensitive in detecting donor HLA antibodies in potential allograft recipients, which were undetected by standard serologic techniques (Amos and antihuman globulin). The flow cytometry crossmatch is performed by incubating donor cells with recipient sera followed by a fluoresceinated (FITC) goat antihuman immunoglobulin. A phycoerythrin (PE) labeled antibody to detect either T or B cells is used to discriminate between the two subpopulations of lymphocytes. Cells are analyzed and results expressed as positive or negative, based on the shift in fluorescence intensity of the test serum with respect to negative serum (Fig. 23–12). To achieve good graft survival rates, centers are investigating more sensitive crossmatch techniques for the detection of donor-specific HLA alloantibodies.

## HLA Molecular Techniques

Human leukocyte antigen class II (HLA-DR, HLA-DQ, HLA-DP) typing is being performed in most laboratories by DNA hybridization techniques.[50] These procedures have currently replaced serologic typing in many laboratories. Human leukocytic antigen class I (HLA-A, HLA-B, HLA-C) typing is also being performed by DNA techniques, however, in a more restricted number of laboratories. The numerous alleles at the three loci, in

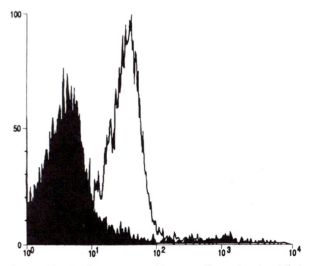

**Figure 23–12.** Flow cytometry histogram illustrating the shift in fluorescence light intensity emitted by a cell population coated with fluorescein-labeled antibody. The vertical ordinate represents increasing fluorescence and the horizontal abscissa represents increasing cell numbers. (From Rodney, GE: HLA Beyond Tears, DeNovo, Atlanta, 1991, p 17, with permission.)

particular HLA-B, make it more difficult and time consuming to perform.

Two of the more common techniques used for class II DNA typing are sequence-specific primers (SSP) and sequence-specific oligonucleotide probes (SSOP), replacing restriction fragment length polymorphism (RFLP) and allele-specific oligonucleotide probes (ASOP). Both use the polymerase chain reaction (PCR), an in vitro technique to amplify specific DNA sequences of interest. This technique provides a rapid and sensitive method to identify specific allelic genes when the sequence of the gene is known. Figure 23–13 illustrates a basic strategy for oligonucleotide typing.

Direct nucleotide sequencing of HLA genes is the next step in molecular typing techniques. Because detection is not based on the use of a sequence-specific oligonucleotide probe and prior knowledge of the nucleotide sequences,[51,52] previously undefined alleles can be detected.

## CLINICAL SIGNIFICANCE OF THE HLA SYSTEM

The identification of HLA antigens was fueled by their potential clinical application to transplantation. The HLA system is still of primary clinical importance in transplantation, but it has recently become of great interest to individuals in the field of human genetics and to investigators of disease associations. Human leukocyte antigens are associated with disease susceptibility to a greater extent than any other known genetic marker in humans, and the HLA system has the highest exclusion probability of any single system in resolving cases of disputed paternity.[53]

### Paternity

Paternity testing involves the analysis of genetic markers from the mother, child, and alleged father to determine whether or not the tested man could be the

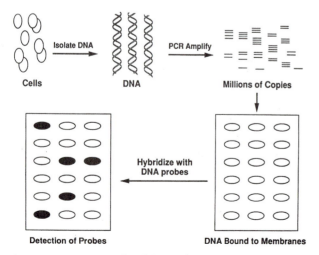

**Figure 23–13.** Strategy for allele-specific oligonucleotide typing.

biologic father of a child. To accomplish this, the laboratory uses a number of techniques to accurately identify the polymorphic genetic markers in a paternity trio. Combinations of various genetic markers are used, including red cell markers and enzymes, serum proteins, HLA typing, and DNA testing. Previously, the most common combination of testing included red cell markers together with HLA typing. However, owing to increased costs of HLA typing reagents and the significantly high power of exclusion when testing multiple DNA loci, DNA methodologies are used increasingly more than HLA typing.

### Disease Association

Recently it was determined that HLA antigens are associated with disease susceptibility to a greater extent than any other known genetic marker.[54] Many genetic markers have been suspected to be associated with disease, the most extensively studied being blood groups, enzymes, and serum proteins. Data from these studies[55] show weak association of disease and relative risks of less than two. Relative risk indicates how many times more frequently the disease occurs in individuals positive for the marker than in individuals negative for the marker. In contrast, the association between HLA-B27 and ankylosing spondylitis has a relative risk ranging from 60 to 100, depending on the population studied. Although many diseases associated with HLA have a relative risk value greater than 2, none exceed the strength of the association of HLA-B27 with ankylosing spondylitis. To date, 530 diseases have been studied.[54] A list of the most significant HLA and disease associations is given in Table 23–8.

The exact cause for the association of HLA to disease is unclear. There is no question that genetic factors coded within or near the HLA complex confer susceptibility for a variety of diseases. This susceptibility may somehow be related to altered immunologic responsiveness in many cases. It is also probable that the diseases in question may be a result of both multiple gene interactions and environmental factors. Although the study of HLA and disease associations is very important in understanding disease susceptibility and manifestation, HLA alone is not clinically useful as a diagnostic tool.

### Platelet Transfusion

Bone marrow transplantation and more aggressive use of chemotherapy in the treatment of malignancies have led to a dramatic increase in platelet transfusions in the past decade. Human leukocyte class I antigens are expressed variably on platelets.[56–60] Alloimmunization to the HLA results in refractoriness to random donor platelet transfusions. Refractoriness is manifested by the failure to achieve a rise in circulating platelet count 1 hour after infusion of adequate numbers of platelets. The refractory state is often associated with lymphocytotoxic HLA antibodies.

**Table 23–8.** Significant HLA Disease Associations

| Disease | HLA | Relative Risk* |
|---|---|---|
| Narcolepsy | DR2 | 129.8 |
| Ankylosing spondylitis | B27 | 69.1 |
| Reiter's syndrome | B27 | 37.1 |
| Dermatitis herpetiformis | DR3 | 17.3 |
|  | B8 | 9.8 |
| Pemphigus vulgaris | DR4 | 14.6 |
|  | A26 | 4.8 |
|  | B38 | 4.6 |
| Goodpasture's syndrome | DR2 | 13.8 |
| Celiac disease | DR3 | 11.6 |
|  | DR7 | 7.7 |
|  | B8 | 7.6 |
| Acute anterior uveitis | B27 | 8.2 |
| Psoriasis vulgaris | Cw6 | 7.5 |
|  | B17 | 5.3 |
|  | B13 | 4.1 |
|  | B37 | 3.9 |
|  | DR7 | 3.2 |
| Idiopathic hemochromatosis | A3 | 6.7 |
|  | B7 | 2.9 |
|  | B14 | 2.7 |
| Sjögren's syndrome | Dw3 | 5.7 |
|  | B8 | 3.3 |
| Juvenile rheumatoid arthritis | B27 | 3.9 |
|  | DR5 | 3.3 |
| Behçet's disease | B5 | 3.8 |
| Rheumatoid arthritis | DR4 | 3.8 |
|  | B27 | 2.0 |
| Grave's disease | DR3 | 3.7 |
|  | B8 | 2.5 |
| Juvenile diabetes mellitus | DR4 | 3.6 |
|  | DR3 | 3.3 |
|  | B8 | 2.5 |
|  | B15 | 2.1 |
| Myasthenia gravis | B8 | 3.3 |
| Multiple sclerosis | DR2 | 2.7 |
|  | B7 | 1.8 |

*Relative risk of the disease in the white population. Frequencies for other races can be found in Tiwari, JL, and Terasaki, PI: HLA and Disease. New York, Springer-Verlag, 1995, p 33.

Considering the highly polymorphic nature of the HLA system, it is impossible to obtain sufficient numbers of HLA-typed donors to provide HLA-matched platelets for all alloimmunized patients. Duquesnoy and associates[61] have demonstrated that platelet transfusions from donors mismatched only for cross-reactive antigens can effectively provide hemostasis for refractory patients. For example, an HLA A1,B7; A11,B22 recipient might benefit from the platelets of an A1,B7; A3,B27 donor, because A3 and A11 and B27 and B22 are cross-reactive. Table 23–9 lists the major cross-reactive groups and the private specificities associated with each. As a result of these observations, the donor pool necessary to sustain an HLA-matched platelet program can be reduced from 8000 to 10,000 to manageable numbers of 2000 to 5000.

Good platelet survival and HLA matching are not absolute. For example, poor transfusion results are sometimes obtained despite a perfect HLA match. Poor recovery may be a result of sensitization to non-HLA antigens, such as platelet-specific antigens. [...] transfusion results are at other times [...] ence of complete HLA mismatch. Go[...] a function of (1) a restricted pattern [...] tion—private versus public antibodies[...] expression of HLA antigens on the pla[...]

Leukocytes are more immunogen[...] platelets, and refractoriness is probably initiated by HLA antigens on the contaminating leukocytes. Evidence for this is based on a study by Brand and others,[62] in which they demonstrated a decreased rate of alloimmunization to random donor platelets when contaminating leukocytes were removed before transfusion. Herzig and colleagues[63] were also able to improve the transfusion response to HLA-matched platelets by removing the leukocytes. This type of approach might be useful for those patients who are unable to produce a response to HLA-matched platelets.

## Transplantation

Clinical transplant immunology is a difficult field. Unlike animal experimentation, in which studies are performed under controlled conditions in selected inbred strains, transplant immunology deals with actual patients with different medical histories and backgrounds. Individuals working in transplant immunology must determine how best to select recipients and donors, when to increase or to decrease immunosuppressive treatment, and how to precondition potential recipients so that their immune systems will accept a graft. Decisions are based on the relative merits of laboratory findings viewed against complex medical histories. Differences of opinion exist from center to center about the significance of immunologic test results and their considerations in clinical treatment protocols.

### Bone Marrow

Bone marrow transplantation is used to treat patients with severe aplastic anemia, immunodeficiency disease, and various forms of leukemia. Since 1980 there has been a change in the proportion of patients treated with bone marrow transplantation for malig-

**Table 23–9.** Major Cross-reactive Groups (CREGs) and Their Private Specificities

| Major CREG | Associated Private Specificities |
|---|---|
| A1 CREG | A1, 36, 3, 9 (23, 34), 10 (25, 26, 34, 66), 11, 19 (29, 30, 31, 32, 33), 28 (68, 69), 74 |
| A2 CREG | A2, 9 (23, 24), 28 (68, 69), B17 |
| B5 CREG | B5 (51, 52), 15 (62, 63, 75, 76, 77), 17 (57, 58), 18, 35, 49, 53, 70 (71, 72), 78 |
| B7 CREG | B7, 42, 22 (54, 55, 56), 27, 40 (60, 61), 13, 41, 47, 48, 81 |
| B8 CREG | B8, 14 (64, 65), 16 (38, 39), 18, 55 |
| B12 CREG | B12 (44, 45), 21 (49, 50), 13, 40 (60, 61), 41, 48 |
| 4c CREG | A9 (23, 24), A25, A32, Bw4 |
| 6c CREG | Bw6, Cw1, Cw3, Cw7 |

nt versus nonmalignant diseases.[64] Before 1980, 72 percent of bone marrow transplants were performed for nonmalignant diseases. Since 1980, 77 percent have been performed for malignant diseases.

Before 1980, bone marrow transplantation was performed only between HLA-identical siblings. This restricted transplantation to 35 to 40 percent of individuals eligible for transplant. Since then an increasing number of transplants has been performed using family members or unrelated donors who are fully or partially HLA-matched with the recipient when no HLA-identical sibling is available. An important application of mismatching for cross-reactive antigens in bone marrow recipients who receive one haplotype-mismatched donor marrow has been reported.[65] A significantly lower incidence of graft-versus-host disease (59 percent) was observed in patients receiving donor marrow with compatible class I cross-reactive public antigens compared with patients receiving public antigen-incompatible donor marrow (89 percent). Another study performed by Hows and associates[66] revealed 58 percent patient survival with unrelated HLA-identical donor transplantation versus 25 percent with related HLA-nonidentical siblings.

**National Marrow Donor Program.** The single most important factor for the potential increase of bone marrow transplantation is expanding the donor pool to include both related and unrelated individuals. To meet the needs of patients who do not have a matched, related donor, the United States Congress authorized a federal contract in 1986 to establish a national marrow donor registry.

In response to a request for proposal, the National Marrow Donor Program (NMDP) was formed with cosponsorship of the American Association of Blood Banks (AABB), American Red Cross (ARC), and the Council of Community Blood Centers (CCBC). The goals were to recruit a large number of informed HLA-typed volunteers to be listed as potential marrow donors, to combine all available donor HLA data into a centralized registry, and to establish a national coordinating center for facilitating donor searches and communication between donor and transplant centers. As of October 1, 1998, the NMDP had facilitated 7200 unrelated marrow transplants throughout the world. The NMDP registry contains information on 804,565 volunteers willing to donate their marrow to patients needing unrelated donors. Recruiting minorities to be volunteer donors continues to be a focus for the NMDP, inasmuch as minorities represent only 606,826 volunteers on the registry.

### Kidney

Kidney transplantation is used to treat end-stage renal disease (ESRD). Transplantation is preferred over dialysis in treating patients with chronic renal failure because it is more cost-effective and it usually returns patients to a state of relatively normal health. The best graft survival rates are obtained when kidneys are ob-

tained from HLA-identical, ABO-compatible siblings, but such donors are available for relatively few patients.[67,68] Three general strategies are employed by transplantation surgeons and immunologists to minimize the graft rejection process: (1) the use of immunosuppressive agents, (2) the reduction of graft "foreignness," and (3) the induction of tolerance.

Immunosuppressive agents such as azathioprine, prednisone, antilymphocyte globulin, and cyclosporine are used to diminish the destructive immunologic responses to the graft. These agents are nonselective and carry risks of serious side effects, especially life-threatening infection.[69]

Extensive efforts are used to minimize graft "foreignness" through matching of donor and recipient antigens. Antigen disparities that most influence graft rejection include the ABO blood group antigens and the HLA antigens. Although it is still not clear what combinations of HLA gene products matching promotes optimal graft survival, it appears that HLA-DR is the most critical for good graft survival.[70-72] In highly sensitized recipients, it is necessary to match for HLA-A and HLA-B because of the presence of class I HLA antibodies. Sanfilippo and colleagues[73] have found that matching based on public cross-reactive antigens can provide the same association with graft outcome as private antigens. When matching for highly sensitized recipients, by either private or public antigens, identification of HLA serum antibodies is important. Oldfather and others[74] have observed that crossmatch results can be predicted in highly sensitized recipients based on careful analysis of serum HLA-antibody specificities.

The third strategy is based upon the induction of tolerance to donor-specific antigens. The evidence that transfusion of blood products before transplantation promotes graft acceptance suggests that tolerance induction may be feasible. In 1973, Opelz and coworkers[75] reported that blood transfusion might promote renal allograft survival in patients receiving kidneys from crossmatch-negative donors. In their retrospective study, graft survival rates at 1 year were significantly improved in patients who had received more than 10 transfusions (66 percent), compared with patients who had received 1 to 10 units (43 percent) or no transfusions (29 percent). Salvatierra and colleagues[76] applied this observation to the potential benefits of donor-specific blood transfusions and transplants between living related individuals. The effects of blood transfusion on the success of renal transplantation are complex and paradoxic. Transfusion of blood usually leads to HLA alloimmunization, and when this leads to HLA antibody production, it is difficult to find compatible donors. Yet graft survival rates are improved when pretransplant blood is given to the recipient with no resulting sensitization. Data on the blood transfusion effect were obtained from recipients treated with azathioprine. There is a question as to whether blood transfusion is or will be necessary with new drug therapies such as cyclosporine and FK506. Indications are that the transfusion effect will be lost with the newer immunosuppressive agents.

### Heart

Heart transplantation is used to treat cardiomyopathies and end-stage ischemic heart disease. Because of the organ's extremely short total ischemic time (3 hours for hearts, compared with 72 hours for kidneys), HLA matching is not feasible. Total ischemic time is the amount of time during which there is no blood flow through the organ. The single most important HLA test performed pretransplant is the HLA-antibody screen. Recipients with no preformed HLA antibodies receive transplants without crossmatching. Those with preformed HLA antibodies require pretransplant crossmatches to determine recipient-donor compatibility.

In a retrospective study by Yacoub and coworkers,[77] an additive effect of class I and II matching on graft survival was observed. Matching for class II antigens had a marked influence on increased graft survival, whereas matching for class I antigens alone had no influence on the outcome. More data need to be analyzed to judge the effect of HLA matching on graft survival. Once conclusive data are found that HLA matching is beneficial to graft outcome, it will be necessary to study methods for increasing the total ischemic time or decreasing the time of test procedures.

### Liver

Liver transplantation is now performed with good 1-year graft survival rates (75 percent) because of the benefits of cyclosporine, the principal immunosuppressive agent. A newcomer, FK506, may increase the success of liver transplantation with reported 1-year survivals exceeding 90 percent.[78]

Immunologic factors in recipient/donor matching for liver transplantation and recipient presensitization have largely been ignored in the past. The consequences of HLA presensitization or ABO incompatibility were recently underlined in two reports.[79-81] In the first, a retrospective analysis of preformed HLA antibodies demonstrated 1-year graft survivals of 40 percent in the presensitized individuals (27) as compared with 83 percent in the nonsensitized individuals. In the second, survival of patients with emergency ABO-incompatible transplants was 30 percent, compared with 76 percent in patients with emergency ABO-compatible grafts and 80 percent in patients with elective ABO-compatible grafts.

It is hoped that advances in organ storage will eliminate the need for ABO-incompatible transplantation and increase cold ischemia times, allowing histocompatibility testing, especially for presensitized patients.

### Lung

An overall review of the indications for lung transplantation during the past several years reveals that em-

physema and cystic fibrosis account for the majority of double-lung transplants. The major indications for single-lung transplantation include pulmonary fibrosis (33 percent) and emphysema (41 percent). In addition, more patients are now undergoing single-lung transplants for primary hypertension, previously treated by heart-lung transplantation.

Short cold ischemic times for lungs, as with hearts, preclude prospective histocompatibility testing. However, the HLA matching between donor and recipient may play an important role in live-donor lung transplantation in an attempt to improve posttransplant conditions and graft survival rates.[82]

### Pancreas and Islet Cell

The primary indication for pancreas transplantation is diabetes. The majority of pancreas transplants performed are simultaneous pancreas/kidney transplants (66 percent), with equal numbers of pancreas following kidney (17 percent) and pancreas alone (17 percent).

Human leukocyte antigen matching, as reported by two large pancreas transplant centers, has a major effect on graft survival.[83,84] Increased long-term survival rates were reported with HLA-DR matching, with significant differences demonstrated between 2 and 0 mismatches. Improved graft survivals were observed in all types of pancreas transplants, based on the number of HLA mismatches, 80 percent survival with 0 to 1 mismatches versus 44 percent with 4 to 6 mismatches.

Because of increased risks of myocardial complications with pancreas transplantation, islet cell transplantation has been actively pursued. Although islet cell transplantation is technically simple, difficulty has been encountered in the achievement of sustained engraftment in humans. Scharp and colleagues[85] have reported on their first nine intraportal islet grafts. The first 6 functioned early, but all were rejected within 2 weeks despite heavy immunosuppression. The last 3, transplanted with pooled islet cells, achieved insulin independence ranging from 15 to 184 days. New in vivo systems can now support islet function for longer than 6 months, an important area for continued technology development.

### United Network for Organ Sharing (UNOS)

In an effort to provide a rare commodity, solid organs, equitably, the United Network for Organ Sharing (UNOS) was established in 1986. This organization received the federal contract to operate the National Organ Procurement and Transplantation Network (OPTN) and to develop an equitable scientific and medically sound organ allocation system. The OPTN is charged with developing policies that maximize use of organs donated for transplantation, ensuring quality of care for transplant patients, and addressing medical and ethical issues related to organ transplantation in the United States.

## SUMMARY CHART: IMPORTANT POINTS TO REMEMBER (MT/SBB)

- The MLR (mixed lymphocyte reaction) is used for HLA-D typing, in which lymphocytes from two different individuals undergo blast transformation and divide when mixed and cultured in vitro; the recipient cells act as responders to foreign HLA-alloantigens, and donor cells act as stimulators carrying those antigens.
- The HLA genetic region is a series of closely linked genes located on the short arm of chromosome 6 that determine major histocompatibility factors, that is, surface antigens or receptors that are responsible for the recognition and elimination of foreign tissues.
- The HLA class I region encodes genes for the classic transplantation molecules, HLA-A, HLA-B, and HLA-C. The class II region encodes genes for the molecules HLA-DR, HLA-DP, and HLA-DQ; the class III region encodes genes for C2, C4, Bf (complement factors), 21-hydroxylase, and tumor necrosis factor.
- The HLA *genotype* represents the association of the antigens on the two C6 chromosomes as determined by family studies, and the term *haplotype*

refers to the antigenic makeup of a single C6 chromosome.
- The majority of HLA alloantibodies are IgG and can be grouped into private antibodies (binding to an epitope unique to one HLA gene product), public antibodies (binding to epitopes shared by more than one HLA gene product), or cross-reactive (binding to structurally similar HLA epitopes).
- Techniques of histocompatibility testing include antigen typing, in which known sera are used to type HLA antigens on test cells; HLA antibody detection and identification, in which recipient serum is tested against a panel of cells; and crossmatching, in which specific donor cells and recipient sera are tested for compatibility.
- The general strategies employed by transplantation immunologists include (1) the use of immunosuppressive drugs, (2) the reduction of graft "foreignness," and (3) the induction of tolerance.
- Platelet refractoriness is manifested by the failure to achieve a rise in circulating platelet count 1 hour after infusion of adequate numbers of platelets.

## REVIEW QUESTIONS

1. The HLA genes are located on chromosome number:
   A. 2
   B. 4
   C. 6
   D. 8
   E. 10

2. The majority of HLA antibodies are:
   A. IgA
   B. IgD
   C. IgE
   D. IgG
   E. IgM

3. The test of choice for HLA antigen testing is:
   A. Agglutination
   B. Inhibition
   C. Cytotoxicity
   D. Fluorescent antibody test
   E. Enzyme-linked immunosorbent test

4. Of the following diseases, which one has the highest relative risk in association with an HLA antigen?
   A. Ankylosing spondylitis
   B. Dermatitis herpetiformis
   C. Juvenile diabetes
   D. Narcolepsy
   E. Rheumatoid arthritis

5. Why is HLA matching not feasible in cardiac transplantation?
   A. No HLAs are present on cardiac cells.
   B. No donors ever have HLA antibodies.
   C. Total ischemic time is too long.
   D. Total ischemic time is too short.
   E. None of the above.

6. DR52 molecules are the product of:
   A. DRA and DRB1
   B. DRA and DRB2
   C. DRA and DRB3
   D. DRA and DRB4
   E. DRA and DRB5

7. In the future, testing of DNA will probably be performed by what technique?
   A. Restriction fragment length polymorphism
   B. Allele-specific oligonucleotide typing
   C. Sequence-specific primer typing
   D. Sequence-specific oligonucleotide typing
   E. Direct nucleotide sequencing

8. The association of the antigens on the two C6 chromosomes as determined by family studies is represented by the:
   A. Haplotype
   B. Genotype
   C. Phenotype
   D. Allotype
   E. Xenotype

## ANSWERS TO REVIEW QUESTIONS

1. C (p 491)

2. D (p 495)

3. C (p 497)

4. A (p 500)

5. D (p 503)

6. C (p 491)

7. E (p 500)

8. B (p 494)

## REFERENCES

1. Dausset, H: Leukoagglutinins. IV. Leukoagglutinins and blood transfusion. J Vox Sang 4:190, 1954.
2. Dausset, J: Iso-leuco-anticorps. Acta Haematol 20:156, 1958.
3. Payne, R: The association of febrile transfusion reactions with leukoagglutinins. J Vox Sang 2:233, 1957.
4. Terasaki, PI, and McClelland, JP: Microdroplet assay of human serum cytotoxins. Nature 204:998, 1964.
5. Terasaki, PI, et al: Microdroplet testing for HLA-A, -B, -C, and -D antigens. Am J Clin Pathol 69:103, 1978.
6. van Rood, JJ, and van Leeuwen, A: Leukocyte grouping: A method and its application. J Clin Invest 42:1382, 1963.
7. World Health Organization: Nomenclature for factors of the HL-A system. Bull WHO 39:483, 1968.
8. Dausset, J, et al: Le deuxieme sublocus du systeme HL-A. Nour Rev Franc Hemat 8:861, 1968.
9. Singal, DP, et al: Serotyping for homo-transplantation. XVII. Preliminary studies of HL-A subunits and alleles. Transplantation 6:904, 1968.
10. Sandberg, L, et al: Evidence for a third sub-locus within the HLA chromosomal region. In Terasaki, PI (ed): Histocompatibility Testing 1970. Munksgaard, Copenhagen, 1970, p 165.
11. Bach, FH, and Hirschhorn, K: Lymphocyte interaction: A potential histocompatibility test in vitro. Science 143:813, 1964.
12. Bain, B, and Lowenstein, L: Genetic studies on the mixed leukocyte reaction. Science 145:1315, 1964.
13. Bach, FH, and Amos, DB: Hu-1: Major histocompatibility locus in man. Science 156:1506, 1967.
14. Bodmer, WF, et al (eds): Histocompatibility Testing 1977. Munksgaard, Copenhagen, 1977.
15. Bodmer, JG, et al: Nomenclature for factors of the HLA system. Hum Immunol 53:1, 1997.
16. Kissmeyer-Nielson, F, et al: Hyperacute rejection of kidney allografts associated with preexisting humoral antibodies against donor cells. Lancet 1:662, 1966.
17. Orr, HT, et al: Complete amino acid sequence of a papain-solubilized human histocompatibility antigen, HLA-B7. 2. Sequence determination and search for homologies. Biochem 18:5711, 1979.
18. Kaufman, JF, and Strominger, JL: Both chains of HLA-DR bind to the membrane with a penultimate hydrophobic region and the heavy chain is phosphorylated at its hydrophilic carboxy terminus. Proc Natl Acad Sci USA 76:6304, 1979.
19. Kaufman, JF, and Strominger, JL: The extracellular region of light chains from human and murine MHC class II antigens consists of two domains. J Immunol 130:808, 1983.
20. Figueroa, F, and Klein, J: The evolution of class II genes. Immunol Today 7:78, 1986.
21. Bjorkman, PJ, et al: Structure of the HLA class I histocompatibility antigen, HLA-A2. Nature 329:506, 1987.
22. Bjorkman, PJ, et al: The foreign antigen binding site and T cell recognition regions of class I histocompatibility antigens. Nature 329:512, 1987.
23. Rodey, GE, and Fuller, TC: Public epitopes and the antigenic structure of HLA molecules. Crit Rev Immunol 7:229, 1987.
24. Kohler, G, and Milstein, C: Derivation of specific antibody producing tissue culture and tumor lines by cell fusion. Eur J Immunol 6:611, 1976.
25. Lee, CC: Population Genetics. University of Chicago Press, Chicago, 1955.
26. Dausset, J, et al: Un nouvel antigene du systeme HL-A (Hu-1), 1' antigene 15 allelle possible des antigenes 1, 11, 12. Nouv Rev Fr Hematol 8:398, 1968.
27. Kissmeyer-Nielsen, F, Svejgaard, A, and Hange, M: Genetics of the HL-A transplantation system. Nature 291:1116, 1968.
28. Svejgaard, A, and Kissmeyer-Nielsen, F: Crossreactive human HL-A iso-antibodies. Nature 219:868, 1968.
29. Legrand, L, and Dausset, J: Histocompatibility Testing 1972. Munksgaard, Copenhagen, 1972, p 441.
30. Rodey, G, et al: ASHI HLA class I public epitope workshop: Phase I report. Transplant Proc 19:872, 1987.
31. Colombani, J, Colombani, M, and Dausset, J: Crossreactions in the HL-A system with special reference to Da 6 crossreacting group. In Terasaki, PI (ed): Histocompatibility Testing 1970. Munksgaard, Copenhagen, 1970, p 79.
32. Legrand, L, and Dausset, J: The complexity of the HLA gene product. II. Possible evidence for a "public" determinant common to the first and second HLA series. Transplantation 19:177, 1975.
33. Scalamogne, M, et al: Crossreactivity between the first and second segregant series of the HLA system. Tissue Antigens 7:125, 1976.
34. Kostyu, DD, Cresswell, P, and Amos, DB: A public HLA antigen associated with HLA-A9, Aw32 and Bw4. Immunogenetics 10:433, 1980.
35. Muller, C, et al: Monoclonal antibody (Tu 48) defining alloantigenic class I determinants specific for HLA-Bw4 and HLA-Aw23, -Aw24 as well as -Aw32. Hum Immunol 5:269, 1982.
36. Belvedere, M, Mattiuz, PL, and Curtoni, ES: An antibody crossreacting with LA and FOUR antigens of the HLA system. Immunogenetics 1:538, 1975.
37. McMichael, AJ, et al: A monoclonal antibody that recognizes an antigenic determinant shared by HLA-A2 and B17. Hum Immunol 1:121, 1980.
38. Ahern, AT, et al: HLA-A2 and HLA-B17 antigens share an alloantigenic determinant. Hum Immunol 5:139, 1982.
39. Claas, F, et al: Alloantibodies to an antigenic determinant shared by HLA-A2 and B17. Tissue Antigens 19:388, 1982.
40. Troup, CM, and Walford, RL: Cytotoxicity test for the typing of human lymphocytes. Am J Clin Pathol 51:529, 1969.
41. Eisen, SA, Wedner, HJ, and Parker, CW: Isolation of pure human peripheral blood T-lymphocytes using nylon wool columns. Immunological Communications 1:571, 1972.
42. Lowry, R, et al: Improved B cell typing for HLA-DR using nylon wool column enriched B lymphocyte preparations. Tissue Antigens 14:325, 1979.
43. van Rood, JJ, van Leeuwen, A, and Ploem, JS: Simultaneous detection of two cell populations by two-color fluorescence and application to the recognition of B cell determinants. Nature 262:795, 1976.
44. Vartdal, F, et al: HLA class I and II typing using cells positively selected from blood by immunomagnetic isolation: A fast and reliable technique. Tissue Antigens 28:301, 1986.
45. Fuller, TC, et al: Antigenic specificity of antibody reactive in the antiglobulin-augmented lymphocytotoxicity test. Transplantation 34:24, 1982.
46. Fuller, TC, and Rodey, GE: Specificity of alloantibodies against antigens of the HLA complex. In Theoretical Aspects of HLA: A Technical Workshop. American Association of Blood Banks, Arlington, VA, 1982, p 51.
47. Lucas, ZG, et al: Early renal transplant failure associated with subliminal sensitization. Transplantation 10:522, 1970.
48. Patel, R, and Briggs, WA: Limitation of the lymphocyte cytotoxicity crossmatch test in recipients of kidney transplants having preformed anti-leukocyte antibodies. N Engl J Med 284:1016, 1971.
49. Thistlewaite, JR, et al: The T cell immunofluorescence flow cytometric crossmatch: Correlation of results with rejection and graft

loss in cadaveric donor renal transplant recipients (abstract). XI International Congress of the Transplantation Society 1:S2.3, 1986.

50. Tiercy, JM, Jannet, M, and Mach, B: A new approach for the analysis of HLA class II polymorphism: HLA oligo typing. Blood Rev 4:9, 1990.

51. Zemmour, J, and Parham, P: HLA class I nucleotide sequences. Hum Immunol 31:195, 1991.

52. Marsh, SGE, and Bodmer, J: HLA class II nucleotide sequences. Hum Immunol 31:207, 1991.

53. Polesky, HF: New concepts in paternity testing. Diagnostic Medicine 1981.

54. Tiwari, JL, and Terasaki, PI: HLA and Disease. New York, Springer-Verlag, 1985.

55. Mourant, AE, Kopec, AC, and Domaniewska-Solczak, K: Blood Groups and Diseases. New York, Oxford University Press, 1978.

56. Colombani, J: Blood platelets in HL-A serology. Transplant Proc 3:1078, 1971.

57. Svejgaard, A, Kissemeyer-Nielson, F, and Thorsby, E: HL-A typing of platelets. In Terasaki, PI (ed): Histocompatibility Testing 1970. Munksgaard, Copenhagen, 1970, p 160.

58. Leibert, M, and Aster, RH: Expression of HLA-B12 on platelets, on lymphocytes and in serum: A quantitative study. Tissue Antigens 9:199, 1977.

59. Aster, RH, Szatkowski, N, and Liebert, M: Expression of HLA-B12, HLA-B8, W4 and W6 on platelets. Transplant Proc 9:1965, 1977.

60. Duquesnoy, RJ, Testin, J, and Aster, RH: Variable expression of W4 and W6 on platelets: Possible relevance to platelet transfusion therapy of alloimmunized thrombocytopenic patients. Transplant Proc 9:1827, 1977.

61. Duquesnoy, RJ, Filip, DJ, and Rody, GE: Successful transfusion of platelet "mismatched" for HLA antigens to alloimmunized thrombocytopenic patients. Am J Hematol 2:219, 1977.

62. Brand, A, van Leeuwen, A, and Eernisse, JG: Platelet immunology with special regard to platelet transfusion therapy. Excerpta Medica International Congress 415:639, 1978.

63. Herzig, RH, Herzig, GP, and Biell, MI: Correction of poor platelet transfusion responses with leukocyte poor HLA-matched platelet concentrates. Blood 46:743, 1975.

64. Bortin, MM, and Rimm, AA: Increasing utilization of bone marrow transplantation. Transplantation 42:229, 1986.

65. Puppo, F, et al: Serum HLA class I antigen levels in allogeneic bone marrow transplantation: A possible marker of acute GVHD. Bone Marrow Transplant 17(5):753, 1996.

66. Hows, JM, et al: Histocompatible unrelated volunteer donors compared with HLA non-identical family donors for marrow transplantation (abstract). XI International Congress of the Transplantation Society 1:S8.1, 1986.

67. Siegler, HF, et al: Comparisons of mixed leukocyte reactions with

68. Hamburger, J, et al: The value of present methods used for the selection of organ donors. Transplant Proc 3:260, 1971.

69. Alexander, JW: Impact of transplantation on microbiology and infectious diseases. Transplant Proc 12:593, 1980.

70. Ichikawa, Y, et al: Significant effect of HLA-DRB1 typing by linkage disequilibrium on kidney graft outcome. Transplant Proc 25(4):2707, 1993.

71. Opelz, G: Effect of HLA matching, blood transfusions, and presensitization in cyclosporine-treated kidney transplant recipients. Transplant Proc 17:2179, 1985.

72. Joysey, VC, Thiru, S, and Evans, DB: Effect of HLA-DR compatibility on kidney transplants treated with cyclosporine A. Transplant Proc 17:2187, 1985.

73. Sanfilippo, F, Vaughn, WK, and Spees, EKL: The effect of HLA-A, -B matching on cadaver renal allograft rejection comparing public and private specificities. Transplantation 38:483, 1984.

74. Oldfather, JW, et al: Prediction of crossmatch outcome in highly sensitized dialysis patients based on the identification of serum HLA antibodies. Transplantation 42:267, 1986.

75. Opelz, G, et al: Effect of blood transfusions on subsequent kidney transplants. Transplant Proc 5:253, 1973.

76. Salvatierra, O, Jr, et al: Deliberate donor-specific transfusions prior to living related renal transplantation: A new approach. Ann Surg 192:543, 1980.

77. Yacoub, M, et al: The influence of HLA matching in cardiac allograft recipients receiving CyA and Imuran (abstract). XI International Congress of the Transplantation Society 1:S7.1, 1986.

78. Fung, J, Abu-Elmagd, A, and Jain, A: A randomized trial of primary liver transplantation under immunosuppression with FK506 versus cyclosporine. Transplant Proc 23:2977, 1991.

79. Karuppan, S, Ericzon, BG, and Moller, E: Relevance of a positive crossmatch in liver transplantation. Transpl Int 4:18, 1991.

80. Gugenheim, J, Samuel, D, and Reynes, M: Liver transplantation across ABO blood group barriers. Lancet 336:519, 1990.

81. Mathew, J, et al: Biochemical and immunological evaluation of donor-specific soluble HLA in the circulation of liver transplant recipients. Transplantation 62(2):217, 1996.

82. Shaw, LR, Miller, JD, and Slutsky, AS: Ethics of lung transplantation with live donors. Lancet 338:461, 1991.

83. Pirsch, JD, et al: The effect of donor age, recipient age and HLA match on immunologic graft survival in cadaver renal transplant recipients. Transplantation 53:55, 1992.

84. So, SKS, et al: Matching improves cadaveric pancreas transplant results. Transplant Proc 22:687, 1990.

85. Scharp, DW, Lacy, PE, and Santiago, JE: Results of our first nine intraportal islet allografts in type 1, insulin-dependent diabetic patients. Transplantation 51:76, 1991.

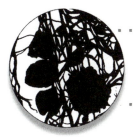

CHAPTER **24**

# PARENTAGE TESTING

Chantal Ricaud Harrison, MD

**OBJECTIVES**

*On completion of this chapter, the learner should be able to:*

1 State the goals of parentage testing.

2 List criteria used in choosing a genetic system for parentage testing.

3 Briefly describe the testing technologies used for the different types of genetic systems.

4 Briefly discuss the advantages and disadvantages of the different types of genetic systems.

5 Define and give examples of false direct and indirect exclusions.

6 List three causes of false direct and indirect exclusions.

7 Define paternity index, probability of paternity, and power of exclusion.

8 List organizations involved and resources available in quality improvement for parentage testing laboratories.

## INTRODUCTION

### Definition

Parentage testing refers to the testing of genetic markers that are inherited to determine the presence or absence of a biologic relationship. This is most commonly applied to answer the question whether a man is or is not the biologic father of a child, but it can also be applied to the determination of maternity or siblingship.

### History

The scientific basis for parentage testing can be traced back to the statistical analysis published by Bernstein[1] in 1924 demonstrating that the ABO blood group frequency distribution in Austria was most compatible with a three-allele theory. The ABO blood group testing results were first used in establishing nonpaternity in Vienna in 1926. As other blood groups were described and their inheritance established, they too were used in paternity studies. Then, in 1955, Smithies[2] described the polymorphism of haptoglobin, opening the door to a new type of genetic system: enzymes and proteins. The next evolution step occurred in 1972, when the extreme polymorphism of the human leukocyte antigen (HLA) system was demonstrated at the Evian workshop organized by Dausset.[3] All these genetic systems were expressed on different elements of the blood (red cells, proteins, and leukocytes) but had one important aspect in common: All were dependent on a complex biochemical expression of the original genes. This group of genetic systems is often termed the *classic systems*. The molecular genetics technology developed in the next decade laid the foun-

dation for a revolution in parentage testing, heralded by the description by Jeffreys[4] in 1985 of a new type of polymorphism in human deoxyribonucleic acid (DNA): hypervariable minisatellites often referred to as variable number tandem repeats (VNTR). New genetic systems, tested by technologies that assess directly the variability of the DNA, have now become the norm. These are called DNA polymorphisms.

## GOALS OF TESTING

The ultimate goal of parentage testing is to confirm a specific biologic relationship with the individual in question, usually a father or a mother or sometimes a sibling. When applied to the usual trio (mother, child, and alleged father), the goals are to exclude all falsely accused men and to provide sufficient inclusionary evidence if a man is not excluded.

## CRITERIA FOR SELECTION OF GENETIC SYSTEMS

In selecting genetic systems to use in parentage testing, one should take into account the following considerations:

1. The system should be polymorphic; that is, it should have multiple alleles, ideally in Hardy-Weinberg equilibrium.
2. Inheritance pattern should be well established and follow Mendel's rules.
3. Mutation rate should be known to be low.
4. Possible genotypes should be easily deducible from the phenotype.
5. Testing methodology should be reliable, reproducible, and available in more than one laboratory.
6. Markers tested should be stable and not affected by environmental factors, age, disease, reagents, or methodology used.
7. Databases of allele frequencies should be available for all ethnic groups that may be tested.
8. Allelic distributions should be of such nature as to provide a high probability of excluding a falsely accused man.
9. Each genetic system should be known to be genetically independent (e.g., no linkage disequilibrium) from all other genetic systems selected by the laboratory.

## TYPES OF GENETIC SYSTEMS AND TECHNOLOGY USED

Table 24–1 lists the most common genetic systems currently in use. In the last few years there has been a significant increase in the number of laboratories performing DNA polymorphisms and more specifically of those using polymerase chain reaction (PCR) technology.

**Table 24–1.** List of Genetic Systems Commonly Used in Parentage Testing

| Red Cell Antigens | DNA-RFLP | DNA-PCR SSP |
|---|---|---|
| ABO | D1S339 | HLA DQA1 |
| Rh | D2S44 | LDLR |
| MNSs | D4S139 | GYPA |
| Kell | D4S163 | HBGG |
| Duffy | D5S110 | D7S8 |
| Kidd | D6S132 | GC |
| | | |
| Red Cell Enzymes/Serum Proteins | D7S467 | DNA-PCR LTR |
| PGM1 | D10S28 | D1S80 |
| ACP | D12S11 | DNA-PCR STR |
| ESD | D14S13 | HUMTHO1 |
| HP | | |
| Gc | | |
| | | |
| Immunoglobulin Allotypes | D17S26 | HUMTPOX |
| Gm | D17S79 | HUMCSF1PO |
| Km | | HUMF13AO1 |
| Am | | HUMVWA13/A |
| | | |
| HLA | | HUMFESPES |
| A and B locus | | |

*not used; historic* (handwritten annotation)

## Red Cell Antigens

Six blood groups have been routinely used in paternity testing: ABO, Rh, MNSs, Kell, Duffy, and Kidd. These systems have been in use for the longest period of time, and their potential pitfalls in interpretation are well known from the vast worldwide experience accumulated. Phenotype determination is based on standard red cell agglutination techniques with regulated reagents and, with some extra built-in quality control steps, is indistinguishable from testing performed daily in most blood bank or transfusion services. This is the reason why, until recently, the majority of laboratories performing parentage testing were associated with a blood bank or a transfusion service. Duplicate testing of each specimen is required. It is recommended that this be done independently by two different individuals using two different sources of antisera. This will minimize the occurrence of inaccurate phenotypes as a result of reagent variability or technical error. Careful attention should be given when selecting positive control cells to ensure that the reagent antiserum can detect weak expressions of the antigen. An example is anti-C, which often contains mostly anti-Ce (rh$_i$) and may not react with the CcDE phenotype. This phenotype is not uncommon in Mexican-Americans, Native Americans, and Asian-Americans, and a false-negative reaction could lead to an erroneous interpretation of exclusion.

## Red Cell Enzymes and Serum Proteins

Currently the red cell enzyme genetic systems still tested by a substantial number of laboratories are phosphoglucomutase 1 (PGM1), acid phosphatase (ACP), and esterase D (ESD). Serum protein genetic systems tested are haptoglobin (Hp) and group-specific component (Gc). Testing methodology consists of separating the different allelic proteins by electrophoresis, followed by staining. Subtyping of the *PGM1* and *Gc* alleles may be done using isoelectric focusing, which allows separation of molecules of similar size, thereby increasing the degree of polymorphism of the system. When isoelectric focusing is used, it is customary to refer to the system with a subscript letter $i$ (e.g., $PGM1_i$ or $Gc_i$).

Phenotypes are identified by the number and respective position of the bands detected and comparison with control specimens expressing at least two known allotypes that are tested in parallel with the unknown specimens. Interpretation of the band patterns must be performed independently by two observers. Rare variants exist in most systems, and the laboratories should maintain a file of variants to permit identification of rare phenotypes.

## Immunoglobulins

Three immunoglobulin chains demonstrate a polymorphism that has been applied to paternity testing. The gamma heavy chain expresses the Gm polymorphism, whereas the kappa light chain expresses Km (also referred to as Inv), and the alpha heavy chain expresses Am. Determination of the phenotype is done by hemagglutination inhibition using indicator red cells coated with antibodies of known phenotype and reagent anti-Gm, anti-Km, or anti-Am. Reagents are not widely available, genetic interpretation is complex, and phenotypic interpretation is often not possible in infants less than 6 months of age because of interference with maternal immunoglobulins. For these reasons few laboratories in the world now use these genetic systems. They are mentioned solely for the sake of completion and historic perspective.

## Human Leukocyte Antigens (HLA)

The HLA complex represents the most polymorphic genetic system in the human genome. As discussed in the previous chapter, it comprises multiple-linked loci expressed as class I and class II antigens. In parentage testing with classic methodology (non-DNA), only antigens expressed by the A and the B loci are considered.

The usual method is termed *microlymphocytotoxicity* and depends on the evaluation of the reactions of live lymphocytes with a panel of cytotoxic antibodies of known specificity in the presence of complement. Testing is performed in 60 or 72 microwell trays preloaded with reagent antisera. A sufficient number of antisera should be used so that all HLA-A and HLA-B specificities recognized by the 1980 HLA Nomenclature Committee of the World Health Organization can be reliably identified. Additional antigens should be tested, if appropriate antisera can be obtained. The greater the number of antigens that can be defined, the more powerful the system becomes; that is, the better it is able to exclude falsely accused men. Because of the large number of antigens existing, no single tray can identify all relevant antigens. Some antigens occur more frequently in specific racial groups, and specially designed trays are available for blacks and Asians. Such trays should be selected when appropriate.

Antisera are either of human origin or monoclonal, and monospecific sera are not available for a large number of antigens. It is required that each antigen be defined by at least two different operationally monospecific sera, by one monospecific and two multispecific sera, or by three multispecific sera. Phenotypes must be verified by reading two full trays or tray sets, each containing antisera for all the HLA-A and HLA-B antigens detected by the laboratory. Each tray or tray set must be read independently.

In interpreting phenotypes, a certain amount of expertise is needed, requiring knowledge of cross-reactivity between antigens and splits of broader reactivity (e.g., A9 splitting into A23 and A24) and familiarity with the unexpected reactivity of the antisera used (false-negative or extra reactions). Because of the variability of HLA antisera, it is recommended that all individuals in a parentage case be tested in the same laboratory.

## DNA Polymorphisms: Restriction Fragment Length Polymorphism (RFLP)

Restriction fragment length polymorphism (RFLP) refers to polymorphisms of the DNA that can be detected through the use of restriction enzymes. These enzymes are endonucleases that recognize specific DNA sequences of 4 to 6 bases and cut the double-stranded DNA at that site. These enzymes have been isolated from bacteria and are named after the bacteria from which they were isolated (e.g., Eco RI from *Escherichia coli* RY13, Hae III from *Haemophilus aegyptius*). After the isolated DNA is incubated with the restriction enzyme (digestion step), it is electrophoresed on a gel to separate the DNA fragments according to length. The DNA is then denatured to dissociate the complementary strands and transferred by blotting (Southern blotting) to a membrane, and hybridization with a labeled probe is performed to reveal the DNA fragments corresponding to the locus tested. Earlier, the probes were labeled with radioactive P[32], but currently detection is often achieved by a colorimetric or chemiluminescent method. Phenotypes are assigned as the length of the DNA fragments in kilobases (kb), measured by comparison with a sizing ladder consisting of DNA fragments of known size. Some variability in migration may occur within a gel, depending on the position of the electrophoretic lane (band shifting), and it is required that mixtures of DNA of each alleged father with each child be electrophoresed together in a single lane to observe for such band shifting and to confirm a match or mismatch in fragment size. Figure 24–1 illustrates this process.

The DNA polymorphisms detected by RFLP may be

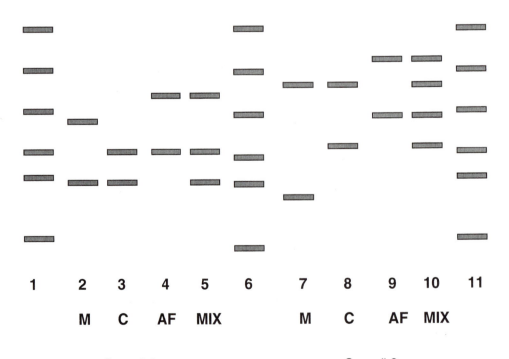

**Figure 24–1.** Schematic representation of RFLP results from two paternity testing trios. Lanes 1, 6, and 11 represent sizing standards of known length used to measure the band size of each individual. Both cases consist of a mother (M), a child (C), an alleged father (AF), and a mixed lane with the child's and alleged father's DNA. In the first case, on the left, the paternal band of the child matches one of the bands of the alleged father and the mixed lane only contains three bands; the alleged father is included. In the second case, none of the alleged father bands matches the child's paternal band and the mixed lane clearly demonstrates four bands; this is a mismatch.

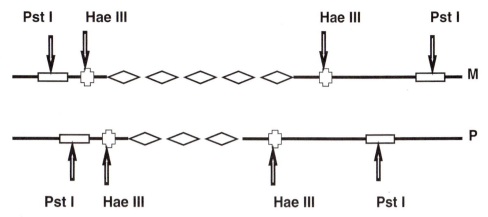

**Figure 24–2.** RFLP fragment lengths are dependent on the number of tandem repeats and on the restriction enzyme used. The maternal allele has 5 repeat units whereas the paternal allele has 3. The fragments cut by Pst I are larger than the fragments cut by Hae III.

of three types. The first type results from mutations, insertions, or deletions between restriction sites. The second type results from single-base mutations causing a new cutting site for the restriction enzyme or deleting a cutting site. The third type of polymorphism relates to the presence throughout the genome of noncoding DNA segments consisting of a variable number of repeats of a core-base sequence. These areas are called variable number tandem repeats (VNTR). They are also referred to as minisatellites, when the size of the core sequence typically ranges from 14 to 70 base pairs. It is this latter type of polymorphism that is widely applied to parentage testing.

As illustrated in Figure 24–2, the fragment size of VNTR loci depends on the number of repeats and on the restriction enzyme utilized. This is an important concept: the phenotype of the same individual at the same locus will differ between two laboratories if each uses a different restriction enzyme. This is why, when reporting RFLP results, it is mandatory to identify not only the locus and probe tested but also the restriction enzyme used. In the United States the most common restriction enzymes used are Hae III and Pst I, whereas in Europe Hinf I is more popular. Table 24–2 illustrates the different band sizes obtained on the same individuals at the same locus when using different restriction enzymes.

Another important concept with VNTR polymorphisms tested by RFLP has to do with the fact that the allele designation is a quantitative entity: a length of DNA in kilobase. As in any quantitative measurement there is a measurement variability; this variability is referred to as sigma ($\sigma$). Another variable is the ability to distinguish between two close alleles (alleles differing by only a few repeats). This ability may vary greatly among laboratories, depending on the methodology used, especially the technical conditions during electrophoresis. This variability is referred to as delta ($\delta$). Because of these two sources of variability, the allele frequency distribution for VNTR polymorphisms

tested by RFLP is a continuous distribution, as opposed to the discrete distribution of allele frequencies in the classic genetic systems. For example, in most laboratories a DNA fragment measured at 1.60 kb cannot be considered different from a fragment measured at 1.57 kb or 1.63 kb. Each laboratory must decide, for each allele size, the range of allele sizes that are considered within matching criteria of the one measured. This range is called a *bin*. The allele frequency used in the statistical calculations is actually the frequency of all the alleles falling into the bin for the allele size measured. Inasmuch as the size of the bin varies with the technical characteristics of the laboratories, the final statistical evaluation result (paternity index, probability of paternity, or probability of exclusion) may differ between two laboratories for the same locus with the same restriction enzyme, even if their band sizes are identical.

These VNTR loci are very polymorphic and thus are very powerful in excluding falsely accused men and in providing inclusionary evidence in true biologic relationships. However, their mutation rate can be up to 2 per 1000, which is small but not negligible.[5]

## DNA Polymorphisms: Polymerase Chain Reaction (PCR)

This new technology has seen a striking increase in popularity for parentage testing since 1994. The DNA

**Table 24–2.** DNA-RFLP Results on a Parentage Testing Trio at the D2S44 Locus Tested with Three Different Restriction Enzymes

|  | Hae III | Hinf I | Pst I |
|---|---|---|---|
| Mother | 3.43, 4.25 | 4.55, 5.36 | 12.68, 13.53 |
| Child | 2.91, 3.43 | 4.03, 4.55 | 12.16, 12.68 |
| Alleged father | 2.91, 3.13 | 4.03, 4.25 | 12.16, 12.46 |

fragment of interest is amplified several million times by the PCR technique, and the resulting product is identified either by hybridization with a set of labeled probes or by its location on a gel after electrophoresis. The exact section of DNA that is amplified is defined by a pair of primers. The variation detected in the amplified products is caused by DNA sequence polymorphisms or by fragment-length polymorphisms.

### Sequence-specific Polymorphism (SSP)

Sequence-specific polymorphisms (SSPs) are the result of specific nucleotide differences at the locus tested. The phenotype is determined by dot blot using sequence-specific oligonucleotide probes. Currently used SSP genetic systems are the *DQA1* locus, which codes for the alpha chain of the HLA class II antigen DQ, and a group of five loci tested together: *LDLR, GYPA, HBGG, D7S8,* and *GC.* It is important to realize that *GYPA* is the locus coding for glycophorin A, which is the red cell transmembrane protein carrying the MN antigens, and that *GC* is the locus coding for the serum protein Gc. A laboratory should not test for these two loci by PCR technology and by classic techniques without realizing that the same genetic system is being investigated. In other words, in the final interpretation they should not be considered as different systems. Similarly, there is very strong linkage between *DQA1* and the *HLA-A* and *HLA-B* loci; thus they cannot be considered genetically independent when calculating overall probability of paternity.

### Amplified Fragment Length Polymorphisms (AmpFLPs)

The fragment length polymorphisms detected by PCR are similar to those detected by RFLP in that they consist of a variable number of repeats of noncoding DNA sequences. However, the core sequence is usually shorter. When the core sequence ranges from 2 to 7 base pairs (bp) and the overall length of the fragment sizes remains less than 350 bp, they are called microsatellites or short tandem repeats (STR). If the core sequence is greater than 7, they are called long tandem repeats (LTR). Only one LTR locus is currently widely used, D1S80. The almost exponential growth in the use of DNA polymorphisms by PCR for parentage testing is entirely caused by the interest in the STR systems, and new genetic systems are being described and put into use every year.

### Mitochondrial DNA

Noncoding segments (the displacement loop) of mitochondrial DNA (mtDNA) are amplified by PCR and then sequenced. The sequence is then compared with a published reference sequence. Any deviation from the published sequence should be inherited from mother to child. Inasmuch as mitochondria are passed on with the cytoplasm of the oocyte and not by spermatozoa,

mitochondrial DNA can verify only maternal lineage. Mitochondrial DNA appears to be stable for extremely long periods of time (thousands of years). These genetic systems have been applied to anthropologic studies aiming at solving human evolution questions. Preserved mitochondrial DNA has been isolated from mummies and fossils.[6] This technique is very useful in demonstrating maternal lineage in long-distance relatives such as a grandmother to a grandchild or a great-granduncle with a great-grandnephew, and it was recently applied to the authentifications of the remains of the family of Tsar Nicholas II of Russia who were assassinated during the Bolshevik uprising.[7]

## INTERPRETATION OF RESULTS

In interpreting the testing results on a classic trio (mother, child, and alleged father), it is always assumed that the mother is the biologic mother. The results are first analyzed to determine whether the alleged father is excluded as the biologic father of the child. If he is not excluded, a statistical analysis is performed to determine his relative probability of being the biologic father of the child as compared to a random man unrelated to him or to the mother.

### Terminology

In the past, when using the classic genetic systems it has been customary to interpret the results in one genetic system as an exclusion, direct or indirect, when the expected inheritance pattern was not observed. It was customary to accept a single direct exclusion as evidence of nonpaternity, whereas an indirect exclusion only suggested the possibility of nonpaternity and required confirmation by additional testing. However, as soon as some experience was accumulated with the newly introduced DNA polymorphisms, it became evident that mutations, which were extremely rare with the classic systems (less than one in a million), were being recognized in these new systems at a higher frequency. There appears to be a significant number of crossover mutations at the level of the tandem repeats. It is also likely that a number of single nucleotide mutations that can be detected at the DNA level may not result in a recognizable change in the final expression product when tested by classic technologies. When an inconsistency in the inheritance pattern is detected in a genetic system result concerning a DNA polymorphism, the term *exclusion* is not used; instead, the term *mismatch* is used to refer to the fact that the bands between the child and the alleged father do not match. *Exclusion* is reserved for the final interpretation of the entire set of genetic systems tested. A minimum of two mismatches is required before an opinion of nonpaternity (or nonmaternity) is rendered.

In the following section, we reserve the terms *direct* and *indirect* exclusion to the interpretation of results in the classic genetic systems.

## Direct Exclusion

A direct exclusion occurs when a marker is detected in the child, but it is absent in the mother and the alleged father. For example, the child has blood group B, the mother has group A, and the alleged father has group O. The B antigen on the child's red cells is the result of the expression of the B gene, which is not present in the mother and thus must have been passed to the child by the child's biologic father. The tested man does not have it. Therefore, a direct exclusion is present.

Another situation that is interpreted as a direct exclusion occurs when the alleged father's phenotype demonstrates two markers and the child has neither one of them. For example, the alleged father's blood group is AB and the child's is O. The alleged father's phenotype implies that he has both the *A* gene and the *B* gene and thus must pass on either one of them to any of his children. The child has neither one of them.

Direct exclusions are considered very strong evidence of nonpaternity because they rely on direct observation of a marker with a known pattern of inheritance, which was not inherited as expected. As discussed later, false direct exclusions in classic genetic systems can occur but are extremely rare. Thus a single direct exclusion in these systems is considered sufficient to render an opinion of nonpaternity as long as appropriate controls to rule out rare situations have been put into place.

## Indirect Exclusion

An indirect exclusion occurs when a single marker is detected in the child and a different single marker is detected in the alleged father. For example, the child is Jk(a+b−) and the alleged father is Jk(a−b+). The indirect exclusion is based on the assumption that if a person expresses only one marker, he must be homozygous for the allele coding for the marker. In the example, the child types as Jk(a+b−) and is thus assumed to be homozygous for the *Jk*a gene, but the alleged father is assumed to be homozygous for the *Jk*b gene. This is interpreted as an indirect exclusion, because the man should pass on a *Jk*b gene to any offspring and the child does not have it. This situation is termed *apparent opposite homozygosity*. The term *apparent* is very important. The homozygosity is assumed and not directly proved. A different allele not detected by the testing performed could be present, and the individual could actually be heterozygous. In fact, a silent allele does exist in the Kidd system, called *Jk*, which has no detectable product. Thus the child could possibly be heterozygous for the *Jk* and the *Jk*a alleles and the alleged father could be heterozygous for the *Jk* and the *Jk*b alleles. In this case there would be no inconsistency in the inheritance pattern and no exclusion. However, this *Jk* gene is very rare and is seen almost only in populations originating in the Western Pacific Islands. Thus, if the individuals tested were North American whites or blacks, these results would be interpreted as an indirect exclusion.

## Causes of False Exclusions

False direct exclusions can occur as the result of mutations that are significant enough to alter the final product, lack of precursor substance, suppressor activity at a locus unlinked to the one tested, or chimeric state of one of the tested individuals.

A classic example of the lack of a precursor substance is the Bombay phenotype, in which an individual is homozygous for the *h* gene and cannot produce H substance, the precursor for the A and B antigens. This person may have the *A* or *B* genes (or even both) and pass it on to an offspring, but he or she cannot express them and will have a phenotype of O. The offspring, more than likely, will inherit an *H* gene from the other parent inasmuch as the *h* gene is very rare, and thus he or she will be able to express the *A* or *B* gene inherited from the first parent. Thus a Bombay phenotype in either parent can explain a trio: mother O, child A, alleged father O. However, Bombay phenotypes are extremely rare and can easily be detected by testing the O individuals with anti-H, or by performing a reverse typing with O cells, inasmuch as all Bombay phenotypes have strong anti-H activity in their serum.

An example of an erroneous direct exclusion caused by a suppressor gene is illustrated in the following trio: alleged father Rh negative, mother Rh negative, child Rh positive. In the Rh system a null phenotype, although extremely rare, does exist. $Rh_{null}$ individuals produce no Rh substances; that is, no D, C, c, E, or e antigens. Most $Rh_{null}$ phenotypes are caused by a suppressor gene at an unknown but unlinked locus. Thus, a person typing D negative may actually have a *D* gene at the Rh locus and pass it to an offspring without passing on the suppressor gene. However, this is a problem only if the trio is tested with anti-D only because a complete Rh phenotype would immediately reveal that one of the Rh-negative individuals is actually $Rh_{null}$.

False indirect exclusions can occur secondary to the presence of silent alleles, alternate alleles that are not tested for, or weak variants not detected with the reagents or technique used. Silent or alternate alleles exist in almost all classic genetic systems, as is evident by the list in Table 24–3. This is why a single indirect exclusion is not sufficient evidence for an interpretation of nonpaternity. In some ethnic groups, a silent allele

**Table 24–3.** Alternate Alleles at Classic Genetic Systems Loci

| Genetic System | Null or Weak Alleles | Other Alleles |
|---|---|---|
| ABO | | cis AB |
| Rh | Rh null (amorph), -D-, CDE, (c)D(E) | e Bantu, Cw |
| MNSs | Su, En, Mk | Mg |
| Kell | Ko, McLeod | |
| Duffy | Fy, Fyx | |
| Kidd | Jk | |
| Hp | Hpo | |

**Table 24–4.** Calculation Results on a Paternity Testing Trio

| | Mother | Child | Alleged Father | X | Y | SI | RMNE |
|---|---|---|---|---|---|---|---|
| D2S44/Hae III | 3.42 | 2.89 | 2.89 | 0.5 | 0.074 | 6.76 | 0.1425 |
| | 4.22 | 3.42 | 3.12 | | | | |
| D6S132/Hae III | 1.84 | 1.84 | 2.79 | 1 | 0.241 | 4.15 | 0.4239 |
| | 3.77 | 2.79 | | | | | |
| D17S79/Hae III | 1.35 | 1.35 | 1.45 | 0.25 | 0.183 | 1.37 | 0.5980 |
| | 1.55 | 1.55 | 1.55 | | | | |
| Allele frequencies: | | | | | | | |
| D2S44/Hae III | 2.89 : 0.074 | | | | | | |
| D6S132/Hae III | 2.79 : 0.241 | | | | | | |
| D17S79/Hae III | 1.35 : 0.149 | | | | | | |
| | 1.55 : 0.217 | | | | | | |

may be very common and should be taken into account in the statistical evaluation of inclusion, without even considering the situation as an indirect exclusion. This is the case for the Duffy system in blacks. A third allele Fy exists that does not produce Fyᵃ or Fyᵇ substance. Over 60 percent of blacks are Fy(a−b−), thus homozygous for the Fy gene. The frequency of this Fy gene in blacks is 0.82. Thus an Fy(a+b−) in a black is more likely to be the result of an FyᵃFy phenotype than Fyᵃ Fyᵃ. A child with an Fy(a+b−) phenotype and alleged father with an Fy(a−b+) phenotype should not lead to an interpretation of indirect exclusion but to a calculation of a paternity index taking into account the relative probability of the Fyᵇ Fyᵇ versus Fy Fyᵇ genotypes in the alleged father. This Fy gene also exists, but not at such a high frequency, in Hispanics, Arabs, and other populations of the Middle East. It is very rare in other whites and if the tested individuals were white, this combination of phenotypes could be interpreted as an indirect exclusion. This example illustrates the importance of having expertise in the existence of alternate alleles and their relative frequency in various populations when interpreting parentage testing results in the classic genetic systems.

## INCLUSIONARY CALCULATIONS

Three types of statistical evaluations can be calculated when the alleged father is not excluded: the paternity index (PI), the probability of paternity, and the probability of exclusion. It is important to realize that all these calculations are based on the assumption that the "random man" with whom the tested man is compared is biologically unrelated to him or to the mother. The standard calculations are not valid if a brother, father, uncle, or other close biologic relative of the tested man is a possible biologic father of the child. Another important aspect of the calculations is the need to have accurate allele frequencies for each genetic system tested, estimated from databases drawn from a suffi-

ciently large sample population of the appropriate ethnic group.

### Paternity Index

The paternity index is a likelihood ratio. It is calculated one genetic system at a time and sometimes referred to as the *system index*. If all the genetic systems tested are genetically independent from each other, the overall final paternity index is the product of all of the system indices calculated. When the paternity index is greater than 100, the evidence for paternity is considered very strong.

This likelihood ratio is the ratio of the chance (X) that the tested man can contribute the obligatory gene or genes to any offspring by the chance (Y) that a random unrelated man of the appropriate ethnic background can contribute the same gene or genes to an offspring. An example of testing results on a trio are listed in Table 24–4. In the first genetic system listed the mother and child share the 3.42 allele, thus the obligatory gene (paternal allele in the child) is 2.89. The alleged father is heterozygous for this allele; thus his chance of passing it on to an offspring is 0.5. The frequency of this allele in the general population is 0.074; thus the system index is X/Y = 0.5/0.074 = 6.76. In the second system listed the alleged father is homozygous for the obligatory gene 2.79; thus his chance of passing it on is 1 and the SI is 1/0.241 = 4.15. In the third system the mother and child are identical; thus there are two possible paternal alleles in the child. The mother's chance of passing the 1.35 allele is 0.5, and it is also 0.5 for the 1.55 allele. If the mother passes the 1.35 allele, the corresponding paternal allele is 1.55. The alleged father's chance of passing this allele is 0.5 and the random man's chance is 0.217. If the mother passes on the 1.55 allele, the corresponding paternal allele is 1.35. The alleged father's chance of passing this allele is 0, and the random man's chance is 0.149. Thus X = 0.5 × 0.5 + 0.5 × 0 = 0.25 and Y = 0.5 × 0.217 + 0.5 × 0.149 =

0.183 and SI = X/Y = 0.25/0.183 = 1.37. The overall paternity index is the product of the three systems indices, or 6.76 × 4.15 × 1.37 = 38.43. This means that the tested man is 38.43 times more likely to pass on the appropriate genes to a child in all three genetic systems simultaneously than a random unrelated man.

### Probability of Paternity

The probability is calculated from the paternity index. It is based on a statistical theory developed by Bayes and requires an estimate of the prior probability of paternity; that is, the probability that the tested man is the father of the child based on nongenetic evidence (e.g., social evidence, such as access to the woman at the right time, whether the man is fertile or not, etc.). Inasmuch as a parentage testing laboratory cannot evaluate such type of evidence, it is customary to assign the value of 0.5 to the prior probability. In other words, this means that before testing, the tested man and another untested man are given equal probability of being the biologic father of the child. If the prior probability is 0.5, the probability of paternity (PP) after testing becomes PP = PI/(PI + 1). In the case illustrated, the probability of paternity would be 38.43/39.43 = 0.975 or 97.5 percent. This result in most states would be considered too low to shift the burden of proof to the man, and additional testing in other genetic systems would be needed.

### Probability of Exclusion

The probability of exclusion is the probability of excluding a falsely accused man given the phenotypes of the mother and the child. This probability is entirely dependent on the mother-and-child phenotype combination and does not require knowledge of the alleged father's phenotype. It is evaluated by first calculating the proportion of men who would not be excluded; this number is called *random men not excluded, or RMNE.* The probability of exclusion is 1 − RMNE. If p is the sum of all the possible paternal alleles, then RMNE = p(2 − p) for each genetic system. The overall RMNE for all the genetic systems tested is the product of all the RMNE and the overall probability of exclusion is 1 − overall RMNE. In the case illustrated in Table 24–4, the overall RMNE is 0.1425 × 0.4239 × 0.5980 = 0.0361 and the probability of exclusion is 0.96. The probability of exclusion represents the proportion of untested men who would have been excluded by the extent of testing performed (96 percent in our case) and is more easily understood by a layperson, such as a jury member or a judge. The probability of paternity is a more accurate way to quantify the situation, inasmuch as it includes all the genetic information available, whereas the probability of exclusion does not take into account the phenotype of the alleged father.

## NONCLASSIC SITUATIONS

The majority of parentage testing cases consist of the classic trio of mother, child, and alleged father. However, nonclassic cases are more and more commonly encountered. This may be because the newer technologies are better able to give reliable answers in these situations. It is not unusual to attempt to establish the presence or absence of a biologic relationship between an alleged father and a child when the mother is unavailable for testing. Special calculation formulas have been developed to apply to such cases.[8] Occasionally the alleged father is dead and a reconstruction of his possible genetic makeup is attempted by testing all available parents, siblings, and children of the alleged father. Other biologic relationships, such as sibling-ship, may be in question in adoption, immigration, or inheritance cases.

## ADVANTAGES AND DISADVANTAGES OF THE DIFFERENT TYPES OF GENETIC SYSTEMS

The classic systems have the advantage of the vast experience accumulated over the decades during which they have been in place in many countries. Phenotypes are well recognized and consistently reproducible from laboratory to laboratory. Potential pitfalls have been thoroughly studied, gene frequency distributions are available for almost every population in the world, and the mutation rate has been shown to be extremely low (less than one in a million). Statistical analyses in inclusion cases give extremely consistent results between laboratories. However, they do have some serious drawbacks when compared with the newer technologies testing DNA polymorphisms. In particular, each genetic system, except for the HLA A and B antigens, has a relatively low average power of exclusion. The highest power of exclusion is achieved by $PGM1_i$ at 0.32, followed by MNSs and $Gc_i$ at 0.31 and Rh 0.27, respectively. Virtually all other systems have power of exclusion below 0.20. In contrast, the HLA A and B antigens, analyzed as a haplotype, have a power of exclusion of 0.87. By testing all the classic systems, one can achieve a high power of exclusion, but it is almost impractical to go beyond 0.99. In addition, to get the full benefit of these systems, one must be competent with a multiplicity of techniques. Fairly rigid restrictions exist on the type, amount, and quality of samples needed. Because of the small number of alleles existing in each system, often no more than two or three, they lack efficacy in nonclassic cases.

The DNA polymorphisms by RFLP are extremely powerful genetic systems with average powers of exclusion almost always above 0.50 and often reaching above 0.90 per genetic system. Thus testing only four different loci by DNA-RFLP ensures very high levels of probability of paternity in nonexcluded men. The samples required are any tissue or body fluid from which sufficient DNA can be extracted. Thus not only peripheral blood but also buccal smears, amniotic fluid, chorionic villi, and tissue biopsies can be analyzed. Once extracted, DNA can be kept frozen for an indefinite period of time. However, the technique is time consuming and labor intensive, and turnaround times are long. The main drawback, however, may be the lack of precise correlation in the final paternity index (PI) value between laboratories testing the same loci. This is because, as previously discussed, the phenotypes consist of measured band sizes, with the unavoidable difficulties caused by a built-in incertitude in measurement. This can be very confusing when results from a case tested in several different laboratories are compared, and they may give a false impression of unreliability to someone who is unfamiliar with the limitations of the methodology.

The DNA polymorphisms by PCR avoid this difficulty because they return to a discrete allele distribution. Even when identifying alleles of a genetic system depending on fragment length polymorphisms, one can actually identify the number of repeats and not a length of DNA subject to an imprecision in measurement. This technique has the least restriction in the amount and type of sample needed but the highest requirement in environmental controls to prevent sample contamination, inasmuch as it is based on high amplification of a very small amount of DNA. A great advantage of DNA-PCR technology is the ability to amplify as many as 10 or even more loci in a single amplification reaction. Current instrument technology allows the resolution of 10 STR loci in real-time analysis within 2 to 5 hours. However, these systems are not as powerful as DNA-RFLP systems, and one needs to run two to three times the number of genetic systems to achieve the same level of probability as with DNA-RFLP systems. Both types of DNA polymorphisms have in common a significantly higher mutation rate than the classic systems have. As previously discussed, this has resulted in abandoning the concept of direct and indirect exclusion that has been so effective in classic systems. A mismatch observed in a DNA polymorphism system should lead to the calculation of a system index, which takes into account the rate of mutation for that system. A single mismatch should never lead to an interpretation of nonpaternity but rather to the testing of additional systems.

## SOCIAL AND LEGAL ISSUES

Currently over 200,000 cases of parentage testing are performed every year in the United States. The great majority of these cases are done in view of establishing paternity for children born out of wedlock with the aim of obtaining child support. Child support enforcement agencies in all states actively pursue the identification of the biologic father of children who are eligible for their Aid to Families with Dependent Children, for the purpose of seeking child support from the biologic father. Contracts with child support agencies account for the great majority of the activity of many parentage testing laboratories. Most of the cases done outside the child support enforcement agencies contracts also have a legal implication, such as child support or custody in divorce cases, inheritance rights, or immigration. Occasionally cases have criminal implications relating to incest or statutory rape.

Every step in the collection, storage, processing, and testing of the samples must be carefully documented as to time of occurrence and person performing the task. An unbroken chain of custody must be maintained. Careful verification of the identification of the individuals tested must be done, and procedures must be in place to ensure that unauthorized persons do not have access to the samples or test results. Without careful attention to these aspects, the results may not be valid in court. If called to testify as to the validity and significance of the testing results, the laboratory director must be able to re-create from the documented evidence every step in the handling of the case.

## ACCREDITATION AND QUALITY ISSUES

Almost 30 years ago, the American Association of Blood Banks (AABB) took the lead in promoting the establishment of standardization and quality in the field of paternity testing and created a standing committee on parentage testing. This committee offered educational opportunities such as workshops and publications. With the participation of the American Medical Association, the American Bar Association, and the Office of Child Support Enforcement, the Committee on Parentage Testing organized an international conference in 1982 at Airlie, Virginia. There a group of international experts in the field established a common base to interpret inclusionary evidence. An accreditation program for parentage testing laboratories was implemented, and the first edition of *Standards for Parentage Testing Laboratories* was published in 1990. A complementary *Accreditation Requirements Manual* followed in 1991. The College of American Pathologists with joint sponsorship by the AABB initiated a proficiency testing program for parentage testing laboratories in 1993. The American Society for Clinical Pathology regularly offers educational activities in the form of workshops, teleconferences, or Check Sample.

Continuing involvement by professional organizations in the promotion of quality improvement and in the provision of opportunities for continuing education in the field of paternity testing is essential to the maintenance of a high level of accuracy and consistency in ascertaining biologic relationships.

---

## SUMMARY CHART: IMPORTANT POINTS TO REMEMBER (SBB)

- Parentage testing refers to the testing of genetic markers that are inherited to determine the presence or absence of a biological relationship.
- The ultimate goal of parentage testing is to confirm a specific biologic relationship with the individual in question, usually a father or a mother or sometimes a sibling.
- The blood group systems used most often in paternity testing are ABO, Rh, MNSs, Kell, Duffy, and Kidd.
- The HLA complex represents the most polymorphic genetic system in the human genome; only antigens expressed by the *A* and *B* loci are considered in non-DNA parentage testing.
- Restriction fragment length polymorphism (RFLP) refers to polymorphisms of the DNA that can be detected through the use of restriction enzymes; polymorphisms detected in parentage testing relates to the presence of variable number tandem repeats (VNTR).
- In the polymerase chain reaction, the DNA fragment of interest is amplified several million times and the resulting product is identified either by hybridization with a set of labeled probes or by its location on a gel after electrophoresis.
- Mitochondrial DNA can verify only maternal lineage.
- A *mismatch* is used to refer to the fact that the bands between the child and the alleged father do not match; a minimum of two mismatches is required before an opinion of nonpaternity (or nonmaternity) is rendered.
- A *direct* exclusion occurs when a marker is detected in the child, whereas it is absent in the mother and the alleged father, or when the alleged father's phenotype demonstrates two markers and the child has neither one of them.
- An *indirect* exclusion occurs when a single marker is detected in the child and a different single marker is detected in the alleged father.
- False direct exclusions can occur as the result of mutations that are significant enough to alter the final product, lack of precursor substance, suppressor activity at a locus unlinked to the one tested, or chimeric state of one of the tested individuals.
- False indirect exclusions occur secondary to the presence of silent alleles (e.g., *Fy*).

## CASE STUDIES

### CASE 1

A black trio consisting of a mother, child, and alleged father is tested in view to establish paternity. The following results are obtained:

| Genetic System | Mother | Child | Alleged Father |
|---|---|---|---|
| ABO | O | B | A |
| Rh | Dce | Dce | DCe |
| MNSs | MSs | MNs | Ns |
| Duffy | Fy(a+b−) | Fy(a+b−) | Fy(a−b+) |
| Kidd | Jk(a+b+) | Jk(a−b+) | Jk(a+b−) |
| HLA | A2,30 B12,42 | A30 B17,42 | A2,B7,35 |

1. Which of the genetic systems tested reveal a direct exclusion?
   a. Rh and MNSs
   b. ABO and HLA
   c. Rh and Kidd
   d. Rh, Duffy, and Kidd
   e. ABO, Rh, Duffy, Kidd, and HLA

2. Which of the genetic systems tested reveal an indirect exclusion?
   a. Rh and MNSs
   b. ABO and HLA
   c. Rh and Kidd
   d. Rh, Duffy, and Kidd
   e. ABO, Rh, Duffy, Kidd, and HLA

3. What is the best interpretation for the results in the Duffy system?
   a. This is a direct exclusion.
   b. This is an indirect exclusion.
   c. In this black trio, this is consistent with the transmission of a silent allele by the alleged father.
   d. In this black trio, this is consistent with the transmission of a silent allele by the mother.
   e. Whatever the racial background of the trio, there is no suspicion of exclusion in this genetic system.

### CASE 2

A white trio consisting of a mother, child, and alleged father is tested in view to establish paternity. The following results are obtained:

| Genetic System | Mother | Child | Alleged Father |
|---|---|---|---|
| ABO | A | O | B |
| MNSs | MNs | MNs | NSs |
| D2S44/Hae III | 3.42, 4.24 | 2.90, 3.42 | 2.90, 3.11 |
| D4S139/Hae III | 4.28, 9.42 | 4.28, 6.50 | 4.28, 7.25 |
| D10S28/Hae III | 1.70, 2.90 | 1.70, 3.32 | 1.05, 3.32 |
| GYPA | A,B | A,B | B |
| HUMTH01 | 6,9 | 6,9 | 6,7 |

4. The third genetic system tested (D2S44/Hae III) represents a:
   a. Red cell antigen system tested by agglutination
   b. Red cell enzyme system
   c. DNA polymorphism by RFLP
   d. SSP-DNA polymorphism tested by PCR
   e. STR-DNA polymorphism tested by PCR

5. The sixth genetic system tested (GYPA) represents a:
   a. Red cell antigen system tested by agglutination
   b. Red cell enzyme system
   c. DNA polymorphism tested by PCR
   d. SSP-DNA polymorphism tested by PCR
   e. STR-DNA polymorphism tested by PCR

6. Among the following statements relating to the interpretation of these results, choose the one that is true:
   a. The alleged father is excluded because of a direct exclusion at D4S139.
   b. The alleged father is excluded because of an indirect exclusion at D4S139.
   c. A mutation may have occurred at D4S139.
   d. The alleged father is excluded because of a direct exclusion in the ABO system.
   e. The final paternity index can be obtained by multiplying together the paternity indices of each of the seven systems tested.

**Answers to Case Studies**

Case 1:

1. b

2. c

3. c

In blacks the silent *Fy* alleles constitute 82 percent of the gene pool; thus an Fy(a − b+) individual is much more likely to be heterozygous *Fy*$^b$*Fy* than homozygous *Fy*$^b$ *Fy*$^b$ and has a high probability of passing on an *Fy* gene.

Case 2:

4. c

5. d

6. c

In DNA polymorphisms the mutation rate can be as high as 2 per 1000; thus, a single mismatch, when all other systems are consistent with paternity, may represent a mutation. A minimum of two mismatches is necessary before an interpretation of exclusion is rendered.

The MN red cell antigens tested by agglutination are a product from the same locus as the *GYPA* locus tested by PCR-SSP; thus, one cannot multiply the PI from each of these two systems together. The best option is to choose the system giving the greatest PI and to ignore the PI of the other system.

## REVIEW QUESTIONS

1. Among the combinations of attributes described below select the one that would NOT be suitable for a genetic system used in parentage testing analysis.
   A. The system has multiple alleles in Hardy-Weinberg equilibrium.
   B. The system has a high mutation rate.
   C. Databases of allele frequencies are available for all ethnic groups tested by the laboratory.
   D. All genetic systems selected are genetically independent from each other.
   E. Testing methodology is available in several laboratories.

2. In which of the following genetic systems is the allele frequency distribution continuous (not discrete)?
   A. DNA polymorphisms by RFLP
   B. DNA polymorphisms by PCR
   C. Red cell antigens
   D. Red cell enzymes
   E. Serum proteins

3. A false direct exclusion in red cell antigen genetic systems can be caused by:
   A. A silent allele
   B. A lack of precursor substance
   C. An alternate untested allele
   D. A weakly expressed variant
   E. Weak reagents

4. Among the following organizations, which one offers an accreditation program for parentage testing laboratories?
   A. AABB
   B. ASCP
   C. CAP
   D. FDA
   E. HCFA

## ANSWERS TO REVIEW QUESTIONS

1. B (p 508)

2. A (pp 510–511)

3. B (p 513)

4. A (p 516)

## REFERENCES

1. Bernstein, F: Ergebnisse einer biostatischen zusammenfassenden Betrachtung über die erblichen Blutstrukturen des Menschen. Klin Wschr 3:1495, 1924.
2. Smithies, O: Zone electrophoresis in starch gels: Group variations in the serum proteins of normal human adults. Biochemical Journal 61:629, 1955.
3. Histocompatibility Testing 1972. Proceedings of the 5th International Conference. Evian. Munksgaard, Copenhagen, 1973.
4. Jeffreys, AJ, Wilson B, and Thein, SL: Hypervariable "minisatellite" regions in human DNA. Nature 314:67, 1985.
5. Walker, RH (ed): Parentage Testing Accreditation Requirements Manual, ed 2. American Association of Blood Banks, Bethesda, MD, 1995, p 66.

6. Krings, M, et al: Neanderthal DNA sequences and the origin of modern humans. Cell 90:19, 1997.

7. Ivanov, P, et al: Mitochondrial DNA sequence heteroplasmy in the grand duke of Russia Giorgig Romanov establishes the authenticity of remains of Tsar Nicholas II. Nat Genet 12:417, 1996.

8. Brenner, CH: A note on paternity computation in cases lacking a mother. Transfusion 33:51, 1993.

## BIBLIOGRAPHY

Allen, RW, Wallhermfechtel, M, and Miller, WV: The application of restriction fragment length polymorphism mapping to parentage testing. Transfusion 30:552, 1990.

Committee on DNA Forensic Science: The Evaluation of Forensic DNA Evidence: An Update. National Academic Press, Washington, DC 1996, pp 53–54.

Parentage Testing Accreditation Requirements Manual, ed 2. American Association of Blood Banks, Bethesda, MD, 1995.

Polesky, HF: Blood groups, human leukocyte antigens and DNA polymorphism in parentage testing. In Henry, JB (ed): Clinical Diagnosis and Management by Laboratory Methods, ed 19. WB Saunders, Philadelphia, 1996, pp 1413–1426.

Standards for Parentage Testing Laboratories, ed 3. American Association of Blood Banks, Bethesda, MD, 1998.

Walker, RH: Molecular biology in paternity testing. Lab Med 23:752, 1992.

# CHAPTER 25

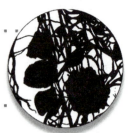

# INFORMATIONAL SYSTEMS IN THE BLOOD BANK

Ann Tiehen, MT(ASCP)SBB

**System Components**
Hardware
- Processing hardware
- Input and output devices
- Information storage hardware

Software
- Application software
- Operating system software
- Interface software

People
- Users
- System managers

**Blood Bank Software Applications**
Donation Facility
- Donor management
- Blood component management

Transfusing Facility
- Blood component management
- Patient management

General System Applications
- Security
- Quality assurance
- Management assistance

**Regulatory and Accreditation Requirements**

**System Management**
Standard Operating Procedures
- Archiving data
- Backup of software programs and data
- Computer downtime
- Hardware maintenance
- Maintenance of security
- Tracking and correction of errors
- Training of personnel

Validation of Software
- Test plan
- Test cases

**Summary Chart: Important Points to Remember**

**Review Questions**

**Bibliography**

*On completion of this chapter, the learner should be able to:*

1 Describe the purpose of an information system in the blood bank.

2 Define the hardware components of a blood bank information system.

3 Describe the functions of the software components of a blood bank information system.

4 List the responsibilities for operating and maintaining a blood bank information system.

5 Identify regulatory and accrediting agency requirements pertaining to blood bank information systems.

6 List the applications available in blood bank information systems.

7 Describe the purpose of a truth table.

8 Name the standard operating procedures needed to manage a blood bank information system.

9 Describe the kinds of testing that should be included in the validation of a blood bank information system.

10 Identify the times at which validation testing must be performed.

11 Define control function and discuss the difference between process control and decision support.

Information processing plays a vital role in blood banking practice. Proper management of information related to blood donors, blood components, and patients receiving transfusions is crucial to ensuring the safety and traceability of blood products. Blood bank personnel are relying more and more on computerized information systems to assist in the handling of this important data. Regulatory and standard setting agencies have put increasing pressure on blood banks to be able to store information in a safe manner and to be able to retrieve it in a timely fashion. It must be possible to track a blood component from the time of its donation, through all of the processing steps, and finally to the patient who received it. It is also essential to be able to perform that trace in reverse order; that is, from the recipient back to the donor. Before computerized information systems were available, all blood bank data were stored on paper, or "hard-copy," records requiring labor-intensive and sometimes error-prone procedures to retrieve it. As blood bank information systems have become more and more sophisticated, they have made recovery of the information much more efficient and have offered the industry a great variety of process controls to reduce errors. Several acronyms unique to the specialty of information systems will be used throughout this chapter and are listed in Table 25–1.

Computerized blood bank information systems are available in many different configurations, but they fall into three general categories. They may take the form of a highly complex system like that found in a community blood center; they may be a small part of a complete clinical laboratory information system (LIS), or they may exist as a "stand-alone" system usually found in a hospital blood bank or transfusion service. The functionality of these systems varies from category to category and from vendor to vendor within each category. Some systems may merely act as record keepers, whereas others have the ability to use the information in such a way as to prevent errors in donor acceptance, blood component release, or patient transfusion. For example, a basic system used in a hospital transfusion service may simply allow the entry of an ABO group and Rh type in a patient's record with subsequent generation of a charge for the test. A more complex system in a hospital blood bank can record the donation of an autologous unit in the donor room and then make the transfusion service technologist aware of its presence when the patient is admitted for a type and screen test at the time of surgery.

## SYSTEM COMPONENTS

A computer system includes three major components: hardware, software, and people. Hardware components are the physical pieces of equipment. Software is a set of instructions written in special computer language that tells the computer how to operate and manipulate the data. The people interface with the hardware to enter the data that are manipulated by the software. Just as there are many different kinds of people who enter data, so there are many different kinds of hardware and software available.

### Hardware

Most of the hardware components of a computer system are readily identifiable because they can be seen and touched, although some are hidden inside a case or a central system unit. Each piece of hardware performs a specific function in the handling of information. The three main functions performed by hardware components are processing, input/output, and storage.

Hardware components include a central system unit, sometimes referred to as the "box," and a number of

**Table 25–1.** Common Acronyms

| | |
|---|---|
| CPU: | Central processing unit |
| HIS: | Hospital information system |
| LIS: | Laboratory information system |
| PC: | Personal computer |
| RAM: | Random access memory |
| ROM: | Read-only memory |
| SOP: | Standard operating procedure |

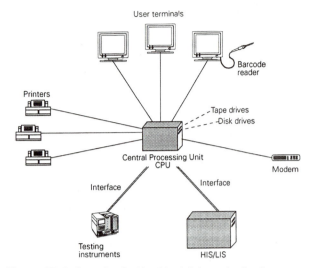

**Figure 25–1.** Example of a blood bank information hardware configuration.

different peripheral devices that send or receive information through the system unit. Peripheral devices include display terminals, keyboards; bar code readers, scanners and wands, pointing devices such as mice, printers, and modems. The hardware components and the way in which they are connected to each other is the system configuration. Figure 25–1 illustrates one such configuration.

### Processing Hardware

The central hardware component of a computer system is the central processing unit (CPU), which is an electric circuit or silicon "chip" that processes information. The CPU, also called a *processor,* is the core of the machine. It controls the interpretation and execution of instructions provided by the software. Other pieces of processing hardware that also exist in the system unit are the ROM and RAM chips. ROM stands for *read-only memory* and contains the "start-up" instructions for the computer. *Random access memory* (RAM) is an array of chips where data are temporarily entered while they are being processed. When a computer is turned on, these chips interact with each other and the operating system software to prepare the computer to accept data and instructions from its users.

### Input and Output Devices

Although users can occasionally be seen shouting at their computer systems, most blood bank information systems cannot recognize voice instructions. Commands and data must be entered in a format that the computer can understand. This requires tools that are connected to the system's CPU such as keyboards, pointing devices, bar code readers, and testing instruments. Keyboards are used to type instructions that tell the computer what to do, or to enter data such as donor demographic information or patient test results. Many

systems also accept bar-coded information from sources such as blood component labels or test tubes. Blood component labels contain many pieces of bar-coded information, including the unit number, blood type, product type, facility identification number, and expiration date. Entry of this information by a bar code reader is much more accurate than manual entry methods. Figure 25–2 shows a blood component label with this bar-coded information. Scanning the bar codes with an optical or laser device allows efficient entry of the blood component data.

The most common output device is the monitor, which displays information as it is typed on the keyboard. Together, the monitor and the keyboard make up the user terminal. The monitor may also display historical information at the request of the user.

Another commonly used output device is the printer, which provides hard-copy output on paper. Printers can produce labels, donor registration records, compatibility tags, management reports, patient chart reports, or donor correspondence. The kind of printer chosen for any of these applications depends on the quality of print desired. For example, a bar code label printer requires a high-resolution printing capability for accurate interpretation by the bar code reader. Management reports, which are usually used internally, can be of lower-quality print.

A modem is an example of a combined input and output device. Modems allow computer systems to communicate with each other over telephone lines. Blood banks can use this mechanism to connect re-

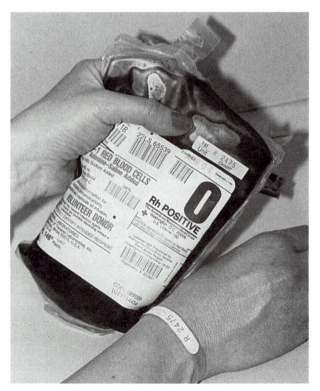

**Figure 25–2.** Barcodes on unit label.

mote facilities to the main computer system so that all sites have access to the system's databases. This configuration is found in blood centers with several collection or testing locations or in a system of hospital affiliates. The technical support staff of software vendors also use modems to investigate and to solve system problems or to transfer files to the customer.

### Information Storage Hardware

All computer systems have hardware that allows long-term storage of data. This is sometimes referred to as "memory" but should not be confused with RAM, which is only temporary and active when the system is turned on. Long-term "memory" is data saved on a medium from which they can later be retrieved, such as a hard disk. Most systems contain a hard disk controlled by a hard drive. The disk is made of metal coated with a magnetic film and contains software applications (programs) and user-entered data. The hard disk is often contained in the main system unit, but it may also be a peripheral device. The information on the disk is accessed by entering commands, usually with a keyboard connected to a display terminal. Other information storage hardware may be used for archiving old information that has been removed from the hard disk.

## Software

Software tells the computer what to do with all of the information it has received. Minimally, every computer system has two kinds of software—namely, operating system software and application software. Some systems may also use interface software, which allows the system to communicate with other computer systems.

### Application Software

An application is software that has been designed to perform specific tasks. Personal computers (PCs) can be equipped with application programs such as word processing, spreadsheets, and databases. In a blood bank information system the application software allows users to perform tasks that are specific to blood bank operations. In a donor setting, some of these tasks might include entry of donor demographic information and test results, confirmation of blood component labeling, and generation of donor recruitment lists. In a transfusion service, the computer may help with tasks such as searching for a blood component of a particular ABO group, entry of blood component modification information, and issuing blood for transfusion. These tasks are very distinctly connected to blood banking and would be difficult, if not impossible, to perform in an application not specifically designed for blood bank use. One of the most important functions performed by blood bank applications is the maintenance of the database of donors, blood components, and transfusion recipients. A database is an organized set of information divided into files and then further subdivided into records. Files exist in one of two ways: they may be static or dynamic. The dynamic files contain records related to a specific donor, patient, or blood component. These records are frequently changed as updated information is added to them. For example, the status of a blood component can go from quarantine to transfused with many intermediate statuses during its shelf life. The static files contain information that is infrequently updated, such as the list of blood products used in the facility. These files, which look different in each blood bank, define the terminology that the blood bank will use. When a new blood bank information system is installed, the static files must be defined before the system can be put into use. One of the most important functions of the static files is to provide a "dictionary" of coded terms that the information system can use to sort and organize the tremendous amount of data entered into it. For example, two static files, one containing codes for physicians and the other for blood products, can allow the system to sort information regarding the crossmatch to transfusion (C:T) ratio of each physician who ordered blood within a particular time frame.

Figure 25–3 shows how the parts of a database relate

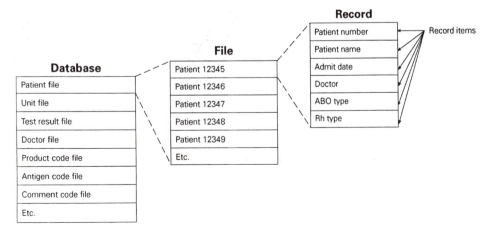

**Figure 25–3.** Database components.

to each other. The database itself can be thought of as a file cabinet containing folders or files that in turn contain specific records. This illustration is of a dynamic file containing patient records. A static file illustrated in this way, for example, for blood product codes, would list a separate file for each blood product code used in the facility. The associated records would include such information as the official name of the blood component, its maximum allowable shelf life, and whether or not it contains red blood cells, thus requiring cross-matching.

### Operating System Software

The tasks performed by the operating system are fairly invisible to users because this software works in the background. It is a set of instructions that controls the computer's hardware, manipulates the application software, and coordinates the flow of data to and from disks and memory. When new data are entered into one of the application programs, it is the operating system that places those data on the disk for storage; when a request for those data is made through the application program, the operating system retrieves them and sends them to the application software for display on a monitor or printed report.

### Interface Software

Frequently, different information systems must be allowed to share data with each other to take full advantage of their functionality. Because different systems communicate in different computer languages, they need an interpreter that will allow data to flow between the two systems in a controlled manner. The interpreter is another set of software called an interface. Interface software may be used to allow data to flow between a hospital information system (HIS) and the blood bank system, or the LIS and the blood bank. For example, an interface between the HIS and the blood bank information system can allow flow of patient demographic information from the HIS to the blood bank system and allow test results and blood component information to flow from the blood bank system to the HIS, where they can be displayed on terminals in patient care areas.

### People

The human components of a blood bank information system are the users and at least one person designated as the system manager. Users have access to the technical applications needed to perform day-to-day blood bank operations. System managers require access to a wider range of applications, including system maintenance functions.

### Users

Entry of commands and data into the system is performed by the users. The success with which a blood

bank computer system can be used depends not only on its ease of use but also on the training provided to its users. Most systems are equipped with both a "live" or production database and a "test" database. The static files in both databases are identical, but their dynamic files contain different information. The production database contains real information, whereas the test database is composed of fictitious records. The test database offers the user an opportunity to practice the applications of the system (and to make mistakes) without corrupting the database containing actual donor and patient information. Users should be trained in every application they will be expected to use.

### System Managers

The configuration and location of the information system will determine the identity and quantity of people performing this task. In a large community blood center there may be an entire staff dedicated to the management of the system. In a hospital blood bank or transfusion service that uses the blood bank module of a complete clinical LIS, the laboratory system manager is likely to have responsibility for the entire system, but there should also be a designated blood bank system manager. In blood banks equipped with a stand-alone blood bank computer, designated system managers may also have other supervisory, technical, or quality assurance duties as part of their job description.

Whatever the identity of the system manager, he or she oversees the maintenance of the system's hardware and software. Some specific duties include adding or deleting items from the static database files, assigning access codes to new users, and implementing software upgrades from the vendor. In addition, the system manager will be called upon to investigate problems encountered by the users and to report them to the system vendor.

## BLOOD BANK SOFTWARE APPLICATIONS

The kinds of data that must be managed by a particular blood bank information system depend on the types of services provided by the blood bank. Most community blood centers focus on donations and distribution of the donated blood components to customer hospitals. In the hospital transfusion service, the primary concern is the transfusion of patients. However, a community blood center or a hospital blood bank with both a transfusion service laboratory and a donation center must address issues of both donor and patient management. Application programs exist for every task, from scheduling donors to assigning a transfused status to a blood component. Many of the typical blood bank information system applications currently available are discussed in this section.

## Donation Facility

### Donor Management

The system should allow the capture of donor demographic information necessary for definitive donor identification, telephone contact for recruitment, and notification in the event that abnormal laboratory testing results are obtained. In addition, the system should have a means for preventing a donation from a deferred individual or from one attempting to donate before the required waiting period between donations.

**Donor Registration.** When a potential donor registers at a donation facility, several pieces of demographic data must be provided, such as social security number, name, date of birth, phone number, and mailing address. When this information is entered into the donor database, the system can search for a previous donation record from the same donor. If none is found, a new donor record is created in the system. If there is a record of a previous donation, the system can review the donor's eligibility status. This would include calculating the length of time elapsed since the last donation and examination of the record for a deferral because of medical history or disease testing results. If the donor is not eligible because of either an inadequate amount of time since the last donation or a previous deferral, the system can alert the registrar and prevent an unsuitable donation from occurring. If the registration is taking place at a location that does not have immediate access to the electronic database, as happens on a mobile blood drive, the registrars can be equipped with a printed list of eligible and ineligible donors. Alternatively, the database can be downloaded to a portable PC and transported to the mobile site.

**Donation Data.** Information regarding the donation event also can be entered into the system. This data entry is usually performed after the donation but can include important information, such as the unique identification number applied to the collection container, the type of donation made (e.g., whole blood or apheresis), the collection time, and the occurrence of a donor reaction. If the donation is intended for a specific recipient, as in the case of an autologous or designated donation, data regarding the intended recipient can be entered.

**Donor Recruitment.** The capture of donor demographic information at registration allows the collecting facility to recruit the donor from a system-generated list of eligible donors. Mailing labels can also be generated for recruitment efforts. Once laboratory testing is associated with the donor's record, lists of donors meeting special needs can be printed. Such lists may include donors with a specific ABO group, other red cell antigen type, or cytomegalovirus (CMV) seronegativity.

### Blood Component Management

**Component Production.** After a whole blood unit has been collected, it is usually delivered to a component-processing laboratory, where it is separated into different components, including red blood cells, fresh frozen plasma, and platelets, and labeled appropriately. The new components created are entered into the system with the unique donation identification number assigned at the time of donation, their new blood product codes, time of preparation, and expiration dates.

**Laboratory Testing.** Samples of the donor's blood that were collected at the time of donation and labeled with the same unique donation identification number are tested for ABO, Rh, atypical antibodies, and markers of transfusion-transmitted diseases such as hepatitis and human immunodeficiency virus. The results of all of these tests are entered into the system so that they are associated with the unique donation identification number as well as with the donor. In larger community blood centers, the results of testing performed on automated instruments can be sent directly from the instrument to the system via an instrument interface.

**Label Application and Verification.** After completion of component production and laboratory testing, the blood products are labeled with the ABO/Rh type. This is a crucial step and must be stringently controlled so that no unsuitable blood products are released into the blood supply. After the label has been applied, the unique donation identification number and ABO/Rh type bar codes on the blood component label can be scanned into the system using a bar code reader. This allows the system to perform a final check on donor suitability and blood type. If the component "passes" this verification, the blood component can be placed in the available inventory.

**Inventory Management and Product Shipping.** The collection facility staff members who are responsible for product distribution to customer hospitals must have access to the entire inventory of available blood products. As transfusion services place requests for quantities and ABO/Rh types of blood components, the distribution staff can monitor and control distribution to optimize blood use within the community. For example, blood products nearing their expiration date can be sent to active transfusion services where there is a high probability of transfusion before expiration. As products are shipped to transfusing facilities, their status is updated in the system, along with the identification of the facility to which they were shipped.

## Transfusing Facility

### Blood Component Management

**Product Receipt and Entry.** When the products are received at the transfusing facility, they are entered into the blood bank information system, where the entire inventory of blood components is maintained. If ABO/Rh confirmation is required, as in the case of components containing red cells, a status of quarantine will be assigned by the system until confirmation testing is completed. Components not requiring ABO/Rh confirmation testing may be assigned a status of available on entry into the system.

**Inventory Management.** A computerized inventory makes it easy for blood bank staff members to monitor inventory levels so that they do not drop below predefined minimums. Most systems sort the inventory by product code, ABO/Rh, and expiration date, and output it to a display monitor or printed report. When a selection list of blood components is indexed in this way, the products that are closer to the end of their shelf lives can be chosen for patients with a high likelihood of transfusion.

**Blood Component Modification.** Many components require modification to meet the special transfusion needs of a particular patient. Modifications include irradiation, leukocyte reduction, aliquoting (dividing), washing, and pooling. As these physical modifications are performed in the blood bank, the steps associated with them are captured by the information system, either by changing the product name or by adding a special attribute to the component. Some of these steps may also require a shortening of the shelf life of the component, and the system can enter the new expiration date and time, if applicable. Attributes may also be added to components that have undergone special testing, such as tests for antibodies to cytomegalovirus (CMV) or specific red blood cell antigens.

**Component Status Tracking.** After blood components are received in the transfusion service they are assigned various statuses, ending with a final disposition of transfused or discarded. Each blood component record in the information system should contain a complete status history. Figure 25–4 illustrates the var-

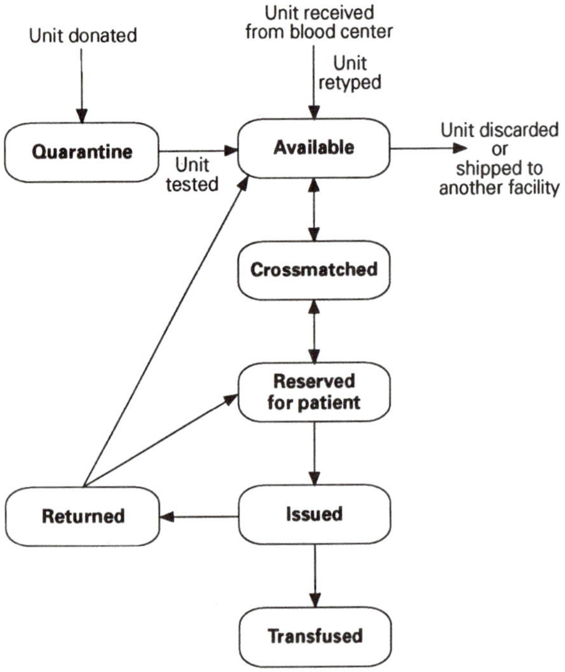

**Figure 25–4.** Various statuses of a blood component on a blood bank information system.

**Table 25–2.** ABO Truth Table

| Anti-A | Anti-B | A$_1$ Cells | B Cells | Interpretation |
|--------|--------|-------------|---------|----------------|
| 0 | 0 | + | + | O |
| + | 0 | 0 | + | A |
| 0 | + | + | 0 | B |
| + | + | 0 | 0 | AB |

ious statuses that a blood component may be ascribed throughout its shelf life.

## Patient Management

**Patient Identification.** A blood bank information system used by a facility issuing blood for transfusion should have the capability of capturing patient demographic information such as name and unique facility identification number. In addition, there are other pieces of information specific to the blood bank that the system should maintain. These include previous ABO/Rh type, transfusion history, previously identified clinically significant antibodies, and transfusion instructions such as the need for irradiated or leukocyte-reduced cellular components.

**Order Entry.** On receipt of a specimen for patient testing, the system can retrieve previous test results and alert the technologist to special transfusion requirements of the patient. For example, the record for a patient with a history of a clinically significant antibody can alert the technologist to the need for specific antigen-negative red cell components. Physician's orders for blood components can also be entered.

**Patient Testing.** Some systems allow direct entry of test results into the system, thus replacing paper worksheets. If appropriate "truth tables" have been set up in the system, the entered test results can be compared with the truth tables for accuracy. Truth tables define the combination of results considered valid for a particular test. This can prevent the release of invalid results such as nonmatching forward and reverse types. Table 25–2 shows how such a truth table might look. Each row represents one combination of individual test results and an interpretation, which the system will allow in its ABO test entry function. In the case of the ABO test, there are only four valid result combinations, and the system warns the user if any other combination is entered. When the results are entered correctly and match one of the valid combinations in the truth table, the results are accepted and verified. Other tests, such as Rh$_0$ (D) and antibody screen, may also have to meet their own truth table requirements. Figure 25–5 illustrates what a user would see on the display monitor when a valid ABO group is entered. Working behind the scenes and invisible to most users is the truth table, which in this figure is highlighted where the valid combination of results has been found to indicate the match with the valid ABO results entered and displayed

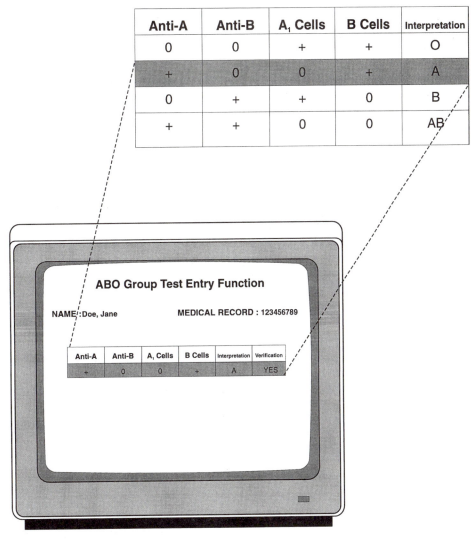

## ABO Truth Table
## Working behind the Scenes

| Anti-A | Anti-B | A₁ Cells | B Cells | Interpretation |
|--------|--------|----------|---------|----------------|
| 0 | 0 | + | + | O |
| + | 0 | 0 | + | A |
| 0 | + | + | 0 | B |
| + | + | 0 | 0 | AB |

**ABO Group Test Entry Function**

NAME: Doe, Jane          MEDICAL RECORD : 123456789

| Anti-A | Anti-B | A₁ Cells | B Cells | Interpretation | Verification |
|--------|--------|----------|---------|----------------|--------------|
| + | 0 | 0 | + | A | YES |

**Figure 25–5.** Display monitor: entry of a valid ABO group.

on the monitor. Truth tables make their presence known when an invalid combination of results is entered. Figure 25–6 illustrates what a user might see when invalid ABO results are entered. In this example, an incorrect result has been entered for the reaction of the patient's plasma or serum with group B reagent red cells. When the technologist attempts to verify the results, the computer responds with a warning message, indicating that it was not able to find a match in the truth table for this particular combination of results.

The most critical test performed in the blood bank is the patient ABO/Rh type, and it is required that previous test results be compared with current results. When this comparison, performed by the system, reveals a discrepancy, a warning is given to alert the technologist to the possibility of a mislabeled specimen or incorrect test results.

**Blood Component Reservation.** The system can aid in the selection of blood components that will satisfy special transfusion needs and that are compatible with the patient's ABO/Rh. Selections may be made by manual entry or bar code entry, or from an indexed selection list. If autologous or designated blood components are available for a patient, the system can alert the user. As blood components are selected and either crossmatched or reserved for a patient, the system links those products to the patient record and prints compatibility tags.

A fairly recent application available on some systems is the "computer crossmatch." It allows electronic veri-

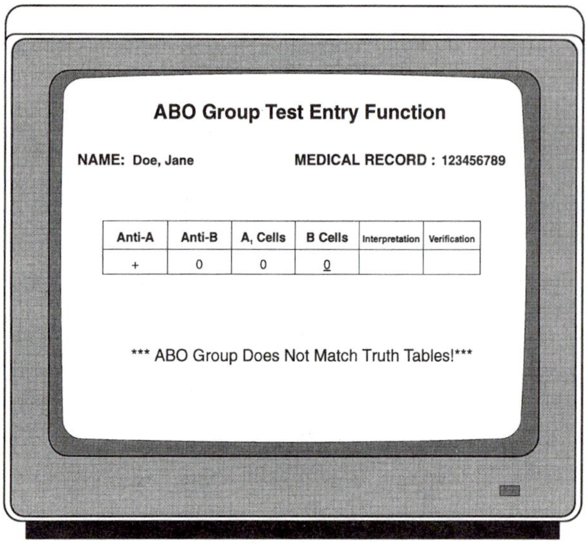

**Figure 25–6.** Display monitor: entry of an invalid ABO group.

fication of recipient and donor compatibility and dispenses with the serologic crossmatch test. A patient is eligible for the computer crossmatch when his or her records indicate that two criteria have been met: (1) there is no current or past history of clinically significant antibodies, and (2) there are at least two concordant ABO grouping test results. In addition, the system must contain the donation identification number, component name, component ABO group and Rh type, the interpretation of the component ABO confirmatory test, and recipient information including ABO group and Rh type. The system must use this information to alert the user when there are discrepancies between donor unit labeling and blood group confirmatory test interpretation and when ABO incompatibilities exist between the recipient and donor unit. Finally, the system must require verification of correct entry of data before release of blood components. These stringent requirements for a computer crossmatch must be in place to prevent the issue of ABO-incompatible components.

**Result Reporting.** Information regarding patient test results and any products linked to the patient should be accessible to the patient's caregivers. This may be in the form of printed reports and/or monitor displays. The status of linked products should be updatable. That is, as the products go from crossmatched or reserved, to issued, to transfused or returned, the status should be reported.

**Blood Component Issue.** When blood components are requested for transfusion, the system can assist in issuing them appropriately. For example, if both an autologous red blood cell (RBC) and an allogeneic RBC have been reserved for the same patient, it is essential that the autologous unit be issued first. Many systems alert the issuer if he or she attempts to issue the allogeneic unit first. In addition, the system can warn if a special transfusion need is not being met by the prod-

uct being issued. Verification of unit inspection before issue can also be recorded in the system. When a product is issued, the system updates its status in the inventory.

## General System Applications

In addition to the requirements specific to a collection or transfusion facility, there are general applications that are found in all blood bank information systems. These functions assist with system security, quality assurance, and management reports.

### Security

It is critical for only authorized users to have access to the information contained in a blood bank computer system. Access is obtained through the use of assigned user codes and passwords, and it is the responsibility of the users to keep their passwords confidential. A second level of security restricts some users to some of the system's functions. This is important for two reasons: donor/patient confidentiality and protection of data from accidental or unauthorized destruction or modification. Sensitive information, such as test results for markers of transfusion-transmitted disease, should be available only to the medical director and selected supervisory personnel. The system manager has access to most or all of the functions, including those that allow modification of the static database files. Technical staff members can access those functions that are specific to their jobs, such as test result entry, labeling, or component production. Clerical staff members may be restricted to inquiry functions that allow them to answer questions from patients or physicians but not to enter or to modify patient data. In addition to providing system security, user codes are used to capture the identity of each person performing each step in the information system.

### Quality Assurance

**Control Functions.** One of the most useful features that a blood bank information system can offer is assistance to users in ensuring safe transfusion. When blood bank personnel depend on this assistance in making decisions at critical points in the selection of donors and release of blood products for transfusion, the system is said to be exerting "control functions." Control functions can be placed in two general categories: (1) process control and (2) decision support. Process control functions are decisions made by the system without human intervention. Decision support control functions occur when the system displays information to the user, who then decides on the next course of action. Table 25–3 shows some examples of control functions.

**Corrected or Amended Results.** Sometimes it is necessary to correct or to amend incorrect or incomplete information that was entered into the system.

**Table 25–3.** Examples of Control Functions

| Application | Process Control | Decision Support |
| --- | --- | --- |
| Donor management | Prevention of registration of permanently deferred donor | Warning of current ABO/Rh not matching previous results |
| Blood component management: Collection facility | Prevention of unit release if testing unacceptable | Calculation of component expiration date |
| Blood component management: Transfusing facility | Prevention of entry of donation identification number which already exists in the system | Warning of entry of an expiration date that exceeds the possible shelf life of a blood component |
| Patient management | Prevention of issue of outdated unit | Warning of product not meeting special transfusion needs |

This need arises when errors are made in testing or when testing is performed on a mislabeled specimen so that results are associated with the wrong patient. When corrections must be made, both the original erroneous results and the corrected results must be clearly specified as such on monitor displays and printed reports. Figure 25–7 illustrates one method for correcting erroneous results. This method of error correction alerts patient caregivers who may have made clinical decisions based on the incorrect results. The information system should make it impossible to simply delete the erroneous result and substitute a corrected result.

**Blood Product Utilization Review.** Transfusion services are required by several accrediting agencies to monitor the utilization of blood products within the facility. This includes both the blood ordering and transfusing practices of physicians. An information system can be of tremendous help in sorting and reporting utilization data. C:T ratios can be reported for individual physicians and for services such as surgery and obstetrics.

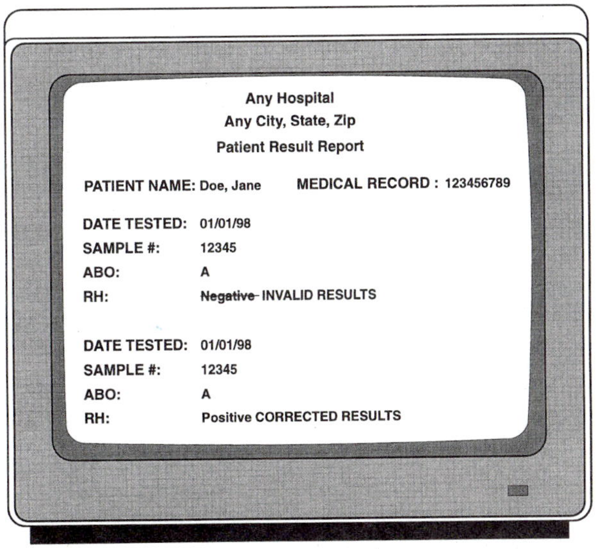

**Figure 25–7.** Display monitor: patient report with corrected result.

### Management Assistance

Enormous amounts of different kinds of data can be entered into the blood bank information system. When appropriate reporting capabilities are designed into the system, they can provide valuable information to assist in management decisions. Reports of the number of donors drawn and deferred or blood products transfused and expired can help evaluate productivity and future resource needs. In addition, patient or hospital billing can be done more accurately and consistently than with manual systems.

## REGULATORY AND ACCREDITATION REQUIREMENTS

Over the last 10 years, blood bank computer systems have been the subject of increasing regulatory oversight. In the late 1980s the Food and Drug Administration (FDA) recognized that unsuitable blood components were being released into the blood supply because of inadequately controlled and validated computer systems. In 1988 and 1989 the FDA issued memoranda to registered blood establishments to provide guidance on the use of computer systems. In 1993 they issued a draft guideline for the validation of blood establishment computer systems, which outlined a validation program in compliance with current good manufacturing practices. After that, in 1994 and 1995, memoranda were sent to blood establishment computer software manufacturers, advising them that the FDA intended to regulate blood bank software as a medical device under the Safe Medical Devices Act of 1990. These regulatory initiatives have had significant impact on the availability and implementation of blood bank information systems. Both software vendors and users must follow prescribed guidelines in the introduction of new software. Vendors must perform thorough validation testing before making software available for purchase, and users must, in turn, document validation procedures on site before using such a system.

Voluntary accreditation agencies such as the Joint Commission on Accreditation of Healthcare Organizations (JCAHO), the American Association of Blood Banks (AABB), and the College of American Pathologists (CAP) also have standards or inspection checklist items that emphasize the responsibilities of operating an information system. A blood bank must have documented evidence of validation of its system as well as written procedures for all aspects of system management to comply with regulatory and accreditation requirements.

## SYSTEM MANAGEMENT

Many responsibilities are associated with the operation and maintenance of a computerized blood bank information system. The bulk of these responsibilities occur when a system is first installed as new standard operating procedures (SOPs) are written, the system is validated, and personnel are trained. After a system is established, routine maintenance procedures are performed to ensure the ongoing operation of the system.

### Standard Operating Procedures

Written procedures for every blood bank operation are required by all regulatory and accreditation agencies, and computer operations are no exception. The computer-related tasks associated with each of the blood bank's technical operations can be incorporated into each technical procedure or can be addressed in a separate section of the procedures manual. In addition, there are a number of computer-specific standard operating procedures that must also be available. The subjects of these are included in the following discussions.

### Archiving Data

As the system's databases grow in size, the hard disk becomes crowded with this stored information. As a result, the response time of the computer reaches an undesirably slow pace, and the hard disk is no longer able to store new data. When this happens, additional hard disks may be added to the system, or old data may be removed from the hard disk and placed in archival storage. Removing old data frees up space on the hard disk so that new data can be placed on it. Old data may be archived to long-term storage media as such as tape, disk, microfiche, or even paper. A procedure for periodic assessment of hard disk space should be instituted so that data can be archived in an orderly fashion before the hard disk becomes full. Procedures for archiving must also be written and should adhere to applicable regulatory and standard-setting agency requirements for data retention. For example, AABB Standards require that each donor's ABO group and Rh type be retained for a minimum of 5 years, and patient records of adverse reactions to transfusion must be retained indefinitely. Written procedures for retrieval of archived data must ensure that records can be retrieved within a reasonable period of time to maintain patient care.

### Backup of Software Programs and Data

Blood banks have come to depend heavily on their information systems, but it must be realized that they are not infallible. Unexpected, and sometimes inexplicable, failures of software or hardware can occur. Worse, a natural disaster such as a fire or flood can destroy parts or all of an information system. Software and databases should be routinely copied to some storage medium, such as tape or another set of disks. The copies can then be used to restore any corrupted or lost information. The frequency with which this backup routine is performed depends on an individual blood bank's data volume and the recommendations of the software vendor. The copies should be stored in a safe location separate from the information system so that they will not be affected by disastrous events such as fire or flooding. There should also be a procedure to identify and restore any information that was not included in the backup copies. This can be done by manually reentering data that was input between the time of the most recent backup and the disaster.

### Computer Downtime

Every computer system, at some period, experiences downtime. Sometimes the downtime is planned, as when the system must undergo maintenance procedures, system backup, or software enhancement. Other downtimes are unplanned and usually unpleasant, because the system is experiencing some difficulty such as a power outage. In either case, there must be a written procedure that will allow blood bank operations to continue. The procedure must address the need for historical patient and donor data as well as systems for recording new data obtained during the downtime. Transfusion service staff must be able to compare current patient test results with previous records before blood components are issued. Donor center staff must have access to permanently deferred donor files. This essential data may be in the form of paper records or may be available to personnel on a PC where the information has been previously downloaded from the blood bank information system. New data generated during downtime—such as test results, blood donations, and distribution or issuance of blood products—can be recorded on hard copy worksheets or forms and then "backloaded" into the computer when it becomes functional.

### Hardware Maintenance

Information system hardware, like all pieces of equipment, requires periodic cleaning, lubrication, and replacement of parts to ensure continued operation. Maintenance procedures usually require that the system be "taken down" or turned off for a period of time. For that reason, regular maintenance procedures should be scheduled and posted so that blood bank staff members can prepare for the downtime. When possible, maintenance should be scheduled to minimize interruption of service, such as during usual periods of low activity.

As the system's databases grow in size, the response time of the computer may reach an undesirably slow pace. Procedures should be established for removing the data from the disk. The software will contain programs for purging and archiving older data. Vendors may also offer support services that can examine the system disk(s) to identify potential problems.

## Maintenance of Security

A procedure for adding users to a system must be established, including the basis on which security levels will be assigned. For example, the list of functions or applications to which a user will have access can be created for each job description. It is also important to have a method for deleting the access codes of users who leave the facility. An additional level of security can be obtained by requiring users to periodically change their passwords; many security applications can be programmed to require this at specified intervals.

## Tracking and Correction of Errors

Error management, required by regulatory and accrediting agencies, has become an integral part of blood bank operations. It includes detection, documentation, investigation, implementation of corrective actions, and reporting to appropriate agencies. Errors in the operation of a blood bank information system may be caused by inadequate training, incomplete or cumbersome written procedures, or system problems. In any case, tracking and categorization of errors is essential if corrective actions are to be taken. Identified information system problems should be reported to the software vendor so that other users can be notified and remedies can be included in a future software revision.

## Training of Personnel

The most elegant and user-friendly information system can be a disaster if staff members are inadequately trained in its use. Training programs should address every function and procedure that each user will be expected to perform. Flowcharts and checklists are useful training tools. Training modules can be designed that will present users with the situations that they will encounter in their work. The competence of each staff person must be documented before allowing routine use of the computer. Competence assessment methods can include direct observation, review of system-generated records, and written examinations. Once initial competence has been demonstrated, an ongoing program of periodic assessment must be established to document the continued competence of blood bank staff to use the information system appropriately. As

previously discussed, it is most beneficial to allow users access to a test database for training purposes. If one is not available, "test data" can be used in the production database.

## Validation of Software

Software validation is the establishment of documented evidence, which provides a high degree of assurance that the system will consistently function as expected. It is the responsibility of the software vendor to validate, to the extent possible, the functionality of a software product before it is marketed to blood banks. However, software vendors cannot simulate the conditions under which each system will be used. Differences in environment, hardware, databases, standard operating procedures, and people require that each blood bank perform on-site validation testing to prove that the system will perform appropriately under those unique conditions.

Validation testing must be performed before a new system can be implemented and whenever new software, databases, or hardware is added to the system. When validation is to be performed on an existing system, the testing should be done in the test database, where it will not affect the production data.

## Test Plan

Proper validation of the system requires careful planning. Each system function that the blood bank will use must be included in the test plan. A test plan should be created for each function or operation that the computer will perform. Test plans should include the following items:

Control functions
Data entry methods (keyboard, bar code reader, instrument interface, LIS, or HIS interface)
Specific test cases
Documentation methods
Acceptance criteria (expected outputs)
Result review
Corrective action (if necessary)
Acceptance

Most of these items will be different in each of the system's applications, so a separate test plan for each application may be necessary. Control functions should be defined by the vendor, but data entry methods will be selected by the user; some applications may have multiple data entry methods. Specific tests cases are discussed below. Screen printouts, written logs, or printed reports can be used to document the testing. After the testing is completed, the results should be compared with the acceptance criteria to determine acceptability. If unacceptable results are obtained, they should be investigated, and corrective action should be implemented. When corrective action is necessary, testing should be repeated until it is found acceptable.

## Test Cases

The validation test cases include the specific steps to be followed by those performing the testing. Test cases should assess the system under normal operating conditions but must also offer challenges to the system. The goal is to make sure that the system repeatedly performs intended functions and does not perform unintended functions. The types of testing that should be performed are normal, boundary, invalid, special, and stress cases.

1. Normal testing uses typical blood bank inputs to produce normal, or routine, outputs.
2. Boundary testing involves forcing the system to evaluate data that are slightly below or slightly above valid ranges. This kind of testing might be used for disease test results.
3. Invalid test cases assess the system's ability to recognize and to reject incorrect inputs. Examples of invalid inputs include entry of Q for an ABO interpretation or entry of a blood product code that has not been defined in the static database file.
4. Special cases are those that make the system react to unusual inputs. A special case could be designed to see how the system responds when more than one person attempts to add or edit special transfusion instructions in the same patient's record.

5. Stress testing involves pushing the system to its physical limits. This might be accomplished by allowing large volumes of data to be entered into the system via all available input devices.

Not every type of test case may be appropriate for each function to be tested. For example, boundary test cases will probably not be applicable in a donor registration function. Another kind of validation testing is parallel testing. This involves running two systems in parallel and comparing the outputs of both. For a blood bank switching from a manual to a computerized system, every procedure would be performed manually and in the computer.

Validation of a blood bank information system is a very lengthy and labor-intensive process, but it provides great benefits if undertaken in a thorough manner. Extensive testing will identify potential problems in the way that the blood bank intends to use the system. Sometimes workarounds have to be created, but when it is done as part of validation testing, staff members can be properly trained before going "live" on the new system or software. The creation and performance of comprehensive and detailed validation test cases require allocation of significant resources to the project, but the end result, a well-validated blood bank information system, is well worth the resource costs.

## SUMMARY CHART: IMPORTANT POINTS TO REMEMBER (MT/SBB)

- Blood bank information systems assist in the management of data and can allow tracing of a blood component through all processing steps from donation through transfusion (final disposition).
- A computer system is composed of three main components: hardware, software, and people.
- Hardware components perform functions related to input and output, processing, and storage of data.
- Software tells the computer what to do with the information it has received.
- Application software allows users to perform tasks that are specific to blood bank operations.
- Donor, patient, and blood component information is maintained in databases, which are divided into files and further subdivided into individual records.
- Static database files define the terminology that the blood bank will use and provides a dictionary of coded terms that the system can use to sort data.
- Operating system software controls the hardware, manipulates the application software, and coordinates the flow of information between the disks and memory.
- The system manager oversees the maintenance of the system's hardware and software, including adding or deleting items from the static database files, assigning access codes to new users, implementing software upgrades from the vendor, and investigating and reporting problems encountered by the users.

- A blood bank information system can have numerous specific applications related to the management of donors, patients, and blood components.
- User codes and passwords prevent unauthorized use of the system and provide a means for capturing the identity of each person who performs a task in the information system.
- Control functions assist in making decisions at critical points in the selection of donors and release of blood components for transfusion.
- When results must be corrected or amended, they must be clearly designated as such on printed reports and monitor displays used by patient caregivers.
- A blood bank must have documented evidence of validation of its system as well as written procedures for all aspects of system management to comply with regulatory and accreditation requirements.
- Blood bank SOPs must address computer tasks related to blood bank technical duties, as well as computer-specific procedures such as computer downtime, backup of software programs and data, system maintenance, security, error management, and personnel training.
- On-site software validation must provide documented evidence that provides a high degree of assurance that the system will function consistently as expected under the unique combination of hardware, databases, environment, SOPs, and people that exist at the site.

## REVIEW QUESTIONS

1. Components of an information system consist of all of the following except:
   A. Hardware
   B. Software
   C. Validation
   D. People

2. Compliance with regulatory and accreditation agency requirements for blood bank information systems requires blood banks to maintain standard operating procedures for all of the following except:
   A. Vendor validation testing
   B. Computer downtime
   C. System maintenance
   D. Personnel training

3. A validation test case that assesses the system's ability to recognize an erroneous input is called:
   A. Normal

   B. Boundary
   C. Stress
   D. Invalid

4. An example of interface software functionality is:
   A. The entry of blood components into the blood bank database
   B. The transmission of patient information from the HIS into the blood bank system
   C. The printing of a workload report
   D. Preventing access to the system by an unauthorized user

5. Backup copies of the information system:
   A. Can be used to restore the information system data and software if the production system is damaged
   B. Are used to maintain hardware components
   C. Are performed once a month
   D. Are created any time changes are made to the system

6. User passwords should be:
   A. Shared with others
   B. Kept confidential
   C. Posted at each terminal
   D. Never changed

7. The prevention of the issue of an incompatible blood component is an example of:
   A. Inventory management
   B. Utilization review
   C. System security
   D. Control function

8. Information is stored in a collection of many different files called the:
   A. Database
   B. Configuration
   C. Hardware
   D. Disk drive

9. Application software communicates with this type of software to retrieve data from the system disks:
   A. Interface
   B. Operating system
   C. Security
   D. Program

10. Validation testing for software should consider all of the following items except:
    A. Data entry methods
    B. Control functions
    C. Performance of testing in production database
    D. Invalid data

## ANSWERS TO REVIEW QUESTIONS

1. C (p 521)

2. A (p 530)

3. D (p 532)

4. B (p 523)

5. A (p 530)

6. B (p 531)

7. D (p 528)

8. A (p 523)

9. B (p 524)

10. C (p 532)

## BIBLIOGRAPHY

American Association of Blood Banks: Blood Bank/Transfusion Service Computer Systems User Validation Guidelines. Association Bulletin #93-2, August 27, 1993.

Butch, SH: Computer software quality assurance. Lab Med 22:18, 1991.

Butch, SH, et al: Electronic verification of donor-recipient compatibility: The computer crossmatch. Transfusion 34:105–109, 1994.

Butch, SH, and Judd, WJ: Letter to the editor. Transfusion 34:187, 1994.

Food and Drug Administration: Recommendation for implementation of computerization in blood establishments: Memo to all registered blood establishments, April 6, 1988.

Food and Drug Administration: Requirements for computerization of blood establishments: Memo to all registered blood establishments, September 8, 1989.

Food and Drug Administration: Draft guideline for the validation of blood establishment computer systems, September 28, 1993.

Food and Drug Administration: Guideline for quality assurance in blood establishments, July 11, 1995.

Hoffstadter, LK: Blood Bank Information Systems. Lab Med 25:110–117, 1994.

Leavitt, J, and Smith, LE (directors): Administrative workshop on quality assurance and the blood bank computer system. American Association of Blood Banks annual meeting, San Diego, November 1994.

Responsibilities in Implementing and Using a Blood Bank Computer System. American Association of Blood Banks. Washington, DC, 1989.

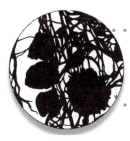

CHAPTER **26**

# MEDICOLEGAL AND ETHICAL ASPECTS OF PROVIDING TRANSFUSION SERVICES

Kathleen Sazama, MD, JD, MS, MT(ASCP)

## OBJECTIVES

*On completion of this chapter, the learner should be able to:*

1 Understand the legal and ethical implications of providing transfusion services.

2 Discuss the legal bases for liability for providing transfusion medicine services.

3 Define the necessity for establishing and following standard operating procedures similar to those of other comparable facilities throughout the United States.

4 Identify and list the evolving legal and ethical concerns likely to accompany the increasing complexity of providing blood during the late 1990s.

5 List the two reasons why patients sue for transfusion injury.

6 List the steps that blood bank professionals can take to avoid litigation.

7 Describe the legal issues related to transfusion-transmitted diseases in laboratory medicine.

## INTRODUCTION

Legal issues involving transfusion medicine in the late 1990s center around transfusion-transmitted viruses, including transfusion-transmitted acquired immunodeficiency syndrome (TTAIDS), first reported in 1982, and the hepatitis viruses, especially hepatitis C (HCV), first identified in 1989. Legal issues also concern transfusion indications, informed consent, and other medically relevant topics. However, even before TTAIDS became the basis for numerous lawsuits (probably more than 800 since 1985) against blood centers, hospitals, and physicians, there was litigation because of death and serious injury caused by transfusion-transmitted hepatitis B virus (HBV)* (*Perlmutter v. Beth David Hospital*, 308 NY 100, 123 N.E.2d 792 [1954]) and a few because of donor injury.[1] The HBV cases stimulated nearly every state legislature to enact protection for blood banks through "blood shield statutes."[2] (California was the first state to enact such protection for blood banks in 1955. Only New Jersey lacks such a law, but it provides similar protection solely through judicial decisions.) Because of these blood shield statutes, most of which extended protection without amendment or modification for TTAIDS as well as for HBV, many TTAIDS lawsuits have been either dismissed or unsuccessful for the person suing (the plaintiff). Recently, however, this premise has come under new challenge in the courts. In addition, because most TTAIDS cases have been unsuccessful in compensating plaintiffs (usually patients or their families), new theories of liability are increasingly being raised. When questions of appropriateness of transfusion, availability of blood

components, and informed consent arise, the ethical bases of transfusion medicine practice are more sharply focused.

Although blood shield statutes generally protect against application of strict liability, tort liability remains the basis for most lawsuits. In this chapter, after a brief discussion of sources of law, theories of liability are discussed with practical hints for reducing likelihood of being found liable, when possible. Emerging concerns for the twenty-first century are also identified. This chapter is not intended as a substitute for legal advice, which is necessary in particular situations; rather, it is intended to provide the reader with some general principles and definitions so that ethically and legally sound practices continue within transfusion medicine.

## SOURCES OF LAW

Laws are created by society through legislation called statutes (passed by either the U.S. Congress or by individual state legislatures) or by court decisions (in federal courts, including the U.S. Supreme Court, or in state courts through their own highest state court).

### Statutes and Regulations

Frequently, federal law (enacted by Congress or by decision in federal courts, including the Supreme Court) supersedes state law, but both can be and often are applied in particular instances. The details of how laws are to be put into action are provided in regulations. Regulations, both federal and state, can be applied only if they have been established according to a formal process called the Administrative Procedure Act (APA).[3] Federal regulations that apply specifically to blood banking are found in the Title 21, Code of Federal Regulations, parts 600–699 and, to some extent, in parts 200–299, published annually on April 1.[4] Blood banks are also federally regulated by provisions of the Clinical Laboratories Improvement Act of 1988 and the Medicare provisions of the Social Security Act.

State legislatures also enact laws and publish explanatory regulations about blood banking, clinical laboratories, and transfusion practices, principally covering licensure of facilities and personnel.

### Case Law

Law is also established by court decisions, sometimes related to interpretations and applications of statutes and regulations. Patients generally believe that medical treatment administered to them (it is hoped with their consent) will, on balance, be beneficial.

---

*The court decided that transactions involving blood were not sales but were incidental to the provision of medical services. The effect of this decision was to preclude application of commercial law, particularly that of warranties, to blood transfusions.

When transfusion causes harm (e.g., through TTAIDS, HBV, or HCV), patients have understandably reacted by seeking redress in the courts. The legal bases for such suits are generally civil (not criminal) actions for tort.

United States civil law depends on each adult person in our society behaving reasonably (i.e., not negligently and not aggressively) toward every other person, respecting other people's rights. Civil lawsuits arise because someone disrespects another's rights by (1) striking or threatening to strike another person (battery and assault), (2) being careless or reckless (negligence), (3) failing to complete an agreement (breach of contract), (4) intruding on another's property or privacy, or (5) misbehaving in other similar ways. Civil suits can also arise because of violation of specific statutes or regulations that require certain types of actions.

## BASIS OF LIABILITY: TORTS

### Intentional Tort of Battery

Any unconsented touching (including deliberate blows and intentional striking) is legally defined as battery. For transfusion medicine, this concept is used when a donor or a patient claims that he or she never agreed to have the needle placed in his or her arm.

### Doctrine of Informed Consent

Particularly in the special circumstances of the practice of medicine, the issue of whether a patient (or, in the case of a blood collection organization, a donor) agreed to undergo the procedure actually performed with full knowledge of the possible benefits, alternatives, and harm that may accompany it has come to be known as the doctrine of informed consent. This doctrine protects the patient (or donor) by requiring that information be provided in a manner understandable to the patient under circumstances that permit the patient to ask questions and to receive answers to any questions or concerns he or she may have (*Canterbury v. Spence*, 464 F.2d 772 [DC Cir 1972]).

For TTAIDS transfusion recipients, this issue first came into sharp focus in the case of *Kozup v. Georgetown University*, 663 F. Supp. 1048 (DC 1987), 851 F.2d 437 (DC Cir 1988), 906 F.2d 783 (DC Cir 1990). In this case, an infant brought by his parents to Georgetown University Hospital for medical care contracted TTAIDS and died. His parents argued that they were insufficiently informed about the harm of the transfusions and did not specifically agree to transfusions as part of the care given their child. The District of Columbia court ruled that their actions in bringing the child to the hospital and not objecting to transfusions at the time of infusion amounted to tacit consent. The issue of whether specific consent is required for transfusion and who should obtain such consent (generally physicians have been held responsible [*Ritter v. Delaney*, 790 S.W.2d 29 (Tex. App.-San Antonio, 1990) and *Howell v.

*Spokane*, 785 P.2d 815 (Wash. 1990)]) remains controversial (*Hoemke v. New York Blood Center*, 90-7182 [2d Cir. 1990] and *Gibson v. Methodist Hospital*, 01-89-00645-CV [Tex. Ct. App. 1991]). However, in 1996, the Joint Commission on Accreditation of Healthcare Organizations (JCAHO) specifically required hospitals to obtain informed consent for transfusion in some situations.[5]

Another arena in which the doctrine of informed consent is the key to resolving disputes is that of donor rights. With the onset of AIDS, the language of donor histories has been subjected to continuing revision and updating to include information about the disease, how it is acquired, and under what circumstances a person should donate blood. Federal and voluntary requirements for the way in which the history is obtained have emphasized more face-to-face oral questioning, not just self-administration of these questionnaires. One part of the donation process has always been for donors to sign a statement of consent to donate.

Until the late 1980s, donors were protected from subpoena in cases of transfusion-transmitted diseases. However, an increasing number of plaintiffs in state courts are insisting that the donor be subject to questioning regarding his or her donation. This questioning may completely or partially protect a donor's identity or may require that donor to appear in open court. Because no one donates blood expecting to have to defend that altruistic act at some future date, the impact of these decisions on the future availability of blood for transfusion is uncertain.

### Intentional Infliction of Emotional Distress

As the phrase suggests, a plaintiff must show that what the defendant did to cause actual and severe emotional distress was intentional, usually some extreme or outrageous conduct that was calculated to deliberately cause real harm to the plaintiff. This can take the form of a claim for wrongful death of the plaintiff's relative, particularly in some TTAIDS cases.

### Negligence

#### Elements

Liability for negligence is found when all of the following factors are satisfied:

1. A duty was owed to the injured party.
2. The duty was not met by the injuring party.
3. Because the duty was not met, the injured party was harmed.
4. Failure to meet the duty owed was directly responsible for or could have been predicted to cause the harm suffered by the injured party.
5. Some measurable (compensable) harm (called "damages") occurred. (Table 26–1)

To be successful in a negligence action, the plaintiff has the responsibility to prove all these factors against the person being sued (the defendant).

**Table 26–1.** Elements of Negligence

Duty owed
Breach of duty
Causation
Damages

### Standard of Care

When the negligence involves ordinary things that everyone encounters (e.g., injuries caused by traffic accidents), a jury (or judge) can consider the facts and decide whether the behavior of the defendant was reasonable; that is, did the defendant meet the standard of care required in the situation? For ordinary or usual negligence, this standard of care depends only on what the average person (e.g., a juror) believes is acceptable in our society. That is, the jury decides whether a reasonable person, in the same circumstances as the defendant, would have acted the same way as or differently from the way the defendant did. If the defendant acted reasonably in the circumstances, the plaintiff will be unsuccessful in the lawsuit and vice versa.

In situations in which larger organizations are involved, the question of who is liable for the actions of employees has been resolved under the doctrine of *respondeat superior*. Under this doctrine, the actions of employees are attributable to the employer or person who directs their actions. This responsible person for transfusion services has been defined by federal regulation and general practice to be a physician, a definition that has been reinforced by judicial decision in many states for blood centers as well as for hospitals. The advantage of having a physician as the responsible employer is that the principles and regulations related to medical malpractice usually apply, including the requirement for establishing a professional standard of care.

**Professional Standard of Care.** When the negligence lawsuit involves professionals such as physicians and scientists, including laboratory professionals, nurses, or other allied health practitioners, the definition of what is reasonable, the "standard of care," depends on expert testimony from other physicians or scientists about what should have been done by other reasonable practitioners (usually of the same specialty). The law makes an extra requirement; that is, that in discharging his or her duty to the plaintiff, the defendant apply the special knowledge and ability he or she possesses by virtue of the profession. This increased "professional standard of care" is not just what the judge or jury would have done but what other professionals (so-called expert witnesses) testify should have been done. The judge or jury is not permitted to decide what they would have done but must depend upon testimony by expert witnesses of the same profession as the defendant who define what that reasonable professional standard of care is. For the complex scientific, technical, and medical issues involved in

TTAIDS litigation, this distinction has been a key element in protecting blood bankers.

### Voluntary and Mandatory Standards

The testimony of experts should generally be supportable by authorities such as statutes, regulations, or other bodies of published knowledge, including published scientific articles and texts. The existence of voluntary standards—particularly those provided by the American Association of Blood Banks (AABB)[6] but also those from the College of American Pathologists, the American Association of Tissue Banks, the American Society for Histocompatibility and Immunogenetics, the Joint Commission on Accreditation of Healthcare Organizations, and other organizations—are helpful in establishing the professional standard of practice for transfusion medicine. In fact, some state and federal regulations cross-reference the AABB standards specifically. Blood bankers and transfusion services that can show that they acted in conformance with these standards are more likely to be found nonnegligent than those who do not follow such guidelines. This safeguard is now being challenged in several states.

### Is Blood Banking a Medical Profession?

The question of whether blood banking is a medical profession is being relitigated in courts today, with conflicting results.[7] One possible chilling result is that collecting, processing, and distributing of blood may be considered differently from the crossmatching, issuance, and transfusion of blood to individual patients. Redefining blood banking as *not* medical practice removes the extra protection provided by the requirement for expert medical testimony to establish the standard of care, leaving defendants to be judged by the ordinary negligence standard. There is little dispute that loss of medical professional stature would significantly alter the practice of blood banking. None of the protections of medical malpractice reform would be available, and blood centers may even find themselves subject to strict liability.

---

**CASE 1**

A 26-year-old woman is critically injured in a two-car collision. She is rushed via helicopter to the nearest trauma center, where 10 units of uncrossmatched O-negative red blood cells, 12 units of crossmatch-compatible A-negative red blood cells, 4 apheresis platelet packs, and 8 units of fresh frozen plasma are administered within the first 24 hours of her care. Soon after her admission, she is taken to the operating room, where splenectomy is performed, liver and left kidney lacerations are repaired, numerous fractures of both lower extremities are reset, and a chest tube is placed for a collapsed left lung. She requires only 4 more units of packed red blood cells during the next several days and recovers sufficiently to be discharged home to recuperate 15 days after the accident. Two years later, during her first prenatal visit for a second pregnancy, she tests positive for HIV. Two weeks later she is told by her obstetrician that the blood center reported that one of the units she received came from a donor who recently had tested positive for HIV.

### Questions:

1. Was the blood center negligent?

2. Was the physician who transfused the patient negligent?

3. Would using an "ordinary" versus a "professional" standard of care yield a different answer?

### Strict Liability

Manufacturers and distributors of goods used in everyday life have been defined by law to have certain responsibilities in their activities to protect consumers. Among other requirements, there are certain warranties that the product you buy—for example, a television set—will actually work and will continue to do so for some fixed period of time, with small risk of harm to you from such things as electric shock or blowing up. These warranties, actual or implied, exist for virtually anything a consumer buys and uses. If a product fails to perform as expected or creates harm when none was expected, the consumer has the right to have a replacement or, if the manufacturer denies responsibility, to sue for negligent manufacturing or distribution.

In addition, for some items (such as dynamite), the danger from proper use is so great that manufacturers are legally liable for *all* harm that occurs, "strict" liability. This means that anyone who is harmed when properly using dynamite does not have to prove that the manufacturer or distributor was negligent; he or she has only to show that he or she was injured while properly using it. Imagine how rare and expensive blood transfusions would become if these theories were allowed to be applied. Instead, states enacted specific protection, the blood shield statutes described previously, to exclude harm from blood transfusions from suit under these legal theories. It is important that blood bankers avoid implying or stating that blood transfusion is completely safe, because such statements may be construed as creating a warranty, invoking these theories of liability.

### Invasion of Privacy

Healthcare providers, including blood bankers, are required to respect personal privacy and to maintain patient and donor confidentiality. Plaintiffs may claim remuneration for loss of privacy under four theories:

1. Intrusion upon plaintiff's seclusion or solitude or into his or her private affairs

2. Public disclosure of embarrassing facts

3. Placing plaintiff in a "false light" in public

4. Appropriation of plaintiff's name or likeness for defendant's benefit

These categories protect a patient or donor from illegal or inadvertent disclosure of his or her personal information, of particular concern with HIV because of the lack of appropriate safeguards to prevent loss of employment, housing, insurance, and other benefits of society. When information is exciting or noteworthy, the media may become aware of and publish private information. Blood banks and transfusion services will be involved in such suits if they are responsible (through negligence or by intention) for release of the data. Great care should be exercised by blood banking professionals to ensure that private information (whether about donors, patients, or relatives) be kept confidential and not released without written authorization. Procedures to safeguard such release should include proper use of copying and facsimile machines as well as direct electronic transfer via information systems.

### CASE 2

A 32-year-old male multitime blood donor is found to test positive for HIV p24 antigen and for antibodies to HIV, having been repeatedly tested negative on prior donations. Before confirmatory testing is completed, he returns to the blood collection center to donate HLA-matched platelets. Before questioning begins, the registering staff person notices that his prior record indicates his deferral status. She informs the donor that he is not eligible to donate the platelets. The donor is shocked and embarrassed by the news and storms out of the center. Two weeks later, the donor sues the blood center for intentional infliction of emotional distress.

### Questions

1. Is the donor likely to be successful?

2. Are there other bases on which suit can be brought?

3. Are there established standards for preventing such an occurrence?

## RESTRICTIONS ON PLAINTIFF SUITS AND RECOVERY

### Statutes of Limitations

Some protection arises because of a statutorily defined limit of time during which a lawsuit can be filed. States often have different limits, depending on the legal requirements for initiating suits. Statutes of limitations for medical malpractice are generally shorter (approximately 2 years from the date that the injury should have been discovered in adults) than limitations for other kinds of negligence (2 to 6 years is common).

## Doctrine of Charitable Immunity

Historically, courts provided immunity for nonprofit organizations such as hospitals from excess liability because they performed charitable acts. Many state legislatures have enacted and continue to support statutes to provide protection for boards of directors and/or volunteers using this common law rationale. A recent decision in New Jersey is redefining the protection (*Snyder v. AABB*, 144 N.J. 269 [1996]). However, many healthcare institutions rely less on this doctrine and more on insurance for protection.

## Tort Reform

State legislatures, recognizing the need to protect some specialties such as obstetrics, have been active in seeking limits on damages against physicians, protecting them from abusive litigation. For transfusion practices, it is vital that these protections be afforded.

## RISK MANAGEMENT AND QUALITY PERFORMANCE

Avoiding liability for TTAIDS and other possible harm from practicing transfusion medicine, whether in hospitals or blood centers, depends on having well-established policies and procedures that comply with recognized authorities, regulations, and statutes and having some measurement of how persons engaged in all activities actually follow those procedures. To avoid being negligent, one must behave reasonably. Reasonable behavior for transfusion medicine practice includes continually obtaining and applying new knowledge from all possible sources that will safeguard the donor during collection, the component during handling and delivery, and the patient before and during transfusion.

## Donor Issues

### Screening

What the AIDS epidemic has taught us is that every person who volunteers to donate does not have an unqualified right to do so. In fact, for several years before March 1985, when a test for HIV in blood was first available, the best safeguard against TTAIDS was improved donor education and more pertinent questioning regarding behaviors that might put that donor at risk for acquiring HIV. Although numerous lawsuits have been filed against blood collection agencies for improper donor screening, few have been successful when collecting facilities could show that they had written procedures and properly trained employees who followed those procedures and that proper docu-

mentation of each screen occurred. Problems occurred only when breaches in procedure, typically failures to follow or to properly document actual practice, were discovered. However, with several state courts now demanding release of donor identity or access to donor for questioning, further attention to the process of donor screening, including consideration of adding information for donors that they may be subject to subpoena if transfusion harm occurs, is required. Balancing the real threat of lack of availability of blood with the serious nature of litigation related to TTAIDS or transfusion-transmitted hepatitis will continue to challenge blood banking professionals.

### Donations Requested by Patients

Several monetary settlements in the range of hundreds of thousands to millions of dollars have resulted from either failing to offer directed donor services or from improperly characterizing them.

### Untimely Notification

When recipients received notification years after blood centers knew (or should have known) the recipient had received an HIV-reactive unit, many of them or their families were angry enough to file suit on the basis that they should have been informed sooner. Procedures for lookback and recipient notification were not well established for several years following application of specific testing in most blood collection organizations until 1996, when the U.S. government, through HCFA and FDA, issued specific regulations for HIV lookback notification by hospitals.

---

**CASE 3**

A 67-year-old woman crippled by degenerative arthritis requests that her own blood and blood from members of her family be used during her hip replacement surgery. The blood center describes its donation procedures, which do not permit directed donations. Although she is disappointed, she agrees to donate for herself. When her first unit is tested, it is repeat reactive for HBsAg. The patient-donor is advised that she may no longer donate and that the unit she has already donated will not be available for her surgery. Surgery proceeds. She receives 4 units of volunteer blood and develops AIDS 3 years later. She sues the blood-collecting organization.

**Questions**

1. On what legal grounds can this suit be brought?

2. What is the current standard of care regarding directed donations?

3. Can healthcare organizations deny autologous donor-patients access to their own test-reactive blood?

### Component Collection

Occasionally lawsuits have occurred from injury to donors during the collection process. Generally, the injuries are more severe than a simple bruise at the needle site and involve such things as nerve damage, slip-and-fall incidents, and severe reactions. The continuing problem of microbial contamination during collection, although infrequently litigated, remains a more serious concern. Although donor deaths continue to be reported at a rate of approximately two per year, these infrequently result in litigation.

## Processing, Labeling, and Distribution

### No Standard Protocol for Implementing Testing

Several successful TTAIDS lawsuits awarded millions of dollars against blood-collecting organizations (*Belle Bonfils Memorial Blood Bank v. Denver District Court*, 723 P.2d 1003 [Colo. 1988]) because they had no standard protocol for implementing new testing to ensure that all available components (including those distributed or in active inventory) were test-negative before transfusion, once the test kits and equipment was received by the collection facility. The lack of a written plan to implement such testing, including training of personnel, validating instrumentation and reagents, and establishing the necessary information service support, was seen as negligent by the jury (even *with* expert testimony to the contrary).

### Failure to Perform Surrogate Testing

Despite concerted efforts, rarely has a plaintiff prevailed when alleging that blood collection facilities should have performed more or different surrogate tests between 1983 and 1985, when a specific test was first available (*Baker v. JK and Susie Wadley Research Institutes and Blood Bank, dba The Blood Center at Wadley*, 86-2728-C [Tex. Jud. Dist. Ct. 1988] and *Clark v. United Blood Services*, CV 88-6981 [Nev. 2d Jud. Dist. Ct. 1990]).

### Failure to Properly Perform Testing

Testing personnel should be constantly alert to proper performance and documentation of all required testing of blood components. Failure to document is as damning as failure to perform at all and must be avoided. Considerable effort has been expended by the U.S. FDA to inform and to enforce requirements for proper testing for virally transmissible diseases in blood components. Private accrediting organizations, likewise, emphasize proper performance and documentation of these activities.

### Informed Consent

In TTAIDS cases arising in the early 1980s, it was frequently alleged that patients were insufficiently warned of the hazards of transfusion because transfusion experts failed to warn hospitals and ordering physicians about them. Few cases were successful because the state of scientific knowledge, established by expert testimony relying on published data, was limited. Also, the early HBV cases had established a record that supported the defense position that transfusions were already known by hospitals and other physicians to be unavoidably unsafe, particularly for transfusion-transmitted viral diseases. Some states (e.g., California) enacted specific legislation about informed consent for transfusion.

## Medical Malpractice

Several multimillion dollar suits, decided for the plaintiff, resulted from successful allegations that either the patient did not need a transfusion at all, could have waited until test-negative blood was available before receiving a transfusion, or required transfusion solely because of something the physician did. In all these cases, the basis for fault was negligence by the treating physician.

---

### CASE 4

A 43-year-old man received a 1-unit transfusion of red blood cells during an emergency coronary artery bypass operation. Three years later, just before his second marriage, he was found to be HIV-positive. He sued his cardiologist and the blood center.

#### Question

1. Which issues are likely to be successful for this plaintiff?

2. Would the result be different if ordinary rather than professional standard of care was applied?

---

## ETHICS AND TRANSFUSION MEDICINE

Biomedical ethical principles that must be balanced when considering appropriateness of and informed consent for transfusion include autonomy, beneficence, and justice (Table 26–2). In transfusion medicine, autonomy is increasingly important as patients become aware of the harm, as well as the benefit, of transfusions and insist on the right to choose the type of therapy and the source of the blood they receive. Autonomy is not unrestricted, but it must form part of the healthcare relationship. When transfusions are offered, patients expect that the treatment will benefit them. When the benefit is marginal or even questionable, and particularly if something harmful occurs, the decision of the healthcare professional may be challenged both legally and ethically. Fortunately, there are only rare instances in which transfusions are inequitably distributed, generally because of shortage of collections. In

**Table 26–2.** Ethical Principles

**Autonomy**

The right of each person to make decisions based on that person's values and beliefs, having adequate information and an understanding of the choices available to him or her, and lacking any compulsion by external or internal forces.

**Beneficence**

In the healthcare setting, professionals seek the well-being of each patient.

**Justice**

Patients should be treated fairly, with equal, need-based access to beneficial treatment.

times of blood shortages, rationing begins with canceling of elective surgical procedures for which transfusion may be indicated and rarely reaches a point at which emergency needs are compromised. An example of balancing ethical principles that has caused legal action is when patients have suffered serious or fatal consequences and were denied access to a choice of donating for themselves or selecting their own blood donors from among family members, church or social groups, or coworkers.

## EMERGING ISSUES

In addition to the concerns listed previously, there are new ones surrounding changing practices of transfusion medicine, such as responsibilities for out-of-hospital (specifically at home) transfusions, issues surrounding provision of autologous services (crossover of unused units, transfusion of reactive components, freezing of unused reactive units, informed consent, etc.), new therapies such as red blood cell substitutes and use of recombinant erythropoietin, standards for provision of perioperative blood collection and reinfusion, and control over use of gene therapy to treat certain transfusion-dependent illnesses. In the TTAIDS area, suits have been filed for reporting false AIDS test results and for fear of AIDS because of exposure through transfusion or via a healthcare worker, plus ongoing concerns over handling of lookback. New concerns about bacterial contamination, fueled by the still-unexplained upsurge in *Yersinia* growth in red blood cells, and newer issues surrounding hepatitis C and other non-A, non-B hepatitis viruses will surface.

## CONCLUSIONS

The lessons learned from transfusion-related litigation underscore the fact that every blood bank/transfusion service needs complete, comprehensive, and current written procedures and policies. When such procedures and policies conform to federal and state statutes and regulations as well as meet private voluntary standards, such as those of the CAP, AABB, JCAHO, the organization can have a higher assurance that it will meet the standard of care required to avoid being found negligent and thus liable for the damages the patient or donor suffered. Patients are demanding on ethical grounds the right to have greater control over the use of human blood for treatment, including appropriate informed consent. Pending and future issues will redefine the legal and ethical aspects of transfusion medicine.

---

## SUMMARY CHART: IMPORTANT POINTS TO REMEMBER (MT/MLT)

- Tort liability is the basis for most lawsuits.
- Federal regulations that apply specifically to blood banking are found in Title 21, Code of Federal Regulations.
- Intentional tort of battery is used in transfusion medicine when a donor or a patient claims that he or she never agreed to have the needle placed into his or her arm.
- The Doctrine of Informed Consent protects the patient (or donor) by requiring that information be provided in a manner understandable to the patient under circumstances that permit the patient to ask questions and to receive answers to any questions or concerns.
- The elements of negligence include (1) a duty was owed to the injured party; (2) the duty was not met by the injuring party; (3) because the duty was not met, the injured party was harmed; (4) failure to meet the duty owed was directly responsible for or could have been predicted to cause the harm suffered by the injured party; (5) some measurable (compensable) harm occurred (damages).

- Under the Doctrine of Respondeat Superior the actions of employees are attributable to the employer or person who directs their actions; that is, in transfusion medicine, a physician.
- The concept of strict liability implies that a warranty exists for virtually any product a consumer buys, and if the product fails to perform or creates harm when none was expected, the consumer has a right to a replacement or, if denied a replacement, to sue for negligent manufacturing or distribution.
- Blood banks may be liable for invasion of privacy suits if confidentiality is breached via public disclosure of embarrassing facts (e.g., HIV-positive results).
- Traditionally, hospitals and other nonprofit organizations are protected under the Doctrine of Charitable Immunity from excess liability because they performed charitable acts.
- Biomedical ethical principles that must be balanced when considering appropriateness of and informed consent for transfusion include autonomy, beneficence, and justice.

## REVIEW QUESTIONS

1. Transfusion-transmitted diseases can result in lawsuits claiming:
   A. Battery
   B. Invasion of privacy
   C. Negligence
   D. A and B
   E. A, B, and C

2. Laws applicable to blood banking and transfusion medicine can arise:
   A. In state and federal courts
   B. In U.S. Congress, state legislatures, and state and federal courts
   C. In state legislatures and courts
   D. In state legislatures and U.S. Congress

3. The reasons patients have sued for transfusion injury include:
   A. Failure to perform surrogate testing
   B. Failure to properly test blood components
   C. Failure to properly screen donors
   D. Unnecessary transfusion
   E. All of the above

4. Blood banking professionals can avoid litigation by:
   A. Knowing the legal bases for liability
   B. Following published regulations and guidelines
   C. Disclosing all information about patients and donors

   D. Practicing good medicine
   E. None of the above

5. All issues about transfusion-transmitted diseases:
   A. Have already been litigated
   B. Always result in plaintiff verdicts
   C. Never have provided for any protection for defendants
   D. Are known and avoidable
   E. Are evolving and will continue to result in litigation in the foreseeable future

## ANSWERS TO REVIEW QUESTIONS

1. E (p 537, 538, 539)

2. B (p 536)

3. E (p 541)

4. B (p 540)

5. E (p 540)

## REFERENCES

1. Randall, CH, Jr: Medicolegal Problems in Blood Transfusion. Joint Blood Council, Washington, DC, 1962. Reprinted by Committee on Blood, American Medical Association, Chicago, 1963.
2. Rabkin, B, and Rabkin, MS: Individual and institutional liability for transfusion-acquired disease: An update. JAMA 256:2242, 1986.

3. Administrative Procedure Act, 60 Statutes 237–244, 5 USC Sections 551–559, 1988.
4. Code of Federal Regulations: Food and Drugs, Title 21, Parts 200–299 and 600–699, Title 42, Part 482. U.S. Government Printing Office, Washington, DC, 1997.
5. Sazama, K: Practical issues in informed consent for transfusion. Am J Clin Pathol 107:572–574, 1997.
6. Klein, HG (ed): Standards for Blood Banks and Transfusion Services, ed 17. American Association of Blood Banks, Bethesda, MD, 1996.
7. Kelly, C, and Barber, JP: Legal issues in transfusion medicine: Is blood banking a medical profession? Clin Lab Med 12:819–833, 1992.

## BIBLIOGRAPHY

Cooper, JS, and Rodrigue, JE: Legal issues in transfusion medicine. Lab Med 23:794–797, 1992.

Crigger, B-J (ed): Cases in Bioethics, ed 2. St. Martin's Press, New York, 1993.

Klein, HG (ed): Standards for Blood Banks and Transfusion Services, ed 18. American Association of Blood Banks, Bethesda, MD, 1997.

Prosser, WL, Wade, JW, and Schwartz, VE: Torts: Cases and Materials, ed 7. Foundation Press, Mineola, NY, 1980.

Rabkin, B, and Rabkin, MS: Individual and institutional liability for transfusion-acquired disease: An update. JAMA 256:2242, 1986.

Stowell, C (ed): Informed Consent for Transfusion. American Association of Blood Banks, Bethesda, MD, 1997.

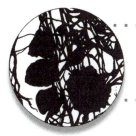

CHAPTER **27**

# ALTERNATIVE TECHNOLOGIES IN ROUTINE BLOOD BANK TESTING

Denise M. Harmening, PhD, MT(ASCP), CLS(NCA), and Phyllis S. Walker, MS, MT(ASCP)SBB

**OBJECTIVES**

*On completion of this chapter, the learner
should be able to:*

1 Define the principles of gel, solid-phase, and
   affinity-column technology.

2 Describe the test reactions and methods of
   grading reactions for each technology.

3 List the tests currently approved by the Food and
   Drug Administration (FDA).

4 List the advantages and disadvantages of each
   technology.

5 Compare the three technologies—gel, solid-phase,
   and affinity-column—in terms of equipment, test
   reactions, procedures, sensitivity, and quality
   control.

## INTRODUCTION

Previous chapters have discussed ABO, Rh, direct antiglobulin test (DAT), antibody screen, and identification procedures based on routine tube testing techniques. Responding to the pressures of current good manufacturing practices (cGMP), three different alternative technologies have emerged to provide accurate, safe, and cost-effective blood bank testing. These include the gel test, solid-phase assays, and affinity-column testing. This chapter will present the history, basic principle, test reactions, tests approved by the Food and Drug Administration (FDA), and the advantages and disadvantages of each technology.

## GEL TECHNOLOGY

### History

In 1985, the gel test was developed by Dr. Yves Lapierre of Lyon, France.[1] Dr. Lapierre investigated this new test methodology in an attempt to develop more stable reaction endpoints for blood bank testing to produce more reproducible results in comparison with traditional tube methodology. Dr. Lapierre investigated alternative methods to traditional tube tests because he was trying to control two specific variables present in the test system: the physical resuspension of red cell buttons after centrifugation and the interpretation of the hemagglutination reactions. His research investigated various media, which included gelatin, acrylamide gel, and glass beads, in an attempt to trap agglutinates during a standardized sedimentation or centrifugation stage.

Gel particles appeared to be the ideal material and led to a patented process for the separation of red cell agglutination reactions. Dr. Lapierre accomplished his goal with his gel test by producing a more reproducible and standardized test result. With the antiglobulin test, Dr. Lapierre found that he could perform this procedure without multiple saline washes before the addition of antihuman globulin (AHG) serum and without the need to add antiglobulin control cells to all negative AHG tests.

Dr. Lapierre aligned with DiaMed A.G., Murten, Switzerland, in 1988 for the commercial development and production of the gel test in Europe. In September 1994, Micro Typing Systems Inc., Pompano Beach, Florida, an affiliated partner of DiaMed A.G., received an FDA license to manufacture and distribute an antiglobulin Anti-IgG gel card and a buffered gel card in the United States. In January 1995, Ortho Diagnostic Systems Inc. (ODSI) and Micro Typing Systems Inc. (MTS) signed an agreement giving ODSI exclusive rights to distribute the gel test in North America. This gel-based test is named the ID-Micro Typing System.[2]

### Principle

The gel test uses the principle of controlled centrifugation of red blood cells through a dextran-acrylamide gel and appropriate reagents predispensed in a specially designed microtube (Fig. 27–1). Each microtube is composed of an upper reaction chamber that is wider than the tube itself and a long, narrow portion referred to as the column (see Figure 27–1). In the gel test, a plastic card with microtubes is used instead of test tubes (Fig. 27–2). A gel card is approximately 5 × 7 centimeters and consists of six microtubes. Each microtube contains predispensed gel, diluent, and reagents if applicable. Measured volumes of serum or plasma and/or red blood cells are dispensed into the reaction chamber of the microtube (Fig. 27–3). If necessary, the card is incubated (Fig. 27–4) and then centrifuged (Fig. 27–5).

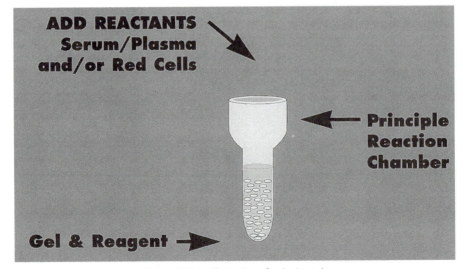

**Figure 27–1.** Illustration of gel microtube.

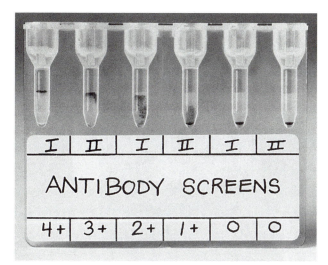

**Figure 27–2.** The gel card (microtubes are used instead of test tubes).

Each chamber is actually a miniature test tube, providing an area for sensitization of red cells (antigen-antibody binding) during incubation. The column of each microtube contains the gel particles suspended in a diluent or reagent. The shape and length provide a large surface area for prolonged contact of the red cells with the gel particles in the test system during the centrifugation phase.

The gel particles are dextran-acrylamide beads and make up 75 percent of the gel-liquid mixture preloaded in each microtube.[2] The gel particles are porous and serve as a reaction medium and filter. The gel performs molecular sieving based on the size of the red cell agglutinates present in the microtube during centrifugation. Large agglutinates are trapped in the gel and are not allowed to travel through the gel during centrifugation of the card (Fig. 27–6). Any agglutinated red cells present remain fixed or suspended in the gel. Unagglutinated red cells may travel unimpeded through the length of the microtube, forming a pellet at the bottom after centrifugation.

Unlike agglutination observed with traditional test tube hemagglutination methods, the gel test reactions are stable, allowing observation or review over an extended period of time.

## Test Reactions

The actual agglutination reactions in the gel test are graded in a fashion similar to that used in test tube hemagglutination (Fig. 27–7).[2]

A 4+ reaction is represented by a solid band of agglutinated red cells at the top of the gel column. Usually no red cells are visible in the bottom of the microtube.

A 3+ reaction is represented by a predominant amount of agglutinated red cells toward the top of the gel column with a few agglutinates staggered below the thicker band. The majority of agglutinates are observed in the top half of the gel column.

A 2+ reaction is characterized by red cell agglutinates dispersed throughout the gel column with few agglutinates at the bottom of the microtube. Agglutinates should be distributed through the upper and lower halves of the gel.

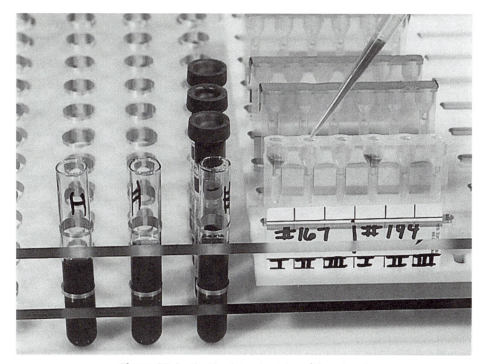

**Figure 27–3.** Pipetting into microtubes of the gel card.

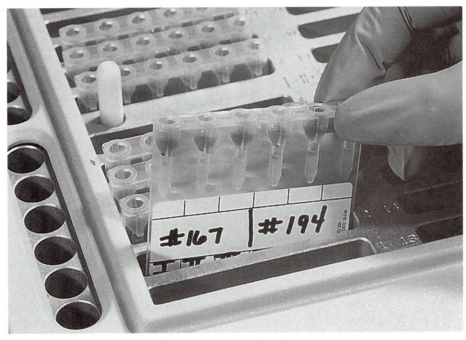

**Figure 27–4.** Incubation of gel cards.

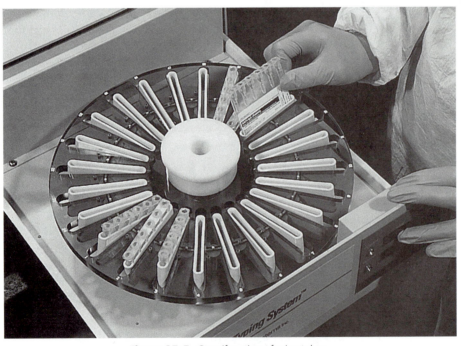

**Figure 27–5.** Centrifugation of microtubes.

A 1+ reaction is characterized by red cell agglutinates predominantly observed in the lower half of the gel column with red cells also in the bottom. These reactions may be weak, with a few agglutinates remaining in the gel area just above the red cell pellet in the bottom of the microtube.

A negative reaction is represented by red cells forming a well-delineated pellet in the bottom of the microtube. The gel above the red cell pellet is clear and free of agglutinates.

Mixed-field reactions may be recognized as a layer of red cell agglutinates at the top of the gel accompanied by a pellet of unagglutinated cells in the bottom of the microtube. Before interpreting reactions as mixed-field, the clinical history of the patient and the type of testing performed should be considered.

Negative reactions may appear mixed-field when incompletely clotted serum samples are used in the gel test. Fibrin strands present in those sera may trap unagglutinated red cells, forming a thin line at the top of

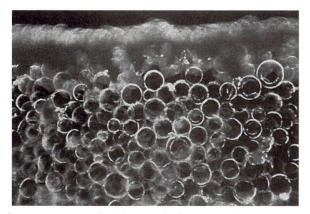

**Figure 27–6.** Magnified photograph of agglutinated red blood cells trapped above the gel matrix.

the gel. Other unagglutinated cells pass through the gel during centrifugation and travel to the bottom of the microtube.

### Tests Approved by the Food and Drug Administration

Gel technology is currently approved for ABO forward and reverse grouping, Rh typing, direct antiglobulin testing, antibody screen, antibody identification, and compatibility testing. The ABO blood grouping card contains gels that include anti-A, anti-B, and anti-A,B for forward grouping, and microtubes with buffered gel are used for ABO reverse grouping.[3] The Rh phenotype card uses microtubes filled with gel containing anti-D.[4] Microtubes filled with gel containing anti-IgG are used for compatibility testing, antibody detection, and identification.[5] The Rh phenotype card contains gel that includes anti-D, anti-C, anti-E, anti-c, anti-e, and a control.[6]

### Advantages and Disadvantages

Gel technology is applicable to a broad range of blood bank tests and offers several advantages over routine tube testing.[7] Standardization is one of the major advantages, inasmuch as there is no tube shaking or resuspension of a red cell button leading to variation among technologists in reading and grading the agglutination reaction. Stable, well-defined endpoints of the agglutination reaction, and simple standardized procedures that include no wash steps and no need to use antiglobulin control cells, lead to more objective, consistent, and reproducible interpretation of test results. This also facilitates easy training, especially for individuals who have been cross-trained to work in the blood bank. Other advantages include the decreased sample volume needed for testing and the enhanced sensitivity and specificity of gel technology. In addition, gel technology offers other significant advantages, including improvement in productivity, standardization, and ability to meet regulatory requirements when compared with traditional tube testing.[8] Table 27–1 defines these three advantages in more detail. The major disadvantage of the gel technology is the need to purchase special incubators and centrifuges to accommodate the microtube cards used for testing. In addition, a specific pipette must be used to dispense 25 $\mu$L of plasma or serum and 50 $\mu$L of a 0.8 percent suspension of red cells into the reaction chambers of the microtubes.[9]

## SOLID-PHASE TECHNOLOGY

### History

Solid-phase immunoassays have been used for many years in immunology and chemistry laboratories. In these test systems (immunoassays), one of the test reactants (either antigen or antibody) is bound to a solid support (usually microtiter wells) before test initiation. The ability of the plastics of the microplate wells (such as polystyrene) to absorb proteins from solution and to bind them irreversibly has made solid-phase serologic assays possible. In 1978, Rosenfield and coworkers[10] were the first to apply these principles to red cell typing and antibody screening tests. Other investigators were quick to follow with the solid-phase red cell adherence (SPRCA) technology first reported in 1984 for the detection of blood antigens and antibodies by Plapp and coworkers.[11,12]

This technology was developed commercially and manufactured under the trade name of Capture by Immucor for the detection of red cell–related and platelet antibodies. Using the Capture technology, tests were adapted to microplate wells, either as full 96-well U-bottomed plates or as 1 $\times$ 8 or 2 $\times$ 8 strips of U-bottomed wells.[13] The first-generation SPRCA assays designed commercially include Capture-R for the detection of red cell antibodies and Capture-P for platelet antibody detection.[13] To perform these tests, a laboratory centrifuge capable of holding 96-well microplates or strip wells is required, along with a microplate incubator and an illuminated reading surface or microplate reader (Fig. 27–8).

Solid-phase immunoassays are currently available to detect antibodies to red cells, platelets, syphilis, and cytomegalovirus (CMV).[14]

### Principle

As mentioned previously, the principle of this technology is based on solid-phase red cell adherence (SPRCA).[11] The first-generation tests use chemically modified microplate test wells in which intact reagent red cells are bound to the microwells before starting the test. Patient serum or plasma and LISS (low ionic strength saline) are added to the red cell–coated microwells and incubated at 37°C. After incubation, the wells are washed free of residual serum proteins, an indicator of anti-IgG–coated red cells is added, and the microplate is then centrifuged. Centrifugation forces the indicator red cells to contact the immobilized sensitized reagent red cells. Positive tests show adherence of indicator red cells to part or all of the well bottom,

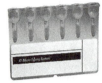

## ID-Micro Typing System™

## Gel Technology Reaction Grading Chart

Agglutinated cells form a cell layer at the top of the gel media.

**4+**

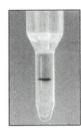

Agglutinated cells disperse throughout the gel media and may concentrate toward the bottom of the microtube.

**1+**

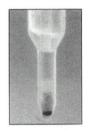

Agglutinated cells begin to disperse into gel media and are concentrated near the top of the microtube.

**3+**

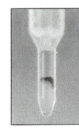

All cells pass through the gel media and form a cell button at the bottom of the microtube.

**Negative**

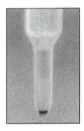

Agglutinated cells disperse into the gel media and are observed throughout the length of the microtube.

**2+**

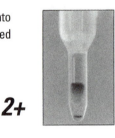

Agglutinated cells form a layer at the top of the gel media. Unagglutinated cells pass to the bottom of the microtube.

**Mixed-Field**

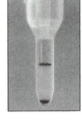

**Figure 27–7.** Gel technology reaction grading chart.

depending on the strength of the reaction (Fig. 27–9 and Fig. 27–10).

In second-generation antibody screening tests, red cell membranes are bound to the microplate test wells and dried during the manufacturing process.

Capture-R (Immucor) for the detection of red cell antibodies is a first-generation solid-phase test, and Capture-R Ready-Screen/Ready-ID (Immucor) are second-generation tests.[13]

Solidscreen (Biotest) is an antibody detection solid-phase test that uses microplate wells coated with poly-specific antihuman globulin.[13]

### Test Reactions

In solid-phase technology, the target antigen (i.e., red cells) is affixed to the bottom of the microplate wells. The patient plasma or serum and LISS are added and incubated at 37°C to allow time for possible antibodies to attach to the antigen in the well. The wells are washed with pH-buffered, isotonic saline to remove unbound plasma or serum, indicator cells are added, and the microplates are centrifuged. The indicator cells are antihuman globulin (AHG)-coated red blood cells. If patient antibody has attached to the antigen, the in-

**Table 27–1.** Advantages of the Gel Technology in Terms of Productivity, Standardization, and Regulatory Issues

| Improves Productivity | Increases Standardization | Addresses Regulatory Issues |
|---|---|---|
| Fewer procedural steps minimize hands-on time | Clearly defined endpoints promote uniform interpretation among technologists | Enhanced cGMP compliance attained through simplified training and standardized procedures |
| Standardized procedures simplify interpretation, reducing repeat and unnecessary testing | Use of precise measurements decreases test performance variability | Minimal handling of reagents and samples increases biosafety |
| Easy-to-perform testing enables optimal utilization of personnel | Elimination of technique-dependent steps improves consistency of test results | Test performance verification and NCCLS-formatted SOPs are provided to ensure easy implementation |

cGMP = current good manufacturing practices; NCCLS = National Committee in Clinical Laboratory Standards; SOPs = standard operational procedures.

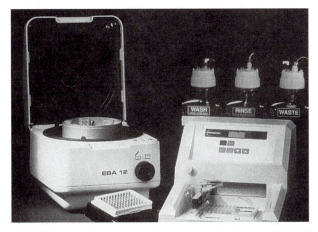

**Figure 27–8.** Equipment for solid-phase red cell adherence (SPRCA) technology.

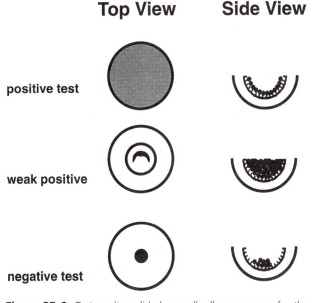

**Figure 27–9.** Test results: solid-phase cell adherence assay for the detection of antigens (illustration).

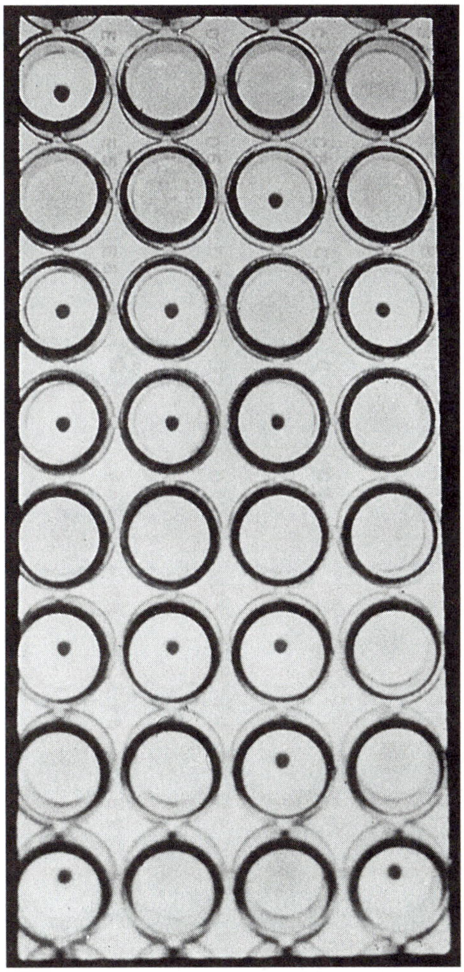

**Figure 27–10.** Test results: solid-phase cell adherence assay for the detection of antigens.

dicator cells will form a monolayer of red blood cells. If patient antibody is not present, nothing will attach to the antigen, and the indicator cells will form a clearly delineated button at the center of the microplate well.

Figure 27–11 compares test results from solid-phase technology with the traditional tube testing reactions.

Solid-phase assays may be performed with either plasma or serum, but plasma is preferable. If serum is used and the sample is incompletely clotted, the serum is difficult to remove during the wash cycle. Residual unbound serum may clot and make the endpoint of the test unreadable. For best results, the manufacturer recommends adding a pH-stabilizing buffer to

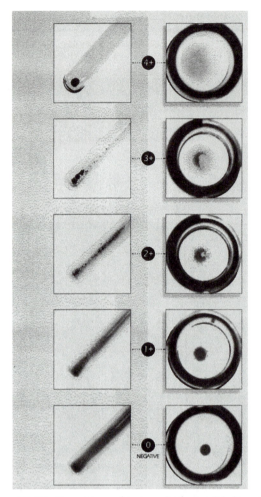

**Figure 27–11.** Comparison of test results from solid-phase technology with the traditional tube testing reactions.

the isotonic saline that is used to wash the microplates. A suitable buffer is available from the manufacturer.[15]

### Tests Approved by the Food and Drug Administration

Solid-phase technology is currently approved for antibody screening, antibody identification, and compatibility testing.

Antibody screening cells are available as a two-cell (I and II) screen, four-cell screens, or as a pool of two cells. The two-cell screen is recommended for recipient antibody detection. Pooled cells are used for donor antibody detection when increased sensitivity is undesirable. A panel is available for red cell antibody identification.

### Advantages and Disadvantages

Standardization is again one of the major advantages of solid-phase technology, inasmuch as there are no tubes to shake and read. Stable, well-defined endpoints

and standardized procedures, which have now been automated, produce objective, consistent, and reproducible test results. This facilitates technologist training or cross-training. Other advantages include the ease of use, because no predilution of reagents is required; the ability to run hemolyzed, lipemic, or icteric samples; and the enhanced sensitivity, which makes the detection of weak alloantibodies easier. In addition, the Immucor Capture technology also has a color change incorporated into the assay to ensure the addition of the patient sample, which is easily visualized for monitoring. Also, enzymes and dithiothreitol (DTT) can be used as well as LISS in the test system.

The major disadvantage is the need for a centrifuge that can spin microplates, a heating block or dry-air 37°C incubator for microplates, and a light source for reading final results. In addition, the increased sensitivity of solid-phase technology may also be a disadvantage, inasmuch as it makes it easier to detect weak autoantibodies.

## AFFINITY-COLUMN TECHNOLOGY

### History

In 1967, Axen and coworkers[16] reported the coupling of proteins to a chemically activated polysaccharide matrix. This represented the first application of affinity chromatography as a routine separation technique. Affinity chromatography allows the purification of biomolecules based on their individual chemical structure or biologic function.

In red cell affinity chromatography, the red cell is specifically adsorbed by a complementary binding substance (ligand) that is covalently bound to an insoluble support (beaded gel matrix).[17] A number of ready-to-use adsorbents are commercially available; namely, protein A (isolated from *Staphylococcus aureus*) and protein G (isolated from group G *Streptococcus*). Both proteins have been extensively used in affinity chromatography applications by being covalently coupled to sepharose gel. These bacterial proteins are now produced by recombinant deoxyribonucleic acid (DNA) technology and are now readily available. Protein G binds specifically to the Fc portion of all four subclasses of the human IgG molecules.[18] (For a review of the structure of the IgG immunoglobulin, refer to Chapter 3.) Protein A binds to the Fc portion of IgG1, IgG2, and IgG4 subclasses, but not to IgG3.[19]

The IgG binding ability of protein G and protein A has been used in the gamma-ReACT (Gamma Biologicals) affinity-column technology designed for the detection of red blood cell (RBC) antibodies. ReACT is an abbreviation for *red* cell *affinity-column technology*.[17]

### Principle

Red cell affinity-column technology is based on the principle of affinity adherence of IgG-sensitized erythrocytes to an immunologically active matrix. The ReACT microcolumn gel consists of a mixture of protein G/sepharose 4B and protein A/sephacryl S200 gels, suspended in a viscous buffer solution containing a preservative (Fig. 27–12).[17] The ReACT system consists of a centrifuge, incubator, view box, and a disposable strip containing an immunoreactive matrix (Fig. 27–13). The strip is available containing six or eight microcolumns, each column being suitable for the performance of one test (Fig. 27–14).

The ReACT test procedure is simple; add reagent red blood cells to serum or plasma in the microcolumn, incubate at 37°C, centrifuge, read, and interpret. IgG-coated cells are available from Gamma to confirm negative tests (as in the Coombs control test). If this option is not exercised, the strip can be sealed to prevent dry-ing and kept under refrigeration for later review of the test results.

When a serum containing IgG antibodies is incubated with red blood cells possessing the appropriate antigen(s), antibodies become attached to the cell surface. During incubation, a viscous barrier separates the test mixture and immunoreactive gel. When the microcolumns are centrifuged, only the red blood cells pass through the viscous barrier. If the cells are coated with IgG antibodies, they adhere to the immunoreactive gel, producing a positive reaction (Fig. 27–15). In the case of a negative reaction, all the red blood cells pass through the gel column and form a button at the bottom of the column.

## Test Reactions

Strongly positive reactions produce a band of red cells at the top of the immunoreactive gel column. Other positives produce a band of red cells at the top of the gel column and a button at the bottom. The thickness of the band of red cells at the top of the gel column is indicative of the strength of the antigen-antibody reaction.

Using an appropriate source of illumination (i.e., a view box), the following reaction patterns can be recorded (Fig. 27–16):

A strong positive reaction: the red cells form a discrete layer at the top of the gel column.

A positive reaction: some red cells form a discrete layer at the top of the gel column, and the rest have passed through the gel column to form a button at the bottom of the microcolumn.

A weak positive reaction: a fine band of red cells is visible at the top of the gel column, and the rest have passed through the gel column to form a button at the bottom of the microcolumn.

A negative reaction: all the red cells have passed through the gel column to form a button at the bottom of the microcolumn.

## ReACT™ Microcolumn

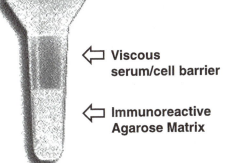

⇐ **Test Chamber**

⇐ **Viscous serum/cell barrier**

⇐ **Immunoreactive Agarose Matrix**

**Figure 27–12.** ReACT Microcolumn.

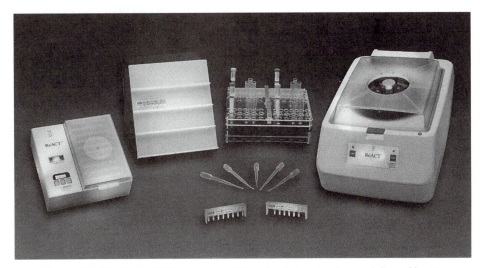

**Figure 27–13.** The ReACT System: a centrifuge, incubator, view box, and disposable strip.

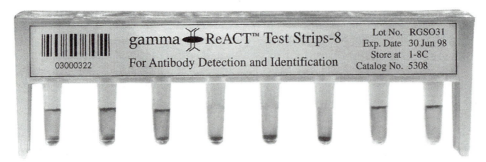

**Figure 27–14.** A ReACT disposable strip containing eight microcolumns.

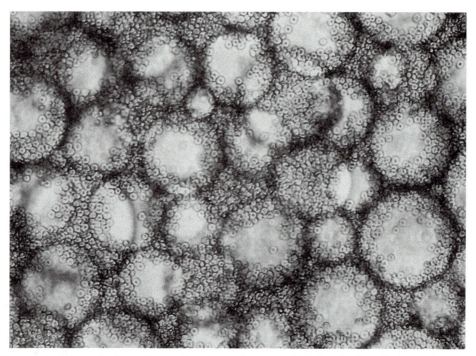

**Figure 27–15.** Microscopic photograph of a positive reaction of red cells coated with IgG antibodies adhering to the immunoreactive gel in a ReACT microcolumn.

# gamma ReACT™

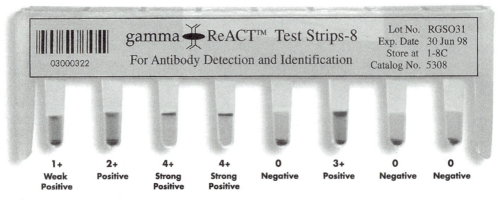

**Figure 27–16.** Graded agglutination reactions for the gamma (ReACT) red cell affinity-column technology.

## Tests Approved by the Food and Drug Administration

Affinity-column technology is currently cleared to be marketed for antibody screening, antibody identification, and compatibility testing under the trade name gamma-ReACT.

Gamma Biologicals has available a line of licensed 0.8 percent reagent red cells for antibody detection and identification in a microcolumn system.[17] The red cells are diluted in a phosphate-buffered, low ionic strength medium that does not interfere with their antigenic reactivity.

## Advantages and Disadvantages

The advantages of affinity-column technology over conventional tube test procedures include prefilled strips, no washing after incubation, ease of use, stable and reproducible results, less than 3 minutes of centrifuge time, and clear differentiation between positive and negative results.

Other advantages include the elimination of subjective interpretation resulting from differences in resuspension technique with conventional tube tests, as well as the decreased sample volume needed for testing.

The major disadvantage is the need to purchase special centrifuges and incubators to accommodate the microcolumn strips used for testing. In addition, automation is not currently available, and an appropriate source of illumination is recommended for reading, such as the gamma ReACT view box.

## COMPARISON OF TECHNOLOGIES

This section compares all three alternative technologies in terms of equipment needed, test reactions and procedures, sensitivity, quality control, and automation.[20] Table 27–2 lists the current tests available for the three alternative technologies.

**Table 27–2.** Current Tests Available for the Three Alternative Technologies*

| Test | Gel Test (Ortho) | Solid-Phase (Immucor) | Affinity-Column (Gamma) |
|---|---|---|---|
| ABO—Forward | Yes | No | No |
| ABO—Reverse | Yes | No | No |
| Rh typing | Yes | No | No |
| Antibody screen | Yes | Yes | Yes |
| Crossmatch | Yes | Yes | Yes |
| Antibody identification | Yes | Yes | Yes |
| Auto-control (IgG only) | Yes | Yes | Yes |
| DAT | No | No | No |

*Gel test (Ortho Diagnostic Systems, Raritan, NJ); solid-phase (Immucor, Norcross, GA); affinity-column (Gamma Biologicals, Houston); IgG indicates immunoglobulin G; DAT = direct antiglobulin testing.

## Equipment

The gel and affinity-column technologies require special incubators and centrifuges to accommodate the cards or strips. The solid-phase technology requires a centrifuge that can spin microplates, a dry-air 37°C incubator or a heat block for incubating microplates, and a light source for reading final results. Semiautomated equipment approved by the FDA is currently available for solid-phase technology.

All three technologies improve safety and decrease hazardous waste, inasmuch as the use of plastic eliminates the danger associated with broken glass, and miniaturized reaction chambers reduce the quantity of hazardous waste.

## Test Reactions and Procedures

All technologies demonstrate reproducible endpoints. The gel test uses a special pipette to precisely measure the quantity of test cells and sera. The solid-phase and affinity-column tests use drops of cells and sera. By standardizing the reactants in the assay and eliminating variation in the tube-shaking technique, it is possible to eliminate the subjectivity associated with interpreting the endpoint of test tube agglutination tests. Quantitation of these assays is also less subjective than conventional test tube technology. The gel test is read as 4+, 3+, 2+, 1+, and negative and is based on agglutination reactions. The ease of quantitating the reactions with the gel test is an advantage when evaluating an antibody identification for multiple antibodies or dosage effects. The ReACT test is based upon immune adherence or affinity adherence. The descriptions of weak positive, positive, and strong positive are generally used, although the reactions can be graded from 1+ to 4+. The solid-phase assays are read as strong positive, positive, and negative reactions.

Mixed-field agglutination produces a characteristic pattern in the gel and affinity-column technology. In the gel technology, the agglutinated population of red cells is trapped in the gel, and the unagglutinated population is pelleted at the bottom of the microtube following centrifugation. The ability to recognize mixed-field reactions is particularly valuable in evaluating a possible transfusion reaction or the survival of a minor population of transfused cells.

The endpoints of all of the new technologies are extremely stable and can be read 2 to 3 days after the test is performed. Such stability is a distinct advantage when less experienced technologists are cross-trained to work in the transfusion service. When interpretation of assays is unclear, it is helpful to be able to retain test results until a supervisor can review them.

It should be pointed out that the ReACT technology does not use antihuman globulin serum for testing, as the gel technology does. Instead, ReACT uses protein G and protein A to bind sensitized red cells to an immunoreactive gel matrix. The gel cards use an immunologically inert gel or matrix.

The procedures for all three technologies parallel steps performed in routine blood bank tube testing, including pipetting, incubating, spinning, and reading. The washing cycle step has been eliminated with these alternative technologies with the exception of the solid phase. Because the endpoint of all the assays detects IgG, it is possible to perform an auto-control to detect IgG-coated cells. An auto-control cannot be substituted for a DAT, however, because none of the technologies currently detects C3d complement–coated cells. Table 27–3 compares the procedural steps of the three technologies.

## Sensitivity

Although the three technologies are LISS-based, their sensitivity varies. The technologies have been shown to detect at least as many IgG antibodies as the conventional test tube methods using the LISS antiglobulin technique. The solid-phase technology is more sensitive than traditional serologic techniques. The sensitivity of all of the technologies can be modified by pretreating the test cells or monolayer with enzymes, dithiothreitol (DTT), or chloroquine. Increased sensitivity is advantageous when a low-titered, clinically significant antibody is present, but it is a disadvantage when a low-titered warm autoantibody is present. Assays that detect only IgG avoid clinically insignificant IgM antibodies, but not the clinically insignificant IgG antibodies such as the high titer–low avidity (HTLA) antibodies.

## Quality Control

In addition to routine quality control (QC) for the 37°C incubator, centrifuge, pipette tips, and pipette dispenser used in testing, the new technologies have other QC features. The gel test uses special dispensers to prepare the red cell suspensions and special pipettes to add a measured volume of plasma/serum and red cells. Each

**Table 27–3.** Procedural Steps of Three Technologies

| | Solid-Phase | | | |
| Procedural Steps | Preloaded Microwells | Selected Cells | Gel Test | Affinity-Column |
|---|---|---|---|---|
| 1. Add RBCs to wells or tubes | N/A | Yes | Yes | Yes |
| 2. Centrifuge plate to form monolayer | N/A | Yes | N/A | N/A |
| 3. Wash away unbound RBCs | N/A | Yes | N/A | N/A |
| 4. Add test serum/plasma | Yes | Yes | Yes | Yes |
| 5. Incubation | 15 min | 15 min | 15 min | 15 min |
| 6. Wash cycle | Yes | Yes | N/A | N/A |
| 7. Add indicator cells | Yes | Yes | N/A | N/A |
| 8. Centrifuge | 2 min | 2 min | 10 min | 3 min |

*Solid-phase (Immucor, Norcross, GA); gel test (Ortho Diagnostic Systems, Raritan, NJ); affinity-column (Gamma Biologicals, Houston); RBC = red blood cells; N/A = not applicable.

**Table 27–4.** Routine Blood Bank Testing: Comparison of Traditional and Alternative Methods

| | Traditional | Gel | Solid-Phase | Affinity-Column |
|---|---|---|---|---|
| Reaction chamber | Tube | Microtube card | Microplate wells | Microcolumn strip |
| Reaction patterns | Agglutination | Agglutination | Solid-phase immune adherence | Immune adherence |
| Reaction matrix | None (cells and serum/plasma) | Immunologically inert dextran-acrylamide gels | Chemically modified polystyrene microplate wells | Immunoreactive sepharose gel |
| Testing detection | AHG (antihuman globulin sera) | AHG (antihuman globulin sera) | Anti-IgG–coated red cells | Protein G and protein A used |
| Washing required | Yes | No | Yes | No |
| Centrifugation required | Yes | Yes | Yes | Yes |
| Reaction readings | Quantitative: 1+ to 4+, MF | Quantitative: 1+ to 4+, MF | Semiquantitative: strong pos, pos, neg, no MF | Semiquantitative: strong pos, pos, weak pos, no MF |
| Stable reactions | No | Yes (2–3 days) | Yes (2 days) | Yes (7 days) |
| Quality control | Positive and negative controls/Coombs' check cells | Lot number of cards and diluent on day of use | LISS color change, pos and neg control | IgG-coated control cells |
| Special equipment | No | Yes | Yes | Yes |
| Automation (FDA-approved) | No | No | Yes | No |

MF = mixed-field.

lot number of cards and diluent should be tested on the day of use to confirm that the test cards and the diluted reagent red cells are reacting as expected. The manufacturer of the solid-phase technology recommends including a positive and a negative control with each batch of tests. In addition, in the solid-phase system, LISS is designed to detect the addition of plasma by a color change from purple to blue when the plasma is added. This feature protects the user from failing to add plasma to a well. Affinity-column technology is limited to the antiglobulin technique. IgG-coated cells can be used to confirm that protein G was active in the columns that demonstrate a negative test result. This is similar to using IgG-coated red blood cells after a negative antiglobulin result in the conventional test tube method.

## Automation

The solid-phase technology has been fully automated, and two models of equipment are awaiting FDA approval. Both models include a bar code scanner, a robotic liquid-handling system, an analyzer, an optical reader, and a computer to monitor the process and to compile results into a comprehensive report.

Automated equipment for the gel test is being used successfully in Europe, and similar equipment is pending FDA approval in the United States. Automation of the affinity-column technology is under development. Table 27–4 compares the features of the three alternative technologies for routine blood bank testing.

---

## SUMMARY CHART: IMPORTANT POINTS TO REMEMBER (MT/MLT)

- The gel test employs the principle of controlled centrifugation of red blood cells through a dextran-acrylamide gel and appropriate reagents predispensed in a specially designed microtube.
- The gel test reactions are stable for observation or review over an extended period of time.
- The principle of solid-phase technology is based on solid-phase red cell adherence (SPRCA).
- Red cell affinity-column technology is based on the principle of affinity adherence of IgG-sensitized erythrocytes to an immunologically active matrix.
- In solid-phase technology, the target antigen (red cells) is affixed to the bottom of the microplate wells. If patient antibody has attached to the antigen, the indicator cells will form a monolayer of red blood cells. If patient antibody is not present, nothing will attach to the antigen, and the indicator cells will form a clearly delineated button at the center of the microplate well.
- Gel technology is currently approved for ABO forward and reverse grouping, Rh typing, direct antiglobulin testing, antibody screening, antibody identification, and compatibility testing.
- Solid-phase technology is currently approved for antibody screening, antibody identification, and compatibility testing.
- Affinity-column technology is currently approved for antibody screening, antibody identification, and compatibility testing under the trade name gamma-ReACT.
- The major advantages of these technologies over routine tube testing are standardization (there is no tube shaking or resuspension of a red cell button leading to variation among technologists),

- stability (there are well-defined endpoints of the agglutination reaction), a decreased sample volume needed for testing, and enhanced sensitivity and specificity.
- One of the major advantages of solid-phase technology is standardization because there are no tubes to shake and read. Other advantages include ease of use because no predilution of reagents is required; ability to run hemolyzed, lipemic, or icteric samples; and enhanced sensitivity, which makes detection of weak alloantibodies easier.
- The major advantages of affinity-column technology over conventional test tube procedures include prefilled strips, no washing after incubation, ease of use, stable and reproducible results, less than 3 minutes of centrifuge time, and clear differentiation between positive and negative results.
- The major disadvantage of the gel technology is the need to purchase a special centrifuge to accommodate the microtube cards used for testing. In addition, a pipette must be used to dispense plasma or serum and suspension of red cells into the reaction chambers of the microtubes.
- The major disadvantage of solid-phase technology is the need for a centrifuge that can spin microplates, a heating block or dry-air 37°C incubator for microplates, and a light source for reading final results.
- The major disadvantage of affinity-column technology is the need to purchase special centrifuges and incubators to accommodate the microcolumn strips used for testing.

## REVIEW QUESTIONS

1. The principle of affinity adherence of IgG-sensitized erythrocytes to an immunologically active matrix is demonstrated by using:
   A. A gel column and microcolumn system in affinity-column technology
   B. Target antigen affixed to microplate wells in solid-phase technology
   C. Gel-filled microtubes containing anti-IgG in gel technology
   D. Antibody affixed to microplate wells in affinity-column technology

2. ABO forward and reverse grouping and Rh typing are currently approved by the FDA in which of the following technologies?
   A. Solid-phase
   B. Gel
   C. Affinity-column
   D. All of the above

3. Antibody screening, antibody identification, and compatibility testing are currently approved by the FDA for which technologies?
   A. Solid-phase and gel
   B. Gel and affinity-column
   C. Affinity-column and solid-phase
   D. Gel, solid-phase, and affinity-column

4. One of the disadvantages of gel, solid-phase, and affinity-column technology (select one for each technology) is:
   A. Decreased sensitivity
   B. Inability to test hemolyzed, lipemic, or icteric samples
   C. Inability to detect C3d complement–coated cells
   D. A and C

5. The major advantage of gel, solid-phase, and affinity-column technology (select one for each technology) is:
   A. No cell washing steps
   B. Cost effectiveness
   C. Easy cross-training
   D. Standardization

## ANSWERS TO REVIEW QUESTIONS

1. A (p 549)

2. B (p 549)

3. D (p 555, Table 27–2)

4. C (p 549, 552, 555)

5. D (p 549, 552, 555)

## REFERENCES

1. Lapierre, Y, et al: The gel test: A new way to detect red cell antigen-antibody reactions. Transfusion 30:109–13, 1990.
2. ID-Micro Typing System Question and Answer Guide. Ortho Diagnostic Systems, Raritan, NJ, 1996.
3. Package insert for MTS Buffered Gel Card. Pompano Beach, FL. Micro Typing Systems, 1995.
4. Package insert for MTS and Anti-D Gel Card. Pompano Beach, FL. Micro Typing Systems, 1995.
5. Package insert for MTS Anti-IgG Card. Pompano Beach, FL. Micro Typing Systems, 1995.
6. Package insert for MTS Anti-IgG, -C3d Card. Pompano Beach, FL. Micro Typing Systems, 1995.
7. Chan, A, et al: The impact of a gel system on routine work in a general hospital blood bank. Immunohematology 12:30–32, 1996.
8. A new era begins: Introducing ID-MTS, ID-Micro Typing System (Product brochure). Ortho Diagnostics Systems, Raritan, NJ, November 1995.
9. Package insert for ID-Pipetor FP-2. Pompano Beach, FL. Micro Typing Systems, 1995.
10. Rosenfield, RE, Kochwa, SE, and Kaczera, Z: Solid phase serology for the study of human erythrocyte antigen-antibody reactions. Proceedings, Plenary Session, 25th Congress, International Society Blood Transfusion. Paris, 1978.
11. Plapp, FV, et al: Blood antigens and antibodies: Solid phase adherence assays. Laboratory Management 22:39, 1984.
12. Moore, HH: Automated reading of red cell antibody detection tests by a solid phase antiglobulin technique. Transfusion 24:218, 1985.
13. Rolih, S, et al: Solid phase red cell adherence assays. La Transfusione del Sangue 36:4, 1991.
14. Haslam, GM, et al: A comparison of two solid phase systems for antibody detection. Immunohematology 11:8–10, 1995.
15. Capture-R (solid phase technology). Package insert for Capture-R Ready Screen and Capture-R Ready-ID. Immucor, Norcross, GA, 1994.
16. Axen, R, Parath, J, and Ernback, S: Chemical coupling of peptides and proteins to polysaccharides by means of cyanogen halides. Nature 214:1302, 1967.
17. ReACT (affinity column technology). Gamma-ReACT product preview. Gamma Biologicals, Houston, 1996.
18. Björck, L, and Kronvall, G: Purification and some properties of streptococcal protein G: A novel IgG-binding agent. J Immunol 133:969–974, 1984.
19. Björck, L, Petersson, BA, and Sjörquist, J: Some physiochemical properties of protein A from *Staphylococcus aureus*. Eur J Biochem 29:572–584, 1972.
20. Walker, PS: New technologies in transfusion medicine. Laboratory Medicine 28:258–262, 1997.

# GLOSSARY

**Abruptio placentae:** Premature detachment of normally situated placenta.

**Absorbed anti-A$_1$:** If serum from a group B individual that contains anti-A plus anti-A$_1$ is incubated with A$_2$ cells, the anti-A will adsorb onto the cells. Removal of the cells then yields a serum containing only anti-A$_1$; thus, absorbed anti-A$_1$.

**Absorption:** Removal of an unwanted antibody from a serum; often used interchangeably with adsorption.

**Acid-citrate-dextrose (ACD):** An anticoagulant and preservative solution that once was used routinely for blood donor collection but is now used only occasionally.

**Acid phosphatase (ACP):** A red cell enzyme used as an identification marker in paternity testing and criminal investigation.

**Adenosine deaminase (ADA):** A red cell enzyme used as an identification marker in paternity testing and criminal investigation.

**Adenosine triphosphate (ATP):** A compound composed of adenosine (nucleotide containing adenine and ribose) and three phosphoric acid groups, which, when split by enzyme action, produces energy that can be used to support other reactions.

**Adenylate kinase (AK):** A red cell enzyme used as an identification marker in paternity testing and criminal investigation.

**Adjuvant:** One of a variety of substances that, when combined with an antigen, enhance the antibody response to that antigen.

**Adsorption:** Providing an antibody with its corresponding antigen under optimal conditions so that the antibody will attach to the antigen, thereby removing the antibody from the serum; often used interchangeably with absorption.

**Affinity-column technology:** Separation and purification of biomolecules based on individual binding specificities and biologic function. Ligands bound to an insoluble matrix facilitate adherence of target protein.

**Agammaglobulinemia:** A rare disorder in which gamma globulin is virtually absent.

**Agglutination:** The clumping together of red blood cells or any particulate matter resulting from interaction of antibody and its corresponding antigen.

**Agglutinin:** An antibody that agglutinates cells.

**Agglutinogen:** A substance that stimulates the production of an agglutinin, thereby acting as an antigen.

**Agranulocytosis:** An acute disease in which the white blood cell count drops to extremely low levels and neutropenia becomes pronounced.

**Albumin:** Protein found in the highest concentration in human plasma; used as a diluent for blood typing antisera and a potentiator solution in serologic testing to enhance antigen-antibody reactions.

**Aldomet:** *See* Methyldopa.

**Alkaline phosphatase (ALP):** A red cell enzyme used as an identification marker in paternity testing and criminal investigation.

**Allele:** One of two or more different genes that may occupy a specific locus on a chromosome.

**Allo-:** Prefix indicating differences within a species (e.g., an alloantibody is produced in one individual against the red cell antigens of another individual).

**Allograft:** A tissue transplant between individuals of the same species.

**Allosteric change:** A change in conformation that exposes a new reactive site on a molecule.

**Alpha-adrenergic receptor:** A site in autonomic nerve pathways wherein excitatory responses occur when adrenergic agents such as norepinephrine and epinephrine are released.

**Alum precipitation:** A method for obtaining an enhanced response when producing antibody; *see also* Adjuvant.

**Amniocentesis:** Transabdominal puncture of the amniotic sac, using a needle and syringe, in order to remove amniotic fluid. The material may then be studied to detect genetic disorders or fetomaternal blood incompatibility.

**Amniotic fluid:** Liquid or albuminous fluid contained in the amnion.

**Amorph:** A gene that does not appear to produce a detectable antigen; a silent gene, such as *Jk, Lu, O.*

**Anamnestic response:** An accentuated antibody response following a secondary exposure to an antigen. Antibody levels from the initial exposure are not detectable in the patient's serum until the secondary exposures, when a rapid rise in antibody titer is observed.

**Anaphylaxis:** An allergic hypersensitivity reaction of the body to a foreign protein or drug.

**Anastomosis:** A connection between two blood vessels, either direct or through connecting channels.

**Anemia:** A condition in which there is reduced oxygen delivery to the tissues; may result from increased destruction of red cells, excessive blood loss, or decreased production of red cells. **Aplastic a.:** Anemia caused by aplasia of bone marrow or its destruction by chemical agents or physical factors. **Autoimmune hemolytic a.:** Acquired disorder characterized by premature erythrocyte destruction owing to abnormalities in the individual's own immune system. **Hemolytic a.:** Anemia caused by hemolysis of red blood cells resulting in reduction of normal red cell lifespan. **Iron-deficiency a.:** Anemia resulting from a greater demand on stored iron than can be met. **Megaloblastic a.:** Anemia in which megaloblasts are found in the blood. **Sickle cell a.:** Hereditary, chronic hemolytic anemia characterized by large numbers of sickle-shaped red blood cells occurring almost exclusively in blacks.

**559**

**Angina pectoris:** Severe pain and constriction about the heart caused by an insufficient supply of blood to the heart.

**Anion:** An ion carrying a negative charge.

**Antecubital:** In front of the elbow, at the bend of the elbow; usual site for blood collection.

**Antenatal:** Occurring before birth.

**Anti-A$_1$ lectin:** A reagent anti-A$_1$ serum produced from the seeds of the plant *Dolichos biflorus*; reacts with A$_1$ cells but not with A subgroup cells such as A$_2$, A$_3$, and so on; reacts weakly with A$_{int}$ cells.

**Anti-B lectin:** A reagent anti-B serum produced from the seeds of the plant *Bandeiraea simplicifolia*.

**Antibody:** A protein substance secreted by plasma cells that is developed in response to, and interacting specifically with, an antigen. In blood banking, it is found in serum, from either a commercial manufacturer or a patient. **Cross-reacting a.:** Antibody that reacts with antigens functionally similar to its specific antigen. **Fluorescent a.:** Antibody reaction made visible by incorporating a fluorescent dye into the antigen-antibody reaction and examining the specimen with a fluorescent microscope. **Maternal a.:** Antibody produced in the mother and transferred to the fetus in utero. **Naturally occurring a.:** Antibody present in a patient without known prior exposure to the corresponding red cell antigen.

**Antibody screen:** Testing the patient's serum with group O reagent red cells in an effort to detect atypical antibodies.

**Anticoagulant:** An agent that prevents or delays blood coagulation.

**Anticodon:** A sequence of three bases that is found on transfer RNA, which also carries an amino acid residue; recognizes its complementary codon on messenger RNA at the ribosome and deposits the amino acid on the ribosome, generating the amino acid sequence of the protein.

**Anti-dl:** An antibody implicated in warm autoimmune hemolytic anemia, which reacts with all Rh cells including Rh$_{null}$ and Rh-deleted cells.

**Antigen:** A substance recognized by the body as being foreign, which can cause an immune response. In blood banking, antigens are usually, but not exclusively, found on the red blood cell membrane.

**Antihemophilic factor:** *See* Hemophilia A.

**Antihemophilic globulin:** *See* Hemophilia A.

**Antihistamine:** Drug that opposes the action of histamine.

**Anti-H lectin:** A reagent anti-H produced from the seeds of the plant *Ulex europaeus*.

**Antihuman globulin** or **antiglobulin:** *See* Antihuman serum.

**Antihuman globulin** or **antiglobulin serum:** *See* Antihuman serum.

**Antihuman globulin test antiglobulin** or **(AGT):** Test to ascertain the presence or absence of red cell coating by immunoglobulin G (IgG) or complement, or both; uses a xenoantibody (rabbit antihuman serum) to act as a bridge between sensitized cells, thus yielding agglutination as a positive result. Also referred to as antiglobulin test. **Direct antihuman globulin test (DAT):** Used to detect in vivo cell sensitization. **Indirect antihuman globulin test (IAT):** Used to detect antigen-antibody reactions that occur in vitro.

**Antihuman serum:** An antibody prepared in rabbits or other suitable animals that is directed against human immunoglobulin or complement, or both; used to perform the antihuman globulin or Coombs' test. The serum may be either polyspecific (anti-IgG plus anti-complement) or monospecific (anti-IgG or anti-complement).

**Anti-M lectin:** A reagent anti-M serum produced from the plant *Iberis amara*.

**Anti-nl:** An antibody implicated in warm autoimmune hemolytic anemia, which reacts with all normal Rh cells except Rh$_{null}$ cells and deleted Rh cells.

**Anti-N lectin:** A reagent anti-N serum produced from the plant *Vicia graminea*.

**Anti-pdl:** An antibody implicated in warm autoimmune hemolytic anemia, which reacts with all normal Rh cells and deleted Rh cells but not with Rh$_{null}$ cells.

**Antipyretic:** An agent that reduces fever.

**Antiserum:** A reagent source of antibody, as in a commercial antiserum.

**Antithetical:** Referring to antigens that are the product of allelic genes (e.g., Kell [K] and Cellano [k]).

**Apheresis:** A method of blood collection in which whole blood is withdrawn, a desired component separated and retained, and the remainder of the blood returned to the donor. *See also* Plateletpheresis and Plasmapheresis.

**Aplasia:** Failure of an organ or tissue to develop normally.

***Arachis hypogaea:*** A peanut lectin used to differentiate T polyagglutination from Tn polyagglutination.

**Asphyxia:** Condition caused by insufficient intake of oxygen.

**Asthma:** Paroxysmal dyspnea accompanied by wheezing caused by a spasm of the bronchial tubes or by swelling of their mucous membrane.

**Atypical antibodies:** Any antibody other than anti-A, anti-B, or anti-A,B.

**Australia antigen:** Old terminology referring to the hepatitis B–associated antigen.

**Auto-:** Prefix indicating self (e.g., an autoantibody is reactive against one's own red cell antigens); usually associated with a disease state.

**Autoabsorption:** A procedure to remove a patient's antibody using the patient's own cells.

**Autologous control:** Testing the patient's serum with his or her own cells in an effort to detect autoantibody activity.

**Autosome:** Any chromosome other than the sex (X and Y) chromosomes.

**Bactericidal:** Destructive to or destroying bacteria.

***Bandeiraea simplicifolia:*** *See* Anti-B lectin.

**Bar code reader:** An optical input device that reads and interprets data from a bar code for entry into a computer system.

**Bilirubin:** The orange-yellow pigment in bile carried to the liver by the blood; produced from hemoglobin of red blood cells by reticuloendothelial cells in bone marrow, spleen, and elsewhere. **Direct b.:** The conjugated water-soluble form of bilirubin. **Indirect b.:** The unconjugated water-insoluble form of bilirubin.

**Bilirubinemia:** Pathologic condition in which excessive destruction of red blood cells occurs, increasing the amount of bilirubin found in the blood.

**Binding constant:** The "goodness of fit" in an antigen-antibody complex.

**Biphasic:** Reactivity occurring in two phases.

**Blood bank information system:** Computer system that has been developed specifically to assist blood bank professionals in the management of the patient, donor, and blood component information.

**Blood gases:** Determination of pH, $P_{CO_2}$, $P_{O_2}$, and $HCO_3$ performed on a blood gas analyzer.

**Blood group–specific substances (BGSSs):** Soluble antigens present in fluids that can be used to neutralize their corresponding antibodies; systems that demonstrate BGSSs include ABO, Lewis, and P blood group systems.

**Bombay:** Phenotype occurring in individuals who possess normal *A* or *B* genes but are unable to express them because they lack the gene necessary for production of H antigen, the required precursor for A and B. These persons often have a potent anti-H in their serum, which reacts with all cells except other Bombays. Also known as $O_h$.

**Bovine:** Pertaining to cattle.

**Bradykinin:** A plasma kinin.

**Bromelin:** A proteolytic enzyme obtained from the pineapple.

**Buffy coat:** Light stratum of a blood clot seen when the blood is centrifuged or allowed to stand in a test tube. The red blood cells settle to the bottom, and between the plasma and the red blood cells is a light-colored layer that contains mostly white blood cells.

**Burst-forming unit committed to erythropoiesis (BFU-E):** A primitive progenitor cell committed to erythropoiesis and thought to be a precursor to the CFU-E.

**C3a:** A biologically active fragment of the complement C3 molecule that demonstrates anaphylactic capabilities upon liberation.

**C3b:** A biologically active fragment of the complement C3 molecule that is an opsonin and promotes immune adherence.

**C3d:** A biologically inactive fragment of the C3b complement component formed by inactivation by the C3b inactivator substance present in serum.

**C4:** A complement component present in serum that participates in the classic pathway of complement activation.

**C5a:** A biologically active fragment of the C5 molecule, which demonstrates anaphylactic capabilities as well as chemotactic properties upon liberation. This fragment is also a potent aggregator of platelets.

**Cardiac output:** The amount of blood discharged from the left or right ventricle per minute.

**Catecholamines:** Biologically active amines, epinephrine and norepinephrine, derived from the amino acid tyrosine. They have a marked effect on nervous and cardiovascular systems, metabolic rate, temperature, and smooth muscle.

**Cathode ray tube (CRT):** A display device in an information system.

**Cation:** An ion carrying a positive charge.

**Central processing unit (CPU):** The part of a computer that contains the semiconductor chips that process the instructions of the computer programs.

**Central venous pressure:** The pressure within the superior vena cava reflecting the pressure under which the blood is returned to the right atrium.

**Chemically modified anti-D:** IgG anti-D reagent antisera in which the immunoglobulin has been chemically modified to react in the saline phase of testing by breaking disulfide bonds at the hinge region of the molecule, converting the Y-shaped antibody structure to a T-shaped form through the use of sulfhydryl-reducing reagents.

**Chemotaxis:** Movement toward a stimulus, particularly that movement displayed by phagocytic cells toward bacteria and sites of cell injury.

**Chimera:** An individual who possesses a mixed cell population.

**Chloroquine diphosphate:** Substance that dissociates IgG antibody from red cells with little or no damage to the red cell membrane.

**Chromogen:** Any chemical that may be changed into coloring matter.

**Chromosome:** The structures within a nucleus that contain a linear thread of DNA, which transmits genetic information. Genes are arranged along the strand of DNA and constitute portions of the DNA.

**Cis position:** The location of two or more genes on the same chromosome of a homologous pair.

**Citrate:** Compound of citric acid and a base; used in anticoagulant solutions.

**Citrate-phosphate-dextrose (CPD):** The anticoagulant preservative solution that replaced ACD in routine donor collection. It has been replaced by CPDA-1 in routine use.

**Citrate-phosphate-dextrose-adenine (CPDA-1):** The anticoagulant preservative solution in current use. It has extended the shelf life of blood from 21 days (ACD and CPD) to 35 days.

**Clone:** A group of genetically identical cells.

**Codominant:** A pair of genes in which neither is dominant over the other; that is, they are both expressed.

**Codon:** A sequence of three bases in a strand of DNA that provides the genetic code for a specific amino acid. The complementary triplets are found on messenger RNA, which is synthesized from the DNA and then proceeds to the ribosomes for protein synthesis.

**Colloid:** A gluelike substance such as protein or starch whose particles, when dispersed in a solvent to the greatest possible degree, remain uniformly distributed and fail to form a true solution.

**Colony-forming unit committed to erythropoiesis (CFU-E):** A progenitor cell that is committed to forming cells of the red blood cell series.

**Colony-forming unit—culture (CFU-C):** Generation of stem cells using tissue culture methods. Current synonym is CFU-GM, which is a colony-forming unit committed to the production of myeloid cells (granulocytes and monocytes).

**Colostrum:** Thin yellowish breast fluid secreted 2 to 3 days after birth but before the onset of true lactation; it contains a great quantity of proteins and calories as well as antibodies and lymphocytes.

**Compatibility testing:** All pretransfusion testing performed on a potential transfusion recipient and the appropriate donor blood, in an attempt to ensure that the product will survive in the recipient and induce improvement in the patient's clinical condition; the crossmatch between recipient's serum and donor's cells.

**Complement:** A series of proteins in the circulation that, when sequentially activated, causes disruption of bacterial and other cell membranes. Activation occurs via one of two pathways, and once activated, the components are involved in a great number of immune defense mechanisms including anaphylaxis, chemotaxis, and phagocytosis. Red cell antibodies that activate complement may be capable of causing hemolysis.

**Complement fixation (CF):** An immunologic test.

**Component therapy:** Transfusion of specific components (e.g., red blood cells, platelets, plasma) rather than whole blood to treat a patient. Components are separable by physical means such as centrifugation.

**Compound antibody:** An antibody whose corresponding antigen is an interaction product of two or more antigens.

**Compound antigen:** Two or more antigens that interact and are recognized as a single antigen by an antibody.

**Configuration:** The physical layout and design of the central processing unit and the peripheral devices of an information system.

**Conglutinin:** A substance present in bovine serum that will agglutinate sensitized cells in the presence of complement.

**Constant region:** The portion of the immunoglobulin chain that shows a relatively constant amino acid sequence within each class of immunoglobulin. Both light and heavy chains have these constant portions, which originate at the carboxyl region of the molecule.

**Convulsion:** Involuntary muscle contraction and relaxation.

**Coombs' serum:** *See* Antihuman serum.

**Coombs' test:** *See* Antihuman globulin test (AGT).

**Cord cells:** Fetal cells obtained from the umbilical cord at birth; may be contaminated with Wharton's jelly.

**Coumarin (Coumadin):** A commonly employed anticoagulant that acts as a vitamin K antagonist that prolongs the prothrombin time.

**Counterelectrophoresis (CEP):** An immunologic procedure.

**Crossmatch:** Testing a patient and prospective donor for compatibility. **Major c.:** Recipient serum tested with donor cells. **Minor c.:** Recipient cells tested with donor serum or plasma.

**Cryoprecipitate:** A concentrated source of coagulation factor VIII prepared from a single unit of donor blood; it also contains fibrinogen, factor XIII, and von Willebrand factor.

**Cryopreservation:** Preservation by freezing at very low temperatures.

**Cryoprotectant:** A substance that protects blood cells from damaged caused by freezing and thawing. Glycerol and dimethyl sulfoxide are examples.

**Cryptantigens:** Hidden receptors that may be exposed when normal erythrocyte membranes are altered by bacterial or viral enzymes.

**Crystalloid:** A substance capable of crystallization; opposite of colloid.

**Cyanosis:** Slightly bluish or grayish skin discoloration resulting from accumulations of reduced hemoglobin or deoxyhemoglobin in the blood caused by oxygen deficiency or carbon dioxide buildup.

**Cytomegalovirus (CMV):** One of a group of species-specific herpesviruses.

**Cytopheresis:** A procedure performed using a machine by which one can selectively remove a particular cell type normally found in peripheral blood of a patient or donor.

**Cytotoxicity:** Ability to destroy cells.

**Cytotoxicity testing:** Procedure commonly used in HLA typing and crossmatching.

**Dane particle:** Hepatitis B virion.

**Database:** An organized group of files in which information is stored in an information system.

**Deglycerolization:** Removal of glycerol from a unit of red cells after thawing has been performed; required to return the cells to a normal osmolality.

**Deletion:** The loss of a portion of chromosome.

**Deoxyribonucleic acid (DNA):** The chemical basis of heredity and the carrier of genetic information for all organisms except RNA viruses.

**Dexamethasone:** A topical steroid with anti-inflammatory, antipruritic, and vasoconstrictive actions.

**Dextran:** A plasma expander that may be used as a substitute for plasma; can be used to treat shock by increasing blood volume. Rouleaux may be observed in the recipient's serum or plasma.

**Diagnosis-related group (DRG):** Classification system that organizes short-term, general hospital inpatients into statistically stable groups based on age and illness.

**Diaphoresis:** Profuse sweating.

**Diastolic pressure:** The point of least pressure in the arterial vascular system; the lower or bottom value of a blood pressure reading.

**Dielectric constant:** A measure of the electrical conductivity of a suspending medium.

**Differential count:** Counting 100 leukocytes to ascertain the relative percentages of each.

**2,3-Diphosphoglycerate (2,3-DPG):** An organic phosphate in red blood cells that alters the affinity of hemoglobin for oxygen. Blood cells stored in a blood bank lose 2,3-DPG, but once infused, the substance is resynthesized or reactivated.

**Diploid:** Having two sets of 23 chromosomes, for a total of 46.

**Disk drive:** A hardware device in an information system that contains a disk(s) on which data are stored; provides for quick access to storing or retrieval of data.

**Disseminated intravascular coagulation (DIC):** Clinical condition of altered blood coagulation secondary to a variety of diseases.

**Dithiothreitol (DTT):** A sulfhydryl compound used to disrupt the disulfide bonds of immunoglobulin M, yielding monomeric units rather than the typical pentameric molecule.

**Diuresis:** Secretion and passage of large amounts of urine.

**Diuretic:** An agent that increases the secretion of urine, either by increasing glomerular filtration or by decreasing reabsorption from the tubules.

**Dizygotic twins:** Twins who are the product of two fertilized ova (also called fraternal twins).

**DNA polymerase:** An enzyme that catalyzes the template—dependent on synthesis of DNA. Also known as the $HB_eAg$ of the hepatitis B virion.

**Dolichos biflorus:** *See* Anti-$A_1$ lectin.

**Domain:** Portions along the immunoglobulin chain that show specific biologic function.

**Dominant:** A trait or characteristic that will be expressed in the offspring even though it is only carried on one of the homologous chromosomes.

**Donath-Landsteiner test:** A test usually performed in the blood bank to detect the presence of the Donath-Landsteiner antibody, which is a biphasic immunoglobulin G antibody with anti-P specificity found in patients suffering from paroxysmal cold hemoglobinuria.

**Donor:** An individual who donates a pint of blood.

**Dopamine:** A catecholamine synthesized by the adrenal gland, used especially in the treatment of shock.

**Dosage:** A phenomenon whereby an antibody reacts more strongly with a red cell carrying a double dose (homozygous inheritance of the appropriate gene) than with a red cell carrying a single dose (heterozygous inheritance) of an antigen.

**Dyscrasia:** An old term now used as a synonym for disease.

**Ecchymosis:** A form of macula appearing in large irregularly formed hemorrhagic areas of the skin; originally blue-black, then changing to greenish brown or yellow.

**Edema:** A local or generalized condition in which the body tissues contain an excessive amount of tissue fluid.

**Electrolyte:** A substance that in solution conducts an electric current; common electrolytes are acids, bases, and salts.

**Electrophoresis:** The movement of charged particles through a medium (paper, agar gel) in the presence of an electrical field; useful in the separation and analysis of proteins.

**Eluate:** *See* Elution.

**Elution:** A process whereby cells that are coated with antibody are treated in such a manner as to disrupt the bonds between the antigen and antibody. The freed antibody is collected in an inert diluent such as saline or 6 percent albumin. This antibody serum then can be tested to identify its specificity using routine methods. The mechanism to free the antibody may be physical (heating, shaking) or chemical (ether, acid), and the harvested antibody-containing fluid is called an eluate.

**Embolism:** Obstruction of a blood vessel by foreign substances or a blood clot.

**Embolus:** A mass of undissolved matter present in a blood or lymphatic vessel, brought there by the blood or lymph circulation.

**Endemic:** A disease that occurs continuously in a particular population but has a *low* mortality; used in contrast to epidemic.

**Endogenous:** Produced or arising from within a cell or organism.

**Endothelium:** A form of squamous epithelium consisting of flat cells that line the blood and lymphatic vessels, the heart, and various other body cavities; derived from mesoderm.

**Endotoxemia:** The presence of endotoxin in the blood; endotoxin is present in the cells of certain bacteria (e.g., gram-negative organisms).

**Engraftment:** The successful establishment, proliferation, and differentiation of transplanted hematopoietic stem cells.

**Enzyme:** A substance capable of catalyzing a reaction; proteins that induce chemical changes in other substances without being changed themselves.

**Enzyme-linked immunosorbent assay (ELISA):** An immunologic test.

**Enzyme treatment:** A procedure in which red blood cells are incubated with an enzyme solution that cleaves some of the membrane's glycoproteins, then washed free of the enzyme, and used in serologic testing. Enzyme treatment cleaves some antigens and exposes others.

**Epistaxis:** Hemorrhage from the nose; nosebleed.

**Epitope:** The portion of the antigen molecule that is directly involved in the interaction with the antibody; the antigenic determinant.

**Equivalence zone:** The zone in which antigen and antibody concentrations are optimal and lattice formation is most stable.

**Erythroblast:** Any form of nucleated red corpuscles, containing hemoglobin, which are not normally seen in the circulating blood.

**Erythroblastosis fetalis:** *See* Hemolytic disease of the newborn (HDN).

**Erythrocyte:** The blood cell that transports oxygen and carbon dioxide; a mature red blood cell.

**Ethylenediaminetetraacetic acid (EDTA):** An anticoagulant useful in hematologic testing and preferable when direct anti-human globulin testing is indicated.

**Euglobulin lysis:** Coagulation procedure testing for fibrinolysins.

**Exogenous:** Originating outside an organ or part.

**Extracorporeal:** Outside of the body.

**Extravascular:** Outside of the blood vessel.

**Factor assay:** Coagulation procedure to assay the concentration of specific plasma coagulation factors.

**Factor VIII concentrate:** A commercially prepared source of coagulation factor VIII.

**Febrile reaction:** A transfusion reaction caused by leukoagglutinins that is characterized by fever; usually observed in multiply transfused or multiparous patients.

**Fibrin:** A whitish filamentous protein or clot formed by the action of thrombin on fibrinogen, converting it to fibrin.

**Fibrinogen:** A protein produced in the liver that circulates in plasma. In the presence of thrombin, an enzyme produced by the activation of the clotting mechanism, fibrinogen is cleaved into fibrin, which is an insoluble protein that is responsible for clot formation.

**Fibrinolysin:** The substance that has the ability to dissolve fibrin; also called plasmin.

**Fibrinolysis:** Dissolution of fibrin by fibrinolysin caused by the action of a proteolytic enzyme system that is continually active in the body but that is increased greatly by various stress stimuli.

**Fibroblast:** Cells found throughout the body that synthesize connective tissue.

**Ficin:** A proteolytic enzyme derived from the fig.

**Ficoll:** A macromolecular additive that enhances the agglutination of red cells.

**Ficoll-Hypaque:** A density-gradient medium utilized for the separation and harvesting of specific white blood cells, most commonly lymphocytes.

**Formaldehyde:** A disinfectant solution.

**Forward grouping:** Testing unknown red cells with known reagent antisera to determine which ABO antigens are present.

**Fresh frozen plasma (FFP):** A frozen plasma product (from a single donor) that contains all clotting factors, especially the labile factors V and VIII; useful for clotting factor deficiencies other than hemophilia A, von Willebrand's disease, and hypofibrinogenemia.

**Freund's adjuvant:** Mixture of killed microorganisms, usually mycobacteria, in an oil-and-water emulsion. The material is administered to induce antibody formation and yields a much greater antibody response.

**Furosemide (Lasix):** An oral diuretic.

**G6PD (glucose-6-phosphate dehydrogenase):** A liver enzyme used to monitor liver function.

**Gamete:** A mature male or female reproductive cell.

**Gamma globulin:** A protein found in plasma and known to be involved in immunity.

**Gamma marker:** Allotypic marker on the gamma heavy chain of the IgG immunoglobulin.

**Gel test:** A blood group serology test method that uses a microtube containing gel (incorporating antisera or antiglobulin sera) that acts as a reaction vessel for agglutination.

**Gene:** A unit of inheritance within a chromosome.

**Genotype:** An individual's actual genetic makeup.

**Gestation:** In mammals, the length of time from conception to birth.

**Globin:** A protein constituent of hemoglobin. There are four globin chains in the hemoglobin molecule.

**Glomerulonephritis:** A form of nephritis in which the lesions involve primarily the glomeruli.

**Glutamic pyruvate transaminase:** A liver enzyme used to monitor liver function; also called serum glutamic pyruvate transaminase (SGPT).

**Gluten enteropathy:** A condition associated with malabsorption of food from the intestinal tract.

**Glycerol:** A cryoprotective agent.

**Glycerolization:** Adding glycerol to a unit of red cells for the purpose of freezing.

*Glycine soja:* Soybean extract or lectin used to differentiate different forms of polyagglutination.

**Glycophorin A:** A major glycoprotein of the red cell membrane. MN antigen activity is found on it.

**Glycophorin B:** An important red cell glycoprotein: SsU antigen activity is found here.

**Glycosyl transferase:** A protein enzyme that promotes the attachment of a specific sugar molecule to a predetermined acceptor molecule. Many blood group genes code for transferases, which reproduce their respective antigens by attaching sugars to designated precursor substances.

**Goodpasture syndrome:** A disease entity that represents a rapidly progressive glomerulonephritis associated with pulmonary lesions. Usually the patients possess an antibody to the basement membrane of the renal glomeruli.

**Graft-versus-host (GVH) disease:** A disorder in which the grafted tissue attacks the host tissue.

**Granulocytopenia:** Abnormal reduction of granulocytes in the blood.

**Hageman factor:** Synonym for coagulation factor XII.

**Half-life:** The time that is required for the concentration of a substance to be reduced by one half.

**Haploid:** Possessing half the normal number of chromosomes found in somatic or body cells; seen in germ cells (sperm and ova).

**Haplotype:** A term used in HLA testing to denote the five genes (*HLA-A, -B, -C, -D, -DR*) on the same chromosome.

**Haptene:** The portion of an antigen containing the grouping on which the specificity depends.

**Haptoglobin:** A mucoprotein to which hemoglobin released into plasma is bound; it is increased in certain inflammatory conditions and decreased in hemolytic disorders.

**Hardware:** Components of an information computer system that are the tangible, physical pieces of equipment that one can see and touch such as the central processing unit, cathode ray tube, and keyboard.

**HB$_c$Ag:** Hepatitis core antigen, referring to the nucleocapsid of the virion.

**HB$_e$Ag:** Hepatitis DNA polymerase of the nucleus of the virion.

**HB$_s$Ag:** Hepatitis B surface antigen.

**Hemangioma:** A benign tumor of dilated blood vessels.

**Hemarthrosis:** Bloody effusion into the cavity of a joint.

**Hematinic:** Pertaining to blood; an agent that increases the amount of hemoglobin in the blood.

**Hematocrit:** The proportion of red cells in whole blood, expressed as a percentage.

**Hematoma:** A swelling or mass of blood confined to an organ, tissue, or space and caused by a break in a blood vessel.

**Hematuria:** Blood in the urine.

**Heme:** The iron-containing protoporphyrin portion of the hemoglobin wherein the iron is in the ferrous ($Fe^{2+}$) state.

**Hemodialysis:** Removal of chemical substances from the blood by passing it through tubes made of semipermeable membranes, which are continually bathed by solutions that selectively remove unwanted material; used to cleanse the blood of patients in whom one or both kidneys are defective or absent and to remove excess accumulation of drugs or toxic chemicals in the blood.

**Hemodilution:** An increase in the volume of blood plasma, resulting in reduced relative concentration of red blood cells.

**Hemoglobin:** The iron-containing pigment of the red blood cells whose function is to carry oxygen from the lungs to the tissues.

**Hemoglobinemia:** Presence of hemoglobin in the blood plasma.

**Hemoglobin-oxygen dissociation curve:** The relationship between the percent saturation of the hemoglobin molecule with oxygen and the environmental oxygen tension.

**Hemoglobinuria:** The presence of hemoglobin in the urine freed from lysed red blood cells, which occurs when hemoglobin from disintegrating red blood cells or from rapid hemolysis of red cells exceeds the ability of the blood proteins to combine with the hemoglobin.

**Hemolysin:** An antibody that activates complement leading to cell lysis.

**Hemolysis:** Disruption of the red cell membrane and the subsequent release of hemoglobin into the suspending medium or plasma.

**Hemolytic disease of the newborn (HDN):** A disease characterized by anemia, jaundice, enlargement of the liver and spleen, and generalized edema (hydrops fetalis) that is caused by maternal IgG antibodies crossing the placenta and attacking fetal red cells when there is a fetomaternal blood group incompatibility (usually ABO or Rh antibodies). Synonym is erythroblastosis fetalis.

**Hemolytic transfusion reaction (HTR):** A reaction from red cell destruction caused by patient's antibody(ies) directed to donor red cell antigen(s).

**Hemophilia A:** A hereditary disorder characterized by greatly prolonged coagulation time. The blood fails to clot and bleeding occurs; caused by inheritance of a factor VIII deficiency, it occurs almost exclusively in males.

**Hemophilia B:** "Christmas disease," which is a hemophilia-like disease caused by a lack of factor IX.

**Hemopoiesis:** Formation of blood cells. Synonym is hematopoiesis.

**Hemorrhage:** Abnormal internal or external bleeding; may be venous, arterial, or capillary; from blood vessels into the tissues or out of the body.

**Hemorrhagic diathesis:** Uncontrolled spontaneous bleeding.

**Hemosiderin:** An iron-containing pigment derived from hemoglobin from disintegration of red blood cells; a method of storing iron until it is needed for making hemoglobin.

**Hemostasis:** Arrest of bleeding; maintaining blood flow within vessels by repairing rapidly any vascular break without compromising the fluidity of the blood.

**Hemotherapy:** Blood transfusion as a therapeutic measure.

**Heparin:** An anticoagulant used for collecting whole blood that is to be filtered for the removal of leukocytes.

**Hepatitis:** Inflammation of the liver.

**Hepatitis-associated antigen (HAA):** Older terminology currently replaced by HB$_s$Ag.

**Hepatitis B immunoglobulin (HBIg):** An immune serum given to individuals exposed to the hepatitis B virus.

**Heterozygote:** An individual with different alleles for a given characteristic.

**Heterozygous:** Possessing different alleles at a given locus.

**High-frequency antigen:** Also known as high-incidence antigen; antigen whose frequency in the population is 98 to 99 percent.

**Histocompatibility:** The ability of cells to survive without immunologic interference; especially important in blood transfusion and transplantation.

**HLA:** Human leukocyte antigen.

**Homeostasis:** State of equilibrium of the internal environment of the body that is maintained by dynamic processes of feedback and regulation.

**Homozygote:** An individual developing from gametes with similar alleles and thus possessing like pairs of genes for a given hereditary characteristic.

**Homozygous:** Possessing a pair of identical alleles.

**Hormone:** A substance originating in an organ or gland that is conveyed through the blood to another part of the body, stimulating it chemically to increase functional activity and increase secretion.

**Hyaluronidase:** An enzyme found in the testes; present in semen.

**Hybridoma:** A hybrid (cross) between a plasmacytoma cell and a spleen (or Ab-producing) cell that produces a monoclonal antibody, resulting in a malignant cell line that can grow indefinitely in culture and can produce high quantities of Ab. This antibody is monoclonal because only one Ab-producing cell combined with the plasmacytoma cell is present.

**Hydatid cyst fluid:** Source of $P_1$ substance.

**Hydrocortisone:** A corticosteroid with anti-inflammatory properties.

**Hydrops fetalis:** *See* Hemolytic disease of the newborn (HDN).

**Hydroxyethyl starch (HES):** A red cell sedimenting agent used to facilitate leukocyte withdrawal during leukapheresis.

**Hypertension:** Increase in blood pressure.

**Hyperventilation:** Rapid breathing that results in carbon dioxide depletion and accompanies hypotension, vasoconstriction, and fainting.

**Hypogammaglobulinemia:** Decreased levels of gamma globulins seen in some disease states.

**Hypotension:** Decrease in blood pressure.

**Hypothermia:** Having a body temperature below normal.

**Hypovolemia:** Diminished blood volume.

**Hypoxia:** Deficiency of oxygen.

*Iberis amara: See* Anti-M lectin.

**Icterus:** A condition characterized by yellowish skin, whites of the eyes, mucous membranes, and body fluids caused by increased circulating bilirubin resulting from excessive hemolysis or from liver damage due to hepatitis. Synonym is jaundice.

**Idiopathic:** Pertaining to conditions without clear pathogenesis, or disease without recognizable cause, as of spontaneous origin.

**Idiopathic thrombocytopenic purpura (ITP):** Bleeding owing to a decreased number of platelets; the etiology is unknown, with most evidence pointing to platelet autoantibodies.

**Idiothrombocythemia:** An increase in blood platelets of unknown etiology.

**Idiotype:** The portion of the immunoglobulin variable region that is the antigen-combining site, which interacts with the antigenic epitope.

**Immune response:** The reactions of the body to substances that are foreign or are interpreted as being foreign. Cell-mediated or cellular immunity pertains to tissue destruction mediated by T cells, such as graft rejection and hypersensitivity reactions. Humoral immunity pertains to cell destruction response during the early period of the reaction.

**Immune serum globulin:** Gamma globulin protein fraction of serum-containing antibodies.

**Immunoblast:** A mitotically active T or B cell.

**Immunodeficiency:** A decrease from the normal concentration of immunoglobulins in serum.

**Immunodominant sugar:** In reference to glycoprotein or glycolipid antigens, the sugar molecule that gives the antigen its specificity (e.g., galactose, which confers B antigen specificity).

**Immunogen:** Any substance capable of stimulating an immune response.

**Immunogenicity:** The ability of an antigen to stimulate an antibody response.

**Immunoglobulin (Ig):** One of a family of closely related though not identical proteins that are capable of acting as antibodies: IgA, IgD, IgE, IgG, and IgM. IgA is the principal immunoglobulin in exocrine secretions such as saliva and tears. IgD may play a role in antigen recognition and the initiation of antibody synthesis. IgE, produced by the cells lining the intestinal and respiratory tracts, is important in forming reagin. IgG is the main immunoglobulin in human serum. IgM is formed in almost every immune response during the early period of the reaction.

**Immunologic memory:** The development of T and B memory cells that have been sensitized by exposure to an antigen and respond rapidly under subsequent encounters with the antigen.

**Immunologic unresponsiveness:** Development of a tolerance to certain antigens that would otherwise evoke an immune response.

**Immunoprecipitin:** An antigen-antibody reaction that results in precipitation.

**Incubation:** In vitro combination of antigen and antibody under certain conditions of time and temperature to allow antigen-antibody complexes to occur.

**Initiation:** The deposition of *N*-formylmethionine on the ribosome, which begins the synthesis of all proteins.

*In Lu:* A rare dominant gene that inhibits the production of all Lutheran antigens as well as i, $P_1$, and $Au^a$ (Auberger). The quantity of antigen on the red cell is markedly reduced in the presence of *In Lu*; it may be virtually undetectable.

**Interface:** Software that allows a computer system to send data to or receive data from another computer system.

**Intraoperative salvage:** A procedure to reclaim a patient's blood loss during an operation by reinfusion.

**Intravascular:** Within the blood vessel.

**In utero:** Within the uterus.

**Inversion:** The breaking of a chromosome during division with subsequent reattachment occurring in an inverted or upside-down position.

**In vitro:** Outside the living body, as in a laboratory setting.

**In vivo:** Inside the living body.

**Ion exchange resin:** Synthetic organic substances of high molecular weight. They replace certain positive or negative ions, which they encounter in solutions.

**Ionic strength:** Refers to the number of charged particles present in a solution.

*Ir genes:* Immune response genes found within the region of the major histocompatibility complex. *Ir* genes in humans are likely to exist; preliminary evidence shows genes at the D-related locus may be analogous to the *Ir* genes of mice.

**Ischemia:** Local and temporary deficiency of blood supply caused by obstruction of the circulation to a cell, tissue, or organ.

**Isogglutinins:** The ABO antibodies anti-A, anti-B, and anti-A,B.

**Isoimmune:** An antibody produced against a foreign antigen in the same species.

**Isotype:** The subclasses of an immunoglobulin molecule.

**Jaundice:** *See* Icterus.

**Karyotype:** A photomicrograph of a single cell in the metaphase stage of mitosis that is arranged to show the chromosomes in descending order of size.

**Kernicterus:** A form of icterus neonatorum occurring in infants, developing at 2 to 8 days of life; prognosis poor if untreated.

**Kinin:** A group of polypeptides that have considerable biologic activity (e.g., vasoactivity).

**Kleihauer-Betke technique:** Quantitative procedure used to determine the amount of fetal cells present in the maternal circulation.

**Km:** Light chain marker on the kappa light chains of IgG (formerly known as InV).

**Labile:** Capable of deteriorating rapidly upon storage.

**Lectin:** Proteins present in plants (usually seeds), which bind specifically to carbohydrate determinants and agglutinate erythrocytes through their cell surface of oligosaccharide determinants.

**Leukemia:** Malignant proliferation of leukocytes, which spill into the blood, yielding an elevated leukocyte count.

**Leukoagglutinins:** Antibodies to white blood cells.

**Ligature:** Process of binding or tying; a band or bandage; a thread or wire for tying a blood vessel or other structure in order to constrict it.

**Linkage:** The association between distinct genes that occupy closely situated loci on the same chromosome, resulting in an association in the inheritance of these genes.

**Linkage disequilibrium:** Genes associated in a haplotype more often than would be expected on the basis of chance alone.

**Locus:** The site of a gene on a chromosome.

**Low-frequency antigen:** Also known as low-incidence antigen; antigen whose frequency in a random population is very low—less than 10 percent.

**Low ionic–polycation test:** A compatibility test that incorporates both glycine (low ionic) and protamine (polycation) in an effort to obtain maximal sensitivity and to minimize the need for antibody screening.

**Low ionic strength solution (LISS):** A type of potentiating medium in use for serologic testing. Reducing the ionic strength of the red cell suspending medium increases the affinity of the antigen for its corresponding antibody such that sensitivity can be increased and incubation time decreased. LISS contains glycine or glucose in addition to saline.

**Lymphocyte:** A type of white blood cell involved in the immune response. Lymphocytes normally total 20 to 45 percent of total white cells. T lymphocytes mature during passage through the thymus or after interaction with thymic hormones; these cells function both in cellular and humoral immunity. Subsets include helper T cells ($T_h$), which enhance B-cell antibody production, and suppressor T cells ($T_s$), which inhibit B-cell antibody production. B-lymphocyte cells are not processed by the thymus. Through morphologic and functional differentiation, they mature into plasma cells that secrete immunoglobulin.

**Lymphoma:** A solid tumor of lymphocyte cells.

**Lysosomes:** Part of an intracellular digestive system that exists as separate particles in the cell. Even though their importance in health and disease is certain, all the precise ways lysosomes effect changes are not understood.

**Macroglobulinemia:** Abnormal presence of high-molecular-weight immunoglobulins (IgM) in the blood.

**Macrophage:** End-stage development for the blood monocyte; these cells can ingest (phagocytose) a variety of substances for subsequent digestion or storage and are located in a number of sites in the body (e.g., spleen, liver, lung), existing as free mobile cells or as fixed cells. Functions include elimination of senescent blood cells and participation in the immune response.

**Major crossmatch:** Compatibility testing procedure using recipient's serum and donor red cells.

**Major histocompatibility complex (MHC):** Present in all mammalian and ovarian species; analogous to HLA complex. HLA antigens are within the MHC at a locus on chromosome 6.

**Malaria:** An acute and sometimes chronic infectious disease caused by the presence of a parasite within red blood cells. The parasite is *Plasmodium* (*P. vivax, P. falciparum, P. malariae, P. ovale*), which is introduced through bites of infected female *Anopheles* mosquitoes or through blood transfusion.

**Meiosis:** Type of cell division of germ cells in which two successive divisions of the nucleus produce cells that contain half the number of chromosomes present in somatic cells.

**Menorrhagia:** Excessive menstrual bleeding, in number of days or amount of blood, or both.

**2-Mercaptoethanol (2-ME):** A sulfhydryl compound used to disrupt the disulfide bonds of immunoglobulin M, yielding monomeric units rather than the typical pentameric units.

**Metastasis:** Movement of bacteria or body cells, especially cancer cells, from one part of the body to another; change in location of a disease or of its manifestations or transfer from one organ or part to another not directly connected. Spread is by the lymph or blood circulation.

**Methemoglobin:** An abnormal form of hemoglobin wherein the ferrous ($Fe^{2+}$) iron has been oxidized to ferric ($Fe^{3+}$) iron.

**Methyldopa (Aldomet):** Common drug used to treat hypertension; frequently the cause of a positive direct Coombs' test result.

**Microaggregates:** Aggregates of platelets and leukocytes that accumulate in stored blood.

**Microglobulin ($\beta_2$):** A protein synthesized by all nucleated cell types; an integral part of the class I MHC antigens.

**Microspherocytes:** Red blood cells, small and spherical, in certain kinds of anemia.

**Minor crossmatch:** Compatibility testing procedure using recipient's red cells and donor's serum.

**Mitosis:** Type of cell division in which each daughter cell contains the same number of chromosomes as the parent cell. All cells except sex cells undergo mitosis.

**Mixed field:** A type of agglutination pattern in which numerous small clumps of cells exist amid a sea of free cells.

**MLC:** Mixed lymphocyte culture.

**MLR:** Mixed lymphocyte reaction.

**Modem:** Hardware device that provides the ability to attach to a computer system via telephone communication lines.

**Monoclonal:** Antibody derived from a single ancestral antibody-producing parent cell.

**Monocytes:** *See* Macrophage.

**Monozygotic twins:** Two offspring that develop from a single fertilized ovum.

**Mosaic:** An antigen composed of several subunits, such as the $Rh_0(D)$ antigen. A mixture of characteristics that may result from a genetic crossover or mutation.

**Multiparous:** Having borne more than one child.

**Multiple myeloma:** A neoplastic proliferation of plasma cells, which is characterized by very high immunoglobulin levels of monoclonal origin.

**Mutation:** A change in a gene potentially capable of being transmitted to offspring. **Point m.:** A change in a base in DNA that can lead to a change in the amino acid incorporated into the polypeptide; identifiable by analysis of the amino acid sequences of the original protein and its mutant offspring. **Frameshift m.:** A change in which a message is read incorrectly either because a base is missing or an extra base is added, which results in an entirely new polypeptide because the triplet sequence has been shifted one base.

**Myelofibrosis:** Replacement of bone marrow by fibrous tissue.

**Myeloproliferative:** An autonomous, purposeless increase in the production of the myeloid cell elements of the bone marrow, which includes granulocytic, erythrocytic, and megakaryocytic cell lines as well as the stromal connective tissue.

**N-acetylneuraminic acid (NANA):** *See* Sialic acid.

**Neonate:** A newborn infant up to 4 months of age.

**Network:** Configuration of personal computers linked together with cables; allows all of the personal computers to access common data and software located on a fileserver.

**Neuraminidase:** An enzyme that cleaves sialic acid from the red cell membrane.

**Neutralization:** Inactivating an antibody by reacting it with an antigen against which it is directed.

**Neutrophil:** A leukocyte that ingests bacteria and small particles and plays a role in combating infection.

**Nondisjunction:** Failure of a pair of chromosomes to separate during meiosis.

**Nonresponder:** An individual whose immune system does not respond well in antibody formation to antigenic stimulation.

**Normal serum albumin:** *See* Albumin.

**O$_h$:** *See* Bombay.

**Oligonucleotide:** A short, approximately 20 nucleotides in length, synthetic segment of DNA used as a probe.

**Oliguria:** Diminished amount of urine formation.

**Opsonin:** A substance in serum that promotes immune adherence and facilitates phagocytosis by the reticuloendothelial system.

**Orthostatic:** Concerning an erect position.

**Osmolality:** The osmotic concentration of a solution determined by the ionic concentration of dissolved substances per unit of solvent.

**Ouchterlony diffusion:** An immunologic procedure in which antibody and antigen are placed in wells of a gel medium plate and allowed to diffuse in order to visualize the reaction by a precipitin line.

**Oxyhemoglobin:** The combined form of hemoglobin and oxygen.

**P$_{50}$:** The partial pressure of oxygen or oxygen tension at which the hemoglobin molecule is 50 percent saturated with oxygen.

**Pallor:** Paleness; lack of color.

**Panagglutinin:** An antibody capable of agglutinating all red blood cells tested, including the patient's own cells.

**Pancytopenia:** A reduction in all cellular elements of the blood, including red cells, white cells, and platelets.

**Panel:** A large number of group O reagent red cells that are of known antigenic characterization and are used for antibody identification.

**Papain:** A proteolytic enzyme derived from papaya.

**Paragloboside:** The immediate precursor for the H and P antigens of the red cell.

**Paroxysm:** A sudden, periodic attack or recurrence of symptoms of a disease.

**Paroxysmal cold hemoglobinuria (PCH):** A type of cold autoimmune hemolytic anemia usually found in children suffering from viral infections in which a biphasic immunoglobulin G antibody can be demonstrated with anti-P specificity. *See also* Donath-Landsteiner test.

**Paroxysmal nocturnal hemoglobinuria (PNH):** An intrinsic defect in the red blood cell membrane rendering it more susceptible to hemolysins in an acid environment; characterized by hemoglobin in the urine following periods of sleep.

**Perfusion:** Supplying an organ or tissue with nutrients and oxygen by passing blood or another suitable fluid through it.

**Perioral paresthesia:** Tingling around the mouth occasionally experienced by apheresis donors, resulting from the rapid return of citrated plasma, which contains citrate-bound calcium and free citrate.

**Peroxidase:** An enzyme that hastens the transfer of oxygen from peroxide to a tissue that requires oxygen; this process is essential to intracellular respiration.

**Phagocytosis:** Ingestion of microorganisms, other cells, and foreign particles by a phagocyte.

**Phenotype:** The outward expression of genes (e.g., a blood type). On blood cells, serologically demonstrable antigens constitute the phenotype, except those sugar sites that are determined by transferases.

**Phenylthiocarbamide (PTC):** A chemical used in studying medical genetics to detect the presence of a marker gene. About 70 percent of the population inherit the ability to taste PTC, which tastes bitter; the remaining 30 percent find PTC tasteless. The inheritance of this trait is due to a single dominant gene of a pair.

**Phlebotomy:** The procedure used to draw blood from a person.

**Phosphoglyceromutase:** A red cell enzyme.

**Phototherapy:** Exposure to sunlight or artificial light for therapeutic purposes.

**Plasma:** The liquid portion of whole blood containing water, electrolytes, glucose, fats, proteins, and gases. Plasma contains all the clotting factors necessary for coagulation, but in an inactive form. Once coagulation occurs, the fluid is converted to serum.

**Plasma cell:** A B lymphocyte–derived cell that secretes immunoglobulins or antibodies.

**Plasmapheresis:** A procedure using a machine to remove only plasma from a donor or patient.

**Plasma protein fraction (PPF):** Also known as Plasmanate; sterile pooled plasma stored as a fluid or freeze-dried and used for volume replacement.

**Plasminogen:** A protein in many tissues and body fluids important in preventing fibrin clot formation.

***Plasmodium:*** *See* Malaria.

***Plasmodium knowlesi:*** A parasite that causes malaria in monkeys.

**Platelet:** A round or oval disc, 2 to 4 $\mu$m in diameter, that is derived from the cytoplasm of the megakaryocyte, a large cell in the bone marrow. Platelets play an important role in blood coagulation, hemostasis, and blood thrombus formation. When a small vessel is injured, platelets adhere to each other and to the edges of the injury, forming a "plug" that covers the area and stops the blood loss.

**Platelet concentrate:** Platelets prepared from a single unit of whole blood or plasma and suspended in a specific volume of the original plasma; also known as random-donor platelets.

**Plateletpheresis:** A procedure using a machine to remove only platelets from a donor or patient.

**Platelet refractoriness:** Failure to yield an increase in recipient's platelet count on transfusion of suitably preserved platelets. HLA alloimmunization is a common cause.

**Polyacrylamide gel:** A type of matrix used in electrophoresis upon which substances are separated.

**Polyagglutination:** A state in which an individual's red cells are agglutinated by all sera regardless of blood type.

**Polyagglutinins:** Naturally occurring immunoglobulin antibodies that are found in most normal human adult sera.

**Polybrene:** A positively charged polymer that causes normal red cells to aggregate spontaneously by neutralizing the negative surface charge contributed by sialic acid.

**Polyclonal:** Antibodies derived from more than one antibody-producing parent cell.

**Polycythemia vera:** A chronic life-shortening myeloproliferative disorder involving all bone marrow elements, characterized by an increase in red blood cell mass and hemoglobin concentration.

**Polymer:** Combination of two or more molecules of the same substance.

**Polymerase chain reaction (PCR):** An in vitro method of amplification of a specific DNA segment.

**Polymorphism:** A genetic system that possesses numerous allelic forms, such as a blood group system.

**Polyspecific Coombs' sera:** A reagent that contains antihuman globulin sera against immunoglobulin G and C3d.

**Polyvinylpyrrolidone (PVP):** A neutral polymeric substance used to increase blood volume in patients with extensive blood loss; also used to enhance antigen-antibody reactions in vitro.

**Portal hypertension:** Increased pressure in the portal vein as a result of obstruction of the flow of blood through the liver.

**Postpartum:** Occurring after childbirth.

**Potentiator:** A substance that, when added to a serum and cell mixture, will enhance antigen-antibody interactions.

**Precipitation:** The formation of a visible complex (precipitate) in a medium containing soluble antigen (precipitinogen) and the corresponding antibody (precipitin).

**Precipitin:** An antibody formed in the blood serum of an animal by the presence of a soluble antigen, usually a protein. When added to a solution of the antigen, it brings about precipitation. The injected protein is called the antigen and the antibody produced, the precipitin.

**Precursor substance:** A substance that is converted to another substance by the addition of a specific constituent (e.g., a sugar residue).

**Primer:** A short segment of single-stranded DNA, usually 17 to 25 nucleotides long, used to initiate DNA replication in PCR.

**Private antigen:** An antigenic characteristic of the red blood cell membrane that is unique to an individual or a related family of individuals and, therefore, is not commonly found on all cells (usually less than 1 percent of the population).

**Probe:** A fragment of DNA which is labeled and hybridized to diagnostic material to locate a complementary strand of DNA.

**Prodrome:** A symptom indicative of an approaching disease.

**Propositus:** The initial individual whose condition led to investigation of a hereditary disorder or to a serologic evaluation of family members. Feminine form is proposita. Synonyms are proband and index case.

**Prospective validation:** Validation testing of software; done before implementation of the computer system.

**Prosthesis:** An artificial substitute for a missing part, such as an artificial extremity.

**Protamine:** A polycation with applications similar to those of polybrene.

**Protamine sulfate:** A substance used to neutralize the effects of heparin.

**Prothrombin complex:** A concentrate of coagulation factors II, VII, IX, and X in lyophilized form.

**Prozone:** Incomplete lattice formation caused by an excess of antibody molecules relative to the number of antigen sites, resulting in false-negative reactions.

**PRP:** Platelet-rich plasma.

**Public antigen:** An antigen characteristic of the red blood cell membrane found commonly among individuals, usually greater than 98 percent of the population.

**Pulmonary artery wedge pressure:** Pressure measured in the pulmonary artery at its capillary end.

**Pulse pressure:** The difference between the systolic and the diastolic pressures.

**Quality assurance (QA):** A set of planned actions to provide confidence that systems and elements that influence the quality of the product or service are working as expected individually and collectively.

**Radioimmunoassay (RIA):** A very sensitive method for determination of substances present in low concentrations in serum or plasma by using specific antibodies and radioactively labeled or tagged substances.

**Rapid passive hemagglutination assay (RPHA):** A third-generation procedure used in hepatitis testing.

**Rapid passive latex assay (RPLA):** A second-generation procedure used in hepatitis testing.

**Raynaud's disease:** A peripheral vascular disorder characterized by abnormal vasoconstriction of the extremities upon exposure to cold or emotional stress. A history of symptoms for at least 2 years is necessary for diagnosis.

**Recessive:** A type of gene that, in the presence of its dominant allele, does not express itself; expression occurs when it is inherited in the homozygous state.

**Recipient:** A patient who is receiving a transfusion of blood or a blood product.

**Refractory:** Obstinate; stubborn; resistant to ordinary treatment; resistant to stimulation (said of a muscle or nerve).

**Respiratory distress syndrome (RDS):** A condition, formerly known as hyaline membrane disease, accounting for more than 25,000 infant deaths per year in the United States. Clinical signs, including delayed onset of respiration and low Apgar score, are usually present at birth.

**Reticulocyte:** Also known as neocyte, the last stage of development before becoming a mature erythrocyte. The reticulocyte has lost its nucleus but retains some residual RNA in its cytoplasm, which is stainable by special techniques. It may be slightly larger than the mature red cell.

**Reticuloendothelial system (RES):** The fixed phagocytic cells of the body, such as the macrophage, having the ability to ingest particulate matter.

**Retrospective validation:** Validation testing of software, which is done after the computer system has been implemented.

**Reverse grouping:** Testing a patient's serum with commercial or reagent A and B red blood cells to determine which ABO antibodies are present.

**Rh immunoglobulin (RhIg):** A concentrated, purified anti-$Rh_0(D)$ prepared from human serum (of immunized donors), which is given to $Rh_0(D)$-negative mothers after they have given birth to an $Rh_0(D)$-positive baby or after abortion or miscarriage. It acts to prevent the mother from becoming immunized to any $Rh_0(D)$-positive fetal cells that may have entered her circulation and thereby prevents formation of anti-$Rh_0(D)$ by the mother.

**$Rh_{null}$:** A rare Rh phenotype in which no Rh antigens are expressed on the red blood cell; may result from the action of an inhibitor gene that is inherited independently from the *Rh* genes or caused by the rare genotype $\bar{r}\,\bar{r}$, which is the *Rh* amorphic gene.

**Ribonucleic acid (RNA):** A nucleic acid that controls protein synthesis in all living cells. There are three different types, and all are derived from the information encoded in the DNA of the cell. Messenger RNA (mRNA) carries the code for specific amino acid sequences from the DNA to the cytoplasm for protein synthesis. Transfer RNA (tRNA) carries the amino acid groups to the ribosome for protein synthesis. Ribosomal RNA (rRNA), which exists within the ribosomes, is thought to assist in protein synthesis.

**Ribosome:** A cellular organelle that contains ribosomal RNA and protein and functions to synthesize protein. Ribosomes may be single units or clusters called polyribosomes or polysomes.

**Rickettsia:** Any of the microorganisms belonging to the genus *Rickettsia*.

**Ringer's lactated injection:** An aqueous solution suitable for intravenous use.

**Rouleaux:** Coinlike stacking of red blood cells in the presence of plasma expanders or abnormal plasma proteins.

**Saline anti-D:** A low-protein (6 to 8 percent albumin) immunoglobulin M anti-D reagent.

***Salvia horminum:*** Plant lectin used in the differentiation of various forms of polyagglutination.

***Salvia sclarea:*** Plant lectin with anti-Tn activity, used in the differentiation of various forms of polyagglutination.

**Screening cells:** Group O reagent red cells that are used in antibody detection or screening tests.

**SD:** Serologically defined antigens.

**Secretor:** An individual who is capable of secreting soluble, glycoprotein ABH-soluble substances into saliva and other body fluids.

**Sensitization:** A condition of being made sensitive to a specific substance (e.g., an antigen) after the initial exposure to that substance. This results in the development of immunologic memory that evokes an accentuated immune response with subsequent exposure to the substance.

**Sepsis:** Pathologic state, usually febrile, resulting from the presence of microorganisms or their toxins in the bloodstream.

**Septicemia:** Presence of pathogenic bacteria in the blood.

**Serologic test for syphilis (STS):** First developed in 1906 by Wassermann, present tests are of three main types based on complement fixation, flocculation, and detection of specific antitreponemal antibodies.

**Serotinin:** A chemical present in platelets that is a potent vasoconstrictor.

**Serum:** The fluid that remains after whole blood has clotted.

**Sex chromosome:** Chromosomes associated with determination of sex.

**Sex linkage:** A genetic characteristic located on the X or Y chromosome.

**Shelf life:** The amount of time blood or blood products may be stored upon collection.

**Shock:** A clinical syndrome in which the peripheral blood flow is inadequate to return sufficient blood to the heart for normal function, particularly transport of oxygen to all organs and tissues. Shock may be caused by a variety of conditions, including hemorrhage, infection, drug reaction, trauma, poisoning, myocardial infarction, or dehydration. Symptoms include paleness of skin (pallor), a bluish gray discoloration (cyanosis), a weak and rapid pulse, rapid and shallow breathing, or blood pressure that is decreased and perhaps unmeasurable.

**Sialic acid:** A group of sugars found on the red cell membrane attached to a protein backbone; the major source of the membrane's net negative charge.

**Sickle trait:** Blood that is heterozygous for the gene coding for the abnormal hemoglobin of sickle cell anemia.

**Siderosis:** A form of pneumoconiosis resulting from inhalation of dust or fumes containing iron particles.

**Single-donor platelets:** Platelets collected from a single donor by apheresis.

**Sodium dodecyl sulfate (SDS):** An anionic detergent that renders a net negative charge to substances it solubilizes.

**Software:** Written instructions for a computer, which result in information being stored, manipulated, and retrieved.

**Solid phase test:** A blood group serology test method that uses RBC adherence on an endpoint instead of agglutination.

**Specificity:** The affinity of an antibody and the antigen against which it is directed.

**Splenomegaly:** Enlargement of the spleen.

**Steatorrhea:** Increased secretion of the sebaceous glands.

**Stem cell:** An unspecialized cell, capable of self-renewal, that gives rise to a group of differential cells such as the hematopoietic cells.

**Steroid hormones:** Hormones of the adrenal cortex and the sex hormones.

**Stertorous:** Pertaining to laborious breathing.

**Storage lesion:** A loss of viability and function associated with certain biochemical changes that are initiated when blood is stored in vitro.

**Stroma:** The red cell membrane that is left after hemolysis has occurred.

**Subgroup:** Antigens within the ABO group that react less strongly with their corresponding antisera than do A and B antigens.

**Survival studies:** A measure of the in vivo survival of transfused blood cells; usually performed with radioactive isotopes. Normal red cells survive approximately 100 to 120 days in circulation.

**Syngeneic:** Possessing identical genotypes, as monozygotic twins.

**Synteny:** Genes that are closely situated on a chromosome but cannot be shown to be linked.

**Systemic lupus erythematosus (SLE):** A disseminated autoimmune disease characterized by anemia, thrombocytopenia, increased immunoglobulin G levels, and the presence of four immunoglobulin G antibodies: antinuclear antibody, antinucleoprotein antibody, anti-DNA antibody, and antihistone antibody; believed to be caused by suppressor T-cell dysfunction.

**System manager:** A specially trained person who is responsible for the maintenance of an information system.

**Systolic pressure:** Maximum blood pressure that occurs at ventricular contraction; upper value of a blood pressure reading.

**Tachycardia:** Abnormally rapid heart action, usually defined as a heart rate greater than 100 beats per minute.

**Tachypnea:** Abnormally rapid respirations.

**Template bleeding time:** The elapsed time a uniform incision made by a template and blade stops bleeding, which is a test of platelet function, assuming a normal platelet count.

**Tetany:** A nervous affliction characterized by intermittent spasms of the muscles of the extremities.

**Thalassemia major:** The homozygous form of deficient beta-chain synthesis, which is very severe and presents itself during childhood. Prognosis varies; however, the younger the child at disease onset, the less favorable the outcome.

**Thermal amplitude:** The range of temperature over which an antibody demonstrates serologic and/or in vitro activity.

**Thrombin:** An enzyme that converts fibrinogen to fibrin so that a soluble clot can be formed.

**Thrombocytopenia:** A reduction in the platelet count below the normal level, which is associated with spontaneous hemorrhage.

**Thrombotic thrombocytopenic purpura (TTP):** A coagulation disorder characterized by (1) increased bleeding owing to a decreased number of platelets, (2) hemolytic anemia, (3) renal failure, and (4) changing neurologic signs. The characteristic morphologic lesion is thrombotic occlusion of small arteries or capillaries in various organs.

**Thymidine:** An essential ingredient used in DNA synthesis and incorporated by T lymphocytes undergoing blast transformation in response to foreign HLA-D antigens in the mixed lymphocyte culture test.

**Titer:** A measure of the strength of an antibody by testing its reactivity at increasing dilutions against the appropriate antigen. The reciprocal of the highest dilution that shows agglutination is the titer.

**Titer score:** A method used to evaluate more precisely than simple dilution by comparing the titers of an antibody. Agglutination at each higher dilution is graded on a continuous scale; the total is the titer score.

**Trait:** A characteristic that is inherited.

**Trans:** The location of two or more genes on opposite chromosomes of a homologous pair.

**Transcription:** The process of RNA production from DNA, which requires the enzyme RNA polymerase.

**Transferase:** An enzyme that catalyzes the transfer of atoms or groups of atoms from one chemical compound to another.

**Transfuse:** To perform a transfusion.

**Transfusion:** The injection of blood, a blood component, saline, or other fluids into the bloodstream. **Cadaver blood t.:** Using blood obtained from a cadaver within a short time after death. **Direct t.:** Transfer of blood directly from one person to another. **Exchange t.:** Transfusion and withdrawal of small amounts of blood, repeated until blood volume is almost entirely exchanged; used in infants born with hemolytic disease. **Indirect t.:** Transfusion of blood from a donor to a suitable storage container and then to a patient. **Intrauterine t.:** Transfusion of blood into a fetus in utero.

**Transfusion reaction:** An adverse response to a transfusion.

**Translation:** The production of protein from the interactions of the RNAs.

**Translocation:** Transfer of a portion of one chromosome to its allele.

**Transposition:** The location of two genes on opposite chromosomes of a homologous pair.

**Trypsin:** A proteolytic enzyme formed in the intestine.

**Type and screen:** Testing a patient's blood for ABO group, Rh type, and atypical antibodies. The sample is then retained in the event that subsequent crossmatching is necessary.

*Ulex europaeus: See* Anti-H lectin.

**Ultracentrifugation:** Rapid and prolonged centrifugation used to separate by density gradient substances of various specific gravities.

**Urticaria:** A vascular reaction of the skin similar to hives.

**User:** A person who uses a computer information system.

**Vaccine:** A suspension of infectious organisms or components of them that is given as a form of passive immunization to establish resistance to the infectious disease caused by that organism.

**Validation:** A systematic process of testing the hardware, software, and user components of an information system to ensure that they are functioning correctly for their intended purpose.

**Valvular:** Relating to or having a valve.

**Variable region:** That portion of the immunoglobulin light and heavy chains where amino acid sequences vary tremendously, thereby permitting the different immunoglobulin molecules to recognize different antigenic determinants. In other words, the variable region determines the antigen against which the antibody will react, thus providing each antibody molecule with its unique specificity. The variable region is located at the amino terminal region of the molecule.

**Vasculitis:** Inflammation of a blood or lymph vessel.

**Vasoconstriction:** Constriction of blood vessels.

**Vasodilatation:** Dilatation of blood vessels, especially small arteries and arterioles.

**Vasovagal syncope:** Syncope resulting from hypotension caused by emotional stress, pain, acute blood loss, fear, or rapid rising from a recumbent position.

**Venesection:** *See* Phlebotomy.

**Venipuncture:** Puncture of a vein for any purpose.

**Venule:** A tiny vein continuous with a capillary.

**Viability:** Ability of a cell to live or to survive for a reasonably normal lifespan.

*Vicia graminea: See* Anti-N lectin.

**Virion:** A complete virus particle; a unit of genetic material surrounded by a protective coat that serves as a vehicle for its transmission from one cell to another.

**von Willebrand factor:** Coagulation factor VIII.

**von Willebrand's disease:** A congenital bleeding disorder.

**WAIHA:** Warm autoimmune hemolytic anemia. A hemolytic anemia caused by the patient's autoantibody that reacts at 37°C.

**Wharton's jelly:** A gelatinous intercellular substance consisting of primitive connective tissue of the umbilical cord.

**X chromosome:** The chromosome that determines female sex characteristics. The normal female has two X chromosomes, and the normal male an X and a Y chromosome.

**Xeno-:** Prefix indicating differing species. For example, a xenoantibody is an antibody produced in one species against an antigen present in another species. Synonym is hetero-.

**Yaws:** An infectious nonvenereal disease caused by a spirochete, *Treponema pertenue*, and found mainly in humid equatorial regions.

**Zeta potential:** The difference in charge density between the inner and outer layers of the ionic cloud that surrounds red cells in an electrolyte solution.

# INDEX

Page numbers followed by *f* indicate figures; those followed by *t* indicate tabular material.

# ANTIGEN–ANTIBODY CHARACTERISTIC CHART*

| | | | ANTIGENS | | | | | |
|---|---|---|---|---|---|---|---|---|
| Antigen System | Antigen Name | ISBT Number | Antigen Freq. % W | Antigen Freq. % B | RBC Antigen Expression at Birth | Antigen Distrib. Plasma/RBC | Demonstrates Dosage | Antigen Modification Enzyme/Other |
| Kidd | Jk$^a$ | JK1 | 77 | 91 | strong | RBC only | yes | Enz. ↑ |
| | Jk$^b$ | JK2 | 73 | 43 | strong | RBC only | yes | Enz. ↑ |
| | | JK3 | 100 | 100 | strong | RBC | no | Enz. ↑ |
| Lewis | Le$^a$ | LE1 | 22 | 23 | nil | Plasma/RBC | no | Enz. ↑ |
| | Le$^b$ | LE2 | 72 | 55 | nil | Plasma/RBC | no | Enz. ↑ |
| †P | P$_1$ | P1 | 79 | 94 | moderate | RBC, platelets, WBC | individual variation | Enz. ↑ AET → ZZAP ↑ |
| | P | | 100 | 100 | moderate | RBC platelets, WBC | no | Enz. ↑ AET → ZZAP ↑ |
| | ‡p$^k$ | | 100 | 100 | ? | RBC, platelets, fibroblast | no | no |
| MNS | M | MNS1 | 78 | 70 | strong | RBC only | yes | Enz. ↓ AET → ZZAP ↓ |
| | N | MNS2 | 72 | 74 | strong | RBC only | yes | Enz. ↓ AET → ZZAP ↓ |
| | S | MNS3 | 55 | 37 | strong | RBC only | yes | Enz. ↓ AET → ZZAP ↓ |
| | s | MNS4 | 89 | 97 | strong | RBC only | yes | Enz. ↓ AET → ZZAP ↓ |
| | U | MNS5 | 100 | 100 | strong | RBC only | no | Enz. → AET → ZZAP ↓ |
| Lutheran | Lu$^a$ | LU1 | 7.6 | 5.3 | poor | RBC only | yes | Enz. → AET → ZZAP ↓ |
| | Lu$^b$ | LU2 LU3 | 99.8 >99.8 | 99.9 | poor | RBC only | yes | ? |

*This chart is to be used for general informaton only. Please refer to the appropriate chapter for more detailed information.

†In the P system, phenotype P contains both P$_1$ and P antigens; phenotype P$_2$ contains only P antigens; phenotype p lacks both P$_1$ and P antigens.

‡The p$^k$ antigen is typically converted to P; therefore there is no p$^k$ antigen detectable on adult cells. There are rare individuals (p$_1^k$, p$_2^k$) where pk antigen is not converted to P.

AET = 2-aminoethylisothiouronium ↑ enhanced reactivity → no effect; HDN = hemolytic disease of the newborn; HTR = hemolytic transfusion reaction; NRBC = non-red blood cell; RBC = red blood cell; WBC = white blood cell; ZZAP = dithiothreitol plus papain ↓ depressed reactivity.